Health Informatics
An Interprofessional Approach

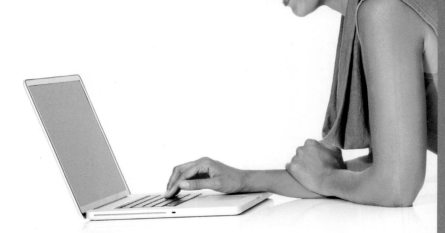

SECOND EDITION

Health Informatics
An Interprofessional Approach

Ramona Nelson, PhD, RN-BC, ANEF, FAAN

Professor Emerita,
Slippery Rock University,
Slippery Rock, Pennsylvania;
President, Ramona Nelson Consulting,
Allison Park, Pennsylvania

Nancy Staggers, PhD, RN, FAAN

President, Summit Health Informatics;
Adjunct Professor, College of Nursing and
Department of Biomedical Informatics,
University of Utah,
Salt Lake City, Utah

ELSEVIER

ELSEVIER

3251 Riverport Lane
St. Louis, Missouri 63043

HEALTH INFORMATICS: AN INTERPROFESSIONAL APPROACH, SECOND EDITION

ISBN: 978-0-323-40231-6

Notices

Knowledge and best practice in this field are constantly changing. As new research and experience broaden our understanding, changes in research methods, professional practices, or medical treatment may become necessary.

Practitioners and researchers must always rely on their own experience and knowledge in evaluating and using any information, methods, compounds, or experiments described herein. In using such information or methods they should be mindful of their own safety and the safety of others, including parties for whom they have a professional responsibility.

With respect to any drug or pharmaceutical products identified, readers are advised to check the most current information provided (i) on procedures featured or (ii) by the manufacturer of each product to be administered, to verify the recommended dose or formula, the method and duration of administration, and contraindications. It is the responsibility of practitioners, relying on their own experience and knowledge of their patients, to make diagnoses, to determine dosages and the best treatment for each individual patient, and to take all appropriate safety precautions.

To the fullest extent of the law, neither the Publisher nor the authors, contributors, or editors, assume any liability for any injury and/or damage to persons or property as a matter of products liability, negligence or otherwise, or from any use or operation of any methods, products, instructions, or ideas contained in the material herein.

Previous edition copyrighted 2014.

International Standard Book Number: 978-0-323-40231-6

Executive Content Strategist: Kellie White
Content Development Manager: Lisa Newton
Senior Content Development Specialist: Danielle M. Frazier
Publishing Services Manager: Jeff Patterson
Senior Project Manager: Jodi M. Willard
Design Direction: Ryan Cook

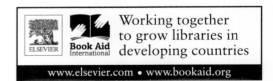

Printed in China

Last digit is the print number: 9 8 7 6 5 4 3 2 1

To my husband, Glenn M. Nelson, who always manages to be there
To my daughters, who managed to pick wonderful husbands,
Dorianne & Michael Hollis and Leslie-Ann & Kristopher Bidelson
and
To my grandchildren, who are today's joy and tomorrow's hope,
Mackenzie, Hope, Ella, and Molly
Ramona Nelson

To my father, Forest Thorpe, who supported education for women
during an age when it was deemed superfluous
and
To my husband, Bob Staggers, who has always been a champion of strong women
Nancy Staggers

Ramona Nelson holds a baccalaureate degree in nursing from Duquesne University and a master's degree in both nursing and information science and a PhD in education from the University of Pittsburgh. In addition, she completed a post-doctoral fellowship at the University of Utah. Prior to her current position as president of her own consulting company, Ramona was a Professor of Nursing and Chair of the Department of Nursing at Slippery Rock University. Today Ramona continues her association with Slippery Rock University in the role of Professor Emerita. Her primary areas of interest include informatics education for health professionals, social media and empowered patients, and the application of theoretical concepts in health informatics practice.

Her past publications include textbooks, monographs, book chapters, journal articles, World Wide Web publications, abstracts, and newsletters. She has been recognized as a Nursing Informatics Pioneer by the American Medical Informatics Association. In addition, she was named a fellow in the American Academy of Nursing in 2004 and in the National League for Nursing Academy of Nursing Education Fellows.

Nancy Staggers is a nursing informatics pioneer who is actively involved in informatics user experience research. Her education was at the University of Wyoming and the University of Maryland School of Nursing, culminating in a PhD with a concentration on informatics and research. Her background includes both health informatics practice and academia. She was a health informatics executive in the Department of Defense and elsewhere, leading enterprise acquisitions and installations of inpatient electronic health records. Her academic career includes professorships at both the University of Utah and the University of Maryland. Nancy's academic work began with developing nursing informatics competencies and later leading teams to revise the American Nurses' Association document on the scope and practice of nursing informatics in the United States in 2002 and 2008. Her research program focuses health IT support and redesign for complex activities such as electronic medication administration records and handoffs/care transitions. Recently she led a team on the user experience community at the Healthcare Information and Management Systems Society to identify nursing user experience issues and solutions for nurses' interactions with health IT. She was elected as a fellow in the American Academy of Nursing in 1999 and received the American Medical Informatics Association Virginia K. Saba nursing informatics award in 2013 for her contributions to informatics. She owns her own health informatics company, which focuses on research consultations and international collaborations. She is also adjunct professor of informatics at the Department of Biomedical Informatics and College of Nursing, University of Utah, and she teaches user experience research methods for the Health Informatics program at the University of Alabama Birmingham. Nancy publishes widely on health informatics topics, concentrating on user experience research.

CONTRIBUTORS

Antonia Arnaert, RN, MPH, MPA, PhD
Associate Professor
Ingram School of Nursing
McGill University
Montreal, Quebec, Canada

Nancy C. Brazelton, RN, MS
Application Service Director
Information Technology Services
University of Utah Health Care
Salt Lake City, Utah

Christine A. Caligtan, RN, MSN
Health Data and Patient Safety
    Clinical Specialist
Health Data Integrity
PatientsLikeMe
Cambridge, Massachusetts

Robin L. Canowitz, AB, JD
Senior Attorney
Vorys, Sater, Seymour and
    Pease, LLP
Columbus, Ohio

Heather Carter-Templeton, PhD, RN-BC
Assistant Professor
Capstone College of Nursing
The University of Alabama
Tuscaloosa, Alabama;
Associate Professor and Reference
    Librarian
Health Sciences Library
University of Tennessee Health Science
    Center
Memphis, Tennessee

Diane Castelli, RN, MS, MSN
Adjunct Clinical Nursing Instructor
Cape Cod Community College
West Barnstable, Massachusetts

Kathleen G. Charters, PhD, RN, CPHIMS
Clinical Information Systems Specialist
Defense Health Agency
Healthcare Operations Directorate
Clinical Support Division
Integrated System Support
Measurements & Clinical Reporting
Falls Church, Virginia

Jon C. Christiansen, BS, JD
Attorney
TechLaw Ventures, PLLC
Salt Lake City, Utah

Helen B. Connors, PhD, RN, DrPS (Hon), FAAN, ANEF
Executive Director
Center for Health Informatics;
Associate Dean
University of Kansas School of Nursing
Kansas City, Kansas

Vicky Elfrink Cordi, PhD, RN
Clinical Associate Professor Emeritus
The Ohio State University
Columbus, Ohio

Mollie R. Cummins, PhD, RN, FAAN
Associate Dean for Research and the PhD
    Program;
Associate Professor
College of Nursing;
Adjunct Associate Professor
Department of Biomedical Informatics
University of Utah
Salt Lake City, Utah

Andrea Day, RN, MS, PMP
Informatics Nurse Consultant
New Market, Maryland

Mical DeBrow, PhD, RN
Associate Director
Health Economics and Outcomes Research
Boehringer Ingelheim Pharmaceuticals
Houston, Texas

Guilherme Del Fiol, MD, PhD
Assistant Professor
Department of Biomedical Informatics
University of Utah
Salt Lake City, Utah

Vikrant G. Deshmukh, PhD, MS, MSc
Adjunct Assistant Professor
Population Health Sciences
University of Utah School of Medicine;
Adjunct Assistant Professor
College of Nursing
University of Utah;
Lead Principal Data Warehouse Architect
Enterprise Data Warehouse
University of Utah Health Care
Salt Lake City, Utah

Patricia C. Dykes, PhD, RN, FAAN, FACMI
Senior Nurse Scientist
Program Director, Center for Patient Safety
    Research and Practice
Program Director, Center for Nursing
    Excellence
Brigham and Women's Hospital
Boston, Massachusetts

William Scott Erdley, DNS, RN, CHSE
Simulation Education Specialist
The Behling Simulation Center
Jacobs School of Medicine and Biomedical
    Sciences
University at Buffalo
Buffalo, NY;
Adjunct Professor
School of Nursing
Niagara University
Niagara University, New York

David L. Gibbs, PhD, CPHIMS, CHPS, CISSP
Assistant Professor
Department of Health Information
    Management
Texas State University
San Marcos, Texas

Bryan Gibson, DPT, PhD
Assistant Professor
Department of Biomedical Informatics
University of Utah
Salt Lake City, Utah

Teresa Gore, PhD, DNP, FNP-BC, NP-C, CHSE-A
Associate Professor and Director of
    Experiential Learning College of Nursing
University of South Florida
Tampa, Florida;
President
International Nursing Association for
    Clinical Simulation and Learning
    (INACSL)
Morrisville, North Carolina

ix

Nicholas R. Hardiker, PhD, RN, FACMI
Professor of Nursing and Health Informatics
School of Nursing, Midwifery, Social Work
    & Social Sciences
University of Salford
Salford, England;
Director, eHealth Programme
International Council of Nurses
Geneva, Switzerland;
Adjunct Professor
College of Nursing
University of Colorado
Denver, Colorado

Angel Hoffman, MSN, RN
Principal/Owner
Advanced Partners in Health Care
    Compliance
Pittsburgh, Pennsylvania

Susan D. Horn, PhD
Adjunct Professor
University of Utah School of Medicine
Health System Innovation and Research
    Program
Salt Lake City, Utah

Valerie M. Howard, EdD, MSN, RN
Dean and University Professor
School of Nursing and Health Sciences
Robert Morris University
Moon Township, Pennsylvania

Sarah J. Iribarren, PhD, RN
Postdoctoral Research Fellow
School of Nursing
Columbia University
New York City, New York

Jonathan M. Ishee, JD, MPH, MS, LLM
Assistant Professor
School of Biomedical Informatics
University of Texas Health Science Center;
Partner
Vorys, Sater, Seymour and Pease, LLP
Houston, Texas

David E. Jones, PhD
Applied Public Health Informatics Fellow
Utah Department of Health
Salt Lake City, Utah

Irene Joos, PhD, MSIS, MN, BSN, RN
Professor & Former Director
Online Learning
Department of Information Technology;
Adjunct Faculty
Department of Nursing
La Roche College
Pittsburgh, Pennsylvania

Kensaku Kawamoto, MD, PhD, MHS
Associate Chief Medical Information Officer
University of Utah Health Care;
Assistant Professor
Department of Biomedical Informatics
University of Utah
Salt Lake City, Utah

Jacob Kean, PhD, MA, BS
Research Speech-Language Pathologist
VA Salt Lake City Health Care System;
Associate Professor
Population Health Sciences
University of Utah School of Medicine
Salt Lake City, Utah

Michael H. Kennedy, PhD, MHA, FACHE
Associate Professor
Department of Health Services and
    Information Management
East Carolina University
Greenville, North Carolina

Tae Youn Kim, PhD, RN
Associate Professor
Betty Irene Moore School of Nursing
University of California, Davis
Sacramento, California

Gerald R. Ledlow, PhD, MHA, FACHE
Chair and Professor
Department of Health Policy and
    Management
Jiann-Ping Hsu College of Public Health
Georgia Southern University
Statesboro, Georgia

Kim Leighton, PhD, RN, ANEF
Assistant Dean
Research & Simulation Faculty
    Development
Institute for Research & Clinical Strategy
DeVry Medical International
Iselin, New Jersey

Louis Luangkesorn, PhD
Research Assistant Professor
Industrial Engineering
University of Pittsburgh
Pittsburgh, Pennsylvania

Ann M. Lyons, PhD, RN
Medical Informaticist
Data Science Service
University of Utah
Salt Lake City, Utah

Kathleen MacMahon, RN, MS, CNP
Telehealth Nurse Practitioner
American Telecare
Minneapolis, Minnesota

Michele P. Madison, JD
Partner
Morris, Manning and Martin, LLP
Atlanta, Georgia

Shannon Majoras, JD
Associate
Vorys, Sater, Seymour and Pease, LLP
Cleveland, Ohio

E. LaVerne Manos, DNP, RN-BC
Faculty
School of Nursing
University of Kansas;
Program Director
Interprofessional Master of Science in
    Health Informatics and Post-Master's
    Interprofessional Certificate in
    Informatics
Center for Health Informatics
University of Kansas;
Director of Nursing Informatics
Center for Health Informatics
University of Kansas
Kansas City, Kansas

Karen S. Martin, RN, MSN, FAAN
Health Care Consultant
Martin Associates
Omaha, Nebraska

Cynthia M. Mascara, RN, MSN, MBA
Principal Clinical Consultant
Strategic Clinical Consulting
Cerner Corporation
Kansas City, Missouri

Susan A. Matney, PhD, RN-C, FAAN
Medical Informaticist
Healthcare Data Dictionary (HDD) Team
3M Health Information Systems
Salt Lake City, Utah

Christine D. Meyer, PhD, RN
Healthcare IT
Independent Consultant
Bridgeville, Pennsylvania

Michele Mills, MBA.PM, PMP, CPHIMS, FHIMSS
Director
Information Technology Services
University of Utah Health Care
Salt Lake City, Utah

Sandra A. Mitchell, PhD, CRNP, FAAN
Research Scientist
Outcomes Research Branch
National Cancer Institute
Rockville, Maryland

Judy Murphy, RN, BSN, FACMI, FHIMSS, FAAN
Chief Nursing Officer
Global Healthcare & Life Sciences
IBM
Washington, DC

Daniel A. Nagel, RN, BScN, MSN, PhD(c)
Lecturer, Department of Nursing & Health Sciences
University of New Brunswick
Saint John, New Brunswick, Canada

Scott P. Narus, PhD
Medical Informatics Director
Intermountain Healthcare Associates;
Professor
Department of Biomedical Informatics
University of Utah
Salt Lake City, Utah

Ramona Nelson, PhD, RN-BC, ANEF, FAAN
Professor Emerita
Slippery Rock University
Slippery Rock, Pennsylvania;
President, Ramona Nelson Consulting
Allison Park, Pennsylvania

Sally Okun, RN, MMHS
Vice President, Advocacy, Policy, and Patient Safety
PatientsLikeMe
Cambridge, Massachusetts

Hyeoun-Ae Park, PhD
Professor
College of Nursing
Seoul National University
Seoul, South Korea

Mitra Rocca, Dipl. Inform. Med.
Senior Medical Informatician
Center for Drug Evaluation and Research
U.S. Food and Drug Administration
Silver Spring, Maryland

Kay M. Sackett-Fitzgerald, BSN, RN, MEd, MSN, EdD
Fitzgerald Consulting
Jenkintown, Pennsylvania

Loretta Schlachta-Fairchild, RN, PhD, FACHE, LTC (Ret.) U.S. Army Nurse Corps
Health Information Sciences Research Program Manager
Joint Program Committee-1 (JPC-1)
U.S. Army Medical Research and Materiel Command/Department of Defense Health Agency
Fort Detrick, Maryland

Rebecca Schnall, PhD, MPH, RN-BC
Assistant Professor
School of Nursing
Columbia University
New York, New York

Kumiko O. Schnock, PhD, RN
Research Fellow
Division of General Internal Medicine and Primary Care
Brigham and Women's Hospital
Boston, Massachusetts

Charlotte A. Seckman, PhD, RN-BC, CNE
Assistant Professor
Course Director
Organizational Systems and Adult Health
School of Nursing
University of Maryland
Baltimore, Maryland

Joyce Sensmeier, MS, RN-BC, CPHIMS, FHIMSS, FAAN
Vice President, Informatics
Healthcare Information and Management Systems Society
Chicago, Illinois

Catherine Janes Staes, BSN, MPH, PhD
Assistant Professor
Department of Biomedical Informatics
University of Utah School of Medicine
Salt Lake City, Utah

Nancy Staggers, PhD, RN, FAAN
President, Summit Health Informatics;
Adjunct Professor
College of Nursing and Department of Biomedical Informatics
University of Utah
Salt Lake City, Utah

Teresa Stenner, MA
Program Manager
Center for Health Informatics
University of Kansas Medical Center
Kansas City, Kansas

Kathleen R. Stevens, RN, MS, EdD, ANEF, FAAN
Professor and Director
Improvement Science Research Network
School of Nursing
University of Texas Health Science Center
San Antonio, Texas

Jim Turnbull, DHA, MBA, BA
Chief Information Officer
University of Utah Health Care
Salt Lake City, Utah

Karen B. Utterback, MSN, RN
Independent Consultant
Homecare
Mitre
Hattiesburg, Mississippi

Dianna Vice-Pasch, MSN, RN, CCM, CTCP
Associate Degree Nursing Faculty
Kentucky Community and Technical College Systems
Lexington, Kentucky

Judith J. Warren, PhD, RN, FAAN, FACMI
Professor Emeritus
School of Nursing
University of Kansas Medical Center
Kansas City, Kansas

Charlene R. Weir, PhD, RN
Associate Professor
Department of Biomedical Informatics
University of Utah School of Medicine;
Associate Director
IDEAS Center of Innovation
Veterans Affairs Salt Lake City
Salt Lake City, Utah

Kathy H. Wood, PhD, FHFMA, CHFP
Assistant Professor
College of Health
Human Services, and Science
Ashford University
San Diego, California

REVIEWERS AND ANCILLARY WRITERS

REVIEWERS

Joanna V. Bachour, MSN, RN
Assistant Professor and Lab Manager
MCPHS University, School of Nursing
Worcester, Massachusetts

Carol J. Bickford, PhD, RN-BC, CPHIMS, FHIMSS, FAAN
Senior Policy Advisor
Department of Nursing Practice & Work Environment
American Nurses Association
Silver Spring, Maryland

Connie B. Bishop, DNP, MBA, RN-BC
Clinical Assistant Professor
College of Health and Human Services
School of Nursing
North Carolina A&T State University
Greensboro, North Carolina

Barbara Blackwell, EdD, RN-BC
Director
School of Nursing (RN and LPN School)
Holy Name Medical Center School of Nursing
Teaneck, New Jersey

Mary T. Boylston, RN, MSN, EdD, AHN-BC
Professor of Nursing
Nursing Department
Eastern University
St. Davids, Pennsylvania

Kathleen M. Burke, PhD, RN
Assistant Dean in Charge of Nursing
Professor of Nursing
Adler Center for Nursing Excellence
Ramapo College of New Jersey
Mahwah, New Jersey

Pat Callard, DNP, RN, CNL
Associate Professor of Nursing
College of Graduate Nursing
Western University of Health Sciences
Pomona, California

Karen Chang, PhD, RN
Associate Professor
School of Nursing
College of Health and Human Services
Purdue University
West Lafayette, Indiana

Amanda Dorsey, MSHI, FHIMSS
Assistant Professor
UAB MS in Health Informatics Program
University of Alabama at Birmingham
Birmingham, Alabama

Judith A. Effken, PhD, RN, FACMI, FAAN
Professor Emerita
College of Nursing
The University of Arizona
Tucson, Arizona

Matthew J. Fox, MSN, RN-BC
Assistant Professor of Nursing
Ohio University-Zanesville
Zanesville, Ohio

Robert L. Garrie, MPA, RHIA
Associate Professor
Health Services Administration
University of Alabama at Birmingham
Birmingham, Alabama

Lynda R. Hardy, PhD, RN
Associate Dean for Research
College of Nursing
University of Tennessee, Knoxville
Knoxville, Tennessee

Gayle McGinty, MSN, RN
Assistant Professor of Nursing
MCPHS University, School of Nursing
Worcester, Massachusetts

Carol M. Patton, PhD, FNP-BC, CRNP, CNE
Informatics Health Certificate, CNE
Associate Clinical Professor
Drexel University
Philadelphia, Pennsylvania

Alison Pittman, RN, MSN, CPN
Clinical Assistant Professor
Texas A&M Health Science Center
College of Nursing
Bryan, Texas

Teresa L. Scherer, MS, RN
Clinical Instructor
School of Nursing
Idaho State University, College of Technology
Pocatello, Idaho

M. Kathleen Smith, MScEd, RN-BC, FHIMSS
Managing Partner
Informatics Consulting and Continuing Education, L.L.C.
Weeki Wachee, Florida

Nadia Sultana, MBA, RN, BC
Clinical Assistant Professor
College of Nursing
New York University
New York, New York

Lindsay Tucker, BA, AAA, CPC
Training and Education Manager
Moses Cone Health System
Adjunct Professor
Guilford Technical Community College
Greensboro, North Carolina

Dorothea M. Winter, PhD, RN
Professor of Nursing
Nursing Department
Salisbury University
Salisbury, Maryland

ANCILLARY WRITER

Jane M. Brokel, PhD, RN, FNI
Adjunct Faculty
College of Nursing
University of Iowa
Iowa City, Iowa;
Section Instructor
School of Nursing and Health Sciences
Simmons College
Boston, Massachusetts

ACKNOWLEDGMENTS

First, we would like to acknowledge Kellie White, Executive Content Strategist, whose overview and coordination of this second edition is greatly appreciated. We also thank Danielle Frazier, Senior Content Development Specialist, who was responsible for providing support during the process of writing and editing; and especially Jodi Willard, Senior Project Manager, whose attention to detail was invaluable during the editing process. Finally, we would like to acknowledge Jeff Patterson, Publishing Services Manager, and Ryan Cook, Designer. Their expertise was imperative for developing a polished and professional product.

Each chapter of this book is supported with Evolve resources. We also wish to acknowledge the support of Umarani Natarajan, Senior Project Manager, and Hariprasad Maniyaan, Multimedia Producer, for the Evolve resources, as well as ancillary writer Jane Brokel and various content experts for their development of these resources.

Finally, we would like to acknowledge the reviewers. Their many suggestions, tips, and comments were invaluable in creating this book.

Ramona Nelson
Nancy Staggers

Health informatics and our current information technology (IT) environment are inherently interdisciplinary. Over our many years of working in health informatics practice and teaching health informatics content, we recognized the need for a health informatics textbook that provides a solid overview of the field using an interdisciplinary approach. Therefore the title, authors, and content of this book reflect the comprehensive nature of contemporary informatics practice. The contributors to this book are leaders in health informatics and represent various disciplines and a wide variety of settings, areas of expertise, and positions.

Health Informatics: An Interprofessional Approach provides readers with a comprehensive understanding of health informatics, its practice, and relevant research on health informatics topics. Each chapter opens with key terms, learning objectives and an abstract that outlines the topics covered within the chapter. Chapter headings give readers a conceptual framework for understanding the content in the chapter. Each chapter ends with conclusions that include thoughts about future directions for the topic. Every chapter includes a set of discussion questions to encourage critical thinking and to encourage the reader to consider how the content in the chapter can be applied in the ever-changing world of healthcare. Case studies with analytic questions demonstrate how informatics applies in real-life practice.

USES OF THE BOOK

This textbook is an excellent resource for use within and across various health disciplines. Every attempt has been made to be culturally sensitive to the various disciplines within healthcare while encouraging readers to recognize themselves as key members of an interprofessional team. This book is written to be used for both intradisciplinary and inter-disciplinary informatics courses. The text can span levels of education depending on the program of study, depth of informatics material needed, and the needs of faculty and students. This book is targeted to students needing introductory health or nursing informatics knowledge. As with the first edition, it is useful at several levels: for upper division or advanced undergraduate courses, for RN to BSN/MSN programs, for introductory health informatics content or courses in master's programs and, particularly, for DNP students.

VENDORS, APPLICATIONS, FOUNDATIONS AND INSTITUTIONS

Vendors, health IT applications, commercial products, and organizations and institutions are discussed throughout the textbook. They are included for information purposes and to provide readers with examples of the variety of resources available. No endorsement of a specific company, product, or organization is intended.

ORGANIZATION OF THE BOOK

The book is organized into nine units. The first unit is *Foundational Information in Health Informatics* and focuses on material that is basic to understanding the discipline as a whole. Content includes the definition and significance of the field, theories and models, evidence-based practice and practice-based evidence, program evaluation, and technical infrastructures for health IT.

The second unit is *Information Systems and Applications for the Delivery of Healthcare.* This unit begins with an overview of electronic health records, followed by a discussion of financial and other administrative applications and clinical decision support systems. Remaining chapters focus on health IT in non–acute care settings: telehealth, home health, and public health informatics. This unit provides readers with content on major health applications in institutions and relevant settings.

The third unit, *Participatory Healthcare Informatics,* recognizes the shift toward patient engagement in recent years. Patients are now more involved in their own healthcare and are equipped with health IT applications. Topics in this unit include epatients, social media, personal health records and, new to the second edition, mHealth (mobile health). Readers are introduced to the impact of this movement on patients, providers, and the patient-provider relationship as well as the partnership between each of these groups and health IT.

The fourth unit is entitled *Managing the Life Cycle of a Health Information System,* and the first chapter outlines strategic planning and selecting an information system. Salient topics are then introduced to readers: project management, contract negotiations, implementing and upgrading a system, and downtime and disaster recovery. This material gives readers the knowledge and skills to lead and participate in health informatics systems projects in every phase of the systems life cycle. The chapters on contract negotiations and project management are new to this edition.

The fifth unit, *User Experience, Standards, Safety and Analytics in Health Informatics,* explains complex interactions among health IT and safety, user experience, and needed standards. This unit introduces concepts and practical uses for data science and analytics, which represent a major focus of health organizational leaders, health professionals, and informatics specialists today. This unit focuses on creating a culture of safety, effective and efficient health IT interactions, and methods for knowledge building. The analytics chapter provides new material on data science.

The sixth unit, *Governance Structures, Legal, and Regulatory Issues in Health Informatics,* deals with local and national structures, laws, and regulations important to health informatics. At the local level, contributors discuss how organizations develop support structures for managing health IT. On a national level, the development of federal programs and regulations dealing with HITECH, MU, MACRA, MIPS, and ACO are carefully explained. Other chapters outline privacy and security concerns and health policy issues and also provide the reader with directions for professional involvement in these activities.

The seventh unit, *Education and Health Informatics*, focuses on the role of education in informatics and the role of informatics in health provider education. It includes chapters that discuss educational applications and issues, educational tools, simulation, distributive education, and informatics in the health curriculum.

The eighth unit, *International Health Informatics Efforts*, contains a chapter on the aspects, initiatives, and progress of health informatics worldwide.

The ninth unit, *Historical Implications and Future Directions in Health Informatics*, provides an overview of the history of health informatics. It then concentrates on future directions and future research needed in the field of health informatics, including a unique section about nanotechnology.

TEACHING AND LEARNING PACKAGE

Health informatics is a fast-changing field. Resources and emerging developments related to each chapter are available on the Evolve website. For example, new government reports and other important documents are posted or referenced for easy student access. These materials are targeted to all faculty, including those newer to the field as well as those with additional experience in the discipline of informatics. Each chapter includes a number of discussion questions and a case study. These questions and case studies are carefully designed to represent the reality of health informatics, including the typical ill-defined problems common in informatics practice. Numerous approaches are available to manage these challenges. Thus the discussion questions and case studies can stimulate discussion, and faculty and students can explore how the material in the chapters can be applied for developing approaches for practice situations. Students should be especially encouraged to consider how these materials apply to their own experiences and situations.

For the Instructor

- **TEACH Lesson Plans** contain objectives and key terms from the text. Topics from the book are mapped to Quality and Safety Education for Nurses (QSEN) standards, American Association of Colleges of Nursing (AACN) Essentials Series, concept-based learning, and American Health Information Management Association (AHIMA) competencies. These lesson plans tie in all of the chapter resources for effective presentation of material and include additional highlights and learning activities tied to content within the chapters. Online Activities for each chapter provide additional assignments to deepen students' understanding of the content of the text.
- **PowerPoint Presentations** are available to accompany the TEACH Lesson Plans. Pulling content and figures from the text, the PowerPoint slides provide students with chapter highlights and provide instructors with additional relevant topics of conversation.
- A **Test Bank** containing more than 300 questions is compliant with the NCLEX® standards and provides text page references and cognitive levels. The ExamView software allows instructors to create new tests; edit, add, and delete text questions; sort questions; and administer and grade online tests.
- The **Image Collection** contains all of the art from the text for use in lectures or to supplement the PowerPoint presentations.

For the Student

- **Student Review Questions** provide additional practice for students trying to master the content presented within the text.
- Most chapters have **Additional Readings** to provide sources of additional research on the subject.

CONTENTS

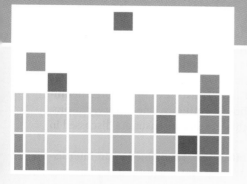

An Introduction to Health Informatics

Ramona Nelson and Nancy Staggers

The ultimate goal of health informatics is to empower populations, communities, families, and individuals with the opportunity to improve the quality and increase the quantity of their days by maximizing the use of technology in healthcare.

OBJECTIVES

At the completion of this chapter, the reader will be prepared to:
1. Define healthcare informatics.

2. Discuss the significance of health informatics within healthcare delivery.
3. Provide an overview of health informatics-related topics.

KEY TERMS

health informaticians, 2
health informatics, 2

ABSTRACT ❖

This chapter provides the reader with an introduction to health informatics as both a discipline and a profession. It begins by introducing the reader to the significance of health informatics. Health informatics is then defined, and example applications are listed. The next section of the chapter provides an overview of the topics inherent in the discipline and profession of health informatics. These topics are organized around the nine units in the book.

INTRODUCTION

Almost 20 years after the Institute of Medicine (IOM) report *To Err Is Human*[1] was released, John T. James published a seminal article on the same topic in *The Journal of Patient Safety*. Using a carefully designed methodology, he analyzed data published from 2008 to 2011 to estimate the number of preventable adverse events occurring in American hospitals. James found that each year, an estimated 440,000 hospitalized Americans experience a preventable adverse event that contributed to their death. In addition, serious harm is estimated to be 10- to 20-fold more common than lethal harm.[2] These findings were reinforced in 2016 when Martin Makary and Michael Daniel published a study in *The BMJ* entitled "Medical Error—The Third Leading Cause of Death in the US."[2a]

The numbers are astounding, but the personal consequences are even greater for the people and the families who suffer such "preventable events." Dr. James, whose distinguished professional career was in healthcare, maintains a website that provides some insight into his strong interest in patient safety.[3] The website is dedicated as follows:

> *This site is dedicated to my 19-year-old son, John Alexander James, who died as a result of uninformed, careless, and unethical care by cardiologists at a hospital in central Texas in the late summer of 2002.*

In 2016, 3 years after publication of the James article, this same journal published another research study in which the question is asked Can electronic health records prevent harm to patients?[4] Key points from this research include the following:

- The investigators analyzed Medicare Patient Safety Monitoring System (MPSMS) patient medical record data for 1351 hospitals from the years 2012 and 2013. They found 347,281 exposures to adverse events. Of these exposures, 7820 adverse events actually took place, resulting in a 2.25% occurrence rate.
- Of the patients, 13% (5876) received care that was captured by an electronic health record (EHR).
- The analysis of these data demonstrated that cardiovascular, surgery, and pneumonia patients whose complete treatment was captured in an EHR were between 17% and 30% less likely to experience in-hospital adverse events.[5]

The studies[2,2a,4] taken together suggest that if EHRs were in use in American hospitals, somewhere between 74,800 and 132,000 preventable fatal hospital-based events each year might never occur.

Going forward, if **health informaticians** and knowledgeable healthcare providers are fully involved in the design, selection, and implementation of health information systems, these numbers are just the beginning of what would be possible in terms of improved healthcare. Improved patient safety is just one of the many reasons why the study of health informatics is imperative for all healthcare professionals. Throughout this book, other vital reasons will become obvious. Competent, compassionate healthcare depends on healthcare providers who understand and can maximize their use of health information technology (IT) and informatics knowledge in providing care to patients. This book provides the foundation required to develop that competence.

DEFINITION OF HEALTH INFORMATICS

Today health informatics is an exciting and well-established field. It is recognized as both a discipline and a profession. As a discipline, it is a field of study in the same sense that medicine, sociology, and pharmacy are fields of study. Core disciplines, including informatics, along with terminal competencies or learning outcomes, provide the framework for developing curricula within the healthcare professions. Learning outcomes include the skills, knowledge, and professional aptitudes expected of all graduates within the profession. In 2003 the IOM identified five core competences that should be achieved by all healthcare professionals:

- Delivering patient-centered care
- Working as part of interdisciplinary teams
- Practicing evidence-based medicine
- Focusing on quality improvement
- Using informatics[6]

Other professional groups and accrediting agencies are now including an informatics-related requirement. For example, the American Association of Colleges of Nursing (AACN) developed a group of documents titled the Essentials Series.[7–9] The Essentials outline the necessary curriculum content and expected competencies of graduates from baccalaureate, master's, and doctor of nursing practice programs. Each of these documents includes a technology or informatics requirement and cites the IOM report as the rationale for this requirement.

Health informatics is also a profession within the healthcare arena. Thousands of informaticians practice the specialty in varied roles that include, for example:

- Installing and evaluating new technologies such as EHRs
- Developing mHealth (mobile health applications) for patients
- Analyzing users' interactions with health IT to create applications that mirror the way clinicians think and do work
- Leading telehealth initiatives in a region or nationally
- Developing and implementing national policies for health IT and informatics
- Building terminologies to support interoperability
- Doing research on the effect of health IT on patients, providers, or organizations

Although the existence of health informatics as both a discipline and as a profession is well accepted, it is interesting to note there is currently no consensus or generally accepted name and standard definition for this profession. Current titles for members of this profession include health informatics specialist, informaticist, or informatician (sometimes spelled *informaticien*). Table 1.1 lists several accepted definitions and the source of those definitions. The history, reasons, and issues presented by this lack of consensus are discussed in detail in Chapter 35.

In this book, **health informatics** is defined as an interdisciplinary professional specialty and scientific discipline that integrates the health sciences, computer science, and information science, as well as a number of other analytic sciences, with the goal of managing and communicating data, information, knowledge, and wisdom in the provision of healthcare for individuals, families, groups, and communities. A review of this definition as well as the definitions in Table 1.1 demonstrates three common themes within each of these definitions. That is, health informatics is:

- An interdisciplinary professional specialty
- Tied to the use of IT in healthcare
- Focused on assisting healthcare providers with tasks related to collecting data, processing information, and applying that information to processes such as problem solving, knowledge development, and decision making

Health IT touches nearly every aspect of healthcare today, even less obvious ones such as providing emotional support to patients. A few examples include:

- **Tele-intensive care units (ICUs).** Patients in ICUs in more remote geographical areas are monitored by experienced ICU nurses and physicians using telehealth technology.

TABLE 1.1	Common Definitions of Health Informatics	
Source	Definition
AHIMA	*Health informatics* is the scientific discipline concerned with the cognitive, information-processing, and communication tasks of healthcare practice, education, and research, including the information science and technology to support these tasks.[28]
HIMSS	*Health informatics* is the interdisciplinary study of the design, development, adoption, and application of IT-based innovations in healthcare services delivery, management, and planning as defined by the U.S. National Library of Medicine.[29]
AMIA	*Biomedical informatics* is the interdisciplinary field that studies and pursues the effective uses of biomedical data, information, and knowledge for scientific inquiry, problem solving and decision making, motivated by efforts to improve human health.[30]
US NLM	*Health informatics* is "the interdisciplinary study of the design, development, adoption, and application of IT-based innovations in healthcare services delivery, management, and planning."[31]

- **Robotics**. DaVinci is a widely used surgical robot guided by a surgeon. It is used to translate hand movements during minimally invasive surgery, using tiny instruments inserted into small incisions.
- **Behavioral health at-a-distance**. The U.S. Army has a telehealth network that spans 50 countries. Behavioral health telehealth makes up 55% of their services, followed by cardiology and dermatology.[10]
- **Sensors**. Sensors in long-term care settings can help monitor residents' health status, detect emergency situations, and contact health providers.[11] In the future, clinicians may monitor patients with wearable sensors, such as clothing, after discharge.[12]
- **Healthcare for islanders**. People living on four islands off the coast of Maine have no available healthcare providers. A 72-foot boat beams health services via live video conferencing with a nurse.

TOPICS AND AREAS OF STUDY IN INFORMATICS

This book is divided into nine units outlining the key topics and areas of study within health informatics. This section of the chapter is built around these nine units. Each subsection presented here focuses on one of the nine units, and begins by describing the theme of the unit. This is followed by an example taken from professional reports, research studies, or a news story. As you read each subsection, you are encouraged to think about how informaticians using information technology could improve the quality of healthcare and the satisfaction of both providers and patients, while decreasing costs.

Unit 1: Fundamental Information in Health Informatics

The content of the first five chapters of the book can be applied to each of the remaining chapters. These chapters introduce the reader to terms, definitions, concepts, theories, and models that are used throughout the book, thereby providing the mental infrastructure for understanding the discipline of health informatics.

Why Informatics Is Needed in Healthcare: An Example

The weblog GeriPal is an online community of interdisciplinary providers interested in geriatrics or palliative care. In August 2013, they published an article titled "Transfers from the hospital to nursing home: an F-grade for quality."[13] The article reviews a study published in *Journal of the American Geriatrics Society*.[14] GeriPal describes the finding from this research as follows: "A rather stunning study in the *Journal of the American Geriatrics Society* suggests the quality of communication between the hospital and the nursing home is horrendous."[13] Patients arrived at skilled nursing facilities (SNF) with missing or inaccurate information on their health status, their medication orders, and their functional abilities. The research found that care was routinely delayed and nursing hours were wasted trying to obtain the required information. Poor-quality discharge communication was identified as the major barrier to safe and effective transitions. Interestingly, nurses from the SNFs in the study identified a specific list of information and components that they need to facilitate a safe, high-quality transition. Nevertheless, the lack of an interoperable healthcare system providing clear, concise patient data/information between institutions makes the situation described in their study a common occurrence in SNFs across the country. Healthcare providers and informaticians who have a mental infrastructure and understand what is possible are the first requirement for building such an interoperable system.

Unit 2: Information Systems and Applications for the Delivery of Healthcare

The Health Information Management Systems Society (HIMSS) provides a searchable website for applications used in healthcare. As of this writing, HIMSS listed 30 categories of applications ranging from Ambulatory to Web/Internet Solutions. Under each of these categories are subcategories: for example, under Operating Room, one can find Peri-Operative Systems, Post-Operative Systems, Pre-Operative Systems, and Scheduling. The point is that an enormous number of applications are used in healthcare and more are being developed every day. As healthcare providers discover and explore different applications used in healthcare, three questions can be used to provide an overview of each application.

- What is the *purpose* of this application? Each healthcare application will have a specific purpose or list of purposes: for example, a scheduling system helps schedule staff or patients within a particular clinical unit.
- What *functions* can this application perform? *Function* is how an application achieves its purpose: For example, can the scheduling system assign staff to work shifts of any length or does it function with predetermined shifts only?
- How is this application internally and externally *structured*? *Internal structure* determines how efficiently and effectively the application actually functions; for example, a poorly designed user interface can increase the number of user errors. *External structure* determines how the application fits into the environment, especially how the application interfaces with other applications.

The six chapters in this unit explore the common applications used across the healthcare settings.

Healthcare Applications Improving Healthcare: An Example

A study conducted in 2008 entitled *The Balancing Act: Patient Care Time Versus Cost* explored how nursing time is distributed in a clinical setting.[15] This research correlated the time spent on various activities with the nurses' wages, thereby measuring the cost of nursing care. The authors reported that $757,000 of nursing wages was spent on tasks such as hunting for equipment. *Nursing Times*, in 2009, published an article based on an online survey of over 1000 nurses[16] entitled "Nurses Waste 'an Hour a Shift' Finding Equipment." A 2011 study from the Robert Wood Johnson Foundation estimated that only 20% to 30% of a nurse's time is actually spent at the

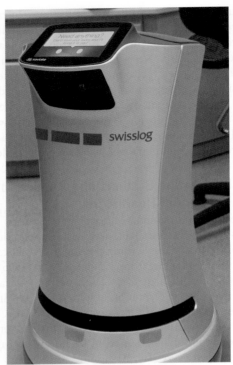

FIG 1.1 RoboCourier® Autonomous Mobile Robot. (Used with permission of Swisslog.)

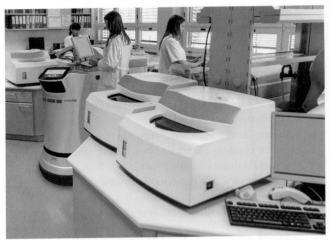

FIG 1.2 RoboCourier® Autonomous Mobile Robot in a healthcare setting with the people and information systems that direct the robot. (Used with permission of Swisslog.)

bedside, and as much as 70% of their time can be spent on documentation, finding supplies, and carrying out other duties, such as tracking down equipment.[17]

One informatics-based solution to this well-documented waste of nursing time is the use of an autonomous mobile robot (AMR) with tracking software, RFID (radio-frequency identification), and barcode technology to manage supplies needed on a clinical unit. One example of such a robot is RoboCourier®, developed by Swisslog (Fig. 1.1). Automated robots such as RoboCourier® can safely and securely transport laboratory specimens, medications, clinical supplies, and other materials throughout the healthcare setting, thereby allowing healthcare professionals to focus on patient care instead of searching for the materials they need to provide that care.[18]

As you consider this technology, think about how the robot would be programed to automatically interface with elevators and doors so the robot can move independently throughout the facility on programmed paths with no human interference. Also consider how the robot would know what supplies to deliver where. To gain the maximum benefit of AMRs, they need to be interfaced with other information systems in the hospital, thus diminishing the human effort needed to maintain needed supplies on a clinical unit. For example, could the pharmacy system be interfaced with the AMR so that new medication orders could be quickly delivered to the clinical unit? Fig. 1.2 demonstrates an AMR in relation to the people and information systems that direct the AMR as well as other institutional systems that might be interfaced with the AMR.

Unit 3: Participatory Healthcare Informatics (Healthcare on the Internet)

Since the beginning of healthcare, providers have been proactive in meeting the needs of patients. Historically, patients and their families have looked to healthcare providers both to assess/diagnosis their health problems and to tell them what was needed. Today patients are no longer exclusively dependent on providers to determine what is wrong and what options they might consider in dealing with their health problem. Patients, whether well or facing problems, are assuming an increasingly proactive role in maintaining or obtaining a higher level of health. These proactive patients are often referred to as ePatients. ePatients are equipped, empowered, engaged, and electronically connected. They are informed about their health and have gained much of that knowledge via the internet. Knowledge is power, and as more patients are becoming ePatients, the traditional relationship between the patient and the provider is shifting from a parent–child-type relationship toward more collegial ones.

Now providers and patients have access to much of the same information. However, both patients and providers are overwhelmed by the amount of quality information they can access. In addition, they differ greatly by the scope of the information that each group needs to access. Providers must focus on a much larger scope of data/information. First, they need to be aware of the growing literature base across their specialty and also the information available to patients. Second, they must be aware of trends and changes across the broad area of healthcare delivery: for example, providers need to be aware of the role that social media plays in healthcare delivery.

Patients and their families can limit research to their own health issues rather than all disorders within a specific specialty. When working together in social media groups, individuals can become experts in every sense of the word about their own expression of their specific health problems.

However, when confronted with this massive amount of information, providers have one significant advantage not available to most patients. Their experience and education makes it much easier to assess the quality of the information and incorporate new findings into their current knowledge. Patients, on the contrary, must often spend a great deal of time and effort correctly interpreting information and determining its significance in terms of their health issues. This is especially true for patients with a new health problem or diagnosis.

The solution may seem obvious. Working together as colleagues, patients and providers can take advantage of each other's strengths in meeting the challenges presented by various healthcare problems. The amount of responsibility for leading this effort will vary at different points in the wellness–illness continuum. As patients move toward a high level of health, they are increasingly responsible for maintaining their own health through diet, exercise, and avoiding poor health habits. As they move toward the other end of the continuum, with, for example, a severe acute episode or illness, the provider has a higher level of responsibility. However, even in these situations, patients and/or their families must sign the consent form and, therefore, must make the final decision.

In Unit 3, the reader will explore the changing relationship between ePatients and health informatics. As an introduction to the unit, these authors suggest that the reader do a quick search of the internet for the term *ePatient* and note the variety of examples presented by searching with this one term.

Unit 4: Managing the Life Cycle of a Health Information System

As the title suggests, Unit 4 is focused on the life cycle of a health information system. Fig. 2.8 provides a model of this life cycle. The systems life cycle (SLC) is one of the oldest and yet still widely used methods for selecting/tailoring or building, implementing, and evaluating software applications in the IT arena. The lifecycle has evolved over the years in response to ever-changing scenarios and paradigm shifts pertaining to the building or acquiring of software; however, its central tenants are as applicable now as they ever were. Lifecycle stages have gone through iterations, with different names and numbers of steps, but the SLC is resilient as a tried and true method in a wide variety of settings including healthcare. Thus, learning about the SLC remains important to students.[18]

Healthcare providers, whether they are informaticians or working in other areas of the healthcare system, play a major role in the life cycle of healthcare information systems. Acquiring new systems is a complicated process that affects the entire facility. In the past, a common mistake has been selecting healthcare systems that affect patient care with little or no input from providers across the healthcare team. Healthcare providers often discover these new applications when they are requested to change their practice to "work around" an issue with a new system in another department. Therefore it is imperative that healthcare providers not only understand the life cycle of healthcare information applications but also be involved in systems selection.

Using the Systems Life Cycle: An Example

A few years ago, Mark McMurtrey, PhD, a faculty member at the University of Central Arkansas, and a colleague were invited to serve as consultants for the selection of a home health software application in a medium-sized regional hospital. The 149-bed facility included an emergency department; a hospice; intensive care, obstetrics, pediatrics rehabilitation, and home units; an imaging center; primary care clinics; a health and fitness center; and a wound healing center. After completing this project, McMurtrey published a paper describing how the use of the systems life cycle provided the project with a systemic and structured process. He concluded the paper with the following statement: "While both researchers hold terminal degrees, each learned quite a bit from the application of principles taught in the classroom to the complexities surrounding real-world utilization of them."[19, p. 23]

Unit 4 contains five chapters exploring the application of life-cycle–related principles to the complexities surrounding their real-world use in healthcare. With this background, the reader is prepared to participate actively and effectively in real-life use of the life cycle in healthcare.

Unit 5: User Experience, Standards, Safety, and Analytics in Health Informatics

This unit is focused on discovering and using information and knowledge to improve the way that healthcare is delivered, and in turn, to improve healthcare outcomes. Currently, there is a large body of knowledge concerning drug-drug and drug-diet interaction. In addition, there is extensive knowledge about lab tests, diet, and drug interactions. The human mind is not designed to remember this type of extensive detail. In addition, when a computer is used for order entry, deciding the specific medications, diagnostic tests, and diet to order for an individual patient can carry a heavy cognitive load, thereby leaving less mental resources for remembering details related to interactions. In such a situation, health providers benefit from using a clinical decision support (CDS) system to analyze the details and offer suggestions. However, a CDS system will not make a difference unless the information the provider needs is presented in a way that meshes with the mental workflow of the provider. In other words, the provider must be able to use the information and knowledge. Therefore this unit begins by discussing usability.

The process of discovering and using knowledge is highly dependent on standards. It is only through standards that technologies interface and interact. For example, it would be impossible to use a computer and a printer if there were no standards on how these two pieces of technology are connected. Every piece of technology becomes an isolated and useless piece of equipment without an agreement on how the pieces of equipment physically and logically communicate. This agreement is called a *standard*. In this unit, current standards and the processes for establishing these standards in healthcare are explored.

Establishing standards, analyzing data, discovering knowledge, and making the information/knowledge useful to healthcare providers is executed with the overall goals of providing safe, effective, quality care. The unit ends with an analysis of methods, programs, and procedures used to ensure safe, effective, quality care.

Using Big Data: A Real-Life Example

Dr. John D. Halamka is the chief information officer of Beth Israel Deaconess Medical Center in Boston. In 2011 his wife, a healthy 49-year-old Korean woman, was diagnosed with breast cancer. Using big-data technology available at all Harvard hospitals, Dr. Halamka was able to ask the big-data questions: Of the last 10,000 Asian women near age 50 who were treated for the same tumor, what medications were used? Was surgery or radiation necessary, and what were the outcomes? From his queries, he was able to ascertain the most effective treatment approach for a person with this history. His wife was treated successfully and is now cancer free.[20] The challenge for informatics is: How do we develop information systems that can provide this level of care to patients in all settings?

Unit 6: Governance Structures, Legal, and Regulatory Issues in Health Informatics

Unit 6 is built on the concept of governance, beginning with health informatics governance at the federal level. The U.S. government and related legal systems have established processes for achieving justice, defense, promotion of the general welfare of citizens, and security. Unit 6 is built around these concepts. The first chapter explains how health informatics-related legislation, programs, and regulations are developed and implemented. Major legislation is analyzed, from the Health Insurance Portability and Accountability Act (HIPAA) to the Health Information Technology for Economic Clinical Health (HITECH) Act, soon to be followed by the Medicare and CHIP Reauthorization Act (MACRA). Healthcare leaders, including informaticians, and health IT users must play active roles in developing these policies, as described in Chapter 28. Finally, this unit concludes by describing how the concepts of governance apply to the management and operation of a Health IT department.

Health Policy in Operation: An Example

The HITECH Act, which provided financial incentives for the adoption of EHRs, was implemented in 2009 with the goal to modernize the IT infrastructure of the U.S. healthcare system.[21]

- As of 2009, only 12% of hospitals had adopted a basic EHR system.[22] By 2014, 75% of U.S. hospitals had adopted at least a basic EHR system, up from 59% in 2013.
- The EHRs also showed significant improvement in functionality. By 2014, hospitals able to meet the stage 2 criteria used in the implementation of the HITECH Act increased to 40.5%, up from 5.8% in 2013.[23]
- By 2013, 63% of physicians had implemented an EHR, and another 20% were in the process of implementing one.[21]

Going forward, healthcare providers must be involved in governance at the institutional, local, state, and federal levels. This unit provides the foundation for that involvement as it relates to health informatics.

Unit 7: Education and Health Informatics

In today's networked healthcare world, all healthcare professionals require a foundational understanding of health informatics. However, a significant number of healthcare professionals currently in the workforce were educated before this was true, and this is especially true for faculty teaching in health education programs today. According to AACN's report on 2013–14 Salaries of Instructional and Administrative Nursing Faculty in Baccalaureate and Graduate Programs in Nursing, the average age of faculty varied from 51.2 to 61.6.[24] The Association of American Medical Colleges (AAMC) reported in 2007 that the average age of medical school faculty is growing older, a finding that held regardless of degree, department type, rank, or demographic characteristic. At that time, the average age of MD faculty teaching in the basic sciences was 52.9.[25] This might explain why the introduction of computers in healthcare has been a slow process, and the introduction of informatics into the curriculum has been even slower. This unit begins by analyzing where informatics fits in the curriculum for healthcare professionals.

The following three chapters in this unit discuss how technology is changing the pedagogy of healthcare education. Initially technology made the educational process more efficient. For example, using a computerized spreadsheet is more efficient than using a paper-and-pencil gradebook and calculating grades by hand. Moreover, technology is changing the teaching and learning process. Distance education often uses more interactive learning experiences in comparison to the more passive process of taking notes during a lecture. Simulation provides the opportunity to analyze one's own performance and try again, and learning the same procedures in the clinical setting does not offer the "do-over" option. Professors are increasingly seen not as authorities or all-knowing experts, but rather as learning coaches encouraging the student to develop their own expertise, knowledge, and skills.

Computerization is changing both healthcare delivery and healthcare education. This Unit explores these changes and their interrelationship. The interrelationship is illustrated in Fig. 1.3.

Curriculi for Health Professions

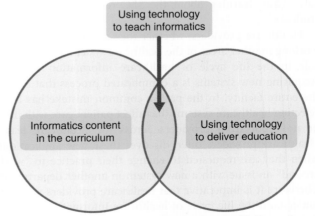

FIG 1.3 The interrelationship of education and informatics.

Safegarding security and privacy likely to become more challenging with the evolving healthcare landscape

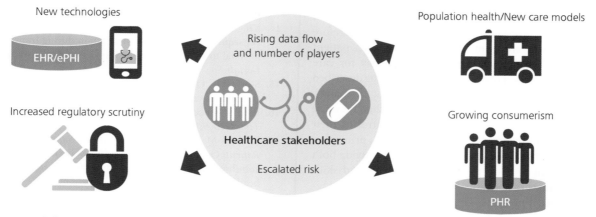

New technologies

EHR/ePHI

Increased regulatory scrutiny

Rising data flow and number of players

Healthcare stakeholders

Escalated risk

Population health/New care models

Growing consumerism

PHR

FIG 1.4 Example of international health trends and driving forces interacting. *EHR*, Electronic health record; *ePHI*, electronic protected health information; *PHR*, personal health record. (Used with permission of Deloitte Touch Tohmastu Limited.)

Unit 8: International Health Informatics Efforts

The need for health information systems that can function around the world cannot be over emphasized. The desire to be in good health and the need to deliver healthcare to those in need is universal. Although countries and regions of the world demonstrate variation in their healthcare needs, as well as how they pay for and deliver healthcare, globally, healthcare needs, costs, and delivery are becoming more similar. With increased travel, infectious diseases can quickly spread around the world. Chronic diseases are a growing global health problem. The Population Reference Bureau, with the mission of informing people around the world about population, health, and the environment, reported in 2013 that global health trends have undergone a dramatic shift since 1990. During this period, chronic diseases, such as heart disease, cancer, and diabetes, have replaced infectious diseases and malnutrition-related childhood illnesses as the leading causes of death and disability across the globe, with the exception of sub-Saharan Africa.[26]

From an international prospective, healthcare delivery systems around the world face a core of common challenges. In 2015, Deloitte, an international consulting company, identified a number of such global challenges:

- Cost was the largest healthcare issue facing most countries in 2015. Across the globe, there is increasing pressure to contain costs and demonstrate value.
- Dynamic market forces, such as the increasing role of government, workforce shortage, demand for improving access to care, and consumerism, are requiring providers and health plans to rethink traditional business models.
- Adoption of new digital health IT advances (e.g., EHRs, mHealth applications, and predictive analytics) are transforming the way physicians, payers, patients, and other healthcare stakeholders interact and function within the healthcare system.
- The increased use of government regulation to protect patient health, safety, and privacy is creating demand for innovative government processes and partnerships.[27]

Fig. 1.4 provides an illustration of how these international health trends and driving forces interact together, influencing the practice of health informatics, which, in turn, through a recursive process, influences international health trends and driving forces.

This unit presents international health informatics initiatives, as well as the international organizations involved in these initiatives and how health practitioners are involved in the activities of these organizations. In addition, international informatics implications are woven throughout each chapter of this book as appropriate.

Unit 9: Historical Implications and Future Directions in Health Informatics

Those who would prefer a better future must take an active role in creating that future. Those healthcare professionals who would prefer future healthcare information systems that are effective, improved, and innovative must take an active role in creating such systems. The work creating these systems requires professionals who understand the past as a foundation for creating a preferred future. The unit begins by using the history of informatics to understand the current status of informatics. The rich history of health informatics presents unique challenges and opportunities. For example, the authors know of no other profession where the educational programs for the discipline are housed in so many different academic departments, schools, and/or colleges, ranging from computer and/or information science to medicine and/or nursing. Establishing a consensus on the level of education required, let alone the competencies of the graduate, is a unique challenge for the profession of health informatics. However, this diversity presents a unique opportunity to define and develop interdisciplinary education.

The unit concludes by presenting the reader with specific research skills for both predicting and creating the future, along with an understanding of the driving forces influencing the future of health informatics.

CONCLUSION AND FUTURE DIRECTIONS

Although health informatics is a young discipline, the use of technology in healthcare is growing exponentially. Therefore all aspects of healthcare from the relations between patient and provider to the financial models used to pay for care are being redesigned by a process that might best be described as disruptive innovation. In this world of rapid change, healthcare students and providers often feel that they are unable to stay current and no longer have control of their own practice. A strong foundation in the concepts, principles, methods, and science of health informatics will provide both future and current providers with the knowledge and skills needed to maximize the benefits of technology, while managing the challenges it presents. The goal of this book is to provide that foundation.

REFERENCES

1. Kohn LT, Corrigan JM, Donaldson MS. In: *To Err Is Human: Building a Safer Health System*. Washington, DC: National Academy Press, Institute of Medicine; 1999.
2. James JT. A new, evidence-based estimate of patient harms associated with hospital care. *J Patient Saf*. 2013;9(3): 122–128.
2a. Makary MA, Daniel M. Medical error—the third leading cause of death in the US. *BMJ*. 2016;353:i2139.
3. *Patient Safety America*. About the author; n.d. http://sandbox. patientsafetyamerica.com/a-sea-of-broken-hearts.
4. Furukawa MF, Eldridge N, Wang Y, Metersky M. Electronic health record adoption and rates of in-hospital adverse events. *J Patient Saf*. 2016; [Epub ahead of print].
5. Helwig A, Lomotan E. *Can Electronic Health Records Prevent Harm to Patients?* 2016. http://www.ahrq.gov/news/blog/ahrqviews/020916.html.
6. Institute of Medicine. *Health Professions Education: A Bridge to Quality*. Washington, DC: The National Academies Press; 2003.
7. American Association of Colleges of Nursing (AACN). *The Essentials of Baccalaureate Education for Professional Nursing Practice*; 2008. http://www.aacn.nche.edu/education-resources/essential-series.
8. American Association of Colleges of Nursing (AACN). *The Essentials of Master's Education for Professional Nursing*; 2011. http://www.aacn.nche.edu/education-resources/MastersEssentials11.pdf.
9. American Association of Colleges of Nursing (AACN). *The Essentials of Doctoral Education for Advanced Practice Nurses*; 2006. http://www.aacn.nche.edu/publications/position/DNPEssentials.pdf.
10. Hall SD. *Army telemedicine programs going mobile. Fierce Mobile Healthcare*; 2013. http://www.fiercemobilehealthcare.com/story/army-telemedicine-programs-going-mobile/2013-05-13.
11. Rantz MJ, Skubic M, Miller SJ, et al. Sensor technology to support aging in place. *J Am Med Dir Assoc*. 2013;14(6): 386–391.
12. Michard F. Hemodynamic monitoring in the era of digital health. *Ann Intensive Care*. 2016;6(1):15.
13. Covinsky K. *Transfers from the Hospital to Nursing Home: An F-Grade for Quality*; 2013. http://www.geripal.org/2013/08/transfers-from-hospital-to-nursing-home.html.
14. King BJ, Gilmore-Bykovskyi AL, Roiland RA, et al. The consequences of poor communication during transitions from hospital to skilled nursing facility: a qualitative study. *J Am Geriatr Soc*. 2013;61(7):1095–1102.
15. Storfjell JL, Omoike O, Ohlson S. The balancing act: patient care time versus cost. *J Nurs Adm*. 2008;38(5):244–249.
16. Ford S. Nurses waste 'an hour a shift' finding equipment. *Nurs Times*. 2009;105(5):1.
17. Robbins M. *Refocusing the Healthcare Supply Chain on the Patient*; October 27, 2014. http://www.beckershospitalreview.com/hospital-management-administration/refocusing-the-healthcare-supply-chain-on-the-patient.html.
18. Swisslog. *RoboCourier® Autonomous Mobile Robot*. http://www.swisslog.com/en/Products/HCS/Automated-Material-Transport/RoboCourier-Autonomous-Mobile-Robot. Retrieved November 17, 2016.
19. McMurtrey M. A case study of the application of the systems development life cycle (SDLC) in 21st century health care: something old, something new? *J South Assoc Inform Syst*. 2013;1(1):14–25.
20. Halamka JD. *Using Big Data to Make Wiser Medical Decisions*; December 2015. https://hbr.org/2015/12/using-big-data-to-make-wiser-medical-decisions.
21. DesRoches C. Progress and challenges in electronic health record adoption: findings from a national survey of physicians. *Ann Intern Med*. 2015;162(5):396.
22. The Office of the National Coordinator for Health Information Technology (ONC). *Report to Congress on Health IT Adoption and HIE 2014*; 2014. https://www.healthit.gov/sites/default/files/rtc_adoption_and_exchange9302014.pdf.
23. Adler-Milstein J, DesRoches CM, Kralovec P, et al. Electronic health record adoption in US hospitals: progress continues, but challenges persist. *Health Aff (Millwood)*. 2015;34(12):2174–2180.
24. American Association of Colleges of Nursing (AACN). *Nursing Faculty Shortage Fact Sheet*; March 16, 2015. http://www.aacn.nche.edu/media-relations/NrsgShortageFS.pdf.
25. Hershel A. The Aging of Full-time U.S. Medical School Faculty: 1967-2007. *Anal Brief*. 2009;9(4). https://www.aamc.org/download/102368/data/aibvol9no4.pdf.
26. Population Reference Bureau (PRB). *Shifts in Country-Specific Health Trends, Growth in Chronic Disease*; 2013. http://www.prb.org/Publications/Articles/2013/global-burden-disease-2010.aspx.
27. Deloitte Limited. *Global Health Care Outlook: Common Goals, Competing Priorities*; 2015. https://www2.deloitte.com/content/dam/Deloitte/global/Documents/Life-Sciences-Health-Care/gx-lshc-2015-health-care-outlook-global.pdf.
28. AHIMA. Defining the basics of health informatics for HIM professionals. *J AHIMA*. 2014;85(9):60–66.
29. 44 HIMSS KOfPICa. *Health Informatics Defined*; 2014. http://www.himss.org/ResourceLibrary/genResourceDetailPDF.aspx?ItemNumber=27767.
30. Kulikowski CA, Shortliffe EH, Currie LM, et al. AMIA board white paper: definition of biomedical informatics and specification of core competencies for graduate education in the discipline. *J Am Med Inform Assoc*. 2012;19(6):931–938.
31. US:NLM. *Health Services Research (HSR) Topic Definitions*; 2009. https://www.nlm.nih.gov/hsrinfo/ahsr/html/health_services_research_definition.html.

DISCUSSION QUESTIONS

1. Health informatics is both a discipline and a profession. Describe how health informatics as a discipline influences health informatics as a profession, as well as how the profession influences the discipline.
2. Describe how health informatics content and related courses fits within the curriculum for your discipline. For example, if you are a nurse or student of nursing, explain how health informatics is integrated into the curriculum for your profession.
3. Develop a definition of *health informatics* that might be used to describe and explain it to a patient with limited literacy.
4. Select three units in the book. Read the abstract for each chapter in each of the three units. Now write a paragraph summarizing each unit. At the end of the three paragraphs, write a fourth paragraph describing the interrelationships you can identify between these units.

CASE STUDY

You are currently employed as a healthcare provider in a community hospital in your local community. The local high school is designing a learning unit for sophomores who have expressed an interest in computers and other technology as a potential future career. The teacher, who has designed this unit, has asked you to attend one of the classes as a guest speaker discussing how computer-related technology is used in healthcare. Design a 20- to 30-minute presentation that you might use in meeting the teacher's request.

Case Study Questions

1. What questions might you ask the teacher to assess the literacy levels of the students?
2. The first 2 minutes of the presentation should be designed to grab the student's interest. What content would you include in these first two minutes?
3. What are the 3 to 5 key points you would want to include in this presentation?
4. What questions do you anticipate the students might ask and how would you prepare to answer their questions?

2

Theoretical Foundations of Health Informatics

Ramona Nelson and Nancy Staggers

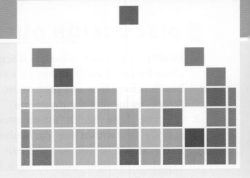

Whether designing effective and innovative technology-based solutions, implementing these approaches, or evaluating them, truly nothing is as useful as a good theory to guide the process.

Judith Effken

OBJECTIVES

At the completion of this chapter, the reader will be prepared to:

1. Explain the technology-related literacies and their relationship to health informatics.
2. Use major theories and models underpinning informatics to analyze health informatics-related phenomena.
3. Use major theories and models underpinning informatics to predict health informatics-related phenomena.
4. Use major theories and models underpinning informatics to manage health informatics-related phenomena.

KEY TERMS

ABSTRACT ❖

This chapter provides an overview of the technology-related literacies, theories, and models useful for guiding practice in health informatics. For both providers and patients, developing knowledge and related skills in health informatics requires first a foundation in technology-related literacies. The chapter begins by exploring these literacies and their relationship to health informatics. Next, the chapter defines and explains components of grand, middle-range, and micro theories. Whether designing effective and innovative technology-based solutions, implementing these approaches, or evaluating them, truly nothing is as useful as a good theory to guide the process. Specific theories relevant to informatics are outlined. Systems and complexity adaptation theory provide the foundation for understanding each of the theories presented. Information models from Blum, Graves, and Nelson outline the data, information, knowledge, and wisdom continuum. The next section of the chapter presents change theories including the diffusion of innovation theory. In the final section of the chapter, the Staggers and Nelson model of the systems life cycle is described, and its application is outlined.

INTRODUCTION

Health informatics is a profession. In turn, the individuals who practice this profession function as professionals. These statements may seem obvious, but there are important implications in these statements that can be easily overlooked. The professionals who practice a profession possess a body of knowledge, as well as values and skills unique to that profession. The body of knowledge, values, and skills guide the profession as a whole, as well as the individual professional, in decisions related directly or indirectly to the services provided to society by that profession. Professional practice is not based on a set of rules that can be carefully followed. Rather, the profession, through its professional organizations, and the professional, as an individual, make decisions by applying their knowledge, values, and skills to the specific situation. The profession and the professional within that profession have a high degree of autonomy, and are therefore responsible for the practice and the decision made within that practice. This chapter provides an overview of the primary technology-related literacies, the theories, and the models useful for guiding the professional practice in health informatics.

Foundational Literacies for Health Informatics

For both providers and patients, developing their knowledge and related skills in health informatics requires a foundation in the technology-related literacies.

The discussion in this chapter focuses on basic literacy and technology-related literacies that relate directly to the work of patients and healthcare providers. Successful use of technology is dependent on basic literacy, computer literacy, information literacy, digital literacy, and health literacy. These specific literacies are both overlapping and interrelated as illustrated in Fig. 2.1.

Definition of Basic Literacy

As illustrated in Fig. 2.1, basic literacy is the foundational skill. Without a basic level of literacy, the other types of literacy become impossible and irrelevant. UNESCO offered one of the first definitions of *literacy*. "A literate person is one who can, with understanding, both read and write a short simple statement on his or her everyday life."[1, p. 12] This definition is still in frequent use today. In 2003 UNESCO proposed an operational definition that attempted to encompass several different dimensions of literacy. "Literacy is the ability to identify, understand, interpret, create, communicate, and compute, using printed and written materials associated with varying contexts. Literacy involves a continuum of learning in enabling individuals to achieve their goals, to develop their knowledge and potential, and to participate fully in their community and wider society."[1] Although other UNESCO publications have provided additional definitions of literacy, the 2003 definition continues to be the more comprehensive definition.

In the United States, the U.S. Department of Education, Institute of Education Sciences, National Center for Education Statistics conducts the National Assessment of Adult Literacy (NAAL). The NAAL definition of *literacy* includes both knowledge and skills. NAAL assesses three types of literacy: prose, document, and quantitative.

- **Prose literacy**: The knowledge and skills needed to search, comprehend, and use continuous texts such as editorials, news stories, brochures, and instructional materials.
- **Document literacy:** The document-related knowledge and skills needed to perform a search, comprehend, and use noncontinuous texts in various formats such as job applications, payroll forms, transportation schedules, maps, tables, and drug or food labels.
- **Quantitative literacy:** The quantitative knowledge and skills required for identifying and performing computations, either alone or sequentially, using numbers embedded in printed materials such as balancing a checkbook, figuring out a tip, completing an order form, or determining the amount.[2]

The focus of both the national and international definitions is the ability to understand and use information in printed or written format. The assumption is that this includes the ability to understand both text and numeric information. Many people assume that if one can read and understand information in

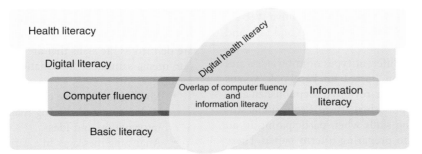

FIG 2.1 Overlapping relationships of technology-related literacies and basic literacy. (Printed with Permission of Ramona Nelson all rights reserved.)

printed format, presumably that individual could read and understand the same information on a computer screen. However, computer literacy involves much more than the ability to read information from a computer screen. In fact, the term *computer literacy* with its limited scope is outdated.

Definition of Computer Literacy/Fluency

Over 15 years ago, the National Academy of Science coined the term FIT persons to describe people who are fluent with information technology. That definition remains current. FIT persons possess three types of knowledge:

- **Contemporary skills** are the ability to use current computer applications such as word processors, spreadsheets, or an internet search engine, using the correct tool for the right job (e.g., spreadsheets when manipulating numbers and word processors when manipulating text).
- **Foundational concepts** are understanding the how and why of information technology. This knowledge gives the person insight into the opportunities and limitations of social media and other information technologies.
- **Intellectual capabilities** are the ability to apply information technology to actual problems and challenges of everyday life. An example of this knowledge is the ability to use critical thinking when evaluating health information on a social media site.[3]

Definition of Information Literacy

The Association of College and Research Libraries (ACRL), a division of the American Library Association (ALA), initially defined information literacy and has led the development of information literacy standards since the 1980s. As part of this effort, they established standards of information literacy for higher education, high schools, and even elementary education. The ALA defines *information literacy* as a set of abilities requiring individuals to recognize when information is needed and have the ability to locate, evaluate, and effectively use the needed information.[4] This definition has gained wide acceptance. However, with the extensive growth of new technologies, including different internet-based information sources and social media, there have been increasing calls to revise the definition and the established standards from over a decade ago. "Social media environments and online communities are innovative collaborative technologies that challenge the traditional definitions of information literacy…information is not a static object that is simply accessed and retrieved. It is a dynamic entity that is produced and shared collaboratively with such innovative Web 2.0 technologies as Facebook, Twitter, Delicious, Second Life, and YouTube."[5, p. 62]

For example, it requires different types of knowledge and skills to evaluate information posted on Facebook, versus Wikipedia, versus an online peer-reviewed prepublished article, versus a peer-reviewed published article. Professional students need different writing skills when participating in an online dialog as opposed to preparing a term paper. There are standards that apply to text messaging, especially if the message is between healthcare colleagues or is being sent to a patient. Developing appropriate policies, procedures, and standards are the challenges facing healthcare leaders in the world of evidence-based practice, social media, and engaged patients. Recognizing the changing world of information creation, access, and use, ACRL has expanded the definition of *information literacy*:

> Information literacy is the set of integrated abilities encompassing the reflective discovery of information, the understanding of how information is produced and valued, and the use of information in creating new knowledge and participating ethically in communities of learning.[6]

In line with the expanded definition, the ACRL developed a Framework for Information Literacy for Higher Education (Framework).[6] The Framework grows out of their belief that information literacy as an educational reform movement will realize its potential only through a richer, more complex set of core ideas. While the Framework does not replace the standards previously developed, it does provide a less prescriptive approach for incorporating information literacy, knowledge, and skills into education, including the education of health professionals. Table 2.1 lists and gives a brief description of the six frames in the Framework. As can be seen from the changing definition of *information literacy* the internet and related apps, as well as technologies, are changing the concept of information literacy. Arising from this change is the concept of digital literacy.

Definition of Digital Literacy

The term digital literacy first appears in the literature in the 1990s. However, to date, there is no generally accepted definition. While there is no generally accepted definition, there are a number of national and international Digital Literacy Centers supporting the development of digital literacy. Some examples include:

- Syracuse University's Center for Digital Literacy at http://digital-literacy.syr.edu/
- University of British Columbia, the Digital Literacy Centre at http://dlc.lled.educ.ubc.ca/
- Microsoft Digital Literacy Curriculum at www.microsoft.com/en-us/DigitalLiteracy
- National Telecommunications and Information Administration Literacy Center at www.digitalliteracy.gov/

There are also a number of books published about digital literacy. Three recognized definitions are published. The earliest of these is provided in a White Paper commissioned by the Aspen Institute Communications and Society Program and the John S. and James L. Knight Foundation, "Digital and media literacy are defined as life skills that are necessary for participation in our media-saturated, information-rich society." These skills include:

- Making responsible choices and accessing information by locating and sharing materials and comprehending information and ideas.
- Analyzing messages in a variety of forms by identifying the author, purpose, and point of view, and evaluating the quality and credibility of the content.

TABLE 2.1 Framework for Information Literacy for Higher Education[6]

Frames	Description
Authority Is Constructed and Contextual	Information resources reflect their creators' expertise and credibility, and are evaluated based on the information need and the context in which the information will be used.
Information Creation as a Process	The iterative processes of researching, creating, revising, and disseminating information vary, and the resulting product reflects these differences.
Information Has Value	Information possesses several dimensions of value, including as a commodity, as a means of education, as a means to influence, and as a means of negotiating and understanding the world.
Research as Inquiry	Research is iterative and depends upon asking increasingly complex or new questions whose answers in turn develop additional questions or lines of inquiry in any field.
Scholarship as Conversation	Communities of scholars, researchers, or professionals engage in sustained discourse with new insights and discoveries occurring over time as a result of varied perspectives and interpretations
Searching as Strategic Exploration	Searching for information is often nonlinear and iterative, requiring the evaluation of a range of information sources and the mental flexibility to pursue alternate avenues as new understanding develops.

- Creating content in a variety of forms, making use of language, images, sound, and new digital tools and technologies.
- Reflecting on one's own conduct and communication behavior by applying social responsibility and ethical principles.
- Taking social action by working individually and collaboratively to share knowledge and solve problems in the family, workplace, and community, and by participating as a member of a community.[7]

The second, and most recognized definition of digital literacy, provided by the ALA's Digital Literacy Task Force, describes it as "the ability to use information and communication technologies to find, understand, evaluate, create, and communicate digital information, an ability that requires both cognitive and technical skills."[8, p. 2]

A digitally literate person:
- Possesses a variety of skills—cognitive and technical—required to find, understand, evaluate, create, and communicate digital information in a wide variety of formats
- Is able to use diverse technologies appropriately and effectively to search for and retrieve information, interpret search results, and judge the quality of the information retrieved
- Understands the relationships among technology, lifelong learning, personal privacy, and appropriate stewardship of information
- Uses these skills and the appropriate technologies to communicate and collaborate with peers, colleagues, family, and, on occasion, the public
- Uses these skills to participate actively in society and contribute to a vibrant, informed, and engaged community[8]

The third definition, published by Springer in a book focused on social media for nurses, defined digital literacy as including:
- Competency with digital devices of all types including cameras, eReaders, smartphones, computers, tablets, and video games boards. This does not mean that one can pick up a new device and use that device without an orientation. Rather, one can use trial and error, as well as a manufacturer's manual, to determine how to use a device effectively.
- The technical skills to operate these devices, as well as the conceptual knowledge to understand their functionality.
- The ability to creatively and critically use these devices to access, manipulate, evaluate, and apply data, information, knowledge, and wisdom in activities of daily living.
- The ability to apply basic emotional intelligence in collaborating and communicating with others.
- The ethical values and sense of community responsibility to use digital devices for the enjoyment and benefit of society.[9]

These three definitions have much in common, and together they demonstrate that digital literacy is a more comprehensive concept than computer or information literacy. The definition goes beyond the comfortable use of technology demonstrated by the digital native. Digital literacy is about understanding the implications of digital technology and the impact it is having, and will have, on every aspect of our lives. "The truth is, though most people think kids these days *get* the digital world, we are actually breeding a generation of digital illiterates. How? We are not teaching them how to really understand and use the tools. *We are only teaching them how to click buttons.* We need to be teaching our students, at all levels, not just how to click and poke, but how to communicate, and interact, and build relationships in a connected world."[10]

Definition of Health Literacy

Although health literacy is concerned with the ability to access, evaluate, and apply information to health-related decisions, there is also not a consistent, generally accepted agreement on the definition of the term. In 2011, a published systematic review of the literature in Medline, PubMed, and Web of Science identified 17 definitions of health literacy and 12 conceptual models. The most frequently cited definitions of health literacy were from the American Medical Association, the Institute of Medicine, and World Health Organization (WHO).[11] Current definitions from the Institute of Medicine, and WHO include:

- The Institution of Medicine uses the definition of health literacy developed by Ratzan and Parker and cited in Healthy *People 2010.* Health literacy is "the degree to which individuals have the capacity to obtain, process, and understand basic health information and services needed to make appropriate health decisions."[12]
- The WHO has defined health literacy as "the cognitive and social skills that determine the motivation and ability of individuals to gain access to, understand, and use information in ways which promote and maintain good health." Health literacy means more than being able to read pamphlets and successfully make appointments. By improving people's access to health information and their capacity to use it effectively, health literacy is critical to empowerment. It is the degree to which people are able to access, understand, appraise, and communicate information to engage with the demands of different health contexts to promote and maintain good health across the life-course.[13]

The focus in each of these definitions is on an individual's skill in obtaining and using the health information and services necessary to make appropriate health decisions. These definitions do not fully address the networked world of the internet. In recognition of this deficiency, Norman and Skinner introduced the concept of eHealth as "the ability to seek, find, understand, and appraise health information from electronic sources and apply the knowledge gained to addressing or solving a health problem."[14, e9] This definition acknowledges the need for computer fluency and the use of information skills to obtain an effective level of health literacy. However, this definition is not especially sensitive to the impact of social media. For example, it does not address the individual as a patient/consumer collaboratively creating health-related information that others could use in making health-related decisions. There is increasing evidence that patients bring to the dialog a unique knowledge base for addressing a number of health-related problems.[15] Creating the comprehensive definition and model for assessment of health literacy levels that includes the social media literacy skills needed for today's communication processes remains a challenge for health professionals. A key resource in meeting the health literacy needs within the clinical setting and the community can be found at http://nnlm.gov/outreach/consumer/hlthlit.html.

While each of the technology-related communication literacies presented here focuses on a different aspect of literacy and has a different definition, they all overlap and are interrelated. Fig. 2.1 demonstrates those interrelationships. In this figure, basic literacy is depicted as foundational to all other literacies. Digital literacy includes computer and

information literacy as well as other social media–related knowledge and skills that were not initially included in the definitions of computer and information literacy. For example, playing online games is not usually considered part of information or computer literacy, but it clearly requires digital literacy. Health literacy now requires both digital literacy and a basic knowledge of health unrelated to automation. All of the literacies require the ability to evaluate online information and, especially, to pay attention to information generated on social media sites.

Understanding these technology-related communication literacies and integrating them into current policies and procedures is the challenge all healthcare providers and informaticians face.

UNDERSTANDING THEORIES AND MODELS

A **theory** explains the process by which certain phenomena occur.[16] Theories vary in scope depending on the extent and complexity of the **phenomenon** of interest. Grand theories are wide in scope and attempt to explain a complex phenomenon within the human experience. For example, a learning theory that attempted to explain all aspects of human learning would be considered a grand theory. Because of the complexity of the theory and the number of variables interacting in dependent, independent, and interdependent ways, these theories are difficult to test. However, grand theories can be foundational within a discipline or subdiscipline. For example, learning and teaching theories are foundational theories within the discipline of education.

Middle-range theories are used to explain specific defined phenomena. They begin with an observation of the specific phenomena. For example, one might note how people react to change. However, why and how does this phenomenon occur? A theory focused on the phenomenon of change would explain the process that occurs when people experience change and predict when and how they will respond in adjusting to the change.

Micro theories are limited in scope and specific to a situation. For example, one might describe the introduction of a new electronic health record (EHR) within a large ambulatory practice and even measure the variables within that situation that could be influencing the acceptance and use of the new system. In the past, micro theories, with their limited scope, have rarely been used to test theory. However, this is changing with the development of Web 2.0 and the application of meta-analysis techniques to automatized natural language processing.

The development of a theory occurs in a recursive process moving on a continuum from the initial observation of the phenomenon to the development of a theory to explain that phenomenon. The process of moving on this continuum can be divided into several stages, including the following:

1. A specific phenomenon is observed and noted.
2. An idea is proposed to explain the development of the phenomenon.
3. Key concepts used to explain the phenomenon are identified, and the processes by which the concepts interact are described.

4. A conceptual framework is developed to clarify the concepts and their relationships and interactions. Conceptual frameworks can be used to propose theories and generate research questions. The conceptual framework can also be used to develop a conceptual model. A conceptual model is a visual representation of the concepts and their relationships.
5. A theory and related hypothesis are proposed and tested.
6. Evidence accumulates, and the theory is modified, rejected, replaced, or it gains general acceptance.

Many of the models used to guide the practice of health informatics and discussed in this chapter can be considered theoretical models or frameworks. Because theoretical frameworks explain a combination of related theories and concepts, they can be used to guide practice and generate additional research questions. With this definition, one can argue that the concept of a theoretical framework can be conceived as a bridge between a middle-range theory and a grand theory. A theoretical model is a visual representation of a theoretical framework. Many of the models in healthcare and health informatics use a combination of theories in explaining phenomena of interest within these disciplines and fit the definition of a theoretical framework.

Even though the terms *theory* and *concept* are consistently defined and used in the literature, the terms *conceptual* and *theoretical framework*, as well as the terms *conceptual* and *theoretical models*, are not. No set of consistent criteria can be applied to determine whether a model is conceptual or theoretical. As a result, researchers and informaticians will often publish models without clarifying that the proposed model is either conceptual or theoretical. In turn, it is possible for one reference to refer to a model as a conceptual framework whereas another uses the term *theory* when it refers to a model as a theoretical framework.

Theories and Models Underlying Health Informatics

Health informatics is an applied field of study incorporating theories from information science; computer science; the science for the specific discipline, such as medicine, nursing, or pharmacy; and the wide range of sciences used in healthcare

delivery. Therefore health professionals and health informatics specialists draw on a wide range of theories to guide their practice. This chapter focuses on selected theories that are of major importance to health informatics and those that are most directly applicable. These theories are vital to understanding and managing the challenges and decisions faced by health professionals and informatics specialists. In analyzing the selected theories, the reader will discover that understanding these theories presents certain challenges. Some of the theories overlap, different theories are used to explain the same phenomena, and sometimes, different theories have the same name. The theories of information are an example of each of these challenges.

The one theory that underlies all of the theories used in health informatics is systems theory. Therefore this is the first theory discussed in this chapter.

Systems Theory

A system is a set of related interacting parts enclosed in a boundary.[17] Examples of systems include computer systems, school systems, the healthcare system, and a person. Systems may be living or nonliving.[18] Systems may be either open or closed. Closed systems are enclosed within an impermeable boundary and do not interact with the environment. Open systems are enclosed within a semipermeable boundary and do interact with the environment. This chapter focuses on open systems, which can be used to understand technology and the people who are interacting with the technology. Fig. 2.2 demonstrates an open system interacting with the environment. Open systems take input (information, matter, and energy) from the environment, process the input, and then return output to the environment. The output then becomes feedback to the system. Concepts from systems theory can be applied in understanding the way people work with computers in a healthcare organization. These concepts can also be used to analyze individual elements such as software or the total picture of what happens when systems interact.

A common expression in computer science is "garbage in garbage out," or GIGO. GIGO refers to the input-output process. The counter-concept implied by this expression is that quality input is required to achieve quality output. Although

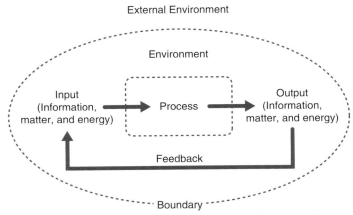

FIG 2.2 An open system interacting with the environment. (Copyright Ramona Nelson. Reprinted with permission. All rights reserved.)

GIGO usually is used to refer to computer systems, it can apply to any open system. An example of this concept can be seen when informed active participants provide input for the selection of a healthcare information system. In this example, garbage in can result in garbage out or quality input can support the potential for quality output. Not only is quality input required for quality output, but the system must also have effective procedures for processing those data. Systems theory provides a framework for looking at the inputs to a system, analyzing how the system processes those inputs, and measuring and evaluating the outputs from the system.

Characteristics of Systems

Open systems have three types of characteristics: purpose, structure, and functions. The purpose is the reason for the system's existence. The purpose of an institution or program is often outlined in the mission statement. Such statements can include more than one purpose. For example, many healthcare institutions have three purposes: (1) provide patient care, (2) provide educational programs for students in the health professions, and (3) conduct health-related research. Computer systems are often referred to or classified by their purpose(s). The purpose of a radiology system is to support the radiology department. An EHR can have several different purposes. One of the purposes is to maintain a census that can be used to bill for patient care.

One of the first steps in selecting a computer system for use in a healthcare organization is to identify the purposes of that system. Having a succinct purpose answers the question "Why select a system?" Many times, there is a tendency to minimize this step with the assumption that everyone already agrees on the purposes of the system. When a system has several different purposes, it is common for individuals to focus on the purposes most directly related to their area of responsibility. Taking the time to specify and prioritize the purposes helps to ensure that the representatives from clinical, administration, and technology agree on the reasons for selecting a system and understand the full scope of the project.

Functions, on the contrary, focus on the question "How will the system achieve its purpose?" Functions are sometimes mistaken for purpose. However, it is important to clarify why a system is needed, and then identify what functions the system will carry out to achieve that purpose. For example, a hospital may maintain patient census data including admissions, discharges, and transfers through a computerized registration system. Each time a department accesses the patient's online record, the name and other identifying information are transmitted from a master file, ensuring consistency throughout the institution. When selecting a computer system, the functions for that system are carefully identified and defined in writing. These are listed as functional specifications. Specifications identify each function and describe how that function will be performed.

Systems are structured to perform their functions. Two different structural models operating concurrently can be used to conceptualize healthcare technical infrastructures. These are hierarchical and web. The hierarchical model is an older architectural model, and the terms, such as *mainframe*, that are used to describe the model reflect that reality.

The location and type of hardware used within a system often follow a hierarchical model; however, as computer systems are becoming more integrated, information flow increasingly follows a web model. The hierarchical model can be used to structure the distribution of the computer processing loads at the same time as the web model is used to structure communication of health-related data throughout the institution. The hierarchical model is demonstrated in Fig. 2.3. Each individual computer is part of a local area network (LAN). The LANs join together to form a wide area network (WAN) that is connected to the mainframe computers. In Fig. 2.3 the mainframe is the lead computer or lead part. This structure demonstrates a centralized approach to managing the computer structure.

When analyzing the hierarchical model, the term *system* may refer to any level of the structure. In Fig. 2.3, an individual computer may be referred to as a system or the whole diagram may be considered a system. Three terms are used to indicate the level of reference. These are subsystem, target system, and supersystem. A subsystem is any system within the target system. For example, if the target system is a LAN, each computer is a subsystem. The supersystem is the overall structure in which the target system exists. If the target system is a LAN, then Fig. 2.3 represents a supersystem.

The second model used to analyze the structure of a system is the web model. The interrelationships between the different LANs function like a web. Laboratory data may be shared with the pharmacy and the clinical units concurrently, just as the data collected by nursing, such as weight and height, may be shared with each department needing the data. The internet is an example of a complex system that demonstrates both hierarchical and web structures interacting as a cohesive unit. As these examples demonstrate, a system includes structural elements from both the web model and the hierarchical model. Complex and complicated systems discussed later in this chapter can include a number of supersystems organized using both hierarchical and web structures.

Boundary, attributes, and environment are three concepts used to characterize structure. The boundary of a system forms the demarcation between the target system and the environment of the system. Input flows into the system by moving across the boundary and output flows into the environment across this boundary. For example, with a web model, information flows across the systems. Thinking in terms of boundaries can help to distinguish information flowing into a system from information being processed within a system. Fig. 2.3 can be used to demonstrate how these concepts can establish the boundaries of a project. Each computer in the diagram represents a target system for a specific project. For example, a healthcare institution could be planning for a new pharmacy information system. The new pharmacy system becomes the target system. However, as the model demonstrates, the pharmacy system interacts with other systems within the total system. The task group selecting the new pharmacy system will need to identify the functional specifications needed to automate the pharmacy and the functional specifications needed for the pharmacy system to interact with the other systems in the environment. Clearly, specifying

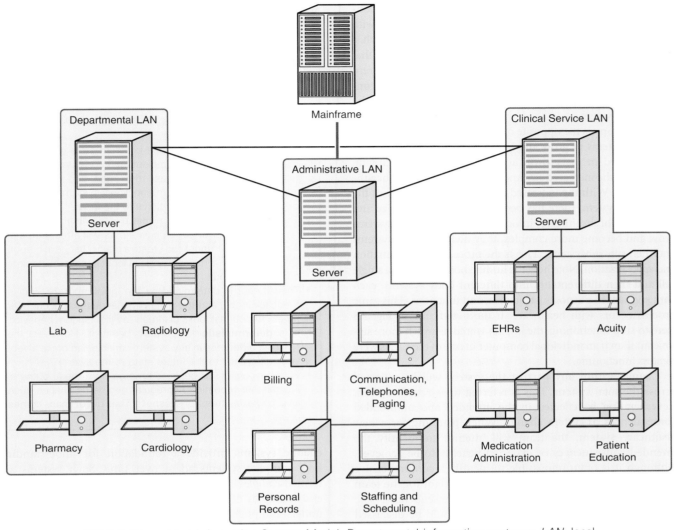

FIG 2.3 Hierarchical Information System Model. Departmental information systems; *LAN*, local area network. (Copyright Ramona Nelson. Reprinted with permission. All right reserved.)

the target system and the other systems in the environment that must interact or interface with the target will assist in defining the scope of the project. By defining the scope of the project, it becomes possible to focus on the task while planning for the integration of the pharmacy system with other systems in the institution. A key example is planning for the impact of a new pharmacy system in terms of the activities of nurses who are administering medications.

In planning for healthcare information systems, **attributes** of the system are identified. Attributes are the properties of the parts or components of the system. When discussing computer hardware, these attributes are usually referred to as *specifications*. An example of a list of patient-related attributes can be seen on an intake or patient assessment form in a healthcare setting. Attributes and the expression of those attributes play a major role in the development of databases. Field names are a list of the attributes of interest for a specific system. The datum in each cell is the individual system's expression of that attribute. A record lists the attributes for each individual system. The record can also be seen as a subsystem of the total database system.

Systems and the Change Process

Both living and nonliving systems are constantly in a process of change. Six concepts are helpful in understanding the change process. These are dynamic homeostasis, equifinality, entropy, negentropy, specialization, and reverberation.

Dynamic homeostasis refers to the processes used by a system to maintain a steady state or balance. This same goal of maintaining a steady state can affect how clinical settings respond when changes are made or a new system is implemented.

Equifinality is the tendency of open systems to reach a characteristic final state from different initial conditions and in different ways. For example, two different clinics may be scheduled for the implementation of a new EHR. One unit may be using paper records and the other unit may have an outdated computer system. A year or two later, both clinical units may be at the same point, comfortably using the new system. However, the process for reaching this point may have been very different.

Entropy is the tendency of all systems to break down into their simplest parts. As it breaks down, the system becomes increasingly disorganized or random. Entropy is demonstrated in the tendency of all systems to wear out. Even with maintenance, a healthcare information system will reach a point where it must be replaced. Healthcare information that is transferred across many different systems in many different formats can also demonstrate entropy, thereby causing confusion and conflict between different entities within the healthcare system.

Negentropy is the opposite of entropy. This is the tendency of living systems to grow and become more complex. This is demonstrated in the growth and development of an infant, as well as in the increased size and complexity of today's healthcare system. With the increased growth and complexity of the healthcare system, there has been an increase in the size and complexity of healthcare information systems. As systems grow and become more complex, they divide into subsystems and then sub-subsystems. This is the process of differentiation and specialization. Note how the human body begins as a single cell and then differentiates into different body systems, each with specialized purposes, structures, and functions. This same process occurs with healthcare. If the mainframe in Fig. 2.3 were to stop functioning, the impact would be much more significant than if an individual computer in one of the LANs were to stop functioning.

Change within any part of the system will be reflected across the total system. This is referred to as reverberation. Reverberation is reflected in the intended and unintended consequences of system change. When planning for a new healthcare system, the team will attempt to identify the intended consequences or expected benefits to be achieved. Although it is often impossible to identify a comprehensive list of unintended consequences, it is important for the team to consider the reality of unintended consequences. The potential for unintended consequences should be discussed during the planning stage; however, these will be more evident during the testing stage that precedes the implementation or "go-live." Many times unintended consequences are not considered until after go-live, when they become obvious. For example, e-mail may be successfully introduced to improve communication in an organization. However, an unintended consequence can be the increased workload from irrelevant e-mail messages. Unintended consequences are not always negative. They can be either positive or negative.

Unintended consequences is just one example of how difficult it is to describe, explain, and predict events and maybe even control outcomes in complex systems such as a healthcare institution. Starting in the 1950s, chaos theory, followed by complexity theory, began to develop and was seen as an approach for understanding complex systems. Both chaos and complexity theory involve the study of dynamic nonlinear systems that change with time and demonstrate a variety of cause-and-effect relationships between inputs and outputs because of reiterative feedback loops. "The quantitative study of these systems is chaos theory. Complexity theory is the qualitative aspect drawing upon insights and metaphors that are derived from chaos theory."[19] Box 2.1 outlines the characteristics of chaotic systems. The characteristics of

BOX 2.1 Characteristics of Chaotic Systems

Chaos is defined as a physical "mathematical dynamic system which is: (a) deterministic (b) is recurrent and (c) has sensitive dependence on the initial state."[20, p.164] In turn, *chaos theory* can be defined as "the qualitative study of unstable aperiodic behavior in deterministic, nonlinear dynamical systems."[21, p.2] Chaotic systems demonstrate the following characteristics:

- They are dynamic systems in a constant state of nonlinear change. In a linear system, the output is consistently proportional to the input. Increase the input and the output increases at the same rate. In a nonlinear system, the output of the system is not proportional to the input.
- The reiterative feedback loop that exists within these systems has a major effect on how inputs will affect outputs. A minor change in input can create a major change in output. On the contrary, a major change in input can result in minor changes in output.
- Their output is determined by the initial input, reiterative feedback loops, and the dynamic changes that occur over time. "Although it looks disorganized like random behavior, it is deterministic-like periodic behavior. However, the smallest difference in any system variable can make a very large difference to the future state of the system."[19, p.15]
- Fractal-type patterns begin to emerge from these outputs. Fractals are repeating nonregular geometric shapes such as snowflakes, trees, or seashells. Thus out of chaos comes order.[22]

chaotic systems provide a foundation for understanding how complex systems adapt over time. Such systems are termed *complex adaptive systems* (CAS). There are now several examples of how the concept of CAS is being use to understand phenomenon of interest in the healthcare literature.[23-30]

Complex Adaptive Systems

A Complex Adaptive System (CAS) is defined as an "entity consisting of many diverse and autonomous parts which are interrelated, interdependent, linked through many interconnections, and behave as a unified whole in learning from experience and in adjusting (not just reacting) to changes in the environment. Each individual agent of a CAS is itself a CAS."[31] This definition is best understood by analyzing the characteristics of a CAS.[32–35]

Characteristics of a CAS.

Change occurs through nonlinear interdependencies. A CAS demonstrates interrelationships, interaction, and interconnectivity of the units within the system and between the system and its environment. A change in any one part of the system will influence all other related parts but not in any uniform manner. For example, a small inexpensive change on a computer screen may make that screen easier to understand and in turn prevent a number of very dangerous mistakes. On the contrary, a major revision of an organization website may have minimal impact on how the user of that site sees the organization or uses the site.

Control is distributed. Within a CAS, there is no single person or group who has full control of the organization. It is the interrelationship and interdependencies that produce a level of coherence that makes it possible for the organization to function and even grow. Thus the overall behavior cannot be predicted by reviewing the activities of one section or part of the organization. Hindsight can be used to explain past events, but foresight is limited in predicting outcomes. Therefore solutions based on past practices may prove ineffective when presented with a new version of a previous problem.

Learning and behavior change is constant. Individuals and groups within a CAS are intelligent agents who learn from each other, probe their environment, and test out ideas. They are constantly learning and changing their ideas as well as their behavior.

Units or parts of a CAS are self-organizing. *Self-organizing* refers to the ability of CAS to arrange workflow and patterns of interaction spontaneously into a purposeful (nonrandom) manner, without the help of an external agency. Individuals and groups within a CAS are unique. Individuals and groups with the CAS will have different and overlapping needs, desires, knowledge, and personality traits. Order results from the feedback inherent in the interactions between individuals and groups as each moves through their own activities. Behavior patterns that were not designed into the system will emerge. As these individuals and groups interact, the emerging patterns of interactions will include some degree of both cooperation and conflict. Therefore these emergent behaviors may range from valuable innovations to severe conflict issues.

The patterns of interaction are for the most part informal yet well established for the individuals functioning in the group. The patterns of behavior will have a major influence on the organization of workflow, but are often not obvious to someone new in the group. In addition, such behaviors are often not documented; for example, in a policy or procedure. However, these emergent behaviors can be key to understanding how a department or group actually functions. In addition, emergent behaviors are constantly changing as both the external and internal environment of the unit changes.

The adaptive process within complex organizations demonstrates infinitely complex, unique emerging patterns. For example, the go-live process within or across complex organizations follows a similar but unique process each time a new system is installed, even when the same software is installed in a similar type of clinical unit in a new site. Sites and units all have different workflows and organizational cultures to which processes need to be tailored.

CASs exist in co-evolution with the environment. The concept of co-evolution refers to the process whereby a CAS is continuously adapting as it responds to its environment and, simultaneously, the environment is constantly adapting as it responds to the changing CAS. They are evolving together in a co-evolutionary interactive process.

The adaptive response of a complex system to environmental change and the resulting environmental change from that adaptation includes an element of unpredictability. The overall pattern of adaptation that emerges from the adaptive changes within each unit is unique to each organization and impossible to predict completely. For example, computerized provider order entry (CPOE) changed the workflow for unit secretaries, nurses, physicians, and hospital departments. Each of these units within the system is creating adaptations at the same time as it is adjusting to changes occurring in the other units. A significant number of these changes (whether they were seen as positive or negative by individuals in the institution) are experienced as unintended consequences.

A CAS includes both order and disorder. A certain level of order is necessary for a CAS to be effective and efficient. However, the more firmly order is imposed, the less flexibility the CAS has to adjust to change. Systems that are too tightly controlled can become fragile. A CAS needs to maintain some slack and redundancy to buffer against environmental changes that are not anticipated. This balance between creating a unified whole and an institution with enough flexibility to adapt to the changing internal and external environment can be a challenge when integrated healthcare institutions attempt to merge hospitals, long-term care facilities, clinics, and other settings into one healthcare system. The larger and more diffuse the organization, the more likely it is to include a degree of order and disorder and, therefore, more potential to survive in some form. For example, individual hospitals, clinics, and third-party payers may go out of business, but the healthcare system as a societal institution will continue to exist in ever-evolving ways.

The characteristics of a CAS interact together in a synergistic manner, ensuring that a certain level of uncertainty is inherent in the management of a CAS. The natural disposition of decision makers in such an environment is to attempt to reduce the uncertainty. However, imposing order and tightly regulating a CAS does not let the system take advantage of the inherent ability to adapt, and, in the end, it creates a CAS that is less resilient and less robust. Resilience is the ability to recover from a failure, and robustness is the ability to resist failure. The more robust a system is, the better able it is to anticipate and avoid a failure. The more resilient a system is, the better able it is to recover quickly from a failure.

That being said, frameworks for understanding how to manage CASs such as organizations and communities continue to evolve. One such framework is the Cynefin Framework.[34-39]

Cynefin Framework for Managing Uncertainly in CAS.
A CAS, such as a healthcare organization, will exist with a constantly fluctuating balance between order and disorder. This can be thought of as a continuum with any one system or part of the system moving between order and disorder. The Cynefin Framework was developed to guide organizational management on this continuum, and it provides a helpful perspective for managing informatics-related projects within a healthcare

The Cynefin Framework

The Cynefin framework helps leaders determine the prevailing operative context so that they can make appropriate choices. Each domain requires different actions. Simple and complicated contexts assume an ordered universe in which cause-and-effect relationships are perceptible and right answers can be determined based on the facts. Complex and chaotic contexts are unordered—there is no immediately apparent relationship between cause and effect, and the way forward is determined based on emerging patterns. The ordered world is the world of fact-based management; the unordered world represents pattern-based management.

The very nature of the fifth context—disorder—makes it particularly difficult to recognize when one is in it. Here, multiple perspectives jostle for prominence, factional leaders argue with one another, and cacophony rules. The way out of this realm is to break down the situation into constituent parts and assign each to one of the other four realms. Leaders can then make decisions and intervene in contextually appropriate ways.

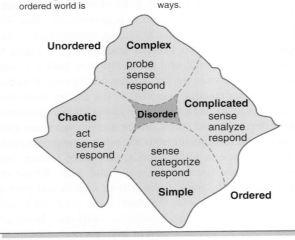

FIG 2.4 The Cynefin framework. (From Snowden DJ, Boone ME. A leader's framework for decision making. *Harv Bus Rev.* 2007;86(11):68–76. Reprinted by permission of *Harvard Business Review.* Copyright © 2007 by the Harvard Business School Publishing Corporation. All rights reserved.)

institution. The Framework consists of five domains, as depicted in Fig. 2.4.[36] The first four domains (simple, complicated, complex, and chaotic) require the leader or manager to determine the level of order or disorder and adjust their management style to that reality. The fifth domain exists when the manager/leader is unclear which of the other four domains are predominant in a specific situation. As a situation moves toward the ordered end on the continuum, one of two domains will predominate. Those are the simple and complicated domains.

Simple Domain. A simple domain is highly ordered. Cause and effect are evident to the people involved in the setting. Processes are carried out using known procedures that are effective and efficient. This process involves (1) sensing or collecting the pertinent data, (2) categorizing the data, and (3) applying the appropriate response. An example would be administering medications on a clinical unit. The procedures are carefully designed to ensure the five rights of the patient are effectively and efficiently met. There are rules about what should be done if a patient refuses a medication, is off the clinical unit, or some other usual issue occurs. With this type of situation, everyone is expected to follow the

procedure carefully. The concept of best practices is most appropriate in these types of situations. Often these types of processes or at least parts of their procedures are excellent candidates for computerization. Because these situations are highly ordered, they have little flexibility. A change in the environment of the unit can lead to chaos because there is no set procedure to be followed. For example, the procedure for administering medication may require that only registered nurses (RNs) open the medication cart. However, what happens in a disaster if no RNs are available? While micromanagement is contraindicated, the leadership in these situations should stay in the information loop, watching for early signs of change and avoiding a move to a chaotic domain.

Complicated Domain. In this domain, the relationship between cause and effect is known but it is not obvious to everyone in the domain. As a result, knowledge and expertise are very important for managing complicated problems. These types of problems are managed by collecting and analyzing data before responding. The expert will know what data are pertinent, as well as different approaches for analyzing these data and different options for responding. There is often more than one right answer. Different experts may solve the problem in different ways. In addition, experts can identify an effective solution but not be able to articulate every detail of the cause-and-effect relationship. For example, health professional or a health informatics specialist may be planning the educational program to accompany a major system implementation in a healthcare setting. In such a situation, there is not one perfect answer but rather several excellent options that can be used to prepare users for the new work environment. In these cases, good practice is a more appropriate approach than best practice because good practice is more flexible and able to tap into the expertise of the expert. Forcing experts to use the "one right approach" usually results in strong resistance.

Because experts are the dominant players, there are problems in the complicated domain that a manager must consider. Innovative approaches offered by nonexperts can be easily dismissed. This can be a significant problem in hierarchical organizations such as healthcare. A group of experts with different approaches can disagree and become bogged down in "analysis paralysis." In addition, all experts are limited in scope of expertise, and experts are not always able to realize when they have drifted out of their scope of expertise. As a situation moves toward the disordered end on the continuum, one of two domains will predominate. These are the complex and the chaotic domains.

Complex Domain. In the complex domain, the cause-effect relationship is not known. If the cause-and-effect relationship is not known, what data are pertinent data is also unknown. Decisions must be based on incomplete data in an environment of unknown unknowns. The difference between a complicated situation and complex situation can be demonstrated in analyzing the difference between a computer and a person. A computer expert can identify all of the parts of a computer and how they interact. The expert can predict with high accuracy how a computer will react in different situations. For example, a bad hard drive can prevent a computer from booting, but the response of a person to different situations cannot be predicted with the same accuracy. Because healthcare organizations are CASs and always in flux, many important situations and decisions are complex. In this domain, problems are not solved by imposing order. Rather than collecting many data, better solutions can emerge if the manager probes by trying small, fail-safe solutions. For example, a large medical center recently purchased a small rural hospital with little to no computerization in the clinical units. Imposing the information systems installed in the medical center could produce significant resistance and probably fail. Success is more likely if small pilot tests are conducted and then used to pull key leaders and users in when analyzing the results. In the analysis, patterns and potential solutions will begin to emerge. Obviously, this process is time consuming and a bit messy but not nearly as messy as failure. However, there are leadership tools to utilize in a complex domain as illustrated in Box 2.2.

Chaotic Domain. In the chaotic domain, there is no discernable relationship between cause and effect; therefore it is impossible to determine and manage the underlying problem. In healthcare, the term *crash* is often used for this situation. For example, a patient is crashing or a computer crashed. In this situation, the goal is to first stabilize the situation and then assess potential causes. CPR will be tried before there is any attempt to determine why the patient would have experienced a cardiac arrest. In a crisis, the manager takes charge and gives orders. In our previous example dealing with medication administration, the health professional or health informatician may decide to unlock the medication cart for all patients and determine if family or other staff may be able to give at least some of the medications. In a chaotic situation, there is no time to seek input or second-guess decisions. However, once the situation begins to stabilize, this can be a unique opportunity for innovation. Organizations and individuals are more open to change after a crisis: note, for example, the number of patients who will change their lifestyle after they have experienced a myocardial infarction. In Fig. 2.4, the fifth domain is the center domain, existing between disorder and order.

Disorder Domain. Showden uses the term *disorder* to name this domain. Each of the other domains is focused

on the type of situation or state of the organization. In the fifth domain, it is not the organization that is in disorder but rather the leader. The leader does not know which domain is predominant. If the leaders are aware of their confusion, they can begin by using the Framework to assess the situation. However, managers do not always realize what they do not know. If they do not realize the need to diagnosis the situation, there is a tendency to continue using their preferred management style.

While CASs are a unique type of system, all systems, whether they are complex or simple, change, and in the process interact and/or co-evolve with the environment. The basic framework of this interaction is shown in Fig. 2.2. Input to the system consists of information, matter, and energy. These inputs are then processed, and the result is output. Understanding this process as it applies to informatics involves an understanding of information theory.

Information Theory

The term *information* has several different meanings. An example of this can be seen in Box 2.3, taken from *Merriam-Webster's Collegiate Dictionary*.[40] Just as the term *information* has more than one meaning, information theory refers to more than one theory.[41] In this chapter, two theoretical models of information theory are examined: the Shannon-Weaver information-communication model and the Nelson data-information-knowledge-wisdom model (DIKW) that evolved from Blum's and Graves's initial work.

Shannon-Weaver Information-Communication Model

Information theory was formally established in 1948 with the publication of the landmark paper "The Mathematical Theory of Communication" by Claude Shannon.[42] The concepts

---

BOX 2.2   Management Tools in Complex Situations[36]

1. Encourage open discussion so people are comfortable both speaking and listening.
2. Set boundaries as clear simple rules: such as, meeting will always end on time.
3. Watch for and use attractors. Listen for ideas that resonate with people to use as potential probes.
4. Encourage and look for new and novel ideas. For example, one provider may notice that clicking on the patient's address may tell that provider how far the patient lives from the healthcare setting. This piece of information may be useful in making decisions about when to discharge or meet with family.
5. Do not look for predetermined results. Let answers emerge.

BOX 2.3   Definition of Information

1. The communication or reception of knowledge or intelligence
2. a. Knowledge obtained from investigation, study, or instruction; intelligence, news; facts, data
   b. The attribute inherent in and communicated by one of two or more alternative sequences or arrangements of something (as nucleotides in DNA or binary digits in a computer program) that produce specific effects
   c. A signal or character (as in a communication system or computer) representing data; (2) Something (as a message, experimental data, or a picture), which justifies change in a construct (as a plan or theory) that represents physical or mental experience or another construct
   d. A quantitative measure of the content of information; specifically, a numerical quantity that measures the uncertainty in the outcome of an experiment to be performed
3. The act of informing against a person
4. A formal accusation of a crime made by a prosecuting officer as distinguished from an indictment presented by a grand jury

Information. *Merriam-Webster's Collegiate Dictionary*. http://www.merriam-webster.com/dictionary/information; 2012.

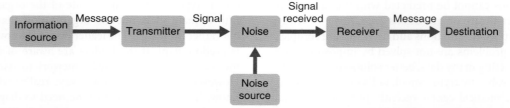

FIG 2.5 Schematic diagram of a general communication system. (Reprinted with corrections from Shannon C, Weaver W. The mathematical theory of communication. *Bell Syst Tech J*. 1948;27:379-423, 623-656. <http://worrydream.com/refs/Shannon%20-%20A%20Mathematical%20Theory%20of%20Communication.pdf>. Reprinted with permission of Alcatel-Lucent USA Inc.)

in this model are presented in Fig. 2.5. The sender is the originator of the message or the information source. The transmitter is the encoder that converts the content of the message to a code. The code can be letters, words, music, symbols, or a computer code. A cable is the channel, or the medium used to carry the message. Examples of channels include satellites, cell towers, glass optical fibers, coaxial cables, ultraviolet light, radio waves, telephone lines, and paper. Each channel has its own physical limitations in terms of the size of the message that can be carried. Noise is anything that is not part of the message but occupies space on the channel and is transmitted with the message. Examples of noise include static on a telephone line and background sounds in a room. The decoder converts the message to a format that can be understood by the receiver. When listening to a phone call, the telephone is a decoder. It converts the signal back into sound waves that are understood as words by the person listening. The person listening to the words is the destination.

Shannon, one of the authors of the Shannon-Weaver Information-Communication theory, was a telephone engineer. He used the concept of entropy to explain and measure the technical amount of information in a message. The amount of information in a message is measured by the extent to which the message decreases entropy. The unit of measurement is a bit. A bit is represented by a 0 (zero) or a 1 (one). Computer codes are built on this concept. For example, how many bits are needed to code the letters of the alphabet? What other symbols are used in communication and must be included when developing a code?

Warren Weaver, from the Sloan-Kettering Institute for Cancer Research, provided the interpretation for understanding the semantic meaning of a message.[42] He used Shannon's work to explain the interpersonal aspects of communication. For example, if the speaker is a physician who uses medical terms that are not known to the receiver (the patient), there is a communication problem caused by the method used to code the message. However, if the patient cannot hear well, he may not hear all of the words in the message. In this case the communication problem is caused by the patient's ear.

The communication-information model provides an excellent framework for analyzing the effectiveness and efficiency of information transfer and communication. For example, a healthcare provider may use CPOE to enter orders.

Is the order-entry screen designed to capture and code all of the key elements for each order? Are all aspects of the message coded in a way that can be transmitted and decoded by the receiving computer? Does the message that is received by the receiving department include all of the key elements in the message sent? Does the screen designed at the receiver's end make it possible for the message to be decoded or understood by the receiver?

These questions demonstrate three levels of communication that can be used in analyzing communication problems.[43] The first level of communication is the technical level. Do the system hardware and software function effectively and efficiently? The second level of communication is the semantic level. Does the message convey meaning? Does the receiver understand the message that was sent by the sender? The third level of communication is the effectiveness level. Does the message produce the intended result at the receiver's end? For example, did the provider order one medication but the patient received a different medication with a similar spelling? Some of these questions require a more in-depth look at how healthcare information is produced and used. Bruce Blum's definition of information provides a framework for this more in-depth analysis.

Blum Model

Bruce L. Blum developed his definition of *information* from an analysis of the accomplishments in medical computing.[44] In his analysis, he identified three types of healthcare computing applications. Blum grouped applications according to the objects they processed. The three types of objects he identified are data, information, and knowledge. Blum defined data as uninterpreted elements such as a person's name, weight, or age. Information was defined as a collection of data that have been processed and then displayed as information, such as weight over time. Knowledge results when data and information are identified and the relationships between the data and information are formalized. A knowledge base is more than the sum of the data and information pieces in that knowledge base. A knowledge base includes the interrelationships between the data and information within the knowledge base. A textbook can be seen as containing knowledge.[44] These concepts are well accepted across information science and are not limited to healthcare and health informatics.[45]

Graves Model

Judy Graves and Sheila Corcoran, in their classic article "The Study of Nursing Informatics," used the Blum concepts of data, information, and knowledge to explain the study of nursing informatics.[46] They incorporated Barbara A. Carper's four types of knowledge: empirical, ethical, personal, and aesthetic. Each of these represents a way of knowing and a structure for organizing knowledge. This article is considered the foundation for most definitions of *nursing informatics*.

Nelson Model

In 1989 Nelson extended the Blum and Graves and Corcoran data-to-knowledge continuum by including wisdom.[47] This initial publication provided only brief definitions of the concepts, but later publications included a model.[48] Fig. 2.6 demonstrates the most current version of this model. Within this model, wisdom is defined as the appropriate use of knowledge in managing or solving human problems. It is knowing when and how to use knowledge in managing patient needs or problems. Effectively using wisdom in managing a patient problem requires a combination of values, experience, and knowledge. The concepts of data, information, knowledge, and wisdom overlap and interrelate as demonstrated by the overlapping circles and arrows in the model. Of note, what is information in one context may be data in another. For example, a nursing student may view the liver function tests within the blood work results reported this morning and see only data or a group of numbers related to some strange-looking tests. However, the staff nurse looking at the same results will see the information and in turn see the implications for the patient's plan of care. The greater the knowledge base used to interpret data, the more information disclosed from that data, and in turn the more data points that may be generated. Data processed to become information can create new data items. For example, if one collects the blood sugar levels for a diabetic patient over time, patterns begin to emerge. These patterns become new data items to be interpreted. One nurse may notice and describe the pattern, but a nurse with more knowledge related to diabetes may identify a Somogyi-type pattern, with important implications for the patient's treatment protocols. The concept of constant flux is illustrated by the curved arrows moving between the concepts. As one moves up the continuum, there are increasing interactions and interrelationships within and between the circles, producing increased complexity of the elements within each circle. Therefore the concept of wisdom is much more complex than the concept of data.

The introduction of the concept of wisdom gained professional acceptance in 2008 when the American Nurses Association included this concept and the related model in *Nursing Informatics: Scope and Standards of Practice*.[49] In this document the model is used to frame the scope of practice for nursing informatics. This change meant that the scope of practice for nursing informatics was no longer fully defined by the

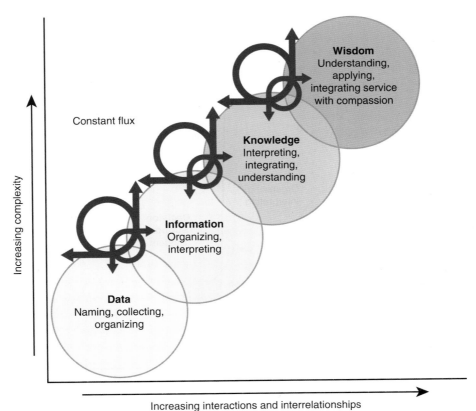

FIG 2.6 Revised Nelson data-to-wisdom continuum. (Copyright 2013 Ramona Nelson. Consulting. Reprinted with permission. All rights reserved.)

functionality of a computer and the types of applications processed by a computer. Rather the scope of practice is now defined by the goals of nursing and nurse-computer interactions in achieving these goals.

Using the concepts of data, information, knowledge, and wisdom makes it possible to classify the different levels of computing. An information system such as a pharmacy information system takes in data and information, processes the data and information, and outputs information. A computerized decision support system uses knowledge and a set of rules for using that knowledge to interpret data and information and output suggested or actual recommendations. A healthcare application may recommend additional diagnostic tests based on a pattern of abnormal test results, such as increasing creatinine levels. With a decision support system, the user decides whether the suggestion or recommendations will be implemented. A decision support system relies on the knowledge and wisdom of the user.

An computerized expert system goes one step further. An expert system implements the decision that has been programmed into the computer system without the intervention of the user. For example, an automated system that monitors a patient's overall status and then uses a set of predetermined parameters to trigger and implement the decision to call a code is an expert system. In this example, the data were converted to information, a knowledge base was used to interpret that information, and the decision to implement an action based on this process has been automated. The relationships among the concepts of data, information, knowledge, and wisdom, as well as information, decision support, and expert computer systems, are demonstrated in Fig. 2.7.

In the model, the three types of electronic systems overlap, reflecting how such systems are used in actual practice. For example, an electronic system recommending that a medication order be changed to decrease costs might be consistently implemented with no further thought by the provider entering the orders. In this example, an application designed as a decision support system is actually being used as an expert system by the provider. Because there are limits to the amount of data and information the human mind can remember and process, each practitioner walks a tightrope between depending on the computer to assist in the management of a situation with a high cognitive load and delegating the decision to the computer application. This reality presents interesting and important practical and research questions concerning the effective and appropriate use of computerized decision support systems in the provision of healthcare.

Effective computerized systems are dependent on the quality of data, information, and knowledge processed. Box 2.4 lists the attributes of data, information, and knowledge. These attributes provide a framework for developing evaluation forms that measure the quality of data, information, and

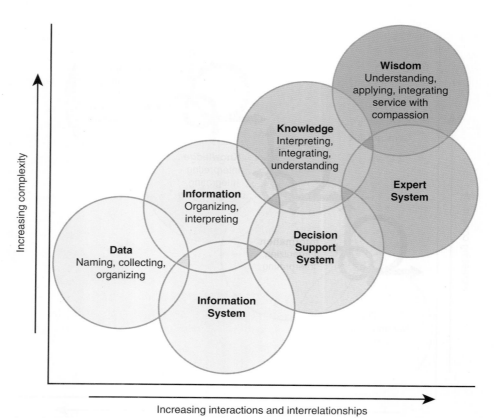

FIG 2.7 Moving from data to expert systems. (Modified from Englebardt S and Nelson R. *Health Care Informatics: An Interdisciplinary Approach*. St. Louis, MO: Mosby; 2002. Modified figure designed by Ramona Nelson Consulting and printed here with her permission. All rights reserved.)

BOX 2.4 Attributes of Data, Information, and Knowledge

Data
- Descriptive qualitative
- Measurable quantitative

Information
Quality
- Accurate
- Coherent
- Comprehensive or complete
- Objective or free from bias
- Verifiable

Usable
- Appropriate or relevant
- Economical
- Clear or understandable

Format
- Quantifiable
- Precise
- Organized for specific use

Available
- Accessible
- Secure
- Timely or current

Knowledge
- Accurate
- Relevant
- Type

BOX 2.5 Databases: Learning Theories

Name of Organization	URLs
Berkeley Graduate Division: GSI Teaching & Resource Center	http://gsi.berkeley.edu/gsi-guide-contents/learning-theory-research/
Learning-Theories.Com	www.learning-theories.com/
InstructionalDesign.org	www.instructionaldesign.org/theories/index.html

knowledge. For example, healthcare data are presented as text, numbers, or a combination of text and numbers. Good-quality health data provide a complete description of the item being presented with accurate measurements. Using these attributes, an evaluation form can be developed for judging the quality (including completeness) of a completed patient assessment form or for judging the quality of a healthcare website. The same process can be used with the attributes of knowledge. Think about the books or online references one might access in developing a treatment plan for a patient or consider a knowledge base that is built into a decision support system. What would result if the knowledge was incomplete or inaccurate or did not apply to the patient's specific problem or if suggested approaches were out of date and no longer considered effective in treating the patient's problem? What if the knowledge was not presented in the appropriate format for use?

Although this section has focused on computer systems, humans are also open systems that take in data, information, knowledge, and wisdom. Learning theory provides a framework for understanding how patients and healthcare providers, as open learning systems, take in, process, and output data, information, knowledge, and wisdom.

Learning Theory

Learning theory attempts to determine how people learn and to identify the factors that influence that process. Learning has been defined in a variety of ways, but for the purpose of this text, learning is defined as an increase in knowledge, a change in attitude or values, or the development of new skills. Several different learning theories have been developed. Each theory reflects a different paradigm and approach to understanding and explaining the learning process. Box 2.5 provides links to three sites that demonstrate the wide range of theories and the various approaches to classifying these theories.

These databases of different learning theories cannot be used to create a comprehensive theory of the learning process. The theories are not mutually exclusive. They often overlap and interrelate, yet they cannot be combined to create a total theory of learning.

Learning theories are important to the practice of health informatics for a variety of reasons. Health professionals and health informatics specialists plan and implement educational programs to teach healthcare providers to use new and updated applications and systems. A well-designed and well-implemented educational program can result in competent healthcare providers when it is able to satisfy all learning styles. Understanding how people learn is especially helpful in developing computer-related procedures that are safe and effective for healthcare providers and in building decision support systems that provide effective and appropriate support for healthcare providers who deal with a multitude of complex problems. Adult learning theories are often used when planning for a system implementation, whereas constructivist theories are often used in planning for a distance-education program. Specific learning theories as they relate to specific topics are presented in other chapters. For a listing of the learning theories included in this book, please check the index under the term *learning theories*. We will discuss four types of learning theories used to demonstrate the major approaches to learning theory.

Cognitive and Constructionist Learning Theories

Learning theories that are included under the heading of information processing theories divide learning into four steps:

1. How the learner takes input into the system
2. How that input is processed and constructed
3. What type of learned behaviors are exhibited as output
4. How feedback to the system is used to change or correct behavior

Data are taken into the system through the senses. First, if there is a sensory organ defect, such as hearing loss, data can be distorted or excluded. Second, data are moving across the semipermeable boundary of the system. There are limits to how much data can enter at one time. For example, if one is listening to a person who is talking too fast, some of the words will be missed. In addition, the learner will screen out data that are considered irrelevant or meaningless, such as background noise. Data limits are increased if the learner is under stress. Individuals who are anxious about learning to use a computer program will experience higher data limits and thereby less learning.

If new information is presented using several senses simultaneously, it is more likely to be taken in. For example, if a new concept is presented using slides that are explained by a speaker, the combination of both verbal and visual input makes it more likely that the learner will grasp the concept. As data enter the system, the learner structures and interprets these data, producing meaningful information. Previous learning has a major effect on how the data are structured and interpreted. For example, if a healthcare provider is already comfortable using Windows and is now learning a new software program based on Windows, he or she will be able to structure and interpret the new information quickly using previously developed cognitive structures. This is one reason why consistency in screen development can be very important for patient safety. In contrast, if the new information cannot be related to previous learning, the learner will need to build interpreting structures as he or she takes in the new information. For example, if a person is reading new information, she may stop at the end of each sentence and think about the content in that sentence. She is building interpretive cognitive structures while importing the data. If this same learner is hearing the new information at the same time she is taking notes, she may have difficulty capturing the content she is trying to record. The more time that is needed to interpret and structure data, the slower the learner will be able to import data. Assessment of the learner's previous knowledge can help the instructor to identify these potential problems. Relating new information to previously learned information will help the learner to develop interpreting structures and in turn learn the information more effectively. Describing learning as a process of building interpretive cognitive structures while learning new content is consistent with constructionist theory explained below. By combining what is known with the new information the learner goes beyond the information that was provided in the learning experience. Using organizing structures such as outlines, providing examples, and explaining how new information relates to previously learned concepts encourages the learner to develop chunks and increases retention. An "aha moment" is the sudden understanding that occurs when the new information fits with previous learning and the student gains a new insight on the discussion.

Social constructivism focuses on how group interaction can be used to build new knowledge.[50] Group discussion in which learners share their perceptions and understanding through peer learning encourages new insight, as well as retention of the newly constructed knowledge. There is limited research on how groups such as interprofessional health teams actually learn via the group construction process. Two studies at Massachusetts Institute of Technology and Carnegie Mellon University found converging evidence that groups participating in problem-solving activities demonstrate a general collective intelligence factor that explains a group's performance on a wide variety of tasks. "This 'c factor' is not strongly correlated with the average or maximum individual intelligence of group members but instead with the average social sensitivity of group members, the equality in distribution of conversational turn-taking and the proportion of females in the group."[51, p. 686] Certain characteristics of the individuals within the group and the group's ability to work together as a whole can influence the effectiveness of the group. "A group's interactions drive its intelligence more than the brain power of individual members."[52] Approaches to assessing and measuring the c facture within a group are now being explored with hopes that this measure could be used to support the effective of groups or teams.[53,54]

Information once taken into the system is retained in several different formats. The three most common formats are episodic order, hierarchical order, and linked. For example, life events are often retained in episodic order. A list of computer commands is also retained in episodic order. Psychomotor commands learned episodically can become automatic. An example of this can be seen in the simple behavior of typing or the more complex behavior of driving a car. Cognitive learning tends to be retained in hierarchical order. For example, penicillin is an antibiotic. An antibiotic is a medication. Finally, information is retained because it is linked or related to other information. For example, the concept "paper" is related to a printer. The process by which information is retained in long-term memory (LTM) can be reinforced by a variety of teaching techniques. Providing the student with an outline when presenting cognitive information helps to reinforce the learner retaining the information in hierarchical order. Telling stories or jokes can be used to reinforce links between concepts. Practice exercises that encourage repeated use of specific keystroke sequences or computer commands assist with long-term retention of psychomotor episodic learning including muscle memory.

While LTM can retain large amounts of information, two processes can interfere with the storage of information in LTM. First, new information or learning may replace old information. For example, healthcare providers may become very proficient with a computerized order-entry system. However, over time they may forget how to use the manual system to place orders. This can be a problem if the manual system is the backup plan for computer downtime. Second, previously learned information can interfere with the learning of new information. This can be seen when a new computer system is installed and new procedures are implemented. Experienced users of the old system must remember *not* to use the old procedures that were part of that system. This can be especially difficult if the previous learning has become automatic psychomotor commands. If the instructor for the new system includes clues to remind the experienced users of the change, the process of replacing old learning with new information can be reinforced.

When planning educational programs for healthcare users, the health professional and health informatics specialist must

TABLE 2.2 Planning for Long-Term Retention of New Information

Principle	Example
Distribute the learning over time	Online learning should be designed so that the content is divided into logical units, with learners encouraged to spread the learning over a period, and not all of the content is available from the beginning.
Plan to retain the information	Before teaching new content, explain to the learners why the information will be important to their performance and when they will need to recall the new information.
Review the materials	When presenting a list of new ideas, stop after each idea is explained, and list each of the ideas that have already been explained. Include practice sessions or self-assessment tools that reinforce the learning.
Increase the time spent on the task	This does not mean increasing the time scheduled for class but increasing the amount of time the learner is actively working on the content to be learned with readings before class or exercises after class.

first plan for intake of the new information via short-term memory (STM) and then for transfer of the new information to LTM. Several factors assist in moving information from STM to LTM. A list of these factors and examples of each can be seen in Table 2.2. Information that is stored in LTM is used in critical thinking, problem solving, decision making, and a number of other mental processes.

Learned behaviors are exhibited as output. Three types of output or behaviors are usually considered: cognitive, affective, and psychomotor. Cognitive behaviors reflect intellectual skills. They include critical thinking, problem solving, decision making, and a number of other mental processes. These are the skills used when designing a protocol for a user of an automated healthcare information system or for troubleshooting a computer system that is not functioning correctly.

Affective skills relate to values and attitudes. Planning for the learning of appropriate values and attitudes is often overlooked, and yet these can have a major impact on the implementation of an automated healthcare information system. Computerizing healthcare delivery requires change. This change can be stressful for healthcare providers. Training programs may focus exclusively on how to use the system without time to discuss how to integrate the new system into patient care. There may be limited discussion of the benefits of change and little support for the development of positive attitudes toward a new system. Development of positive values and attitudes can also be important to the ongoing maintenance of automated systems in healthcare.[74] Positive attitudes encourage users to suggest new and innovative uses for computer systems.

Psychomotor skills involve the integration of cognitive and motor skills. These types of skills require time and practice to develop. When new healthcare information systems are implemented, the institution is interested in measuring the impact of the new system. However, while new users are in the process of developing the psychomotor skills that are part of using the new system, it is ineffective to measure either the impact of a new system or user satisfaction. During this period, the focus should be on supporting the users' adjustment, tracking, and troubleshooting problems. Any decision to make significant changes to a new system based on user feedback must be evaluated carefully.

Adult Learning Theories

In 1970, Knowles coined and defined the term *andragogy*.[55] Andragogy is the art and science of helping adults to learn. Knowles's model proposed that adults share a number of similar learning characteristics and that these characteristics can be used in planning adult educational programs. Table 2.3 lists a number of these characteristics and provides examples of how they can be used to plan for teaching adult users.[50,56-58]

Learning Styles

All learners are not alike. They learn in different ways. They vary in how they take in and process information. There are preferential differences in seeing and hearing new information. Some learners process information by reflecting, whereas others process it by acting. Some learners approach reasoning logically, whereas others are intuitive. Some learners learn by analyzing, whereas others learn by visualizing. Learning theories concerning learning styles attempt to explain these differences. Experiential learning theory is one example.[59] The first stage of Kolb's theory involves concrete experience. For example, the learner may view a demonstration of a new healthcare information system.

As the learner begins to understand how the system works, he begins to think about how the system would work in his healthcare setting. This is the second stage, or reflection. In this stage, the learner reflects or thinks about the concrete experience. As the learner continues to think, he begins to form abstract conceptualizations of how the system functions. This is the third stage. Finally, the learner is ready to try using the system: this is the fourth stage, when the learner uses his abstract conceptualization to guide action. In Kolb's model, these four stages exist on two intersecting continuums. These are Concrete Experience–Abstract Conceptualization (CE-AC) and Reflective Observation–Active Experimentation (RO-AE). There are individual differences in how learners use each of these four stages in their individual learning

TABLE 2.3   Adult Learning Characteristics and Related Applications

Learning Characteristics	Application
Adults are self-directed.	If they do not see the relevance of new information, learners will not focus on remembering that information. Explain in practical terms when and how the new information will be used.
Adults have accumulated a number of life experiences and cognitive structures. These are used to interpret new learning.	When teaching a new system, ask the learners to provide examples from their experience and use these examples to correct misconceptions, as well as to reinforce how the new system will function.
Adults are practical and look for immediate application of learning.	Orientation to a new system should occur no more than 4 weeks before actual implementation.
Adults are more interested in learning how to solve problems than in retaining facts.	When teaching adults about computer applications, use real-life examples and scripts that can be expected to occur on the clinical unit.
Adult learners expect to be treated with respect and have their previous learning acknowledged.	When explaining a new system, ask the learners what they already know about the new system. Listen to their comments and concerns about the screen design and how it will or will not support safe practice.

BOX 2.6   Theory-Based Learning Principles

- Each learner is an individual with his or her own approach to learning.
- Making new information meaningful to the individual learner supports retention.
- Only so much input or new information can be handled at one time.
- Scheduling learning over time and ensuring adequate time on task improves learning.
- Active engagement and participation in the learning task supports long-term retention.
- Conceptual learning is enhanced with concrete realistic examples.
- Learning is enhanced when the teaching method includes the cognitive, affective, and psychomotor domains in concert.
- Learning takes place intentionally and unintentionally.
- Learning is contagious. A core of knowledgeable users creates a learning environment.

continuums is then used to form a composite picture of the learner's individual learning style.

A health professional and health informatics specialist plan and implement educational programs for a variety of groups within the healthcare delivery system. These may include physicians, nurses, unlicensed personnel, administrators, and others. These groups vary widely in learning ability, education, motivation, and experience. However, a great deal of variation exists among the learners within each group. Learning styles help to explain these differences and are helpful in planning instructional strategies that are effective for individual learners within a group. Each of the four types of learning theories discussed in this chapter provides insights into effective approaches to teaching. Box 2.6 lists examples of principles that can be derived from these theories.

Change Theory

Each of the theories presented in this chapter includes an element of change. Change theory is the study of change in individuals or social systems such as organizations. Understanding change theory provides a framework for effectively planning and implementing change in social systems and organizations. Healthcare information systems have a major impact on the structure and functions of healthcare delivery systems. They bring about significant change. The approach to managing the change process may result in a more effective and efficient healthcare delivery system or it may result in increased dissatisfaction and disruption. Health professionals and health informatics specialists play a major role in planning for, guiding, and directing these changes.

The change process can be analyzed from two perspectives. The first perspective is demonstrated by Kurt Lewin's theory, which focuses on how a change agent can guide the change process. This is referred to as planned change. The second perspective focuses on the process by which people and social systems make changes. Research in this area has demonstrated that people in various cultures follow a similar

approaches, but all learners ultimately learn by doing. Using this model, Kolb developed a learning-assessment tool to identify individual learning styles. The intersection of the two continuums forms four quadrants, Diverger, Assimilator, Converger, and Accommodator, representing four individual learning styles. The learner plots a score along the CE-AC scale and along the RO-AE scale to identify which quadrant reflects his or her learning style.

A second, more widely used measure of individual learning styles is the Myers–Briggs Type Indicator.[60] This theory uses four continuums: Thinking–Feeling, Sensing–Intuition, Extroverted–Introverted, and Judging–Perceptive. A series of questions is used to determine where the learner falls on each of the four continuums. For example, a learner may be Thinking, Sensing, Extroverted, and Judging. The combination of where the learner falls on each of the four pattern when incorporating innovation and change. Both of these perspectives provide a framework for understanding how people react to change and guiding the change process.

Planned Change

Kurt Lewin is frequently recognized as the father of change theory.[61] His theory of planned change divides change into three stages: unfreezing, moving, and refreezing.[62] As demonstrated in the discussion of homeostasis, systems expend energy to stay in a steady state of stability. A system will remain stable when the restraining forces preventing change are stronger than the driving forces for change. Initiating change begins by increasing the driving forces and limiting the restraining forces, thereby increasing the instability of the system. This is the unfreezing stage. The first stage in the life cycle of an information system involves evaluating the current system and deciding what changes, if any, need to be made. The pros and cons for change reflect the driving and restraining forces for change. If changes are to be made, the restraining forces that maintain a stable system and resist change must be limited. At the same time, the driving forces that encourage change must be increased. For example, pointing out to users the limitations and weaknesses with the current information management system increases the driving force for change. Also pointing out the advantages offered by a new system can increase driving forces for change.

Asking for user input early in the process before decisions have been made can decrease the restraining forces. However, this is true only if the users believe they are heard and accept that their representative is really representing their interests. If, however, the users believe their representatives are only "going through the motions of asking," resistance to change will be increased. In addition, at this point when questions are being asked, it can be very effective to anticipate who the objectors might be and include them in the process. Once a decision is made to initiate change, the second stage, moving, begins.

The moving stage involves the implementation of the planned change. By definition, this is an unstable period for the social system. Anxiety levels can be expected to increase. The social system attempts to minimize the impact or degree of change. This resistance to change may occur as missed meetings, failure to attend training classes, and failure to provide staff with information about the new system. If the resistance continues, it can cause the planned change to fail. Health professionals and health informatics specialists as change agents must anticipate and minimize these resistive efforts. This can be as simple as providing food at meetings or a planned program of recognition for early adopters. For example, an article in the institution's newsletter describing and praising the pilot units for their leadership will encourage the driving forces for change. It is important at each stage of the change process to evaluate and make needed changes to the initial plans; however, it is especially important during the moving phase to identify changes in the system and procedures that need to be modified. The goal is to avoid in the next phase "refreezing" a bad procedure or system.

Once the system is in place or the change has been implemented, additional energy is needed to maintain the change. This is the refreezing stage, and it occurs during the maintenance phase of the information system life cycle. If managed effectively by the change agent, this phase is characterized by increased stability. In this stage, the new system is in place, and forces resistant to change are encouraged. Examples include training programs for new employees, a yearly review of all policies and procedures related to the new system, and continued recognition for those who become experts with the new system.

In the current healthcare environment, several new information applications may be implemented at the same time. Not all of these implementations will affect everyone to the same degree. Different individuals and clinical units can be at different stages of change with different implementations. Taken together, the overall scope of change will create a sense of anxiety or excitement throughout the organization. It is important for health professionals and health informatics specialists to monitor the amount of change and the resulting tension in placing and planning for ongoing implementations.

Health professionals and informaticians may find helpful newer change models that have been built on Lewin's premises. For example, Conner's book *Managing at the Speed of Change* outlines key concepts to facilitate change in complex organizations:

- Create a burning platform for change (the burning need for change).
- Identify key stakeholders and clearly define their roles in the change.
- Hold managers responsible and accountable for specific elements of change.
- Assess organizational culture, capacity, resistance, and responsiveness to create an effective plan for change.[63]

Find out how change has taken place in the past. Determine what worked in specific areas and what did not. Build on what has worked in the past. Understanding the culture and communication patterns of various units is critical to successful change management.

Diffusion of Innovation

The diffusion of innovation theory, developed by Everett Rogers, explains how individuals and communities respond to new ideas, practices, or objects.[64-66] Diffusion of innovation is the process by which an innovation is communicated through certain channels over time among members of a social system. Innovations may be either accepted or rejected. Healthcare automation, with new ideas and technology, involves ongoing diffusion of innovation. By understanding the diffusion of innovation process and the factors that influence this process, health professionals and health informatics specialists can assist individuals and organizations in maximizing the benefits of automation.

Social systems consist of individuals within organizations. Both the individuals and the organization as a whole vary in how they respond to innovations. Based on their responses, individuals can be classified into five groups—innovators, early adopters, early majority, late majority, and laggards—with the number of individuals in each group following a normal distribution. Innovators are the first 2.5% of individuals within a system to adapt to an innovation. These individuals tend to be more cosmopolitan. They are comfortable with uncertainty and above average in their understanding of complex technical concepts. These are the individuals who test out a new technology; however, they are too far ahead of the social group to be seen as leaders by other members of the social system. Some of their ideas become useful over time, whereas others are just passing fads. Therefore they are not usually able to sell others on trying new technology. This is the role of the early adopters.

Early adopters are the next 13.5% of individuals in the organization. They are perceived by others as thoughtful in their adoption of new ideas and, therefore, serve as role models for others. Because of their leadership role within the organization, the support of early adopters is key when introducing new approaches to automation. If the early adopters accept an innovation, the early majority are more likely to follow their example. The early majority are the next 34% of individuals in an organization. Members of the early majority are willing to adapt to innovation but not to lead. However, acceptance by the early majority means that the innovation is becoming well integrated in the organization. This is sometimes referred to as the tipping point.

The late majority is the next group to accept an innovation. The late majority makes up 34% of the individuals within the organization. Most of the uncertainty that is inherent in a new idea must be removed before this group will adapt to an innovation. They adopt the innovation, not because of their interest in the innovation, but rather because of peer pressure.

The late majority is followed by the last 16% of individuals in the organization. These are the laggards. Laggards focus on the local environment and on the past. They are resistant to change and will change only when there is no other alternative. They are suspicious of change and change agents. Change agents should not spend time encouraging laggards to change but rather should work at establishing policies and procedures that incorporate the innovation into the required operation of the organization.

Just as individuals vary in their response to innovation, organizations also vary. Five internal organizational characteristics can be used to understand how an organization will respond to an innovation.[67]

- *Centralization:* Organizations that are highly centralized, with power concentrated in the hands of a few individuals, tend to be less accepting of new ideas and, therefore, less innovative.
- *Complexity:* Organizations in which many of the individuals have a high level of knowledge and expertise tend to be more accepting of innovation. However, organizations of this type can have difficulty reaching a consensus on approaches to implementation.
- *Formalization:* Organizations that place a great deal of emphasis on rules and procedures tend to inhibit new ideas and innovation. However, once a decision has been made to move ahead, this tendency toward rules and procedures does make it easier to implement an innovation.
- *Interconnectedness:* Organizations in which there are strong interpersonal networks linking the individuals within the organization are better prepared to communicate and share innovation. This can be seen, for example, in organizations in which Web 2.0 tools are an integral part of organizational communication.
- *Organizational slack:* Organizations with uncommitted resources are better prepared to manage innovation. These resources may be people and/or money. With the current emphasis on cost control, healthcare institutions have ever decreasing organizational slack.

These characteristics help to explain how an organization as a whole will respond to innovation; however, they can be analyzed at both an individual and an organizational level. For example, adapting to new software involves a certain degree of complexity. Think about what is involved when an individual must select a new e-mail application. Now think about what is involved if an organization decides to select a new clinical documentation application.

The perceived attributes of the innovation, the nature of organizational communication channels, the innovative decision process, and the efforts of change agents influence the possibility that an innovation will be adapted, as well as the rate of adoption. Five attributes can be used to characterize an innovation.

- *Relative advantage:* Is the innovation seen as an improvement over the current approach? For example, has the need to standardize with one patient documentation system forced certain clinical units to give up certain functionality? Alternatively, is the new system seen as an upgrade with new functionality?
- *Compatibility:* Does the innovation fit with existing values, workflow, and individual expectations? For example, will the new application cause certain tasks to be shifted from one department to another?
- *Complexity:* Is the innovation easy to use and understand? If yes, the innovation can be seen as a minor change. If no, the innovation will be seen as a major change.
- *Trialability:* Can the innovation be tested or tried before individuals must make a commitment to it? Although trialability can be an advantage in encouraging innovation, it can be difficult to conduct a trial of a computer application in a large, complex organization such as a healthcare institution.
- *Observability:* Are the results of using the innovation visible to others?

If each of these five questions related to the five innovative attributes can be answered with a "yes," it is more likely that the innovation will be adopted and that the adoption will occur at a rapid rate. If, on the contrary, an innovation is not gaining acceptance, these characteristics can be used as a framework for evaluating the source of the problem. For example, it may take more time to document a patient assessment with the new system compared with the previous system. Thus nurses will prefer the previous system because of the relative advantage.

The decision of individuals and organizations to accept or reject an innovation is not an instantaneous event. The process involves five stages.[68] These stages can be demonstrated when a healthcare institution considers using blogs and wikis to support internal communication for all professional staff. The first stage of the innovation decision process is knowledge. In the knowledge stage, the individual or organization becomes aware of the existence of the innovation. Managers become aware of other institutions that are using these tools and begin to learn about the possible advantages. Mass communication channels are usually most effective at this stage. For example, the institution's newsletter may carry a story about blogs and wikis and how staff might use these tools to support patient care and institutional goals. If the change agent does not have access to formal mass communication channels to reach all professional staff, the knowledge stage can be significantly delayed. Although personal information moves quickly via informal communication channels, cognitive information involving the processing of information and knowledge does not move as quickly through these types of channels.

Once individuals become aware of an innovation, they begin to develop an opinion or attitude about it. This is the persuasion stage. During the persuasion stage, interpersonal channels of communication are more important, and early adopters begin to play a key role. In the persuasion stage, attitudes are not fixed but are in the process of being formed. The health professional and health informatics specialist should work closely with early adopters in developing and communicating positive attitudes to others in the organization.

Once these attitudes become more fixed, individuals make a decision to accept or reject the innovation. This is the decision stage. It is at this point that individuals will decide to try these tools for themselves. For each person this decision can occur at a different point. The early adopters will decide to try the system before the early majority. In testing out the system, most people begin to discover new features or functions of the system. They also begin to discover potential problems. As they gain a better understanding of how to use the new functions, they also discover challenges, modifications, and adjustments that need to be made. Readers and health professional and health informatics specialist needs to be sensitive to these modifications because they will take on an added significance when formal and informal policies and procedures are developed. For example, workarounds can begin to develop at this point.

Once the decision has been made to accept the innovation, the implementation stage begins. The development of formal policies and procedures related to the innovation is a clear indication that the implementation stage is in place. The final stage is confirmation. At this point, the innovation is no longer an innovation. It has either been rejected or

become the standard procedure. For example, certain key interinstitutional communication will depend on staff using these tools.

Using Change Theory

Effective change requires a champion or champions with a clear vision, a culture of trust, an organizational sense of pride, and the intense involvement of the people who must live with the change. Ongoing, visible support from leaders for these champions is critical. The champion must have the institutional resources to support the change process. These resources include leadership skills; personnel, including change agents; money; and time. The change agent uses change theory to understand and manage reactions to change throughout the change process. Reactions to change may be negative, such as resistance, frustration, aggression, acceptance, indifference, ignoring, and organized resistance. Alternatively, the reaction to change can be positive, such as an increase in excitement and energy, a sense of pride, supporting and encouraging others, involvement in demonstrating how the innovation improves the organization, and overall acceptance. Change agents usually encounter both positive and negative reactions during the change process. It is usually more effective to support the positive reactions to change than it is to spend time and effort responding to the negative reactions.

The Systems Life Cycle Model

The most common change for health professionals and informaticians is the introduction of or upgrade to a health information system. A commonly used model of the stages within this change is the systems life cycle (SLC) model. This model is used in project management to describe stages or phases of an informatics project and it guides system implementation from initial feasibility through a more completed stage of maintenance and evaluation of the products. Most authors use the title "systems development life cycle" to describe the model. However, the term *development* is too limiting in health informatics because we often purchase systems or applications from vendors and customize them rather than developing them from scratch.

Various iterations of the systems life cycle have been published, and no agreement exists about the numbers and types of stages in the life cycle. The number of stages ranges from three (preimplementation, implementation, and postimplementation) to at least seven. Project managers may even sort and combine phases to suit their needs according to the complexity and type of project being planned. Deficiencies in past models include:

- The depiction of the life cycle as a circular process, beginning with analysis, cycling through planning, develop/purchase/implement, maintain/evaluate, and returning to analysis. This would indicate a return to the original baseline, which is not the case after implementation. Instead, a new life cycle builds on previous installations and organizational learning.

- The development step does not indicate a choice to purchase a system, a common strategic choice today.
- Evaluation is listed only at the postimplementation phase. Instead, evaluation should be built into the process at the beginning of the cycle, and each phase should include evaluation.[69]
- Testing is de-emphasized as one aspect of the implementation process. This step is critical in any upgrade or implementation, so it should be a separate step.

An entire life cycle can last many years. The average life cycle is about a decade, but some systems may be in place for longer periods; for example, the original inpatient system in the military is being replaced after two decades. Other systems may evolve continually for several decades with upgrades, module additions, and technology platform changes.

Staggers and Nelson Systems Life Cycle Model

The Staggers and Nelson systems life cycle model (SLCM) depicted in Fig. 2.8 incorporates the steps listed above; combines them with previous work from Thompson, Snyder-Halpern, and Staggers; and expands the steps to include a new, important consideration, the depiction of the cycle as a spiral.[70] Once an organization completes the SLCM, it does not return in circular fashion to the assessment stage. Instead, reassessment occurs based on the organization's development into a new operating baseline (see Fig. 2.8). Two notions are used from work first published by Thompson and colleagues outlining an expanded SLC.[70] The first is a step divided into

purchase or development. The second is that evaluation occurs at every stage of the SLC versus relegating evaluation to the end of the cycle. The steps of the life cycle are outlined as follows:

1. *Analyze.* The existing environment and systems are evaluated. Major problems and deficiencies are identified using informal or formal methods. A readiness assessment may be done. The feasibility of the system is determined, and system requirements are defined. Analysts or informaticians may interview key system users or potential users and consult with information technology (IT) personnel. A part of the initial analysis is to understand the organizational culture, how the organization handled change in the past, and to determine the number of other changes the organization is encountering to understand how a technology change will fit (or not) into their priorities. Formal research projects (e.g., observing users interacting with applications, determining workflow in specialty areas such as the operating room) or formal surveys or focus groups may be conducted to determine needs. Workflow analyses are important to perform even though they are time consuming. Deficiencies in the existing system are addressed with specific proposals for improvement. Benefits include engaging staff in the change process, and potential problems in processes can be identified. Gaps are noted, and current capabilities and limitations are outlined. Initial user and system requirements are formulated.

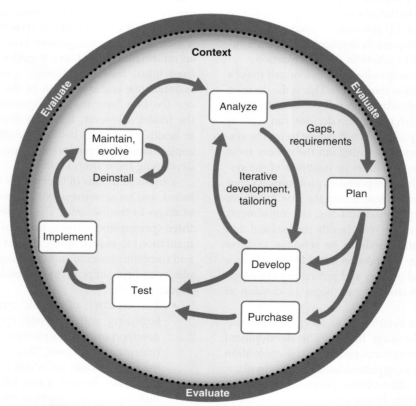

FIG 2.8 The Staggers and Nelson systems life cycle model.

2. *Plan.* The proposed system is comprehensively planned. Planning includes strategic levels, such as whether the system will be developed internally, purchased, and tailored or designed and developed jointly with a vendor. The analysis and planning phases are the most time consuming of any project and are often estimated to require about 70% of a project's time and resources from start to initial implementation. Workflow analyses and process reengineering may be completed as a basis for determining the scope of system functions and the flow of information and activities within care processes. This is time intensive but worth the effort. In this process, the staff becomes involved, and everyone begins to see where the bottlenecks and other issues are. Potential problems can often be avoided through this analysis. Other topics to consider in this step include planning for project governance, key stakeholders, hardware, operating systems, databases, interface engines, programming (if needed), tailoring methods, marketing and communications, support for go-live, support for extensive testing, project maintenance, evaluation and success factors, security and privacy, and systems integration and IT support, such as integration into the call center, on-call support for clinicians, and physical construction.

3. *Develop or purchase.* At this stage, the system is purchased or new system development begins. New components and programs are obtained and installed. For vendor-supported solutions, extensive tailoring occurs. This step may not be distinct from steps 1 and 2, depending on the type of development and tailoring the organization decides to employ. For instance, the organization may use user-centered techniques that include iterative design and evaluation with actual end users. Training is designed but may be carried out as part of the implementation stage.

4. *Test.* In this stage, extensive testing occurs just before implementation and go or no-go decisions are made about deadlines. The system should be tested intensively before implementation in as close to normal situations as possible. Simulated units are ideal. Ideally, adjustments are made at this stage to correct gaps in the scope of system functions or work processes.[71] Toward the end of this step, marketing and communication efforts are accelerated to make users aware of the impending change.

5. *Implement or go-live.* The system is implemented using a selected method best suited to the organization and its tolerance for risk. Communication and training plans are executed. Mass user training is completed. The plan for conversion or go-live is implemented. For larger projects, the go-live can include a command center to coordinate activities for the few days or weeks. Users begin to use the system for their activities such as patient care.

6. *Maintain and evolve.* Once the system has been formally acknowledged as passing user acceptance testing, typically at 90 or 120 days after going live, it enters a maintenance stage. Here, the project is considered routine and is integrated into normal operations in IT, clinical, and business areas. However, the system is not static: it evolves over time. For example, a project in the maintenance stage should have regular upgrades to maintain software currency and have system change requests completed.

7. *Evaluate.* Evaluation occurs at each step of the SLCM, as may be seen in Fig. 2.8. The evaluation stage actually begins in the planning stage of the project. The system should be tested intensively before implementation in as close to normal situations as possible. A simulated unit is ideal. Ideally, adjustments are made at this stage to correct gaps in the scope of system functions or work processes. Evaluation techniques are discussed in Chapter 4.

8. *Return to analyze.* Unlike the methods depicted in most systems, in life cycle models, the organizational baseline has matured and does not return to the preimplementation baseline. Thus the SLCM is typically a spiral of ongoing analysis, refinement with installation of upgrades and enhancements, and new projects building on the initial work. Atypically, a project may have a formal end through deinstallation or replacement with a new system. If that occurs, it would be at this step in the SLCM.

ADDITIONAL INFORMATICS-RELATED MODELS

Although informatics is a new discipline, various models have proven useful to leaders within this field. An overview of several key models and theories used within the discipline has been provided. Currently there is no single comprehensive, generally accepted theoretical or conceptual model of health or nursing informatics. A number of models have been introduced, some defining an overall model of informatics and some dealing with a specific aspect of informatics. For example, Graves and Corcoran, discussed earlier, defined an overall model, whereas Garcia-Smith proposed an integrated model to predict a successful clinical information system (CIS) implementation.[72] Selected models are included in Table 2.4.

CONCLUSION AND FUTURE DIRECTIONS

Healthcare is an information-intensive service. Computerization and the use of technology provide an effective and efficient means to manage large volumes of data and information with knowledge and wisdom. However, the move to an electronic healthcare system is changing every aspect of healthcare. With this degree of change come excitement, anxiety, resistance, and conflict. Health professionals and health informatics specialists function at the very core of this change. They play a major role in implementing, managing, and leading healthcare organization as they move forward with automation. To play this role, they work directly with the clinical, administrative, and technical people in the organization. For health professionals and health informatics specialists to provide effective leadership, they must understand the institution's vision and values and the people and processes within these organizations. The theories presented in this

TABLE 2.4   Selected Models of Nursing Informatics

Name	Author	Major Concepts	Reference
The NI Pyramid Model	Patricia M. Schwirian, PhD, RN Professor Emerita School of Nursing The Ohio State University	The four primary concepts are raw nursing information, the technology, the users, and the goal or objective, arranged in a pyramid with a triangular base. Although the stated purpose was to describe concepts in NI, the model probably better describes human-computer interaction concepts.	Schwirian PM. The NI pyramid: a model for research in nursing informatics. *Comput Nurs.* 1986;4(3):134-136.
Turley's Nursing Informatics Model	James Turley, PhD, RN Associate Professor School of Health Information Sciences University of Texas Health Science Center at Houston	The five primary concepts are cognitive science, information science, computer science, informatics, and nursing science. The concepts of cognitive science, information science, and computer science are depicted as three overlapping circles, with informatics at the junction of all three. Nursing science surrounds and provides a context for the overlapping circles.	Turley J. Toward a model for nursing informatics. *Image J Nurs Sch.* 1996;28 (4):309-313.
Goosen's Framework for Nursing Informatics Research	William T.F. Goosen, RN, PhD Director Results 4 Care Netherlands	Goosen's model builds on and extends the Graves model. The concepts of data, information, knowledge, decision, action, and evaluation are depicted as six boxes, with each of these concepts progressing to the next. Each of these six concepts interacts with the seventh concept in the model: Nursing Management and Processing to Patient Care.	Goosen W. Nursing informatics research. *Nurs Res.* 2000;8(2):42-54. Goosen W. Nursing information management and processing: a framework and definition for systems analysis, design and evaluation. *Int J Biomed Comput.* 1996;40(3):187-195.
IRO Model	Judith Effken, PhD, RN, FACMI, FAAN Associate Professor, Nursing College of Nursing The University of Arizona	This model includes two component models. First is a five-phase systems development life cycle depicted as a circle in the center of the IRO model. This is surrounded by the process of evaluation, which occurs throughout the life cycle. The outer ring includes four constructs that interact with each other and the inner circle. These are (1) the client, (2) NI interventions, (3) outcomes, and (4) the cultural, economic, social, and physical context.	Effken J. An organizing framework for nursing informatics research. *CIN—Comput Inform Nu.* 2003;21(6):316-323.

IRO, The Informatics Research; *NI,* nursing informatics.

chapter provide a foundation for supporting and managing the enormous degree of change experienced by the healthcare system and the people within any healthcare system.

Informatics incorporates a number of other disciplines and, therefore, theories from those disciplines have been effectively used to guide research within the field of informatics. This chapter is an introduction to the use of theory in informatics and not a comprehensive analysis of theories that have or can be used to deal with questions of importance to informatics. Several theoretical and conceptual models used in health informatics are described elsewhere in this book and are not repeated in this section. For example, the model of biomedical

informatics developed by the American Medical Informatics Association is included in Chapter 35 Staggers's model of human-computer interaction is included in Chapter 21. In the future, one can expect to see additional models developed as the field of informatics continues to mature and as developments in healthcare and technology continue to evolve.

REFERENCES

1. UNESCO Education Section. *The Plurality of Literacy and its Implications for Policies and Programmes: Position Paper;* 2004: 1-32. http://unesdoc.unesco.org/images/0013/001362/136246e.pdf.

2. Three Types of Literacy. *National Assessment of Adult Literacy (NAAL)*; 2003. http://nces.ed.gov/naal/literacytypes.asp.

3. Committee on Information Technology Literacy NRC. *Being Fluent with Information Technology*. Washington, DC: National Academy Press; 1999.

4. American Library Association. *Information Literacy Competency Standards for Higher Education*; 2000. http://www.ala.org/acrl/standards/informationliteracycompetency.

5. Mackey TP, Jacobson TE. Reframing information literacy as a metaliteracy. *Coll Res Libr*. 2011;72(1):62–78.

6. Association of College and Research Libraries (ACRL). *Framework for Information Literacy for Higher Education*; 2016. http://www.ala.org/acrl/standards/ilframework.

7. Hobbs R. *Digital and Media Literacy: A Plan of Action*; 2010. http://www.knightcomm.org/wp-content/uploads/2010/12/Digital_and_Media_Literacy_A_Plan_of_Action.pd.

8. The American Library Association (ALA). *Office for Information Technology Policy (OITP). Digital Literacy, Libraries and Public Policy*; 2013. http://connect.ala.org/files/94226/2012_OITP_digilitreport_1_22_13.pdf.

9. Nelson R, Joos I. An introduction: social media and the transforming roles and relationships in health care. In: Nelson R, Joos I, Wolf DM, eds. *Social Media for Nurses: Educating Practitioners and Patients in a Networked World*. New York, NY: Springer Publishing Company; 2013.

10. Murphy S. *Digital Literacy is in Crisis. Social Media Today*; 2011. http://www.socialmediatoday.com/content/digital-literacy-crisis.

11. Sorensen K, Van den Broucke S, Fullam J, et al. Health literacy and public health: a systematic review and integration of definitions and models. *BMC Public Health*. 2012;12:80.

12. The IOM Committee on Health Literacy Medicine. *Health Literacy: A Prescription to End Confusion*; 2004. http://iom.nationalacademies.org/Activities/PublicHealth/RtblHealthLiteracy.asp.

13. World Health Organization. *Track 2: Health Literacy and Health Behaviour*. http://www.who.int/healthpromotion/conferences/7gchp/track2/en/.

14. Norman CD, Skinner HA. eHealth literacy: essential skills for consumer health in a networked world. *J Med Internet Res*. 2006;8(2):e9.

15. Hartzler A, Pratt W. Managing the personal side of health: how patient expertise differs from the expertise of clinicians. *J Med Internet Res*. 2011;13(3):e62.

16. Hawking SW. *A Brief History of Time*. New York, NY: Bantam Books; 1988.

17. Von Bertalanffy L, Ruben BD, Kim JY, eds. *General Systems Theory and Human Communication*. Rochelle Park, NJ: Hayden Book Company; 1975.

18. Joos I, Nelson R, Lyness A. *Man, Health and Nursing*. Reston, VA: Reston Publishing Company; 1985.

19. Kernick D. *Complexity and Healthcare Organizations: A View From the Street*. Oxon, United Kingdom: Radcliffe-Medical Press Ltd; 2004.

20. Smith L, Smith L. *Chaos: A Very Short Introduction*. New York, NY: Oxford University Press; 2007.

21. Kellert S. *In the Wake of Chaos: Unpredictable Order in Dynamical Systems*. Chicago, IL: University of Chicago Press; 1993.

22. Walker R. *Quotations from Friedrich Nietzsche [1844–1900]. Working Minds*; 2012. http://www.working-minds.com/FNquotes.htm.

23. Holden LM. Complex adaptive systems: concept analysis. *J Adv Nurs*. 2005;52(6):651–657.

24. McDaniel RR, Lanham HJ, Anderson RA. Implications of complex adaptive systems theory for the design of research on health care organizations. *Health Care Manage Rev*. 2009;34(2):191–199. http://www.ncbi.nlm.nih.gov/pmc/articles/PMC3667498/pdf/nihms107789.pdf.

25. Van Beurden EK, Kia AM, Zask A, Dietrich U, Rose L. Making sense in a complex landscape: how the Cynefin Framework from Complex Adaptive Systems Theory can inform health promotion practice. *Health Promot Int*. 2013;28(1):73–83.

26. Ellis B, Herbert SI. Complex adaptive systems (CAS): an overview of key elements, characteristics and application to management theory. *Inform Prim Care*. 2011;19(1):33–37.

27. Rouse W. Health care as a complex adaptive system: implication design and management; *Bridge*. 2008;38(1):7–25. https://www.nae.edu/Publications/Bridge/EngineeringandtheHealthCareDeliverySystem/ HealthCareasaComplexAdaptiveSystemImplicationsforDesignandManagement.aspx.

28. Chandler J, Rycroft-Malone J, Hawkes C, Noyes J. Application of simplified complexity theory concepts for healthcare social systems to explain the implementation of evidence into practice. *J Adv Nurs*. 2016;72(2):461–480. http://dx.doi.org/10.1111/jan.12815.

29. Sturmberg JP, Martin CM, Katerndahl DC. Systems and complexity thinking in the general practice literature: an integrative, historical narrative. *Ann Fam Med*. 2014;12(1):66–74.

30. Essén A, Lindblad S. Innovation as emergence in healthcare: unpacking change from within. *Soc Sci Med*. 2013;93:203–211.

31. *BusinessDictionary.com*. Complex adaptive system (CAS). http://www.businessdictionary.com/definition/complex-adaptive-system-CAS.html; n.d. Accessed May 26, 2016.

32. Chan S. Complex adaptive systems. ESD.83 Research Seminar in Engineering Systems. <http://web.mit.edu/esd.83/www/notebook/Complex%20Adaptive%20Systems.pdf>; 2001.

33. Jell-Mann M. Complex adaptive theory. Santa Fe Institute, and Los Alamos National Laboratory <http://tuvalu.santafe.edu/~mgm/Site/Publications_files/MGM%20113.pdf>; n.d. Accessed May 26, 2016.

34. Hasan H, Kazlauskas A. The Cynefin framework: putting complexity into perspective. In: Hasan H, ed. *Being Practical with Theory: A Window into Business Research*. Wollongong, NSW: THEORI; 2014:55–57. http://eurekaconnection.files.wordpress.com/2014/02/p-55-57-cynefin-framework-theori-ebook_finaljan2014-v3.pdf. Accessed May 26, 2016.

35. Hasan HM, Kazlauskas A. Making sense of IS the Cynefin framework. In: *Proceedings of the Pacific Asia Conference on Information Systems (PACIS)*, Hyderabad, India: Indian School of Business; 2009. http://aisel.aisnet.org/pacis2009/47/.

36. Snowden DJ, Boone ME. A leader's framework for decision making. *Harv Bus Rev*. 2007;85(11):68–76. 149.

37. Snowden DJ. Good fences make good neighbors[1]. *Inf Knowl Syst Manag*. 2011;10:135–150 [Chapter 8].

38. Snowden DJ. *The Cynefin Framework YouTube*; 2010. https://www.youtube.com/watch?v=N7oz366X0-8.

39. Snowden DJ. *Managing Under Conditions of Uncertainty State of the Net 2014. YouTube*; 2014. https://www.youtube.com/watch?v=APB_mhpsQp8.

40. Information. *Merriam-Webster's Collegiate Dictionary*; 2012. http://www.merriam-webster.com/dictionary/information.

41. Robertson J. *The Fundamentals of Information Science: an Online Overview*; 2004. http://jamescrobertson.com/infosci/.

42. Shannon C, Weaver W. The mathematical theory of communication; *Bell Syst Tech J*. 1948;27:379–423. http://worrydreamcom/refs/Shannon%20-%20A%20Mathematical%20Theory%20of%20Communication.pdf. Accessed May 26, 2016.

43. Hersh W. *Information Retrieval: A Health Care Perspective*. 3rd ed. New York, NY: Springer Science; 2009.

44. Blum B. *Clinical Information Systems*. New York, NY: Springer-Verlag; 1986.

45. Clarke R. *Fundamentals of "information systems."* Xamax Consultancy Pty Ltd; 1999. http://www.rogerclarke.com/SOS/ISFundas.html.

46. Graves J, Corcoran S. The study of nursing informatics. *Image*. 1989;21(4):227–230.

47. Nelson R, Joos I. On language in nursing: from data to wisdom. *PLN Vis*. 1989;6. Fall.

48. Nelson R. Major theories supporting health care informatics. In: Englebardt S, Nelson R, eds. *Health Care Informatics: An Interdisciplinary Approach*. St. Louis: Mosby; 2002:3–27.

49. American Nurses Association. *Nursing Informatics: Scope and Standards of Practice*. Silver Spring, MD: Nursesbooks.org; 2008.

50. Harapnuik D. *Inquisitivism or "the HHHMMM??? What Does this Button Do?" Approach Learning: the Synthesis of Cognitive Theories into a Novel Approach to Adult Education*; 1998. https://archive.org/stream/ERIC_ED427704#page/n1/mode/2up.

51. Woolley A, Chabris C, Pentland A, Hashmi N, Malone T. Evidence for a collective intelligence factor in the performance of human groups. *Science*. 2010;330:686–689.

52. Marshall J. *How to Measure the Wisdom of a Crowd. Discovery News*; 2013. http://news.discovery.com/human/group-intelligence-wisdom-crowd.htm.

53. Aggarwal I, Woolley AW. Do you see what I see? The effect of members' cognitive styles on team processes and errors. *Organ Behav Hum Decis Process*. 2013;122(1):92–99.

54. Woolley AW, Bear JB, Chang JW, DeCostanza AH. The effects of team strategic orientation on team process and information search. *Organ Behav Hum Decis Process*. 2013;122(2):114–126.

55. Knowles M. *The Modern Practice of Adult Education: Andragogy Versus Pedagogy*. New York, NY: Association Press; 1970.

56. Harriman G. *Adult Learning. E-learning Resources*; 2004. http://www.grayharriman.com/adult_learning.htm.

57. Conner M. Introduction to adult learning. <http://marciaconner.com/resources/adult-learning>; n.d. Accessed March 19, 2016.

58. Conner ML. *Learning: The Critical Technology—A Whitepaper on Adult Education in the Information Age*. St. Louis: Wave Technologies International; 1996.

59. Kolb D. *Experiential Learning: Experience as the Source of Learning and Development*. Englewood Cliffs, NJ: Prentice-Hall; 1984.

60. Myers IB, McCaulley MH. *Manual: A Guide to the Development and Use of the Myers Briggs Type Indicator*. Mountain View, CA: Consulting Psychologists Press; 1985.

61. Greathouse J. *Kurt Lewin: 1890–1947*. Muskingum College, Psychology Department; 1997. http://www.muskingum.edu/~psychology/psycweb/history/lewin.htm.

62. Schein E. *Kurt Lewin's Change Theory in the Field and in the Classroom*. Purdue University, College of Technology; 1999. (1999). http://dspace.mit.edu/bitstream/handle/1721.1/2576/SWP-3821-32871445.pdf.

63. Conner D. *Managing at the Speed of Change*. New York, NY: Random House; 2006.

64. Rogers EM. *Diffusion of Innovation*. 4th ed. New York, NY: The Free Press; 1995.

65. Rogers EM, Scott KL. *The Diffusion of Innovations Model and Outreach from the National Network of Libraries of Medicine to Native American communities*. National Network of Libraries of Medicine; 1997. http://www.au.af.mil/au/awc/awcgate/documents/diffusion/rogers.htm.

66. Sapp S. *Diffusion of Innovation: Part 1 and Part 2*. Iowa State University, Department of Sociology; 2012. http://www.soc.iastate.edu/sapp/soc415read.html.

67. Trujillo MF. *Diffusion of ICT Innovations for Sustainable Human Development: Problem Definition*. Tulane University Law School, Payson Center for International Development; 2000. http://payson.tulane.edu/research/E-DiffInnova/diff-prob.html.

68. Rogers EM. *Diffusion of Innovation*. 5th ed. New York, NY: The Free Press; 2003.

69. Rouse M. *Systems Development Life Cycle (SDLC)*. TechTarget; 2009. http://searchsoftwarequality.techtarget.com/definition/systems-development-life-cycle.

70. Thompson C, Synder-Halpern R, Staggers N. Analysis, processes, and techniques: case study. *Comput Nurs*. 1999;17(5):203–206.

71. Kushniruk AW, Borycki EM, Kuwata S, Kannry J. Emerging approaches to usability evaluation of health information systems: towards in-situ analysis of complex healthcare systems and environments. *Stud Health Technol Inform*. 2011;169:915–919.

72. Garcia-Smith D. *Testing a Model to Predict Successful Clinical Information Systems* [doctoral dissertation]. The University of Arizona, College of Nursing; 2007. http://arizona.openrepository.com/arizona/handle/10150/195846.

DISCUSSION QUESTIONS

1. Describe the technology-related literacies and explain their relationship to health informatics.

2. Using Shannon and Weaver's model of information as a framework, describe several ways in which miscommunication can occur between healthcare providers working together in a clinical setting. Use this same framework to suggest how technology could be used to decrease this miscommunication.

3. Use Blum's model of information to explain the process used by healthcare providers for diagnosing and managing or treating healthcare problems. Identify the implication of this model for the development of decision support systems to support the patient care process.

4. Some have argued that the data-to-wisdom continuum cannot be used to define the scope of clinical practice

because computers cannot process wisdom. Identify and describe whether this is a fallacy.

5. This chapter includes four types of learning theories. Use each of these types of learning theories to explain how to design and implement a staff education program to support a go-live implementation in a major medical center.

6. The responses of individuals to innovation have been classified into five groups. List and describe the five groups.

Now describe how each group should be managed when planning for a major change within a healthcare institution.

7. List and explain the five internal organizational characteristics that can be used to predict how an organization will respond to a change in automation. Now use these same characteristics to predict how the U.S. healthcare system will respond to the automation of healthcare over the next 5 years.

CASE STUDY

A good friend of yours is director of patient services at a 220-bed community hospital. Last year the hospital merged with a much larger medical center. One of the upsides, as well as one of the challenges, is the rapid introduction of new health information systems. The goal is to bring the hospital "up to speed" within 3 years. At present, CPOE is being implemented. The general medical and surgical units went live last month. The intensive care unit and pediatrics and obstetrics units are scheduled to go-live next month. The plan is to work out any kinks or problems on the general units and then go-live in the specialty units.

Most of the physicians, nurse practitioners, and physician assistants initially complained but are now becoming more comfortable with the computers and are beginning to integrate the CPOE process into their daily routines. Several physicians are now requesting the ability to enter orders from their offices, and others are looking into this option.

However, three physicians have not commented during this process but are clearly resisting. For example, after performing rounds and returning to their offices, they called the unit with verbal orders. After being counseled on this behavior,

they began to write the orders on scraps of paper and put these in the patient's charts or leave them at the nurses' station. When they were informed that these were not "legal orders," they began smuggling in order sheets from the non-activated units. In addition, they have been coercing the staff nurses on the units to enter the orders for them. This has taken two forms. Sometimes they sign in and then ask the nurses to enter the orders. Other times they ask the nurses to put the orders in verbally and then they confirm the orders. The nurses feel caught between the hospital's goals and the need to maintain a good working relationship with these physicians.

Discussion Questions

1. How would you use the theories presented in this chapter to diagnosis the problems demonstrated in this case. List your diagnoses and explain your analysis.

2. What actions would you recommend to your friend and what reason (theories) would you use as a basis for your recommendations?

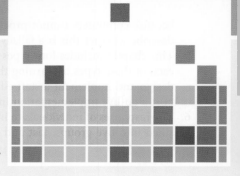

3

Evidence-Based Practice, Practice-Based Evidence, and Health Informatics

Kathleen R. Stevens, Susan D. Horn, Jacob Kean, Vikrant G. Deshmukh, Sandra A. Mitchell, and Ramona Nelson

High-quality cost-effective care requires health information systems that present the evidence needed for providers to make best-practice decisions at the point of care and then capture the data by which the effectiveness of those decisions can be measured.

OBJECTIVES

At the completion of this chapter, the reader will be prepared to:

1. Explore trends in evidence-based quality improvement.
2. Discuss the implications of evidence-based quality improvement for various levels and types of healthcare organizations as well as across multiple professions.
3. Review effective models in structuring evidence-based practice (EBP) initiatives.
4. Define the goals and analyze processes employed in practice-based evidence (PBE) designs.
5. Analyze the strengths and weaknesses of observational designs in general and of PBE specifically.
6. Identify the roles and activities of the informatics specialist in PBE in healthcare environments.
7. Discuss the synergistic role of EBP and PBE in developing informatics-based solutions for managing patients' care needs.

KEY TERMS

ABSTRACT ❖

This chapter links evidence-based practice (EBP) and practice-based evidence (PBE) with informatics by exploring the central, shared construct of knowledge. The discussion offers a foundation for understanding EBP and PBE, as well as their interrelationships. It describes how EBP and PBE are supported and integrated through a variety of current informatics applications. The chapter concludes by exploring opportunities for applying informatics solutions to maximize the advantages offered by the synergistic implementation of EBP and PBE in providing cost-effective, safe, quality healthcare for individuals, families, groups, and communities.

INTRODUCTION

Informatics solutions and tools hold great potential for enhancing evidence-based clinical decision making and for measuring the effectiveness of those decisions in real time. The field of informatics and the concepts of evidence-based practice (EBP) and practice-based evidence (PBE) intersect at the crucial junction of knowledge for clinical decisions, with the goal of transforming healthcare to be reliable, safe, and effective.

A foundational paradigm for informatics is the framework of data, information, knowledge, and wisdom discussed in Chapter 2. This framework indicates that as data are organized into meaningful groupings, the information within those data can then be seen and interpreted. The organization of information and the identification of the relationships between the facts within the information create knowledge. The effective use of knowledge, such as the process of providing personalized care to manage human healthcare needs, is wisdom. Computerization offers the opportunity to collect, organize, label, and deliver efficiently and effectively evidence-based information and knowledge at the point of decision making, thereby making it possible for clinicians to apply concepts from EBP at the point of care. As that care is delivered, patient-specific data can be captured through documentation in the patient's electronic health record (EHR), thereby providing a feedback loop for evaluating the effectiveness of those patient-care decisions. In addition, these data can be aggregated across patients, demonstrating the effectiveness of evidence-based decisions across groups of patients in a variety of different settings.

A prime challenge to achieve this ideal is the complexity of issues surrounding standardized terminology in healthcare and the lack of a common framework across the field of EBP and PBE. Standardized terminology is requisite for naming, classifying, tagging, locating, and then analyzing evidence to use that evidence in practice.

EVIDENCE-BASED PRACTICE

Knowledge is at the heart of EBP. Within the EBP paradigm, knowledge must be transformed through a number of forms to increase its utility at the point of care.[1] The ultimate goal of EBP is improving systems and microsystems within healthcare, with these improvements based on science. Using computerized methods and resources to support the implementation of EBP holds great potential for improving healthcare. Delivering evidence to the point of patient care can align care processes with best practices that are supported by evidence.

The evolution of EBP underscores its potential impact on quality of care and health outcomes. In a well-known report, *To Err Is Human*, experts noted that almost 100,000 patients were being harmed annually by the healthcare system.[2] When this report was issued, 100,000 deaths was seen as unbelievably high. Today experts consider 100,000 deaths as a severe underestimation.[3] One of the latest estimates published in 2013 reported 400,000 deaths resulting from preventable medical error, with serious harm 10 to 20 times more common than lethal harm.[4]

As an immediate response to the Institute of Medicine (IOM)* report, national leaders identified the gap between what is known about best care and what is widely practiced in the 2001 report titled *Crossing the Quality Chasm (Chasm)*.[5]

In the *Chasm* report, more than 100 surveys of quality of care were cited, showing that scores on the "report card" for healthcare performance were poor. Box 3.1 presents findings from these surveys, comparing current care to what was deemed the best care or standards of care. These results indicated that significant improvement was needed if every patient is to receive high-quality care at all times. To achieve this goal, the report pointed to EBP as a critical solution to redesigning and improving healthcare.

Another set of reports demonstrating this challenge is the National Healthcare Quality Report (NHQR) and the National Healthcare Disparities Report (NHDR) produced

---

*Effective July 1, 2015, the National Academy of Science, Engineering, and Medicine voted to change the name of the Institute of Medicine to the National Academy of Medicine. In March 2016 the National Academy of Sciences announced that the division of the National Academies of Sciences, Engineering, and Medicine (the Academies) that focuses on health and medicine was renamed the Health and Medicine Division (HMD) instead of using the name Institute of Medicine (IOM). In this textbook you may see any of these three names used depending on the date of the publication or report.

BOX 3.1 Institute of Medicine Findings on 2001 Level of Current Care Compared With Standards of Care

- 47% of myocardial infarction patients did not receive beta blockers
- 50% of children with asthma did not receive written instructions
- 48% of elderly did not receive annual influenza vaccine
- 63% of smokers were not advised to quit smoking
- 84% of Medicare patients with diabetes were not tested with the A1c blood test

Data from Institute of Medicine. Crossing the quality chasm: A new health system for the 21st Century [Committee on Health Care in America & Institute of Medicine]. Washington, DC: National Academies Press; 2001.

---

by the Agency for Healthcare Research and Quality (AHRQ). These reports, published annually since 2003, have provided an annual snapshot of the quality of care across the country.[6] Beginning in 2014, findings on healthcare quality and healthcare disparities were integrated into a single document titled the *National Healthcare Quality and Disparities Report* (QDR). This report highlights the importance of examining quality and disparities together to gain a more comprehensive picture of healthcare. "The report demonstrates that the nation has made clear progress in improving the health care delivery system to achieve the three aims of better care, smarter spending, and healthier people, but there is still more work to do, specifically to address disparities in care."[6] For example, patient safety improved, as demonstrated by a 17% reduction in rates of hospital-acquired conditions between 2010 and 2013. However, across a broad range of measures, recommended care is delivered only 70% of the time.

Solutions to the healthcare quality gap are offered in the *Chasm* report.[5] The IOM expert panel issued recommendations for urgent action to redesign healthcare so that it is safe, timely, effective, efficient, equitable, and patient centered, often referred to as the STEEEP principles.[5] Each of the STEEEP redesign principles is described further in Table 3.1.

The *Chasm* report continues to be a major influence, directing national efforts targeted at transforming healthcare. For example, the STEEEP recommendations are now reflected in health profession education programs. The American Association of Colleges of Nursing (AACN) educational competencies include requirements for programs to prepare nurses who contribute to quality improvement.[7] AACN *Essentials* specify that professional nursing practice be grounded in translation of current evidence into practice and further point to the need for knowledge and skills in information management as being critical in the delivery of quality patient care.[7] Likewise, the Accreditation Council for Graduate Medical Education (ACGME) requires medical education in quality improvement.[8] The STEEEP principles are also reflected in clinical practice resources, such as the AHRQ Health Care Innovations Exchange, in which the elements of STEEEP are employed as selection criteria for inclusion in this unique clearinghouse.[9]

TABLE 3.1 Descriptions of the STEEEP Principles for Redesigning Healthcare

Principle	Description
Safe	Avoid injuries to patients from the care that is intended to help them.
Timely	Reduce wait time and sometimes-harmful delays for both those who receive and those who give care.
Effective	Provide services based on scientific knowledge to all who could benefit, and refrain from providing services to those not likely to benefit.
Efficient	Avoid waste, including waste of equipment, supplies, ideas, and energy.
Equitable	Provide care that does not vary in quality because of personal characteristics such as gender, ethnicity, geographic location, and socioeconomic status.
Patient centered	Provide care that is respectful of and responsive to individual patient preferences, needs, and values, and ensure that patient values guide all clinical decisions.

Adapted from Institute of Medicine. Crossing the quality chasm: A new health system for the 21st Century (Committee on Health Care in America & Institute of Medicine). Washington, DC: National Academies Press; 2001:39-40.

Quality of care and EBP are conceptually linked, and they form the hub of healthcare improvement. The descriptions and definitions of each reflect the overlap of these concepts and offer reference points against which to expand the understanding of them. In particular, the focal point of both is the use of knowledge in practice.

The definition of *quality of care* includes two key connections to EBP and knowledge that in turn provide a strong linking point for informatics. First, quality healthcare services increase the likelihood that the goals of care or desired outcomes will be reached. This implies that processes of EBP must assist clinicians in knowing which options in health services are effective. The strongest cause-and-effect knowledge is discovered through formal research. Second, EBP is connected to quality insofar as healthcare is consistent with current knowledge. *Using knowledge* presumes accessibility to it at the point of care. The overlap of EBP and knowledge is further underscored by the definition of the STEEEP principle "effective." In the STEEEP framework, *effectiveness* is defined as evidence-based decision making, suggesting, "Patients should receive care based on the best available scientific knowledge."[5, p. 62] *Knowledge* is the point of convergence across the areas of EBP, informatics, and improvement. Using informatics approaches can make evidence available and accessible at the point of care.

EBP is put into action during clinical decision making. The primary impetus for EBP in healthcare is that clinicians should select the option that is most likely to be effective in improving the patient's health problem. This option is supported by best available research evidence. Clients present a plethora of actual and potential health problems that need to be managed or resolved (e.g., living with asthma, succeeding in the face of learning disabilities, and preventing obesity). Currently, many clinical actions are not based on best available scientific knowledge and, therefore, offer the client care that is not as effective as it could be.[5] The essential role of the healthcare provider is to select and apply interventions having the greatest potential to improve the client's situation and to implement the most effective strategies for changing the microsystem or system of care. Clinicians choose from and interpret a huge variety of clinical data and information while facing pressure to decrease uncertainty, risks to patients, and costs. Knowledge underlies these decisions and plays a primary role in the care provided.

Evidence-based clinical decision making can be described as a prescriptive approach to making choices in diagnostic and intervention care, based on the idea that research-based care improves outcomes most effectively. Research-based care provides evidence about which option is most likely to produce the desired outcome. EBP is seen as a key solution in closing the gap between what is known and what is practiced.

However, important questions lie between accepting this as true and the clinician's and system's ability to enact it: How do clinicians know which interventions will most likely diminish or resolve the health problem and help the client reach his or her health goal? What resources are available to apply EBP principles directly in clinical decision making? Answering these questions begins with analyzing the different models of EBP.

EVIDENCE-BASED PRACTICE MODELS

A number of EBP models are useful in understanding various aspects of EBP and elucidating connections between informatics and EBP. An overview of models in the field reflects several challenges for developing informatics approaches. The primary challenge is the lack of a common framework that could be used to consistently organize and implement EBP principles.

Prominent EBP models can be grouped into three categories of models for designing and implementing systematic approaches to strengthen evidence-based clinical decision making.[10] Table 3.2 describes the critical attributes and provides examples in three categories.

The first category includes models that focus on EBP, research use, and knowledge transformation principles. These models emphasize a systematic approach to synthesizing knowledge. The models specify a series of processes designed to:

1. Identify a question, topic, or problem in healthcare.
2. Retrieve relevant evidence to address the identified issue.
3. Critically appraise the level and strength of that evidence.
4. Synthesize and apply the evidence to improve clinical outcomes.

TABLE 3.2 Models for Evidence-Based Practice

Focus	Description	Examples of Models
EBP, research use, and knowledge transformation processes	Direct a systematic approach to synthesizing knowledge and transforming research findings to improve patient outcomes and the quality of care. Address both individual practitioners and healthcare organizations. Focus on increasing the meaningfulness and utility of research findings in clinical decision making.	• Stevens Star Model of Knowledge Transformation[1] • Advancing Research and Clinical Practice through Close Collaboration (ARCC) Model of Evidence-Based Practice in Nursing and Healthcare[11] • Johns Hopkins Nursing Evidence-Based Practice Model and Guidelines[12] • Iowa Model of Evidence-Based Practice[13] • Stetler Model of Research Utilization[14]
Strategic and organizational change theory to promote uptake and adoption of new knowledge	Trace mechanisms by which individual, small group, and organizational contexts affect diffusion, uptake, and adoption of new knowledge and innovation. Premise is that interventions, outcomes evaluations, and feedback are important methods to promote practice change.	• Promoting Action on Research Implementation in Health Services (PARiHS)[15-17] • Vratny and Shriver Model for Evidence-Based Practice[18] • Pettigrew and Whipp Model of Strategic Change[14] • Outcomes-Focused Knowledge Translation[19] • Determinants of Effective Implementation of Complex Innovations in Organizations[20] • Ottawa Model of Research Use[21,22]
Knowledge exchange and synthesis for application and inquiry	Structure ongoing interactions among practitioners, researchers, policy-makers, and consumers to facilitate the generation of clinically relevant knowledge and the application of knowledge in practice; all parties are engaged in bidirectional collaboration across the translation continuum.	• Collaborative Model for Knowledge Translation between Research and Practice Settings[23] • Framework for Translating Evidence into Action[24] • Knowledge Transfer and Exchange[25] • Canadian Institutes of Health Research Knowledge Translation within the Research Cycle Model or Knowledge Action Model[26-28] • Interactive Systems Framework for Dissemination and Implementation[29]

From Mitchell SA, Fisher CA, Hastings CE, et al. A thematic analysis of theoretical models for translational science in nursing: mapping the field. *Nurs Outlook.* 2010;58(6):287-300. Used with permission.

Some models in this category emphasize the process by which research findings can be developed into a more useful form, such as a clinical practice guideline or standards of care, which can then be used to guide clinical decision making in the practice arena. Other models reflect a PBE approach by addressing outcomes evaluation to determine whether the EBP change has produced the expected clinical outcomes or to compare actual practice and ideal practice (thereby identifying unacceptable practice variation).

The second category includes models that offer an understanding of the mechanisms by which individual, small group, and organizational contexts affect the diffusion, uptake, and adoption of new knowledge, as well as innovation, which is essential to the design of EBP initiatives. These models propose that specific interventions serve to accelerate the adoption of practices that are based on best evidence. Examples of such interventions include:

- Facilitation
- Use of opinion leaders
- Real-time feedback about patient outcomes

- Audit feedback about clinicians' variation from established practice standards

Thus within these models, feedback regarding both patient and practitioner outcomes is seen as a change strategy.

A third category of models and frameworks postulates that formalized, bidirectional, and ongoing interactions among practitioners, researchers, policy-makers, and consumers accelerate the application of new discoveries in clinical care. This ongoing interaction increases the likelihood that researchers will focus on problems of importance to clinicians. Such models simultaneously address the generation of new knowledge (discovery) and uptake. This collaboration supports the exchange of expertise and knowledge to strengthen decision making and action for all involved parties.[10]

Each EBP model described previously has perspectives that may prove valuable in designing and advancing informatics approaches to EBP. The following section examines the application of one of these models, the Stevens ACE Star Model of Knowledge Transformation,[1] which will be used to demonstrate how an EBP model can:

1. Guide the transition from the discovery of new information and knowledge to the provision of care that is based on evidence.
2. Identify how computerization and informatics principles can be used to make this transition realistically possible in a world in which information and knowledge are growing at an explosive rate.

STEVENS STAR MODEL OF KNOWLEDGE TRANSFORMATION

The Star Model provides a framework for converting research knowledge into a form that has utility in the clinical decision-making process. The model articulates a necessary process for reducing the volume and complexity of research knowledge, evolving one form of knowledge to the next, and incorporating a broad range of sources of knowledge throughout the EBP process.

The model addresses two major hurdles in employing EBP: (1) the volume of current professional knowledge and (2) the form of knowledge that healthcare professionals attempt to apply in practice. In both instances, informatics-based solutions have been created. The Star Model explains the key concept of knowledge transformation. Knowledge transformation is defined as the conversion of research findings from discovery of primary research results, through a series of stages and forms, to increase the relevance, accessibility, and utility of evidence at the point of care to improve healthcare and health outcomes by way of evidence-based care.[1]

When considering the *volume* of knowledge, experts point out, "no unaided human being can read, recall, and act effectively on the volume of clinically relevant scientific literature."[5, p. 25] It is estimated that in medicine, more than 10,000 new research articles are published annually. Even the most enthusiastic clinician or researcher would find it challenging to stay abreast of this volume of literature. When considering the *form* of knowledge as a barrier, it is clear that most research reports are not directly useful in a clinical setting but must be converted to a form applicable at the point of care. Research results, often presented in the form of statistical results, exist in a larger body of knowledge. The complexity and lack of congruence across all studies on a topic create a barrier when using this as a basis for clinical decision making. The Stevens Star Model addresses the transformation that is necessary for converting research results from single-study findings to guidelines that can be applied and measured for effect. Discussion of this model is expanded in the next section, with specific electronic resources for each form of knowledge identified and described.

In the Star Model, individual studies move through four cycles, ending in practice outcomes and patient outcomes. The knowledge transformation process occurs at five points, which can be conceptualized as a five-point star as shown in Fig. 3.1. These five points are discovery research, evidence summary, translation to guidelines, practice integration, and evaluation of process and outcome.[1] A description of

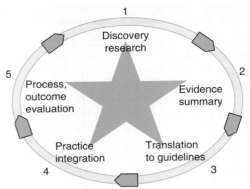

FIG 3.1 ACE Star Model of Knowledge Transformation. (Copyright Stevens KR. *ACE Star Model of EBP: Knowledge Transformation.* San Antonio, TX: Academic Center for Evidence-Based Practice, University of Texas Health Science Center at San Antonio; 2004. Used with expressed permission.)

each point is provided below, along with identification and descriptions of computerized resources and examples.

Point 1: Discovery Research

Primary research on Point 1 represents the knowledge produced through primary discovery. In this stage, knowledge is in the form of results from single research studies. Over the past 3 decades, health-related research has produced thousands of research studies on a wide variety of health-related issues. However, the clinical utility of this form of knowledge is low. The cluster of primary research studies on any given topic may include both strong and weak study designs, small and large samples, and conflicting or converging results, leaving the clinician to wonder which study is the best reflection of cause and effect in selecting effective interventions. Point 1 knowledge is less useful in clinical decision making because there may be hundreds of research studies on a given topic, with the overall collection being unwieldy. Further, the group of studies does not necessarily converge on a consensus of the intervention most likely to produce the desired outcome. Instead, one study may show that the intervention was successful, whereas another shows no difference between control and experimental conditions.

Initially, health sciences researchers focused on applying results from primary research studies directly in patient care, detailing ways to move a single study into practice. However, since there may be multiple studies on a given topic, this strategy is no longer considered appropriate for most interventions. Table 3.3 illustrates part of the challenge in moving research into practice with this approach. In this example, the clinician seeks to locate current evidence about falls prevention in the elderly. A CINAHL literature search on the topic "falls prevention" returned more than 14,000 articles to consider. Even when the search strategy was limited to "research," more than 6500 articles remained on the list. This volume of literature is far too great to have clinical utility.

From Mulrow CD. Rationale for systematic reviews. *Br Med J.* 1994;309(6954):597-599. Reproduced with permission from BMJ Publishing Group Ltd.

TABLE 3.3 Literature Search and Knowledge Forms on "Falls Prevention"

Star Point form of Knowledge	Search	Results
Point 1: Discovery research	CINAHL search for "falls"	14,627 citations
	Limit search to "research"	6991 citations
Point 2: Evidence summary	Limit search to "systematic reviews"	250 citations
Focus on "prevention in elderly"	Limit to prevention in elderly	6 systematic reviews

Point 2: Evidence Summary

Table 3.3 illustrates the striking advantage of knowledge management through knowledge transformation stages, in particular evidence summaries. Evidence summaries include evidence synthesis, systematic reviews (SRs), integrative reviews, and reviews of literature, with SRs being the most rigorous approach to evidence summary. Before evidence summaries were developed, the clinician was left to deal with the many articles located via a bibliographic database search: in this case, thousands of articles. However, if the research knowledge has been transformed through evidence synthesis, the resulting SR will contain this comprehensive knowledge base in a single article. The EBP solution to the complexity and volume of literature seen in Point 1 is the Point 2 evidence summary. In this second stage of knowledge transformation, a team locates all primary research on a given clinical topic and summarizes it into a single document about the state of knowledge on the topic. This summary step is the main knowledge transformation that distinguishes EBP from simple research application and research use in clinical practice. The importance of this transformation cannot be overstated: SRs are described as the central link between research and clinical decision making.[30] Key advantages of SRs are summarized in Box 3.2. Returning to Table 3.3 and our example on

BOX 3.2 Advantages of Systematic Reviews

A rigorous systematic review:
- Reduces information into a manageable form
- Establishes generalizability—participants, settings, treatment variations, and study designs
- Assesses consistencies across studies
- Increases power in cause and effect
- Reduces bias and improves true reflection of reality
- Integrates information for decisions
- Reduces time between research and implementation
- Offers basis for continuous updates

falls, once the literature search is transformed into "systematic reviews," the volume of located sources is decreased to 250 citations. Once a narrowed clinical topic is applied, the search yields six SR on falls prevention in the elderly, thereby transforming over 14,000 pieces of knowledge into manageable resource.

An SR combines results from a body of original research studies into a clinically meaningful whole to produce new knowledge through synthesis and can use the statistical procedure meta-analysis to combine findings across multiple studies. Evidence summaries communicate the latest scientific findings in an accessible form that can be readily applied in making clinical decisions; that is, evidence summaries form the basis upon which to build EBP. When developing an evidence summary, one must keep in mind that nonsignificant findings can be as important to practice as positive results. However, nonsignificant findings tend not to be published and so are underrepresented in the literature.

Conducting sound evidence summaries requires scientific skill and extensive resources: often more than a year's worth of scientific work. Therefore evidence summaries are often conducted by scientific and clinical teams that are specifically prepared in the methodology. The dominant methodology for SRs is published in the *Cochrane Handbook for Systematic Reviews of Interventions.*[31]

The process of narrowing down the publications for computerization is facilitated by computerized methods using Covidence (available at: https://www.covidence.org/) to screen publications and by using reference managers such as EndNote. The state of the science in informatics points to the fact that the field is nascent; as such, research conducted on key aspects remains in the descriptive and correlational phases of scientific development: causal studies that test interventions are scarce. This can preclude the use of the SR method to summarize effect sizes across multiple studies. In fact, Weir et al. contend that researchers rushed to perform experimental studies for computerized provider order entry (CPOE) before the phenomenon was understood.[32,33] With newer fields such as informatics, qualitative and descriptive studies are needed first. Then causal and comparative research and subsequent integrative reviews and SRs can be conducted to summarize the science of health informatics.

Resources and Examples

Major computerized resources for locating SRs include the Cochrane Database of Systematic Reviews, the AHRQ, as well as the general professional literature. The Cochrane's primary strategy is the production and dissemination of SRs of healthcare interventions. This group established the "systematic review" as a literature review, conducted using rigorous approaches that synthesize all high-quality research evidence to reflect current knowledge about a specific question. The scientific methods are specified by the Cochrane Collaboration, and its design is considered the gold standard for evidence summaries. As of March 2016, the Cochrane Database of Systematic Reviews included 6471 SRs.[34] Using an example of falls prevention, the most accessed *Cochrane Review* in 2014 is entitled "Interventions for Preventing Falls in Older People Living in the Community." The findings from this SR are summarized in Box 3.3. The evidence summary offers powerful knowledge about what interventions are likely to be most successful. Note that in this example 62 trials (Point 1 studies) were located, screened for relevance and quality, and meta-analysis was used to consolidate results into a single set of conclusions. However, the recommendations for practice from the SR are not yet action-oriented. For this to happen, it is necessary to translate a conclusion into an actionable recommendation by moving knowledge to Point 3 on the Star model.

Point 3: Translation to Guidelines

In the third stage of EBP, translation, experts are called on to consider the evidence summary, fill in gaps with consensus expert opinion, and merge research knowledge with expertise to produce clinical practice guidelines (CPGs). This process translates the research evidence into clinical recommendations. The IOM defines clinical guidelines as "systematically developed statements to assist practitioner and patient decisions about appropriate healthcare for specific clinical circumstances."[35]

CPGs have evolved during the past 20 years from recommendations based largely on expert judgment to recommendations grounded primarily in evidence. Expert consensus is used in guideline development when research-based evidence is lacking.[36] CPGs are commonly produced and sponsored by a clinical specialty organization. Such guidelines are present throughout all organized healthcare in the form of clinical pathways, nursing care standards, and unit policies. An exemplar of the development of CPGs in nursing is Putting Evidence into Practice in Oncology.[37] This program engages scientists and expert clinicians in examining evidence, conducting evidence summaries, generating practice recommendations, and developing tools to implement the guidelines. These online guidelines are accessible to clinicians and are also published in nursing literature.[38]

Crucial criteria for well-developed CPGs are (1) the evidence is explicitly identified and (2) the evidence and recommendation are rated. To assist in rating evidence, several taxonomies have been developed. One such taxonomy was developed by the Center for Evidence Based Medicine in the United Kingdom. This rating system identifies SRs as the uppermost strength of evidence.[39]

Also included and counted as evidence is *consensus of expert opinion*, which is rated the weakest strength of all levels of evidence. However, if no other evidence exists, this may serve to support clinical decision making. Well-developed CPGs and care standards share several characteristics: a specified process is followed during guideline development; the guideline identifies the evidence upon which each recommendation is made, whether it is research or expert opinion; and the evidence is rated using a strength-of-evidence rating scale. Fig. 3.2 illustrates a strength-of-evidence rating hierarchy.[40] The higher the evidence is placed on the pyramid, the more confident the clinician can be that the intervention will cause the targeted health effect.

A number of EBP approaches emphasize the usefulness of CPGs in bridging the gap between primary research findings and clinical decision making.[30] CPGs are systematically developed statements to assist practitioners and patients in decisions about appropriate healthcare for specific clinical circumstances.[35] CPGs are seen as tools to help move scientific evidence to the bedside. To increase the likelihood that the recommended action will have a positive impact on the clinical outcome, it is imperative that guidelines are based on best available evidence, systematically located, appraised, and synthesized (i.e., evidence based).

Resources and Examples

Today the AHRQ provides the National Guideline Clearinghouse, a searchable database of more than 2500 CPGs entered by numerous sources. Although this knowledge management database can be easily used to locate a wide variety of CPGs, the user must examine the information presented with the CPG to determine that the CPG is current, was developed systematically, and is based on best evidence.

Other guidelines can be located on the U.S. Preventive Services Task Force (USPSTF) segment of the AHRQ website.[41]

**Strength of Evidence
Rating**

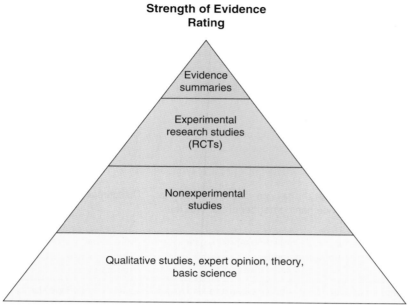

FIG 3.2 Strength-of-evidence hierarchy. *RCT,* Randomized controlled trial. (From *Stevens KR, Clutter PC.* Strength of evidence rating. Academic Center for Evidence-Based Practice. http://www. ACESTAR.uthscsa.edu; 2007. Used with permission.)

These recommendations focus on screening tests, counseling, immunizations, and chemoprophylaxis and are based on evidence summary work performed by the AHRQ.

Critical appraisal of the various forms of knowledge is important. However, for clinical decision making, appraisal of guidelines is crucial for effective clinical care. A number of standards for critical appraisal of CPGs are available and can be used to examine CPGs as clinical agencies consider adoption into practice. An excellent example of a systematic approach is the instrument used to assess practice guidelines developed by the Appraisal of Guidelines for Research and Evaluation (AGREE) enterprise.[42] The 23-item AGREE II instrument developed by this international collaboration is reliable and valid. It outlines primary facets of the CPG to be appraised: scope and purpose, stakeholder involvement, rigor of development, clarity and presentation, application, and editorial independence. Even though the instrument is not easily used by the individual clinician, it is helpful to groups and organizations charged with adoption of specific CPGs. Box 3.4 identifies key elements to be examined when appraising a CPG.

Recommendations flowing from evidence are rated in terms of strength. The USPSTF uses a schema for rating its evidence-based recommendations.[41] It grades strength of recommendations according to one of five classifications (A, B, C, D, and I). The recommendation grade reflects the strength of evidence and magnitude of net benefit (benefits minus harms). Table 3.4 defines each grade and indicates the suggestion for practice.

Professional groups within the agency can move forward with confidence that all research evidence has been systematically gathered and amassed into a powerful conclusion of what will work. The evidence summary is vetted through

> **BOX 3.4   Critically Appraising a Clinical Practice Guideline**
>
> 1. Why was this guideline developed?
> 2. What was the composition (expertise and disciplinary perspective) of the panel that developed the guideline?
> 3. What entity provided financial sponsorship?
> 4. What decision-making processes were used in developing the guideline?
>   a. What clinical question was the guideline developed to address?
>   b. How was the evidence used in the guideline gathered and evaluated?
>   c. Were gaps in the evidence explicitly identified?
>   d. How explicitly is the available evidence linked to the recommendations in the guideline?
>   e. If lower levels of evidence were incorporated (e.g., expert opinion) in the guideline, are these instances labeled explicitly, and are the reasons for the inclusion of expert opinion, the line of reasoning, and the strength of extrapolation from other data clearly identified?
>   f. How are patient preferences incorporated into the guideline?
>   g. Is cost effectiveness considered?
>   h. What is the mechanism and interval for updating the guideline?

clinical experts, and interpretations are made for direct clinical application. In instances where there is a gap in the evidence summary, the experts consider evidence of lower rating and finally add their own expertise into the fully developed CPG. Box 3.5 presents an example of Point 3 in the form of a CPG for preventing falls in the elderly. Note that both the evidence and the recommendation are rated.

TABLE 3.4   U.S. Preventive Services Task Force Grade, Definition, and Suggestion for Practice

Grade	Definition	Suggestion for Practice
A	The USPSTF recommends the service. There is high certainty that the net benefit is substantial.	Offer/provide this service.
B	The USPSTF recommends the service. There is high certainty that the net benefit is moderate or there is moderate certainty that the net benefit is moderate to substantial.	Offer/provide this service.
C	The USPSTF recommends selectively offering or providing this service to individual patients based on professional judgment and patient preferences. There is at least moderate certainty that the net benefit is small.	Offer or provide this service for selected patients depending on individual circumstances.
D	The USPSTF recommends against the service. There is moderate or high certainty that the service has no net benefit or that the harms outweigh the benefits.	Discourage the use of this service.
I	Evidence is lacking, of poor quality, or conflicting, and the balance of benefits and harms cannot be determined.	If the service is offered, patients should understand the uncertainty about the balance of benefits and harms.

US Preventive Services Task Force. Grade definitions. http://www.uspreventiveservicestaskforce.org/Page/Name/grade-definitions; October 2014. Reprinted with permission of the Agency for Healthcare Research and Quality.

BOX 3.5   Example of Stevens Star Point 3: Clinical Practice Guidelines for Preventing Falls in the Elderly

Multifactorial Interventions

Strong—All older people with recurrent falls or assessed as being at increased risk of falling should be considered for an individualized multifactorial intervention. (Evidence level I)

Strong—In successful multifactorial intervention programs, the following specific components are common (Evidence level I):
- Strength and balance training
- Home hazard assessment and intervention
- Vision assessment and referral
- Medication review with modification/withdrawal

From *National Collaborating Centre for Nursing and Supportive Care.* CPG for the Assessment and Prevention of Falls in Older People. London, United Kingdom: National Institute for Clinical Excellence. <https://www.nice.org.uk/guidance/cg161>; 2004; Updated 2013, Reviewed January 2016.

A number of available rating scales convey the strength of the recommendation. Coupled with strength of evidence, the clinician can use "Level 1" evidence and "Grade A" recommendations to support clinical decisions. The USPSTF adopted a system linking strength of evidence with strength of recommendation as follows: strength of the evidence as "A" (strongly recommends), "B" (recommends), "C" (no recommendation for or against), "D" (recommends against), or "I" (insufficient evidence to recommend for or against).[43] Box 3.6 presents three examples of USPSTF recommendations, along with the grade of each recommendation.

As evidenced by the discussion, the translation of guidelines into practice is a labor-intensive process involving a significant cognitive load. In the busy world of healthcare, clinicians cannot routinely take the time to search out CPGs and then translate their application to individual patients. However, using CPGs to design clinical decision support (CDS) systems in EHRs can make it possible for busy clinicians to access evidence-based guidelines that have been individualized to the patient's needs and status at the point of care.

Point 4: Practice Integration

Once guidelines are produced, the recommended actions are clear. Next, the challenge is to integrate the clinical action into practice and thinking. This integration is accomplished through change at individual clinician, organizational, and policy levels. Integration inevitably involves change and integration of evidence into a myriad of health IT tools such as CDS, Infobuttons, order sets in EHRs, and evaluation of compliance using data warehouses or other big data sources. As advances and best practices emerge, it is essential that all members of the healthcare team be actively involved in making quality-improvement and health IT changes. Healthcare providers are called on to be leaders and followers in contributing to such improvement at the individual level of care, as well as at the system level of care, together with other disciplines.[44]

Patient preference must be taken into account at the point of integration, with patient and family circumstances guiding individualized EBP. Integration may not be straightforward because underlying evidence and science of healthcare is yet incomplete. In addition, computerized tools may not be available to assist in the process. As EHRs increasingly include social and behavioral determinants of health and as personal health records expand, health IT should be able to integrate patient preferences in a more electronic and systematic manner. In reviewing the USPSTF's highly developed, well-grounded recommendations presented in Box 3.6, it becomes clear that clinical judgment must be used, and

---

BOX 3.6 Examples of Star Point 3 USPSTF Clinical Recommendations and Grades

Ocular Prophylaxis for Gonococcal Ophthalmia Neonatorum

Release Date: July 2011

Summary of Recommendation

- The USPSTF recommends prophylactic ocular topical medication for all newborns for the prevention of gonococcal ophthalmia neonatorum.

Grade: A Recommendation

From *US Preventive Services Task Force (USPSTF)*. Ocular prophylaxis for gonococcal ophthalmia neonatorum. USPSTF. <http://www.uspreventiveservicestaskforce.org/uspstf/uspsgononew.htm>; 2011.

Prevention of Falls in Community-Dwelling Older Adults

Current Recommendations

Release Date: May 2012

- The USPSTF recommends exercise or physical therapy and vitamin D supplementation to prevent falls in community-dwelling adults aged 65 years or older who are at increased risk for falls.

Grade: B Recommendation

- The USPSTF does not recommend automatically performing an in-depth multifactorial risk assessment in conjunction with comprehensive management of identified risks to prevent falls in community-dwelling adults aged 65 years or older because the likelihood of benefit is small. In determining whether this service is appropriate in individual cases, patients and clinicians should consider the balance of benefits and harms based on the circumstances of prior falls, comorbid medical conditions, and patient values.

Grade: C Recommendation

From *US Preventive Services Task Force (USPSTF)*. Prevention of falls in community-dwelling older adults. USPSTF. <http://www.uspreventiveservicestaskforce.org/uspstf/uspsfalls.htm>; 2012.

Screening for Prostate Cancer

Current Recommendation

Release Date: May 2012

- The USPSTF recommends against prostate-specific antigen-based screening for prostate cancer.

Grade: D Recommendation

This recommendation applies to men in the general U.S. population, regardless of age. This recommendation does not include the use of the prostate-specific antigen test for surveillance after diagnosis or treatment of prostate cancer; the use of the prostate-specific antigen test for this indication is outside the scope of the USPSTF.

From *US Preventive Services Task Force (USPSTF)*. Screening for prostate cancer. USPSTF. <http://www.uspreventiveservicestaskforce.org/Page/Document/RecommendationStatementFinal/prostate-cancer-screening>; 2012. From National Collaborating Centre for Nursing and Supportive Care. CPG for the Assessment and Prevention of Falls in Older People. London, United Kingdom: National Institute for Clinical Excellence. <http://www.nice.org.uk/>; 2004.

---

individualization to patient circumstances and preferences occurs in moving the evidence-based recommendations into practice. It is at this point in the transformation of knowledge that the whole of the EBP definition becomes clear: *EBP is the integration of best research knowledge, clinical expertise, and patient preference to produce the best-practice decisions.*

Resources and Examples

The AHRQ Health Care Innovations Exchange provides a venue for sharing "what works at our place" along with the evidence of how the innovation was tested.[9] The Health Care Innovations Exchange was created to speed the implementation of new and better ways of delivering healthcare. This online collection of more than 700 innovation profiles supports the AHRQ's mission to improve the quality of healthcare and reduce disparities. The Health Care Innovations Exchange offers frontline health professionals a variety of opportunities to share, learn about, and hasten adoption of tested innovations. It also contains more than 1500 quality tools suitable for a range of healthcare settings and populations. Innovation profiles and quality tools are continuously entered into the Exchange. Box 3.7 presents an example of an innovation profile.

Increasingly, agencies are raising the standard of excellence in local policies and procedures by moving toward EBP guidelines. Health IT approaches to integrate EBP guidelines into care hold promise of placing such best practices into

BOX 3.7 Example of Star Point 4: An Innovation

Fall-Prevention Tool Kit Facilitates Customized Risk-Assessment and Prevention Strategies, Reducing Inpatient Falls

What They Did

Periodic assessment, specific risk factors, and customized interventions

Computerized program produces tailored prevention recommendations

Individualized care plan, educational handout, and bedside alert poster

Did It Work?

Significantly reduced falls, particularly in in persons aged >65

Evidence Rating

Strong: Cluster randomized study comparing fall rates

AHRQ, Agency for Healthcare Research and Quality. Adapted from Dykes P. *Interprofessional Nursing Quality Research Initiative.* AHRQ Health Care Innovations Exchange. http://www.innovations.ahrq.gov/content.aspx?id=3094.

point-of-care decision making. For example, as clinical summaries and evidence-based order sets can be available in EHRs, credible practice guidelines can be linked and available via CDS applications.

Point 5: Evaluation

The fifth stage in knowledge transformation is evaluation. Practice changes are followed by evaluation of the impact on a wide variety of outcomes, including safety, effectiveness of the care in producing desired redesign of care, patient outcomes, population outcomes, efficiency and cost factors in the care (short term and long term), and satisfaction of both healthcare providers and patients. Evaluation of specific outcomes is at a high level of public interest.[5,6] As a result, quality indicators are being established for healthcare improvement and public reporting. Additional information on how EHRs and computerization can be used to provide evaluation data is discussed under PBE later in this chapter and in Chapter 23. Chapter 10 provides detailed information about integrating EBP into CDS applications.

Resources and Examples

Among the significant entities establishing quality indicator sets is the AHRQ, through its National Healthcare Quality & Disparities Report (QDR), introduced at the beginning of this chapter.[6] These reports provide a comprehensive overview of the quality of healthcare received by the U.S. population, as well as disparities in care experienced by different racial, ethnic, and socioeconomic groups. The reports are based on more than 250 measures of quality and disparities covering a broad array of healthcare services and settings. Key selection criteria include measures that are the most important and scientifically supported. With these measures the QDR present in summary statements and chart form a snapshot of how our healthcare system is performing and the extent to which healthcare quality and disparities have improved or worsened over time.

Selected examples of summary statements include:

- Access improved—after years without improvement, the rate of uninsured patients among adults ages 18-64 decreased substantially during the first half of 2014.
- Quality improved for most NQS priorities—healthy living improved, led by doubling of selected adolescent immunization rates from 2008 to 2012.

Fig. 3.3 is a summary chart showing trends across the NQS priorities from the QDR.

Another influential entity establishing quality measures is the National Quality Forum (NQF). This nonprofit organization brings together a variety of healthcare stakeholders, including consumer organizations, public and private purchasers, physicians, nurses, informaticians, hospitals, accrediting and certifying bodies, supporting industries, and healthcare research and quality improvement organizations. The NQF's mission includes consensus building on priorities for performance improvement, endorsing national consensus standards for measuring and reporting on performance, and education and outreach.[45] An example of an NQF-endorsed measure for patient safety is presented in Box 3.8.

An important collection of quality measures is assembled in the National Quality Measures Clearinghouse (NQMC), an initiative of the AHRQ.[46] The NQMC is a database and website

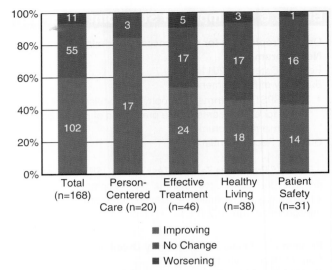

FIG 3.3 Example of Star Point 5. Summary of trends across national quality strategy priorities. Number and percentage of all quality measures that are improving, not changing, or worsening through 2012 overall and by NQS priority. (Source: http://www.ahrq.gov/research/findings/nhqrdr/2014char tbooks/patientsafety/ps-chartbook.html.)

BOX 3.8 Example of Star Point 5 From the National Quality Forum

Patient Safety Measure
#0674: Percent of Residents Experiencing One or More Falls with Major Injury (Long Stay) (Centers for Medicare & Medicaid Services):

Description: This measure reports the percentage of residents who have experienced one or more falls with major injury during their episode of nursing home care ending in the target quarter (3-month period). *Major injury* is defined as bone fractures, joint dislocations, closed head injuries with altered consciousness, or subdural hematoma. Long-stay residents are identified as residents who have had at least 101 cumulative days of nursing facility care.

Measure Type: Outcome
Level of Analysis: Facility
Setting of Care: Post-Acute/Long-Term Care Facility: Nursing Home/Skilled Nursing Facility
Data Source: Electronic Clinical Data

Adapted from *National Quality Forum (NQF)*. Patient Safety 2015 Final Report. February 2016. http://www.qualityforum.org/Publications/2016/02/Patient_Safety_2015_Final_Report.aspx; 2016.

---

for information on evidence-based healthcare quality measures and measure sets. Its purpose is to promote widespread access to quality measures by the healthcare community and other interested individuals. The key targets are practitioners, healthcare providers, health plans, integrated delivery systems, purchasers, and others. The aim is to provide an accessible mechanism for obtaining detailed information on quality measures and to further their dissemination, implementation, and

BOX 3.9 **Example of Star Point 5 From the National Quality Measures Clearinghouse**

Fall Risk Management
The percentage of Medicare members 65 years of age and older who had a fall or had problems with balance or walking in the past 12 months who were seen by a practitioner in the past 12 months and who received fall risk intervention from their current practitioner.

From National Quality Measures Clearinghouse (NQMC). *Measure Summary: fall risk management.* https://www.qualitymeasures.ahrq.gov/summaries/summary/43758; 2015.

use to inform healthcare decisions. Box 3.9 presents a measure from the NQMC. Computerized tools for analyzing the big data in these national databases and teasing out the factors influencing healthcare outcomes will provide a basis for evidence in the search for other levels of EBP.

INFORMATICS AND EVIDENCE-BASED PRACTICE

Informatics and IT hold great promise for achieving full integration of EBP into all care, for every patient, every time. The EBP frameworks provide a foundation upon which informatics solutions can be constructed to move evidence into practice. As seen in the examples addressing each point in the Stevens ACE Star Model, knowledge can be sorted and organized into its various forms. The national efforts cited here resulted in the availability of a number of significant web-based information resources to support each point on the Star Model. New and innovative knowledge management tools are still being developed.

Informatics can greatly add to support of EBP, patient-centered care, and transitions of care across settings. Such technology can greatly assist in the exchange of health information for continuity and quality of care. Health informatics is also essential in improving healthcare decision making by using integrated datasets and knowledge management.

The success of improvement through best (evidence-based) practice could be boosted with greater understanding of the context in which such changes are being made. Once the knowledge is transformed into recommendations (best practices), integration of EBP into practice requires change at levels that include the patient and family, individual provider, microsystem, and macrosystem. The good intentions of an individual provider to use practice guidelines in decision making can be either supported or thwarted by the clinical information systems at the point of care.

Successful models for integrating EBP into practice are emerging. For example, the national team performance training, Team Strategies and Tools to Enhance Performance and Patient Safety (TeamSTEPPS), has been promoted across military healthcare since 1995, with a "civilian" rollout initiated in 2006.[47] The program is built on a solid evidence base from human factors engineering and solves urgent problems arising from team-based care. The program demonstrated improvements in communication and teamwork skills among healthcare professionals leading to improvements in patient care.

In an AHRQ report, the role of health IT in quality measurement was described.[48] Past quality processes were conducted via manual chart entry, manual chart abstraction, and analysis of administrative claims data. In locations with existing health IT, advances are seen. As information systems are created and expanded, the ability to pull meaningful data from the point of care is increasingly computerized. A major potential for health IT is to evolve existing measures into electronic measures and computerized data collection.[48]

The long-term goal for improving health IT–enabled quality measurement is to achieve a robust information infrastructure that supports national quality measurement and reporting strategies. Key goals include interoperability that ensures that EHRs can share information for care coordination, patient-centered care, and cost savings. Such interoperability relies on harmonizing standards. Information exchange, integrating interoperability standards into vendor products, and data linkage are critical for advancement.[48]

A number of challenges must be overcome to achieve the next generation of health IT–enabled quality measurement. First, consensus among quality stakeholders is required to move forward on topics such as the purpose of measurement; achieving patient-centricity in a fragmented health delivery system; alignment of incentives; ownership and funding; increased information exchange; and ensuring privacy, security, and confidentiality. Second, measurement challenges to be overcome include measures valuable to consumers, measures to assess value, measures for specialty uses, and accounting for variations in risk in measurement. Third, technology challenges to be overcome include expansion of eMeasures; advancement in measure capture technologies; advancement in patient-focused technologies, health information exchange, interoperability, and standards; internet connectivity; and aggregation and analysis. Importantly, the report concludes with a call for stakeholder input to inform pathways to achieving the next generation of quality improvement, an important opportunity in which healthcare providers can engage.[48]

The health informatics research agenda published in 2008 includes an expansion to interdisciplinary teams and reflects farsighted goals related to research needed in evidence-based quality improvement.[49] The shifting emphasis on performance improvement and EBP results in the need for research that tests innovations in real-world settings. When the conditions for standardization and interoperability of EHRs are satisfied, patient-specific data can be connected across healthcare settings. Once this occurs, knowledge discovery about coordination and care processes can be expanded using data generated routinely from care settings using PBE principles. By organizing the informatics approach of data, information, knowledge, and wisdom into the EBP knowledge transformation and application in real-world settings, the field of quality improvement and EBP translation into practice can be advanced.

RELATIONSHIP OF EBP AND PBE

The goal of EBP is to achieve safe, cost-effective quality outcomes by using research-based evidence to direct patient-care decisions. However, to be fully effective, EBP requires the feedback loop provided by practice to determine if the goals of EBP have been achieved in the real world of healthcare delivery. Because evidence should drive practice and the data from the practice environment is the ultimate test of the evidence that was used, models of EBP and PBE often overlap. Leaders need to foster a shared learning culture where evidence drives practice, and the real world of the practice setting provides the ultimate evidence for improving healthcare. With the increasing interoperability of health IT, a shared learning culture extends beyond the local department or institution with the opportunity to create generalizable knowledge to improve care worldwide. Typical PBE questions are:

- Are treatments used in daily practice associated with intended outcomes?
- Can we predict adverse events in time to prevent or ameliorate them?
- What treatments work best for which patients?
- With limited financial resources, what are the best interventions to use for specific types of patients?
- What types of individuals are at risk for certain conditions?

Answers to these questions can help clinicians, patients, researchers, healthcare administrators, and policy-makers learn from and improve real-world, everyday clinical practice. An important emerging approach to knowledge building, including knowledge about the effectiveness of EBP guidelines, can be obtained from clinical data through the application of PBE research design techniques.

EHRs and PBE Knowledge Discovery

Increased adoption of EHRs and other health information systems has resulted in vast amounts of structured and textual data. Stored on servers in a data warehouse (a large data repository integrating data across clinical, administrative, and other systems), the data may be a partial or complete copy of all data collected in the course of care provision. The data can include billing information, physician and nursing notes, laboratory results, radiology images, and numerous other diverse types of data. In some settings, data describing individual patients and their characteristics, health issues, treatments, and outcomes have accumulated for years, forming longitudinal records. The clinical record can also be linked to repositories of genetic or familial data.[50–52] These data constitute an incredible resource that is underused for scientific research in biomedicine and nursing.

The potential of using these data stores for the advancement of scientific knowledge and patient care is widely acknowledged. However, clinical concepts are typically represented in the EHR in a way that supports healthcare delivery but not necessarily research. For example, pain might be qualitatively described in a patient's note and EHR as "mild" or "better." This may meet the immediate need for documentation and care, but it does not

allow the researcher to measure differences in pain over time and across patients, as would measurement using a pain scale. Clinical concepts may not be adequately measured or represented in a way that enables scientific analysis. Data quality affects the feasibility of secondary analysis.

Knowledge Building Using Health Information Technology

PBE studies are observational studies that attempt to mitigate the weaknesses traditionally associated with observational designs. This is accomplished by exhaustive attention to determining patient characteristics that may confound conclusions about the effectiveness of an intervention. For example, observational studies might indicate that aerobic exercise is superior to nonaerobic exercise in preventing falls. Nevertheless, if the prescribers tend to order nonaerobic exercise for those who are more debilitated, severity of illness is a confounder and should be controlled in the analysis.

PBE studies use large samples and diverse sources of patients to improve sample representativeness, power, and external validity. In general, there are 800 or more subjects. PBE uses approaches similar to community-based participatory research by including frontline clinicians and patients in the design, execution, and analysis of studies, as well as their data elements, to improve relevance to real-world practice. Finally, PBE uses detailed standardized structured documentation of interventions, which is ideally incorporated into the standard electronic documentation.

This method requires training and quality-control checks for reliability of the measures of the actual process of care. Statistical analysis involves correlations among patient characteristics, intervention process steps, and outcomes. PBE can uncover best practices and combinations of treatments for specific types of patients while achieving many of the presumed advantages of randomized controlled trials (RCTs), especially the presumed advantage that RCTs control for patient differences through randomization. Frontline clinicians treating the study patients lead the study design and analyses of the data prospectively based on clinical experience. The characteristics of PBE are summarized in Table 3.5.

PRACTICE-BASED EVIDENCE

Practice-Based Evidence Features and Challenges

PBE is an innovative prospective research design that uses data gathered from current practice to identify what care processes work in the real world. *EBP is about using evidence to guide practice. PBE is about obtaining evidence from practice.*

PBE studies mitigate the weaknesses usually associated with traditional observational designs in four main ways:

1. Exhaustive attention to patient characteristics to address confounds or alternative explanations of treatment effectiveness.
2. Use of large samples and diverse sources of patients to improve sample representativeness, power, and external validity.

TABLE 3.5 Characteristics of Practice-Based Evidence

Characteristic	Practice-Based Evidence
Description	Participatory research approach requiring documentation of predefined processes and outcome data and analysis
Goal	Determine the effectiveness of multiple interventions on multiple outcomes in actual practice environment
Design classification	Observational (descriptive)
Temporal aspects	Prospective
Typical sample size	800-2000 +

3. Use of detailed standardized structured documentation of interventions with training and quality-control checks for reliability of the measures of the actual process of care.
4. Inclusion of frontline clinicians and patients in the design, execution, and analysis of studies and their data elements to improve ecological validity.

PBE studies require comprehensive data acquisition. By using bivariate and multivariate associations among patient characteristics, process steps, and outcomes can be identified. At the same time PBE study designs are structured to minimize the potential for false associations between treatments and outcomes. These studies focus on minimizing biasing effects of possible alternative factors or explanations when estimating the complex associations between treatments and outcomes within a specific context of care.[53] However, the identified associations between treatment and outcome are not considered causal links. To the extent that the research design can measure and statistically control for these confounders or alternative explanations, the associations still inform causal judgments.

In other words, the PBE approach does not infer causality directly like RCTs, but several sources indicate the strength of the evidence that a causal link exists. First, alternative hypotheses regarding possible causes are tested using the large number of available variables to identify additional potential variables that may be influencing outcomes. Results can be used to drill down to discover potential alternative causes and to generate additional specific hypotheses. Analyses continue until the project team is satisfied that they cannot think of any other variables to explain the outcomes. Second, one can test the predictive validity of significant PBE findings by introducing findings into clinical practice and assessing whether outcomes change when treatments change, as predicted by PBE models. Third, studies can be repeated in different healthcare settings and assessed to determine if the findings remain the same.

Underlying the common criticism of observational studies (that they demonstrate association but not causation) is an unchallenged assumption that the evidence for causation is dichotomous; that is, something either is or is not the cause.

Instead, the evidence for causation should be viewed as a continuum that extends from mere association to undeniable causation. While observational studies cannot prove causation in some absolute sense, by chipping away at potential confounders and by testing for predictive validity in follow-up studies, we move upward on the continuum from mere association to causation. PBE studies offer a methodology for moving up this continuum.

Research design involves a balance of internal validity (the validity of the causal inference that the treatment is the "true" cause of the outcome) and external validity (the validity that the causal inference can be generalized to other subjects, forms of the treatment, measures of the outcome, practitioners, and settings). Essentially, PBE designs trade away the internal validity of RCTs for external validity.[54] PBE designs have high external validity (generalizability) because they include virtually all patients with or at risk for the condition under study, as well as potential confounders that could alter treatment responses. PBE designs attempt to minimize threats to internal validity by trying to collect information on all patient variables—demographic, medical, nursing, functional, and socioeconomic—that might account for differences in outcome. By doing so, PBE designs minimize the need for compensating statistical techniques such as instrumental variables and propensity scoring to mitigate selection bias effects, unknown sources of variance, and threats to internal validity.

PBE study designs attempt to capture the complexity of the healthcare process presented by patient and treatment differences in routine care; PBE studies do not alter or standardize treatment regimens to evaluate the efficacy of a specific intervention or combination of interventions, as one usually does in an RCT or other types of experimental designs.[55,56] PBE studies measure multiple concurrent interventions, patient characteristics, and outcomes. This comprehensive framework provides for consequential analyses of significant associations between treatment combinations and outcomes, controlling for patient differences.

Steps in a PBE Study

Table 3.6 outlines the steps involved in conducting a PBE study and gives a brief description of what each step involves. Once a clinical issue is identified, PBE methods begin with the formation of a multidisciplinary team, often with representatives of multiple sites. Participation of informaticians on the team is critical to ensure that the electronic documentation facilitates data capture for the research and clinical practice without undue documentation burden.

Create a Multisite, Multidisciplinary Project Clinical Team

One factor that distinguishes PBE studies from most other observational studies is the extensive involvement of frontline clinicians and patients. Frontline clinicians and patients are engaged in *all* aspects of PBE projects; they identify data elements to be included in the PBE project based on initial study hypotheses, extensive literature review, and clinical experience and training, as well as patient experience. Many relevant details

TABLE 3.6 Steps in a Practice-Based Evidence Study

Step	Description
1. Create a multisite, multidisciplinary PCT	PCT (a) identifies outcomes of interest, (b) identifies individual components of the care process, (c) creates a common intervention vocabulary and dictionary, (d) identifies key patient characteristics and risk factors, (e) proposes hypotheses for testing, and (f) participates in data collection, analyses, and dissemination of findings. The PCT builds on theoretical understanding, research evidence to date, existing guidelines, and clinical expertise and experience about factors that may influence outcomes.
2. Control for differences in patient severity, including comorbidities, treatment processes, and outcomes	Comprehensive severity measure should be an age- and disease-specific measure of physiologic and psychosocial complexity. It is used to control for selection bias and confounding by indication. An example is the CSI that is disease- and age-specific and composed of more than 2200 clinical indicators.
3. Implement intensive data collection and check reliability	Capture data on patient characteristics, care processes, and outcomes drawn from medical records and study-specific data collection instruments. Data collectors are tested for interrater reliability.
4. Create a study database	Study database consists of merged, cleaned data and is suitable for statistical analyses.
5. Test hypotheses successively	Hypotheses are based on questions that motivated the study originally, previous studies, existing guidelines, and, above all, hypotheses proposed by the PCT. Bivariate and multivariate analysis approaches include multiple regression, analysis of variance, logistic and Cox proportional hazard regression, hierarchical mixed models, and other methods consistent with measurement properties of key variables.
6. Validate and implement study findings	Implement findings in practice to test predictive validity. In this step, findings from the first five steps are implemented and evaluated to determine whether the new or modified interventions replicate results identified in earlier phases and outcomes improve as predicted. After the validation of specific PBE findings, the findings are ready to be incorporated into routine care and clinical guidelines.

CSI, Comprehensive Severity Index; *PCT*, project clinical team.

about patients, treatments, and outcomes may be recorded in existing EHRs; however, the project clinical team (PCT) often identifies additional critical variables that must be collected in supplemental standardized documentation developed specifically for the PBE study. Clinicians and patients also participate in data analyses leading to publication. Front-to-back clinician and patient participation fosters high levels of clinician and patient buy-in that contribute to data completeness and clinical ownership of study findings, even when findings challenge conventional wisdom and practice. Such ownership is essential to knowledge translation and best practice.

Control for Differences in Patient Severity of Illness

Controls for Patient Factors. PBE designs require recording the treatment that each subject receives as determined by clinicians in practice rather than randomizing subjects to neutralize the effect of patient differences. PBE studies address patient differences by *measuring* a wide variety of patient characteristics that go beyond race, gender, age, payer, and other variables that can be exported from administrative, registry, or EHR databases, and then accounting for patient differences through statistical control.

The goal is to measure all variables contributing to outcomes to have the information needed to control for patient differences. This is the major reason for including frontline clinicians and patients in PBE study design and implementation. There always remains the possibility that some patient characteristic may be overlooked, but PBE's exhaustive patient characterization minimizes significantly the chances of not being able to resolve unknown sources of variance because of patient differences.

One critical component of the PBE study design is the use of tools for measuring the degree of illness such as the Comprehensive Severity Index (CSI).[53,57-66] In PBE studies, the CSI can be used to measure how ill a patient is at the time of presentation for care, as well as over time. *Degree of illness* is defined as extent of deviation from "normal values." CSI is "physiologically-based, age- and disease-specific, independent of treatments, and provides an objective, consistent method to define patient severity of illness levels based on over 2,200 signs, symptoms, and physical findings related to a patient's disease(s), not just diagnostic information, such as ICD-9-CM coding alone."[67, p. S132] The validity of CSI has been studied for over 30 years in various clinical settings and conditions such as inpatient adult and pediatric conditions, ambulatory care, rehabilitation care, hospice care, and long-term care settings.[58,65] Patient diagnosis codes and data management rules are used to calculate severity scores for each patient overall and separately for each of a patient's diseases (principal and each secondary diagnosis).

CSI and other measures of patient key characteristics, such as level and completeness of spinal cord injury, severity of stroke disability, or severity of traumatic brain injury, control for patient differences. Using these patient differences can help to account for treatment selection bias or confounding by indication in analyses.

Controls for Treatment and Process Factors. Treatment in clinical settings is often determined by facility standards, regional differences, and clinician training. Therefore, like patient differences, treatment differences must be recorded during a PBE study. The goal is to find measurable factors that describe each treatment to be compared. Examples include the medications dispensed and their dosage; rehabilitation therapies performed and duration on each day of treatment; content, mode, and amount of patient education; and nutritional consumption.

PBE identifies better practices by examining how different approaches to care are associated with outcomes of care, while controlling for patient variables. PBE does not require providers to follow treatment protocols or exclude certain treatment practices. However, characteristics of treatment, including timing and dose, require detailed documentation. These characteristics must be defined by the PBE team and measured in a structured, standard manner for all participating sites and their clinicians. Consistency is critical for minimizing variation in data collection and documentation.[67]

The level of detail found in routine documentation of interventions may be insufficient. Each PBE team must assess the level of detail afforded by routine documentation and determine whether supplemental documentation is necessary.[67] Further, point-of-care documentation or EHR data are pilot tested to ensure complete representation of variables. Pilot testing ensures that point-of-care documentation or EHR data collection captures all elements that clinicians suggest may affect the outcomes of their patients. *If a variable is not measured, it cannot be used in subsequent analyses.*

Controls for Outcome Factors. Multiple outcomes can be addressed in a single PBE project; projects are not limited to one primary outcome, as is the case in other study designs. In particular, PBE studies incorporate widely accepted, standard measures. For example, the Braden Scale for Risk of Pressure Ulcer Development is commonly collected in PBE studies, and it has been used as both a control and an outcome variable.[65-67] Although PBE projects incorporate as many standard measures as possible, they also include outcome measures specific to the study topic. Additional patient outcomes commonly assessed in PBE studies are condition-specific complications, condition-specific long-term medical

outcomes (based on clinician assessment or patient self-report), condition-specific patient-centered measures of activities and participation in society, patient satisfaction, quality of life, and cost.[68]

Some outcomes (e.g., discharge destination [home, community, and institution], length of stay, or death) are commonly available in administrative databases. Other outcome variables (e.g., repeat stroke, deep vein thrombosis, pain, electrolyte imbalance, and anemia) are found in traditional paper charts or EHR documentation but typically are available only up to discharge from the care setting.

Implement Intensive Data Collection and Check Reliability

Using the data elements identified in step 2, historical data are collected from the EHR. Direct care providers document the specific elements of treatment at point of care. For example, if the treatment includes physical therapy, the type, intensity, and duration are precisely recorded during each therapy session. If the healthcare provider offers patient counseling or education, the teaching methods, instructional materials, topical content, and duration of each teaching session are recorded. The informatics specialist is a critical partner in designing the data capture to prevent the need for parallel documentation. If the documentation is too burdensome, clinicians will not comply with documentation requirements and the data will be incomplete. Therefore the design of the data collection is critical to the success of this research approach. The fact that these data collection formats are defined by the frontline clinicians helps to ensure that the data collection formats are specifically designed so that data can be documented easily and quickly.

Create a Study Database

The elements of data collected are compiled into a study-specific database with the assistance of informatics personnel. Data sources include existing or new clinician documentation of care delivered. Patients drop out of a PBE study if they leave the care setting before completion of treatment or drop out during follow-up.[68] Patients who withdraw from a treatment do not distort results of PBE study findings because PBE studies follow patients throughout the care process, taking date and time measurements on all therapies. Hence, if a patient withdraws from care of the study, investigators can use the existing data in the analyses, controlling for time in the study. PBE studies have a huge advantage because of their large sample size, number of information points, and more complete comparison of subjects who complete therapy and subjects who withdraw.

Successively Test Hypotheses

PBE studies use multivariable analyses to identify variables most strongly associated with outcomes. Detailed characterization of patients and treatments allows researchers to specify direct effects, indirect effects, and interactions that might not otherwise become apparent with less detailed data. CSI (overall, individual components, or individual severity indicators) can be used in data analysis to represent the role of comorbid and co-occurring conditions along with the principal diagnosis. If a positive outcome is found to be associated with a specific treatment or combination of treatments, the subsequent methodological approach is to include confounding patient variables or combinations of variables in the analysis in an attempt to "disconfirm" the association. The association may remain robust or variables may be identified that explain the outcome more adequately.

In PBE studies, data include many clinical and therapeutic variables, and a selection procedure is applied to decide on significant variables to retain in regressions. Only variables suggested by the team based on the literature and team members' education and clinical experience and with frequencies equal to or greater than 10 to 20 patients in the sample are usually allowed.

Analyses conducted using PBE databases are iterative. Counterintuitive findings are investigated thoroughly. In fact, counterintuitive and unexpected findings often lead to new discoveries of important associations of treatments with outcomes.

Large numbers of patients (usually >1000 and often >2000) and considerable computing power are required to perform PBE analyses. When multiple outcomes are of interest and there is little information on effect size of each predictor variable, sample size is based on the project team's desire to find small, medium, or large effects of patient and process variables.

Validate and Implement Findings

See the exemplar in Box 3.10 showing how a PBE study of stroke rehabilitation culminated in validation studies and changes in the standard of care in a healthcare system. Because PBE studies are observational, the conclusions require prospective validation before they can be incorporated into clinical guidelines and standards of care. Validation of PBE findings can use a continuous quality improvement approach consisting of systematic implementation of the interventions found to be better in conjunction with monitoring of their outcomes. If the findings from the outcome assessment replicate the findings of the initial retrospective stage in multiple settings and populations, the intervention would be a candidate for incorporation into clinical guidelines as a care process that has established efficacy and effectiveness. This is in contrast to interventions that only have RCT evidence, which generally indicates only efficacy.

Limitations and Strengths of Practice-Based Evidence Studies

PBE methods work best in situations where one wishes to study existing clinical practice. However, there are no limitations related to conditions or settings for use of PBE study methods. Of course, the technique can be time consuming in terms of conducting the initial PBE steps, as well as data

extraction. Although the relevant variables may change, PBE study designs have been found to work in various practice settings, including acute and ambulatory care, inpatient and outpatient rehabilitation, hospice, and long-term care, and for adult and pediatric patients.

INFORMATICS AND PRACTICE-BASED EVIDENCE

As more healthcare systems move toward EHRs, data elements needed for PBE, and especially for CSI, can be captured in structured, exportable formats, while also being used for clinical documentation of care. This concept is implemented already in health systems in Israel and in various PBE studies in the United States.[69] However, transitioning to EHRs presents its own challenges, especially for data-intensive PBE studies. EHRs can facilitate data acquisition, but they are not always research-friendly because many desired data elements are in text, such as clinical notes, and cannot be exported easily. If EHR data cannot be exported directly, they must be abstracted manually or alternatively, processed using Natural Language Processing (NLP) methods.[70] Whereas manual abstraction from EHR can be more labor intensive than abstracting paper charts are, when relying on NLP methods, a bulk of the effort is spent on training the computer algorithms to extract the needed data elements. In addition, EHR modifications for optimization of point-of-care data documentation and abstraction are costly and time consuming, potentially slowing down planning and implementation of PBE studies based on routine electronic data capture. With HITECH, EHRs have become pervasive in clinical practice.[71] Over time, new EHR exporting and reporting software are emerging and making EHR data abstraction less labor intensive.

Examination of CSI elements themselves may show a reduced set that differentiates severity, as well as the full set. It is possible that two valid data elements would each contribute clinically unique information but be fully redundant with respect to their ability to differentiate severity in a population. For example, unresponsive neurological status and fever ≥ 104 degrees are clinically unique indicators of severity in pneumonia. If these indicators differentiate only the same most gravely ill pneumonia patients from the rest of the population, they provide redundant information with respect to the severity of pneumonia. In this case, it may be possible to use only one of the two indicators in CSI scoring, reducing the information burden to compute a CSI score and increasing efficiency.

PBE requires a multidisciplinary team approach for comparative effectiveness research and ensures inclusion of a wide spectrum of variables so that differences in patient characteristics and treatments are measured and controlled statistically.[67]

The next step for comparative effectiveness research is to conduct more rigorous, prospective large-scale observational cohort studies. National efforts such as the Patient-Centered Outcomes Research Institute's (PCORI) Clinical Data

BOX 3.10   Practice-Based Evidence Exemplar: Stroke Rehabilitation

An integrated healthcare system determined that outcomes were highly variable for patients following a stroke. Rehabilitation professionals in the geographic region were polled to determine the local standards of care, and the interventions were quite diverse. A regional task force was convened representing 8 hospitals from 2 care-delivery systems, as well as an independent hospital. The task force was led by a rehabilitation nurse and a physical therapist. A PBE study was initiated to determine what combinations of medical devices, therapies (e.g., physical therapy, occupational therapy, and speech therapy), medications, feeding, and nutritional approaches worked best for various subtypes of stroke patients in real-world practices. A multidisciplinary project clinical team was convened of physicians, nurses, social workers, psychologists, physical therapists, occupational therapists, recreational therapists, and speech-language therapists. Poststroke patients and caregivers were also invited to participate.

The first decisions of the group addressed the outcome variables, including the Functional Independence Measure (FIM) scale score, length of stay in rehabilitation, discharge disposition, mortality, and morbidity (contracture, deep vein thrombosis, major bleeding, pulmonary embolism, pressure ulcer, and pneumonia). Each profession identified possible interventions and developed documentation for the components of the intervention and the intensity (e.g., number of repetitions for each exercise maneuver and time required). Documentation was incorporated into the standard EHR documentation. Over a 2-year period, 1461 patients were studied ranging from 18.4 to 95.6 years of age. Collected patient-related data included age, gender, race, payer, stroke risk factors, and FIM scores. Detailed process and outcome data were collected. Severity of illness was determined using the CSI scale. There were significant differences in the average severity of illness at the 8 sites. There was also heterogeneity in the intensity of therapies, use of tube feedings, and use of psychotropic and opioid medication. Following control for severity of illness, univariate and multivariate analysis of the data determined that factors were positively and negatively associated with the FIM scores at discharge.

Categories of Factors	Positive Association With FIM Score (↑ Independence)	Negative Association With FIM Score (↓ Independence)
Patient factors	Bed motility in first 3 hour (h) Advanced gait activity in first 3 h Home management by OT	Age Severe motor and cognitive impairment at admission
Therapy factors	Bed motility in first 3 h Advanced gait activity in first 3 h	Days until rehabilitation onset
Nutrition	Enteral feeding	
Medications	Atypical antipsychotics Neurotropic pain treated with medications	Tricyclic antidepressants Older SSRIs

OT, Occupational therapist; *SSRIs*, selective serotonin reuptake inhibitors.

After additional studies to replicate findings, the participating hospitals initiated the following policy changes in the treatment of stroke patients. Several of these are novel interventions that would not have been identified without the PBE study method. Continuous quality improvement monitoring was implemented to document adherence and outcomes:

- *Early rehabilitation admission:* patients are admitted to rehabilitation as soon as possible, and therapies begin in the intensive care unit if possible
- *Early gait training by physical therapy:* patients are put in a harness on a treadmill for safety, but gait training is initiated as soon as possible, even in the most affected patients
- *Early feeding:* if patients are not able to eat a full diet, early enteral feedings (nutritional supplements, tube feeding) are initiated
- *Opioids for pain:* opioids are ordered at admission for any time the patient misses therapy because of pain

Source: Horn SD, DeJong G, Smout RJ, Gassaway J, James R, Conroy B. Stroke rehabilitation patients, practice, and outcomes: is earlier and more aggressive therapy better? *Arch Phys Med Rehab.* 2005;86(12 suppl 2):S101-S114.

Research Networks (CDRN) can enable comparative effectiveness research and PBE by providing informatics solutions for sharing data across multiple institutions.[72] From a PBE perspective, rigor entails controlled measurement of outcomes related to multiple intervention combinations and a variety of patient characteristics in diverse clinical settings.[67] PBE studies address questions in the real world where multiple variables and factors can affect the outcomes; they can fit seamlessly into everyday clinical documentation and, therefore, have the potential to influence and improve the evidence in EBP in real-world clinical environment of patient care.

CONCLUSION AND FUTURE DIRECTIONS

Healthcare continues to be a dangerous experience for many patients. Moreover, many healthcare providers and other healthcare decision makers continue to underuse interventions demonstrated to be effective at improving health outcomes.[6,73] The problem is not uncaring disinterested providers, but a lack of organizational infrastructure and information systems designed to support the implementation of EBP and PBE. Green is well recognized for asking the question "If it is an EBP, where's the practice-based evidence?"[74] Going forward, only by creating well-designed healthcare information systems that present the evidence needed for providers to make best-practice decisions at the point of care, and then capturing the patient-care data by which the effectiveness of those decision can be measured, will we have information systems that truly support high-quality cost-effective care.

REFERENCES

1. Stevens KR. *Stevens Star Model of EBP: Knowledge Transformation.* San Antonio, TX: Academic Center for Evidence-Based Practice, University of Texas Health Science Center in San Antonio; 2015.
2. Institute of Medicine. *To Err Is Human: Building a Safer Health System.* Washington, DC: National Academies Press; 2000.
3. McCann E. Deaths by medical mistakes hit records. *Healthcare IT News*; July 18, 2014. http://www.healthcareitnews.com/news/deaths-by-medical-mistakes-hit-records.
4. John TJ. A new, evidence-based estimate of patient harms associated with hospital care. *J Patient Saf.* 2013;9(3):122–128. (2013). http://journals.lww.com/journalpatientsafety/Fulltext/2013/09000/A_New,_Evidence_based_Estimate_of_Patient_Harms.2.aspx.
5. Institute of Medicine. *Crossing the Quality Chasm: A New Health System for the 21st Century.* Washington, DC: National Academies Press; 2001.
6. Agency for Healthcare Research and Quality. *The 2014 National Healthcare Quality & Disparities Report.* Rockville, MD: Agency for Healthcare Research and Quality; 2015. http://www.ahrq.gov/research/findings/nhqrdr/nhqdr14/index.html.
7. American Association of Colleges of Nursing (AACN). *The Essentials of Baccalaureate Education for Professional Nursing Practice.* Washington, DC: AACN; 2008.
8. Accreditation Council for Graduate Medical Education (ACGME). *Common Program Requirements.* Chicago, IL: ACGME; 2007.
9. Agency for Healthcare Research and Quality (AHRQ). *AHRQ Health Care Innovations Exchange. AHRQ.* <http://www.innovations.ahrq.gov/>; n.d. Accessed March 17, 2016.
10. Mitchell SA, Fisher CA, Hastings CE, Silverman LB, Wallen GR. A thematic analysis of theoretical models for translational science in nursing: mapping the field. *Nurs Outlook.* 2010;58(6):287–300.
11. Melnyk BM, Fineout-Overholt E, Mays MZ. The evidence-based practice beliefs and implementation scales: psychometric properties of two new instruments. *Worldviews Evid Based Nurs.* 2008;5(4):208–216.
12. Newhouse RP, Dearholt SL, Poe SS, Pugh LC, White KM. *Johns Hopkins Nursing Evidence-Based Practice Model and Guidelines.* New York, NY: Sigma Theta Tau International Honor Society of Nursing; 2007.
13. Titler MG, Kleiber C, Steelman VJ, et al. The Iowa model of evidence-based practice to promote quality care. *Crit Care Nurs Clin North Am.* 2001;13(4):497–509.
14. Stetler CB, Ritchie J, Rycroft-Malone J, Schultz A, Charns M. Improving quality of care through routine, successful implementation of evidence-based practice at the bedside: an organizational case study protocol using the Pettigrew and Whipp model of strategic change. *Implement Sci.* 2007;2(1):3.
15. Kitson AL, Rycroft-Malone J, Harvey G, McCormack B, Seers K, Titchen A. Evaluating the successful implementation of evidence into practice using the PARiHS framework: theoretical and practical challenges. *Implement Sci.* 2008;3:1.
16. Rycroft-Malone J. The PARiHS framework: a framework for guiding the implementation of evidence-based practice. *J Nurs Care Qual.* 2004;19(4):297–304.
17. Rycroft-Malone J, Kitson A, Harvey G, et al. Ingredients for change: revisiting a conceptual framework. *Qual Saf Health Care.* 2002;11(2):174–180.
18. Vratny A, Shriver D. A conceptual model for growing evidence-based practice. *Nurs Adm Q.* 2007;31:162–170.
19. Doran DM, Sidani S. Outcomes-focused knowledge translation: a framework for knowledge translation and patient outcomes improvement. *Worldviews Evid Based Nurs.* 2007;4(1):3–13.
20. Weiner BJ, Lewis MA, Linnan LA. Using organization theory to understand the determinants of effective implementation of worksite health promotion programs. *Health Educ Res.* 2009;24(2):292–305.
21. Graham ID, Tetroe J. Some theoretical underpinnings of knowledge translation. *Acad Emerg Med.* 2007;14(11):936–941.
22. Logan J, Graham ID. Toward a comprehensive interdisciplinary model of health care research use. *Sci Commun.* 1998;20(2):227–246.
23. Baumbusch JL, Kirkham SR, Khan KB, et al. Pursuing common agendas: a collaborative model for knowledge translation between research and practice in clinical settings. *Res Nurs Health.* 2008;31(2):130–140.
24. Swinburn B, Gill T, Kumanyika S. Obesity prevention: a proposed framework for translating evidence into action. *Obes Rev.* 2005;6(1):23–33.
25. Mitton C, Adair CE, McKenzie E, Patten SB, Perry BW. Knowledge transfer and exchange: review and synthesis of the literature. *Milbank Q.* 2007;85(4):729–768.
26. Armstrong R, Waters E, Roberts H, et al. The role and theoretical evolution of knowledge translation and exchange in public health. *J Public Health.* 2006;28(4):384–389.
27. Brachaniec M, Tillier W, Dell F. The Institute of Musculoskeletal Health and Arthritis (IMHA) Knowledge Exchange Task Force: an innovative approach to knowledge translation. *J Can Chiropr Assoc.* 2006;50(1):8–13.
28. Graham ID, Logan J, Harrison MB, et al. Lost in knowledge translation: time for a map? *J Contin Educ Health Prof.* 2006;26:13–24.
29. Wandersman A, Duffy J, Flaspohler P, et al. Bridging the gap between prevention research and practice: the interactive systems framework for dissemination and implementation. *Am J Community Psychol.* 2008;41(3-4):171–181.
30. Institute of Medicine. *Knowing What Works in Health Care: A Roadmap for the Nation.* Washington, DC: National Academies Press; 2008.
31. Higgins JPT, Green S, eds. *Cochrane Handbook for Systematic Reviews of Interventions Version 5.1.0 [updated March 2011].* The Cochrane Collaboration; 2011. http://handbook.cochrane.org/.
32. Weir C, Staggers N, Laukert T. Reviewing the impact of computerized provider order entry on clinical outcomes: the quality of systematic reviews. *Int J Med Inform.* 2012;81:219–231.
33. Weir C, Staggers N, Phansalkar S. The state of the evidence for computerized provider order entry: a systematic review and

analysis of the quality of the literature. *Int J Med Inform.* 2009;78 (6):365–374.

34. The Cochrane Collaboration. *The Cochrane Database of Systematic Reviews*; 2016. http://www.cochranelibrary.com/ cochrane-database-of-systematic-reviews/index.html.

35. Institute of Medicine (IOM). *Clinical Practice Guidelines We Can Trust.* Washington, DC: National Academies Press; 2011.

36. Clancy CM, Cronin K. Evidence-based decision making: global evidence, local decisions. *Health Aff.* 2005;24(1):151–162.

37. Oncology Nursing Society (ONS). In: *Putting Evidence into Practice.* ONS; June 19, 2015. https://www.ons.org/sites/default/ files/Using%20the%20PEP%20website.pdf.

38. Mitchell SA, Beck SL, Hood LE, Moore K, Tanner ER. Putting evidence into practice: evidence-based interventions for fatigue during and following cancer and its treatment. *Clin J Oncol Nurs.* 2009;11(1):99–113.

39. *Center for Evidence-Based Medicine (CEBM).* The 2011 Oxford CEBM Levels of Evidence: Introductory Document. CEBM. <http://www.cebm.net/wp-content/uploads/2014/06/CEBM-Levels-of-Evidence-Introduction-2.1.pdf>; n.d. Accessed March 17, 2016.

40. Stevens KR, McDuffie K, Clutter PC. Research and the mandate for evidence-based practice, quality, and patient safety. In: Mateo MA, Kirchhoff KT, eds. *Research for Advanced Practice Nurses: From Evidence to Practice.* New York, NY: Springer Publishing Company; 2009:43–70. [Chapter 3].

41. US Preventive Services Task Force (USPSTF). *US Preventive Services Task Force ratings* USPSTF; 2011. http:// uspreventiveservicestaskforce.org/uspstf07/ratingsv2.htm.

42. Appraisal of Guidelines, Research, and Evaluation (AGREE). *About the AGREE Enterprise* AGREE; 2010. http://www. agreetrust.org/.

43. Harris RP, Helfand M, Woolf SH, et al. Current methods of the U.S. Preventive Services Task Force: a review of the process. *Am J Prev Med.* 2001;20(suppl 3):21–35.

44. Institute of Medicine. *The Future of Nursing: Focus on Scope of Practice.* Washington, DC: National Academies Press; 2010.

45. *National Quality Forum (NQF).* http://www.qualityforum.org/ Home.aspx. Accessed March 17, 2016.

46. Agency for Healthcare Research and Quality (AHRQ). *National Quality Measures Clearinghouse (NQMC).* Bethesda, MD: Agency for Healthcare Research and Quality; 2014.

47. TeamSTEPPS®. *National Implementation.* Rockville, MD: Agency for Healthcare Research and Quality; April 2015. http://www.ahrq.gov/professionals/education/curriculum-tools/teamstepps/national-meeting/index.html.

48. Anderson KM, Marsh CA, Flemming AC, Isenstein H, Reynolds J. *Quality Measurement Enabled by Health IT: Overview, Possibilities, and Challenges.* Rockville, MD: Agency for Healthcare Research and Quality; 2012 [AHRQ Publication No. 12–0061-EF].

49. Bakken S, Stone PW, Larson EL. A nursing informatics research agenda for 2008–18: contextual influences and key components. *Nurs Outlook.* 2008;56:206–214.

50. Duvall SL, Fraser AM, Rowe K, Thomas A, Mineau GP. Evaluation of record linkage between a large healthcare provider and the Utah Population Database. *J Am Med Inform Assoc.* 2012;19(e1):e54–e59.

51. Slattery ML, Kerber RA. A comprehensive evaluation of family history and breast cancer risk: the Utah Population Database. *J Am Med Assoc.* 1993;270(13):1563–1568.

52. Hu H, Correll M, Kvecher L, et al. DW4TR: a data warehouse for translational research. *J Biomed Inform.* 2011;44 (6):1004–1019.

53. Horn SD, DeJong G, Ryser DK, Veazie PJ, Teraoka J. Another look at observational studies in rehabilitation research: going beyond the holy grail of the randomized controlled trial. *Arch Phys Med Rehabil.* 2005;86(12 suppl 2):S8–S15.

54. Mitchell M, Jolley J. *Research Design Explained.* 4th ed. New York, NY: Harcourt; 2001.

55. Horn S, Gassaway J. Practice-based evidence study design for comparative effectiveness research. *Med Care.* 2007;45(suppl 2): S50–S57.

56. Horn SD, Gassaway J. Practice-based evidence: incorporating clinical heterogeneity and patient-reported outcomes for comparative effectiveness research. *Med Care.* 2010;48(6 suppl 1):S17–S22.

57. Horn SD, Sharkey PD, Kelly HW, Uden DL. Newness of drugs and use of HMO services by asthma patients. *Ann Pharmacother.* 2001;35:990–996.

58. Averill RF, McGuire TE, Manning BE, et al. A study of the relationship between severity of illness and hospital cost in New Jersey hospitals. *Health Serv Res.* 1992;27:587–606. discussion 607–612.

59. Clemmer TP, Spuhler VJ, Oniki TA, Horn SD. Results of a collaborative quality improvement program on outcomes and costs in a tertiary critical care unit. *Crit Care Med.* 1999;27:1768–1774.

60. Horn SD, Torres Jr. A, Willson D, Dean JM, Gassaway J, Smout R. Development of a pediatric age- and disease-specific severity measure. *J Pediatr.* 2002;141:496–503.

61. Willson DF, Horn SD, Smout R, Gassaway J, Torres A. Severity assessment in children hospitalized with bronchiolitis using the pediatric component of the Comprehensive Severity Index. *Pediatr Crit Care Med.* 2000;1:127–132.

62. Ryser DK, Egger MJ, Horn SD, Handrahan D, Gandhi P, Bigler ED. Measuring medical complexity during inpatient rehabilitation after traumatic brain injury. *Arch Phys Med Rehabil.* 2005;86:1108–1117.

63. Horn SD, Sharkey PD, Buckle JM, Backofen JE, Averill RF, Horn RA. The relationship between severity of illness and hospital length of stay and mortality. *Med Care.* 1991;29:305–317.

64. Gassaway JV, Horn SD, DeJong G, Smout RJ, Clark C. Applying the clinical practice improvement approach to stroke rehabilitation: methods used and baseline results. *Arch Phys Med Rehabil.* 2005;86(12 suppl 2):S16–S33.

65. Carter MJ, Fife CE, Walker D, Thomson B. Estimating the applicability of wound care randomized controlled trials to general wound-care populations by estimating the percentage of individuals excluded from a typical wound-care population in such trials. *Adv Skin Wound Care.* 2009;22(7): 316–324.

66. Rosenbaum PR. *Observational Studies.* New York, NY: Springer; 2002.

67. Horn SD, DeJong G, et al. Practice-based evidence research in rehabilitation: an alternative to randomized controlled trials and traditional observational studies. *Arch Phys Med Rehabil.* 2012;93(suppl 8):S127–S137.

68. Deutscher D, Horn SD, Dickstein R, et al. Associations between treatment processes, patient characteristics, and outcomes in outpatient physical therapy practice. *Arch Phys Med Rehabil.* 2009;90(8):1349–1363.

69. Deutscher D, Hart DL, Dickstein R, Horn SD, Gutvirtz M. Implementing an integrated electronic outcomes and electronic health record process to create a foundation for clinical practice improvement. *Phys Ther.* 2008;88(2):270–285.

70. Spyns P. Natural language processing: an overview. *Methods Inf Med.* 1996;35(4):285–301.

71. Mennemeyer ST, Menachemi N, Rahurkar S, Ford EW. Impact of the HITECH act on physicians' adoption of electronic health records. *J Am Med Inform Assoc.* 2016;23(2):375–379. http://dx.doi.org/10.1093/jamia/ocv103 [Epub 2015 Jul 30].

72. Amin W, Tsui FR, Borromeo C, et al. PaTH: towards a learning health system in the Mid-Atlantic region. *J Am Med Inform Assoc.* 2014;21(4):633–636.

73. Stevens KR, Staley JM. The Quality Chasm reports, evidence-based practice, and nursing's response to improve healthcare. *Nurs Outlook.* 2006;54(2):94–101.

74. Green LW. Making research relevant: If it is an evidence-based practice, where's the practice-based evidence? *Fam Pract.* 2008;25(suppl 1):i20–i24.

DISCUSSION QUESTIONS

1. Review the three categories of EBP models and discuss how these models might be used to guide the development of EBP.
2. Discuss why computerization is required if EBP is to become reality in clinical settings.
3. How can the design of a healthcare information system support or thwart the use of EBP guidelines at the point of care? Give examples from your own experience if possible.
4. Explore the AHRQ Health Care Innovations Exchange at www.innovations.ahrq.gov/index.aspx. Discuss how automation and informatics-based tools could be used to bring resources from this site to the point of care.
5. Analyze the following statement and determine whether you do or do not support it: "With the development of a fully integrated national health information system, big data reflecting patient outcomes will replace the role of research studies in developing EBP guidelines."
6. Why is the informatician a critical member of the PBE team? What essential skills should this team member have?
7. You are a member of a PBE team that will study the prevention and management of ventilator-associated pneumonia. Describe how you would apply the steps of PBE to this problem.

EBP CASE STUDY

You are consulting with the education and practice development team in a large tertiary care hospital serving a region comprising mostly rural communities. The team is responsible for strengthening the implementation of EBP based on outcomes. Over the next 2 years, it must set performance objectives to (1) strengthen screening for pain, depression, and adverse health behaviors (smoking, excess alcohol intake, and body mass index [BMI] greater than 30) at intake for all adult admissions; (2) implement comprehensive geriatric assessment for all those over age 65 hospitalized for more than 7 days or readmitted within less than 3 days following discharge; and (3) promote care-team performance. The hospital has 200 adult admissions each week and has implemented an electronic health record. Guideline dissemination generally occurs through educational venues or via the electronic policy and procedure manual. The method of documentation for narrative notes is documentation by exception using subjective, objective, assessment, and plan (SOAP) and the hospital has made extensive use of checklists to complement the documentation system.

Discussion Questions
1. Using clinical guidelines and standards of care, identify what data elements should be included in the EHR assessment and evaluation screens if these goals are to be achieved.
2. Identify how information system defaults and alerts could be used to achieve these goals.
3. Once screening has been improved, what are the next steps in improving patient outcomes?
4. How could the electronic health record be designed to support these outcome-related goals?

PBE CASE STUDY

Pressure Ulcer Case Study*
A PBE study involving 95 long-term care facilities in the United States determined that nursing interventions for pressure ulcer (PrU) prevention and management were highly variable among facilities and that nearly 30% of patients at risk for developing a PrU developed an ulcer during the 12-week study. Characteristics and interventions associated with higher and lower likelihood of PrU development are summarized in the following table.

Research findings were used to develop PrU prevention protocols that included standardized documentation of important data elements and CDS tools. Four long-term care facilities that participated in the study and shared a common EHR (all members of the same provider network) took the first step in changing practice by sharing study findings with clinical staff, who spend the most one-on-one treatment time with nursing home residents and thus are often the first members of the care team to observe changes in residents' nutritional intake, urinary incontinence, and mood state. Concurrently, local study leaders worked with their software vendor to incorporate standard documentation for nurses and the CDS tools for staff.

Negative Association With Likelihood of Developing a Pressure Ulcer (Less Likely)

Patient Factors
Patient new to long-term care
Treatment Factors
Use of disposable briefs for urinary incontinence for > 14 days
Nutrition
Use of oral medical nutritional supplements for >21 days
Tube feeding for >21 days
IV fluid supplementation
Medications
Antidepressant medication
Facility Staffing Patterns
RN hours ≥0.5 h/resident/day
CNA hours ≥2.25 h/resident/day
LPN turnover rate <25%

Positive Association With Likelihood of Developing a Pressure Ulcer (More Likely)

Patient Factors
Higher admission severity of illness
History of PrU in previous 90 days
Significant weight loss
Oral eating problems
Treatment Factors
Use of urinary catheter
Use of positioning devices

Discussion Questions
1. What are the steps of the PBE process related to this case study?
2. As the health professional or informatics specialist working with the clinical team in the four long-term care facilities, identify the following:
   a. Elements to incorporate into the documentation that address factors identified in the original study.
   b. CDS tools that could be incorporated into computer systems.
3. How can the cost effectiveness of the new documentation requirements and standards of care be efficiently evaluated?

This case study is fictional; factors are consistent with findings reported in Sharkey S, Hudak S, Horn SD, Spector W. Leveraging certified nursing assistant documentation and knowledge to improve clinical decision making: the on-time quality improvement program to prevent pressure ulcers. Adv Skin Wound Care. 2011;24(4):182-188.

CNA, Clinical nursing assistant; CDS, clinical decision support; IV, Intravenous; LPN, licensed practical nurse; PBE, practice-based evidence; PrU, pressure ulcer; RN, registered nurse.

4

Models, Theories, and Research for Program Evaluation

Charlene R. Weir

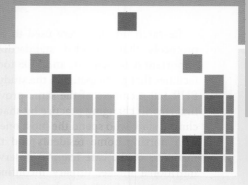

Evaluation of health information technology (health IT) programs and projects can range from simple user satisfaction for a new menu or full-scale analysis of usage, cost, compliance, patient outcomes, and observation of usage to data about patient's rate of improvement.

OBJECTIVES

At the completion of this chapter, the reader will be prepared to:

1. Identify the main components of program evaluation.
2. Discuss the differences between formative and summative evaluation.
3. Apply the three levels of theory relevant to program evaluation.
4. Discriminate program evaluation from program planning and research.
5. Synthesize the core components of program evaluation with the unique characteristics of informatics interventions.

KEY TERMS

ABSTRACT ❖

Evaluation is an essential component in the life cycle of all health information technology (health IT) applications and a key to successful translation of these applications into clinical settings. In planning an evaluation, the central questions must be asked regarding purpose, scope, and focus of the system. This chapter focuses on the larger principles of program evaluation with the goal of informing health IT evaluations in clinical settings. The reader is expected to gain sufficient background in health IT evaluation to lead or participate in program evaluation for applications or systems.

Formative evaluation and summative evaluation are discussed. Three levels of theory are presented, including scientific theory, implementation models, and program theory (logic models). Specific scientific theories include social cognitive theories, diffusion of innovation, cognitive engineering theories, and information theory. Six implementation models are reviewed: Predisposing, Reinforcing, and Enabling Constructs in Educational Diagnosis and Evaluation-Policy, Regulatory, and Organizational Constructs in Educational and Environmental Development (PRECEDE-PROCEED); Promoting Action on Research Implementation in Health Services (PARiHS); Reach Effectiveness Adoption Implementation Maintenance (RE-AIM); Consolidated Framework for Implementation Research (CFIR); Sociotechnical Model; and quality improvement. Program theory models are discussed with an emphasis on logic models.

A review of methods and tools is presented. Relevant research designs are discussed for health IT evaluations, including time series, multiple baseline, and regression discontinuity. Methods of data collection specific to health IT evaluations, including ethnographic observation, interviews, and surveys, are then reviewed.

INTRODUCTION

The outcome of program or project **evaluation** is information that is both useful at the program level and generalizable enough to contribute to the building of science. In the applied sciences, such as informatics, evaluation is critical to the growth of both the specialty and the science. In this chapter **program evaluation** is defined as the "systematic collection of information about the activities, characteristics, and results of programs to make judgments about the program, improve or further develop program effectiveness, inform decisions about future programming, and/or increase understanding."[1] Health information technology (health IT) interventions are nearly always embedded in the larger processes of care delivery and are unique for three reasons. First, stakeholders' knowledge about the capabilities of health IT systems may be limited at the beginning of a project. Second, the health IT product often changes substantially during the implementation process. Third, true implementation often takes 6 months or longer, with users maturing in knowledge, skills, and external influences, such as new regulations or organizational initiatives, occurring over that period. Identification of the unique contribution of the health IT application, therefore, is often difficult and evaluation goals frequently go beyond the health IT component alone. In this chapter the health IT component of evaluation is integrated with overall program evaluation; unique issues are highlighted for evaluating health IT itself.[2] The chapter is organized into three sections: (1) purposes of evaluation, (2) theories and frameworks, and (3) methods, tools, and techniques.

PURPOSES OF EVALUATION

The purpose of evaluation determines the methods, approaches, tools, and dissemination practices for the entire project being evaluated. Therefore identifying the purpose is a crucial first step. Mark, Henry, and Julnes provided four main evaluation purposes as listed in Box **4.1**.

Usually an evaluation project is not restricted to just one of these purposes. Teasing out which purposes are more important is a process for the evaluator and the involved stakeholders. The following sections represent a series of questions that can clarify the process.

Formative Versus Summative Evaluation

Will the results of the evaluation be used to determine whether the goals of the program have been met? This question refers to a common classification of evaluation activities that fall into two types: (1) formative evaluation and (2) summative evaluation. The difference is in how the information is used. The results of the formative evaluation are used as feedback to the program for continuous improvement.[3,4] The results of the summative evaluation are used to evaluate the merit of the program. Formative evaluation is a term coined by Scriven in 1967 and expanded on by a number of other authors to mean an assessment of how well the program is being implemented and to describe the early experiences of participants.[5] Topics for formative evaluation include the fidelity of the intervention, the quality of implementation, the characteristics of the organizational context, the resources involved, the usability of a particular design, and the types of

personnel. Needs assessments and feasibility analyses are also included in this general category. Box **4.2** outlines several questions that fall into the category of formative evaluation for health IT.

In contrast, summative evaluation refers to an assessment of the outcomes and impact of the program. Effectiveness, direct outcomes, and adverse events analyses are the types of measures included in this category. Some questions that fall into the summative evaluation category are listed in Box **4.3**.

Dividing the evaluation process into the formative and summative components is somewhat arbitrary because they can be, and often are, conducted concurrently. They do not necessarily differ in terms of methods or even in terms of the content of the information collected. Formative evaluation is especially important for health IT products where the overall goal is improvement. Because health IT products are "disruptive technologies," they both transform the working environment and are themselves transformed during the process of implementation.[6] Many writers in the informatics field have noted the paucity of information on implementation processes in published studies. In a meta-analysis of health IT by researchers at RAND, the authors noted:

> In summary, we identified no study or collection of studies, outside of those from a handful of health IT leaders that would allow a reader to make a determination about the generalizable knowledge of the system's reported benefit. This limitation in generalizable knowledge is not simply a matter of study design and internal validity. Even if further randomized, controlled trials are performed, the generalizability of the evidence would remain low unless additional systematic, comprehensive, and relevant descriptions and measurements are made regarding how the technology is utilized, the individuals using it, and the environment it is used in.[7, p. 4]

Although written in 2006, this statement is still relevant today.

BOX 4.1 Main Purposes of Program Evaluation

- Program and organizational improvement
- Assessment of merit or worth
- Knowledge development
- Oversight and compliance

Adapted from Mark M, Henry G, Julnes G. *Evaluation: An Integrative Framework for Understanding, Guiding and Improving Policies and Programs.* San Francisco, CA: Jossey-Bass; 2000.

BOX 4.2 Questions to Pose During Formative Evaluation

- What is the nature and scope of the problem that is being addressed by health information technology?
- What is the extent and seriousness of the need?
- How well is the technology working, and what is the best way to deliver it?
- How are participants (and users) experiencing the program?
- How did the intervention change after implementation?

BOX 4.3 Questions to Pose During Summative Evaluation

- To what degree were the outcomes affected by the product?
- What is the cost effectiveness of the product?
- What were the unintended consequences of the product?

Generalizability and Scope

Will the results of the evaluation be used to inform stakeholders of whether a particular program is "working?" This question refers to issues of the generalizability and scope of the project. It is also a question of whether the evaluation is more of a program evaluation or a research study as the criteria regarding "working" varies by this approach. An evaluation of a locally developed project usually would be considered a program evaluation. In contrast, if the program was designed to test a hypothesis or research question and described, measured, or manipulated variables that could be generalized to a larger population, then the results of the evaluation study are more like research. However, both approaches use systematic tools and methods. For example, if the program to be evaluated is a local implementation of alerts and decision support for providers at the point of care to evaluate skin breakdown, then the stakeholders are the administrators, nurses, and patients who are affected by use of the decision support program. The evaluation questions would address the use of the program, the impact on resources, satisfaction, and perhaps clinical outcomes. The evaluation would likely use a before-and-after design and a more informal approach to assess whether the decision support "worked." However, if the evaluation question is whether or not computerized guidelines affect behavior in general and under what conditions, then the specific stakeholders matter less and the ability to generalize beyond the contextual situation matters more. A more formal, research-based approach is then used. This question is really about what is to be learned. Vygotsky called these two approaches "patterning" versus "puzzling."[8] In the patterning approach, the comparison is between what went before at the local level and in the new program, whereas in the puzzling approach, the task is to understand why the two options work and to puzzle through the differences.

Another way to address this issue is to imagine that evaluation activities fall along a continuum from "program evaluation" to "evaluation research." Program evaluation tends to have a wide scope, using multiple methods with a diverse range of outcomes. Evaluation research tends to be more targeted, using more selected methods and fewer outcomes. On the program-evaluation end of the continuum, evaluation can encompass a range of activities including but not limited to needs assessment, program model development, tracking and performance monitoring, and continuous quality improvement. On the research end of the continuum, activities include theory testing, statistical evaluation of models, and hypothesis testing. However, at both ends of the continuum and in between, evaluators can use a variety of research designs, rigorous measurement methods, and statistical analyses.

Program Continuance Versus Growth

Will the results of the evaluation be used to make a decision about continuing the program as is or about expanding it to a larger or different setting if it has generalizable knowledge? Answering the question of whether a program will be continued requires a focus on the concerns and goals of stakeholders, as well as special attention to the contextual issues of cost, burden, user satisfaction, adoption, and effectiveness.

Answering this question also requires an assessment about the manner in which the program was implemented and its feasibility in terms of resources and efforts. Does the program require ongoing and intense training of staff and technicians? Does it require unique hardware requirements that are a one-time or ongoing cost? Does the program have "legs" (i.e., can it exist on its own once implemented)? Are the benefits accrued available immediately or is it a long-term process?

One specific example to determine whether the program should be continued is to assess whether or not it contributes to the institution being a "learning organization."[9,10] This approach focuses on performance improvement and the following four areas of concern (modified for health IT):

1. What are the mental models and implicit theories held by the different stakeholders about the health IT product?
2. How does the health IT product promote mastery or personal control over the work environment?
3. What is the system-level impact of the health IT product? How does the intervention support a system thinking approach?
4. How does the health IT product create a unified vision of the information environment?

Addressing these questions requires understanding of how individuals view the future computerized environment and whether or not they have come to a shared system-level vision.

THEORIES AND FRAMEWORKS

The use of theory in evaluation studies is controversial among evaluators, as well as in the informatics community. On the one hand, some authors note that evaluation studies are local, limited in scope, and not intended to be generalizable. On the other hand, other authors argue that theory is necessary to frame the issues adequately, promote generalizable knowledge, and clarify measurement. This author argues that theory should be used for the latter reason. Theoretical perspectives clarify the constructs and methods of measuring constructs and bring forward an understanding of the mechanisms of action.

For the purposes of this chapter, theoretical perspectives will be divided into three levels of complexity. At the most complex level are the *social science, cognitive engineering,* and *information science theories.* These theories are well established, have a strong evidence base, use validated measures, and have well-understood mechanisms of action. This chapter discusses some well-known social science theories, as well as two health IT–specific adaptations of these theories that have had significant validation. At the next level are the *program implementation models,* which are less complex and consist of a conceptual model. The models are often used to describe processes, but few studies attempt to validate the models or test models against each other. Finally, at the most basic level are the *program theory models,* which are program specific and intended to represent the goals and content of a specific project. *All* evaluations for health IT products should develop a program theory model to guide the evaluation process itself. The descriptions below are brief and are intended to provide an overview of the possibilities at each level.

Social Science Theories

There are myriad theories relevant to both the design of interventions and products and the structure of an evaluation. A short description is provided here for the purpose of context. These social science theories include social cognitive theories, diffusion of innovation theory, cognitive engineering theories, and information theories.

Social Cognitive Theories

The social cognitive theories include the theory of planned behavior[11]; its close relative, the theory of reasoned action[12]; and social cognitive theory.[13] These theories predict intentions and behavior as functions of beliefs about the value of an outcome, the likelihood that the outcome will occur given the behavior, and the expectations of others and self-efficacy beliefs about the personal ability to engage in the activity. The empirical validation of these theories is substantial, and they have been used to predict intentions and behavior across a wide variety of settings.

Diffusion of Innovations Theory

Another very commonly used model in informatics is diffusion of innovations theory by Rogers.[14,15] In this model, characteristics of the innovation, the type of communication channels, the duration, and the social system are predictors of the rate of diffusion. The central premise is that diffusion is the process by which an innovation is communicated through certain channels over time among the members of a social system organization. Individuals pass through five stages: knowledge, persuasion, decision, implementation, and confirmation. Social norms, roles, and the type of communication channels all affect the rate of adoption of an innovation. Characteristics of an innovation that affect the rate of adoption include relative advantage as compared with other options; trialability, or the ease with which it can be tested; compatibility with other work areas; complexity of the innovation; and observability, or the ease with which the innovation is visible.

Cognitive Engineering Theories

The cognitive engineering theories are also widely used in informatics, particularly naturalistic decision making (NDM),[16-18] control theory,[19] and situation awareness (SA).[20] These theories focus more on the interaction between the context and the individual and are more likely to predict decision making, perception, and other cognitive variables. NDM is a broad and inclusive paradigm. SA is narrower and is particularly useful in supporting health IT design.

SA combines the cognitive processes of orientation, attention, categorization or sense making, and planning into three levels of performance. These activities are thought to be critical to human performance in complex environments. Endsley refers to a three-level system of awareness: (1) perception, (2) comprehension, and (3) projection. She defines shared SA as the group understanding of the situation.[20] For example, in one study of health IT, higher SA was significantly associated with integrated displays for intensive care unit (ICU) nursing

TABLE 4.1 Levels of Situational Awareness

Level	Description
Perception of the elements in the environment	What is present, active, salient, and important in the environment? Attention will be driven by task needs.
Comprehension of the current situation	Classification of the event is a function of activation of long-term memory. The cognitive processes of classification and task identification drive meaning.
Projection of future status	Expectations of outcomes in the future, are driven by implicit theories and knowledge about the causal mechanisms underlying events.

staff.[21,22] Table **4.1** presents the core components of SA and associated definitions.

Information Theory

One of the most influential theories is Information Theory, published in 1948 by Claude Shannon.[23] Shannon focused on the mathematical aspects of the theory. Weaver, an oncologist, focused on the semantic meaning of the theory.[24] Information theory identifies the degree of uncertainty in messages as a function of the capacity of the system to transmit those messages given a certain amount of noise and entropy. The transmission of information is broken down into *source, sender, channel, receiver,* and *destination*. Because information theory is essentially a theory of communication, information is defined relative to three levels of analysis:

1. At the *technical* or statistical level, information is defined as a measure of entropy or uncertainty in the situation. The question at this level is: How accurately are the symbols used in the communication being transmitted?
2. At the *semantic* level, information is defined as a reduction of uncertainty at the level of human meaning. The question here is: How well do the symbols that were transmitted convey the correct meaning?
3. At the *effectiveness* level, information is defined as a change in the goal state of the system. The question here is: How well does the perceived meaning effect the desired outcome?[25]

This simple framework can provide an effective evaluation model for any system that evaluates the flow of information. For example, Weir and McCarthy used information theory to develop implementation indicators for a computerized provider order entry (CPOE) intervention.[26]

Information Foraging Theory

Information foraging theory is a relatively new theory of information searching that is very useful for analyzing web searching.[27] Information foraging theory is built on foraging theory, which studies how animals search for food. Pirolli and Card noticed similar patterns in the processes used by animals

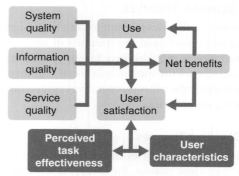

FIG 4.1 A model of information system success. (Adapted from *J Manag Inf Syst.* 1993;19(4):9-30. Copyright © 1993 by M.E. Sharpe, Inc. Reprinted with permission. All Rights Reserved.)

to search for food and the processes used by humans to search for information on the internet. The basic assumption is that all information searches are goal directed and constitute a calibration between the energy cost of searching and the estimated value of information retrieved. The four concepts listed in Box **4.4** are important to measure. Empirical work on foraging theory has validated its core concepts.[28]

Information Technology Theories

Two well-developed information technology theories are specifically used in the IT domain. As is true of many IT theories, they are compiled from several existing theories derived the basic sciences to improve their fit in an applied setting.

Information System Success

Information System Success is an IT model that integrates several formal theories is DeLone and McLean's multifactorial model of IT success developed with the goal of improving scientific generalization.[29] Their theory was originally developed in 1992 and revised in 2003 based on significant empirical support. The model is based on Shannon and Weaver's communication theory[24] and Mason's information "influence" theory.[30] DeLone and McLean used Shannon and Weaver's three levels of information: (1) technical (accuracy and efficiency of the communication system), (2) semantic (communicating meaning), and (3) effectiveness (effect on the receiver). These three levels correspond to DeLone and McLean's constructs of (1) "system quality," (2) "information quality," and (3) effects listed as use, user satisfaction, and net benefits or outcomes. DeLone and McLean revised the model in 2003 to include recent literature and added a fourth level—"service quality"—referring to the degree to which users are supported by IT staff. Fig. **4.1** depicts an adaptation of the updated 2003 model that adds user satisfaction, user characteristics, and task effectiveness to the original model.

Unified Theory of Acceptance and Use of Technology

Unified theory of acceptance and use of technology (UTAUT) is an adaptation of the social cognitive theories within the field of informatics.[31] UTAUT is depicted in Fig. **4.2**, and explains users' intentions to use an information system as a function of performance expectancy or self-efficacy beliefs, effort expectancies, social influence, and facilitating conditions. Significant moderators of these variables of intentions are gender, age, and the degree to which usage is mandated.

This model integrates social cognitive theory,[13] theory of reasoned action,[12] and diffusion of innovations theory.[14]

Venkatesh and Davis conducted a systematic measurement meta-analysis that tested eight major models of adoption to clarify and integrate the adoption literature.[32] All of the evaluated models were based to some degree on the social cognitive models described above but adapted to the question of IT adoption and use. Empirical studies showed that UTAUT explained around 70% of the variance in intention to use, significantly greater than any of the initial models alone did. Two key findings of this work are important. First, Venkatesh et al. found that the variables associated with initial intentions to use are different from the variables associated with later intentions.[31,33,34] Specifically, the perceived work effectiveness constructs (perceived usefulness, extrinsic motivation, job fit, relative advantage, and outcome expectations) were found to be highly predictive of intentions over time. In contrast, variables such as attitudes, perceived behavioral control, ease of use, self-efficacy, and anxiety were predictors only of early intentions to use.

Second, the authors found that the variables predictive of intentions to use are not the same as the variables predictive of usage behavior itself.[31] They found that the "effort factor scale" (resources, knowledge, compatible systems, and support) was the only construct other than intention to significantly predict usage behavior. Finally, these authors found that the model differed significantly depending on whether usage was mandated or by choice. In settings where usage was mandated, social norms had a stronger relationship to intentions to use than the other variables.

Program Implementation Models

Program implementation models refer to generalized, large-scale implementation theories that are focused on performance improvement and institution-wide change. Six models are reviewed here: Predisposing, Reinforcing, and Enabling Constructs in Educational Diagnosis and Evaluation-Policy, Regulatory, and Organizational Constructs in Educational and Environmental Development (PRECEDE-PROCEED), Promoting Action on Research Implementation in Health Services (PARiHS), Reach Effectiveness Adoption Implementation

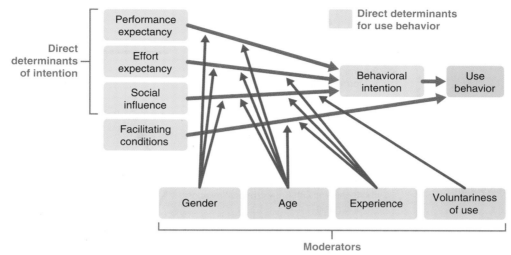

FIG 4.2 An example of unified theory of acceptance and use of technology. (From Venkatesh V, Morris M, Davis G, Davis F. User acceptance of information technology: toward a unified view. *MIS Quart.* 2003;27(3):425-478.)

Maintenance (RE-AIM), Consolidated Framework for Implementation Research (CFIR), Sociotechnical Model, and Quality Improvement.

PRECEDE-PROCEED Model

The letters in the PRECEDE-PROCEED model represent the following terms: PRECEDE Predisposing, Reinforcing, and Enabling Constructs in Educational Diagnosis and Evaluation; PROCEED Policy, Regulatory, and Organizational Constructs in Educational and Environmental Development. This model was originally developed to guide the design of system-level educational interventions, as well as for evaluating program outcomes. It is a model that addresses change at several levels, ranging from the individual to the organization level. According to the model the interaction between the three types of variables produces change:

- *Predisposing factors* that lay the foundation for success (e.g., electronic health records or strong leadership)
- *Reinforcing factors* that follow and strengthen behavior (e.g., incentives and feedback)
- *Enabling factors* that activate and support the change process (e.g., support, training, computerized reminders, and templates or exciting content)

The model has been applied in a variety of settings, ranging from public health interventions, education, and geriatric quality-improvement and alerting studies.[35] Fig. **4.3** illustrates the model applied to a health IT product.

Promoting Action on Research Implementation in Health Services

The PARiHS framework outlines three general areas associated with implementation (Fig. **4.4**):

1. *Evidence:* Establishing the efficiency and effectiveness of the intervention through expert contribution, literature reviews, surveys, usability testing, and cognitive task analyses.

2. *Context:* Enhancing leadership support and integrating with the culture through focus groups and interviews.

3. *Facilitation of the implementation process:* Skill level and role of facilitator in promoting action, as well as frequency of supportive interactions.[36]

These three elements are defined across several subelements, with higher ratings suggestive of more successful implementation. For instance, a high level of evidence may include the presence of randomized controlled trials (i.e., the gold standard in research), high levels of consensus among clinicians, and collaborative relationships between patients and providers. Context is evaluated in terms of readiness for implementation, including consideration of the context's culture, leadership style, and measurement practices. High ratings of context may indicate an environment focused on continuing education, effective teamwork, and consistent evaluation and feedback. Finally, the most successful facilitation is characterized by high levels of respect for the implementation setting, a clearly defined agenda and facilitator role, and supportive flexibility.[37] Successful implementation (SI) is thus conceptualized as a function (f) of evidence (E), context (C), and facilitation (F), or $SI = f(E, C, F)$.[38] The PARiHS framework suggests a continuous multidirectional approach to evaluation of implementation. Importantly, evaluation is viewed as a cyclic and interactive process instead of a linear approach. The concept of facilitation has been gaining significant traction.[39]

Reach Effectiveness Adoption Implementation Maintenance

RE-AIM was designed to address the significant barriers associated with implementation of any new intervention, and it is particularly useful for informatics. Most interventions meet with significant resistance, and any useful evaluation should measure the barriers associated with the constructs (Reach, Effectiveness, Adoption, Implementation, and Maintenance).

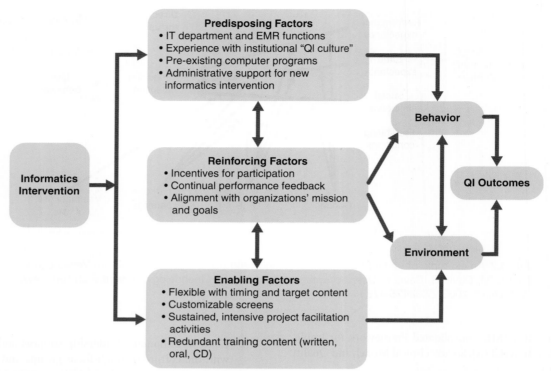

FIG 4.3 An adaptation of the PRECEDE-PROCEED model for a health IT product. (From Green LW, Kreuter MW. *Health Program Planning: An Educational and Ecological Approach.* 4th ed. Mountain View, CA: McGraw-Hill; 2005. Reprinted with permission of McGraw-Hill Companies Inc.)

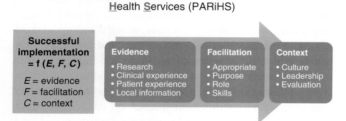

FIG 4.4 The PARiHS model. (From Kitson AL, Rycroft-Malone J, Harvey G, McCormack B, Seers K, Titchen A. Evaluating the successful implementation of evidence into practice using the PARiHS framework: theoretical and practical challenges. *Implement Sci.* 2008;3:1.)

These constructs serve as a good format for evaluation.[40,41] First, did the intervention actually *reach* the intended target population? In other words, how many providers had the opportunity to use the system? Alternatively, how many patients had access to a new website? Second, for *effectiveness*, did the intervention actually do what it was intended to do? Did the wound care decision support actually work as intended every time? Did it identify the patients it was supposed to identify? Or, did the algorithms miss some key variables in real life? Third, for *adoption*, what proportion of the targeted staff, settings, or institutions actually used the program? What was the breadth and depth of usage? Did they use it for all relevant patients or only for some? Fourth, for *implementation*, was the intervention the same across settings and time? With most health IT products there

is constant change to the software, the skill level of users, and the settings in which they are used. These should be documented and addressed in the evaluation. Finally, for *maintenance*, time should be identified a priori to assess maintenance, as well as whether usage continues, and by whom and in what form. For health IT interventions, it is especially useful to look for unintended consequences, as well as workarounds during implementation and maintenance in particular.

Consolidated Framework for Implementation Research

The authors of the CFIR reviewed dozens of implementation theories and consolidated the constructs having evidence of effect on implementation.[42] The consequent model is an overarching consolidated framework, consisting of five major domains: intervention characteristics, outer setting, inner setting, individual characteristics, and implementation processes. About 38 constructs were identified across the five major domains, and they include many of the constructs identified in the preceding theories. Although the model is thought to apply to health services implementations broadly, it is particularly applicable to informatics interventions. Readers may be interested in a step-by-step guide for use of this model, sample studies, and more details about the model which are available at http://cfirguide.org/constructs.html.

Sociotechnical Model for Informatics Interventions

The sociotechnical model described by Sittig and Singh describes eight areas to be addressed in a sociotechnical implementation and evaluation. These include (1) hardware and software, (2) people, (3) clinical content, (4) human-computer interface, (5) workflow and communication, (6) internal organizations features, (7) external rules and regulations, and (8) measurement and monitoring. These categories are a compilation of other models and serve as a general taxonomy to organize an evaluation.[43]

Quality Improvement

Evaluation activities using a quality-improvement framework are often based on Donabedian's classic structure-process-outcome (SPO) model for assessing healthcare quality.[44,45] Donabedian defines *structural measures of quality* as the professional and organizational resources associated with the provision of care, such as IT staff credentials, CPOE systems, or staffing ratios. Process measures include the tasks and decisions imbedded in care, such as the time to provision of antibiotics or the proportion of patients on deep vein thrombosis (DVT) prevention protocols. Finally, *outcomes* are defined as the final or semifinal measurable outcomes of care, such as the number of amputations due to diabetes, the number of patients with DVT, or the number of patients with drug-resistant pneumonia. These three categories of variables are thought to be mutually interdependent and reinforcing. A model for patient safety and quality research design (PSQRD) expands on this well-known, original SPO model.[46] For more details on this model, see Chapter 24.

Program Theory Models

Program theory models are the most basic and practical of the evaluation models. They are the implicit theories of stakeholders and participants of the proposed program. A detailed program theory identifies variables, the timing of measures and observations, and the key expectations that reflect their understandings. Most importantly, a program theory model serves as a shared vision between the evaluator team and the participants, creating a unified conceptual model that guides all evaluation activities.

Six Steps

Program theory evaluation is recommended practice for all program evaluations and an important approach regardless of whether the program is the implementation of a new documentation system or an institution-wide information system. Invariably, various participants will have different ideas about what the program is and why it works.[47] Creation of a program theory model serves to align the various stakeholders into a single view. The Centers for Disease Control and Prevention's six-step program evaluation framework is one of the best examples in current use.[48] It recommends the following six steps:

1. *Engage stakeholders* to ensure that *all* partners have contributed to the goals of the program and the metrics to measure its success.
2. *Describe the program systematically* to identify goals, objectives, activities, resources, and context. This description process involves all stakeholders.
3. *Focus the evaluation design* to assess usefulness, feasibility, ethics, and accuracy.
4. *Gather credible evidence* by collecting data, conducting interviews, and measuring outcomes using a good research design.
5. *Justify conclusions* using comparisons against standards, statistical evidence, or expert review.
6. *Ensure use and share lessons learned* by planning and implementing dissemination activities.

Logic Models

A logic model is a representation of components and mechanisms of the program as noted by the authors of the W.K. Kellogg Foundation's guide to logic models:

> Basically, a logic model is a systematic and visual way to present and share your understanding of the relationship among the resources you have to operate your program, the activities you plan, and the changes or results you hope to achieve. The most basic logic model is a picture of how you believe your program will work. It uses words and/or pictures to describe the sequence of activities thought to bring about change and how these activities are linked to the results the program is expected to achieve. [49,p.1]

The basic structure of a logic model is illustrated in Fig. **4.5**. The logic model starts with a category of "inputs," which include staff, resources, prior success, and stakeholders. In health IT the inputs are the programs, software, the IT staff, hardware, networks, and training. "Outputs" include the activities that are going to be conducted, such as training, implementation, software design, and other computer activities. Participation refers to the individual involved. Outcomes are divided into short, medium, and long outcomes or short-term versus long-term outcomes. The goal is to make sure that the components of the program are easy to see and the mechanisms are made explicit.

The specific methods used to apply a model are not prescribed although creating a logic model is recommended. Use of a wide range of methods and tools is encouraged. Engaging the stakeholders is the first step, and that process could involve needs assessment, functionality requirements analyses, cognitive task analyses, contextual inquiry, and ethnographic observation, to name a few approaches. In all cases, the result is the ability to provide a deep description of the program, the expected mechanisms, and the desired outcomes. Once there is agreement on the characteristics of the program at both the superficial level and the deeper structure, designing the evaluation is straightforward. Agreement among stakeholders is needed not only to identify concepts to measure, but also to determine how to measure them meaningfully.

Leaders and managers should agree on health IT goals and metrics early in the implementation process. Because health IT products are unique, creating a shared vision and a common understanding of the meaning of the evaluation can be challenging. Using an iterative process for implementation

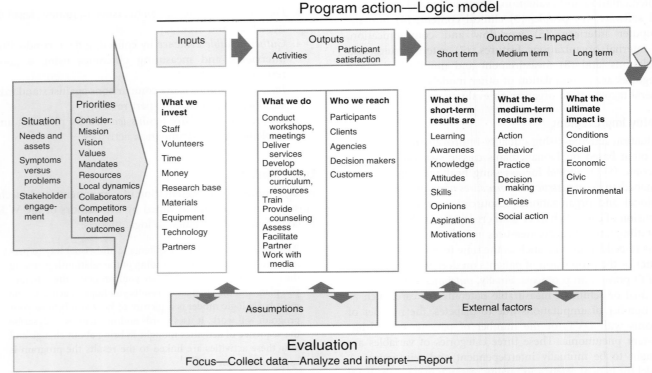

FIG 4.5 Example of a logic model structure. (From University of Wisconsin–Extension, Cooperative Extension, Program Development and Evaluation website. Logic model. <http://www.uwex.edu/ces/pdande/evaluation/evallogicmodel.html>; 2010.)

can mitigate the problem where design and implementation go hand in hand and the stakeholder's vision is addressed repeatedly throughout the process.

METHODS, TOOLS, AND TECHNIQUES

The need for variety in methods is driven by the diversity in population, types of projects, and purposes that are characteristic of research in informatics. Many evaluation projects are classified as either qualitative or quantitative. This division may be somewhat artificial and limited, but using the terms *qualitative* and *quantitative* to organize methods helps to make them relatively easy to understand. A central thesis of this section is that the choice of method should fit the question and multiple methods are commonly used in evaluations.

Quantitative Versus Qualitative Questions

Because evaluation is often a continuous process throughout the life of a project, the systems life cycle is used to organize this discussion. Evaluation activities commonly occur during the planning, analysis, implementation, and maintenance stages of a project (see Chapter 2 for more details about these stages and others in the systems life cycle). At each stage, both quantitative and qualitative questions might be asked. At the beginning of a project, the goal is to identify resources,

feasibility, values, extent of the problem to be solved, and types of needs. The methods used to answer these questions are essentially local and project specific. During the project, evaluation questions focus on the intensity, quality, and depth of the implementation as well as the evolution of the project team and community. Finally, in the maintenance phase of the project, the questions focus on outcomes, cost-benefit value, or overall consequences.

Table **4.2** presents a matrix that outlines the different stages of a project and the types of questions that might be asked during each stage. The questions are illustrations of possible evaluation questions and loosely categorized as either qualitative or quantitative.

Qualitative Methods

Many individuals believe that qualitative methods refer to research procedures that collect subjective human-generated data. However, subjective data can be quantitative, such as the subjective responses to carefully constructed usability questionnaires used as outcome end points. Diagnostic codes are another example of quantitative forms of subjective data. Qualitative methods, rather, refer to procedures and methods that produce narrative or observational descriptive data that are not intended for transformation into numbers. *Narrative data* refers to information in the form of stories, themes, meanings, and metaphors. Collecting this information requires the use of systematic procedures where the purpose

TABLE 4.2   Evaluation Research Questions by Stage of Project and Type of Question

Stage of Project	TYPES OF QUESTIONS	
	Qualitative	Quantitative
Planning	What are the values of the different stakeholders? What are the expectations and goals of participants?	What is the prevalence of the problem being addressed by the health IT product? What are the resources available? What is the relationship between experiencing a factor and having a negative outcome? What are the intensity and depth of use of health IT tools?
Implementation	How are participants experiencing the change? How does the health IT product change the way individuals relate to or communicate with each other?	How many individuals are participating? What changes in performance have been visible? What is the compliance rate? How many resources are being used during implementation (when and where)?
Maintenance	How has the culture of the situation changed? What themes underscore the participants' experience? What metaphors describe the change? What are the participants' personal stories?	Is there a significant change in outcomes for patients? Did compliance rates increase (for addressing the initial problem)? What is the rate of adverse events? Is there a significant change in efficiency? Is there a correlation between usage and outcomes?

Health IT, Health information technology.

is to understand and explore while minimizing bias. There are several very good guides to conducting qualitative research for health IT evaluation studies.[50] The BioMed Central editors now require authors in most informatics journals to self-evaluate their qualitative articles based on the RATS criteria, which also provide good advice for reporting. RATS guidelines are (1) relevance of the study question, (2) appropriateness of qualitative method, (3) transparency of procedures, and (4) soundness of interpretive approach. More detail on these guidelines is available.[51,52]

Structured and Semi-Structured Interviews

In-person interviews can be some of the best sources of information about an individual's unique perspectives, issues, and values. Interviews vary from a very structured set of questions conducted under controlled conditions to a very informal set of questions asked in an open-ended manner. Typically, evaluators audio-record the interviews and conduct thematic or content coding on the results. For example, user interviews that focus on how health IT affects workflow are especially useful. Some interviews have a specific focus, such as in the critical incident method.[53] In this method, an individual recalls a critical incident and describes it in detail for the interviewer. In other cases the interview may focus on the individual's personal perceptions and motivations, such as in motivational interviewing.[54] Finally, cognitive task analysis (CTA) is a group of specialized interviews and observations where the goal is to deconstruct a task or work situation into component parts and functions.[55-57] A CTA usually consists of targeting a task or work process and having the participant walk through or simulate the actions, identifying the goals, strategies, and information needs. These latter methods are useful for user experience studies outlined in Chapter 21.

Observation and Protocol Analysis

An interview may not provide enough information, and, therefore, observing users in action at work is necessary to understand fully the interactions of context, users, and health IT. Observation can take many forms, from using a video camera to a combination of observation and interview where individuals "think aloud" while they work. The think-aloud procedures need to be analyzed both qualitatively for themes and quantitatively for content, timing, and frequency.[58] This method is integral to usability evaluations as outlined in Chapter 21.

Interviews, CTAs, and observation are essential in almost every health IT evaluation of users. Technology interventions are not uniform and cannot simply be inserted into the workflow in a "plug and play" manner. In addition, the current state of the literature in the field lacks clarity about the mechanisms of action or even delineating the key components of health IT. Thus understanding the user's response to the system is essential. For more information about the user experience, see Chapter 21.

Ethnography and Participant Observation

Ethnography and participant observation are derived from the field of anthropology, where the goal is to understand the larger cultural system through observer immersion. The degree of immersion can vary, as can some of the data collection methods, but the overall strategy includes interacting with all aspects of the context. Usually ethnography requires considerable time, multiple observations, interviews, and living and working in the situation if possible. It also includes reading historical documents, exploring artifacts in current use (e.g., memos and minutes), and generally striving to understand a community. These methods are particularly useful in a clinical setting, where understanding the culture is essential.[50,59]

Less intensive ethnographic methods are also possible and reasonable for health IT evaluations. Focused ethnography is a method of observing actions in a particular context. For example, nurses were observed during patient care handoffs and their interactions with electronic health records were recorded. From these observations, design implications for handoff forms were derived.[60,61]

Quantitative Methods
Research Designs

Quantitative designs range from epidemiologic, descriptive studies to randomized controlled trials. Three study designs presented may be particularly useful for health IT and clinical settings. Each of these designs takes advantage of the conditions that are commonly found in health IT projects, including automatically collected data, the ubiquitous use of pre-post design, and outcome-based targets for interventions.

Time Series Analysis

This design is an extension of the simple pre-post format but requires multiple measures in time prior to and after an intervention such as health IT. Evidence of the impact is found in the differences in mathematical slopes between measures during the pretest and posttest periods. This design has significantly more validity than a simple pre-post one-time measure design and can be very feasible in clinical settings where data collection is automatic and can be done for long periods with little increase in costs. For example, top-level administrators might institute a decision support computerized program to improve patient care for pain management. A straightforward design is to measure the rate of compliance to pain management recommendations during several periods about 12 months before and several periods up to 12 months after implementation, controlling for hospital occupancy, patient acuity, and staffing ratios. This design is highly recommended for health IT implementations where data can be captured electronically and reliably over long periods.[62,63]

Regression Discontinuity Design

A regression discontinuity design is similar to a time series analysis, but it is a formal statistical analysis of the pattern of change over time for two groups. This design is particularly suited to community engagement interventions, such as for low vaccination rates in children or seat belt reminders. Participants are divided into two nonoverlapping groups based on their prescores on the outcome of interest. The example used above of compliance with pain management guidelines in an inpatient surgical unit may also be applicable. Providers with greater than 50% compliance to pain guidelines are put in one group and those with less than 50% compliance with pain guidelines are in the other group. Those with the lowest compliance receive a decision support intervention such as a computerized alert and a decision support system to assess and treat pain, whereas the rest do not. Post measures are taken some time after the intervention, and the difference between the predicted scores of the low compliance group and their actual scores as compared to the nonintervention group is noted.

The validity of this design is nearly as high as a randomized controlled trial, but this design is much easier to implement because those who need the intervention receive it. However, this design requires large numbers, which may not be available except in a system-wide or multisite implementation.[64]

Multiple Baseline With Single Subject Design

This design adds significant value to the standard pre-post comparison by staggering implementation systematically (e.g., at 3-month intervals) over many settings but the measurement for *all* settings starts at the same time. In other words, measurement begins at the same time across five clinics, but implementation is staggered every 3 months. Fig. **4.6** illustrates the pattern of responses that might be observed. The strength of the evidence is high if outcomes improved after implementation in each setting and they followed the same pattern.[65] Readers may also find other quasi-experimental research designs useful for health IT research in the comprehensive textbook by Shadish and colleagues.[65]

Instruments

Data are commonly gathered by using instruments. User satisfaction, social network analyses, and cost-effectiveness tools are discussed briefly next.

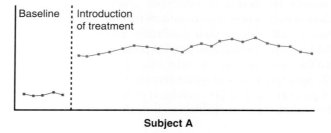

Subject A

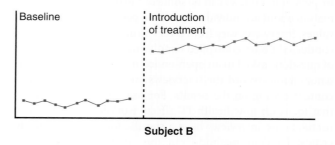

Subject B

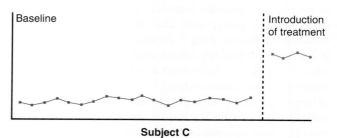

Subject C

FIG 4.6 Example of a multiple baseline study.

User-Satisfaction Instruments

User satisfaction is commonly measured as part of health IT evaluations but is a complex concept. It is thought to be a proxy for adoption; however, it is used as a proxy for system effectiveness. In the first conception, the constructs of interest would be usability and ease of use, as well as whether others use it (usability and social norms). In the second conception, the constructs of interest would refer to how well the system helped to accomplish task goals (usefulness). One of the most common instruments for evaluating user satisfaction is the UTAUT.[32] This well-validated instrument assesses perceived usefulness, social norms and expectations, perceived effort, self-efficacy, ease of use, and intentions to use. Reliability for these six scales ranges from 0.92 to 0.95.

A second measure of user satisfaction focuses on service quality (SERVQUAL) and assesses the degree and quality of IT service. Five scales have been validated: reliability, assurance, tangibles, empathy, and responsiveness. These five scales have been found to have reliability of 0.81 to 0.94.[66]

A third measure is the system usability scale (SUS), which is widely used outside health IT.[67] It is a 10-item questionnaire applicable to any health IT product. Bangor et al. endorsed the SUS above other available instruments because it is technology agnostic (applicable to a variety of products) and easy to administer, and the resulting score is easily interpreted.[68] The authors provide a case study of product iterations and corresponding SUS ratings that demonstrate the sensitivity of the SUS to improvements in usability.

Social Network Analysis

Methods that assess the linkages between people, activities, and locations are likely to be very useful for understanding a community and its structure. Social network analysis (SNA) is a general set of tools that calculates the connections between people based on ratings of similarity, frequency of interaction, or some other metric. The resultant pattern of connection is displayed as a visual network of interacting individuals. Each node is an individual and the lines between nodes reflect the interactions. Although SNA uses numbers to calculate the form of the networked display, it is essentially a qualitative technique because the researcher must interpret the patterns of connections and describe them in narrative form. Conducting an SNA is useful if the goal is to understand how an information system affected communication between individuals. It is also useful to visualize other connections, such as the relationship between search terms or geographical distances.[69] For example, researchers used SNA to examine patient care handoffs from the emergency department to inpatient areas, finding that each handoff entailed 11 to 20 healthcare providers.[70]

Cost-Effectiveness Analysis

Cost-effectiveness analysis (CEA) attempts to quantify the relative costs of two or more options. Simply measuring additional resources, start-up costs, and labor would be a rudimentary cost analysis. A CEA is different from a cost-benefit analysis, which gives specific monetary analysis.

A simple CEA shows a ratio of the cost divided by the change in health outcomes or behavior. For example, a CEA might compare the cost of paying a librarian to answer clinicians' questions as compared with installing Infobuttons per the number of known questions. Most CEA program evaluations will assess resource use, training, increased staff hiring, and other cost-related information. A full economic analysis requiring a consultation with an economist is not necessarily needed. The specific resources used could be delineated in the logic model, unless it was part of hypothesis testing in a more formal survey. The reader is directed to a helpful textbook if further information is needed.[38]

CONCLUSION AND FUTURE DIRECTIONS

Evaluation of health IT programs and projects can range from simple user satisfaction for a new menu to full-scale analysis of usage, cost, compliance, patient outcomes, observation of usage, and data about patients' rate of improvement. Starting with a general theoretical perspective and distilling it to a specific program model is the first step in evaluation. Once overall goals and general constructs have been identified, then decisions about measurement and design can be made. In this chapter, evaluation approaches have been framed, focusing on health IT program evaluation to orient the reader to the resources and opportunities in the evaluation domain. Health IT evaluations are typically multidimensional, longitudinal, and complex. Health IT interventions and programs present a unique challenge, as they are rarely independent of other factors. Rather, they are usually embedded in a larger program. The challenge is to integrate the goals of the entire program while clarifying the effect and importance of the health IT component. In the future, health IT evaluations should become more theory driven and the complex nature of evaluations will be acknowledged more readily.

As health IT becomes integrated at all levels of the information context of an institution, evaluation strategies will necessarily broaden in scope. Outcomes will not only include those related to health IT but also span the whole process. The result will be richer analyses and a deeper understanding of the mechanisms by which health IT has its impact. The incorporation of theory into evaluation will also result in knowledge that is more generalizable and the development of health IT evaluation science. Health practitioners and informaticians will be at the heart of these program evaluations because of their central place in healthcare, IT, and informatics departments.

REFERENCES

1. Patton MQ. *Utilization-Focused Evaluation*. 4th ed. London: SAGE; 2008.
2. Ammenwerth E. Evidence-based health informatics: How do we know what we know? *Methods Inf Med*. 2015;54(4):298–307.
3. Ainsworth L, Viegut D. *Common Formative Assessments*. Thousand Oaks, CA: Corwin Press; 2006.
4. Fetterman D. *Foundations of Empowerment Evaluation*. Thousand Oaks, CA: SAGE; 2001.

5. Scriven M. The methodology of evaluation. In: Stake R, ed. *Curriculum Evaluation.* Chicago: Rand McNally; 1967. American Educational Research Association, Monograph Series on Evaluation; vol 1.

6. Christensen C. *The Innovator's Dilemma.* New York, NY: Harper Business; 2003.

7. Shekelle P. *Costs and Benefits of Health Information Technology.* Santa Monica, CA: Southern California Evidence-Based Practice Center; 2006.

8. Vygotsky L. *Mind and Society.* Cambridge, MA: Harvard University Press; 1978.

9. Preskill H, Torres R. Building capacity for organizational learning through evaluative inquiry. *Evaluation.* 1999;5(1):42–60.

10. Senge P. *The Fifth Discipline: The Art and Practice of the Learning Organization.* New York, NY: Doubleday; 1990.

11. Ajzen I. The theory of planned behavior. *Organ Behav Hum Decis Process.* 1991;50:179–211.

12. Fishbein M, Ajzen I. *Belief, Attitude, Intention, and Behavior: An Introduction to Theory and Research.* Reading, MA: Addison-Wesley; 1975.

13. Bandura A. Human agency in social cognitive theory. *Am Psychol.* 1989;44:1175–1184.

14. Rogers EM. *Diffusion of Innovations.* New York, NY: Free Press; 1983.

15. Cooper RB, Zmud RW. Information technology implementation research: a technological diffusion approach. *Manag Sci.* 1990;36:123–139.

16. Klein G. An overview of natural decision making applications. In: Zsambok CE, Klein G, eds. *Naturalist Decision Making.* Mahwah, NJ: Lawrence Erlbaum Associates; 1997.

17. Kushniruk AW, Patel VL. Cognitive and usability engineering methods for the evaluation of clinical information systems. *J Biomed Inform.* 2004;37(1):56–76.

18. Zsambok C, Klein G. *Naturalistic Decision Making.* Mahwah, NJ: Lawrence Erlbaum; 1997.

19. Åström K, Murray R. *Feedback Systems: An Introduction for Scientists and Engineers.* Princeton, NJ: Princeton University Press; 2008.

20. Endsley M, Garland D. *Situation Awareness Analysis and Measurement.* Mahwah, NJ: Lawrence Erlbaum; 2000.

21. Koch S, Weir C, Haar M, et al. Intensive care unit nurses' information needs and recommendations for integrated displays to improve nurses' situational awareness. *J Am Med Inform Assoc.* 2012;19:583–590. [E-pub 2012 March 21].

22. Koch SH, Weir C, Westenskow D, et al. Evaluation of the effect of information integration in displays for ICU nurses on situation awareness and task completion time: a prospective randomized controlled study. *Int J Med Inform.* 2013;82(8):665–675. http://dx.doi.org/10.1016/j.ijmedinf.2012.10.002.

23. Shannon C. A mathematical theory of communication. *Bell Syst Tech J.* 1948;27:379–423. 623–656.

24. Shannon C, Weaver W. *The Mathematical Theory of Communication.* Urbana, IL: University of Illinois Press; 1949.

25. Krippendorf K. *Information Theory: Structural Models for Qualitative Data.* Thousand Oaks, CA: SAGE; 1986.

26. Weir CR, McCarthy CA. Using implementation safety indicators for CPOE implementation. *Jt Comm J Qual Patient Saf.* 2009;35(1):21–28.

27. Pirolli P, Card S. Information foraging. *Psychol Rev.* 1999;106 (4):643–675.

28. Pirolli P. *Information Foraging Theory: Adaptive Interaction with Information.* Oxford: Oxford University Press; 2007.

29. DeLone W, McLean E. The DeLone and McLean model of information systems success: a ten-year update. *J Manag Inform Syst.* 2003;19(4):9–30.

30. Mason R. Measuring information output: a communication systems approach. *Inf Manag.* 1978;1(5):219–234.

31. Venkatesh V, Morris M, Davis G, Davis F. User acceptance of information technology: toward a unified view. *MIS Quart.* 2003;27(3):425–478.

32. Venkatesh V, Davis F. A theoretical extension of the technology acceptance model: four longitudinal field studies. *Manag Sci.* 2000;46(2):186–204.

33. Agarwal R, Prasad J. A conceptual and operational definition of personal innovativeness in the domain of information technology. *Inform Syst Res.* 1998;9(2):204–215.

34. Karahanna E, Straub D, Chervany N. Information technology adoption across time: a cross-sectional comparison of pre-adoption and post-adoption beliefs. *MIS Quart.* 1999;23 (2):183–213.

35. Green L, Kreuter M. *Health Program Planning: An Educational and Ecological Approach.* 4th ed. Mountain View, CA: Mayfield Publishers; 2005.

36. Stetler CB, Damschroder LJ, Helfrich CD, Hagedorn HJ. A guide for applying a revised version of the PARiHS framework for implementation. *Implement Sci.* 2011;6:99. http://dx.doi.org/10.1186/1748-5908-6-99.

37. Kitson A, Harvey G, McCormack B. Enabling the implementation of evidence based practice: a conceptual framework. *Qual Health Care.* 1998;7(3):149–158.

38. Kitson AL, Rycroft-Malone J, Harvey G, McCormack B, Seers K, Titchen A. Evaluating the successful implementation of evidence into practice using the PARiHS framework: theoretical and practical challenges. *Implement Sci.* 2008;3:1.

39. Stetler CB, Legro M, Rycroft-Malone J, et al. Role of "external facilitation" in implementation of research findings: a qualitative evaluation of facilitation experiences in the Veterans Health Administration. *Implement Sci.* 2006;1:1–23.

40. Gaglio B, Glasgow R. Evaluation approaches for dissemination and implementation research. In: Brownson R, Colditz G, Proctor E, eds. *Dissemination and Implementation Research in Health: Translating Science to Practice.* New York, NY: Oxford University Press; 2012:327–356.

41. Glasgow R, Vogt T, Boles S. Evaluating the public health impact of health promotion interventions: the RE-AIM framework. *Am J Public Health.* 1999;89(9):1922–1927.

42. Damschroder LJ, Aron DC, Keith RE, Kirsh SR, Alexander JA, Lowery JC. Fostering implementation of health services research findings into practice: a consolidated framework for advancing implementation science. *Implement Sci.* 2009 Aug 7;4:50. http://dx.doi.org/10.1186/1748-5908-4-50.

43. Sittig DF, Singh H. A new sociotechnical model for studying health information technology in complex adaptive healthcare systems. *Qual Saf Health Care.* 2010 Oct;19(Suppl 3):i68–i74. http://dx.doi.org/10.1136/qshc.2010.042085.

44. Donabedian A. *Explorations in Quality Assessment and Monitoring: The Definition of Quality and Approaches to Its Assessment*, Vol. 1. Ann Arbor, MI: Health Administration Press; 1980.

45. Donabedian A. The quality of care: how can it be assessed? *JAMA.* 1988;260:1743–1748.

46. Brown C, Hofer T, Johal A, et al. An epistemology of patient safety research: a framework for study design and interpretation. Part 1: conceptualising and developing interventions. *Qual Saf Health Care.* 2008;17(3):158–162.

47. Friedman C. Information technology leadership in academic medical centers: a tale of four cultures. *Acad Med.* 1999;74 (7):795–799.

48. Centers for Disease Control and Prevention. Framework for program evaluation in public health. *MMWR.* 1999;48 (RR11):1–40.

49. Kellogg Foundation WK. *Using Logic Models to Bring Together Planning, Evaluation, and Action: Logic Model Development Guide.* Battle Creek, MI: WK Kellogg Foundation; 2004.

50. Patton M. *Qualitative Research and Evaluation Methods.* 3rd ed. Newberry Park, CA: SAGE; 2001.

51. Clark JP. How to peer review a qualitative manuscript. In: Godlee F, Jefferson T, eds. *Peer Review in Health Sciences.* 2 ed. London: BMJ Books; 2003:219–235.

52. RATS Guidelines. *RATS guidelines at BioMed Central Instructions to Authors*; 2015. http://www.biomedcentral.com/authors/rats.

53. Flanagan JC. The critical incident technique. *Psychol Bull.* 1954;51(4):327–358.

54. Miller WR, Rollnick S. *Motivational Interviewing: Preparing People to Change.* 2nd ed. New York, NY: Guilford Press; 2002.

55. Crandall B, Klein G, Hoffman R. *Working Minds: A Practitioner's Guide to Cognitive Task Analysis.* Cambridge, MA: MIT Press; 2006.

56. Hoffman RR, Militello LG. *Perspectives on Cognitive Task Analysis.* New York, NY: Psychology Press Taylor and Francis Group; 2009.

57. Schraagen J, Chipman S, Shalin V. *Cognitive Task Analysis.* Mahway, NJ: Lawrence Erlbaum Associates; 2000.

58. Ericsson K, Simon H. *Protocol Analysis: Verbal Reports as Data.* Rev. ed. Cambridge, MA: MIT Press; 1993.

59. Kaplan B, Maxwell J. Qualitative research methods for evaluating computer information systems. In: Anderson JG, Aydin CE, Jay SJ, eds. *Evaluating Health Care Information Systems: Approaches and Applications.* Thousand Oaks, CA: SAGE; 1994:45–68.

60. Staggers N, Clark L, Blaz J, Kapsandoy S. Nurses' information management and use of electronic tools during acute care handoffs. *Western J Nurs Res.* 2012;34(2):151–171.

61. Staggers N, Clark L, Blaz J, Kapsandoy S. Why patient summaries in electronic health records do not provide the cognitive support necessary for nurses' handoffs on medical and surgical units: insights from interviews and observations. *Health Inform J.* 2011;17(3):209–223.

62. Harris A, McGregor J, Perencevich E, et al. The use and interpretation of quasi-experimental studies in medical informatics. *J Am Med Inform Assoc.* 2006;13:16–23.

63. Ramsay C, Matowe L, Grill R, Grimshaw J, Thomas R. Interrupted time series designs in health technology assessment: lessons from two systematic reviews of behavior change strategies. *Int J Technol Assess.* 2003;19(4):613–623.

64. Lee H, Monk T. Using regression discontinuity design for program evaluation. In: *American Statistical Association— Proceedings of the Survey Research Methods Section.* ASA; 2008. http://www.amstat.org/sections/srms/Proceedings/.

65. Shadish WR, Cook TD, Campbell DT. *Experimental and Quasi-Experimental Designs for Generalized Causal Inference.* Boston, MA: Houghton Mifflin; 2002.

66. Pitt L, Watso NR, Kavan C. Service quality: a measure of information systems effectiveness. *MIS Quart.* 1995;19(2):173–188.

67. Sauro J. Measuring usability with the system usability scale (SUS). *Measuring Usability LLC*; February 2, 2011. http://www.measuringusability.com/sus.php.

68. Bangor A, Kortum P, Miller JT. An empirical evaluation of the system usability scale. *Int J Hum-Comput Interact.* 2008;24 (6):574–594.

69. Durland M, Fredericks K, eds. *New Directions in Evaluation: Social Network Analysis.* Hoboken, NJ: Jossey-Bass/AEA; 2005.

70. Benham-Hutchins MM, Effken JA. Multi-professional patterns and methods of communication during patient handoffs. *Int J Med Inform.* 2010;79(4):252–267.

DISCUSSION QUESTIONS

1. Of the levels of theory discussed in this chapter, what level would be most appropriate for evaluation of electronic health records? Would the level of theory be different if the intervention was for an application targeting a new scheduling system in a clinic? Why?

2. What is the difference between program evaluation and program-evaluation research?

3. Assume that you are conducting an evaluation of a new decision support system for preventative alerts. What kind of designs would you use in a program evaluation study?

4. Using the life cycle as a framework, explain when and why you would use a formative or summative evaluation approach.

5. What are the basic differences between a research study and a program evaluation?

6. Review the following article: Harris A, McGregor J, Perencevich E, et al. The use and interpretation of quasi-experimental studies in medical informatics. *J Am Med Inform Assoc.* 2006;13:16-23. Explain how you might apply these research designs in structuring a program evaluation.

CASE STUDY

A 410-bed hospital has used a homegrown provider order-entry system for 5 years. Leaders recently decided to put in bar code administration software to scan medications at the time of delivery in order to decrease medical error. The administration is concerned about medication errors, top-level administration is concerned about meeting the Joint Commission accreditation standards, and the IT department is worried that the scanners may not be reliable and may break, increasing their costs. The plan is to have a scanner in each patient's room; nurses will scan the medication when they get to the room and scan their own badges and the patient's armband. The application makes it possible to print out a list of the patients with their scan patterns, and the nurses sometimes carry this printout because patient's armbands can be difficult to locate or nurses do not want to disturb patients while they are sleeping. The bar code software was purchased from a vendor and the facility has spent about a year refining it. The IT department is responsible for implementation and has decided that it will implement each of the four inpatient settings one at a time at 6-month intervals.

The hospital administration wants to conduct an evaluation study. You are assigned to be the lead on the evaluation.

Discussion Questions
1. What is the key evaluation question for this project?
2. Who are the stakeholders?
3. What level of theory is most appropriate?
4. What are specific elements to measure by stakeholder group?

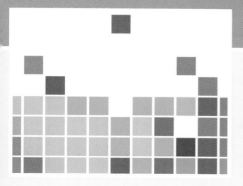

5

Technical Infrastructure to Support Healthcare

Scott P. Narus

A sound understanding of the technical attributes of health IT components, as well as how they interact, is essential for successful system implementations to support the needs of clinician users and the safe, effective care of patients.

OBJECTIVES

At the completion of this chapter, the reader will be prepared to:
1. Describe the key technical components of electronic health records and their interrelationships.
2. Define interoperability and its major elements.
3. Contrast networking arrangements such as regional health information organizations (RHIOs), health information

exchanges (HIEs), and health information organizations (HIOs).
4. Provide information about newer technical models such as cloud computing and application service providers (ASPs).
5. Synthesize current challenges for informatics infrastructure.

KEY TERMS

application service provider (ASP), 83
architecture, 75
clinical data repository (CDR), 76
cloud computing, 84
data dictionary, 79
electronic health record (EHR), 75
health information organization (HIO), 82
infrastructure, 75

interface engine (IE), 81
interoperability, 78
knowledge base, 80
master person index (MPI), 77
regional health information
  organization (RHIO), 82
service-oriented architecture (SOA), 86

ABSTRACT ❖

This chapter introduces the technical aspects supporting electronic health records (EHRs) and related infrastructure components. Complementing the functional components discussed elsewhere, this chapter introduces terms such as *clinical data repository, master person index, interface engine,* and *data dictionary,* as well as other technical components necessary for EHRs to function. Recent material about national efforts related to the infrastructure and electronic data sharing, such as eHealth Exchange and local information exchange networks, is also reviewed.

INTRODUCTION

Understanding the information technology (IT) architecture underlying a healthcare organization's information systems is foundational to understanding how that system actually functions. Decisions about the technical infrastructure have

important consequences for the overall system, in terms of both functional capabilities and support for clinical workflow. Many aspects of a clinical IT infrastructure are unique to the healthcare setting or have different properties or priorities. Understanding the needs of a clinical data repository (CDR) or health data interface network as compared with their counterparts in other industries can mean the difference between successful and failed implementations.

ELECTRONIC HEALTH RECORD COMPONENT MODEL

The electronic health records (EHR) may be thought of as a collection of several key components.[1] Each of these components contributes to overall system functionality. In older EHRs, these components were often bundled, making it difficult if not impossible to separate components from each other. Components of modern technologies are often developed separately but may follow a common architectural design philosophy so that the components can be integrated

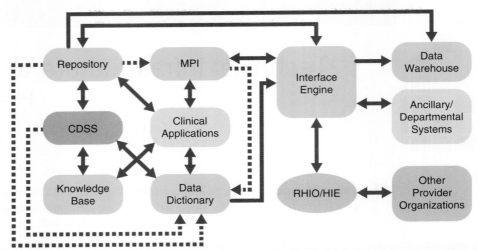

FIG 5.1 The electronic health-record component model. *CDSS,* Clinical decision support system; *HIE,* health information exchange; *MPI,* master person index; *RHIO,* Regional Health Information Organization. Dotted lines denote "foreign key" relationships. For example, the dotted line between the Repository and the MPI denotes that a patient whose data exists in the Repository must first exist in the MPI.

easily. Each component could also be enhanced independent of the others as long as the component integration design was followed. Often the technical responsibility of the informatician is to manage the component design and implementation life cycle, so understanding the component model and integration strategy is essential (Fig. 5.1). The following sections describe common EHR components and important considerations for each component.

Clinical Data Repository

The **clinical data repository (CDR)** is the storage component for all instance data of patient clinical records. By *instance data,* we mean actual pieces of information collected by manual or automated means for a specific patient at a point in time. Data stored in a repository may be lab results, medication orders, vital signs, and clinical documentation. The data may be stored as free text or unstructured documents or as coded and structured elements (e.g., as columnar data in a relational database or as elements of a detailed model within an object-oriented database). Data within the repository are considered the most essential aspect of the EHR: without these data, the other components of the EHR are meaningless. Therefore important aspects of the repository include accessibility, reliability, and security.

Accessibility means the ability to efficiently retrieve data stored within the repository. The repository must provide access methods that allow users of the repository (through, e.g., clinical applications and decision support rules) to find information using criteria that are meaningful to the users. For example, the repository should be able to distinguish data based on patient characteristics such as a patient identifier or encounter number. Data should also be classified by type, such as lab results, medications, and allergies, to permit easy and quick retrieval of a specific category of data. Other important data attributes that help with accessibility include dates (e.g., date recorded and date observed), data owners and entry personnel (e.g., ordering physician, charting nurse, and case manager), and location of service or data entry. The access methods for the repository should be robust enough to support current and future users' access needs.

Repository reliability refers to the dependability and consistency of access to the repository. In a critical healthcare setting, a repository needs to support its users on a 24/7 basis. There is little tolerance for downtime. Inconsistent repository performance—for instance, longer wait times for data retrieval during high usage times of the day—also affects the reliability of the repository. Because of its importance to the functions of all EHR components, the repository reliability is a major factor in determining the perceived reliability of the EHR. Various architectural and procedural models, including redundancy of storage hardware and access routes, system backup policies, and regular performance reviews and maintenance, may be employed to increase the reliability of the repository.

Security is essential to the repository because of both the sensitive nature of the data within and the critical role data play in the healthcare environment. Regulations, such as the Health Insurance Portability and Accountability Act (HIPAA),[2] and sound ethical practices demand that organizations provide a high level of privacy and security for the health information they handle. The repository must incorporate security measures, such as data encryption, secure access paths, user authentication, user and role-based authorization, and physical security of the repository itself, to prevent, to the extent possible, inadvertent and intentionally inappropriate access to data. Some security methods may conflict with accessibility and reliability goals, such as when a measure interferes with needed access to a patient's data.

(Chapter 26 discusses both privacy and security in more detail.) EHR implementers must weigh the benefits and costs of each, but good system design can mitigate conflicts while supporting the needs of the healthcare setting.

Central Versus Distributed Storage

One characteristic that can be used to distinguish repository models is central versus distributed storage. In the central storage model, a single repository is used to store all (or most) clinical data, and it is used as the primary source for reviewing data. There may still be departmental or function-specific clinical information systems, as well as automated data collection devices, that are used to gather data. Some of these systems may even store copies of their information in their own repositories, but these data are also forwarded to the central repository and stored there. In the case of a healthcare enterprise with multiple facilities, potentially consisting of inpatient and outpatient areas, the central model could store information from each of these facilities in one repository. This model improves the ability of a single application to display data from multiple original sources and locations, and it provides the capability to perform clinical decision support (CDS) more efficiently across multiple data types (e.g., combining lab results with medication administration and nutrition data to provide input for medication ordering). Central storage usually requires that data collected from secondary systems be transformed (mapped) to a common storage model and terminology before being stored in the repository. This model does not imply that data cannot be replicated to other locations for safety and disaster recovery purposes.

In the distributed storage model, each data collection application stores its information in its own repository, and data are federated (joined) through a real-time data access methodology. In this case, a results review application may have to access separate repositories for the lab, microbiology, or radiology, for example, to provide a composite view of information. In the previous example of an enterprise with multiple facilities, each facility might store its own data in a facility-based repository. The distributed model provides some reliability to the EHR because, for example, if one repository goes down, the user may still be able to access information from the other repositories. It also allows the most efficient storage and access for particular data types and lessens the complexity of having to map data from one system to another. However, the distributed model produces many single points of failure for each repository, limits performance because of the multiple data access paths that may be required, and makes integrated tasks such as CDS much more difficult.

Encounter-Based Versus Longitudinal-Based Storage

Another characteristic that can be used to distinguish repository models is encounter-based versus longitudinal-based storage. Encounter-based (or episodic) storage was typically used in older, hospital-based EHRs. In this model, data are collected according to the current patient encounter (e.g., clinic visit or hospital admission) and then are usually purged or archived from the repository when the patient is discharged. If the patient has a future encounter with the facility, data may need to be collected completely anew, including patient history, allergies, and previous medications. Encounter-based storage is very efficient in terms of system performance for supporting the current encounter because the data in the repository are always the most current and reflect only what has been collected as relevant to the present circumstances. In this case, the repository's storage space can be quite small. However, because data are purged, some duplication of effort is inherent in this model: data collected during a previous visit may still be relevant and will need to be collected again. There is also a chance that pertinent information from a previous encounter may be lost if a clinician omits collecting it in a subsequent visit.

A longitudinal-based repository, on the contrary, stores data across all encounters. It is often referred to as a "cradle to grave" or "womb to tomb" repository because data may extend over the entire lifespan of an individual. Advantages of the longitudinal-based repository are that clinicians have access to all data collected on a patient from all clinical interventions, and data that do not change and are relevant across all encounters, such as allergies, family medical history, and past procedures, do not need to be reentered at each visit. As with the central (versus distributed) storage model, the longitudinal record may contain data from multiple facilities and health enterprises as well. Access to historical data may be helpful in automated CDS. The disadvantage is that a patient's record (and therefore the entire repository) can grow tremendously large with data that become less relevant over time.

Master Person Index

The master person index (MPI), also known as the master patient index or master member index, is the repository for the information used to uniquely identify each person, patient, or customer of a healthcare enterprise. One or more registration systems may be used at each visit to collect identifying information about the patient, which is then sent to the MPI to match against existing person records and resolve any conflicting information. The MPI stores demographic information about the patient, such as names, addresses, phone numbers, date of birth, and sex. Other organizational identifiers, such as social security number, driver's license number, and insurance identification, also may be stored. Identifiers from within the healthcare enterprise, such as individual facility medical record numbers, are stored as well. (This is often a vestige of paper medical record systems that used facility-specific identifiers for each patient.)

The MPI record is updated as any information added. The MPI then serves as both the master of all information collected, forming what is often referred to as the "golden record" for a person, and the source for distinguishing a patient from all other patients in the system. The latter point is important because it helps to ensure that clinical and administrative data are attributed to the correct patient during healthcare encounters. Each MPI record will have a unique patient identifier or number that is used in the repository to associate a clinical record with the appropriate patient and is used by applications to properly retrieve and store information for the right patient. The MPI will typically support standard access methods for storing and retrieving data (e.g., Health Level Seven [HL7] Admit/Discharge/Transfer messages) so that systems that need to use the MPI can rely on a common interface mechanism. A user-facing patient selection application connected to the MPI is typically provided in the EHR so that EHR users can search for and find a particular patient for use in clinical documentation, review, and patient management applications.

Clinical Applications

Clinical applications provide the user-facing views of the EHR to clinicians. When clinicians think and talk about the EHR, they usually are referring to these applications. Applications are provided in a variety of technologies and user-interface paradigms, including web-based applications, "rich clients" installed on a user's desktop, and mobile apps. A "rich client" (also called a fat, heavy, or thick client) is a client-server architecture or network that provides rich functionality independent of the central server. In contrast, a "thin client" refers to a client-server architecture that is heavily dependent on a server's applications.

When supplied by a single vendor, applications are typically "wrapped" inside a single desktop framework that provides global EHR functions, such as user authentication and patient selection, and then launches the individual applications as part of a clinical workflow. When supplied by different vendors, applications can still share user patient context by using technologies such as Clinical Context Object Workgroup (CCOW), provided the vendor supports such functionality.[3,4] CCOW is an HL7 standard protocol designed to enable different applications to work together in real time at the user interface level. The CCOW standard exists to facilitate interoperability across disparate applications.

Clinical applications can be divided into four broad areas of functionality: review and reporting, data collection, patient management, and clinician productivity. For more information on individual applications in the patient care setting, refer to Chapters 6, 7, and 8.

Review and Reporting

One of the most widely used functions of an EHR is review and reporting of clinical data in the repository. In general, a *review* application is typically focused on one area of clinical data (e.g., a lab results review application or a vital signs review module). On the contrary, a *reporting* application often has a broad range of clinical data that displays to the user (e.g., a 24-hour rounds report that combines lab, vitals, medications, intake and output [*I/O*], invasive line status, assessments, and plan in one view). A reporting application also typically allows much more user customization for

selecting content and layout. A review and reporting application is optimized for display of data and does not necessarily allow direct data entry. However, to improve clinical workflow the application may provide a simple, one-click shortcut to a data collection application to edit or enter new data. A more sophisticated review and reporting application may also provide links from displayed data to more detailed information about that data, such as might be found with an *Infobutton*.[5-9] In more complex graphical user interface environments, the review and reporting application might provide functionality for graphing results, creating timeline associations between data points, and incorporating baseline, average, and goal parameters. The ability of the review and reporting application to support more advanced data display functions will depend significantly on the granularity of data stored in the repository; primarily text-based storage will limit the amount of functionality, whereas highly coded and structured data will allow increased possibilities. The performance and overall display capabilities of the applications are affected by the repository's central versus distributed and encounter-based versus longitudinal-based storage characteristics.

Data Collection

The ability of clinical applications to collect data in the healthcare environment has improved dramatically as new technologies have become available. Older clinical information systems were typically text-based screens that required heavy use of a computer keyboard or 10-key pad for navigation and data entry. More modern graphical user interfaces allow a variety of input and screen navigation possibilities. Some systems may even allow direct collection of information from devices such as blood pressure monitors and weight scales, even by use of wireless (Wi-Fi) connections. Data are usually collected one patient at a time, and stored in the repository. Data may be collected in narrative form as unstructured notes or in a much more granular form as coded and structured data. For example, a vital signs assessment is typically collected in a structured format so that blood pressure, heart rate, and temperature may be used in a variety of reporting and CDS applications. The need for standardized terms and languages are discussed in detail in Chapter 22.

Data collection applications often are linked to review functions so that the clinician can see the status of the patient and then add new or updated information. More advanced clinical workflows such as activity documentation (e.g., medication administration) may involve computerized decision support and computerized documentation flow processes to improve data collection. As with review and reporting applications, links to detailed information about the data to be collected (Infobuttons) may be provided to assist the clinician with evidence-based and regulatory and accreditation requirements for documentation. For example, in a medication administration application, an Infobutton linked to a particular drug might provide information on potential side effects, adverse effects, and therapeutic effects to assess for a particular patient.

Patient Management

Some clinical applications fit within a category that deals with clinician cognitive tasks, particularly around therapeutic and care delivery responsibilities. Ordering and care planning are examples of patient management responsibilities that are increasingly being supported by health information technology (health IT) applications. Each of these responsibilities requires an elevated cognitive load to process the amount of available patient information, as well as the number of potential decisions a clinician can make. Successful EHRs will provide appropriate capabilities within patient management applications to support clinicians' abilities to appropriately adopt these applications and support their cognitive tasks.[10] Quite often patient management applications will provide in-line access to review and reporting applications to improve the ordering and care planning process. The use of standard terminologies from a central data dictionary (discussed below) within these applications ensures that appropriate items are used by clinicians and communicated to other members of the care team. CDS systems and access to knowledge resources (discussed below) may also be employed to enhance decision making.

Clinician Productivity

EHRs often provide clinicians with functionality to assist with care process tasks that cut across many patients and address clinical workflow. Examples include care coordination and physician signature applications, as well as interclinician messaging and notification functions. Point-of-care analytic applications that address quality issues are also becoming popular, particularly because of national health IT initiatives such as Meaningful Use.[11,12] These applications, often called "dash boards," provide information on a clinician's patient population to monitor care and outcomes according to desired goals, and can compare progress over time or against either standard criteria or other similar clinicians. For example, this type of application might report that one physician's patients with a specific diagnosis average an extra day in the hospital but also show a lower average readmission rate compared with other patients with the same diagnosis.

Data Dictionary

A key component of many modern EHRs is a data dictionary that contains the medical vocabulary terms used to store data within the repository. These same terms are used by the EHR applications to collect and display clinical data. (The data dictionary and/or its content may also be referred to as "master reference data" in some systems.) In its simplest form, the data dictionary can be viewed as a list of the health terms and their definitions needed by the EHR, which is usually stored in one or more database tables. The dictionary might contain information such as terms for diagnoses, medications, lab tests, and clinical exam measures. Each of the terms may be assigned a specific code that is independent of how the term is represented to a user. For example, a diagnosis of dyspnea might be assigned a code of 1234. The actual representation for the term *dyspnea* (medical concept) could be "dyspnea" (English medical text representation), "shortness of breath" (English common text name), or "SOB" (English abbreviation of shortness of breath). In this case, all of the representations would have the same definition and dictionary code because they are equivalent. Medical concepts from standard terminologies such as International Classification of Diseases (ICD)-9, ICD-10, or Systematized Nomenclature of Medicine (SNOMED) are also added to the data dictionary so that these terms can be used in applications and in the repository.

The data dictionary is particularly useful in the EHR because it is the central source for defining all terms and their corresponding codes used by the EHR. Instead of hard-coding these terms and codes within applications, the data dictionary allows more flexibility at application runtime to access new and updated terms as they become available over the lifetime of the EHR. For example, as new medications and diagnoses are created, they can be added easily to the data dictionary and made accessible to all applications within the EHR. If instead these terms were hard-coded within an application, the programs would have to be updated and recompiled to make the terms available. In addition, all instances where the terms are used would potentially have to be updated (e.g., if two or more applications were exposing medication information). This leads to a greater maintenance burden for the EHR and can potentially lead to errors if term sources are not kept synchronized.

The data dictionary also provides the ability to create term relations. These relations take the form of hierarchical or associative relations. Hierarchical relations are the most common and can be used to describe domains and subdomains for terms. For example, a domain term for "diagnosis" can be created, and then subdomains of "cardiovascular diagnosis," "respiratory diagnosis," and "endocrine diagnosis" could be defined. Within each of these subdomains, additional subdomains may be defined for more granular categorization, but eventually the domains would list individual diagnosis terms, such as "hypertension" or "pneumonia." The domain relationships are useful in applications and decision support logic when, for example, a user wants to narrow a disease search in a problem list application to just cardiovascular diseases or when a decision support rule broadly defines an inclusion statement such as "IF Ordered_Drug Is_A Cardiovascular_Drug THEN …," where "Ordered_Drug" is an instance of a drug ordered for a patient, "Cardiovascular_Drug" is defined as the domain for all cardiovascular drugs, and "Is_A" is the relationship used by the data dictionary to define hierarchical domain relationships between parent and child terms.

Associative relations can be used to define other useful, nonhierarchical relationships between terms. For example, we could associate the diagnosis term *hypertension* with the drug-domain term *beta blocker*, by creating a relationship called "can be treated by." In this case, because "beta blocker" is a domain, we can assume that all terms within this domain would inherit the "can be treated by" relationship with hypertension. Another example of an associative relationship is a link created between two different coding systems that might describe similar terms. For example, a local laboratory information system (LIS) might contain its own coding for all lab tests it performs. However, the EHR and other external systems might use a standard lab terminology such as Logical Observation Identifiers Names and Codes (LOINC).[13-15] In this case, the dictionary could define a mapping relationship between the terms in each of the systems so that information could be shared between the systems while maintaining the semantic meaning of the terms.

One final note about data dictionaries concerns the desire or need to provide a unique code for each term in the dictionary. The unique code is necessary because the same term representation might be used to describe different concepts. For example, the word *temperature* might be used by a patient to describe having a "high temperature" (chief complaint), whereas a nurse might use this word to chart a physical measurement of "body temperature" (observation). These are different concepts, and the concept codes ensure that they remain distinct. Other reasons to use unique codes are because term representations may change over time or multiple representations for the same term may be allowed depending on the user or display context. In these cases, the code would remain the same. Last, it is usually much faster to search for codes rather than representations within a repository when they follow a strict numeric or alphanumeric syntax. This makes the repository and thus applications more responsive to user access, although the overhead of translating stored codes to user-readable term representations must be considered.

Knowledge Base

A knowledge base (or knowledge repository) is a component within the EHR that stores and organizes a healthcare enterprise's information and knowledge used by the enterprise for clinical operations. This information might range from simple material such as lists of orderable items, available services, or policy documents, to richer content such as order sets and searchable medical subject matter, to highly complex knowledge such as clinical guidelines and decision support rule sets.

Knowledge base content is usually organized by attaching *metadata* (information describing the content) to content items, allowing categorization of the knowledge content based on contextual need. The content itself usually follows a defined *metadata model* (detailed data format description) so that it can be consumed easily by applications. In some cases, the content may be human readable, such as content consisting of medical journal articles that are indexed by subject matter. In other cases, the content may be machine consumable; that is, the content may be read by a computer program and used to automatically produce an output, such as a logic statement that might be executed by a decision support engine to produce a suggestion or alert from a clinical guideline. Often the data dictionary is used to supply coded content and index information within the knowledge base. This ensures that the knowledge base remains synchronized with the patient data repository and clinical applications.

The knowledge base's content (often known as knowledge "artifacts") allows an EHR to become a "content-driven" system as opposed to a system whose knowledge is hard-coded in software programs. When knowledge such as treatment protocols, drug-drug interaction rules, and descriptive content is hard-coded in clinical applications, it is much more difficult and costly to update those applications. By separating the knowledge artifacts from the software and providing access through linkage services, clinical programs can keep pace with the rapidly changing and expanding medical environment, as represented by approaches such as evidence-based practice and precision medicine.

One example of a knowledge-based environment is use of the Infobutton standard: the Infobutton allows clinical applications to link dynamically to contextually relevant content located either within or outside a provider organization.[5] The content provider may update this content as newer information is discovered or produced, but the applications that link to the content through the Infobutton do not need to be changed because the interface (link) remains the same, providing a more robust EHR. Content-driven systems can also use local knowledge about a healthcare enterprise's operations to optimize workflows and enhance clinician interactions with the EHR.

As the content within a knowledge base grows, knowledge management tools become necessary to maintain the information.[16] Authoring tools that allow knowledge content to be created and updated and then facilitate the review process are particularly useful.[17,18] In addition, governance policies and procedures must be instituted to ensure the integrity of and promote and coordinate the use of the knowledge within the repository.

Clinical Decision Support System

A CDS system, discussed in detail in Chapter 10, provides the technical means to combine general medical and health knowledge with specific data about a patient and current clinical context to assist a clinician in making appropriate treatment choices and to alert healthcare providers about relevant information and important events. For example, during the ordering process, a clinician might be alerted about a potential drug-drug interaction that was found by the CDS system when a newly submitted prescription was compared with the patient's current medications. The CDS system also might be used to advise a clinician on the preferred treatment actions for a diabetic patient, based on the institution's best practice guidelines and the patient's current medical state. In addition, a hospital staff member might be alerted about a critically abnormal lab result that could affect medical care.

The CDS system typically consists of (1) an inference engine that runs rules or logic (programs), (2) methods for receiving or pulling data from clinical sources, and (3) a communication system for notifying users or other systems about decision support results. The CDS system may be tied to a knowledge base to receive its rules, in which case the rules can be updated as needed without having to change or recompile CDS code. The CDS system also may contain hard-coded rules that must be changed by recompiling code, or the logic may be based on machine-learning algorithms that dynamically update as new information is processed by the system.

Data services may be used by the CDS system to access clinical data in the repository. Sometimes these data are automatically sent to the CDS system by a "data drive" mechanism that automatically triggers a feed to the CDS system whenever data are stored in the repository. Clinical applications also may supply data directly to the CDS system for real-time decision support; for instance, when a clinician is in the process of performing an action and needs assistance from the CDS system before making a final judgment. Quite often, even if data are automatically sent to the CDS system through a data drive mechanism or directly from an application, the rules to process the data require additional information from the repository. In this case, the CDS system may use data access services to retrieve the needed repository data.

The CDS system may need a queuing mechanism to support rules that will be triggered later. For example, a rule processed on a lab result might trigger an output that says to wait for a new lab value in 24 hours before making a final recommendation to the clinician. If another lab result is not found within 24 hours, the rule will provide a different output recommendation, such as "order a new lab X." Another use for the queue is to support "stateful" clinical protocols, that is, protocols that remember the state of the patient from a previous point in time and use this information to make recommendations later.

Once a rule is run, the output result must be communicated to the appropriate recipients. The CDS system might store a decision support result in the data repository if the rule was triggered without direct user input so that a clinician can see the result later. There might also be a mechanism for notifying a specific user of a result through e-mail, text message, or other communication pathway. When accessing the CDS system directly from a clinical application, the CDS system must have a method for communicating its results back to the application, usually through a service or application programming interface (API). CDS systems are explained in additional detail in Chapter 10.

SYSTEM INTEGRATION AND INTEROPERABILITY

The EHR is often only one piece of a larger health information system environment within a healthcare enterprise. In fact, larger institutions may run two or more EHRs. Because no single EHR today can provide all of the functionality needed in most healthcare facilities, the ability to share information between systems is necessary. Departmental and ancillary systems for the lab, pharmacy, radiology, registration, and billing, for example, must be able to pass information to and receive information from the EHR. Integrating these systems is typically the responsibility of an interface engine (IE) (see the "Interface Engine" section). The different methods for storing and communicating data used by health information systems now necessitate interoperability standards to ensure proper communication.

Interface Engine

Older intersystem communication methodologies used point-to-point connections to allow different systems to share data and information; that is, a specialized interface was created between one system (A) and another system (B). The interface between systems A and B only knew how to translate between these two systems and could not be used to "talk" to another system. This method is fine if there are few systems in the network. However, as the number of systems grows, the number of connections multiplies rapidly. For a network with N systems where all of the systems are interconnected, there are $N \times (N-1)/2$ connections; for example, a network with six systems would have $6 \times (6-1)/2 = 15$ connections. Each system in the network must individually expose $N-1$ interfaces to be fully interconnected with all other systems in the network. In practice, this means that for a network with 6 systems and 15 connections, 30 interfaces must be maintained. If a system in the network is replaced, all of its $N-1$ interfaces must be replaced, too.

Because of the cost and complexity of point-to-point interfaces, modern information systems often employ an interface engine (IE). An IE allows each network data source to have one *outbound* interface that can then be connected to any receiving system on the network. The IE is able to queue the messages from a data source, transform the messages to the proper format for the receiving systems, and then transmit the messages to appropriate systems. Acknowledgment and return messages also can be routed as appropriate by the IE.

IEs use proprietary software or standard programming languages such as Java to write routines for translating one system's data message model into another system's model. Most of today's IEs support standard messaging interfaces such as HL7 and X12. The IE must also translate terminology between systems because, quite often, systems will use different vocabularies or coding methods to represent comparable concepts. Sophisticated IEs will use external sources such as a standard data dictionary to provide the necessary terminology translation services. This allows the IE to remain up to date on the latest coding conventions and translations for the systems on the network.

The following scenario explains how an IE could be used to integrate an EHR with various ancillary systems. At the beginning of a clinical encounter, the patient is registered in the facility's registration system. The collected demographic information and encounter identifiers are transmitted by the registration system to the IE, which then transforms and forwards this information to the EHR and the LIS. During the patient's visit, the physician uses the EHR to order a laboratory test. The lab order message is appended with the correct patient identifiers and routed through the IE to the LIS. The EHR uses a proprietary coding system for lab tests that the physician orders; these are mapped to LOINC codes that the LIS uses. When the lab completes processing of the test, the lab results are returned by the LIS to the EHR via the IE. The IE also branches LIS administrative information for the test to the facility's billing system for reimbursement purposes.

This scenario describes a somewhat simple network of five interfaces. In reality, the registration system may be tied to many more systems that need demographic and patient identifier information. The EHR will provide order messages not only to an LIS but also to departmental systems for radiology, pharmacy, and nutrition, for example. Each department system's results may need to be routed to several receiving systems for storage, processing, and reporting; the EHR will typically need an inbound interface from each of these diagnostic systems. The effect when one or more of the systems on the network is replaced must be considered. An IE greatly improves the ability to address this complicated network environment in an efficient and usually less costly manner.

Interoperability Standards

System and data sharing or interoperability has long been a problem for EHRs. Most EHRs and departmental and ancillary systems have been written using proprietary programming and data storage schema. This has made it difficult to share data between systems. When trying to connect two systems, integrators must first agree on a common exchange mechanism and message format (called syntactic interoperability). Then, to ensure that the data passed between the two systems are understandable by the receiving system, the content of the message must be mapped to a comparable and comprehensible model and terminology in the receiving system (called semantic interoperability).

Some of the most widely used clinical messaging standards are produced by the HL7 organization.[19] Virtually all major clinical information systems in the United States support at least part of the HL7 version 2.x message standard, providing a common method for connecting EHRs and departmental and ancillary systems. The version 2.x standard specifies the format for messages but does not specify a standard for the content. The HL7 version 3 standard uses a much more formal specification to define messages, and it is based on the Reference Information Model (RIM). The RIM and the Clinical Document Architecture (CDA) can be used to ensure better semantic interoperability between systems. Version 3, initially published in 2005, is not as widely implemented in clinical information systems in the United States as is version 2.x because of its added complexity and significant implementation costs. Most clinical interface engines support the HL7 standards.

Many national and international terminology standards have been developed to support the exchange of clinical data and promote the semantic interoperability of systems. Most of these standards were started around a specific clinical domain but may have been expanded to cover additional domains as the terminology was adopted. For example, LOINC was originally developed to describe clinical laboratory data, but it has been expanded to cover other clinical observations such as vital signs. SNOMED CT was originally developed as a nomenclature for pathology. It has been extended to become a highly comprehensive terminology for use in a wide variety of applications, including EHRs. Other terminology standards include ICD-9 and ICD-10, Current Procedural Terminology (CPT), RxNorm, and nursing terminologies such as Nursing Interventions Classification (NIC), Nursing Outcomes Classification (NOC), and North American Nursing Diagnosis Association (NANDA). For additional information on terminology standards, refer to Chapter 22.

NETWORKING SYSTEMS

In the previous section, we discussed system interoperability within the walls of a single institution. However, there is a growing desire and need to share patient information between institutions for quality, financial, and regulatory purposes. In fact, sections of the Meaningful Use criteria in the 2009 Health Information Technology for Economic and Clinical Health (HITECH) Act specifically call for sharing of clinical data between healthcare providers and with public health organizations.[11] Various organizational models for sharing data have been developed at the local, regional, and national level.

Regional Health Information Organization, Health Information Exchanges, and Health Information Organizations

One of the earliest models for a data sharing network was the regional health information organization (RHIO). An RHIO is typically characterized as a quasi-public, nonprofit organization whose goal is to share data within a region. RHIOs were quite often started with grant or public funding. Health information exchanges (HIEs) followed RHIOs, and they are differentiated from them by having an anchor provider organization and, usually, by being started because of financial incentives. The anchor organization often provides a data-sharing mechanism to affiliated providers. In practice, the operating characteristics of RHIOs and HIEs may be quite similar, and the distinctions are only in the terminology used.

Health information organizations (HIOs) are the latest models, and they support the 2009 HITECH Act mandate for health information sharing between EHRs. The role of the HIO is to facilitate data exchange according to nationally recognized standards. This may mean that the HIO only provides guidance to the organizations in an information exchange network or that the HIO assumes the technical responsibility for providing the exchange mechanism.

To facilitate data sharing, the information exchange network is designed as either a centralized or a distributed data architecture (although hybrids of the two are also sometimes deployed). In the centralized model, the participants on the networks push their data to a central repository housed in one location. Organizations then retrieve data from the repository as needed. In a distributed model, the network participants keep their data and provide a mechanism to answer requests for specific data. In either model, the network must provide the ability to match patients between organizations correctly. Without this matching functionality, the network participants are unable to share information accurately.

The network may use a global MPI that can map patient identifiers between organizations. In addition, to provide syntactic and semantic interoperability of the data, the network participants must agree on standards for information exchange. These standards may be similar to those discussed in the previous section on interoperability standards. Last, the exchange network must provide appropriate security mechanisms to authenticate and authorize appropriate use, prevent unwanted access, and accommodate necessary auditing and logging policies.

To connect to the information exchange network, participants may simply treat the network as another interface on their local IEs. This allows participants to use existing methods for sharing data, particularly if a centralized model is used and data are pushed to the central repository. In the case where a distributed model is used and participants must accept ad hoc, asynchronous data requests, some additional effort may be required to effect data sharing. Another model for linking to the exchange network is to provide a service layer that accepts ad hoc requests for data. The data request services are accessible by network participants, often in the same way that web pages are made available as URLs on the World Wide Web. This method is becoming more popular and is particularly advantageous in the distributed exchange model because it better supports pulling data from an organization as it is needed.

eHealth Exchange

The Office of the National Coordinator (ONC) for Health Information Technology facilitated the development of a national "network of networks" whose purpose was to enable healthcare provider organizations and consumers to share information across local information exchange networks. The eHealth Exchange (formerly known as the Nationwide Health Information Network [NwHIN]) created a set of policies and national standards that allows trusted exchange of health information over the internet.[20] The effort is now managed by a nonprofit industry coalition called The Sequoia Project (formerly HealtheWay). The Exchange includes organizations from all 50 states and four federal agencies (Department of Defense [DoD], Veterans Health Affairs [VHA], Health and Human Services [HHS], and Social Security Administration [SSA]) and allows sending and requesting health information from participating organizations. An initial implementation of the information exchange architecture called CONNECT was demonstrated in 2008, with participation by various public and private entities,[21] and it includes components for core services (e.g., locating patients, requesting documents, and authentication), enterprise services (e.g., MPI, consumer preferences management, and audit log), and a client framework (application components for building test and user interfaces to CONNECT). A simplified implementation of the exchange architecture called Direct allows two organizations to share medical information through common methods, such as e-mail-like protocols.[22] These methods require a provider directory to ensure secure, point-to-point routing of messages.

ONC has developed a Shared Nationwide Interoperability Roadmap[23] that gives further direction for the technical and operational infrastructure that must be developed to advance true system-wide interoperability. This Roadmap addresses not only data syntax and semantic standards but also identity resolution, data security, access authorization, directories, and resource locators. Most recently, ONC released an Interoperability Standards Advisory, whose purpose is to "coordinate the identification, assessment, and determination of the 'best available' interoperability standards and implementation specifications...[to meet] clinical health IT interoperability needs."[24] Readers may view the entire document at: www.healthit.gov/sites/default/files/2016-interoperability-standards-advisory-final-508.pdf. New material from the ONC's Standard Advisory panel may be viewed at: www.healthit.gov/providers-professionals/standards-interoperability or by browsing for "interoperability standards," inputting the current year and "ONC."

OTHER INFRASTRUCTURE MODELS

The previous sections on the EHR component model and system integration focused on technical infrastructure that may be deployed locally within an organization. Other models exist that can also supply this infrastructure, but from sources outside an organization's walls.

Application Service Provider

Rather than purchasing and installing an EHR, some institutions opt to partner with an application service provider (ASP) for their clinical application needs. An ASP is a company that hosts an EHR or departmental system solution for a healthcare enterprise and provides access to the application via a secure network. Users of the application are usually unaware that they are connecting to a vendor's offsite computing facilities. An ASP model relieves the healthcare enterprise from having to host and support the technical components of the EHR, which may lead to lower capital infrastructure costs. This obviously helps smaller facilities that lack funding for a complete IT shop, but it also may be financially beneficial for larger facilities because of the economies of scale that an ASP vendor can provide over many customers.

On the contrary, the ASP model implies some loss of control of the EHR. ASP customers must be content with their data being stored at the vendor's offsite location. They must also accept that versions of application software, functionality, configurations, and levels of support typically will be what the majority of the other ASP customers are using. Last, it may be more difficult to integrate with other IT systems at the local site because the ASP vendor may not support interfaces for a healthcare enterprise's entire portfolio of departmental and ancillary systems. Interfaces may be more difficult to develop and maintain because the ASP vendor controls its half of each interface and may not prioritize projects in sync with the customer's needs.

Cloud Computing

A growing trend in IT is the concept of cloud computing. Although the term *cloud computing* is somewhat new, the basic idea behind it goes back decades. It can be traced to early suggestions that computing would someday be like other public utilities, and IT consumers would plug into networks of applications and physical resources in the same way that electricity and phone lines are accessed. Computing resources would be supplied by either public organizations or a few private enterprises and shared by the consumer community.

The term *cloud* was attached to this concept because early networking diagrams enclosed these "public" computing resources within a figure of a cloud to represent resources outside of an organization's physical walls and because of the ability for these resources to change location without affecting the consumer's ability to access them. Although we often still consider clouds as being available in a public space (i.e., accessible by many consuming individuals and organizations), a cloud may also be private (i.e., deployed within the walls of single organization for use by that organization's various entities). Cloud computing can be separated into three models: software as a service (SaaS), infrastructure as a service (IaaS), and platform as a service (PaaS).[25]

In the SaaS model, service providers run applications (services) at one or more locations and make these applications available to consumers. Consumers connect to the services through a cloud client, often something as simple as a web browser. This eliminates the need for consumers to host and support the applications themselves. The SaaS provider can also use economies of scale to provide multiple servers and sites that host applications, potentially increasing the efficiency, performance, and reliability of the applications. SaaS applications may be as simple as a service that provides a single function, such as Google Maps, or an application that covers an entire set of workflow requirements. The ASP model described in the previous section may be considered a type of SaaS. In clinical computing, SaaS might be used to provide an entire EHR or EHR function (e.g., scheduling and lab results review from a lab services provider) or more focused functions within an EHR application such as drug-drug interaction checking during the ordering process, information retrieval for clinical descriptions of diagnoses and abnormal lab results, or terminology mapping between coding systems.[26]

The most utility-like example of cloud computing is IaaS. In this model, the cloud provider makes computing machinery available to consumers from large pools of resources. The IaaS provider can scale the computing resources to the needs of the consumer. This practice has become simpler with the growing use of *virtual machines*, which can be installed as multiple instances on physical hardware and simulate most of the characteristics of an operating system and its environment. The consumer is responsible for deploying the operating system, applications, databases, and tools, for example, and then supporting those installed assets. Users may connect to the assets deployed on the IaaS resources through the internet or via a virtual private network. The IaaS provider can help organizations to lessen the cost of ownership of physical resources and offload the need to employ local technical personnel to maintain equipment.

The PaaS model is a simplification of the IaaS model, in which the cloud provider deploys an entire platform for running the customer's computing needs. This may include the operating system, application server, web server, and database, for example. The consumer then installs or develops software on the resources provided. The PaaS provider supports the computing resources supplied by its cloud, while the cloud user supports the assets built on top of it.

CURRENT CHALLENGES

Even though most of the technologies discussed so far have existed for decades, many technical challenges and barriers remain for implementation in the clinical environment. For the EHR repository, primary challenges remain around the robustness of storage architectures. With transitions to patient-centered longitudinal records, the size and content scope of the repository has grown considerably. Additionally, as new data types are added to the EHR to capture information about clinical encounters and patient health that is more detailed (particularly to meet the expanding requirements of Meaningful Use), the repository must be able to handle new information that was not anticipated in its original design. These facts demand that the database and storage mechanisms be flexible.

Databases must be able to scale in size to accommodate large amounts of online data. As they grow in size, they must retain performance characteristics that do not slow down the workflow of the clinical environment. Some database architectures and their storage services require new designs and recompilations as new data types are added. Some are not designed for the volumes of information that may be stored. Careful consideration of repository architecture must be performed before system selection to ensure that the system will meet the ongoing needs of the healthcare organization. Consider that patient data will have a lifetime measured in decades, whereas the technology will be enhanced or replaced on a 5- to 10-year, or less, life span. There must be a graceful way to transition the data in the repository to new technology without loss of information.

Data integration and interoperability remain the most difficult challenges in health information systems. The lack of standards, or the lack of implementation of standards, is a significant barrier. Expanding federal requirements around data exchange are forcing EHR vendors to abandon proprietary data architectures and adopt accepted standards for many types of data, but considerable work still needs to be accomplished to ensure semantic interoperability of data. This issue, coupled with older, outdated repository architectures, may leave some health IT vendors, and, therefore, their customers, without a path forward for their systems.

Some underlying system architectures make the EHR component model described earlier in the chapter difficult, impractical, or impossible to implement. Component APIs and services may be inflexible and require considerable effort to add new components, particularly if a different development group or vendor supplies those components. This issue reflects a lack of system integration standards (to accompany the lack of data integration standards discussed previously). Because of this, quite often, a health IT vendor must supply all pieces of the component model, locking customers into a single solution that may lack the needed robustness in one or more of the components.

Finally, one of the most vexing challenges for health IT has been the ability for clinical applications to integrate well with clinical workflow. Informatics professionals address these workflow issues during system analysis and usability activities to improve application adoption by clinicians. Additional information for understanding usability activities is included in Chapter 21. Still, a thorough analysis and usability assessment may not ensure acceptance in all environments. Some amount of application adaptability is often necessary to tailor the system to specific settings and for specific individuals. On the contrary, allowing for application customization at the facility, department, and user level may be quite difficult to accomplish and support (depending on the system architecture and technical abilities of the application support staff), and it can lead to nonstandard implementations that may prove costly to operate and maintain. Upgrades to nonstandard and highly tailored applications can also be extremely challenging. How well application providers support customization is an important consideration in system selection. It can have significant consequences on overall clinical IT systems infrastructure. Too little customization may mean that multiple applications must be added to the infrastructure to address the specific needs of each department or unit. More liberal customization, besides adding user complexity, may force larger manual and automated governance structures on the organization to ensure that individual solutions still support organizational policies and goals. In either case, the underlying technology of the clinical applications has a profound effect on the ability of users to do customization. In some cases, a programmer must change or add source code to make local adaptations. In other cases, tools supplied with the application allow configuration changes that can be incorporated more easily and quickly in the application, but obviously with limits to the scope of customization.

CONCLUSION AND FUTURE DIRECTIONS

The technical infrastructure of a health information system includes several key components that are unique to the healthcare environment. A sound understanding of the attributes of these components, as well as how they interact, is essential for a successful system implementation that supports the needs of the clinician users. No single off-the-shelf system today can support all needs of the healthcare environment. Therefore it is critical that the technical architecture be capable of supporting multiple system connections and data interoperability. More functionality will also become available

from third-party vendors, and infrastructures should be designed to support linking these capabilities directly to the clinical workflow. It should also be expected that the desire, and requirement, to share data outside an institution's walls would expand. The informatics role will continue to grow as the need to understand new technologies, as well as how they can be combined with existing systems and exploited in the healthcare environment, gains heightened importance.

Many new technologies are being explored or contemplated for health IT infrastructure. Most of these technologies are not new to other industries; healthcare has been much slower to adopt IT in general. In some cases, these technologies have been implemented in organizations that possess strong informatics experience and/or financial resources, but they have not been employed more widely. Certainly, the increasingly technology-savvy clinicians practicing at healthcare institutions are demanding functionality that looks more like what they use daily in web-based applications, smartphones, and tablet computers.

Mobile Apps

The growing use of mobile electronic devices has resulted in an explosion of smarter technologies for operating systems, user interfaces, and applications. Apple advertised more than 1.5 million apps available for its iPhone and iPad as of July 2015. Google advertises 1.6 million apps for its Android operating system, which is used in smartphones and tablets. Over 165,000 of the available mobile apps can be categorized as mobile health (mHealth) applications, and that number is growing (see Chapter 15 for detailed information). The apps range from personal health and fitness, to medical reference materials, to radiology image and diagnostic results viewers, to robust clinical documentation tools.

A valuable aspect of these apps is that they are easily installed on a user's device. They are typically much cheaper than applications that run on laptop and desktop computers. The ability to "carry" the app anywhere the user goes and remain connected to an institution's network (through a cellular or wireless network) is appealing to clinicians who roam to several locations throughout their workday. The volume, ease of installation, and low cost of apps can provide a much more "democratic" user voice in the selection of apps that are most useful or appealing to the user. The lightweight nature of mobile apps and the use of common user interface and application programming interface standards may make it easier for healthcare institutions to develop their own apps, customized to local needs.

There are challenges, however, to the use of mobile apps in the healthcare setting. First, the small screen factor of mobile devices limits the amount of information that may be displayed or collected. This can mean scrolling or paging through many screens to eventually get to the information needed by the clinician. It also may be easier to miss important information on the screen because of the smaller font and image sizes. Wireless networking may be another challenge for healthcare institutions. The increasing number of mobile devices in a healthcare facility, coupled with the "chatty" nature of many mobile apps, may overwhelm a hospital or clinic network. Organizations may need to develop support for virtual private networks to accommodate users who wish to use their mobile devices and apps outside the institution's walls. IT departments also must be able to handle devices brought into a facility by clinicians who are not employed by the organization, leading to potentially significant support and security issues. Finally, although the "democratization" of apps referred to earlier may seem at first blush to be a positive trait, a healthcare institution must be concerned with the support, data, process standardization, and security issues that may ensue. If clinicians are free to choose any app (e.g., for charting vital signs or ordering), will those apps be able to access and store data in the institution's required format, run decision support rules required for patient safety and quality reporting, and share information with co-workers and referral partners?

Service-Oriented Architecture

There has been much hype for years in the IT industry in general about service-oriented architecture (SOA), and healthcare has certainly been an active topic area in the discussion. SOA can be described as an architecture design pattern in which services are business oriented, loosely coupled with other services and system components, vendor and platform independent, message based, and encapsulated with internal architecture and program flow that are hidden from the service user. SOA services are most evident today as web-based (URL) services that are accessed through Hypertext Transfer Protocol (HTTP). Extensible Markup Language (XML) and JavaScript Object Notation (JSON) are commonly used as the message formats. The interface to a web service, including its allowed input parameters and return data, is often described using the Web Services Description Language (WSDL).[27] SOA fits in the SaaS category of cloud computing, but it has much more highly defined design and implementation patterns.

What this means to IT is potentially a more decentralized approach to system design in which solution providers concentrate on specific aspects of a business need. System architects can pull together many business services to meet the larger application needs of the organization without having to worry about the complexity inside the service code. Reuse is a key benefit of SOA because services may be used by different consumers for a variety of applications. Because the services are loosely coupled with each other and with other aspects of the service user's system, service code may be changed and enhanced without necessarily having to change other aspects of the overall consuming system. Changes can easily be communicated to service users through updates in a service's WSDL.

The SOA design philosophy has been researched in healthcare for a number of years. A joint effort by HL7 and the Object Management Group (OMG) to develop standards for healthcare services has resulted in the Healthcare Services Specification Project (HSSP).[28,29] HSSP has been investigating several health IT functional areas that could become the building blocks for EHR services. One example is CDS.[30] By exposing

CDS services over the web, users would be able to access CDS content from a variety of sources without having to maintain the content locally. Other areas being pursued by HSSP include services for terminology mediation and clinical data access and update.

Because no single vendor product can meet all needs of a healthcare enterprise, vendors and market segments (e.g., pharmacy fulfillment and HIE) are also incorporating SOA principles in their architectures in order to more easily and quickly provide functionality to users. Whether a major EHR product will ever be entirely composed of SOA services supplied by third-party providers is an open question, but it is likely that health IT infrastructures will provide increased support for services as standards continue to emerge and service providers become more numerous and relevant to the healthcare community.

One emerging technology that is capturing the attention of the provider, vendor, and standards communities is Fast Healthcare Interoperability Resources (FHIR).[31] Currently a draft HL7 standard, FHIR combines features from HL7 v2, v3, and CDA with a foundation in existing web messaging standards such as HTTP, XML, JSON, and REST (representational state transfer). As its name implies, it is designed to provide a faster path to system interoperability. The common building blocks of FHIR are called "Resources." Resources describe a specific type of exchange, which includes the type of information being exchanged (e.g., patient demographics, conditions, and medications) and the type of interaction (e.g., search, read, and update). The ease of use of the standard has encouraged several major electronic medical record (EMR) vendors to begin building FHIR interfaces to their systems, demonstrating a long-sought desire for open, nonproprietary services that others may use to access data and build third-party applications.

Open Source Software

Open source software (OSS) can be defined as software whose source code is made available to users, who then may be able to examine, change, and even redistribute the code according to the software's open source license. OSS is often developed in a public forum in which many programmers from different organizations, or acting as independent agents, contribute to the code base. There is typically a central code repository where all contributors place their updates and where users can download the latest versions of code or compiled objects. Users may also keep a list of bug reports and feature requests. Open source advocates believe that OSS may be more secure, bug-free, interoperable, and relevant to specific user needs than proprietary (vendor) software is because a more heterogeneous group of individuals with varying uses for the software has direct access to the source code. Some noted examples of OSS are the Apache HTTP web server, the Linux and Android operating systems, the Eclipse software development platform, the Mozilla Firefox web browser, and the OpenOffice software suite.

Several examples of OSS exist in the healthcare arena. EHR applications include OpenMRS, a multi-institution project led by the Regenstrief Institute and Partners In Health, a Boston-based philanthropic organization,[32] and OpenEHR, an ONC-certified ambulatory EHR.[33] The U.S. Department of Veterans Affairs is seeking to develop an open source version of its VistA EHR.[34] The openEHR Foundation is developing open clinical archetypes (standard data models) to promote sharable and computable information.[35] Open source, standards-based CDS tools and resources are being developed as part of OpenCDS.[36,37] Mirth Connect is an OSS IE that is built for HL7 integration.[38] Apelon provides its terminology engine, Distributed Terminology System (DTS), as an open source platform[39]; 3 M Health Information Systems has announced that it has made its health data dictionary available through open source.[40,41] FHIR (described above) is another example of OSS. These examples, and the many more in development or production, point to a future health IT infrastructure environment with wider clinician collaboration and less expensive software licensing costs. However, organizations need to be aware that "open source" does not mean *free*; they must budget for local customization, implementation, training, support, and hardware costs.

SMART

Through its Strategic Health IT Advanced Research Projects (SHARP), the ONC funded the Harvard-based Substitutable Medical Applications, Reusable Technologies (SMART) Platforms project.[42] The goal of SMART is to provide a health IT platform based on core services that allows apps to be substituted easily. Inspired by the boom in mobile apps for cell phones and tablets, researchers have developed an application ecosystem in which data can be accessed easily and presented to apps constructed for specific purposes. The apps can be bundled to provide an entire health IT solution. Institutions can decide which apps their "containers" will deploy for their clinicians based on local needs and specific app aspects such as security capabilities. The API is open source, allowing anyone to develop new applications, which can then be provided to the user community as open or closed source code. A government-funded effort initially, it will be interesting to see whether the SMART platform will be adopted widely by the healthcare provider and vendor community or if a similar effort may compete with SMART. A recent initiative with FHIR, SMART on FHIR,[43] has combined the open application technology of SMART with the open-exchange standard in FHIR, to provide interesting new possibilities for health application development.

REFERENCES

1. Clayton PD, Narus SP, Huff SM, et al. Building a comprehensive clinical information system from components: the approach at Intermountain Health Care. *Methods Inf Med.* 2003;42(1):1–7.
2. Gostin L. Health care information and the protection of personal privacy: ethical and legal considerations. *Ann Intern Med.* 1997;127(8 Pt 2):683–690.
3. Marietti C. The eyes have it: CCOW (Clinical Context Object Workgroup) brings both cooperation and competition together to tackle visual integration. *Healthc Inform.* 1998;15(6):39.
4. Berger RG, Baba J. The realities of implementation of Clinical Context Object Workgroup (CCOW) standards for integration of vendor disparate clinical software in a large medical center. *Int J Med Inform.* 2009;78(6):386–390.
5. Cimino JJ, Li J, Bakken S, Patel VL. Theoretical, empirical and practical approaches to resolving the unmet information needs of clinical information system users. *Proc AMIA Symp.* 2002;170–174.
6. Reichert JC, Glasgow M, Narus SP, Clayton PD. Using LOINC to link an EMR to the pertinent paragraph in a structured reference knowledge base. *Proc AMIA Symp.* 2002;652–656.
7. Cimino JJ, Li J. Sharing Infobuttons to resolve clinicians' information needs. *AMIA Annu Symp Proc.* 2003;815.
8. Collins S, Bakken S, Cimino JJ, Currie L. A methodology for meeting context-specific information needs related to nursing orders. *AMIA Annu Symp Proc.* 2007;155–159.
9. Del Fiol G, Huser V, Strasberg HR, Maviglia SM, Curtis C, Cimino JJ. Implementations of the HL7 context-aware knowledge retrieval ("Infobutton") standard: challenges, strengths, limitations, and uptake. *J Biomed Inform.* 2012;45(4):726–735.
10. Weir CR, Nebeker JJ, Hicken BL, Campo R, Drews F, Lebar B. A cognitive task analysis of information management strategies in a computerized provider order entry environment. *J Am Med Inform Assoc.* 2007;14(1):65–75.
11. Centers for Medicare & Medicaid Services (CMS). *Electronic Health Records (EHR) Incentive Programs;* 2015. https://www.cms.gov/Regulations-and-Guidance/Legislation/EHRIncentivePrograms/index.html?redirect=/ehrincentiveprograms.
12. Anderson C, Sensmeier J. Alliance for nursing informatics provides key elements for "Meaningful Use" dialogue. *Comput Inform Nurs.* 2009;27(4):266–267.
13. Forrey AW, McDonald CJ, DeMoor G, et al. Logical Observation Identifier Names and Codes (LOINC) database: a public use set of codes and names for electronic reporting of clinical laboratory test results. *Clin Chem.* 1996;42(1):81–90.
14. Huff SM, Rocha RA, McDonald CJ, et al. Development of the Logical Observation Identifier Names and Codes (LOINC) vocabulary. *J Am Med Inform Assoc.* 1998;5(3):276–292.
15. Logical Observation Identifier Names and Codes (LOINC). *Regenstrief Institute;* 2015. http://loinc.org.
16. Sittig DF, Wright A, Simonaitis L, et al. The state of the art in clinical knowledge management: an inventory of tools and techniques. *Int J Med Inform.* 2010;79(1):44–57.
17. Hulse NC, Rocha RA, Del Fiol G, Bradshaw RL, Hanna TP, Roemer LK. KAT: a flexible XML-based knowledge authoring environment. *J Am Med Inform Assoc.* 2005;12(4):418–430.
18. Rocha RA, Bradshaw RL, Bigelow SM, et al. Towards ubiquitous peer review strategies to sustain and enhance a clinical knowledge management framework. *AMIA Annu Symp Proc.* 2006;654–658.
19. *Health Level Seven International (HL7).* http://www.hl7.org; 2015.
20. eHealth Exchange. *The Sequoia Project;* 2015. http://sequoiaproject.org/ehealth-exchange/.
21. *CONNECT Community Portal.* http://www.connectopensource.org/; 2015.
22. *The Direct Project.* http://wiki.directproject.org; 2015.
23. Office of the National Coordinator for Health Information Technology. *Connecting Health and Care for the Nation:*

A Shared Nationwide Interoperability Roadmap; 2015. https://www.healthit.gov/sites/default/files/hie-interoperability/nationwide-interoperability-roadmap-final-version-1.0.

24. Office of the National Coordinator for Health Information Technology. *2016 Interoperability Standards Advisory;* 2016. https://www.healthit.gov/sites/default/files/2016-interoperability-standards-advisory-final-508.pdf.

25. Glaser J. Cloud computing can simplify HIT infrastructure management. *Healthc Financ Manage.* 2011;65(8):52–55.

26. Paterno MD, Maviglia SM, Ramelson HZ, et al. Creating shareable decision support services: an interdisciplinary challenge. *AMIA Annu Symp Proc.* 2010;602–606.

27. Web Services Description Language (WSDL). *1.1. W3C;* 2001. http://www.w3.org/TR/wsdl.

28. Kawamoto K, Honey A, Rubin K. The HL7-OMG Healthcare Services Specification Project: motivation, methodology, and deliverables for enabling a semantically interoperable service-oriented architecture for healthcare. *J Am Med Inform Assoc.* 2009;16(6):874–881.

29. *Healthcare Services Specification Program.* http://hssp.wikispaces.com; 2015.

30. Kawamoto K, Lobach DF. Proposal for fulfilling strategic objectives of the U.S. roadmap for national action on clinical decision support through a service-oriented architecture leveraging HL7 services. *J Am Med Inform Assoc.* 2007;14(2):146–155.

31. Welcome to FHIR. *HL7;* 2015. https://www.hl7.org/fhir/.

32. Mamlin BW, Biondich PG, Wolfe BA, et al. Cooking up an open source EMR for developing countries: OpenMRS—a recipe for successful collaboration. *AMIA Annu Symp Proc.* 2006;529–533.

33. Kalra D, Beale T, Heard S. The open EHR Foundation. *Stud Health Technol Inform.* 2005;115:153–173.

34. Mosquera M. VA's VistA open source agent to launch in August. *Government Health IT [serial online];* 2011. http://www.govhealthit.com/news/vas-vista-open-source-agent-launch-august.

35. Garde S, Hovenga E, Buck J, Knaup P. Expressing clinical data sets with openEHR archetypes: a solid basis for ubiquitous computing. *Int J Med Inform.* 2007;76(suppl 3):S334–S341.

36. OpenCDS. *OpenCDS.org;* 2015. http://www.opencds.org/.

37. Kawamoto K, Del Fiol G, Strasberg HR, et al. Multi-national, multi-institutional analysis of clinical decision support data needs to inform development of the HL7 virtual medical record standard. *AMIA Annu Symp Proc.* 2010;377–381.

38. Mirth. *Mirth Connect.* Quality Systems Inc; 2015. https://www.mirth.com/Products-and-Services/Mirth-Connect.

39. Apelon. *Terminology Tooling Products: DTS* Apelon; 2015. (2015). http://www.apelon.com/solutions/terminology-tooling/dts.

40. HDD Access. *3 M;* 2012. https://www.hddaccess.com/.

41. Goedert J. *3 M health data dictionary going open source. Health Data Management [serial online];* 2012. http://www.healthdatamanagement.com/news/3M-data-dictionary-open-source-interoperability-coding-44468-1.html.

42. Mandl KD, Mandel JC, Murphy SN, et al. The SMART Platform: early experience enabling substitutable applications for electronic health records. *J Am Med Inform Assoc.* 2012;19(4):597–603.

43. *Something New and Powerful: SMART on FHIR.* SMART Health IT. http://smarthealthit.org/smart-on-fhir/; 2015.

DISCUSSION QUESTIONS

1. Describe the role of the informatician in designing and implementing the EHR technical infrastructure as outlined by the component model discussed in the chapter.

2. How does a data dictionary influence the design and implementation of an EHR? How does the data dictionary enhance and restrict the EHR?

3. In what circumstances might a clinical infrastructure based on either third-party service providers or mobile applications be desirable? What cautions would we place on these technologies in the same circumstances?

4. How do incentive programs such as Meaningful Use affect, both positively and negatively, technical infrastructures in healthcare settings?

5. Assume that you are leading a group developing a CDS system for your organization. Choose a particular clinical environment and set of clinical problems you want to address and describe the types of interfaces you would need with other components in the clinical infrastructure in order to be successful.

6. What would be potential areas of concern for an EHR that heavily used third-party services to supply critical clinical functionality, such as decision support or medical reference links?

7. Meaningful Use criteria mandate that healthcare organizations be able to share data with other healthcare providers and public health organizations. These mandates have expanded over time. Describe how you would design the technical infrastructure to support this expansion so that new data-sharing criteria are easily incorporated into the system.

8. Vendors often design "closed" infrastructures to lock customers into their products. What would be positive and negative aspects, from the healthcare organization's viewpoint, of having such an infrastructure?

9. As opposed to the closed infrastructure of most vendor systems, open source systems may allow multiple groups to contribute to the underlying system code and architecture. Describe the positive and negative aspects of this approach for the healthcare organization. Contrast this with the SMART or SMART on FHIR approach.

10. The Infobutton standard for access to knowledge resources is receiving growing interest from health IT vendors and users. If more medical knowledge resources are made available through this standard, how might this change the nature of EHR applications, CDS systems, and local knowledge development and storage?

CDS, Clinical decision support; *EHR,* electronic health record; *FHIR,* Fast Healthcare Interoperability Resources; *SMART,* Substitutable Medical Applications, Reusable Technologies.

CASE STUDY

An integrated delivery network (IDN) serving a large urban and rural demographic area is using separate EHR systems in its inpatient and outpatient settings. Some of the specialty departments have also purchased their own systems for documentation. Unfortunately, this means that information collected in the inpatient setting is not available when patients are seen in the IDN's outpatient clinics (and vice versa). The clinicians need this information to be better informed about their patients and to provide optimal care. In addition, Meaningful Use requirements for problems, medications, and allergies, as well as new chronic disease care initiatives that the IDN is implementing for its patient population, are being hindered by the separate systems. The clinicians have been given accounts on both EHRs, but this is cumbersome for the users because they must be trained on multiple systems, they use valuable time logging into different systems and navigating for information, and there is a potential safety issue if the user selects different patients on the two EHRs. A coordinated decision support environment has also been difficult to implement because the two EHRs use different coding systems and do not share most of their information. This means, for example, that admission rules for congestive heart failure patients cannot be linked to the ambulatory medication list and recent vital signs measurements to run the IDN's standard care process models.

The IDN realizes that it will not be able to replace either EHR in the near future and that, even if it could, there will still be issues with integrating information from the specialty care systems. It decides on a strategic plan to create a CDR that is fed with high-value data from each of the clinical systems. The outpatient EHR's MPI already was being used as the master unique identifier for most of the IDN's systems, so it can be incorporated with the new CDR. A robust IE is implemented to supply data from the clinical systems to the CDR. To normalize the different terminologies used on their various systems, the IDN engages a terminology-services vendor to provide a central data dictionary for the CDR and map the concepts from the current systems to the central standard terminology. The IE uses the terminology services to normalize inbound data to the CDR from the other systems.

The second phase of the strategic plan is to build a CDS system on top of the CDR to develop and maintain enterprise patient-care rules. As rules are executed, their results will be both sent through the IE to the existing EHRs and stored in the CDR; storing the decision support results in the CDR provides a link to supporting data from all clinical systems, which can help with rule triage and maintenance. Another effort in this phase is to provide clinician views into the CDR. The IDN plans to build data services, possibly based on FHIR resources, that can be called by third-party EHRs to display longitudinal, enterprise-wide patient data from within the EHRs. Several simple web- and mobile-based viewing applications using the data services will also be developed and will be available in a stand-alone mode or as callable modules within the current EHRs. The IDN will use SMART to provide the user and patient context from the EHR to these viewing apps so that the clinicians will not have to log in twice and find the patient.

Discussion Questions

1. Describe the advantages and disadvantages of the situation in the case study.
2. You are the chief medical informatics officer for the organization. You are asked to comment about how the technical plans will affect clinicians. Based on the case study, how do you respond?
3. The organization receives a $3 million gift from an informatics benefactor. You are an informatician in the organization. What would your technical priorities be to remedy the issues in the case study?

CDR, Clinical data repository; *CDS,* clinical decision support; *EHR,* electronic health record; *IDN,* integrated delivery network; *IE,* interface engine; *SMART,* Substitutable Medical Applications, Reusable Technologies.

6

Electronic Health Records and Applications for Managing Patient Care

Charlotte A. Seckman

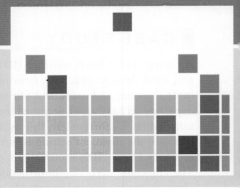

In the future, the electronic health record (EHR) will play a pivotal role in personalized medicine as a medium for data, information, knowledge and wisdom exchange, and exploration.

OBJECTIVES

At the completion of this chapter, the reader will be prepared to:

1. Analyze terms and definitions associated with the electronic health record (EHR).
2. Describe the essential components and attributes of an EHR.
3. Define *federal requirements* in the context of EHR adoption and the impact on health practitioners.
4. Examine EHR applications used in the clinical setting.
5. Analyze the benefits of an EHR related to cost, access, quality, safety, and effectiveness.
6. Evaluate stakeholder perspectives and key issues that affect EHR adoption.
7. Explore future directions for EHR adoption and integration.

KEY TERMS

ABSTRACT ❖

The electronic health record (EHR) is one of the most significant innovations introduced in healthcare over the past several decades. Today almost all healthcare providers are using computerization to share patient data and information across facilities locally, nationally and, eventually, internationally. Although there is concern about how to establish a nationwide interoperable system, and many issues still need to be resolved related to EHR implementation and adoption, the long-term benefits to organizations, healthcare providers, patients, and consumers cannot be ignored. This chapter explores the evolving nature of the EHR to include essential components and functions, how these components are used in the clinical setting, and the benefits related to cost, access, quality, safety, and efficiency of care. A discussion of key issues that influence the implementation and adoption of these systems and future directions concludes this chapter.

INTRODUCTION

The complex nature of the current U.S. healthcare system has created a challenging environment for managing patient data and information. Traditional paper systems can be easier to use for documenting a single episode of care, but access to these records is limited, reporting is extremely cumbersome, and trending of data across patient visits or types over time is nearly impossible. Provider specialty practices create treatment silos that often hinder continuity of care. Healthcare providers and hospitals endeavor to keep current with billing regulations to receive optimal reimbursement. This requires vigilant monitoring of private insurance contracts and changes in governmental mandates. Some clinicians find it difficult to maintain competencies and gain access to information about the latest medical techniques and research. Add to this the introduction of personal computers, mobile devices, and the internet, which have boosted consumer demands and a variety of healthcare delivery concerns.

The robust nature of the electronic health record (EHR) has the potential to address many of these issues and transform the way we collect, store, access, process, manage, and report patient data. Government and financial incentives are being offered to expedite the implementation and expansion of EHR systems. However, despite all of the attention on this technology, different views still exist about what an EHR is, what it does or should do, and how it should be used.

Early Terms and Definitions

Multiple labels and definitions have been used throughout the years to refer to electronic systems used in healthcare. Early terms focused on using the words *computer* and *record* to merge the idea of a paper chart with technology, but computers provided much more functionality than did traditional methods. These early terms were not sufficient to describe this emerging phenomenon. For example, specific terms and acronyms such as computer patient records (CPRs), computer-based patient records (CBPRs), and computer health records (CHRs) were used to identify systems that contained select automated components of the patient's medical record. The acronym CPR was not popular in the health community because it also represents the term *cardiopulmonary resuscitation*. Generic names such as *hospital information system* (HIS) or *medical information system* (MIS) were adopted to represent the management of a larger body of data and information throughout a specific hospital or healthcare system.

Later definitions for electronic systems in healthcare often focused on the system's distinctive purpose, content, ownership, and functional differences. This is especially true for technology used in specialty areas such as nursing, pharmacy, laboratory, radiology, and other support departments. For example, a laboratory information system (LIS) would be used to collect, store, process, and manage laboratory data and would be controlled by the laboratory department personnel, whereas a pharmacy system would provide medication inventory, control, and dispensing for pharmacy personnel. Specific clinical departmental systems will be discussed in more detail later in the chapter. Acronyms such as *CBPR* or *CPR* referred to a larger collection of information about the patient, such as orders, medications, treatments, laboratory and diagnostic test results, and other information related to overall patient care. Although the terms imply a patient-owned record, access and input to the record are typically controlled by the healthcare provider. As computer technology continued to progress and more functionality became available, a need surfaced for clarity and refinement in terms and definitions relating to EHR systems.

Electronic Medical Record Versus Electronic Health Record

More recently, terms such as electronic medical record (EMR) and electronic health record (EHR) have emerged. These are often used interchangeably, but it is important to understand the differences between them. Sewell and Thede defined the *EMR* as "an electronic version of the traditional record used by the healthcare provider."[1] Hebda and Czar described the EMR as an electronic information resource used in healthcare to capture patient data.[2] In essence, an EMR can be viewed as the electronic version of a patient's paper chart. The EMR is what most clinicians think of as the automated medical record system used in the clinical setting, and it represents an episodic view of patient encounters. This type of system, seen in hospitals, hospital corporations, and clinician practices, is predominately controlled by the healthcare provider. The EMR is not just one system but may integrate and/or interface with multiple other systems and applications used by the facility, such as registration, patient scheduling, order entry, clinical documentation, radiology, laboratory, and other departmental systems. The patient usually does not interact with or provide input into the EMR, although software vendors are working to incorporate portals that provide patient access to test results, scheduling features, e-mail interaction with clinicians, and the ability to add, correct, and update health information.

How is this different from an EHR? In 2008, the National Alliance for Health Information Technology (NAHIT), as a division of the U.S. Department of Health & Human Services (HHS), convened to clarify and define key health information technology (health IT) terms. The EHR was defined as "An electronic record of health-related information on an individual that conforms to nationally recognized interoperability standards and that can be created, managed, and consulted by authorized clinicians and staff across more than one healthcare organization."[3] This suggests the availability and use of communication standards, such as nomenclatures, vocabularies, and coding structures, to share patient data across multiple organizations, facilities and providers.[4] In comparison, the EMR is limited to information exchange within a single organization or practice, whereas the EHR has the ability to exchange information outside the healthcare delivery system.[5]

The Healthcare Information and Management Systems Society (HIMSS) provides a similar definition of the EHR as a longitudinal electronic record of patient health information produced by encounters in one or more care settings.[6] The implication is that every person will have a birth-to-death (and even prenatal and postmortem) record of health-related information in electronic form from multiple sources, such as physician office visits, inpatient and outpatient hospital encounters, medications, allergies, and other medical services that support care, as well as personal input from the consumer perspective. This means that components of the EMR would ultimately be part of the larger EHR. Other definitions stress the importance of the EHR as a way to automate and streamline workflow for healthcare providers, support patient care activities, and provide decision support, quality management, and outcomes reporting.[7-11] Despite the clarification provided by these definitions, many are still using the terms *EMR* and *EHR* interchangeably. In addition, these definitions are often directed toward the needs of the healthcare provider and lack reference to patient and consumer interaction or integration of personal health records (PHRs).

At this point, it is important to mention the PHR as a component of the EHR. This type of record is primarily patient or consumer controlled and is discussed in more detail in Chapter 14. The ultimate goal is that PHR development conform to nationally recognized standards and be integrated into larger systems, allowing the individual to view, manage, and share personal health information with providers. As part of the EHR, this could provide a more comprehensive record of a person's medical history and overall health.

In summary, *EHR* has become the preferred term for the lifetime patient record that would include data from a variety of healthcare specialties and provide interactive access and input by the patient. The term *EHR* is distinct in meaning from the term *EMR*. As with other expressions in the past, the term *EMR* may eventually fade away. Although some disagreement exists on exactly what the terms *EHR* and *EMR* mean or how an interoperable lifetime patient record will work, the EHR is clearly a complex tool that will continue to grow and evolve.[12]

ELECTRONIC HEALTH RECORD COMPONENTS, FUNCTIONS, AND ATTRIBUTES

Present-day electronic systems in most organizations typically include patient demographics, financial data, order information, laboratory and diagnostic test results, medications and allergies, problem lists, and clinical documentation. Beyond these basic features, an EHR should also incorporate clinical events monitoring, preventive care recommendations, and decision support tools that enhance the quality, safety, efficiency, and effectiveness of patient care. In 2003, the HHS formed a group called the EHR Collaborative, to support rapid adoption and to develop standards for EHR design in preparation for this initiative.[13] This group included sponsors from the following organizations:

- American Health Information Management Association (AHIMA)
- American Medical Association (AMA)
- American Nurses Association (ANA)
- American Medical Informatics Association (AMIA)
- College of Healthcare Information Management Executives (CHIME)
- eHealth Initiative (eHI)
- HIMSS
- National Alliance for Health IT (NAHIT), later disbanded

The EHR Collaborative held forums and gathered input from stakeholder communities such as healthcare providers, insurance companies, HIT vendors, researchers, pharmacists, public health organizations, and consumers. EHR Collaborative organizations, along with the Institute of Medicine (IOM) and Health Level Seven (HL7), were tasked to design a standard for EHRs. As a result, the IOM released a report on July 31, 2003, called *Key Capabilities of an Electronic Health Record System*.[14] This report identified eight essential care delivery components for an EHR, with an emphasis on

functions that promote patient safety, quality, and efficiency. These essentials still apply today. In recent years, the U.S. Department of Defense added dentistry and optometry records as EHR components needed to provide a more comprehensive picture of overall health status.[15] See Table **6.1** for a list of essential EHR components and their descriptions. Each component of an EHR incorporates unique functions and attributes that contribute to the integration of a comprehensive patient record.

In addition to the various components and functions, there are 12 key attributes prescribed by the IOM[14] as the gold standard components of an EHR. These attributes serve as guidelines to organizations and vendors involved in the design and implementation of EHRs and include the information shown in Box **6.1**.

TABLE 6.1 **Summary of the Electronic Health Record Essential Components and Functions for Care Delivery**

Component	Essential Functions	Application Examples
Administrative processes	Ability to conduct all financial and administrative functions associated with institutional operations and patient management	Admissions/ registration Scheduling Claims processing Administrative reporting
Communication and connectivity	Provides a medium for electronic communication between healthcare providers and patients	E-mail Mobile devices Text/web messaging Integrated health records Telemedicine
Decision support	Provides reminders, alerts, and resource links to improve the diagnosis and care of the patient	Medication dosing, allergies Risk screening/ prevention Clinical guidelines Resource links
Dentistry and optometry	Ability to incorporate dental records and vision prescriptions	Dental records Vision records
Health information and data	Ability to enter and access key information needed to make clinical decisions	Patient demographics Problem lists Medical/nursing diagnoses Medications/ allergies Results reporting

Continued

TABLE 6.1 Summary of the Electronic Health Record Essential Components and Functions for Care Delivery—cont'd

Component	Essential Functions	Application Examples
Order-entry management	Ability to enter all types of orders via the computer system	Laboratory Pharmacy Radiology Other orders
Patient support	Provides patient education and self-monitoring tools	Discharge instructions Computer-based learning Telemonitoring
Results management	Provides the ability to manage current and historical information related to all types of diagnostic reports	Laboratory tests Radiology reports Other procedures
Population health management	Provides data collection tools to support public and private reporting requirements	Public health system Disease surveillance Bioterrorism

Adapted from Institute of Medicine, Committee on Data Standards for Patient Safety: Board of Health Care Services. *Key Capabilities of an Electronic Health Record System: Letter Report.* Washington, DC: The National Academies Press; 2003.

BOX 6.1 The Institute of Medicine's Key Attributes of an Electronic Health Record

1. Provides active and inactive problem lists for each encounter that link to orders and results; meets documentation and coding standards.
2. Incorporates accepted measures to support health status and functional levels.
3. Ability to document clinical decision information; automates, tracks, and shares clinical decision process/rationale with other caregivers.
4. Provides longitudinal and timely linkages with other pertinent records.
5. Guarantees confidentiality, privacy, and audit trails.
6. Provides continuous authorized user access.
7. Supports simultaneous user views.
8. Access to local and remote information.
9. Facilitates clinical problem solving.
10. Supports direct entry by physicians.
11. Cost measuring/quality assurance.
12. Supports existing/evolving clinical specialty needs.

Adapted from Institute of Medicine, Committee on Data Standards for Patient Safety: Board of Health Care Services. Key Capabilities of an Electronic Health Record System: Letter Report. *Washington, DC: The National Academies Press; 2003.*

SOCIOTECHNICAL PERSPECTIVES

Since the late 1990s, the design, implementation, and adoption of EHR systems has received a great deal of attention as a method to reduce medical errors, increase patient safety, and improve the quality of care.[16-18] The underlying assumption is that an EHR will save time, provide real-time access to patient information at the point of care, facilitate the work of the clinician, provide decision support capabilities, support clinical care and research, and improve quality and safety of care.[9,19-22] This section explores factors that influence EHR adoption, federal requirements using MU as an example, and the health practitioner's role in EHR adoption.

Electronic Health Record Adoption

More recently, new regulations have emerged to guide adoption of EHRs in the United States. Numerous strategies and incentives are being used to expedite implementation, adoption, and MU of EHR systems. This section will explore requirements for MU, the EHR Adoption Model, and the health practitioner role in both EHR adoption and MU.

Federal EHR Requirements

National mandates and guidelines from collaborative working groups were not enough to accelerate the development and adoption of health IT. In 2009 the American Recovery and Reinvestment Act was passed, and it included a critical component addressing healthcare technology called the Health Information Technology for Economic and Clinical Health (HITECH) Act. The HITECH Act authorized programs designed to improve healthcare quality, safety, and efficiency using health IT.[23] More details about the HITECH Act and MU criteria, as well as other related legislation can be found in Chapter 27. Of importance to this chapter, the provision was targeted to stimulate the adoption of EHRs and the development of secure health information exchange (HIE) networks. It includes incentives for healthcare providers through MU of certified EHRs. The purpose of MU is more than just implementing an EHR; it is also to leverage the technology to improve quality, safety, and efficiency in patient care. MU objectives are being implemented in three stages. Criteria for each stage vary based on whether the EHR system is implemented in ambulatory practices or hospitals. The first stage began in 2011 and focused on electronic data capture and tracking of key clinical conditions, communication, data sharing and coordination of care, reporting public health information and quality measures, and engaging patients and families.[24,25] A set of core and optional objectives along with clinical quality measures must be meet in order to receive incentive payments.

Requirements for Stage 2 MU were released by the Federal Register in August 2012, with reporting that began as early as fiscal year 2014. The focus of this stage is to encourage patient engagement and the robust use of health IT through continuous quality improvement efforts, HIE networks, and structured data capture. Along with employing Stage 1 objectives, healthcare providers and hospitals need to address an additional set of core, optional, and clinical quality measures. In a broader sense, the expectation for Stage 2 involves expanded EHR functionality to support quality improvement, patient safety, structured information exchange, population health, and research.[24,26] Stage 3 criteria were released for comment in late 2015, but implementation was delayed until 2017. Stage 3 will combine and expand on the objectives for the first two stages to support further quality initiatives; improve safety, efficiency, and patient outcomes; address population health requirements; provide enhanced decision support; and promote patient-centered HIE.[24]

Electronic Medical Record Adoption Model

In 2005, the HIMSS Analytics group developed an EMR Adoption Model (EMRAM) to track the progress of health IT adoption rates in hospitals and, more recently, ambulatory facilities.[27] The systems and functions required for each stage for U.S. hospitals are shown in Table 6.2. Although originally developed for the United States, the EMRAM is also being used in Europe and Canada.[28,29] This model provides realistic and achievable measures in seven stages that coincide with MU requirements. The model assists organizations by

TABLE 6.2   HIMSS Analytics United States Electronic Medical Record Adoption Model 2005–12

Stage	Cumulative Capabilities
Stage 7	Complete EMR; CCD transactions to share data; data warehousing in use; data continuity with emergency department, ambulatory, outpatient; data analytics
Stage 6	Physician documentation (structured templates); full CDS system (variance and compliance); closed-loop medication administration (pharmacy-CPOE-barcode-eMar)
Stage 5	Full radiology-PACS
Stage 4	CPOE; CDS system (clinical protocols)
Stage 3	Clinical documentation to include flow sheets, vitals, nursing notes, eMar; CDS system (error checking); PACS available outside Radiology
Stage 2	CDR with Controlled Medical Vocabulary, CDS system; may have document imaging; health information exchange
Stage 1	Major ancillary systems installed that include Laboratory, Radiology, and Pharmacy
Stage 0	No ancillary systems installed

Adapted from *Healthcare Information and Management Systems Society* (*HIMSS*) *Analytics*. HIMSS Analytics EMR Adoption Model (EMRAM). <http://www.himssanalytics.org/research/emram-stage-criteria/>; 2015.
CCD, Continuity of care document; *CDR*, clinical data repository; *CDS*, clinical decision support; *CPOE*, computerized provider order entry; *eMar*, electronic medication administration record; *EMR*, electronic medical record; *PACS*, picture archiving and communication system.

providing a sequenced implementation structure for IT adoption to align with business strategies, benchmarking data to compare progress with other facilities, and an approach that maps to MU objectives. EMRAMs for physician practice and ambulatory facilities are similar, with modifications specific to those settings.

Health Practitioner Role in Electronic Health Record Adoption and Meaningful Use

Healthcare users play an important role in EHR adoption and MU. Interdisciplinary participation is important throughout the systems life cycle, from identifying strategic needs to selecting a system (see Chapters 16 and 17) to implementing (see Chapter 19) to maintaining systems (see Chapter 20). Practitioners can serve various roles as they may lead efforts, serve on key committees, participate in tailoring a system to local workflow, participate in testing systems, or be super users during implementations or upgrades. Once a system change is implemented, clinical users have a responsibility to report any issues with functionality, usability, workflow, or effect on patient care.

A typical EHR is designed to allow access and input by a variety of healthcare providers as a way to manage care. In the same way, fulfillment of the MU objectives requires active involvement and contributions from multiple disciplines to produce high-quality patient outcomes. Although early incentives were directed toward hospitals, clinics, and physician practices, all health practitioners are integral to the collection of MU data through the use of EHR technology.[30] For example, nursing care is a primary reason for hospitalization, so nurses' roles in addressing the MU objectives should not be underestimated. Nurses are the single largest group of employees in the hospital setting, where labor costs are often bundled with room and supply fees.[31] With the threat of a nursing shortage, executives are pressured to find ways to increase productivity while they struggle to recruit and retain qualified healthcare personnel. The adoption of an EHR system can enhance access to patient information, provide more accurate and complete documentation, improve data availability, and provide decision support capabilities, often leading to increased staff productivity and satisfaction.[2,21,32]

Many health practitioners are involved in providing care coordination and patient education, key objectives of the MU requirements. Health practitioners assist in designing clinical decision support (CDS) systems that can be used to enhance patient adherence to disease management. Other activities include developing data set standards to improve outcomes, increase patient safety, and evaluate quality of care. Many are engaged in local, regional, and national strategic initiatives to improve care coordination using EHRs and an HIE.[25,33,34] Although the initial incentives have resulted in expanding the installed base of EHRs in the United States, how the HITECH Act will affect the role of each group of health professionals in the future is yet to be determined. What is clear is that patient care should be a collaborative effort guided by interdisciplinary teams that work together with the patient to provide the best possible outcomes.

ELECTRONIC HEALTH RECORD APPLICATIONS USED IN THE CLINICAL SETTING

An EHR is composed of multiple applications. In different settings, an EHR may vary in terms of integration between the components, data presentation, usability, and clinical workflow. This section discusses the various applications currently used in the clinical setting, including computerized provider order entry (CPOE), Electronic Medication Administration Record (eMAR), Bar Code Medication Administration (BCMA), clinical documentation, specialty applications, and CDS.

Computerized Provider Order Entry

Computerized provider order entry (CPOE) is a component of the larger EHR system. The "P" in CPOE initially stood for *physician*, but because advanced practice registered nurses, physician assistants, and other healthcare providers also write orders, this "P" refers to *prescriber*, *practitioner*, or *provider*. CPOE is software designed to allow clinicians to enter a variety of orders, such as medications, dietary services, consults, admission and discharge orders, nursing orders, lab requisitions, and other diagnostic tests, via a computer.

For many years, handwritten orders were interpreted and entered into the computer system by unit secretaries, nurses, and pharmacists. Transcription errors such as a misplaced decimal point and illegible handwriting were major causes of error. Incomplete orders were a problem that caused additional steps in the nursing workflow. The idea behind CPOE was for prescribers, such as physicians, dentists, osteopathic doctors, anesthesiologists, nurse practitioners, and physician assistants, to enter orders directly into the computer. During the ordering process, alerts, such as drug allergy warnings, and other decision support rules should be available to assist the healthcare provider. Once an order is entered, the CPOE system interfaces or integrates with other EHR components, such as a laboratory or pharmacy system, to process the order. In fact, the term *order entry* can be misleading, as CPOE is truly an orders management system that allows orders to be entered, processed, tracked, updated, and completed.

The 1999 IOM report *To Err Is Human: Building a Safer Health System*[18] and demands from special interest groups put pressure on physicians and other prescribers to enter their orders directly into EHRs. Financial incentives offered through the HITECH Act and MU objectives in all stages were designed to enforce the use of CPOE and systematic adoption of EHR functionality. The mandate for EHR adoption, and specifically CPOE, as a means of reducing medical and medication errors continues to receive much attention.[17,18,35] Studies have consistently demonstrated the benefits of CPOE on reducing medication errors. Early landmark studies found that the implementation of CPOE decreased the length of hospital stay, lowered costs, improved quality of care, improved the appropriateness of drug dosing, and decreased the number of allergic reactions.[35-38] Mekhjian et al.[39] conducted a pre- and post-CPOE implementation comparison study at a large university medical center and found significant reductions in transcription errors, faster medication turnaround times, and timely reporting of results. Bates et al.[40] went further by evaluating the effect of CPOE with decision support tools on different types of medication errors and reported a significant reduction in overall errors. Other studies that focused on CPOE implementation suggest that medical and medication errors can be reduced along with improving data integrity, accuracy, workflow, and patient outcomes.[41-44] In essence, CPOE combined with CDS capabilities such as checking for drug interactions, drug-allergy interactions, and dosing ranges can significantly reduce many serious medication errors.[45]

Physician resistance, financial constraints, and other issues make CPOE compliance challenging. In a landmark study, Ash et al.[17] identified unintended consequences of CPOE that lead to medical errors related to (1) the process of entering and retrieving information and (2) methods of communication and coordination. Koppel et al.[46] also researched CPOE-related factors that may increase the risk of medication errors and found that new errors were reported because of fragmented data and processes, lack of integration among systems, and human-computer interaction issues.

Using CPOE can be time consuming during order entry, and design efficiencies are needed to entice clinicians to enter their own orders. For example, before CPOE, many providers used standard handwritten order sheets for their patient population. Order sets were developed to include all or most of the information required to process multiple orders at one time. In a study comparing the use of traditional order entry methods and standardized order sets, researchers reported that using order sets had the potential to reduce errors, decrease order-entry time, and eliminate variations in order presentation.[47]

The lack of decision support or overuse of alerts was another issue. In an early study, Payne et al.[48] found that in 42,641 orders generated, there was an 88% override rate for critical drug interaction alerts and a 69% override rate for drug-allergy interaction alerts among ordering practitioners. This prompted concern that too many alerts could cause the ordering healthcare provider to become immune to the warnings and ignore them. Recommendations to address unintended consequences, user resistance, and decision support issues focused on providing education to healthcare providers and consumers, designing systems that support communication and clinical workflow, early user participation in the implementation process, continuous safety monitoring, and the use of qualitative multidisciplinary research methods to provide deeper insight into the benefits and issues surrounding CPOE and EHRs.[49,50]

Electronic Medication Administration Record

The electronic medication administration record (eMAR) provides a medium to view and document medication use for individual patients. This system takes the place of using medication cards or a Kardex. When medication orders are entered into the CPOE system, this information is sent to the pharmacy system for verification and dispensing by the pharmacist. New orders appear on the patient's medication list in the eMAR and include information about the drug name, administration time, dose, and route. Usually the eMAR contains all types of medication and intravenous fluid orders, with the ability to sort the list in a variety of ways. For example, users can display scheduled, as needed (prn), pending, past due, or completed medications and can query the list for specific entries. Some systems will color code medication order types for quick sorting and identification. Efforts to decrease medication administration errors use an eMAR in combination with bar coding devices. An example of an eMAR screen is shown in Fig. **6.1.**

Bar Code Medication Administration

Bar Code Medication Administration (BCMA) is a method used to address patient safety and reduce errors that occur during the actual administration of medicines. This system is most effective when combined with CPOE, a pharmacy dispensing system, and the eMAR. Although CPOE has been successful in reducing transcription-related medication errors, it was not designed to prevent errors that may occur during the actual administration of a drug to the patient. In 2004, the U.S. Food and Drug Administration (FDA) indicated that the use of BCMA had the potential to reduce medication errors and recommended that bar coding become standard on patient identification bands and medication labels.[51] Bar codes can then be read by optical scanners or bar code readers. Research findings in the area of BCMA support advantages such as easy to use, improved satisfaction with medication documentation, a reduction in medication error rates, and avoidance of potential adverse drug events.[52-56]

The medication administration process with BCMA in the clinical setting starts with the nurse scanning his or her badge, the patient's wristband bar code, and the medication bar code. The scanner verifies the five "rights" of medication administration—right patient, right drug, right dose, right time, and right route—and documents the actual administration in the eMAR.

Radio frequency identification (RFID) is also being used for medication administration. This technology uses electronic tags embedded in an identification badge or band to track and monitor activities. Passive RFID works in a similar way to regular bar coding with the use of a scanner. Active RFID does not require a scanner; rather, it automatically transmits signals to a computer or wireless device without disturbing the patient. This technology is becoming more common in hospitals to track patient care activities, including medication dispensing and administration.[57]

Clinical Documentation

Clinical documentation applications provide a medium for recording, managing, and reporting patient care activities by a variety of disciplines. The format for documenting

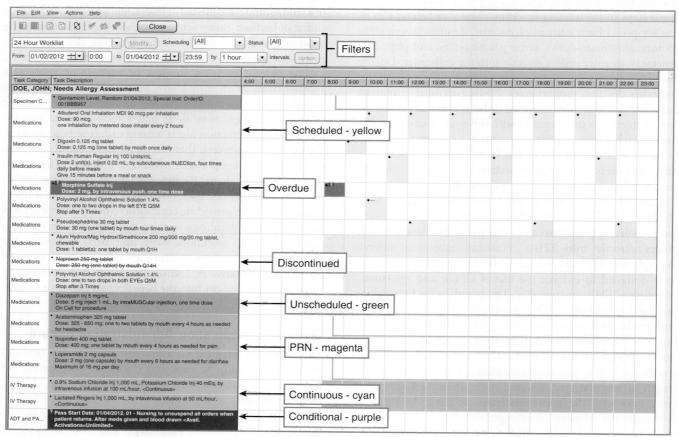

FIG 6.1 Example of an eMAR. (Copyright 2012 Allscripts. Used with permission.)

may differ by application and organizational preference. Although many clinicians still embrace the richness of narrative notes, advantages exist to using standardized vocabularies and taxonomies for documenting patient care, as discussed in detail in Chapter 22. Structured notes using standardized language may come in the form of pull-down menus, decision trees, or key words embedded in a sentence. Some systems contain functionality to store and retrieve predefined notes of normal findings. Some organizations may use "charting by exception," wherein normal values and entries are predefined and selected according to established guidelines so clinicians need to document only abnormal findings.

Clinical documentation systems should have functionality to support workflow processes and the creation of plans of care. Often electronic flow sheets or grids are used to record vital signs and other procedures quickly. An effective documentation system includes decision support rules that alert the clinician about abnormal values, missing content, or additional assessments that are needed. Rules can also be written to remind healthcare providers to verify essential information (e.g., new orders, or allergies). Many systems provide the ability to graph numeric data, such as vital signs and lab values. Problem lists, allergies, medications, and other critical information about a patient can be extracted and displayed on a single summary screen to assist the busy clinician. Depending on the type of data collected, various clinical, administrative, and research reports can be generated.

Overall, clinical documentation systems should support better communication between healthcare providers, promote professional accountability, and streamline workflow. Access to literature sources, policies and procedures, clinical guidelines, and standards of care can be functionally incorporated to support evidence-based practice (EBP) using applications such as Infobuttons or the EBP InfoBot (discussed under Clinical Decision Support section). Additional information about EBP is included in Chapter 3. Electronic documentation makes it easier to search, query, and extract data for reports. This information can be used for quality-improvement initiatives, critical-incident reviews, resource management, long-term planning, clinical research, and to address the requirements of the accreditation process.

Specialty Applications

Many of the basic EHR components, such as CPOE, eMAR, and clinical documentation, are available to all healthcare providers, but in most settings, there is a need for unique functionality beyond what is provided in these applications. Specialty or niche applications are software programs created to address the requirements of specific departments and groups of users. Although many niche applications can function as stand-alone systems, integration with or interface to the hospital-wide EHR is preferred to decrease redundancy, enhance communication, and provide a more comprehensive patient record. Some examples of specialty department systems include perioperative or surgical services, maternity care, neonatal intensive care, and the emergency department (ED).

A surgical information system (SIS) incorporates functionality to improve clinical, operational, and financial outcomes throughout the entire perioperative experience. Functionality may include operating room scheduling; management of equipment, supplies, and inventory; documentation for nurses and anesthesiologists; patient and specimen tracking; and administrative reporting capabilities.

A maternity care information system (MCIS) is another type of niche system used to address the needs of obstetrics staff. An MCIS is used to support clinical protocols for maternity care, track mother and baby progress, capture fetal-uterine monitoring data, and record results of Doppler blood flow and other diagnostic tests. Key features of this system include electronic forms for documenting and reporting all aspects of antenatal, intrapartum, and postnatal care, as well as normal, healthy, or adverse pregnancy outcomes. Likewise, a neonatal information system (NIS) that interfaces with the EHR would contain much of the same information found in the primary system. Unique to an NIS would be growth charts, nutritional calculations, monitor parameters, and coding structures specific to the needs of critically ill newborns. Clinical staff in these specialty units can benefit from user-defined logbooks, resource utilization, quality improvement, and statistical reports designed for their specific needs.

The ED has unique computer needs related to clinical workflow, documentation of triage and patient encounters, tracking of patient location and treatment progress, charge capture and reimbursement management, clinical rules for risk mitigation, and patient education and referral. Once again, not unlike other niche systems, the emergency department information system (EDIS) is designed to improve clinical, operational, and financial outcomes throughout the entire ED experience. However, EDISs are often integrated into a facility's EHR because EDs are the portal into acute care; these integrated data are then readily available to acute care providers and areas.

Clinical Decision Support

CDS systems are tools and applications that assist the healthcare provider with some aspect of decision making. These applications are discussed in detail in Chapter 10. Of importance here, CDS systems are crucial components of EHRs, linked to at least CPOE in the form of alerts related to duplicate orders, allergies, and medication dosing errors. A CDS system could also provide alerts related to changes in a patient's condition and reminders about important tasks such as follow-up visits, preventive care, immunizations, and updates to critical patient information.[58]

Some EHRs may contain external web links to resources to assist with clinical decision making (see, for example, the discussion of Infobuttons in Chapter 10). Many healthcare systems also have internal intranets that provide links to policies and procedures, clinical guidelines, and evidence-based protocols. In 2006, the National Institutes of Health (NIH) in collaboration with the National Library of Medicine (NLM) developed a personalized decision support application called the EBP InfoBot.[59] This system was designed to augment a patient's EHR automatically by searching various literature sources and providing information that could be used to develop plans of care and assist with decision making. Operating behind the scenes are rule sets programmed to extract key data from the patient's medical record, map free text data to standardized terminology, and create a series of EBP-type queries from extracted data. These questions are used to search multiple NLM databases, internal standards of care and guidelines, and other external clinical resources, and then provide a summary of the information based on clinical user-group preference directly into the EHR. The application functions in real time and provides flexibility to adapt to the requirements of the decision maker. Overall, the EBP InfoBot decreased provider search time, reduced information overload, and provided current and timely resources to support decision making at the bedside. An example of the EBP Info-Bot summary screen is shown in Fig. **6.2**. Ideally, at a minimum, the CDS in EHRs should be accurate, be available to the clinician at the point of care, provide timely and up-to-date information, and be incorporated easily into daily care processes and workflow.

Ancillary Systems

An ancillary system usually refers to software applications used by patient care support departments such as laboratory, radiology, and pharmacy. Other departments such as cardiology, respiratory, physical therapy, and material management may have their own software applications as well. LISs and radiology information systems (RISs) were available long before the concept of EHR systems was introduced. Both LISs and RISs are designed to address the specific needs of the department related to collecting, processing, and reporting test results along with managing resources and costs. The LIS consists of several components related to the laboratory subdepartments, including hematology, chemistry, microbiology, blood bank, and pathology. The LIS may also interface with other devices, such as blood analyzers, for direct input of blood test results. Coding structures are used to track and identify resources and provide cost data for billing. Logical Observation Identifier Names and Codes (LOINC) is a universal coding system used to identify laboratory and other clinical observations, whereas the Systematized Nomenclature of Medicine (SNOMED) coding structure is commonly used in pathology. These standard languages are discussed in more detail in Chapter 22.

The RIS is similar to the LIS in that it incorporates data from multiple services that include X-rays, fluoroscopy, mammography, ultrasound, magnetic resonance imaging (MRI) scans, computed tomography (CT) scans, and other special procedures. It also uses coding structures such as Current Procedural Terminology (CPT) or International Classification of Diseases (ICD) to identify procedures, resources, and billing. However, the global standard for the transmission, storage, and display of medical imaging information is Digital Imaging and

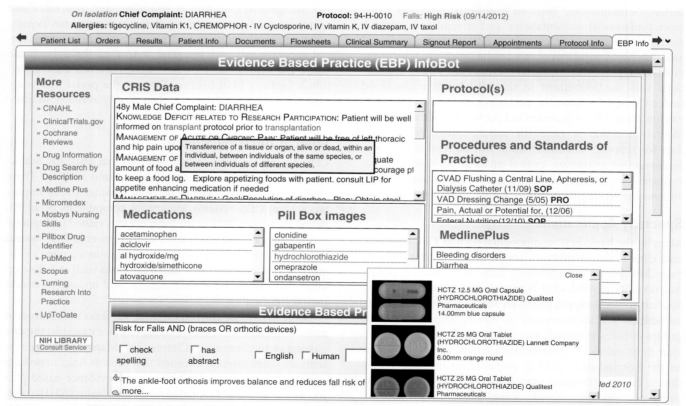

FIG 6.2 EBP InfoBot. (EBP Infobot developed by the National Library of Medicine (NLM) in collaboration with the National Institutes of Health, Clinical Center (NIHCC) Patient Care Services. Screenshot used with permission from NLM.)

Communications in Medicine (DICOM). The RIS may integrate data from a picture archiving and communication system (PACS), which stores digital versions of diagnostic images for display in the EHR.

The pharmacy department typically has a system to assist with inventory, prescription management, billing, and dispensing of medications. The FDA requires that all drugs be registered and reported using a National Drug Code (NDC). The NDC and SNOMED C axis are examples of coding structures that would be used in a pharmacy system. RxNorm is another standard mandated by the Office of the National Coordinator for Health related to MU reporting and data exchange. Clinical screening can be done by monitoring medication usage throughout the hospital and identifying potential adverse drug events. Prescriptions can be tracked along with printing of labels and medication instructions for patients or staff. The pharmacy system can provide patient drug profiles that include current and past medications, allergies, and contraindications. These features are designed to enhance patient safety. A closed-loop medication management system connects the pharmacy system to the CPOE, eMAR, and bar coding systems.

ELECTRONIC HEALTH RECORD BENEFITS

Most health policy initiatives are designed to address a triad of concerns that focus on cost, access, and quality. For example, concerns regarding the increasing cost of prescription drugs became the focus of Medicare reform legislation in 2003. Recent policy directed toward the adoption of EHR systems also highlights these concerns. The HITECH Act (2009) and the Patient Protection and Affordable Care Act (2010) addressed the need for EHR adoption to improve the quality, safety, and efficiency of care. With this in mind, the benefits of an EHR will be presented in terms of cost, access, and quality, safety, and efficiency of care delivery.

Cost

Cost savings is always a big motivator, especially if a healthcare provider or institution wants to stay in business. Numerous studies focusing on direct cost savings related to EHR use reported a positive financial return on investment for the healthcare organization.[60-64] Other cost benefits include increased productivity, efficiency in billing, improved reimbursement rates, improved verification of coverage, faster turnaround for accounts, lower medical record costs, support for pay-for-performance bonuses, and enhanced regulatory requirement compliance.[61,64-66] Benefits to patient care were also seen related to lower costs associated with disease management and decreased length of stay.[65,67]

Access

An EHR provides better and faster access to patient care information. Looking for paper charts that mysteriously disappear from the nurses' station or waiting for medical records to retrieve an old record are events of the past. An EHR allows simultaneous access to patient records and restricts users'

access to only the information that they are permitted to view. Many systems contain functionality such as graphs and charts that trend on demand and tools that facilitate comparison of current and past data. Another benefit is that clinicians have access to drug information, decision support tools, and resources to supplement patient care. Alerts and triggers that warn users of drug interactions and allergies can prevent medication errors. Clinical research often involves reviewing chart data, and can be a cumbersome process if done manually. The EHR provides a more effective and efficient method to access and aggregate data for research. As EHR adoption continues to expand, this will improve data access across multiple facilities and provide better continuity of care.

Quality, Safety, and Efficiency of Care Delivery

One of the main reasons to adopt an EHR is the potential to improve the quality, safety, and efficiency of care delivery. *Quality* is an ambiguous term that has a variety of meanings. Quality as it relates to EHR technology is fostered through better management of health information and improved data integrity. This may take the form of providing data that are readable, organized, accurate, and complete. *Quality* could also refer to increased staff and patient satisfaction, improved care coordination, and support for benchmarking. Safety and efficiency are much easier to quantify. Reducing medication errors has been a major focus of CPOE implementation and BCMA. Systems that support clinical decision making and provide early warnings of changes in patient status can be used to avert medical errors. Diagnosis and treatment options can be explored using decision support technology. Clinical and operational efficiencies in communication, workflow, documentation, and administrative functions are reported benefits of EHR adoption.

STAKEHOLDER PERSPECTIVES

In most organizations, the implementation of an EHR will affect multiple groups or stakeholders that share a stake in the outcome of this endeavor. Stakeholders may have similar concerns about the technology but different needs and approaches for resolution. It is important to consider many perspectives; essential stakeholders may include consumers, nurses and other healthcare providers, healthcare administration and organizations, insurance payers, and state and national governments.

Consumers

Healthcare consumers or patients have a unique vantage point for evaluating the effect of EHRs. They see multiple providers in a variety of settings and recognize gaps in care coordination. They often provide the same information repeatedly and are aware of tests being duplicated because the results were lost or inaccessible. They notice when individual arrangements must be made to hand carry a CD-ROM or paper record from one setting to another.

In 2011, the National Partnership for Women & Families conducted a national survey to determine patients' expectations regarding EHRs and health IT. The survey included patients who met two criteria: (1) they had an ongoing relationship with a main doctor and (2) they knew if their physician was using either electronic or paper record system. The survey was repeated in 2014 with 2045 adults, representing 68% of the adult population in the United States after the data were weighted to represent the demographics of the national adult population.[68] Consumers quickly and intuitively recognized that health IT can contribute directly to fewer medical errors, lower costs, and better health outcomes.[69,70] They see the benefits that technology has brought to other areas of their lives and understand how private and secure health IT can improve our nation's healthcare system.[68] The key findings from the 2014 survey are provided in Box **6.2**.

Nurses

Nurses constitute one of the largest groups of users of the EHR, and their perspective is critical to the successful integration of current and future technology. There are mixed reviews on user satisfaction related to individual systems, but nurses must, in most cases, embrace the EHR as a way to enhance consistency and quality of care.[71-73] Several studies reported that nurses' perception of an EHR was positive and that, overall, the system increased productivity, improved performance, enhanced effectiveness, was easy to use, and supported clinical care and research.[71,74,75] Other reported benefits involve improvements related to centralized access to patient information, clinical documentation, monitoring patient status, and resources for patient education.

Nurses are responsible for distributing medications to patients under their care. Because the EMR and EHR usually

interface with a pharmacy system, eMAR, and bar coding technology, the potential exists to decrease administration-related medication errors. Knowledge-based systems may include functionality that integrates clinical guidelines or protocols to assist nurses in the development of critical pathways and plans of care.

Nurse leaders struggle to measure quality outcomes required by the Joint Commission (TJC), the Centers for Medicare & Medicaid Services (CMS), and other regulatory agencies. The EHR provides the ability to access data and compare across institutions for benchmarking. Stefan[76] suggested several quality metrics that nurse leaders should evaluate when implementing an EHR, including timely access and documentation of patient information, EBP alerts, effect on length of stay, discharge follow-up with patients, and accuracy of documentation for reimbursement and regulatory agencies.

Healthcare Providers

In a recent study of EHR use in primary care practices, physicians and staff reported increased efficiencies related to billing and care coordination, access to current and past medical records, storing of patient information, and overall office operations.[77] Doyle et al.[78] concurred with these findings and concluded that EHRs used in the healthcare provider's examination room facilitate a partnership between physician and patient through collaboration of treatment plan options, and increase patient teaching by sharing of online medical information. In other studies, physicians also reported improvements in prescribing and medication safety when ePrescribing and decision support tools were available.[79,80] EHRs that provide tools for comprehensive documentation, warnings for changes in patient status, medication alerts, and follow-up and preventive care reminders improve decision making, which can reduce liability for the physician.[81] In addition, automated reporting capabilities enhance compliance to quality and regulatory requirements.[82]

Overall, healthcare providers reported favorable opinions about the EHR, citing many potential benefits related to clinical, organizational, and consumer outcomes.[65] Clinical benefits are often seen through the reduction of medical and medication errors, better health and disease management, and enhanced quality of care. Financial needs of the physician practice are streamlined and more efficient with electronic access to payer information and reporting to facilitate compliance with regulatory requirements. Workflow, communication, and coordination of care activities improve when there is easier access to records and other resources. Consumers also benefit from EHR technology when there is collaborative interaction between patients and physicians, more timely access to personal health information, and online access to educational materials.[70]

Healthcare Organizations

A current question for healthcare organizations is how to stay financially viable in a healthcare environment determined to control escalating healthcare costs. Added to this burden is the mandate to implement comprehensive EHR systems to meet MU criteria and reap the benefits of available incentives. Depending on the size and complexity of each organization, costs for implementing EHR technology are a significant investment. Beyond the initial expense for the hardware and software are fees associated with consultants and programmers to assist with implementation, licensing, maintenance, and providing staff time away from regular duties to participate in the process. For the healthcare executive, implementing EHR systems has the potential to improve operational efficiency, strengthen communication throughout the organization, increase patient safety, support compliance with regulatory requirements, improve medical record security and storage, improve care coordination, enhance the quality of care, and provide faster turnaround for procedure authorization, billing, and claims submission.

Healthcare executives and leaders must look at leveraging this technology not only to control costs but also to improve the quality of care. The successful implementation of information systems requires an understanding of the technical, cultural, and organization factors that influence change. Healthcare executives must also reflect beyond single-facility implementation to the possible benefits of system integration that will foster collaboration at local, national, and international levels.

Insurance Payers

The EHR provides several benefits for insurance companies through better disease management and reporting of services. Pay-for-performance requirements are supported and can be submitted in a timely manner. Claims that are incorrectly coded or that lack coding standards can confuse payers when they attempt to reimburse organizations for services. Systems that integrate patient data with coding and billing structures can provide data to control costs and manage expensive procedures.

State and National Governments

Over the past 20 years, the cost of healthcare in the United States has risen to nearly $2.6 trillion, and it is expected to grow faster than the national income.[83] One proposed measure for cost containment focuses on improving coordination and quality of care. The implementation of a nationwide interoperable EHR is recommended as a solution that would significantly reduce medical errors, improve care quality, and save the U.S. healthcare system major expense.[18,84] The United States is behind other developed nations in deploying technology of this magnitude. A major challenge is how to support the sharing of patient data across multiple organizations, requiring a nationwide technology infrastructure and communication standards, such as standardized nomenclatures, vocabularies, and coding structures.[4] Although the initial expenditures for such a system would be high, the anticipated benefits to our nation would be the ability to identify and address safety issues in a timely fashion, notify patients and populations at risk for disease or environmental exposure, detect epidemics, and prepare for bioterrorism

attacks.[85] A clinical dataset of essential information would be available, allowing researchers to explore preventive and curative solutions that address the nation's health and healthcare issues. Ultimately, the adoption of a nationwide EHR system would assist government agencies to improve overall healthcare for all U.S. citizens.

KEY ISSUES

The actual and potential benefits of an EHR are promising, but challenges also exist. This section focuses on several issues associated with EHR adoption related to cost, ownership, data integrity, privacy and confidentiality, standards, organizational culture, user experience, patient access, and patient-generated health data (PGHD).

Cost

The cost to implement and maintain an EHR is a major barrier. There are basically five financial components to consider when purchasing a system: (1) hardware, (2) software, (3) design and implementation assistance, (4) training, and (5) ongoing maintenance.[86] Physicians in a large private practice can expect to spend an estimated $162,000 or more to purchase and implement a certified EHR along with first-year maintenance expenses around $85,000.[87] This does not include the ongoing maintenance costs or hiring of technical staff to keep the system running on a daily basis. If a practice is using paper records, additional staff may be needed to enter previous patient data into the new system. Providers with a noncertified EHR will need to replace or update the system to meet standards, and data conversion may be necessary to move from the old system to the new system.

For hospitals and healthcare corporations, EHR technology expenses can range from $1 million to $100 million or more depending on the size of the facility, software vendor selection, and functionality purchased. Annual maintenance is an added expense that can be approximately 18% to 20% of the purchase price. In both scenarios, financial planning for initial and ongoing training, technical support, and software upgrades must be considered. The bottom line is that implementing and maintaining an IT system is very expensive. Currently, each healthcare organization purchases its own EHR; connections to other facilities are less common, although this trend is changing with the use of HIE. It is unclear who will be responsible for the electronic links that will form the infrastructure for local, regional, or national EHRs of the future.

Ownership

Ownership of the patient record is another issue. Traditional health records have always been the property of the service institution. Patient access to this record could be permitted, but sometimes at a cost. A comprehensive, interoperable EHR would cross institutional boundaries and include patient interaction, making ownership more complex. Because healthcare providers use many of the same data, many questions are currently unanswered: for example, What data will be shared? How will users access these data? Who will be responsible for updating and ensuring data accuracy? Who will store the shared data? Should the concept of ownership and access be completely separate concepts so that those responsible for storing, updating, and ensuring data accuracy are considered data stewards as opposed to the owners of these data? For example, the patient may own the data but the responsibilities of data stewardship may reside with a healthcare institution. Would patients and consumers have access to the data or a subset of the data? What role would the government play in monitoring the access, quality, security, privacy, and confidentiality of patient records?

Consumer consent and access are critical elements of the EHR adoption initiative that has significant implications for healthcare organizations and the issue of ownership. Some healthcare providers may be uncomfortable with the prospect of patients reading their notes and may alter what and how they document to accommodate consumer access. Consumer consent is required for health professionals to retrieve or share patient records to ensure that personal information is not accessed inappropriately. This rule could affect quality of care if the consumer is concerned about confidentiality and denies permission. Ultimately, ownership may be driven by who has control and access to the data; or ownership may become irrelevant as access becomes the driving force in answering these many questions.

Data Integrity

Data integrity refers to the accuracy and consistency of stored and transmitted data that can be compromised when information is entered incorrectly or deliberately altered or when the system protections are not working correctly or suddenly fail. As EHR adoption expands to include data from multiple healthcare entities, more opportunities for human error exist. Poor screen designs that are confusing and cumbersome and lack of system training often lead to data entry errors. How this will be monitored and who is responsible for correcting inaccurate information will be an issue. Critical patient information, such as allergies, medical history, and medications, should always be validated and updated at each episode of care. Education on how to use the EHR should be provided to all staff before implementing a new system, when changes are made to an existing system, and during orientation for new employees. Stringent security measures that include audit trails, penalties for fraudulent activities, and detailed policies and procedures are other measures that protect data integrity.

Data integrity can also be affected if a system is not working correctly or suddenly fails. Unfortunately, users do not always recognize when a feature is not functioning, such as a broken alert or incorrect calculations, and this leads to inaccuracies in data. When an interface from one application to another is not working, this also may not be readily noticeable. For example, a physician is able to enter orders using CPOE, but the interface to the pharmacy department system fails and medication orders are not received or dispensed, or orders do not arrive in the laboratory and the blood is not drawn. A healthcare provider may discover the problem only when it is time to administer medications or when test results are not available. These kinds of problems ultimately affect patient care. If the interface resumes functioning, the orders may cross over, but depending on the time the order was placed, some data may be lost or corrupted or a new order may have been placed. Support mechanisms, such as the customer help desk maintaining automated, sortable records of issues reported, along with rigorous system testing, is extremely important to ensuring data integrity.

Privacy and Confidentiality

Despite advances in technology and robust software that limits access to computerized health information, privacy and confidentiality continue to be major concerns for both the healthcare professional and consumer. With the expansion of the EHR and HIE as a driving force to automate and share health information, clinicians may find government and regulatory requirements for controlled access to patient information too restrictive or an invasion of privacy. In this respect, providers may be less inclined to use the EHR or more cautious when documenting patient care to avoid litigation. As with facilities, consumers can also be bombarded with computer breaches, such as viruses, spyware, and hackers. Some consumers do not trust that health IT will be any different from traditional healthcare. They fear that a large-scale EHR system could allow access to personal data without adequate protection against unauthorized use of information. Some consumers prefer that sensitive health information (such as psychiatric care) never be shared, which creates problems because this can represent critical information missing from a medical record. Before a nationwide interoperable EHR can be fully implemented, major issues related to privacy and security need to be addressed. This topic is discussed in more detail in Chapter 26.

Standards

In a famous commentary on hospitals in 1863, Florence Nightingale wrote, "In attempting to arrive at the truth, I have applied everywhere for information, but in scarcely an instance have I been able to obtain hospital records fit for any purposes of comparison. If they could be obtained they would enable us to decide many other questions besides the ones alluded to. They would show subscribers how their money was being spent, what amount of good was really being done with it, or whether the money was not doing mischief rather than good."[88, p. 176] Over 150 years later, these same issues with extracting data for comparisons still exist. Healthcare professionals have been discussing the need for standardized vocabularies and terminologies for many decades. Implementation has been hindered by numerous factors related to disagreement on which terminologies to use, lack of standards to harmonize multiple coding structures, cultural and language barriers, interpretation of meaning, threats to autonomy, and user resistance. The benefits of standardization allow for a mutual understanding of terms and improved communication among healthcare professionals along with a common way to collect and aggregate data. A universal language would allow us to consistently capture, represent, access, and communicate clinical data, information, and knowledge across all settings. Although progress is underway, standards continue to be an issue for EHR adoption.

Organizational Culture

The healthcare environment is filled with many cultures, subcultures, and traditions, and the implementation of an EHR is almost always disruptive to the sociocultural system. A disruptive technology is an innovation that replaces long-held traditional ideas and ways of doing things. This type of technology can improve or replace a product in ways that are unexpected and often opens up new market demand, which leads to lower-priced products or products designed for a different set of consumers. Cell phones, e-mail, Twitter, and Facebook have significantly changed our interpersonal, professional, and business communications. In this respect, a disruptive technology such as the EHR may challenge and/or alter social and cultural norms. How these cultures respond to change will vary based on belief systems, values, roles within the healthcare team, and computer knowledge.

Healthcare organizations are challenged with issues surrounding the evolving nature of EHR technology, one of the most important of which is user acceptance. Whether in a hospital setting or private practice, nurses, physicians, and other caregivers are required to use an EHR as part of their daily routine, but some find it difficult to comply. Reasons for this vary from lack of computer skills to complexity of application, poorly designed systems, lack of available hardware, or difficulty adjusting to change. Caregivers often indicate that documenting in the computer interferes with routine workflow or takes away from valuable time with patients. When CPOE was enforced by some institutions, physicians complained that entering orders in the computer was a task beneath them because this was traditionally secretarial work. This also had an effect on the role of nurses because they no longer had to interpret and validate handwritten orders. Physicians entered these orders in isolation, and the computer forced them to be more specific during the entry process. Nurses' workflow changed because they no longer had a paper form to alert them when new orders became available. Although the computer can provide new order alerts, it requires frequent access to the electronic record. Checking the computer more often was disruptive to care, and new procedures were needed to avoid mistakes and delays. These types of reasons for resistance must be addressed for an EHR adoption to be successful. Acceptance of this technology is dependent on effective leadership, user involvement, the ability of the system to integrate with workflow, the ability of the users to adapt and change workflow processes, and timely education and technical support.

User Experience

A significant amount of time is spent by all healthcare providers in processing and documenting patient-related data, but using an EHR system for these activities can be perceived as a frustrating experience.[89] Research on human-computer interaction has identified several issues related to the usability of EHRs. In an early study by Despont-Gros et al.[90] on human-computer interaction models, they reported user acceptance to be a reliable concept to reflect evaluation of clinical information systems. Problems with usability related to complex human-computer interfaces, poorly designed decision support tools, and lack of training are recognized as obstacles that lead to significant medical errors and resistance to accept the technology.[17,89,91,92]

The complexities of EHR technology add concerns that new types of errors are beginning to emerge. Many clinicians complain that information systems increase their workload, which decreases productivity and efficiency. In a landmark study, Ash et al.[17] reported that EMR systems could have a negative effect on communication and teamwork because of the linear processing of computer systems, which conflicts with the more fluid iterative and interruptive nature of providing care. They also concluded that cognitive workload increased with unnecessary clerical tasks, overly structured data entry requirements, and fragmented patient data retrieval formats. Addressing issues related to user experience is complex and requires early user involvement and attention to system design and testing.[92] User experience concepts are discussed in detail in Chapter 21.

Patient Access to the Electronic Health Record

Consumer demand for access to personal protected healthcare information (PHI) is increasing. The EHR has the potential to enhance patient-provider communication and outcomes through electronic messaging, scheduling, reminders, access to laboratory and test results, tracking of progress, and educational resources. Despite these advancements, barriers still exist related to providing consumer access to all data stored in the EHR, such as clinical notes. Cost is a major issue because most hospitals and private practices may lack funding and/or technology resources and support to implement a system for full patient access.[93] The EHR was not originally created for consumer use, and it requires a great deal of redesign and financial investment to allow outside access.

Another consideration is that patients are often seen in a variety of hospitals, other healthcare entities, and by multiple providers. Information is not usually centrally located in one system but fragmented across several different facilities and practices. The technical infrastructure to integrate (or interface) data from these disparate systems is difficult, as well as costly.[94]

Recent reports of health insurance and government data violations fuel concerns over privacy, confidentiality, and security of personal health data. The Health Information Portability and Accountability Act (HIPAA) security rules for electronic health data were established to require entities to take appropriate "administrative, physical, and technical safeguards to ensure the confidentiality, integrity, and security of electronic protected health information."[95] Providers are at risk for lawsuits if strict precautions are not taken and patient data is compromised.[93,96] Caine and Tierney reported that privacy concerns can cause patients to lose trust in providers, withhold important information, or avoid seeking care.[96] This is especially true for patients with sensitive problems such as mental health issues or HIV. Capturing patient preferences related to who can access specific information within an EHR can be difficult to manage and administer.[97]

Consumers have a legal right to request access to PHI, but, as mentioned earlier, control of the data is still debatable. Even if access to PHI is available, consumers may be restricted from viewing certain entries, such as physician notes, and the ability to easily update or correct information is rare. Some providers resist allowing patients real-time access to health records but defend their own right to access all PHI to provide comprehensive care.[93,94] In addition, providers are concerned that patients may not have the knowledge or skills to interpret the information in the health record. In a pilot study of 688 veterans who used a PHR, physicians reported that sharing notes and other health information with patients can be "confusing or harmful," and they were less likely to encourage the use a PHR.[98]

Tension between provider and consumer expectations with EHR access is evident. There is concern that patient access to EHR data will be interpreted as unlimited access to providers. Disagreements related to e-mail use and what can be addressed online versus routine office visits can lead to dissatisfaction with care.[93,94,96] The fear of increased workload or workflow interruptions may hinder online engagement by clinicians. Some clinicians are concerned that consumers may find mistakes in the record, which could prompt legal action, or that patient access to their data would lead to unnecessary worry. Consumer expectations related to data access also filters into the clinical setting. In a recent study of hospitalized patients who were provided real-time access to select EHR data reported positive results related to patient empowerment and clinician optimism. Findings indicated that concerns related to increased workload, identifying mistakes, and patient confusion were unsupported.[99] Other studies have reported that patients are more comfortable during office visits when the physician shares online data and invites interaction with computer.[100]

Consumers who lack computer skills may have difficulty accessing and using EHR systems. A common practice is to provide patients with a link to an EHR portal without any training on how to navigate the site. Chronic illnesses, debilitating diseases, or pain can hinder interest or ability to access a portal. Once access is achieved, consumers may lack the knowledge to interpret the medical results or information provided. Some providers prefer to delay release of test results in a portal until after they discuss findings with the patient verbally. Advocates for immediate and timely access to data contend that there is a need to provide information to consumers in a format that does not require medical training.[94] Despite the need for more effective communication, the task of translating complex interprofessional language into common terms may lead to resistance by healthcare professionals.

Patient-Generated Health Data

Patient-generated health data (PGHD) are defined as "health-related data created, recorded, or gathered by or from patients (or family members or care givers) to help address a health concern" (para 1).[101] Although most EHR systems that provide a patient portal "push" data for viewing, few offer the flexibility and functionality to capture PGHD to augment care. Traditional methods of gathering PGHD through daily logs and journals are common but are rarely directly entered into an EHR by patients. Technology has a pivotal role in the collection of large amounts of PGHD using mobile devices such as smartphones, laptops, and computers, to wearable items such as wristbands, clothing, belt clips, and patches.[102-104] PGHD transmitted or entered into an EHR portal provides an opportunity to monitor and track progress and actively engage patients in care management. Despite these benefits, use of PGHD is met with some scrutiny by healthcare professionals.

There are several major concerns associated with PGHD related to volume, quality of data, privacy, and security.[102,105] The volume of data reported by patients can be overwhelming to providers, leading to information overload and workflow concerns. Discerning which data are pertinent or not could be very time consuming. Detailed data might be useful in gaining insight into a patient problem but could also hinder effective analysis because of challenges associated with screening large amounts of data. This also raises questions about who is responsible for checking the data, when and how often, and what are the liabilities if timely review and response to data does not occur.

Patients may provide more detail than needed, as well as deviate from the actual problem to include experiences of others or data unrelated to their condition.[105] Patients may not be aware of which data should be included when reporting an issue or decide not to report a change because they think it is not important to their condition. Some patients may try to manipulate data to force a certain outcome such as obtaining certain prescription medications. In addition, personal opinions or inappropriate comments could be problematic and cause discomfort for healthcare providers. In a study of patients with diabetes, a significant number of errors related to underreporting of glucose readings, overreporting or adding readings that were not measured, and recording values incorrectly were found.[106] Underreporting and overreporting indicated a need for patients to fill in the blanks to comply with the health provider's directions. Incorrect data entry was a concern because treatment options may be unrelated to status and cause harm or ineffective disease management.

As with patient access to EHR data, privacy and security is a major concern with PGHD as well. Whether direct entry into a portal or transmitted through a device, assurance is critical that the data is from an authenticated source and linked to the correct patient through a secure portal.[102] Some EHR vendors are beginning to integrate data from PGHD sources directly or through questionnaires, but there is still a need for technologies with the ability to transform and filter PGHD into meaningful information to improve decision making and clinical outcomes.[102,107]

CONCLUSION AND FUTURE DIRECTIONS

EHR has become the preferred term for the lifetime patient record that would include healthcare data from the consumer and a variety of provider sources. The IOM identified eight essential care delivery components for all EHRs: (1) administrative processes, (2) communication and connectivity, (3) decision support, (4) health information and data, (5) order entry management, (6) patient support, (7) results management, and (8) population health management.[14] Dentistry and optometry records were added to this list by the Department of Defense.[15]

Common EHR applications used in the clinical setting include CPOE, eMAR, BCMA, clinical documentation, specialty applications, and CDS. The HITECH Act (2009) established programs to accelerate EHR adoption, one of which offers financial incentives for hospitals and healthcare providers who adopt certified EHR technology and comply with federal MU objectives. How the HITECH Act followed by the MACRA Act will address the needs of health practitioners is unclear, but many are actively involved in local, regional, and national initiatives to improve the quality, safety, and efficiency of care using technology. Current research findings indicate that EHR benefits related to cost, access, quality, safety, and efficiency of care delivery support healthcare policy initiatives driving adoption. Despite the many advances in technology, there are still numerous issues to resolve associated with implementation costs, ownership, data integrity, privacy and confidentiality, organizational culture, user experience, patient access, PGD, and the development of an infrastructure to support a nationwide EHR. Future directions are promising for the EHR for personalizing care, supporting research efforts, and mobilizing care coordination across national and international boundaries.

In the future, the EHR will play a pivotal role in personalized medicine as a medium for data, information, knowledge exchange, and exploration. Advanced computing and systems integration will provide powerful evaluation tools to facilitate healthcare providers and consumers in the decision-making process. Genetic testing, along with access to an interoperable EHR, can be used to diagnose, prevent, and treat preexisting and potential health issues based on our unique biological responses, resulting in highly individualized care. Genomics and phenotyping will likely hold the key to disease detection and treatment with the promise of designer medications that target the unique characteristics of each individual.[108,109] In the future, an individual's genome sequence may be part of a comprehensive medical record, not unlike recording medications and allergies.[108]

Customized medications will likely eliminate prescribing drugs or doses that do not work, minimize side effects, and decrease costs. Other treatments, such as diet and exercise, can be personalized to avoid much guesswork and trial and error. For example, if a patient's genetic code reveals a risk for colon cancer, then preventive measures can start earlier. More frequent exams, colonoscopies, and diets that promote colon health can be the focus of care. In addition to personalizing care, the EHR will contain a wealth of information related to disease, interventions, and treatment responses that can be used for research. The emergence of dental informatics and the development of dental repositories will provide data for a more comprehensive EHR record.[110,111] Data mining of these huge databases can reveal patterns and predictions on how to reverse or prevent disease.

The EHR continues to be an evolving concept with global and national implications. In 2014, the Office of the National Coordinator for Health Information Technology (ONC) reported that three out of four (76%) hospitals had adopted at least a basic EHR system. This represented an increase of 27% from 2013 and an eightfold increase since 2008.[112] As of early 2015, using the HIMSS EMRAM, EHR adoption rates in U.S. hospitals were progressing with approximately 32.3% at Stage 5 and another 23.6% at Stage 6 or above.[27] The rate of adoption by physician practices and clinics was much lower, with 33.98% at Stage 1 and 28.68% at Stage 2. Although hospitals may be in a better position to fulfill MU objectives, additional support and guidance may be needed to achieve nationwide implementation goals. Many other countries, such as Canada, Australia, England, and Finland, have focused their efforts on building an infrastructure and developing systems that support health information at a national level.[113] The European Commission has launched several initiatives to improve the safety and quality of care through information sharing at an international level, such as the eHealth Action Plan that supports standardization of EHR content and structure, and the Smart Open Services (SOS) project that recommends allowing healthcare provider access to critical medical information for consumers traveling abroad.[113-115] EHR adoption has the potential to reach beyond the borders of this nation to meet the needs of a mobile society.

REFERENCES

1. Sewell J, Thede L. *Informatics and Nursing: Opportunities and Challenges.* 3rd ed. Philadelphia, PA: Lippincott, Williams, & Wilkins; 2013.
2. Hebda T, Czar P. *Handbook of Informatics for Nurses and Healthcare Professionals.* 5th ed. Boston, MA: Pearson; 2012.
3. National Library of Medicine (NLM). *Medline/PubMed Search and Electronic Health Record Information Resources.* NLM; 2015. http://www.nlm.nih.gov/services/queries/ehr.html/.
4. Seckman C, Romano C. Electronic health record. In: Feldman H, ed. *Nursing Leadership: A Concise Encyclopedia.* 2nd ed. New York, NY: Springer; 2012:126–128.
5. National Alliance for Health Information Technology. *Defining Key Health Information Technology Terms;* 2008. https://www.nachc.com/client/Key%20HIT%20Terms%20Definitions%20Final_April_2008.pdf.
6. Healthcare Information and Management. *Electronic Health Record.* HIMSS; 2015. http://www.himss.org/library/ehr/.
7. Barey E, Mastrian K, McGonigle D. The electronic health record and clinical informatics. In: McGonigle D, Mastrian K, eds. *Nursing Informatics and the Foundation of Knowledge.* 3rd ed. Burlington, MA: Jones & Bartlett; 2014:249–265.

8. Alexander S. The Electronic Health Record. In: Alexander S, Frith KH, Haley H, eds. *Applied Clinical Informatics for Nurses.* Burlington, MA: Jones & Bartlett; 2015:199–221.

9. Keyhani S, Hebert P, Ross J, Federman A, Zhu C, Siu A. Electronic health record components and the quality of care. *Med Care.* 2008;46(12):1267–1272.

10. Dowding D, Turley M, Garrido T. The impact of an electronic health record on nurse sensitive patient outcomes: an interrupted time series analysis. *J Am Med Inform Assoc.* 2012;19(4):615–620.

11. Kelley T, Brandon D, Docherty S. Electronic nursing documentation as a strategy to improve quality of patient care. *J Nurs Scholarsh.* 2011;43(2):154–162.

12. Weaver C, Ball M, Kim G, Kiel J. The evolution of EHR-S functionality for care and coordination. *Healthc Inf Manag Syst.* 2016;73–99. http://dx.doi.org/10.1007/978-3-319-20765-0_5.

13. Gunter TD, Terry NP. The emergence of National Electronic Health Record architectures in the United States and Australia: models, costs, and questions. *J Med Internet Res.* 2005;7(1):e3. http://www.jmir.org/2005/1/e3/?trendmd-shared=1/.

14. Institute of Medicine. *Key Capabilities of an Electronic Health Record System: Letter Report from the Committee on Data Standards for Patient Safety: Board of Health Care Services;* 2003. http://www.nap.edu/catalog/10781/key-capabilities-of-an-electronic-health-record-system-letter-report/.

15. Anderson H. EHR pioneers try to stay out front. *Health Data Manag.* 2007;15(5):26–34.

16. Bates W, Teich J, Lee J, et al. The impact of computerized physician order entry on medication error prevention. *J Am Med Inform Assoc.* 1999;6(4):313–321.

17. Ash JS, Berg M, Coiera E. Patient care information systems-related errors. *J Am Med Inform Assoc.* 2004;11(2):104–112.

18. Kohn LT, Corrigan JM, Donaldson MS. *To Err Is Human: Building a Safer Health System.* Washington, DC: Institute of Medicine; 2000.

19. Campanella P, Lovato E, Marone C, et al. The impact of electronic health records on healthcare quality: a systematic review and meta-analysis. *Eur J Public Health.* June 30, 2015. http://dx.doi.org/10.1093/eurpub/ckv122.

20. Adler-Milstein J, Everson J, Lee SY. EHR adoption and hospital performance: time-related effects. *Health Serv Res.* 2015;1751–1771. http://dx.doi.org/10.1111/1475-6773.12406.

21. American Association of Colleges of Nursing. *Nursing Shortage;* April 24, 2014. http://www.aacn.nche.edu/media-relations/fact-sheets/nursing-shortage. updated.

22. Parsons A, McCullough C, Wang J, Shih S. Validity of electronic health record–derived quality measurement for performance monitoring. *J Am Med Inform Assoc.* 2012. http://dx.doi.org/10.1136/amiajnl-2011-000557.

23. HealthIT.gov. *Health IT Legislation.* Department of Health and Human Services; 2015. https://www.healthit.gov/policy-researchers-implementers/select-portions-hitech-act-and-relationship-onc-work/.

24. HealthIT. *EHR Incentives & Certification: How to Attain Meaingful Use.* Department of Health and Human Services; 2015. https://www.healthit.gov/providers-professionals/how-attain-meaningful-use.

25. Murphy J. HITECH programs supporting the journey to meaningful use of EHRS. *Comput Inform Nurs.* 2011;29(2):130–131. http://dx.doi.org/10.1097/NCN.0b013e318210f0fc.

26. Centers for Medicare and Medicaid Services.. *CMS Fact Sheet: EHR Incentive Programs in 2015 and beyond;* 2015. https://www.cms.gov/Newsroom/MediaReleaseDatabase/Fact-sheets/2015-Fact-sheets-items/2015-10-06-2.html/.

27. HIMSS Analytics. *Ambulatory EMR Adoption Model;* 2014. https://app.himssanalytics.org/emram/AEMRAM.aspx/.

28. HIMSS Analytics Europe. *Be Prepared For What's Next;* 2015. http://www.himssanalytics.eu/emram/.

29. Hoyt J. *State of the Industry: Informatics Perspectives on the EMR Adoption Model.* Healthcare Information and Management Systems Society; 2012. http://www.himss.org/News/NewsDetail.aspx?ItemNumber=6610/.

30. Greenwood K, Murphy J, Sensmeier J, Westra B. Nursing profession reengineered for leadership in landmark report: special report for the Alliance for Nursing Informatics member organizations. *Comput Inform Nurs.* 2011;29(2):66–67.

31. Farrell A, Taylor S. Electronic health record vendor applications. In: Saba V, McCormick K, eds. *Essentials of Nursing Informatics.* 5th ed. New York, NY: McGraw-Hill; 2011:317–339.

32. Cipriano P. The future of nursing and health IT: the quality elixir. *Nurs Econ.* 2011;29(5):286–289.

33. Harrison RL, Lyerla F. Using nursing clinical decision support systems to achieve Meaningful Use. *Comput Inform Nurs.* 2012;30(7):380–385. http://dx.doi.org/10.1097/NCN.0b013e31823eb813.

34. Westra BL, Subramanian A, Hart CM, et al. Achieving "meaningful use" of electronic health records through the integration of the nursing management minimum data set. *J Nurs Adm.* 2010;40(7-8):336–343. http://dx.doi.org/10.1097/NNA.0b013e3181e93994.

35. Nuckols TK, Smith-Spangler C, Morton SC, et al. The effectiveness of computerized order entry at reducing preventable adverse drug events and medication errors in hospital settings: a systematic review and meta-analysis. *Syst Rev.* 2014;3:56. http://www.biomedcentral.com/content/pdf/2046-4053-3-56.pdf/.

36. Bates DW, Leape LL, Cullen DJ, et al. Effect of computerized physician order entry and a team intervention on prevention of serious medication errors. *JAMA.* 1998;280(15):1311–1316.

37. Evans RS, Pestotnik SL, Classen DC, et al. A computer-assisted management program for antibiotics and other anti-infective agents. *N Engl J Med.* 1998;338(4):232–238. http://dx.doi.org/10.1056/NEJM199801223380406.

38. Gandhi TK, Weingart SN, Seger AC, et al. Outpatient prescribing errors and the impact of computerized prescribing. *J Gen Intern Med* 20(9):837-841. http://dx.doi.org/10.1111/j.1525-1497.2005.0194.x.

39. Mekhjian HS, Kumar RR, Kuehn L, et al. Immediate benefits realized following implementation of physician order entry at an academic medical center. *J Am Med Inform Assoc.* 2002;9(5):529–539.

40. Bates DW, Cohne M, Leape LL, Overhage M, Shabot MM, Sheridan T. Reducing the frequency of errors in medicine using information technology. *J Am Med Inform Assoc.* 2001;8(4):299–308.

41. Spalding SC, Mayer PH, Ginde AA, Lowenstein SR, Yaron M. Impact of computerized physician order entry on ED patient length of stay. *Am J Emerg Med.* 2011;29(2):207–211. http://dx.doi.org/10.1016/j.ajem.2009.10.007.

42. Altuwaijri MM, Bahanshal A, Almehaid M. Implementation of computerized physician order entry in National Guard

hospitals: assessment of critical success factors. *J Family Community Med.* 2011;18(3):143–151. http://dx.doi.org/10.4103/2230-8229.90014.

43. Chapman AK, Lehmann CU, Donohue PK, Aucott SW. Implementation of computerized provider order entry in a neonatal intensive care unit: impact on admission workflow. *Int J Med Inform.* 2012;81(5):291–295. http://dx.doi.org/10.1016/j.ijmedinf.2011.12.006.

44. Adam TJ, Waitman R, Jones I, Aronsky D. The effect of computerized provider order entry (CPOE) on ordering patterns for chest pain patients in the emergency department. *AMIA Annu Symp Proc.* 2011;38–47.

45. Hughes RG, ed. *Patient Safety and Quality: An Evidence-Based Handbook for Nurses.* Rockville, MD: Agency for Healthcare Research and Quality; 2006.

46. Koppel R, Metlay J, Cohen A, et al. Role of computerized physician order entry systems in facilitating medication errors. *J Am Med Inform Assoc.* 2005;293(10):1197–1203.

47. Seckman C, Romano C, Defensor R, Benham-Hutchins M. Design efficiencies and satisfaction of computerized physician order entry: a comparison of two order entry methods. Presented at the 16th Annual Summer Institute in Nursing Informatics held July 19-22, 2006 at the University of Maryland School of Nursing.

48. Payne TH, Nichol WP, Hoey P, Savarino J. Characteristics and override rates of order checks in a practitioner order entry system. *Proc AMIA Symp.* 2002;602–606.

49. Ash JS, Bates DW. Factors and forces affecting EHR system adoption: report of a 2004 ACMI discussion. *J Am Med Inform Assoc.* 2005;12(1):8–12.

50. Ash J, Sittig D, Dykstra R, Campbell E, Guappone K. The unintended consequences of computerized provider order entry: findings from a mixed methods exploration. *Int J Med Inform.* 2009;78S:S69–S76.

51. U.S. Food and Drug Administration (FDA). *Medication Errors*; 2015. http://www.fda.gov/drugs/drugsafety/medicationerrors/.

52. Poon EG, Keohane CA, Yoon CS, et al. Effect of bar-code technology on the safety of medication administration. *N Engl J Med.* 2010;362(18):1698–1707. http://dx.doi.org/10.1056/NEJMsa0907115.

53. Chou S, Yan H, Huang H, Tseng K, Kuo S. Establishing and evaluating bar-code technology in blood sampling system: a model based on human centered design method. In: *Proceedings from the NI2012: 11th International Congress on Nursing Informatics.* Montreal, Canada; 2012:79–82.

54. Tseng K, Feng R, Chou S, Lin S, Yan H, Huang H. Implementation and evaluation of the effectiveness of the bar-coded medication administration system in a medical center. In: *Proceedings from the NI2012: 11th International Congress on Nursing Informatics, Montreal, Canada*; 2012:416.

55. Seibert HH, Maddox RR, Williams CK. Effect of barcode technology with electronic medication administration record on medication accuracy rates. *Am J Health Syst Pharm.* 2014;73(3):209–218.

56. Dwibedi N, Sansgiry SS, Frost CP, et al. Effect of bar-code-assisted medication administration on nurses' activities in an intensive care unit: a time-motion study. *Am J Health Syst Pharm.* 2011;68(11):1026–1031. http://dx.doi.org/10.2146/ajhp100382; 10.2146/ajhp100382.

57. Versel N. *Emergency room patients tracked with RFID tags. Information Week;* 2011. http://www.informationweek.com/healthcare/electronic-medical-records/emergency-room-patients-tracked-with-rfi/231901224?queryText=emergency room patients tracked with RFID tags/.

58. Coiera E, Lau Y, Tsafnat G, Sintchenko V, Magrabi F. The changing nature of clinical decision support systems: a focus on consumers, genomics, public health and decision safety. *IMIA Yearb Med Inform.* 2009;84–95.

59. Demner-Fushman D, Seckman C, Fisher C, Thoma G. Continual development of a personalized decision support system. *Int Med Inform Assoc Proc.* 2013;175–179. http://www.nlm.nih.gov/medlineplus/connect/overview.html/http://dx.doi.org/10.3233/978-1-6499-289-9-175.

60. Forrester SH, Hepp A, Roth JA, Wirtz HS, Devine EB. Cost-effectiveness of a computerized provider order entry system in improving mediation safety ambulatory care. *Value Health.* 2014;17(4):340–349. http://dx.doi.org/10.1016/j.jval.2014.01.009 DOI:10.1016/j.jval.2014.01.009#doilink.

61. Li K, Naganawa S, Wang K, et al. Study of the cost-benefit analysis of electronic medical record systems in general hospital in China. *J Med Syst.* 2012;36(5):3283–3291. http://dx.doi.org/10.1007/s10916-011-9819-6.

62. Howley M, Chou EY, Hansen N, Dalrymple PW. The long-term financial impact of electronic health record implementation. *J Am Med Inform Assoc.* 2014;22(2):443–452. http://dx.doi.org/10.1136/amiajnl-2014-002686/.

63. Adler-Milstein J, Salzberg C, Franz C, Orav J, Newhouse JP, Bates DW. Effect of electronic health records on health care cost: longitudinal comparative evidence from community practices. *Ann Intern Med.* 2013;159:97–104.

64. Sockolow PS, Bowles KH, Adelsberger MC, Chittams JL, Liao C. Impact of homecare electronic health record on timeliness of clinical documentation, reimbursement, and patient outcomes. *Appl Clin Inform.* 2014;5(2):445–462. http://dx.doi.org/10.4338/ACI-2013-12-RA-0106.

65. Menachemi N, Collum TH. Benefits and drawbacks of electronic health record systems. *Risk Manag Healthc Pol.* 2011;4:47–55.

66. Uslu A, Stausberg J. Value of the electronic patient record: an analysis of the literature. *J Biomed Inform.* 2008;41:675–682.

67. Miskulin DC, Weiner DE, Tighiouart H, et al. Computerized decision support for EPO dosing in hemodialysis patients. *Am J Kidney Dis.* 2009;54(6):1081–1088. http://dx.doi.org/10.1053/j.ajkd.2009.07.010.

68. National Partnership for Women & Families. *Engaging Patients and Families: How Consumers Value and Use Health It.* Washington, DC; December 2014. Available from, http://www.nationalpartnership.org/research-library/health-care/HIT/engaging-patients-and-families.pdf/.

69. Undern T. *Consumers and Health Information Technology: A National Survey.* Oakland, CA: California Healthcare Foundation; April 2010. http://www.chcf.org/publications/2010/04/consumers-and-health-information-technology-a-national-survey/.

70. Pushpangadan S, Seckman C. Consumer perceptive of personal health records. *Online J Nurs Inform.* 2015;19(1). Available from: http://www.himss.org/ResourceLibrary/GenResourceDetail.aspx?ItemNumber=39756/.

71. Judd M, Sackett KM. *Evidence Leveling: Electronic Health Record (HER) Choice for Perceived Nursing Benefit, Usability, Acceptance and Satisfaction.* In: *Sigma Theta Tau International 26th International Nursing Research Congress I San Juan, Puerto Rico*; July 24, 2015. https://stti.confex.com/stti/congrs15/webprogram/Paper72813.html/.

72. HealthIT.gov. *Benefits of EHR's*; 2004. https://www.healthit. gov/providers-professionals/electronic-medical-records-emr/.

73. Cherry BJ, Ford EW, Peterson LT. Experiences with electronic health records: early adopters in long-term care facilities. *Health Care Manage Rev.* 2011;36(3):265–274. http://dx.doi. org/10.1097/HMR.0b013e31820e110f; 10.1097/ HMR.0b013e31820e110f.

74. Chisolm DJ, Purnell TS, Cohen DM, McAlearney AS. Clinician perceptions of an electronic medical record during the first year of implementation in emergency services. *Pediatr Emerg Care.* 2010;26(2):107–110. http://dx.doi.org/10.1097/ PEC.0b013e3181ce2f99.

75. Seckman C, Mills M, Friedmann E, Romano C. Clinicians' perception of usability of an electronic health record over time. *Comput Inform Nurs.* 2009;27(5):331.

76. Stefan S. Using clinical EHR metrics to demonstrate quality outcomes. *Nurs Manag.* 2011;42(3):17–19. http://dx.doi.org/ 10.1097/01. NUMA.0000394062.30819.61.

77. Goetz Goldberg D, Kuzel AJ, Feng LB, DeShazo JP, Love LE. EHRs in primary care practices: benefits, challenges, and successful strategies. *Am J Manag Care.* 2012;18(2):e48–e54.

78. Doyle RJ, Wang N, Anthony D, Borkan J, Shield RR, Goldman RE. Computers in the examination room and the electronic health record: physicians' perceived impact on clinical encounters before and after full installation and implementation. *Fam Pract;* 2012. http://dx.doi.org/10.1093/ fampra/cms015.

79. Abramson EL, Barron Y, Quaresimo J, Kaushal R. Electronic prescribing within an electronic health record reduces ambulatory prescribing errors. *Jt Comm J Qual Patient Saf.* 2011;37(10):470–478.

80. Kaushal R, Kern LM, Barron Y, Quaresimo J, Abramson EL. Electronic prescribing improves medication safety in community-based office practices. *J Gen Intern Med.* 2010;25 (6):530–536. http://dx.doi.org/10.1007/s11606-009-1238-8.

81. Mangalmurti SS, Murtagh L, Mello M. Medical malpractice liability in the age of electronic health records. *N Engl J Med.* 2010;363(21):2060–2067.

82. Bell B, Thornton K. From promise to reality: achieving the value of an EHR. *Healthc Financ Manage.* 2011;65(2):50–56.

83. Kaiser Family Foundation. *U.S. health care costs. KaiserEDU. org;* 2015. http://www.kaiseredu.org/issue-modules/us-health-care-costs/background-brief.aspx/.

84. Kumar S, Aldrich K. Overcoming barriers to electronic medical record (EMR) implementation in the U.S. healthcare system: a comparative study. *Health Informatics J.* 2010;16(4):306–318. http://dx.doi.org/10.1177/1460458210380523.

85. Office of the National Coordinator. *EHR Benefits for Our Country's Health. HealthIT.gov;* 2013. http://www.healthit.gov/ patients-families/ehr-benefits-our-countrys-health. Updated.

86. HealthIT.Gov. *How Much Is This Going To Cost Me?* Department of Health and Human Resources; 2014. https:// www.healthit.gov/providers-professionals/faqs/how-much-going-cost-me/.

87. Fleming NS, Culler SD, McCorkle R, Becker ER, Ballard D. The financial and nonfinancial cost of implementing electronic health records in primary care practices. *Health Aff.* 2011;30 (3):481–489.

88. Nightingale F. *Notes on Hospitals.* London, United Kingdom: Longman, Green, Longman, Roberts, and Green; 1863. http:// archive.org/stream/notesonhospital01nighgoog#page/n218/ mode/2up/.

89. Gillespie G. EHR game changer focuses on taking invisible path to change. *Health Data Manag.* 2012;20(6):48–49.

90. Despont-Gros C, Mueller H, Lovis C. Evaluating user interactions with clinical information systems: a model based on human-computer interaction models. *J Biomed Inform.* 2004;38:244–255.

91. Gardner E. EHR success all in the details. *Health Data Manag.* 2012;20(5):30–32.

92. Pelayo S, Ong MS. *Human Factors and Ergonomics in the Design of Health Information Technology: Trends and Progress in 2014.* IMIA Yearbook of Medical Informatics; 2015:75–77. Retrieved from, http://www.ncbi.nlm.nih.gov/pmc/articles/ PMC4587043/pdf/ymi-10-0075.pdf/.

93. Zuniga AV. Patient access to electronic health records: strengths, weaknesses and what's needed to move forward. *iSchool Student Res J.* 2015;5(1). Available from: http:// scholarworks.sjsu.ed.slissr/vol5/iss1/1/.

94. Beard L, Schein R, Morra D, Wilson K, Keelan J. The challenges in making electronic health records accessible to patients. *J Am Med Inform Assoc.* 2012;19:116–120. http://dx.doi.org/10.1136/ amiajnl-2011-000261.

95. US Department of Health & Human Services. *HHS.gov. Health Information Privacy;* 2015. http://www.hhs.gov/ocr/privacy/ hipaa/administrative/securityrule/index.html/.

96. Caine K, Tierney WM. Point and counterpoint: patient control of access to data in their electronic health record. *J Gen Intern Med.* 2015;30(suppl 1):S38–S41. http://dx.doi.org/10.1007/ s11606-014-3061-0.

97. Leventhal JC, Cummins JA, Schwartz PH, Martin DK, Tierney WM. Designing a system for patients controlling providers' access to their electronic health records: organizational and technical challenges. *J Gen Intern Med.* 2014;30(suppl 1):S17–S24. http://dx.doi.org/10.1007/s11606-014-3055-y.

98. Nazi KM, Hogan TP, McInnes K, Woods SS, Graham G. Evaluating patient access to electronic health records: results from a survey of veterans. *Med Care.* 2013;51(suppl 1): S52–S56.

99. Mendu ML, Lundquist A, Aizer AA, et al. Patient access to electronic health records during hospitalization. *JAMA Internal Medicine.* 2015;175(5):856–858.

100. White A, Danis M. Enhancing patient-centered communication and collaboration by using the electronic health record in the examination room. *JAMA.* 2013;309 (22):2327–2328.

101. HealthIT.gov. *Consumer e-Health: Patient-Generated Health Data;* 2015. https://www.healthit.gov/policy-researchers-implementers/patient-generated-health-data/.

102. Chung AE, Basch EM. Potential and challenges of patient-generated health data for high quality cancer care. *J Oncol Pract;* 2015. http://dx.doi.org/10.1200/JCP.2015.003715.

103. Wood WA, Bennett AV, Basch E. Emerging uses of patient generated data in clinical research. *Mol Oncol.* 2015;9:1018–1024. http://dx.doi.org/10.1016/j. molonc.2014.08.006.

104. Nundy S, Lu CY, Hogan P, Mishra A, Peek ME. Using patient-generated health data from mobile technologies for diabetes self-management support: provider perspectives from an academic medical center. *J Diabetes Sci Technol.* 2014;8 (1):74–82. http://dx.doi.org/10.1177/1932296813511727.

105. Huba N, Zhang Y. Designing patient-centered personal health records (PHRs): health care professionals' perspective on

patient-generated data. *J Med Syst.* 2012;36:3893–3905. http://dx.doi.org/10.1007/s10916-012-9861-z.

106. Given JE, O'Kane MJ, Bunting BP, Coates VE. Comparing patient-generated blood glucose diary records with meter memory in diabetes: a systematic review. *Diabetic Med.* 2013;901–913. http://dx.doi.org/10.111/dme.12130.

107. Sands DZ, Wald JS. Transforming health care delivery through consumer engagement, health data transparency, and patient-generated health information. *IMAI Yearb Med Inform.* 2014;170–176. http://dx.doi.org/10.15265/IY-2014-0017/.

108. NIH News in Health. *Personalized medicine: matching treatments to your genes.* U.S. Department of Health and Human Services National Institutes of Health; 2013. https://newsinhealth.nih.gov/issue/dec2013/feature1/.

109. Pathak J, Kho AN, Denny JC. Electronic health records-driven phenotyping: challenges, recent advances, and perspectives. *J Am Med Inform Assoc.* 2013;20:e206–e211.

110. Walji MF, Kalenderian E, Stark PC, et al. BigMouth: a multi-institutional dental data repository. *J Am Med Inform Assoc.* 2014;21:1136–1140. http://dx.doi.org/10.1136/amiajnl-2013-002230.

111. Boland MR, Hripcsak G, Albers DJ, et al. Discovering medical conditions associated with periodontitis using linked electronic health records. *J Clin Periodontol* 40:474-482. http://dx.doi.org/10.1111/jcpe.12086.

112. Dustin C, Meghan G, Talisha S. *Adoption of Electronic Health Record Systems Among U.S. Non-Federal Acute Care Hospitals: 2008–2014*; 2015. ONC data brief no. 23, https://www.healthit.gov/sites/default/files/data-brief/2014HospitalAdoptionDataBrief.pdf/.

113. European Commission. *eHealth Initiatives to Support Medical Assistance While Traveling and Living Abroad.* Europa; 2008. http://europa.eu/rapid/pressReleasesAction.do?reference=IP/08/1075&format=HTML&aged=0&language=EN&guiLanguage=en/.

114. The European Files. *eHealth in Europe. ICT for Health European Commission*; 2009. http://www.google.com/url?sa=t&rct=j&q=&esrc=s&source=web&cd=2&ved=0CCYQFjABahUKEwibmOT3nNzIAhUDeT4KHXkBs0&url=http%3A%2F%2Fec.europa.eu%2Finformation_society%2Fnewsroom%2Fcf%2Fdae%2Fdocument.cfm%3Fdoc_id%3D611&usg=AFQjCNGgCw8Vsbd2g3klzo7rs8UG9NwU7g/.

115. European Commission. *Digital Agenda for Europe: a Europe 2020 initiative*; 2015. http://ec.europa.eu/digital-agenda/en/newsroom/.

DISCUSSION QUESTIONS

1. It is anticipated that EHR functionality will expand to allow consumers to enter data into the system along with direct input of other types of PGD. What are some benefits and challenges associated with this change from the perspective of consumers, providers, and healthcare organizations?

2. Historically, patient records maintained by healthcare institutions did not contain financial data such as charges or incident reports. Should this segregation of patient data be maintained with the implementation of EHRs?

3. Increasingly, patients expect full access to their EMRs and EHRs. What limitations, if any, would be in the best interest of patients? For example, should healthcare providers have access to new test results for 3 full business days before these are posted for patient viewing?

4. How does the introduction of a CPOE system affect communication between healthcare providers (e.g., between pharmacists and physicians or nurses, or between nurses and physicians)? What modifications, if any, should be made in the workflow of the different healthcare providers to adjust for this change in communication patterns?

5. Discuss the advantages and disadvantages associated with implementing and using a regional and national EHR.

CPOE, Computerized provider order-entry; *EHR,* electronic health record; *EMR,* electronic medical record.

CASE STUDY

A large healthcare enterprise in the Mid-Atlantic region that was created by a merger owns two acute care hospitals, a rehabilitation center, an outpatient surgical center, and three long-term care facilities. Each of these institutions uses a different EMR system. Admitting privileges extend to 550 physicians, who have office systems that interface with at least one of the acute care EMR systems. The vision is to create an environment to support communication, care coordination, and data sharing across the organization in preparation for a regional EHR system. The organization is moving quickly to take advantage of the incentives offered by the government and meet mandatory requirements. Executives decided to focus on the acute care facilities first and use lessons learned there to integrate the other centers later. Hospital A uses certified EHR applications and has implemented ancillary systems, CPOE, and clinical documentation, whereas Hospital B has a highly customized, beloved old mainframe computer that is outdated and no longer supported by the vendor. Instead of selecting a new system for both hospitals, the software programs used in Hospital A are being implemented in Hospital B.

Discussion Questions

1. You are the vice president of Patient Care Services for both acute care hospitals. Who would you identify as

stakeholders in the implementation and why? What steps would you take to minimize user resistance?

2. According to the U.S. EMR Adoption Model, at what stage of implementation would you classify Hospital A? After both hospitals are using the same system, what would you recommend implementing next?

3. The EHR is not fail-proof, and human error is an issue. Discuss potential decision support tools and functionality that could be implemented to increase patient safety.

CPOE, Computerized provider order entry; *EHR*, electronic health record; *EMR*, electronic medical record.

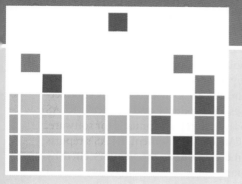

7

Administrative Applications Supporting Healthcare Delivery

Michael H. Kennedy, Kathy H. Wood, and Gerald R. Ledlow

If a health care system cannot effectively track the total cost of all materials used to treat an individual patient and aggregate data to determine the cost of treating groups of patients, managing the cost of health care is not possible.

OBJECTIVES

At the completion of this chapter, the reader will be prepared to:

1. Outline the evolution of financial information systems (FISs) in healthcare organizations.
2. Discuss the basic FISs and their application in healthcare organizations.
3. Compare and contrast practice management systems (PMSs) and integrated healthcare systems.
4. Describe and explain the attributes of an efficient supply chain (materials management) system in a healthcare organization.
5. Appraise how a quality supply chain system supports the operation and management of clinical systems.
6. Describe the human resources management actions associated with the subsystems typically deployed with a human resources information system.
7. Define *business intelligence.*
8. Distinguish between enterprise-level and application-level business intelligence.

KEY TERMS

accountable care organization (ACO), 118
accounts payable, 113
accounts receivable, 113
assets, 113
business intelligence (BI), 127
charge description master file, 122
claims denial management, 114
claims processing and management, 114
financial information system (FIS), 112
fixed asset management, 115
general ledger, 113
incentive management, 126

materials management, 121
open shift management, 126
patient accounting, 114
pay for performance (P4P), 118
payroll, 113
practice management systems (PMSs), 119
predictive scheduling, 126
supply chain management (SCM), 114
supply-item master file, 122
transaction history file, 122
vendor master file, 122

ABSTRACT ❖

This chapter addresses the administrative applications within health information systems that are designed to facilitate the delivery of healthcare, such as financial, practice management, supply chain and materials management, human resources, and business intelligence systems.

INTRODUCTION

Health information systems are "complexes or systems of processing data, information and knowledge in healthcare environments."[1, p. 270] These environments comprise a variety of settings, including hospitals, ambulatory settings, long-term care facilities, and managed care organizations.

Typically, the applications within health information systems are categorized as clinical or administrative. This chapter focuses on the administrative applications within health information systems designed to facilitate the management of healthcare delivery. The chapter considers in turn financial, practice management, supply chain management (SCM), human resources, and business intelligence (BI) systems.

Vendor Resource Guides

The applications required to process information in healthcare settings are primarily provided by vendors. The vendor market for hospital information systems alone in 2013 had total revenues of almost $14 billion, with the top five vendors in terms of revenue being McKesson ($3.4 billion), Cerner ($2.9 billion), Siemens ($1.8 billion), Epic Systems Corporation ($1.7 billion), and Allscripts (almost $1.4 billion). These revenue statistics were based upon published earnings reports, direct contact with vendors, research of websites, and estimates for privately held companies or to exclude nonhealth revenues.[2]

The Healthcare Information and Management Systems Society (HIMSS) (www.himss.org) prepares an annual comprehensive report of healthcare IT applications titled "Essentials of the U.S. Hospital IT Market" based upon the HIMSS Analytics Database. Quarterly "Essential Briefs" (www.himssanalytics.org/research-list) address emerging health technology interest areas.

Vendors that deploy a comprehensive suite of applications are referred to as enterprise vendors. Specialized applications are provided by niche vendors and are listed separately. When specialty vendors and vendors targeting nonhospital markets are included, the health information system marketplace becomes a confusing morass of products whose capabilities are difficult to assess. Fortunately, professional organizations such as the HIMSS, hard copy and online content publishers such as Health Data Management (www.healthdatamanagement.com), and trade and technology research companies such as Gartner (www.gartner.com) and KLAS (www.klasresearch.com) help stakeholders assess their options and make informed decisions.

HIMSS provides an online product and directory service (www.himss.org/product-and-service-directory/) in the form of a searchable database with an exhaustive list of healthcare IT companies, products, and services. Clicking on a product category results in the retrieval of vendor names, contact information, and brief descriptions for featured products and services offered. HIMSS Analytics (www.himssanalytics.org) is a wholly owned not-for-profit subsidiary of HIMSS that offers services to providers and healthcare IT companies. Hospitals and other providers that participate in an annual study gain access to the HIMSS Analytics Database and a number of benefits free of charge, including an Electronic Medical Record Adoption Model Score, benchmarking reports, and hospital profiles. The HIMSS Analytics Database is available by subscription to healthcare IT companies, which may also purchase ad hoc data reports.

In addition to publishing a monthly magazine of the same name and maintaining an extensive website, Health Data Management maintains a resource guide (http://marketplace.healthdatamanagement.com) by subject category. Similar to the HIMSS online conference exhibitor guide, clicking on a subject category returns vendor names, contact information, and brief descriptions of the products and services offered.

Gartner and KLAS provide fee-based ratings services. Gartner states, "We deliver the technology-related insight necessary for our clients to make the right decisions, every day."[3] KLAS declares, "Healthcare technology is rapidly changing, and KLAS is dedicated to being the source that holds vendors accountable and amplifies the voice of your peers."[4] This is done by monitoring vendor performance based on feedback from healthcare providers and by conducting independent analyses of products and services. KLAS publishes a *Best in KLAS Awards* report annually for software, professional services, and medical equipment. KLAS's reports should be used with some caution, as the vendors cited by KLAS represent the rankings of just one ratings service, but they do serve as a resource. Additional information about these services is included in Chapter 19.

MAJOR TYPES OF APPLICATIONS

Financial Systems

A **financial information system (FIS)** is a system that stores and records fiscal (financial) operations within an organization that are then used for reporting and decision making. Healthcare organizations, like any other business, must perform various "financial" types of functions to remain viable. These involve the following components:

- A customer (patient) purchasing the product (receiving the service).
- Salespeople (healthcare personnel) providing the service or product.
- A facility to receive the service or product (healthcare facility).
- Supplies needed for a procedure (materials management).
- Payment received by the healthcare organization for the product (service) received (receivables).
- Monies received to be deposited in accounts (accounting).
- Payment made to healthcare personnel and support staff for services performed (payroll).
- Expenses paid (payables) to external constituents that made it possible to perform a procedure (e.g., mortgage and utilities).

The architecture of a typical FIS is illustrated in Fig. **7.1**. As Rogoski noted, FISs can no longer be regarded as "back-office" systems.[5] Although it is true that financial functions are usually not a matter of life or death for the patient, an ill-fitted FIS can be life or death for the fiscal viability of the organization. Therefore one must choose wisely and update the FIS often to keep up with the ever-changing regulations and variations that affect the revenue and profitability of the organization.

Evolution of Healthcare Financial Information System

Automated FISs were the first type of systems used in many healthcare facilities. The main purpose of these initial FISs was basic bookkeeping and payroll. Basic accounting systems were then put into place to help with the billing function. As Latham quotes, "Cash is king, so cash flow is the lifeblood of the kingdom."[6, p. 1] To get cash flow, charges must be captured and collected from the patient or the patient's third-party payment system. Entering charges and creating claims to send to insurance companies and patients were some of the first,

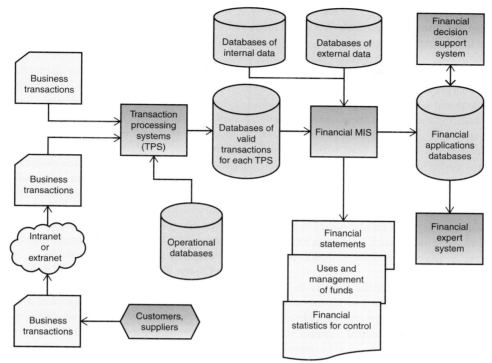

FIG 7.1 Financial information system architecture. (Healthcare Financial Management Association Certification Professional Practicum PowerPoint.)

and easiest, functions for an FIS. Payroll was also a very simple function for an FIS to perform. There was no need for analytics or importing to spreadsheets, and reporting functions were limited.[6] Healthcare organizations embraced the basic financial functions to remain financially viable. Fig. **7.1** shows how financial transactions fit within the FISs.

Some of the basic financial systems required by healthcare organizations and other businesses are general ledger, payroll, patient accounting, claims processing, claims denial management, contracts management, and fixed asset management.

General Ledger. The general ledger consists of *all* financial transactions made by the healthcare organization. This is similar to a personal checking ledger where any checks written or deposits made are recorded in the account. Numerous financial areas need to be tracked. Therefore a healthcare organization will maintain various subsidiary ledgers. Each of these ledgers tracks customer and vendor names, dates of transactions, types of transactions, and balances remaining. The FIS managing the general ledger must be able to track and report information in a variety of ways to meet the needs of the decision makers. Types of financial data that need to be tracked include:

- *Assets:* Assets are property items that can be converted easily into cash. Assets are classified as tangible and intangible. Tangible assets include current and fixed assets such as inventory or buildings and equipment. Intangible assets include nonphysical resources such as copyrights or computer systems.
- *Accounts payable:* Accounts payable are the monies that are owed to vendors and suppliers for items

purchased on credit (very similar to using a personal credit card and then paying back the amount on a monthly basis). These usually occur in the form of invoices or statements. This would fall under the category of disbursements in many systems. Because many vendors offer discounts when paid by a certain date, the FIS needs to be able to track the dates that payments need to be made in order to receive the discount or avoid the penalties that may be applied for late payments.

- *Accounts receivable:* The opposite of accounts payable, accounts receivable are monies that are owed to the institution. The vast majority of the dollars owed to the healthcare organization come in the form of patient-generated revenues. Once claims have been submitted to insurance companies (if the patient is covered by insurance), the remaining balance is sent to the patient for payment. The FIS has to be able to track the amount owed by the insurance, minus any negotiated rate such as managed care contracting, and the remaining balance owed by the patient. Ideally, the system estimates the amounts owed up front so the collection process can begin at the time of the visit.

Payroll Application. The application that handles compensation payments to employees is the payroll system. This is also referred to as a disbursement system. The FIS application must be able to deduct taxes, benefits, possibly savings amounts, and other deductions. At the onset of FISs for payroll, the minimal functions could be performed. In advanced systems, automatic payroll deposits and much more can be performed. In addition, overtime pay, pay rates, and payroll histories must be tracked and reported. At the end of the calendar year, the system must be able to generate W2 forms for the employee to use in income tax preparation.

Patient Accounting Application. A patient accounting application tracks the accounting transactions related to patient services. All charges incurred because of the patient visit need to be tracked and added to the patient's financial record. This can include inpatient fees if the patient is hospitalized, healthcare provider (e.g., physicians and nurse practitioners) and medication fees associated with the treatment, and procedure costs, including surgeries, radiology, and whatever else is necessary for the care of the patient. The procedural and diagnostic codes also become part of the patient billing record in order to complete the information necessary for the insurance payer to submit payment for the claim. Without critical information such as charges and coding, the claim process is delayed, resulting in reduced cash flow for the healthcare organization.

The collection process can begin at the time of the visit. This statement implies that the patient can receive services without paying anything up front. This is the reality in emergencies. Because of the Emergency Medical Treatment and Active Labor Act (EMTALA), patients must be treated in the case of emergency regardless of their ability to pay. This can lead to hundreds of thousands of dollars outstanding that the healthcare facility will try to collect after the service has been performed. Therefore the collection process in healthcare is much different from the process in a traditional business that requires payment before the product or service is provided. The FIS also needs to be able to track outstanding balances and assist in tracking these for the patient accounts personnel who will be attempting to collect the balances. The older the balances are, the more difficult they are to collect. The FIS needs to be able to differentiate the balances based on several factors, including, but not limited to, amount, payer, age of the account, and so forth. The features needed in FISs are now much more complex than in the past. For example, managers now may need to track the revenue generated by staff as a measure of productivity.

Claims Processing and Management System. As patients present for registration and admission, a single healthcare facility must be prepared to bill numerous insurance companies (third-party payers) representing hundreds of coverage and payment plans across government and private insurance. Some patients have primary coverage and supplemental coverage (e.g., Medicare as primary insurer and another insurer for supplemental coverage). Other patients receiving charity care or those with no insurance are categorized as private pay patients.

Claims processing and management is the submission of the insurance claim or bill to the third-party payer, either manually or electronically, and the follow-up on the payment from the payer. The application must be able to keep each of the payer types separate and know the requirements of how to bill the claims, who to bill for the balances, or if the balances need to be written off and not billed to anyone. Collections can be very challenging for the healthcare facility. Many

new standards have been adopted for claims processing, but numerous different standards and requirements must be followed for the various insurance companies and plans.

Sending "clean" claims is the key to getting payment quickly. Clean claims are those claims that contain all critical information such as patient demographics, charges, procedures performed, procedural and diagnostic coding, and other information required by the insurance company to remit prompt payment. Timely claims processing and collection are key to the fiscal health of institutions so they can meet the financial obligations in their disbursements and accounts payable functions. The claims-processing application must review the claim before it is submitted to ensure that all necessary data fields are complete and accurate. If the claim is not clean, it will be denied, creating a delay and generating increased labor costs to correct errors before payment can be received for the service provided.

Claims Denial Management Application. Denials from insurance companies are tracked, and they require follow-up. The claims denial management application can prevent denials imposed by the insurance carrier in a variety of ways. For example, the application can issue an alert on a request by clinical personnel for a patient to stay an additional day in his or her current patient status (i.e., observation, inpatient) if that request is likely to be denied by the insurer. The submitted insurance claim for a patient's stay may also be denied for improper coding or missing information. When the denial occurs, the application must track the update and the progress on having the denial reversed. Because a claim or request was denied initially does not mean that the decision cannot be reversed. Persistence and proper documentation can be the deciding factors leading to reversal. Documentation must be detailed and included with the denial reversal request to be effective.[7] In addition, the communications that took place between each area of patient care must be documented, collected, and stored in an orderly manner for the proof to be shown. This is just one example of why the FIS must be carefully integrated with the clinical systems.

Contract Management Application. Healthcare organizations have a variety of contracts they must track, including those for supply chain management (SCM) and managed care. These types of contracts affect the bottom line of the organization, so the contracts must be tracked and managed for the organization to obtain maximum financial gain. SCM contracts include group purchasing, where healthcare systems negotiate a price for using a standard vendor. Vendor price comparisons and usage need to be tracked, and the system must ensure that employees are adhering to the purchasing policies. Additional SCM functions can include providing incentives for healthcare providers to reduce the cost of their preferred supplies. For example, some surgeons may have particular instruments or supplies they prefer for surgical procedures. These supplies may be much more expensive than an alternative brand. The FIS could help the organization track the supply costs and the costs for procedures and provide reports for physicians to accompany requests for their assistance in reducing those costs.

Managed care contracting can be very challenging and complex. The contracts can be numerous, and each contract can have different terms. The FIS needs to be able to track these contracts and manage the terms and results of each contract individually. For example, when a patient is covered by a nongovernmental insurance plan, the insurance company may have negotiated an agreed-upon amount for reimbursement per service or per patient. The insurance and patients need to be billed according to that contract's terms, and any negotiated discount should not be billed.

Fixed Asset Management Application. Fixed asset management applications manage the fixed assets in a healthcare facility that cannot be converted to cash easily, sold, or used for the care of a patient, such as land, buildings, equipment, fixtures, fittings, motor vehicles, office equipment, computers, software, and so forth. Each fixed asset must be tracked by location, person, age, and other factors. In a healthcare organization, the assets can be issued to a person, a procedure room, a department, and others. Therefore the FIS must handle the vast number of assets and the various areas in which the assets can be located. This system tracks depreciation, maintenance agreements, warranties related to the assets, and when assets will need to be replaced.

Even though healthcare FISs during the first decade of the twenty-first century supported a number of improvements in the business processes, including patient scheduling, laboratory and ancillary reporting, medical record keeping and reporting, and billing and accounting, many opportunities still remain to improve efficiency, productivity, and quality, such as fiscal decision support.[8]

Financial Reporting

One of the primary functions of an FIS is providing the reports that demonstrate the financial condition of the organization. The most common reports for healthcare organizations are summarized in Table 7.1. Note that the titles may vary depending on whether the organization is for profit or not for profit.

The income statement or statement of operations is a good representation of the bottom line, or money left over (net income or loss), of the organization (Table 7.2). This report lists all revenues (monies coming in) and expenses (monies going out), and these are often compared with those of prior years and with the budget plan.

The balance sheet or statement of financial position shows a glimpse of the organization's financial condition at any given point in time (Table 7.3). The FIS needs to pull the financial data from assets, liabilities, and equity to present the report so the organization can determine whether the numbers in the categories are balanced. Balance sheet data

are based on a fundamental accounting equation (Assets = Liabilities + Owner's equity), so each side must "balance" to show the financial condition of the organization.

The cash flow statements show whether the organization will be successful in paying its bills (have more money than it owes). Table 7.4 provides an example of a cash flow statement. Fig. 7.2 illustrates how the cash flow statement reconciles with the income statement.

A healthcare organization keeps track of certain financial ratios to help it evaluate its financial condition; these can be important when borrowing for future capital investments. The FIS must be able to calculate and report ratios on demand so that at any given time the organization can assess its financial condition. Ratios are classified into several categories, such as solvency, debt, management or turnover, profitability, and market value. Several ratios are unique to the healthcare industry (Table 7.5), such as length of stay and bed occupancy. Average length of stay in the United States for most procedures is 4.8 days. Decision makers can analyze the length of stay for their hospitals to determine whether they are on track for most procedures. Keep in mind, however, that a shorter length of stay does not necessarily mean lower costs. Bed occupancy provides a quick glance at how many inpatient beds are being used. The occupancy is typically higher during flu season and other epidemics. The other ratios reported in Table 7.5 are typical of financial ratios for any organization. Accounts receivable days in a healthcare organization are generally higher than in other organizations because the services are provided before payment is made by the patient or insurance company.

Challenges with Financial Information Systems

One of the challenges that large healthcare organizations face with the implementation of FISs is ensuring that the various systems in place at numerous locations are integrated. Larger healthcare organizations can include 20 or more facilities. Within each of these facilities can be numerous sub-facilities. The different financial systems, applications, and SCM systems can become very complicated when they are merged and the information systems do not interface well.[5]

The purpose of healthcare organizations is to provide quality patient care. While generating maximum revenue is not its

TABLE 7.1 Financial Statements

For Profit	Not for Profit
Balance sheet	Statement of financial position
Income statement	Statement of operations
Statement of cash flows	Statement of cash flows

TABLE 7.2 Income Statement

Revenue	$1,195,450.25	100.00%
Cost of goods sold	870,175.83	72.79%
Gross margin	$325,274.42	27.21%
Overhead	29,879.65	2.50%
Net ordinary income (loss)	$295,394.77	24.71%
Interest expense	1269.08	0.11%
Interest income	5387.08	0.45%
Net income (loss)	$299,512.77	25.05%

From Healthcare Financial Management Association Certification Professional Practicum PowerPoint.

TABLE 7.3 Balance Sheet

Assets		Claims on Assets	
Current Assets		**Current Liabilities**	
Cash	$123,000	Accounts payable	$100,000
Marketable securities	$200,000	Notes payable	$150,000
Accounts receivable	$345,000		
Inventories	$100,000	*Total Current Liabilities*	$250,000
		Long-term note	$300,000
Total Current Assets	$768,000		
		Total Liabilities	$550,000
Long-Term Assets		Owner's equity	$843,000
Building (gross)	$350,000		
Accumulated depreciation	$(50,000)	**Total Claims**	$1,393,000
Net building	$300,000		
Land	$325,000		
Total Long-Term Assets	$625,000		
Total Assets	$1,393,000		

From Healthcare Financial Management Association Certification Professional Practicum PowerPoint.

TABLE 7.4 Statement of Cash Flows

Cash Flow from Operations	**$1800.00**
Net income	**$ 259.00**
Adjustments	**$1541.00**
Depreciation expense	$(100.00)
Accounts payable	$130.00
Credit card account	$50.00
Patient credits	$0.00
Sales tax payable	$1.23
Accounts receivable	$986.77
Inventory asset	$473.00
Cash Flow from Investing	**$(1000.00)**
Equipment	$(1000.00)
Cash Flow from Financing	**$1500.00**
Opening balance equity	$2000.00
Owner's equity	$(500.00)
Draw	$(500.00)
Investment	$0.00
Net Change in Cash	**$2300.00**

From Healthcare Financial Management Association Certification Professional Practicum PowerPoint.

defining purpose, an organization must generate income to stay in business and advance new programs and services. What this means is that patient care systems can be seen by some as a higher priority compared with FISs. Decision makers may have a more challenging time realizing the return on investment or understanding the importance of the investment in FISs because IT software applications such as patient accounting or revenue are considered an intangible asset. The key is to ensure the integration of the various applications.[9] If an information system meets the requirements needed for patient care and includes integrated applications such as patient accounting, the organization will have the best of both worlds. True integration supports the effective transfer of captured data across all applications. This leads to improved efficiency and enhanced cash flow, and the total cost of ownership is lower.[9]

Analyzing Accountable Care Organizations and Pay for Performance. Historically healthcare was financed using a "fee-for-service" approach. With this approach, each time a service (e.g., an office visit, an injection, delivery of a baby, or surgery) is completed, payment is provided. There are two key problems with this approach. First, such an approach encourages the provider to increase the amount of services performed. For example, a healthcare system that does more procedures is able to make more money compared with a healthcare system that is more conservative. Second, such an approach does not consider the quality of the service provided. With a fee-for-service approach, a postoperative infection provides the healthcare institution with additional income because they can now charge to treat that infection. "The predominant fee-for-service system under which providers are paid leads to increased costs by rewarding providers for the volume and complexity of services they provide. Higher intensity of care does not necessarily result in higher quality care, and can even be harmful."[10, p. 1] As healthcare costs have increased and problems with healthcare safety have become more obvious, there have been increasing efforts to use a different approach to funding healthcare.

During the 1990s, a managed care approach was introduced to reduce excessive and unnecessary care. By paying providers a lump sum per patient to cover a given set of services, there was no advantage for increasing the amount of service provided. In addition, poor quality could increase the institution's cost with no financial gain. However, this approach presented new concerns because a managed care approach motivated payers to control costs by restricting services. Concerns about compromised quality and constraints on patients having access to providers of their choice led to a backlash.[10]

The most recent regulation affecting healthcare finance to date is the Affordable Care Act (ACA). Officially called the Patient Protection and Affordable Care Act (PPACA), and sometimes called ObamaCare, the ACA is a U.S. law aimed at reforming both the healthcare delivery system and the

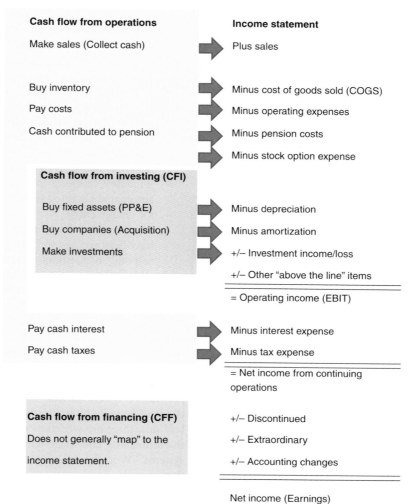

FIG 7.2 Statement of cash flows and reconciliation with income statement. (Healthcare Financial Management Association Certification Professional Practicum PowerPoint.)

TABLE 7.5   Sample of Financial Ratios

Ratio Measure	Hospital #1	Hospital #2	Hospital #3	Hospital #4
Sample size (n)	248	577	450-480	561
Average length of stay (days)	N/A	4.15	4.41	N/A
Maintained bed occupancy (%)	N/A	59.13	57.73	N/A
Operating margin (%)	2.6	2.64	2.93	2.4
Excess margin (%)	3.9	5.11	3.71	4.0
Debt services coverage (x)	3.5	3.05	N/A	3.7
Current ratio (x)	N/A	2.30	2.3	N/A
Cash on hand (days)	180.5	150.70	N/A	164.6
Cushion ratio (x)	13.6	6.06	N/A	14.2
Accounts receivable (days)	43.8	46.38	50.1	44.5
Average payment period (days)	63.4	49.88	N/A	56.8
Average age of plant (years)	10.2	9.51	N/A	10.0
Debt to capitalization (%)	42.1	34.17	50.74	38.1
Capital expense (%)	N/A	6.85	3.25	N/A

Healthcare Financial Management Association Certification Professional Practicum PowerPoint.
x, Denotes ratios whose result commonly is greater than 1.

health insurance industry. The ACA includes a number of provisions designed to encourage improvements in patient outcomes as a basis for payment. For example, Medicare's Hospital Readmissions Reduction Program reduces payments by 1% to hospitals that have excessively high rates of avoidable readmissions for patients experiencing heart attacks, heart failure, or pneumonia.[10]

Another key aspect of the ACA is the concept of pay for performance. The concept of pay for performance ties payment to the quality of the care provided or to patient outcomes as opposed to the service delivered. The most familiar program that pay for performance (P4P) is the voluntary accountable care organization (ACO). An ACO is a network of doctors and hospitals that share responsibility for providing care to a specific group of patients and in return receives bonuses when these providers keep costs down and meet specific quality benchmarks.[10]

Three other P4P programs include value-based purchasing, physician quality reporting, and Medicare Advantage plan bonuses.[10] These programs are intended to provide financial incentives for physicians and healthcare organizations to have accountability over controlling costs while gaining more efficiency and higher quality in their operations. Healthcare organizations are also going beyond the clinical aspect of healthcare by looking at social determinants (e.g., age, gender, geographical location, socioeconomic position, nutritional habits, drug uses or abuses, and work environment) that may cause health issues in certain populations.

Since the inception of the ACA in 2010, over 440 Medicare ACOs have been created nationwide. Of the Medicare ACOs initiated, 54% lowered expenditures and generated $383 million in net savings for Medicare, resulting in significant shared savings payments for the ACOs. Public reporting is one of the requirements for the Medicare Shared Savings Program (MSSP).[11] As ACOs continue to grow in numbers, their overall financial viability will be determined.

There are challenges to the participants in these P4P programs. One of the key challenges is determining the quality "perceived" by patients because this can vary tremendously because of opinions and expectations. In addition, complying with the structural suggestions such as adding health information technology can be costly, so the participants would need to know how much they are receiving in incentives to determine if the costs of the structural changes result in an overall positive gain financially.

As regulations and financial incentives continue to be put into place, healthcare organizations need a means to track the effect of such regulations. Tracking demographics and social determinants will allow any trends to be discovered. The FIS will provide tools to help the healthcare organizations and the ACOs analyze the feasibility and results of the shared savings in the P4P incentive, as well as to track information for the prevention of health issues.

Financial Information Systems Integration

Financial systems matured much faster than clinical systems (CSs) did[12]; therefore the degree of integration of the FIS with

CSs was somewhat limited. However, there are several advantages to integration within the FIS and across CSs. For example, this approach eliminates duplication of effort, which also reduces the number of potential errors. Williams points out the following benefits of integration:

- A transition is provided between front-end and back-end operations.
- Information required for billing such as demographics and insurance can be gathered and verified at the point of service or admission so that the information is immediately available for patient care and financial personnel.
- Eligibility checking for insurance can be done online; automated charging is supported, eliminating the need for charge entry.
- Availability of clinical records with detailed charges that have been secured through proper access allows staff to respond to questions from patients, payers, or others without having to access paper charts.[12]

All of these features of integration improve the bottom line, which is the aim in healthcare finance. In addition to the basic accounting systems, such as general ledger, accounts payable, and accounts receivable, FISs handle functions that are more complex such as activity or project management. Advanced revenue cycle IT, or new generation, is often referred to as integrated "bolt-ons."[9] TechTarget describes a bolt-on as a product or system similar to an add-on but one that can be attached *securely* to an existing system.[13] Besides integrated bolt-ons, there are workflow rules engines, advanced executive scorecards, and single-database clinical and revenue cycle systems.[9] Workflow rules engines help to manage workflow. For example, documents can be stored in a document management system and e-mail or event reminders can be automatically sent to the people involved with the tasks. Advanced executive scorecards are strategic management tools that aggregate data from electronic health records (EHRs) in concert with an FIS, thereby providing a snapshot of how the healthcare institution is performing in certain areas. For example, the snapshot may show a quarterly increase in the hospital's cost to deliver a baby. Investigating these data may demonstrate an increase in C-sections or a decrease in babies delivered by midwifes. These "scores" can then be compared with the data of other hospitals offering obstetrical services. A single-database clinical and revenue cycle system is a system used to ensure accuracy, availability, and data integrity for patient care and billing for the healthcare organization. When changes are made to information contained within the database, those changes are managed throughout the system. In other words, the user does not need to make the change in multiple locations; the database management system will do that for the user to ensure that all necessary changes have been made. This is particularly important when dealing with procedures, documentation for those procedures, and the charges that accompany those procedures. In line with the original accounting systems, these advanced systems are designed to improve billing by reducing billing errors, improving the timeliness of billing to cash collected, decreasing the cost of collections, providing real-time

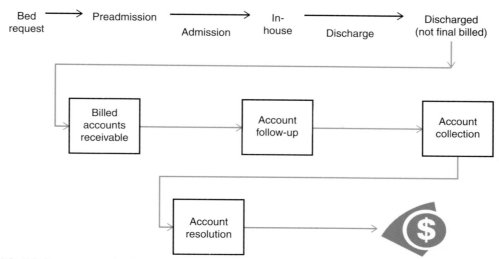

FIG 7.3 Revenue cycle function. (Healthcare Financial Management Association Certification Professional Practicum PowerPoint.)

eligibility for services, and providing improvements to current operational efficiencies via other functions.[9]

Improvement in cash flow has remained a constant goal since the onset of FIS. Adaptability and flexibility in healthcare is the key to successful patient care and quality, and the same applies to FIS choices. An example of the revenue cycle is provided in Fig. **7.3**.

One of the more recent IT tools used to positively affect the revenue cycle is a communication management system. The variety of communications (e.g., patient care, insurance coverage, and patient admission), the method of communication (e.g., face to face, phone, fax, and internet), and the number of people engaged in communications make organizing and tracking communications a complex process. As Cruze points out, communications surrounding care of the patient and payment can be very difficult to track and retrieve.[7] A centralized management tracking system could assist in this area. An audit trail needs to be very detailed, and include all communications that capture and travel with the patient, as well as the authorizations associated with each step. In other words, these communications need to be captured, indexed, and archived for future retrieval.[7]

Efficiency Tools

Decision makers need tools to capture productivity for various activities within the financial services area of the organization. For example, collecting balances from the patient may fall within the responsibilities of a handful of employees. At the front end (before services are received), patients who have been preregistered can be asked for payment on the estimated amount owed. At the back end (after services have been received), patients who have a remaining balance after insurance has paid will need to pay that balance. How does an organization know which employees are having success at collecting payments? The reporting tools must provide a snapshot of the data so the decision makers can immediately analyze financial events within a particular area.

In addition to reporting tools, the application needs to be able to assist end users with the questions that need to be asked, and when. For example, if a patient has an outstanding balance from a previous visit, the patient access personnel may need to know whether they should request payment. Information needed should be readily available and easy to access. When adaptable and flexible designs between clinical and financial systems are combined, powerful analytics are deployed via the web to every desktop; many activities are self-service, freeing up valuable time and resources for the healthcare organization.[9]

Managing services has become more complex. For example, capturing charges has increased in complexity just as medical care has.[9] As a result, there needs to be a seamless flow of charges as a natural by-product of the care process to help reduce lost, late, or duplicate charges. These new functions require an investment in an upgraded system to handle revenue cycle management.[14] A dashboard provides users with a visual analysis of specific data points so an organization can gauge how it is performing in certain areas (it is called a *dashboard* because it resembles the visual data points provided on an automobile dashboard). Efficiency may be improved by applications that allow for coding edits or overriding default values as needed, that are easy to use, and that include executive dashboards capabilities.[14]

Practice Management Systems

Practice management systems (PMSs) are very similar to the information systems supporting integrated healthcare systems, only on a smaller scale. These applications focus on the services provided in a healthcare provider's office compared with the services provided in a large healthcare system or hospital. Similar to the hospital revenue cycle management system, the PMS is designed to collect patient demographic and insurance information, manage appointment scheduling, document the reason for the visit and patient care procedures performed for the patient, post charging information for the billing process, and manage collection and follow-up. As with inpatient or acute care systems, PMSs require integration. The primary differences between PMSs and information systems supporting hospitals are specific provider scheduling templates and types of visits, transaction or line-item provider billing compared with account-driven hospital billing, and provider-based medical record content (orders, referrals, provider documentation, and problem lists) that differs from the typical comprehensive hospital medical record.[15] The charges from a medical practice office are connected to codes used for practice management billing and include Healthcare Common Procedure Coding System (HCPCS) and Current Procedural Terminology (CPT). Therefore the information system must be able to generate claims using this type of coding, usually through an electronic submission. Electronic medical records (EMRs) have become much more common modules within a PMS as the U.S. government has implemented incentives supporting EHRs (discussed in Chapter 27). An explanation of the difference between an EMR and an EHR can be found at www.healthit.gov/buzz-blog/electronic-health-and-medical-records/emr-vs-ehr-difference/. Information on the episodes of care maintained in the EMR can be passed along to the hospital or health center should the patient need to be admitted. Sharing this information helps to ensure that the information in the EMR becomes part of the EHR. However, this is often not a "plug and play" environment. Creating a successful interface to share data between the EMR of a practice and a hospital or health center information system is a complex process. Chapter 5 includes additional information on health information exchanges (HIEs) and health information organizations (HIOs) and the issues involved with these.

In outpatient settings, healthcare providers can spend much of their time documenting the details of the patient visit. There are a variety of ways to accomplish this, including documenting and recording what is being said and done while the patient is in the examination room, dictating and transcribing based on written notes, or using voice recognition software during or after the visit. Traditionally, visit notes were often transcribed by a third party, leaving room for error through misreading of handwriting or mishearing of dictation. There is also a time delay until the documentation becomes part of the patient record because of the multiple processes required. The healthcare provider is required to review and sign off on the final documentation, but time constraints can encourage the provider to rush and perhaps overlook some details.

A method using more enhanced technology and providing quicker turnaround is voice recognition. Voice recognition software capabilities have greatly improved over the last few years. Voice recognition eliminates the need for a third party and allows healthcare providers to input information themselves, saving steps, time, and money. The application allows text to be viewed in real time, and providers can edit and approve it immediately. The time savings can result in much more timely billing and improved cash flow versus waiting for dictated notes to be approved after being transcribed.

Patient Outreach System

Some practices specialize in providing preventive care to manage patients with chronic illnesses. In these practices, an electronic registry of the clinic's entire patient population can be used in a patient outreach system. The registry includes the demographic and medical record information needed to notify patients, and an automated reminder capability.[16] Patient outreach systems should incorporate evidence-based, specialty-specific protocols—or recommended care guidelines—for chronic and preventive care. Then, once the outreach system identifies patients due for preventive screenings and follow-up care for chronic diseases, the patients are contacted via an automated phone messaging system or another computerized method.

Online Billing and Payment Tool

Collections in a practice can be just as challenging as collections in a hospital, except that few emergency cases occur in a provider practice setting, allowing office staff to determine the acceptability of denying services to a patient until a payment plan has been established. In addition to routine collection practices, implementing an online billing and payment tool (e.g., using a credit card to pay online) can help to improve the management and collection of fees owed by patients. Conley states that the healthcare facility can realize increased patient satisfaction and improved staff efficiencies by implementing an online payment tool.[17] Benefits for the patient and the provider's office are outlined in Box **7.1**.

Hospital–Healthcare Provider Connection

PMSs integrated with the hospital information system can be more efficient for healthcare providers in a clinic or private practice. According to Cash, physicians, nurse practitioners, physician assistants, and others with staff privileges who

---

BOX 7.1　Benefits of Implementing an Online Payment Tool for Patients and Provider Offices

- Self-management of their open accounts
- Ability to pay outstanding balances
- Secure communication on a 24/7 basis with the business office (the practice will determine the turnaround time of communications to the patient)
- Ability to update address or demographic changes
- Ability to update changes to insurance coverage (which often occur annually)
- Preregister for services or appointments
- Enhanced customer service capabilities
- Ability for staff to accept payments in person or over the phone
- Ability for staff to view the patient statement exactly as submitted to the patient, which helps to improve communications and efficiencies for payment collection

Data from Conley C. Improve patient satisfaction and collections with efficient payment processes. Emdeon Express Winter Edition, <http://emdeonexpress.blogspot.com/2009/02/its-no-secret-that-health-care-is.html>; 2009.

participate in the hospital network have certain expectations about the IT, including that it should:

- Provide a single sign-on to an integrated information system from all key system entry points.
- Automate the provider's day as much as possible using mobile access (automation means that access is available wherever the clinician is and that the information is in a useful format).
- Have 24/7 support for any device, anywhere.
- Provide a dashboard to view critical clinical and financial information with the ability to act on it immediately.[18]
- Healthcare provider dissatisfaction can occur if the information system:
  - Slows performance of the task
  - Reduces the ability to bill insurance or the patient
  - Adds more administrative duties to clinical responsibilities

A Matter of Perspective

All healthcare providers have patient care as a top priority. Whereas the provider's focus may be on care of the patient, office personnel must focus on receiving maximum payment for the care of that patient. The records stored at the practitioner level must be accessible and transferable to the hospital in the case of an admission or referral. HIEs are making this possible for referrals, consultations, admissions, discharges, and transfers. IT solutions such as EMRs, digital storage of patient data, voice recognition software, and e-mailing of correspondence can offer efficiency, cost savings, and improved patient care, which should be the priorities of practice management.[19]

Supply Chain Management

SCM includes the acquisition of materials of care and the logistics or movement of those materials to caregiving facilities and organizations. Routinely, health systems deploy information system solutions to support the functions of SCM.

Healthcare Supply Chain and Informatics

What is a supply chain? The Council of Supply Chain Management Professionals defines *supply chain* in two ways: (1) starting with unprocessed raw materials and ending with the final customer using the finished goods, the supply chain links many companies together, or (2) the material and informational interchanges in the logistical process stretching from acquisition of raw materials to delivery of finished products to the end user. All vendors, service providers, and customers are links in the supply chain.[20]

A supply chain is much more than procurement of materials. Many times, the potential advantages of SCM are missed because the term is thought to relate only to the supply side of an organization or to the purchasing of materials. In addition, SCM is not:

- Inventory management
- Logistics management

- Forming partnerships with suppliers
- A strategy for shipping
- A logistics pipeline
- A computer system

The healthcare supply chain is complex, with requirements that go across, for example, the equipment for operating suites, pharmaceuticals, and medical and surgical supplies for all settings. In any health system with hospitals, clinics, and employees ordering from the supply chain, thousands of transactions occur daily across hundreds of vendors. Medical and surgical supplies, pharmaceuticals, and equipment are the "technology" that enables the delivery of healthcare services. These technologies couple with clinician knowledge and expertise within an appropriate healthcare facility function to provide efficacious services to patients.

Materials management in healthcare is the storage, inventory control, quality control, and operational management of supplies, pharmaceuticals, equipment, and other items used in the delivery of patient care or the management of the patient care system. As such, materials management is a subset of the larger function of SCM. It should be noted that the *term materials management* is also sometimes used as a synonym for the healthcare supply chain.

Typically, an organization named Materials Management or Central Supply in the hospital bears the burden of having the right item at the right place at the right time. The leading professional association, the Association for Healthcare Resource and Materials Management or AHRMM, lists common functions of the supply chain in healthcare. Several of these functions occur in the Purchasing Department, which is a key department within Materials Management.

As a department within Materials Management, Purchasing traditionally controls or participates in several functions[21]:

- Budgeting
- Replenishing inventory
- Evaluating and selecting capital
- Negotiating
- Maintaining the Materials Management Information System (MMIS)
- Reviewing product use and analyzing value
- Maintaining vendor relationships
- Monitoring the product selection process to ensure selection is competitive
- Coordinating with Finance to ensure reimbursement of products
- Providing information to end users regarding product use, costs, and alternatives

All of these items can be a part of the SCM strategy, but the misconceptions behind what is considered SCM have slowed implementation. As healthcare institutions increasingly need to understand and control actual costs, SCM and in turn materials management is now an area of growth because of the potential for cost savings.[22] Because the acquisition, logistics, and management of materials in healthcare are complex, a sophisticated information system is required to provide effective, efficient, and efficacious materials as needed.

The sophistication in automating this process has increased tremendously since the late 1990s. Applications now include electronic catalogs; information systems such as enterprise resource planning (ERP) systems from vendors such as Infor (www.infor.com) or McKesson (www.mckesson.com); warehousing and inventory control systems from vendors such as TECSYS (www.tecsys.com) and Manhattan (www.manh.com); exchanges from vendors such as Global Health Exchange (GHX) (www.ghx.com); and integration with other systems such as clinical, revenue management, and finance. An innovative technology in this area is radio frequency identification (RFID); more information can be found at www.advantech-inc.com/index.html.

With increased automation, these systems have improved supply chain performance and management in healthcare, with more innovations expected in the future. The healthcare supply chain is an untapped resource of financial savings and revenue enhancement opportunities.[23] Recognizing these opportunities, HIMSS advocated for more improvements in a white paper titled *Healthcare ERP and SCM Information Systems: Strategies and Solutions*. HIMSS indicated that ERP systems will be tools for quality and safety because they integrate capabilities such as procure-to-pay, order-to-cash, and financial reporting cycles. These functions should help institutions match needed materials with care in a more timely and cost-effective manner.[24]

Integrated Applications in Supply Chain Management

The importance of these ERP and SCM systems should be apparent, including the technology associated with them, such as bar code scanners and electronic medication cabinets (e.g.,

Pyxis [www.carefusion.com/our-products/medication-and-supply-management/medication-and-supply-management-technologies/pyxis-medication-technologies/pyxis-medstation-system] and Omnicell [www.omnicell.com]). The basic components of an integrated healthcare supply chain system include the following:

- **Supply item master file**: A list of all items used in the delivery of care for a healthcare organization that can be requested by healthcare service providers and managers. This file typically contains between 30,000 and 100,000 items. Fig. **7.4** shows a supply-item master file.
- **Charge description master file**: A list of all prices for services (e.g., Diagnosis-Related Groups [DRGs], HCPCS, and CPT) or goods provided to patients that serves as the basis for billing.
- **Vendor master file**: A list of all manufacturers or distributors (vendors) that provide the materials needed for the healthcare organization along with the associated contract terms and prices for specific items. This file typically contains 200 to 500 different vendors or suppliers.
- **Transaction history file**: A running log of all material transactions of the healthcare organization. In a computerized system, it is a running list of all supplies and materials being used to deliver care or manage the operations of the institution.

These four files must be integrated to support the operations and management of the supply chain. The integration necessary in the modern healthcare organization is illustrated in Fig. **7.5** as a diagram of interfaces across supply chain, clinical, and financial systems.[25]

	B	C	F	G	H	I
1	Description	Vendor	Qty On Hand	Qty On Order	Min-Max	Packaging
2	INDICATOR CHEM PARACETIC ACID LIQ CSC	3M MED PROD DIV-ALL	51.00 PO	8.00 PO	56.00PO / 21.00CS	CS 4.00 PO 50.00 EA
3	BLADE CLIPPER DISP CSC	3M MED PROD DIV-ALL	21.00 CS	14.00 CS	23.00CS / 35.00CS	CS 50.00 EA
4	CARD MONITORING COMPLY RECORD SYSTEM CSC	3M MED PROD DIV-ALL	12.00 BX	0.00 BX	8.00BX / 3.00CS	CS 4.00 BX 250.00 EA
5	TAPE CLOTH ADH 1INX10YD CSC	3M MED PROD DIV-ALL	13.00 BX	0.00 BX	4.00BX / 1.00CS	CS 10.00 BX 12.00 RL
6	TAPE INDIC STEAM W/DISPENSER 1IN CSC	3M MED PROD DIV-ALL	18.00 RL	38.00 RL	40.00RL / 3.00CS	CS 18.00 RL
7	TAPE INDIC GAS .75X60YD CSC	3M MED PROD DIV-ALL	75.00 RL	0.00 RL	2.00RL / 1.00CS	CS 24.00 RL
8	TAPE PLAS TRANSPORE .50INX10YD CSC	3M MED PROD DIV-ALL	28.00 BX	0.00 BX	21.00BX / 3.00CS	CS 10.00 BX 24.00 EA
9	TAPE PLAS TRANSPORE 1INX10YD CSC	3M MED PROD DIV-ALL	413.00 BX	41.00 BX	573.00BX / 86.00CS	CS 10.00 BX 12.00 EA
10	TAPE SILK DURAPORE 2INX10YD CSC	3M MED PROD DIV-ALL	353.00 BX	671.00 BX	803.00BX / 121.00CS	CS 10.00 BX 6.00 RL
11	TAPE SILK DURAPORE 1INX10YD CSC	3M MED PROD DIV-ALL	611.00 BX	0.00 BX	619.00BX / 93.00CS	CS 10.00 BX 12.00 RL
12	TAPE PAPER MICROPOR DISPNSR 1X10YD CSC	3M MED PROD DIV-ALL	21.00 BX	0.00 BX	19.00BX / 3.00CS	CS 10.00 BX 12.00 RL
13	WRAP COBAN NS 1INX5YD CSC	3M MED PROD DIV-ALL	37.00 CS	0.00 CS	32.00CS / 49.00CS	CS 6.00 PK 5.00 RL
14	DRESSING STRIP STER 1/8X3IN CSC	3M MED PROD DIV-ALL	6.00 BX	0.00 BX	5.00BX / 2.00CS	CS 4.00 BX 50.00 EA
15	DRESSING STRIP STER .25 X 4IN CSC	3M MED PROD DIV-ALL	29.00 BX	0.00 BX	20.00BX / 8.00CS	CS 4.00 BX 50.00 EA
16	SPLINT CONFORMABLE 5INX30IN CSC	3M MED PROD DIV-ALL	9.00 CS	0.00 CS	6.00CS / 9.00CS	CS 10.00 EA
17	DRESSING STRIP STER .5X4IN CSC	3M MED PROD DIV-ALL	64.00 BX	15.00 BX	84.00BX / 32.00CS	CS 4.00 BX 50.00 EA
18	SPLINT CONFORMABLE 2INX10IN CSC	3M MED PROD DIV-ALL	1.00 CS	1.00 CS	2.00CS / 3.00CS	CS 10.00 EA
19	DRESSING TEGADERM 2.375X2.75IN CSC	3M MED PROD DIV-ALL	235.00 BX	0.00 BX	233.00BX / 87.00CS	CS 4.00 BX 100.00 EA
20	DRESSING TEGADERM 4X4.75IN CSC	3M MED PROD DIV-ALL	113.00 BX	0.00 BX	122.00BX / 46.00CS	CS 4.00 BX 50.00 EA
21	DRESSING TEGADERM 4X10IN CSC	3M MED PROD DIV-ALL	11.00 BX	3.00 BX	17.00BX / 6.00CS	CS 4.00 BX 20.00 EA
22	DRESSING TEGADERM 6X8IN CSC	3M MED PROD DIV-ALL	0.00 BX	3.00 BX	11.00BX / 2.00CS	CS 8.00 BX 10.00 EA
23	INDIC BIOLOG FLASH 1HR 270 DEG. CSC	3M MED PROD DIV-ALL	30.00 BX	0.00 BX	28.00BX / 10.00CS	CS 4.00 BX 50.00 EA
24	INDIC BIOLOG STEAM CSC	3M MED PROD DIV-ALL	11.00 BX	0.00 BX	7.00BX / 3.00CS	CS 4.00 BX 100.00 EA
25	WRAP COBAN NS 2INX5YD CSC	3M MED PROD DIV-ALL	775.00 RL	0.00 RL	688.00RL / 29.00CS	CS 36.00 RL
26	FILM NO STING BARRIER SWAB CSC	3M MED PROD DIV-ALL	6.00 BX	0.00 BX	4.00BX / 2.00CS	CS 4.00 BX 25.00 EA

Sample Item Master | Vendors | Volumetric Table

Ready   100%

FIG 7.4 Extract sample of a supply item master file. (Dr. Jerry Ledlow, personal files.)

Supply Cost Capture

As a survey of supply chain progress[26] demonstrates, "In all industries, not just healthcare, three out of four chief executive officers consider their supply chains to be essential to gaining competitive advantage within their markets."[27, p. 2] According to Moore, if the trend in the cost of the healthcare supply chain continues to grow at the current rate, supply chain could equal labor cost in annual operating expenses for hospitals and health systems between 2020 and 2025.[28] Clearly, maximizing efficiency of the healthcare supply chain is an increasing concern.

Consider supply charge capture events in which patient-specific supplies are ordered for the care of that patient and the items are then billed separately to the patient. "Every year, hospitals lose millions of dollars when items used in the course of a patient's care somehow slip through the system without ever being charged or reimbursed."[29, p. 1] Point-of-use technology, or capturing charges when supplies or materials are used, allows healthcare institutions to increase productivity, increase accountability, and reduce downtime through improvements in their internal supply chain. Automated dispensing machines for medications or supplies can be used to decentralize store operations, capture charges, and bring supplies and materials to employees without compromising security and accountability.[30] These systems, if integrated with a solid business process, can enhance efficiency and effectiveness of the healthcare supply chain.

Strategic factors associated with supply success and enhancement are important as well. These include the following[27]:

- Information system usefulness, electronic purchasing, and integration
- Leadership supply chain expertise

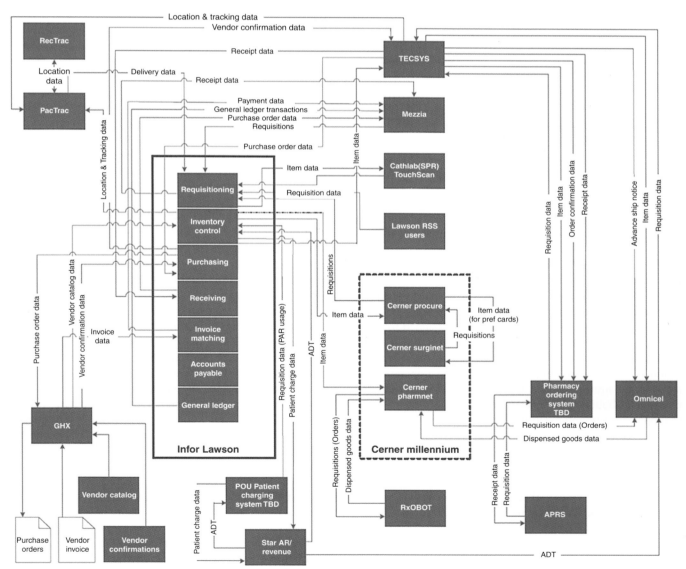

FIG 7.5 Wire diagram of healthcare supply chain information systems. (Dr. Jerry Ledlow, personal files.)

BOX 7.2   Process Standardization

Process Standardization in Conjunction with Utilization of an Information System
- Develop standard (or *more standardized*) processes for:
  - Item master and charge description master maintenance and synchronization
  - Supply stock selection, reduction, compression, and management
  - Supply charge item capture (accurate and timely)
  - Accountability measures for Central Supply and clinical units
  - Standardize clinical/floor stocked supplies replenishment processes
  - Daily reconciliation of pharmaceuticals and medical/surgical supply items, especially supply charge capture items
- Taking into consideration:
  - Clinical unit needs
  - Physical layout variations may require modification to an accepted standard
  - The business process must be efficient before a technological solution can be integrated into the process
  - "One-size" solution will not fit all

Process Standardization in Process Improvement: Balancing Trade-Offs
- Competing goals exist between various stakeholder groups; trade-offs will be required to find the proper balance that best meets all needs
- Clinician Goals
  - Does not impede caregivers or patient care delivery
  - Minimize rework
  - Right supplies, right place, right time
- Supply Chain Managers/Central Supply Goals
  - Improve accuracy for supplies consumed
  - Improve timeliness for supply consumption
  - Efficient use of labor
- Revenue and Cost Avoidance Goals
  - Procure and acquire material wisely with contracted compliance goals
  - Efficient management of materials considering utilization rates, preferences, expiration dates and Food and Drug Administration requirements
  - Reduce number of supply charge capture items
  - Improve accuracy for charge capture
  - Improve timeliness for charge capture
  - Improve charge capture rate

From Ledlow JR, Stephens JH, Fowler HH. Sticker shock: an exploration of supply charge capture outcomes. *Hosp Topics.* 2011;89(1):9. Reprinted by permission of the publisher (Taylor & Francis Ltd, http://www.tandf.co.uk/journals).

- Supply chain expenditures
- Provider level of collaboration
- Nurse and clinical staff level of collaboration
- Leadership team's political and social capital
- Capital funds availability

This section has provided a high-level overview of technology in materials management. Box **7.2** details specific considerations for automating SCM and materials management.[31]

Human Resources Information Systems

Human resources information systems (HRISs) leverage the power of IT to manage human resources. They integrate "software, hardware, support functions and system policies and procedures into an automated process designed to support the strategic and operational activities of the human resources department and managers throughout the organization."[32, p. 58] The authors distinguish between operational, tactical, and strategic HRISs. Operational HRISs collect and report data about employees and the personnel infrastructure to support routine and repetitive decision making while meeting the requirements of government regulations. Tactical HRISs support the design of the personnel infrastructure and decisions about the recruitment, training, and compensation of persons filling jobs in the organization. Strategic HRISs support activities with a longer horizon such as workforce planning and labor negotiations. In contrast, Targowski and Deshpande state that generic HRISs typically include the following subsystems defined by function: recruitment and selection from among candidates; administration of personnel processes; time, labor, and knowledge management; training and career development; administration of compensation and benefits for active workers and pensions for retirees; payroll interface; performance evaluation; transitioning and outplacement; labor relations; organization management; and health and safety.[33]

Human Resources Information Systems as a Competitive Advantage

Khatri argues that the management of human resources in healthcare organizations is a central function because the healthcare and administrative services delivered are based on the knowledge of staff delivering these services.[34] Human resources management should focus on employee training, as well as developing and refining the work systems to improve the work climate and the quality of service to customers. Although healthcare organizations should include the effective management of human resources as part of strategic planning, most fail to do so. Khatri offers three reasons why many healthcare organizations do not employ optimal human resource practices. First, he argues that the responsibilities and activities of human resources personnel are institutionalized and undervalued in many healthcare organizations. Second, the provider culture of healthcare focuses on the clinical delivery of care with less attention paid to the effective management of resources. Finally, lack of expertise and low skills in the human resource function have limited the ability of human resource managers to engage effectively in strategic and operational planning. Khatri's premise is that improving human resource capabilities should help human resource managers engage more effectively in managing human resources.[34]

Khatri further proposed five dimensions of human resources capability. The first four are a competent human resources executive in the C-suite, a skilled human resources staff, an organizational culture that elevates human resources to a central function, and commitment to continuous learning. An integrated, computerized HRIS is the final capability.[34]

Human Resources Information Systems Vendors

Vendors may offer comprehensive or component human resource information system applications to healthcare organizations. Three examples of vendors with comprehensive human resource information system solutions are listed alphabetically in Box **7.3**. Vendors offering component solutions that provide some but not all of the components of a complete human resources information system compete with those of the enterprise human resources suites for the component services that they offer. Two examples of vendors offering component solutions are:

- API Healthcare (www.apihealthcare.com)
- Kronos Workforce HR/Payroll (www.kronos.com)

Human Resources Subsystems

The human resources subsystems described below reflect a modification of the subsystems described by Targowski and Deshpande, and they represent a taxonomy of functions typically described by the vendor websites for HRISs.[33]

Personnel Administration. The centralized and integrated management of employee data is a key feature of HRISs. Personnel records are maintained and updated with information such as employee identification and demographics, dates of service, position and job code, location code, and employment status (permanent or temporary, full time, or part time). Systems also maintain records of licensure, credentials, certifications, and skill proficiency levels. Increasingly, self-service capabilities allow employees to maintain a personal profile with the ability to access and modify personal information such as name, address, contact information, marital status, and information about dependent family members.

Managing Human Resources Strategically and Operationally. HRISs can be used to address, in whole or in part, the challenge of managing human resources from a strategic and operational perspective. First, strategic management of human resources can be accomplished by accurately reflecting the organizational structure of the healthcare institution. This can be accomplished by using a wiring diagram to illustrate the hierarchy of positions in the organization, the job descriptions associated with each position, and whether the positions are filled or vacant. This analysis is then used to support the recruiting process for vacant positions. Functions that support this process include posting job announcements and application forms; providing status reports for submitted applications; maintaining interview schedules; and providing selection tools such as dynamic interview guides, multistage testing, computer adaptive testing, and mini simulations. Once a decision is made, the formal job offer letter and new employee benefits can be viewed online. Vendors who offer these types of functionality include Kronos (http://www.kronos.com/hiring-software/hiring.aspx) and Oracle's PeopleSoft (www.oracle.com/us/products/applications/peoplesoft-enterprise/human-capital-management/053291.html).

HRISs should also have the capability to assist employees in transitioning out of the organization when discharged, displaced by reductions in the workforce, or retiring.[33]

Staffing and Scheduling. Staffing and scheduling replaces the subsystem "time, labor, and knowledge management" as a more accurate representation of the activities supported by this HRIS subsystem. Staffing and scheduling are two different activities. Staffing involves the assignment of personnel to job positions while ensuring that they are qualified by virtue of degree, licensure, certification, training, and experience. Scheduling involves the assignment of qualified personnel to a scheduling template within a work area in the organization to fulfill the mission of that organization. Scheduling of personnel such as nursing staff is extremely challenging, so much so that nurse scheduling can be considered a definitive representative of the archetypal multishift scheduling problem found in operations research and management sciences literature.

Each of the vendors discussed in Box **7.3** offers both staffing and scheduling modules. Other modules manage scheduling for staff development and facilitate self-scheduling in conjunction with temporary staff management to fill openings in the schedule. Key requirements for staffing and scheduling include cost-effective staffing while meeting constraints imposed by required qualifications, scheduling visibility, and matching the level and number of caregivers to patient classification and acuity levels as mandated by law or regulation. An example of an enterprise staffing and scheduling product focused on nurse scheduling is McKesson's ANSOS One-Staff. Functions provided by these systems include:

- Staff schedules derived from patient acuity and workload data collected by the software.
- Hospital schedules automatically generated to meet core coverage goals while enforcing scheduling rules customized to meet schedule constraints and accommodate individual scheduling preferences.
- Synchronous staffing data provided to managers to ensure that nurse-to-patient staff ratios are met.
- Web-based self-scheduling.
- Productivity and labor cost reporting.[35]

BOX 7.3 **Sample Vendors Offering Comprehensive Human Resources Information Systems**

- Infor Healthcare Human Capital Management (www.infor.com/solutions/hcm/)
- McKesson Human Capital Management (www.mckesson.com/providers/health-systems/department-solutions/enterprise-resource-planning/mckesson-human-capital-management/)
- Oracle PeopleSoft Human Capital Management (www.oracle.com/us/products/applications/peoplesoft-enterprise/human-capital-management/overview/index.html)

Once scheduled, employees' time and attendance are tracked. Key elements include accurate time collection, implementation of user-defined pay rules, compliance with a variety of labor laws, and expeditious identification of productivity or overtime issues.

Just as schedules must be explicitly developed, time-off policies must be proactively managed because of their effect on the schedule. These time-off policies are designed to meet the requirements of federal labor laws such as the Family and Medical Leave Act (FMLA) and state and local laws. In addition to meeting legal and regulatory constraints, time-off policies must enforce organizational policy for vacation, maternity leave, and sick leave. The software used to do this is referred to as "leave management" or "absence management" and is typically a rules-based application designed to manage absence requests while interfacing with workload scheduling.

Because of the difficulty of scheduling in healthcare, flexible scheduling solutions are becoming increasingly common. API Healthcare provides software incorporating three solutions representative of many scheduling systems:

- **Open shift management**: This is a web-based self-scheduling solution in which the nurse manager broadcasts openings in the schedule to qualified staff via a number of instant communication tools. Staff members respond by tendering schedule and shift requests for consideration and approval.
- **Incentive management**: This involves the use of monetary and point-based rewards for staff who volunteer to fill openings in the schedule.
- **Predictive scheduling**: Predictive modeling is used to forecast bed demand while accounting for variables such as bed turnover, changes in patient acuity, workload distribution, and variability caused by shift, day of the week, month, and seasonality.[36]

Another vendor, CareSystems (www.caresystemsinc.com/), is a relatively new entry into the healthcare staffing and scheduling arena, with a suite of products that manage time and attendance, assess patient acuity and estimated nurse workload, and employ intelligent scheduling algorithms to create optimal nursing schedules.

Training and Development. The three comprehensive vendors featured in Box **7.3** also addressed staff training and development. IT solutions should be able to be used as the infrastructure to plan and manage employee training, to serve as the delivery mechanism synchronously and online, and to link training with the developmental plan for each employee by identifying shortfalls in skills and competencies and then recording when those shortfalls have been remediated.[33]

Compensation, Benefits, and Pension Administration-Payroll Interface

Compensation and benefit plans can vary from company to company. They include various plans like flexible and non-flexible healthcare plans, short- and long-term disability plans, saving plans, retirement plans, pension plans and Flexible Spending Accounts.[33, p. 46]

When coupled with personnel administration and staffing and scheduling systems and supported by timekeeping and absence management software, the management of compensation, benefits, and pension administration becomes more accurate and less time consuming.

One example of a vendor offering integrated compensation, benefits, and payroll applications is Oracle's PeopleSoft   (www.oracle.com/us/products/applications/peoplesoft-enterprise/human-capital-management/053949.html). The PeopleSoft Enterprise eCompensation system permits managers to view and update employees records online; receive alerts and decision support when changes in salary and benefits are being considered; receive reports on individuals, as well as groups of employees; and permit employees to view and maintain their own records as appropriate.

Performance Evaluation. *Talent management* and *performance management* are terms used by several vendors. From the healthcare provider's perspective, the focus is on recruiting and training employees and developing competencies required to fulfill institutional goals and objectives. The individual career goals of employees are also considered. Information capabilities in this area include:

- Profiling employee competencies and any gaps.
- Identifying when employee and organizational goals are met.
- Identifying top performers.
- Managing dashboards to display unit performance.

Infor's Human Capital Management suite includes modules for talent acquisition, goal management, and performance management.[37]

Underrepresented Subsystems. Labor relations and health and safety have received less attention from vendors developing information for managing human resources, whereas web-based expense and travel applications have become more prevalent in healthcare organizations. These areas may represent future directions for ERP systems.

Business Intelligence Systems

Since the late 1990s, healthcare institutions have been building data warehouses and integrating data. Along with the technical aspects, data warehousing includes improving data quality, developing protocols for governance, and facilitating the employment of appropriate analytic measures. This is difficult because of practice variation and changes to the standards of practice over time. As quoted in an article by Erickson,[38] Dick Gibson, the CIO of Legacy Health, notes,

We generate and use data like any other industry, but health care does not lend itself to the use of discrete data because the outcomes are necessarily fuzzy and ongoing. Airlines have seats, schedules and know if you landed on time. In health care, we know if you are alive but the big money goes to broad sets of descriptive terms around patient care that are very qualitative.[38, p. 29]

These descriptive terms can be captured more succinctly by the use of diagnostic and procedural codes, but data quality and integration is a problem because of the number of procedures and number of providers engaged in the delivery of care.[38]

Many organizations are turning to business intelligence (BI) software to provide tools to effectively manage and use their massive amounts of data. BI software is purported to lead to an improvement in financial (particularly revenue cycle) and operational performance, as well as patient care.[39] Implementing BI in healthcare that successfully integrates financial and clinical data is regarded as one of the four pillars of the Value Project undertaken by the Healthcare Financial Management Association.[40] **Business intelligence (BI)** is defined as the "acquisition, correlation, and transformation of data into insightful and actionable information through analytics, enabling an organization and its business partners to make better, timelier decisions."[41, p. 142] However, Glaser and Stone warn that for the BI to be most effective, the BI tools must be placed in the hands of the people who actually do the work, training must be done initially and throughout the project so that users will have time to use the basic functions and expand their knowledge, questions that arise throughout the analysis must be reviewed and answered, and the BI should be used for long-term planning.[39] Glaser and Stone describe the BI platform as "a stack—one technology on top of another."[39, p. 69] Their description was used to construct Fig. **7.6**. Effective management of this stackable technology involves making the business case for BI, establishing implementation targets, enlisting BI champions, governing effectively, and establishing BI roles to include data stewards, data owners, business users, and data managers.[39]

As with the other information systems discussed in this chapter, BI systems may be part of an enterprise system, provided as component software, or employed at application level. Most of the major healthcare information system vendors have BI software imbedded in their products. For example, McKesson has Enterprise Intelligence; Cerner has Knowledge Solutions; and Allscripts has EPSi Integrated Performance Management.

KLAS lists the following vendors in this category of software, but they are not part of an enterprise healthcare information system. Instead, they provide BI solutions intended to support analytics in conjunction with enterprise software or they provide analytics for a segment of the healthcare marketplace.

- Dimensional Insight (www.dimins.com) provides a BI platform specific to healthcare called HealthcareAware BI (www.dimins.com/healthcare-analytics/) and targeted solutions for physician and surgical management, Meaningful Use, and general ledger cost analysis.
- IBM Cognos (www-01.ibm.com/software/analytics/cognos/) offers a tailored line of analytic solutions, with Cognos Analytics providing large-scale capabilities and Cognos Express targeting midsize companies and work groups.

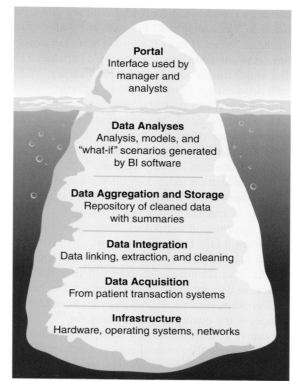

FIG 7.6 Business intelligence platform. (Data from Glaser J, Stone J. Effective use of business intelligence. *Healthc Financ Manag.* 2008;62(2):68-72.)

- Information Builders WebFOCUS Business Intelligence and Analytics Platform (www.informationbuilders.com/products/intelligence) advertises capabilities similar to Dimensional Insight and IBM Cognos.
- Greenway Health (www.greenwayhealth.com/solution/analytics-data-insight/) offers analytic solutions for improving the management of ambulatory practices.

Given the cost, time, and complexity of the large-scale implementation of enterprise BI, application-level BI should be employed strategically to address "key processes, functions, or service lines."[42, p. 95] Application-level BI software provides some of the data integration and visualization of enterprise packages, analyzes existing data that may be overlooked in traditional reporting, and creates actionable knowledge. However, some caution is necessary. Glaser and Stone note that ad hoc, smaller-scale analysis may lead to the creation of data silos, inefficient or repetitive management of data, and unnecessary duplication.[39] These are appropriate cautions, but application-level BI can complement the development of enterprise BI by producing results in the interim as the enterprise capabilities are developed.[42]

CONCLUSION AND FUTURE DIRECTIONS

Given the magnitude of the investment in health information systems, and that administrative applications are more mature than clinical applications, a salient question is whether these administrative applications have made healthcare delivery more productive. In "Unraveling the IT Productivity Paradox—Lessons for Healthcare," Jones, Heaton, Rudin, and Schneider explore the paradoxical relationship between "the rapid increase in IT use and the simultaneous slowdown in productivity."[43, p. 2243] Several lessons emerge from the authors' analysis:

- Mismeasurement partially contributed to the paradox. The authors suggest, "assessment of the value of healthcare outputs could be improved through the more sophisticated use of clinical data to understand access, convenience, and health outcomes."[43, p. 2244]
- New information technology often requires redesign of the processes that were previously tailored to the technology or manual system just replaced.
- New information technology compromises productivity when it fails to be user centered.
- Finally, healthcare organizations can no longer afford to have an abundance of untapped data that fails to improve decision making. Improvements in healthcare information systems, BI, and analytics must continue to improve the quality of decision making.[43]

Administrative systems in this chapter were listed as separate applications because they evolved independently of CSs. Many of the future benefits will accrue from integrating data from all systems. For example, if a healthcare system cannot effectively track the total cost of all materials used to treat an individual patient and aggregate data to determine the cost of treating groups of patients, managing the cost of healthcare is not possible. As new information becomes available for decision making, healthcare professionals on both the administrative and the clinical sides of the organization will need to learn new interprofessional approaches to using these data in making decisions.

REFERENCES

1. Haux R. Health information systems—past, present, and future. *Int J Med Inform.* 2006;75:268–281.
2. Ciotti V, Alcaro B. Top 2013 HIS vendors by revenue. *Health Data Manag.* 2014;22(6):16.
3. Gartner, Inc. *Why Gartner?* http://www.gartner.com/technology/why_gartner.jsp. Accessed June 13, 2016.
4. *KLAS.* Our story. http://www.klasresearch.com/about-us/our-story. Accessed June 13, 2016.
5. Rogoski RR. Counting on efficiency: healthcare organizations in growth mode need financial information systems that can accommodate expansion. *Health Manag Technol.* 2006;27 (3):10–12. 14.
6. Latham H. The healthcare CFO: squeezing more from IT. *Health Manag Technol.* 2009;30(1):10–11.
7. Cruze G. Saying it isn't so: how documentation can decrease denials. *Healthc Financ Manag.* 2008;62(2):84–89.
8. Thompson S, Dean MD. Advancing information technology in health care. *Commun ACM.* 2009;52(6):118–121.
9. Hammer D, Franklin D. Beyond bolt-ons: breakthroughs in revenue cycle information systems. *Healthc Financ Manag.* 2008;62(2):52–60.
10. James J. *Health policy brief.* http://healthaffairs.org/healthpolicybriefs/brief_pdfs/healthpolicybrief_78.pdf. Accessed June 13, 2016.
11. Schulz J, DeCamp M, Berkowitz SA. Medicare shared savings program: public reporting and shared savings distributions. *Am J Manag Care.* 2015;21(8):546–553.
12. Williams B. Gaining with integration: three healthcare organizations use integrated financial-clinical systems to achieve ROI, process improvement and patient care objectives. *Health Manag Technol.* 2002;23(6):10. 12–13, 15.
13. *TechTarget.* WhatIs. http://whatis.techtarget.com. Accessed June 13, 2016.
14. Moore R. Rural healthcare system drops AR days and cleans up claims. *Health Manag Technol.* 2010;31(7):16–17.
15. Sorrentino PA, Sanderson BB. Managing the physician revenue cycle. *Healthc Financ Manag.* 2001;65(12):88. -90, 92, 94.
16. Curtis E, Schelhammer S. Patient outreach system helps clinic boost care visits, revenues. *Healthc Financ Manag Assoc;* 2011. http://www.hfma.org/Leadership/E-Bulletins/2011/August/Patient_Outreach_System_Helps_Clinic_Boost_Care_Visits,_Revenues/.
17. Conley C. *Improve Patient Satisfaction and Collections with Efficient Payment Processes.* Emdeon Express Winter Edition 2009. http://emdeonexpress.blogspot.com/2009/02/its-no-secret-that-health-care-is.html.
18. Cash J. Technology can make or break the hospital-physician relationship. *Healthc Financ Manag.* 2008;62(12):104–109.
19. Gates P, Urquhart J. The electronic, "paperless" medical office: has it arrived? *Intern Med J.* 2007;37:108–111.
20. *Glossary 2013 01 080513. Council of Supply Chain;* 2013. http://cscmp.org/sites/default/files/user_uploads/resources/downloads/glossary-2013.pdf.
21. Blount D, Chaney V, Fohey L, Goodhue R, Greiner T, Hinkle D. Materials Management Review Guide. 4th ed. Chicago, Illinois: Association for Healthcare Resource & Materials Management of the American Hospital Association; 2012:12.
22. Lummus RR, Vokurka RJ. Defining supply chain management: a historical perspective and practical guidelines. *Ind Manag Data Syst.* 1999;99(1):11–17.
23. Roark DC. Managing the healthcare supply chain. *Nurs Manag.* 2005;36(2):36–40.
24. HIMSS. Healthcare ERP and SCM Information Systems: Strategies and Solutions. In: *A White Paper by the HIMSS Enterprise Information Systems Steering Committee;* 2007.
25. Corry AP, Ledlow GR, Shockley S. *Designing the Standard for a Healthy Supply Chain.* Montgomery Research; 2005.
26. Poirer C, Quinn F. A survey of supply chain progress. *Supply Chain Manag Rev.* 2004;8(8):24–31.
27. Ledlow G, Corry A, Cwiek M. *Optimize Your Healthcare Supply Chain Performance: A Strategic Approach.* Chicago, Illinois: Health Administration Press; 2007.
28. Moore V. *Clinical Supply Chain.* Chicago, Illinois: Paper presented at American College of Healthcare Executives National Congress; 2008.
29. Bacon S, Pexton C. *Improving Patient Charge Capture at Yale-New Haven.* iSixSigma; 2010. http://www.isixsigma.com/index.php?option=com_k2&view=item&id=997:&Itemid=49.
30. Evahan Technology. *Point of Use Technology in the Supply Chain.* Ferret; 2005. http://www.ferret.com.au/c/Evahan/Point-of-use-technology-in-the-supply-chain-n698823.
31. Ledlow JR, Stephens JH, Fowler HH. Sticker shock: an exploration of supply charge capture outcomes. *Hosp Top.* 2011;89(1):9.
32. Chauhan A, Sharma S, Tyagi T. Role of HRIS in improving modern HR operations. *Rev Manag.* 2011;1(2):58–70.

33. Targowski AS, Deshpande SP. The utility and selection of an HRIS. *Adv Competitiveness Res.* 2001;9(1):42–56.
34. Khatri N, Building HR. capability in health care organizations. *Health Care Manag Rev.* 2006;31(1):45–54.
35. McKesson. *ANSOS One-Staff.* McKesson; 2013. http://www.mckesson.com/providers/health-systems/department-solutions/capacity-and-workforce-management/ansos-one-staff/.
36. *API Healthcare.* Staffing and Scheduling. API Healthcare. http://www.apihealthcare.com/staffing-scheduling. Accessed June 14, 2016.
37. *Infor.* Talent Management Brochure. http://www.infor.com/product-summary/hcm/talent-management/. Accessed June 14, 2016.
38. Erickson J. BI's march to health care. *Inform Manag.* 2009;19(7):29–34.
39. Glaser J, Stone J. Effective use of business intelligence. *Healthc Financ Manag.* 2008;62(2):68–72.
40. Clarke R. Rethinking business intelligence. *Healthc Financ Manag.* 2012;66(2):120.
41. Giniat EJ. Using business intelligence for competitive advantage. *Healthc Financ Manag.* 2011;65(9):142–146.
42. Hennen J. Targeted business intelligence pays off. *Healthc Financ Manag.* 2009;63(3):92–98.
43. Jones SS, Heaton PS, Rudin RS, Schneider EC. Unraveling the IT productivity paradox—lessons for healthcare. *New Engl J Med.* 2012;366(24):2243–2245.

DISCUSSION QUESTIONS

1. Explain why healthcare facilities would require the use of a financial information system, and provide examples of this type of system.
2. Describe how a decision maker would use the financial information system reporting function to make decisions, and provide a summary of what the various reports tell the decision maker.
3. Explain the importance of physicians using a practice management system, and provide examples of tools that can be used at the point of care.
4. Describe and defend three principles of a quality supply chain management system with regard to patient care and support of clinicians providing care.
5. Discuss how self-service applications are typically deployed in human resources information systems.
6. Discuss the advantages and disadvantages of using business intelligence at the application level as opposed to the enterprise level.

CASE STUDY

Michael H. Kennedy, Kim Crickmore,[a] and Lynne Miles[a]

Managing the flow of patients and bed capacity is challenging for any hospital, especially for unscheduled admissions. For Zed Medical Center, a large regional referral center in the South and a member of the University Health System Consortium, the challenge is even greater. As the flagship hospital for a multihospital system with more than 750 licensed beds and a Level 1 trauma center with 50-plus trauma beds, approximately 70% of annual admissions are unscheduled.

The vice-president for Operations has a PhD in Nursing, is a fellow of the Advisory Board Company, and has more than 20 years' tenure at Zed Medical Center. Three of the ten departments under her purview (Patient Care Coordinator, Bed Control, and Patient Transfers) are directly engaged in managing patient flow and bed capacity. The division is also responsible for system-wide care coordination for patients discharged to skilled nursing facilities, to home health, and to home without planned service delivery. Current operational goals include (1) decreasing the current length of stay by 0.3 days from 5.7 to 5.4 days and (2) "ED to 3"—a slogan incorporating the intention to place patients from the emergency department into a bed within 3 hours of the decision to admit. With the Centers for Medicare & Medicaid Services clarifying penalties for readmissions within 30 days, Zed Medical Center has been preparing to effectively manage readmissions based on CMS guidelines.

The eight staff members assigned to Patient Transfers coordinate with hospitals within the region wanting to transfer patients to Zed Medical Center. They take calls, connect outside transfers with accepting physicians, and arrange transport. The accepting physician determines the patient's needed level of care, special care needs (e.g., diabetic), and the time frame for transfer. The Patient Transfer Department uses the TransferCenter module of TeleTracking (www.teletracking.com) to manage the transfer and admission of patients. After a patient has been accepted for admission by the admitting physician, Bed Control makes the bed assignment. The staff members of Bed Control assign incoming patients to specific beds once the Patient Placement Facilitators from the Patient Care Coordinator Department identify the nursing unit to which patients should be assigned. This determination is made based on the level of care required, physician preferences in choice of nursing unit, and the scope of care supported by the nursing units. The Bed Control Department uses the Capacity Management Suite of the TeleTracking software. The PreAdmitTracking module keeps track of bed status with an "electronic bedboard," which provides a graphical user interface through which planned admissions, transfers, and discharges can be annotated. The status of a bed freed by patient discharge for which a cleaning request has been made is also noted (dirty, in progress, or cleaned). The Bed Tracking module uses the medical center's

---

[a]*Kim Crickmore and Lynne Miles are past Advisory Board members for the East Carolina University Health Services Management Program.*

paging network to notify the environmental services staff of a cleaning request and the unit director of the unit that a patient is incoming. The TransportTracking module automatically dispatches patient transport requests via phone or pager.

Discussion Questions

1. How are patients prioritized for bed assignment?
2. Describe some of the advantages and disadvantages of this new software. Include the stated organizational goals in your answer.
3. Discuss how this software might share data with other institutional applications to provide a dashboard view of census-type activity.

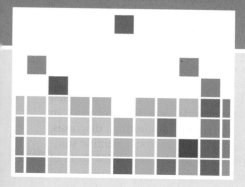

8

Telehealth and Applications for Delivering Care at a Distance

Loretta Schlachta-Fairchild, Mitra Rocca, Vicky Elfrink Cordi,
Andrea Day, Diane Castelli, Kathleen MacMahon,
Dianna Vice-Pasch, Daniel A. Nagel, and Antonia Arnaert*

Growth in telehealth could result in a future where access to health care is not limited by geographic region, time, or availability of skilled health care professionals.

OBJECTIVES

At the completion of this chapter, the reader will be prepared to:
1. Discuss the historical milestones and leading organizations in the development of telehealth.
2. Explain the two overarching types of telehealth technology interactions and provide examples of telehealth technologies for each type.
3. Describe the clinical practice considerations for telehealth-delivered care for health professionals.
4. Analyze operational and organizational success factors and barriers for telehealth within healthcare organizations.
5. Discuss practice and policy considerations for health professionals, including competency, licensure and interstate practice, malpractice, and reimbursement for telehealth.
6. Describe the use of telehealth to enable self-care in consumer informatics.
7. Discuss future trends in telehealth.

KEY TERMS

digital literacy, 147
telehealth, 131
telehealth competency, 137

telemedicine, 131
telenursing, 131
uHealth, 148

ABSTRACT ❖

Rapid advances in technology development and telehealth adoption are opening new opportunities for healthcare providers to leverage technology for improved patient outcomes. Telehealth provides access to care and the ability to export clinical expertise to care for patients regardless of their geographic location. This chapter presents telehealth technologies and programs, as well as telehealth practice considerations such as licensure and malpractice challenges. As telehealth advances, healthcare providers will require competencies and knowledge to incorporate safe and effective clinical practice using telehealth technologies into their daily workflow.

*The views, opinions, and/or findings contained in this publication are those of the author and do not necessarily reflect the views of the Department of Defense and should not be construed as an official DoD/Army position, policy, or decision unless so designated by other documentation. No official endorsement should be made. Reference herein to any specific commercial products, process, or service by trade name, trademark, manufacturer, or otherwise, does not necessarily constitute or imply its endorsement, recommendation, or favoring by the U.S. Government.

INTRODUCTION

Rapid advances in technology development and telehealth adoption are opening new opportunities for healthcare providers to use technology for improved patient outcomes. Before we discuss these technologies and outcomes, it is important to explore the definitions of telehealth-related terminology.

Telehealth encompasses a broad definition of telecommunications and information technology–enabled healthcare services and technologies. Often used interchangeably with the terms *telemedicine, eHealth,* or *mHealth* (mobile health), telehealth is "the use of electronic information and telecommunications technologies to support long-distance clinical health care, patient and professional health-related education, public health, and health administration."[1] Telehealth is being used in this text to encompass all of these other terms. Telemedicine is the use of medical information exchanged from one site to another via electronic communications for the health and education of the patient or healthcare provider and for improving patient care, treatment, and services.[2] Telenursing is the use of telehealth technology to deliver nursing care and conduct nursing practice.[3,4]

Telehealth enables the delivery of clinical care regardless of the geographic location of the patient or the healthcare provider. Well-established telehealth programs and evidence-based research supports the effective use of telehealth across most disciplines and specialties within healthcare (i.e., teleradiology, teledermatology, telepathology, and telenursing).[5–10] Telehealth services provide access to health assessment, diagnosis, intervention, consultation, supervision, and information across distance.[11] As a result, telehealth is now being integrated into routine care delivery of patients around the globe. Fig. 8.1 depicts how telehealth can change healthcare delivery. Telehealth services can be classified as clinical or nonclinical. Clinical telehealth services include, for example, diagnosis; patient communication and education; disease management, triage and advice; remote monitoring; caregiver support; and provider-to-provider teleconsultations. Examples of nonclinical telehealth services include distance education for healthcare consumers or clinicians, video conferencing or conference call meetings, research, healthcare administration, and healthcare management.

Providing care to underserved populations is a challenge, especially in rural areas or in areas with a shortage of healthcare professionals. Patients may face physical, financial, geographic, and other barriers to accessing care. However, telehealth can overcome many of these barriers. Telehealth proponents seek to improve the quality, access, equity, and affordability of healthcare in the United States and globally by using telehealth.[11] Healthcare professionals using telehealth can export their clinical expertise to patients regardless of geographic location.

Telehealth technologies include a simple telephone conversation between a healthcare provider and a patient or a sophisticated robotic surgery on a patient across continents. Telehealth technologies include but are not limited to telephones; facsimile machines; e-mail systems; cellphones; mobile apps; video conferencing; web-based, remote patient-monitoring devices; transmission of still images; and internet applications (eHealth) including patient portals, remote vital signs monitoring, continuing medical education, and direct consumer applications such as online physician consultations via the internet.

Telehealth is used in a variety of settings, among which are rural hospitals, home health agencies, and with patients at home, in prisons, at dialysis centers, and in nursing homes; telehealth is also used to provide care to astronauts in space.[11,12] The benefits of remote monitoring, diagnosis, and intervention are recognized in numerous scientific studies and include increased access to care, decreased costs of healthcare, increased healthcare provider productivity, and a high level of patient satisfaction.[3,13] Further, the advantages of telehealth to patients are numerous, and they include:

- Decreased travel time or distance and removal of travel barriers
- More immediate access to care
- Early detection of disease processes or health issues
- Ownership of healthcare and feelings of empowerment
- Long-term health and independence
- Caregiver reassurance
- Patient satisfaction with healthcare

Examples of Successful Telehealth Programs

The following four examples of telehealth programs demonstrate the wide range of such programs currently providing services to patients at a distance.

- Rochester General Health System, Rochester, New York, developed a clinic-based telehealth program in 2008. Its healthcare providers use a video conferencing system for live patient consults with remote physician specialists. They have the capability to send video images and 12-lead digital ECGs. The Director of Telehealth coordinates and schedules 34 physicians and 5 midlevel healthcare providers who see patients remotely.
- The Department of Defense (DOD), and in particular, the U.S. Army, has been using telemedicine since 1992. Its Telehealth Network spans 50 countries and territories from America Samoa to Afghanistan, across 19 time zones. It has 22 service lines available, with behavioral health telehealth making up 55% of telemedicine services, followed by cardiology, teledermatology, infectious diseases,

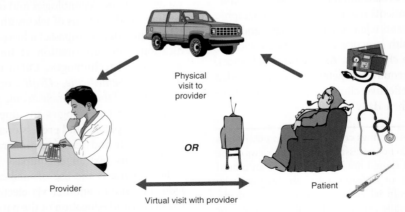

Physical visit to provider

OR

Provider

Virtual visit with provider

Patient

Telehealth enables the export of clinical expertise virtually to patients who need it

FIG 8.1 How telehealth changes healthcare delivery. (Copyright 2010 iTelehealth Inc. All Rights Reserved.)

neurosurgery, pain management, and orthopedic surgery. Although commonly implemented in day-to-day military healthcare settings, limited resources and austerity of the environment are among the challenges the DOD faces in providing telemedicine in field or operational settings. [14]

- Sea Coast Mission Telehealth Program, Bar Harbor, Maine, provides seagoing health services to islanders living on four islands with no healthcare providers available. Daily use of live video conferencing from a 72-foot boat, the *Sunbeam V,* occurs with the support of a boat crew that includes a nurse. The telehealth nurse has developed excellent clinical and technical skills to work proficiently in an austere environment. The goal is to diagnose sick patients in a timely manner so that they can be transferred off the island for access to a higher level of medical care on the mainland. Maine Sea Coast Mission's most recent project has been to implement health centers with video conferencing systems on four islands (Frenchboro, Matinicus, Swan's Island, and Isle au Haut), providing access to remote health/education services year round (Sharon Daley, registered nurse (RN), personal communication, March 2010).
- University of Miami, Miller School of Medicine, Miami, Florida, provides both live video conferencing and store-and-forward capability via its telehealth program, which provided medical support after the 2010 Haiti earthquake. One unique aspect is the Teledermatology Program for private cruise ships that uses expert dermatologists to evaluate an array of skin problems such as lesions, burns, infections, and rashes seen by physicians aboard cruise ships. The Clinical Telehealth Coordinator provides online training to cruise ship staff to use digital cameras to capture and transmit images via a dermatology software application. Images are then reviewed by the dermatologist and patient reports with diagnosis and recommendations are sent back electronically to the cruise ship physician within a specific time frame. [15]

Telehealth Historic Milestones

In contrast to the common perception that telehealth is new and futuristic, it actually has a long history. The first documented report of healthcare delivery at a distance dates back to 1897 in *The Lancet,* when a case of croup was diagnosed over the telephone. In the United States, modern telehealth programs began in 1964, with a closed-circuit television link between the Nebraska Psychiatric Institute and the Norfolk State Hospital for teleconsultations. Shortly thereafter, in 1965, a cardiac surgeon in the United States transmitted a live video feed of a surgical case to spectators in Geneva, Switzerland, via satellite. The surgeon discussed his case and answered live questions from the spectators in Geneva. [16]

The National Aeronautics and Space Administration (NASA) led telehealth initiatives in the 1960s with the transmission of physiologic signals from astronauts in space to command centers on Earth. NASA also funded several telehealth research programs in the late 1960s and early 1970s that contributed to the profession as a whole. [17] A landmark

study completed by Kaiser Permanente in 1997 concluded that "technology in healthcare can be an asset for patients and providers and has the potential to save costs; therefore, this technology must be a part of continuous planning for quality improvement,"[18, p. 45]. The researchers were emphatic about the benefits of telehealth, inspiring many of today's telehealth programs.

From July 2003 to December 2007, the U.S. Department of Veterans Affairs (VA) conducted a home telecare program analysis to coordinate care of chronically ill veterans and reduce long-term care admissions. The program evaluation was highly successful, realizing a reduction in long-term care bed days and inpatient hospital admissions among participants. Further, the veteran participants reported a high level of satisfaction. Costs to provide the program were and are substantially less than other VA programs or nursing home care. The program is now known as Care Coordination/Home Telehealth and is a routinely offered VA service to support aging veterans with chronic conditions. [19]

To determine the effectiveness of telehealth, the Whole System Demonstrator program in the United Kingdom was launched by the National Health Service in 2008. At the time, the study was the largest randomized controlled trial of telehealth in the world, involving more than 6000 participants. The study confirmed that telehealth promotes well-being and should be a part of any complete healthcare system. [20]

In 2011, the Alaska Native Tribal Health Consortium (ANTHC) met a significant milestone, seeing their 100,000th telehealth case since the beginning of the statewide program in 2001. Originally developed as a care supplement to Alaskans in rural areas, the telehealth solution developed by ANTHC has been adopted by the Indian Health Service throughout the United States, in the Maldives, as well as by Canada in an international space station. [21]

Today, telehealth has advanced well beyond that first phone call in 1897, to become more widespread with the ubiquitous use of mobile technology and the introduction of parity laws providing for reimbursement of telehealth services at the same rate as in-person services.

Leading Telehealth Organizations

Starting in the 1990s, a number of professional, industry, and government organizations provided the leadership needed to initiate effective telehealth programs. These leaders include the American Nurses Association (ANA), United States federal government agencies, the American Telemedicine Association (ATA), and the International Council of Nurses (ICN).

American Nurses Association

With the advent of technology and rapidly emerging telehealth practice in the twentieth century, healthcare professionals sought guidance on incorporating telehealth into their care offerings. Multidisciplinary standards were needed to create a cohesive unity for telehealth across professions. To address the expansion and to create unified definitions and policies and a standard of care, the ANA brought together the Interdisciplinary Telehealth Standards Working Group. This group was composed of 41 representatives from different healthcare organizations and professional associations. The report of the interdisciplinary team, *Core Principles on Telehealth*, represents a "sense of the profession" as a whole.[22] The purpose of the core principles is to create a baseline standard of quality telehealth care.

United States Federal Government Agencies

NASA, the VA, the U.S. DOD, and other government agencies have continued to lead the United States in telehealth research and programs. As an early adopter of telehealth, the VA operates the nation's largest telehealth program. The widespread adoption and positive research findings regarding telehealth led the U.S. government to establish the Office for the Advancement of Telehealth (OAT), a division of the Office of Rural Health Policy within Health Resources and Services Administration (HRSA) at the U.S. Department of Health & Human Services (HHS). OAT promotes the use of telehealth technologies for healthcare delivery, education, and health information services, and it increases the use and quality of telehealth delivery through:

- Fostering partnerships within HRSA and with other federal agencies, states, and private sector groups to create telehealth projects
- Administering telehealth grant programs
- Providing technical assistance
- Evaluating the use of telehealth technologies and programs
- Developing telehealth policy initiatives to improve access to quality health services
- Promoting knowledge exchange about "best telehealth practices"[1]

American Telemedicine Association

The ATA is a nonprofit organization founded in 1993 and headquartered in Washington, DC. The mission of ATA is to "promote professional, ethical and equitable improvement in healthcare delivery through telecommunications and information technology" through education, research, and communication.[23] ATA is a mission-driven, nonprofit organization that seeks to incorporate telehealth seamlessly into healthcare so that it is not necessarily a separate program but integrated into healthcare delivery as a whole. The ATA has published a number of telemedicine practice guidelines that form a foundation for telehealth practice that are based on empirical and clinical practice evidence.[24]

International Council of Nurses

Representing more than 130 national nursing organizations, including the ANA, Canadian Nurses Association, and associations of more than 134 countries, the ICN initiated the Telenursing Network in 2008. As telenursing advances, this virtual collaboration is serving to share competencies and other jointly developed telenursing resources.

TELEHEALTH TECHNOLOGIES

Telehealth technologies enable the exchange of all types of data (i.e., voice, video, pictures of wounds, pathology or radiology images, and device readings) between patients and healthcare providers or between healthcare providers on behalf of patients. Early telehealth technologies were "stand-alone" systems in which a telehealth encounter occurred and data were stored in a telehealth system database. With the increasing adoption of electronic health records (EHRs), telehealth technologies are being increasingly integrated with the EHRs. Telehealth services can be delivered using two overarching types of technologies: synchronous (or real-time) technologies or asynchronous (or store-and-forward) technology.

Synchronous or "Real-Time" Technologies

Synchronous, real-time telehealth uses live, two-way interactive telecommunications technology and/or patient monitoring technologies to connect a healthcare provider to a patient for direct care, to other healthcare providers for consultation and collaboration, or to a combination of the two. The most commonly used synchronous telehealth employs video conferencing or telephone-based interaction.

Video Conferencing

Video conferencing integrates audio, video, computing, and communications technologies to allow people in different locations to collaborate electronically face to face, in real time, and to share information, including data, documents, sound, and picture. Interactive video conferencing in telehealth enables patient-provider consultations, provider-specialist discussions, and health education. The technology requires live presence of the healthcare provider and patient or provider and medical specialist in an interactive environment.

A real-time live environment can include:

- Video conferencing units with a codec (*compressor-decompressor*) capable of encoding and decoding the video conferencing data stream.
- Peripheral cameras such as high-definition cameras with remote control pan, tilt, and zoom.
- Video display devices such as computer monitors, television sets such as ultra–high density plasma or LCD displays, and LCD projectors are used to show the images received from the video conferencing codec.
- Audio components (microphones and speakers), a network connection, and the user interface—before the availability of high-bandwidth internet connections, signals were carried over point-to-point connections established via Integrated Services Digital Network (ISDN) lines and plain old telephone service (POTS). The internet has now simplified some of the connectivity issues and the high-bandwidth requirement of video conferencing.

Patient Monitoring Technologies

Patient monitoring technologies, including home telehealth (also known as telehomecare), use devices to remotely collect

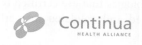

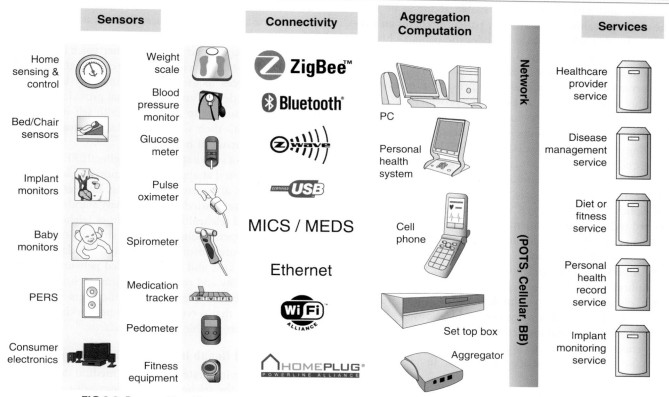

FIG 8.2 Personal health ecosystem. *BB,* Broadband; *PERS,* personal emergency response system; *POTS,* plain old telephone service. (Copyright 2010 Continua Health Alliance. All Rights Reserved.)

and send biometric data to a home health agency or a remote diagnostic testing facility for interpretation by a healthcare provider. Such applications might include a specific vital sign device, such as blood glucose monitor, digital scale, thermometer, heart electrocardiogram (ECG), blood pressure monitor, pulse oximeter, or peak flow meters, or a variety of monitoring devices for homebound patients. Such services can be used to supplement the use of visiting nurses.[25] Use of monitoring devices will also allow patients to become more involved in, and in many cases to oversee, the monitoring process.

Patient monitoring technologies for home telehealth consist of two major components: hardware and software. The hardware includes a base station where the patient interacts by entering data and answering questions, and it applies various medical devices that are used to gather patient data. The software enables healthcare providers and technicians to configure the hardware, receive data, and monitor the patient.

Telecommunications can be *wired,* such as POTS or direct service line (DSL), or *wireless,* such as cellular (sometimes seen as code division multiple access, broadband, satellite, Bluetooth, infrared (IrDA), Wi-Fi (or IEEE Standard 802.11), mobile broadband wireless access (IEEE Standard 802.20), or Worldwide Interoperability for Microwave Access (IEEE Standard 802.16). *mHealth* and *mobile health* are

umbrella terms that incorporate mobile or wireless telecommunications for transmitting telehealth-related data and services. Both the telecommunication and the hardware can be incorporated in the medical device.

Fig. 8.2 provides a diagram of the components of a telehealth system:

1. Personal health devices monitor basic vital signs such as blood pressure, weight, pulse, oxygen level, and blood sugar values and transmit data via a wired or wireless connection via devices or sensors.
2. The aggregation and computation manager is a critical component of the connected health system, enabling individual monitoring devices to log data in an EHR for personal and clinician review. The aggregation manager collects and transmits data from an individual's personal health devices to a server using wired or wireless connections. The aggregation manager itself can be a cell phone, a personal computer (PC), a dedicated device, or a personal health record (PHR).
3. The health service center is a physical location where a patient's digital information is collected, stored, analyzed, and distributed. It can be the doctor's office, the home of a family member, or another type of healthcare-related facility.

Asynchronous or "Store-and-Forward" Technology

"Store-and-forward" technology transmits telehealth-related information, video, images, and audio files when healthcare providers and patients are not available at the same time. The sending healthcare provider or patient prepares an electronic consult package, which includes the patient's history, related diagnoses, and digital images such as x-rays, video, and photos. This package is either e-mailed or placed on a web server for the receiving healthcare provider to access when his or her schedule allows. The receiving provider reviews the package, follows up with clarification questions, and provides a diagnosis, recommendations, and a treatment plan. The receiving provider's response is transmitted electronically back to the sending provider or patient. Store-and-forward technologies can be used in dermatology, radiology, pathology, dentistry, cardiology, wound care, home monitoring, pediatrics, and ophthalmology, as well as other areas. A store-and-forward technical environment can include:

- A personal desktop, laptop computer, tablet, or smartphone for the sender
- A personal desktop, laptop computer, tablet, or smartphone for the receiver
- Telecommunication technologies such as local area network (LAN) and wireless communications
- Digital peripheral medical devices such as digital cameras, x-ray equipment, glucometers, vital sign monitors, and wearable sensors embedded in T-shirts or wristwatches
- Software such as a web-based application, encrypted e-mail, specially designed store-and-forward software, an EHR, a PHR, and an electronic data repository

Technical Standards in Telehealth

Until recently, the demand for telehealth-based medical devices was not sufficient to create unified, global technical standards. However, technical standards that were developed for associated markets have benefited telehealth. For example, use of American National Standards Institute (ANSI) H.32x standards enabled wide-scale video conferencing interoperability, which led to further growth in non-healthcare businesses. Not only has telehealth benefited from the video conferencing standards, but it is also benefiting from a reduction in the cost of equipment, as well as the improved ability to conduct interactions between parties independent of the particular hardware used. In addition, development of Health Level Seven (HL7), which provides global interoperability standards for health information technology (health IT), and Digital Imaging and Communications in Medicine (DICOM) standards for imaging has also been of great benefit for telehealth.[26]

In 2006, a group of healthcare technology companies formed the Continua Health Alliance (CHA) to establish interoperable personal telehealth solutions and technical design guidelines. The goal is to agree on a set of common technical guidelines to build interoperable sensors, home networks, telehealth platforms, and health and wellness services. CHA also has developed a technical certification program based on these guidelines. Technologies that are certified by CHA have been technically tested and validated to work together and be interoperable.[26]

In February 2014, the CHA announced a partnership with the mHealth Summit to create a new global entity, the Personal Connected Health Alliance (PCHA), under the Health Information Management Systems Society (HIMSS) corporate umbrella, to represent the consumer voice in connected health. PCHA brings together a unique combination of expertise and resources focused on plug-and-play interoperable personal health devices and services that provide new opportunities for consumers to engage in health self-improvement and connect with their social networks and healthcare providers in the pursuit of better health.[27]

An example of such a standard is ZigBee/IEEE 802.15. This standard is targeted at applications requiring a low data rate, long battery life, and secure networking. ZigBee/IEEE 802.15 has become a useful wireless connectivity standard for home or facility-based telehealth. ZigBee allows telehealth devices and sensors to operate longer and with smaller power sources, enabling miniature sensors to transmit health data. ZigBee is also a very low cost and easily installed network capability, providing usability and requiring minimal technical support. The ZigBee Alliance offers two specifications (ZigBee and ZigBee RF4CE) that serve as the base networking system to facilitate its interoperable market standards.[28]

Telehealth and Health Information Technology

A need exists to integrate all relevant medical device images and data from the telehealth technology with the patient's EHR. The interoperability of these systems could dramatically streamline a healthcare provider's workflow and improve the healthcare. The need to increase the adoption and effective use of telehealth and mHealth technologies has been identified as a major goal in the Federal Health IT strategic plan (2015–20).[29]

A key to telehealth success is healthcare providers' access to patients' health records at the time of a telehealth encounter—just as it is with in-person care. Telehealth networks serve to establish a link between provider EHRs and securely move clinical information that is exchanged among patients, hospitals, and healthcare providers. Telehealth health information exchange (HIE) is expected to lead to the next generation of health IT interoperability across and among healthcare enterprises. Existing telehealth infrastructure will also serve as a highway for EHRs and information exchange between and among rural and remote areas.[30]

TELEHEALTH CLINICAL PRACTICE CONSIDERATIONS FOR HEALTHCARE PROFESSIONALS

Healthcare providers have used the telephone as a communication tool for patient interaction for decades. Adding to the complexity of remote care delivery now, it is increasingly common to use computers, remote monitoring devices, and interactive audio and video conferencing for patient interactions. With expanding telehealth technology capability, new and more efficient models of care are facilitated, allowing for removal of time and distance barriers.

Equal To or Better Than In-Person Care?

Telehealth is considered to be so effective that in 1997, the World Health Organization (WHO) announced that it has become part of the WHO's "health for all" strategy and should be made available to all people.[31] Provider-patient encounters via telehealth were examined and found to be as effective as standard face-to-face visits held in a provider's office or clinic. In 2008 Dr. Gregory Jicha, assistant professor of neurology at the University of Kentucky's Sanders-Brown Center on Aging, led a study called Telemedicine Assessment of Cognition in Rural Kentucky.

> The goal of the project was to adapt and validate the UDS [National Institute on Aging's Uniform Data Set, a standard set of questions asked of every patient being screened for Alzheimer disease] and other measures for diagnosing mild cognitive impairment (MCI) and early dementia in the telemedicine setting. An important aspect of the goal was to determine whether the telemedicine consultations were as effective as face-to-face meetings with a doctor.[32, p. 32]

Jicha stated, "developing and validating this telemedicine approach for diagnosing and treating MCI and early dementia will become a model for clinician-researchers at other centers serving rural populations."[32, p. 32] Per Jicha's perception of using telemedicine to expand healthcare resources, "the bottom line is, our goal is to ensure that though telemedicine is not *better* than an in-person evaluation, it's *as good as* an in-person evaluation."[32, p. 34]

Two studies from 2012 (one in the United Kingdom and the other in Quebec, Canada) concluded that "telemedicine is increasingly seen as an efficient and cost-effective means for improving clinical outcomes and increasing patient involvement in their own care."[33, p. 59] Both studies demonstrated two important factors that influence healthcare professionals' acceptance of telemedicine: training and support.

Telehealth Clinical Competency

As healthcare providers' use of broader technological tools increases, so does the need to ensure telehealth competency to provide safe and optimal patient care. As healthcare further embraces telehealth to gain efficiencies, improve access to care, and reduce costs, there must be a focus on educating and preparing healthcare providers in telehealth technology, techniques, skills, coordination, and "on camera" communications. A telehealth clinical encounter involves multiple new components and competencies, including coordinating healthcare provider and patient scheduling, telepresenting skills (i.e., steps needed to facilitate a telemedicine encounter between a patient and remote healthcare provider), the exchange of prior medical record and new telehealth information, and an understanding of video and audio technology.

From initial academic preparation through ongoing continuing education requirements, healthcare providers practice in a dynamic field with ongoing changes in care delivery. All healthcare providers are required and expected to maintain and update clinical competency in the care they render to patients. Telehealth also requires competency for optimal healthcare delivery. A number of professional associations identified specific competencies required. As described earlier in this chapter, the ANA and 41 major healthcare provider organizations developed and endorsed core principles for telehealth delivery beginning in 1998.[22] A year later the ANA created and published *Competencies for Telehealth Technologies in Nursing.*[34] In 2001, with further expansion in telehealth, the ANA endorsed the development of telehealth protocols.[35] These protocols were developed to encompass the needs and concerns of both clients and practitioners. On an international level, the ICN published the research-based, validated *International Competencies for Telenursing* based on an international survey of practicing telenurses in 36 countries around the globe.[4]

The *National Initiative for Telehealth Framework of Guidelines* (NIFTE Guidelines) was a critical milestone in development of telehealth not just for those who authored the guidelines in Canada, but globally.[36] This highly important and superbly designed framework was developed in Canada by a multistakeholder interdisciplinary group. The NIFTE Guidelines are designed to assist individuals and organizations to develop telehealth policies, standards, and procedures. NIFTE examines and offers principles and suggested guidelines for five overarching content areas related to telehealth:

- Clinical standards and outcomes
- Human resources
- Organizational readiness
- Organizational leadership
- Technology and equipment

Canadian nurses have also provided over a decade of telenursing leadership and developed extensive practice guidelines for nurses who are becoming or presently in telenurse roles.[37]

In November 2011, the ATA developed an expert opinion consensus document on interactive video conferencing. The Expert Consensus Recommendations for Videoconferencing-Based Telepresenting defines requirements for serving as a telepresenter in a live, synchronous telehealth encounter. As with all patient interactions, processes for patient registration, consent, clinical information, reimbursement information, and privacy are applicable to telehealth encounters.[38] The ATA also developed Telemedicine Standards and Guidelines for Diabetes, Telemental Health, Teledermatology, Home Telehealth, and Telepathology.

Confidentiality, Privacy, and Informed Patients

Patient confidentiality and privacy are paramount when using technology for the transmission of health data and live video presentation of the patient to geographic environments at a distance from the patient's location. The requirements for ensuring confidentiality, privacy, and informing patients receiving care via telehealth are the same as for in-person care.

This is particularly true when the possibility exists of others being present in a room but off camera. Attending to the presence of others at either the sending or receiving locations is an additional, important privacy task for healthcare providers using telehealth. Another important concern is ensuring that patients are being adequately informed and educated regarding telehealth consultation, assessment, and evaluation via video conferencing technology.[4,35]

Scope of Clinical Practice

For healthcare professionals the use of technology does not alter the practitioner's inherent standards of practice, ethics, scope of practice, or legalities of practice.[35,37] Healthcare professionals may use telehealth for patient consultations or for consultation with other healthcare providers. When telehealth is used for patient consultations, the healthcare professional's credentialing and clinical privileges must be completed at the site where the patient is located. The practitioner will need education, training, and technical support for the necessary technologies before, during, and after telehealth consultations.

The decision to refer a patient to a healthcare professional for consultation via telemedicine or telehealth is determined by multiple factors:

1. Does the service requested provide telemedicine or telehealth access as an option?
2. What is the level of the practitioner's expertise and comfort with telemedicine or telehealth?
3. Is the patient's diagnosis appropriate for telemedicine or telehealth consultation?
4. Going forward, who will manage the patient's plan of care and how will this be managed?

As with any in-person patient encounter, documentation is of major importance. Appropriate documentation for telemedicine consults at both the sending and the receiving sites is essential for providing accurate and optimal continuity of care for the patient. Both sites need current patient demographic information, billing information, and consultant notes. Referring practitioners need consultant notes in a timely manner to carry out the patient's plan of care. After a telehealth consult, evaluation of telehealth processes and patient satisfaction is essential. The quality assurance and evaluation processes identify how to improve telehealth procedures, safety, effectiveness, and quality of care.[35]

Types of Clinical Telehealth Applications

In the past 15 years, telehealth specialty areas, such as telecardiology, teledentistry, teledermatology, home telehealth and remote monitoring, teleICU, telemental health, teleopthalmology, telepediatrics, teleradiology, telestroke, telewoundcare, and teletrauma, have been successfully developed and implemented in a variety of healthcare settings. Other telehealth programs outside the hospital setting include emergency preparedness, disaster response, correctional telemedicine, forensic telemedicine, telerehabilitation, and school telehealth.

A complete remote physical examination can be achieved by viewing images and hearing sounds. Healthcare providers can assess and treat a variety of healthcare problems such as cardiac or respiratory illnesses by listening to digital heart, lung, or bowel sounds live; by sending the data over a video conferencing system; or by using a computer with internet connection to the computer of another clinician, who can then assess the information. The healthcare provider can use video scopes to conduct ear, nose, throat, oral cavity, eye, pelvic, or rectal exams; cameras or microscopes for skin examinations; radiology images to diagnose orthopedic injuries; and computed tomography (CT) scans of the head to rule out bleeding, brain injuries, or skull fractures. Teleradiology is one of the most commonly used and accepted telehealth applications, where digital images are captured and transmitted to the radiologist, who makes a diagnosis, sends a report, and stores the image. Healthcare providers can send complete readings for a 12-lead digital ECG to a cardiologist to diagnose heart problems or send a digital spirometry reading to a pulmonologist to diagnose respiratory lung capacity.

TELEHEALTH OPERATIONAL AND ORGANIZATIONAL SUCCESS FACTORS AND BARRIERS

Despite the advancements in telehealth technologies, significant barriers and gaps exist in the successful implementation of robust, integrated healthcare technology delivery systems.

B.E.L.T. Framework

In planning for implementation of telehealth technology, four main components must be considered: bandwidth, education, leadership, and technology (B.E.L.T.). The B.E.L.T. framework (Fig. 8.3) is a metaphoric representation of these four interrelated components, and it may be used to guide planning at macro, meso, or micro levels of implementation.

Bandwidth includes elements of telecommunication technology, including information transmission and connectivity to move and store digital data. Infrastructure and telecommunication architecture in some geographic areas may limit use

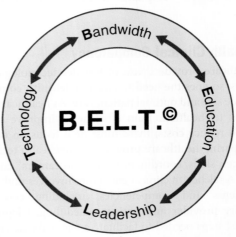

FIG 8.3 The B.E.L.T. framework. (Copyright McGill University School of Nursing. Montreal, Quebec.)

of telehealth applications and have direct implications for access to and delivery of healthcare. This is particularly problematic for rural, isolated, and underserved regions.[39]

Education encompasses the preparation of both the existing workforce and future healthcare providers in developing competencies in the adoption and use of telehealth technologies. Although research was done in some areas of competency development, particularly in healthcare informatics and telenursing, scant research has been completed about the broader use of telehealth technology to inform curriculum development and education of healthcare providers.[4,40] Patient safety in telehealth technology use is one aspect of healthcare delivery that is essential to professional practice and relates to competencies in clinical decision making.

Leadership reflects a broad range of management, change theory, and policy aspects that affect operationalizing telehealth technologies. Barriers to successful telehealth adoption frequently relate to factors such as resistance to technology, lack of interoperability, information security, stakeholder support, reimbursement, and financial commitment.[39,40]

Technology and interoperability spans a large number of considerations such as the choices and types of telehealth software, hardware, and devices available for care. To date, telehealth platforms have limited capacity to address the range of health conditions experienced across the population lifespan, resulting in a narrow focus on overall individual health, fragmentation of care, and duplication of effort for data retrieval and documentation. Because many current telehealth technologies are not interoperable and cannot be integrated into a single environment to support holistic care, data silos are created where information on the same individual may be contained in different systems and cannot be accessed in an efficient, seamless manner. This further fragments care, leads to duplication of services (e.g., repeat of blood work, diagnostics), and creates unnecessary cost. Another limitation is that most current telehealth technologies focus on direct delivery of clinical services to individuals and do not readily support the broader goals of primary healthcare, such as enhancing health promotion, prevention opportunities, or generating necessary epidemiologic data needed to evaluate and inform healthcare delivery.

Operationalizing Telehealth

Several critical steps exist for success of telehealth programs and services. The first is planning, which includes a needs assessment and analysis to define patient populations and healthcare problems in which telehealth services can have a positive impact. A work environment with staff prepared to implement telehealth using specific standards and guidelines is the second important factor for success. Technology preparedness is a third factor for telehealth success. User-friendly technology that enables quality clinical decision making, as well as responsive and accessible technical support, are also crucial factors.[41] The final, critical step is learning how to implement, manage, and support a telehealth project or program. This becomes more complicated when clinical specialties are involved. New telehealth programs should begin with

one focused specialty application, such as teledermatology, and not add other specialties until the initial program has been implemented successfully. Specific procedures are listed in Table 8.1, and project steps are outlined below.

Telehealth Acceptance and Training

As with other educational trends, telehealth technology education has moved toward online courses or certificate education programs in the United States and globally. Online and on-site telehealth training courses are available through several federally funded Telehealth Resource Centers. Additional information about the resource centers can be found at www.telehealthresourcecenter.org/. The ATA, located at www.americantelemed.org/, provides annual meetings with scientific research presentations, special interest groups, educational webinars, educational products, training program accreditations, white papers, and policies.

According to Duclos et al., the success of any telehealth program by providers relates to its acceptance by providers who use it.[42] Healthcare providers who use telehealth in their practice should know how telehealth technologies work and should understand their capabilities in providing patients with better access to healthcare services.

Opportunities abound for clinicians to become adept with telehealth technologies, beginning with a basic proficiency in using room-based video conferencing systems on PCs and mobile video conferencing systems on iPads and smartphones. It is advantageous for healthcare providers to learn to use medical devices with video scopes attached for patient assessments, and video or digital cameras for exams. Providers need to be comfortable using a variety of audio, video, and medical device tools, video conferencing systems, and computer hardware and software applications. New technical challenges often emerge for clinicians, such as using a video ophthalmoscope to view retinal images inside the eye and on a display monitor. Another challenge can be hearing new heart sounds from a digital stethoscope with different high- and low-pitched sounds because of magnification. Clinicians may encounter workflow changes with telehealth software applications in paperless environments. Digital literacy training may also be required for clinicians, which includes knowledge of basic computer skills and communication technologies, basic skills to navigate the internet for up-to-date health information, and the ability to access web-based telehealth software applications. For example, healthcare providers who are fluent in using digital cameras to take dermatology images and who are internet savvy can access online resources to identify a skin lesion or obtain the latest treatment for the lesion.

In the 2005 International Telenursing Survey, telenurses were found to have various job skills and to work in more than 30 clinical telehealth settings, ranging from nurse call centers to urban and rural hospitals, public and private health clinics, schools, prisons, community health centers, military facilities, native tribe reservations, and private physician and nurse practitioner practices.[43] Specific telehealth knowledge regarding equipment, workflow, clinical processes, and technology training is different for each clinical setting.

TABLE 8.1   Telehealth Procedures

Preparation	Provider and Patient "Real-Time" Telehealth Encounter	Follow-Up, Quality, and Safety
Provider credentialing completed at patient site and remote site	Provider is knowledgeable and competent in healthcare needs being addressed during patient-to-provider telemedicine visit	Review plan of care conveyed by provider or consultant and instructions provided regarding treatment plans, with time for patient and family questions and answers
Referral reviewed as appropriate for specialty service and accepted by telespecialist	Introduce patient to all individuals that will be in the patient room and to any individuals at the evaluating physician's location	Complete any necessary forms (e.g., patient consent to treat form; Health Information Portability and Accountability Act [HIPAA] forms) and share reimbursement information with both patient and physician sites
Knowledgeable regarding scheduling procedures and policies of facility and scheduling resources	Identify camera and microphone locations to patient and explain any potential for audio or video delay	Provide patient and family with consulting physician contact information, as needed for follow-up
Obtain and review preconsult clinical information and testing	Presenting site provider is knowledgeable of exam requirements, including patient preparation, patient positioning, and use of peripheral devices (i.e., electronic stethoscopes, Doppler, digital cameras, etc.)	Schedule follow-up appointments, treatments, etc. as ordered by physician
Obtain reimbursement information, such as copies of insurance cards, Medicare cards, etc.	Provide support to patient and family and be alert to nonverbal body language	Provide the referring primary care provider with the telemedicine encounter documentation
Provide patient with the appropriate forms for "consent to treat" and HIPAA compliance information	Provide time within the clinical visit for patient and family questions and answers	Evaluate outcomes of the telemedicine encounter, quality of encounter, and patient satisfaction and assess for improvements for future telemedicine encounters; clinical effectiveness is one of the factors associated with success in telemedicine
Contact patient to explain a telemedicine encounter and provide directions to the telemedicine site	Educate patient and family of their right and ability to terminate the telemedicine clinical visit at any time	
Ensure that equipment and technology has been tested and is in safe working order, provider and patient have clear audio and video of each other, extraneous noises are reduced, and any necessary peripheral devices and supplies are accessible at time of encounter		
Assess and prepare for cultural, language, or disability issues		
Establish a backup plan and be prepared to enact it in the event of technical problems		

Scheduling dedicated time for healthcare providers' telehealth training is an obstacle and is one of the major barriers to a successful telehealth program. Actual hands-on training is beneficial, using telehealth case scenarios similar to those the healthcare provider would typically encounter. As mentioned earlier, clinical workflow is modified when telehealth technologies are implemented. Healthcare providers can adjust by continuing to use the same patient exam rooms for the telehealth patient, using similar medical devices for in-person and telehealth exams, training with telehealth technologies, and interacting with the same physicians and specialists for telehealth consultations as for in-person referrals.

BOX 8.1 Telehealth Preimplementation Steps

- Identify remote physician specialists and other clinical consultants who are willing to provide remote assessment and advice for treatment
- Meet standards and requirements for safe use of telemedicine equipment: installation in designated telehealth rooms; biomedical and electrical engineering help may be required
- Select appropriate telehealth equipment to use for telehealth examinations, including disposable accessories such as nonlatex gloves, gel, measurement tapes, alcohol wipes, gowns and cover sheets, and extra camera batteries
- Identify electrical and cable sources for power outlets and secure internet access
- Designate telehealth exam rooms or areas
- Identify 24/7 technical support for clinicians at both sending and receiving sites
- Develop policies and procedures
- Train interdisciplinary team and staff end users on telehealth equipment
- Set up and test telehealth scenarios before beginning telehealth consultation

Telehealth Implementation

There are three phases for successful telehealth program implementation: preimplementation, implementation, and postimplementation.

Preimplementation Phase

Implementing telehealth technologies in any clinical setting is no different than implementing other twenty-first century technologies (see Chapter 17 on project management and Chapter 19 on systems implementation). As with any informatics project, a team effort is critical to its success. Clinicians will first need to decide what types of telehealth programs provide access to remote healthcare specialists for their patients. Important preimplementation steps are listed in Box 8.1. Forming an administrative or executive team is advisable to oversee the project goals, budget, progress, and growth. The facility may already have a formal committee in place to oversee all IT projects and, if so, can tailor the governance to incorporate telehealth. The executive team should include the following:

- Hospital or facility administrator
- Clinical director (often a physician)
- Chief Information Officer
- Director of information technology and/or director of education
- Telehealth and telecommunications administrator
- Vendor account managers (may be only at the operational level below)

A second level of management for the telehealth program is an operational interdisciplinary team including the following:

- Project manager
- Clinical champion (often a physician)
- Telehealth director or program manager
- Information technology engineer or support technician
- System administrator (if software is involved)

Super users and vendor trainers will also initiate, train, and support new staff for the telehealth project. The interdisciplinary teams are the change agents that assist in developing policies, procedures, evaluation criteria, and permission forms before beginning to use telehealth.

Implementation Phase

Once the equipment is configured or tailored, the implementation phase involves equipment and software testing with mock telehealth patients and remote specialists, and then piloting the project by identifying a patient needing a teleconsult. Equipment testing with mock patients should encompass all staff testing all of the telehealth equipment available. Equipment testing should also be conducted periodically after the initial implementation. After identifying differences between standard and telehealth patient encounters, daily use of telehealth equipment for routine patient exams is recommended so that providers become knowledgeable and comfortable using the various telehealth examination tools (electronic stethoscope, video otoscope or ophthalmoscope, digital ECG or spirometry software, video exam camera, telehealth software applications, and audio or video conferencing systems). The goal is for a clinician to present a patient, capture and send patient data, retrieve patient information from stored telehealth software applications, and respond to cases and add patient encounters if needed.

Postimplementation Phase

As with any other informatics project, evaluation criteria address adequacy of training; implementation, equipment, technology, or training issues; and program outcomes. A program of quality assurance and process improvement should be part of the evaluation process so that iterative progress toward implementation-phase telehealth program success can be achieved.

Telehealth programs of any size experience similarities in success and failure. Table 8.2 lists common success factors and barriers to successful telehealth program implementation.

TELEHEALTH CHALLENGES: LICENSURE AND REGULATORY ISSUES FOR HEALTHCARE PROFESSIONALS

Telehealth enables physicians, advanced practice registered nurses (APRNs), nurses, pharmacists, and other allied health professionals to offer their clinical services remotely. State lines and geographic boundaries have no effect on the potential of the technology to deliver telehealth services. For example, radiologists can read x-ray reports from other countries; mental health professionals can provide care telephonically or with real-time video; and chronically ill patients can be monitored from a distance with telehealth. Despite technological advances, legal and regulatory challenges exist. Provider licensure and the credentialing and privileging processes in facilities remain the biggest hurdles to telehealth adoption in the United States.

TABLE 8.2   Success Factors and Barriers to Telehealth Implementation

Key Success Factors for Telehealth	Barriers to Successful Telehealth Implementation
High-level organizational members (board of directors, administrator, medical director, champion physician, nurse administrator, nurse educator, program director) who have identified a need for telehealth and are able to provide support and finances throughout all phases of implementation, training, and maintenance of the telehealth program	No designated or dedicated project manager; not enough time or resources dedicated to manage project
Designated and dedicated telehealth project manager or coordinator	Interdisciplinary team not designated or prepared properly
Designated interdisciplinary telehealth team	Funding limited
Adequate facility network infrastructure to support the telehealth system or method selected and prepare setup for the telehealth program prior to installation	Lack of communication between administrative management, interdisciplinary team, and participants
Project management to include and allow time for professional telehealth education and refresher training classes, including participation for professional telehealth conferences, telehealth webinars, telehealth video training, and provision of telehealth resource information	Failure to identify remote clinical partners to whom to refer patients or to provide telehealth services; may be due to reimbursement issues, lack of understanding as to how telehealth works, practice and licensing issues in that state
Initiate telehealth program at local facility and then introduce to affiliated remote facilities	Poor telehealth equipment selection for specialty; poor quality and usability of telehealth equipment purchased
Provide staff with educational tools such as workflow diagrams, charts, digital photos, manuals, and descriptive pathways for how to initiate an urgent or nonurgent telehealth consult	Missing parts of equipment and supplies during installation or patient encounter
Provide education, training, and program development for teleconsultants	No designated telehealth area due to limited room availability
Schedule appointments for follow-up teleconsults with dates and times for physician and patient	Ergonomically poor placement of equipment, limited connectivity or lighting in telehealth area, poor cable management, limited counter size, small room, no storage cart for equipment, equipment not secure
Patient privacy and confidential information forms should be completed prior to teleconsult	No pretraining on telehealth system prior to telehealth installation
Provide on-site dedicated technical support throughout all phases of implementation and provide online support for main site, remote site, and teleconsultants	Healthcare providers not familiar with computer literacy (i.e., basic use of keyboard, personal computer, mouse, navigating software, data, or handling images captured) Training not formalized, no schedule confirmed to allow for all participants to be trained, not enough time provided for hands-on training or practice of case scenarios Staff resistant to training, no incentives, and no understanding of telehealth or technology advantages Off-hour shifts not trained or invited to participate in training sessions

Licensure

Both the 1997 and 2001 Telemedicine Reports to Congress by OAT identified licensure as a major barrier to the development of telemedicine and telehealth.[44] The cost and procedural complexity of current professional licensing policies preclude widespread adoption of telehealth. Currently, many health professionals must attain separate licenses in each state where services are rendered. Licensure authority defines who has the legal responsibility to grant a health professional the permission to practice his or her profession.[45] Under Article X of the U.S. Constitution, states have the authority to regulate activities that affect the health, safety, and welfare of their citizens.[45] Regulating the delivery of healthcare services is one such activity. Exceptions to state licensure requirements include physician-to-physician consultations, educational and medical training programs, border state recognition programs, government employees practicing in military or federally funded facilities such as VA hospitals and clinics, and natural disaster and emergency situations.[45]

Legislation such as the 2011 service members' Telemedicine and E-Health Portability Act (STEP Act) facilitates the provision of telemedicine and telehealth services. The STEP Act removes the individual state licensing requirements to allow a licensed medical professional in one state to treat a

TABLE 8.3	**Telehealth Professional Licensure Options**
Licensure Option	**Description**
Endorsement	Allows a state to grant licenses to health professionals licensed in other states that have equivalent standards. States may require additional documentation or qualifications before endorsing a license issued by another state.[45–48]
Mutual recognition	The distant state's licensing board accepts the licensing policies of the health professional's home state.[47] Federal healthcare agencies operate under this type of system. An analogous licensing system would be the mutual recognition of driver's licenses between states.
Reciprocity	A process in which two states voluntarily enter into a reciprocal agreement to allow the health professional to practice in each state without having to become licensed in both states. It does not involve additional review of the health professional's credentials, as endorsement does, and it does not require the participating states to agree to a standardized set of rules or procedures, as mutual recognition does. The negative aspect of this model is that it leaves the healthcare provider subject to different regulations in each state and therefore subject to different sets of laws. This can lead to legal issues of liability and wider exposure to potential malpractice opportunity.[49]
Registration	The health professional licensed in one state informs the authorities of other states that he or she wishes to practice in those states part time. The provider is licensed in the home (originating) state but still is accountable to uphold the legal stipulations and regulations of the guest (distant) states. Similar to reciprocity, the provider would still be subject to the guest state's malpractice rules as well as the home state's rules and regulations.
Limited licensure	The health professional obtains his or her medical licensure in the home state and then obtains a second "limited" licensure in the guest state. The limited license allows for specific scope of services to be delivered under particular circumstances.[49]
National licensure	Individual states would voluntarily incorporate the same set of national standards into their laws. Given that most medical professionals pass the same national exam within their particular discipline, it stands to reason that standards of care and practice guidelines should not differ from state to state. Regulatory processes could be retained at the state or national level. For example, the American Medical Association could take full responsibility for the licensing of all physicians at a national level and similarly nurses could be licensed to practice nationally by their national organization, and likewise with other health professions (e.g., pharmacists, dentists, physical therapists). However, disciplinary actions or other procedural activities could be administered at the state level.

patient in another.[46] As of this writing, the STEP Act rules apply only to military and federal personnel, although it is a beginning in terms of advancing telehealth services into the mainstream. Fortunately, major advancements are occurring to streamline licensure requirements. These regulatory alternatives include licensure by endorsement, state compacts and mutual recognition, reciprocity, registration, and limited licensure (Table 8.3).

Nursing has been the most successful healthcare provider group to adopt the mutual recognition model, referred to as the multistate Nurse Licensure Compact.[47] The Nurse Licensure Compact law became effective on January 1, 2000, with three states initially participating. As of early 2016, 25 compact states existed. Compact status applies only to RN licensure. If RNs hold a license in one of the compact states, they may practice in *any* of the 25 compact states, greatly facilitating telehealth interactions across state boundaries. The latest list of compact states is available at: www.ncsbn.org/nurse-licensure-compact.htm. International nurses on a visa who apply for licensure in a compact state may declare either the country of origin or the compact state as the primary place of residency. If the foreign country is declared as the primary place of residency, a single-state license will be issued by the compact state.[48] A mutual recognition model is being discussed for APRNs at the time of this writing. However, currently, APRNs who practice using telehealth across state boundaries

must first apply for RN licensure (or endorsement) in the distant state and then apply for advanced practice status, which involves extensive credentialing and privileging processes.[47]

Credentialing and Privileging

Credentialing is the process of establishing the qualifications of licensed professionals and assessing their background and legitimacy. For example, if a physician does a telehealth consult from a hospital in State X but the patient resides in a skilled nursing facility in State Y, that physician must be credentialed by both facilities (i.e., the hospital and skilled nursing facility) and must also be licensed in both States X and Y. Each facility could have very different processes and rules for becoming credentialed. Similar to the need for licensing in multiple states, the need for credentialing in multiple, separate healthcare facilities is an obstacle to telehealth services. In May 2011, the Centers for Medicare & Medicaid Services (CMS) modified the existing credentialing and privileging regulations effective July 5, 2011. The new rule under part 42 CFR 410.78 of the CMS regulations allows hospitals or Critical Access Hospitals (CAHs) to use information from a distant-site hospital or other accredited telemedicine entity when making credentialing or privileging decisions for the distant-site physicians and practitioners.[45] Regarding the legal risks and liabilities associated with these changes, the governing body of each hospital and CAH must weigh the risks and benefits of opting for this more streamlined process of credentialing and privileging telemedicine providers.[45] Modifications still need to be made to allow Medicare and Medicaid beneficiaries who reside in urban or metropolitan areas to be eligible to receive the same services.

Reimbursement

Telemedicine is often viewed as a cost-effective alternative to the more traditional face-to-face method of providing medical care.[45] As such, states in the United States have the option to determine whether or not to cover telemedicine- and telehealth-delivered care, what types of telehealth to cover, where in the state it can be covered, how it is provided and covered, what types of telehealth practitioners and providers may be covered and reimbursed (as long as such practitioners and providers are "recognized" and qualified according to Medicare and Medicaid statute and regulation), and how much to reimburse for telemedicine services (as long as such payments do not exceed the Federal Upper Limits).[49]

Reimbursement by insurance companies for medical services is based on Medicare's Current Procedural Terminology (CPT) codes billing system. As of 2012, Medicare telehealth services can be furnished only to an eligible telehealth beneficiary from an eligible originating site. In general, originating sites must be located in a rural Health Professional Shortage Area (HPSA) or in a county outside of a Metropolitan Statistical Area (MSA). The originating sites authorized by the statute include hospitals, skilled nursing facilities, offices of physicians or licensed healthcare practitioners, rural health clinics, community mental health centers, CAHs, CAH-based dialysis centers, and federally qualified health centers.[50] Medicaid reimbursement for telehealth varies by state, with some states electing not to reimburse for telehealth services. Internationally, in countries that provide government-based universal healthcare, telehealth adoption is flourishing, and reimbursement has become a national budgetary decision. Providing more access to more citizens while at the same time reducing costs and more efficiently distributing clinical expertise using technology is a desired goal for any country's health service. Thus countries such as Canada, those in the European Union, Japan, China, and India are all expanding their telehealth capabilities and services.

Malpractice and Liability

Legal issues of liability and malpractice are a burden for the telemedicine practitioner, as they face additional vulnerability and uncertainty related to malpractice exposure in multiple states. They likely face additional expenses for malpractice insurance and for legal defense if a suit were filed in a distant state.[51] Legal issues involve traditional jurisdictional issues, including:

- The place of treatment dilemma (is this the patient's location or the provider's?)
- Lack of an established, bona fide doctor-patient relationship similar to the situation with cybermedicine (medical care via the internet)

- Violating a particular state's specific regulations related to standards of care
- Failing to secure appropriate informed consent from a patient
- Negligence that may arise from technical glitches such as distorted images or poor sound quality of a particular device resulting in injury or misdiagnosis[45]

The traditional concepts of negligence, duty of care, and practicing within one's scope of legal license still apply to telehealth as they do in traditional face-to-face encounters. Initial case law in telemedicine and telehealth to date is limited, primarily involving telephone triage and teleradiology. In telephone triage, if advice was given and a poor patient outcome occurred, the triage service and professionals are at risk for malpractice. In teleradiology (as is the case with in-person and in-house radiology readings), if a diagnosis of a lump or a mass is missed on an image, the radiology service and professional would be at risk for malpractice. As telehealth usage increases, further legal cases will illuminate and clarify these issues.

TELEHEALTH AND DIRECT PATIENT HEALTH SERVICES

While telehealth applications typically involve provider-to-provider teleconsults, patients and other healthcare consumers can use telehealth directly to support their healthcare decision making. Specifically, applications facilitate direct, online patient telemedicine care; provide remote patient telehealth visits and monitoring; and link consumers with online healthcare information.[52] As the technology used to deliver telehealth services becomes easier to use and more affordable, the technology is increasingly being used by patients in interaction with their healthcare providers and at times in directing their own care.

Patient-to-Provider Telehealth-Delivered Care

Increasingly, individuals find it difficult to obtain timely care for urgent health concerns from their healthcare provider. Even though more Americans have expanded health insurance coverage under the Affordable Care Act, more people are going to hospital emergency rooms (ER) for care because they are unable to get an appointment with primary care.[53] Online telehealth direct care is one growing solution, and the use of video conferencing for telehealth visits is increasing. Manhattan Research's Taking the Pulse US v11.0 study indicated that nearly 7% of physicians use online video conferencing to communicate with their patients.[52] In the study, physicians consider telehealth a method for consulting with patients about nonurgent issues or connecting with geographically dispersed patient populations that may not have nearby access to specialists. The study also found that certain specialty healthcare providers, such as psychiatrists and oncologists, are more likely to use video conferencing.

IHS Technology (formerly Information Handling Services Technology) predicts there will be cumulative growth of nearly 25% a year over the next 5 years to 5.4 million video consultations between primary care providers and their patients by 2020 from 2015's 2 million video consultations.[54] Adapt TeleHealth is an example of this healthcare delivery approach. Once a community or clinic identifies a need for psychiatric services, it contracts with Adapt TeleHealth to meet its mental health needs. It purchases a consistent number of hours per week, which are fulfilled by an Adapt Tele-Health mental health provider.[55] Other direct patient care technologies focus more on providing a platform for a healthcare provider's office to provide care via telemedicine. Companies such as Secure Telehealth,[56] TelaDoc,[57] and Online Care Anywhere[58] are examples of platforms for direct online medical care.

Asynchronous applications using store-and-forward technologies or online diagnostic surveys are gaining in popularity. Virtuwell[59] (at www.virtuwell.com) originated with HealthPartners in Minnesota and offers online, 24/7 direct care in 11 states. First, an online survey asks consumers to identify their chief concern. Responses are sent to a nurse practitioner who reviews the information and responds within 30 minutes via text or e-mail with a diagnosis, potential remedies, and tips for preventing the condition in the future. If a prescription is needed, the nurse practitioner can send it to a local pharmacy. Forty common conditions, including bladder and yeast infections, are treated by Virtuwell's nurse practitioners.

Another asynchronous telemedicine company is Relay-Health,[60] providing an online solution to connect consumers with their healthcare providers. Their Medical Home support package provides a secure patient portal to facilitate easy online clinical communications, enabling patients to benefit from care coordination, including patient visits and consultations, prescription renewal, appointment scheduling, PHR management, delivery of lab results, referral requests, and access to medically reviewed information.

Delivering Direct Care Using Health Monitoring Tools and Biometric Sensors

A number of healthcare applications use information and communication core components to help patients stay safe in their homes and communicate vital healthcare data to providers (Box 8.2).[61] Peripheral health monitoring tools such as blood glucose monitors, pulse oximeters, blood pressure and ECG monitors, and electronic scales, already described as components of a telehomecare visit, fit this definition. They are the backbone of a viable remote disease management program. More recently, a group of assistive technology devices dubbed "sensor technologies" emerged, adding a layer of connectedness between patients and their healthcare providers through monitoring patients' activity levels and physiologic parameters. Both forms of biometric sensors are described further.

Remote Telehealth Home Visits and Monitoring Devices

Telehealth systems previously used interactive video conferencing between healthcare providers and patients; however, the ability to self-manage care is a driving fiscal concern.[61,62]

BOX 8.2 Biometric Sensor and Monitoring Device Overview

Purposes
- Detect changes in patterns that signal improvement or early failings
- Signal need for urgent or emergency help
- Integrate with websites or mobile units to promote communication
- Have ubiquitous monitoring for peace of mind for older adult and family
- Keep an inventory of supply levels for medications and other resources
- Coach and monitor exercise effectiveness and participation in games

Information Potentials
- Physical: motion, location, and activity
- Physiologic/medical: pulse, temperature, sweat, and blood chemistry
- Social: telephone or web interaction counts or identification
- Memory support: monitoring cooking stoves and adherence to regimens
- Communication safety issues: stove use, fire, and unsecured doors

Communication
- Devices and protocols networked to connect to computers
- Statistical and computational paradigms for analysis
- Applications for interaction with emergency rescuers, healthcare providers, and social networks

Monitoring Target Examples
- Restlessness as indicator of disturbed sleep
- Gait changes as indicator of drug side effect or physical debility
- Extended bedrest as indicator of depression or physical debility
- Pill counts as indicator of adherence or side effect issues

---

The prevalence of chronic health conditions and multiple chronic health conditions has risen in the United States. More than 25% of all Americans and more than 65% of all older Americans are estimated to have at least two chronic physical or behavioral health problems. Treatment for people living with these multiple chronic conditions accounts for nearly 66% of the nation's healthcare costs. As the U.S. population ages, the number of these patients continues to grow. This growing challenge has become a major public health issue that is linked to lower health outcomes and rising healthcare costs.[63] Use of telehealth technologies for remote home care and digital monitoring instruments are gaining momentum to address chronic illnesses and to promote safety for seniors living independently.

As mentioned earlier, the most widespread U.S. telehealth program is the VA Coordinated Care Home Telehealth (CCHT).[64] Built upon Wagner's Chronic Care Model, CCHT is characterized by "the use of health informatics, disease management and home telehealth technologies ... with the specific intent of providing the right care in the right place at the right time."[65] The range of technologies for CCHT includes videophones, messaging devices, biometric devices, digital cameras, and telemonitoring devices.[61] The videophones and video telemonitors facilitate synchronous face-to-face encounters with a healthcare provider through regular telephone lines or through computer links and the internet. Digital monitoring devices such as Bluetooth blood pressure cuffs and glucometers and digital images are also part of the comprehensive CCHT system and transmit timely healthcare data via asynchronous store-and-forward technologies.

The most common VA home telehealth devices connect a patient to a VA hospital using messaging devices that collect information about symptoms and vital signs from the patient's home. Care coordinators then link patients to treatment, hospitalization, or clinic appointments. In addition, the VA now employs an interactive patient portal and electronic PHR called MyHealtheVet,[66] which is discussed in detail in Chapter 14.

Other initiatives in the public sector involve the use of telehealth technologies with patients who are receiving care through home health agencies, senior living facilities, and other community-based delivery sites. For example, Suncrest Home Health Agency in Nashville, Tennessee, used Philips-developed telemonitoring devices to create a comprehensive heart failure home care program.[67] Provider telestations allowed vital sign collection, health assessment surveys, and tracking symptoms, medications and compliance with care protocols.[68] Within 8 months of implementing their Heart Failure telehealth program, Suncrest Home Health Agency was able to reduce hospital heart failure readmission rates by 50%.[67]

Sensor Technology

Like monitoring devices, sensor technology has the potential to manage disease and promote a safe and healthy environment for seniors.[68] A sensor is a device that detects and responds to some type of input from the physical environment. The specific input could be light, heat, motion, moisture, pressure, or any one of a great number of other environmental phenomena. The output is generally a signal that is converted to human-readable display at the sensor location or transmitted electronically over a network for reading or further processing.[69] The use of sensor technology has increased as the acute medical care paradigm evolves to wellness and a focus on public health. Wellness mobile devices enable healthcare professionals to have access to comprehensive real-time patient data at the point of care or anywhere there is cellular network coverage. Recently, a growing interest has developed for proactive wellness products and health-related smartphone applications.[70]

At the 2014 International Consumer Electronics Show, LG and Garmin introduced devices that track bodily functions ranging from heart rate and blood pressure to a patient's oxygen saturation. It is believed that by 2018, 130 million wearables will be acquired by the public.[71] For example, the Apple Watch, Google Glass, and Fitbit are on the leading edge of consumer "wearables"—technology that combines electronic sensors with everyday apparel. Now shirts, socks, and other accessories are being reimagined to collect, analyze, and use personalized data. Smart clothing, also known as e-textiles, is developed for use in a number of applications. They can measure and report vital signs for inpatient or outpatient healthcare, fitness training, or the handling of hazardous materials. They can track the status and position of soldiers on the battlefield, or monitor the alertness of drivers, air traffic controllers, or construction workers. The following smart clothing products are soon to be available or on the market:

1. AiQ Smart Clothing Company produces a line of smart apparel, including conductive gloves for smudge-free touchscreen use and clothes that give off evenly distributed heat.
2. The line of designer Pauline Van Dongen offers a Wearable Solar Clothing Collection. These coats and dresses integrate solar cells that can charge a smartphone or other electronic device.
3. SmartSox help prevent amputations in diabetes patients who have lost sensation in their feet. They incorporate fiber optics and sensors to monitor temperature, pressure, and the angles of joints in the feet, and alert the wearer or caregiver of any developing problems.
4. Exmobaby is designed for newborn and infants. Sensors monitor vital signs and movement and send this information to 3G.
5. Researchers in Spain have developed an intelligent hospital gown that wirelessly measures body temperature, heart rate, patient location, and whether the patient is sitting, standing, lying down, walking, or running. Although currently in use only in hospitals, the development includes the mobile units, which would move with the patients.
6. OMSignal uses a small data module to create real-time connectivity and data acquisition through fitness shirts. Even fashion icon Ralph Lauren has used the technology in a line of polos, with plans to add dress shirts.[72]

Other nontextile sensor applications being developed for healthcare include Google's Project Iris, a smart contact lens that can monitor glucose levels in diabetics. Fitness devices such as Nike's FuelBand can track steps taken and coach users to push a workout further. Even ingestible computers (capsules with minuscule sensors) are available such as the one from Proteus Digital Health, to help track a patient's responses to various medications.[71]

Additionally, several examples exist for current sensor technology to promote a safe and healthy environment in the smart home. A smart home or intelligent house[61] would use radio frequency identification (RFID) technology.[73] RFID technology uses a microchip to uniquely identify and track objects, record and update information, and make all of this accessible through a global network.[74] Depending on their use, RFIDs can be active or passive and are capable of being ingested, implanted, or attached externally. Although concerns about potential privacy and security breaches exist, RFID benefits include unlimited sight connection and rapid information processing, predicting better utility than other technologies such as bar coding. Monitoring hand-washing practices, transmitting neuromuscular stimulation data, and authenticating medications have the potential to transition from the hospital to the smart home.

Telehealth Technology and Healthcare Consumers

The proportion of American adults seeking information about a health concern from a source other than their physician dropped to 50% in 2010, down from 56% in 2007.[75] At first glance, readers may assume that consumers are not seeking information about their healthcare needs; however, the drop is actually attributed to an 18% decline in their use of print sources: books, magazines, and newspapers. Adults, especially the elderly and those with chronic disease conditions, have increased their internet use for seeking health information, contributing to their engagement in self-care. The Pew Internet and American Life Project noted that 59% of Americans go online every year to search for healthcare information.[76] Online healthcare resources aid consumers by supporting shared decision making with healthcare providers, providing personalized self-management tools and resources, building social support health networks, delivering tailored accurate health information, and increasing health literacy.[77]

Health information websites have been available to consumers since the mid-1990s.[78] Websites such as WebMD, a publicly traded company, and the National Institutes of Health's MedlinePlus, a federal government site, have provided healthcare information to a broad population of consumers, including the public, employers, employees, health plans, and healthcare providers. More recently, however, some health websites have moved beyond one-way communication and developed innovative features and interactive tools that enable consumers to greatly increase their self-knowledge and promote greater safety and independence. Tools such as drug interaction checkers, symptom checkers, various health-related calculators, pill identifiers, patient forums, fitness trackers, and PHRs are becoming more prevalent and helping consumers to gain more control over their health.[78]

Everyday Health (at www.everydayhealth.com) is another example of an interactive, consumer-based website. Everyday Health collaborated with professional experts from Harvard University, Cleveland Clinic, and the American Association of Family Practitioners and commercial enterprises to provide consumers with healthcare information. They have also developed interactive consumer-oriented tools that include websites, mobile applications, and social media assets, designed to provide consumers and healthcare professionals with access to the most trusted health and wellness content tailored to meet their daily needs. For example, consumers can use assessment and tracking tools and online calculators, speak live with a pharmacist, find drugs and treatments, and create a personal health plan. Additional information concerning interactive consumer-oriented resources is included in Chapters 12, 13, and 14.

eHealth Literacy: Critical Element for Telehealth Adoption

The proliferation of online healthcare resources has prompted the need to develop a national and international quality standards agenda to help health professionals and consumers alike access and evaluate high-quality online health information that is accurate, current, valid, appropriate, intelligible, and free of bias.[79–81] Health consumer advocates indicate the need for eHealth literacy (an extension of digital literacy) as a way of evaluating the information and services delivered using IT tools. *eHealth literacy* is defined as "a set of skills and knowledge that are essential for productive interactions with technology-based health tools."[82]

Experts identified six skills for eHealth literacy.[83] These skills are:

- Traditional literacy—ability to read text, understand written passages, and speak and write a language coherently.
- Computer literacy—ability to operate a computer.
- Information literacy—ability to obtain and apply relevant information.
- Media literacy—means of critically thinking about media content, and defined as a process to develop metacognitive reflective strategies by means of study.
- Health literacy—skills required to interact with the health system and engage in self-care.
- Scientific literacy—understanding of the nature, aims, methods, application, limitations, and politics of creating knowledge in a systematic manner.

Taken together, these six literacy types combine to form the foundational skills required to optimize consumers' experiences with eHealth.[83] Nelson, Joos, and Wolf added to this list a broad overarching competency for interacting with all things digital. They noted that consumers need digital literacy or competency with digital devices of all types; technical skills to operate devices and conceptual knowledge to understand their functionality; ability to creatively and critically use devices to access, manipulate, evaluate, and apply data, information, knowledge, and wisdom in activities of daily living; ability to apply basic emotional intelligence in collaborating and communicating with others; ethical values and sense of community responsibility to use digital devices for the enjoyment and benefit of society.[84]

Digital literacy skills are critical for future telehealth adoption for both consumers and healthcare providers. As the internet, telehealth, and other technology-based applications become a consistent part of healthcare, viewing these tools in light of the skills required for people to engage them becomes essential if the power of information technology is to be used to promote health and deliver effective healthcare. Additional information about the types and effects of literacy in health informatics is included in Chapter 2.

CONCLUSION AND FUTURE DIRECTIONS

Currently, telehealth services are being provided in diverse settings from islands off the coast of Maine to across the United States for remote care of military veterans. Two major types of telehealth exist: asynchronous and synchronous. Applications include teleradiology, teleconsulting, telepathology, telesensors, and remote home visits. Telehealth has the potential to decrease care costs and speed treatments, but the field also has challenges, including issues regarding licensure, standards, reimbursement, credentialing and privileging, and lack of integration with other health IT, especially EHRs.

Growth in telehealth could result in a future where access to healthcare is not limited by geographic region, time, or availability of skilled health professionals. The potential to realize comprehensive, integrated, and seamless delivery of healthcare services through virtual environments capable of spanning a broad range of prevention and health promotion interventions has already been made possible through advances in telehealth technology. Conditions exist for expanding telehealth to other sectors for sustainable telehealth, including rising healthcare costs, increasing prevalence of chronic diseases, an aging population, demands for improved access to healthcare, and global shortages of health professionals.[39,40,85-88] Creation of telehealth ecosystems and novel healthcare models requires interdisciplinary and intersectoral approaches spanning technology, education, and health management (Fig. 8.4).

The Canada-India Centre of Excellence for uHealth Research and Education (CuRE) framework in Fig. 8.4 depicts the CuRE. It provides a uHealth (ubiquitous health) view for operationalizing future global collaboration in advancing telehealth.

Policy decisions to adopt and implement telehealth technology in healthcare delivery are influenced by many drivers, such as global socioeconomic contexts, political motivations, capacity of technology to address healthcare needs, and

fundamental understandings of telehealth capabilities.[85,89] Inconsistencies in telehealth research methods and data reporting have had an effect on empirical data available to evaluate telehealth technology in the areas of cost benefit, effectiveness, and patient engagement.[86,87] Issues of authentication, data security, and practical aspects of telecommunication infrastructure remain critical challenges for the adoption and broader use of telehealth technologies.[90,91]

A consistent and coordinated approach in tracking healthcare technology use is lacking; therefore the effectiveness of telehealth is difficult to determine. Much available information on use and trends has been generated through industry and market analysis rather than through independent research. Significant challenges exist in tracking telehealth technology use and trends in healthcare, including:

1. How telehealth is defined: terms such as *telehealth*, *telemedicine*, and *informatics* are frequently and inconsistently used interchangeably in the literature.
2. The variety in modalities of telehealth technologies being used and the capacity to which they are used.
3. The vastly different contexts in which telehealth may be employed, such as varying models and settings for healthcare delivery, geographic regions, and cultural settings.[85,89,91]

Telehealth Industry Growth

One market research firm valued the market for remote patient monitoring, one form of telehealth care, in the United States at about $7.1 billion in 2010, and anticipated market growth to $22.2 billion by 2015.[92] Healthcare technology usage in Canada during 2010 includes delivery of 260,000 telehealth encounters and 2500 patients enrolled in telehomecare services, reflecting a 35% annual growth during the previous 5 years.[93] In Europe, outpatient telehealth services are provided by either public or private hospitals. A report provided to the European Commission in 2011 indicated that 8% of hospitals provided telemonitoring to patients.[93] Continued global growth in telehealth is anticipated as technology evolves and the need for cost-effective healthcare delivery increases in both developed and developing countries.[39,40,85,94]

Rapid advances in technology continue to expand the reach of healthcare delivery and the potential services available. Initially telehealth relied on internet connections; however, a shift to mHealth formats has occurred, particularly in developing countries. Growth in the mobile phone industry in countries such as China and India has increased 321% compared with 46% in developed countries.[95] In India, use of cellular phones is estimated at 742 million phones, with many of these new "mobile citizens" living in poorer and rural areas with scarce infrastructure and facilities, low literacy levels, and low internet access.[96] mHealth capabilities now provide a wide range of wireless monitoring opportunities to transmit information for a variety of health conditions, such as diabetes and cardiovascular diseases. mHealth has also increased access to healthcare for persons and communities in rural and isolated regions.[85] A recent endorsement of 4G standards in wireless telecommunications by the International

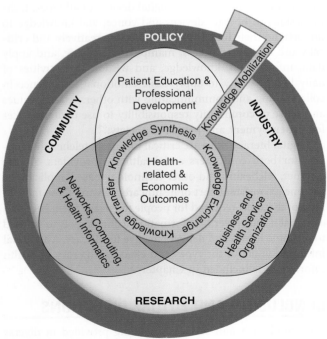

FIG 8.4 The CuRE framework. (Copyright 2012 Daniel Nagel and Antonia Arnaert. All Rights Reserved.)

Telecommunications Union, a branch of the United Nations, will have significant implications for speed and quantity of data transmission and for the future capacity of mHealth technologies in health care delivery.

Telehealth to uHealth

At present, a lack of integrated, secure technology "spaces" exists to facilitate migration of data between the various telehealth platforms, eHealth technologies, and mHealth devices for effective and efficient support of healthcare delivery. This gap in interoperability largely reflects industry strategies to protect proprietary rights; however, the lack of interoperability between technologies limits sharing of health information and the ability to implement a cohesive model of healthcare delivery in a virtual environment.[39]

Advancements in "cloud computing" technology, a more integrated wireless telecommunication architecture that supports accessible and seamless transmission and storage of digital data, may make it possible to facilitate a connection between healthcare information systems and to expand the capacity of healthcare delivery.[90,91]

Further research and development has focused on *ubiquitous* (*uHealth*) technologies that integrate core components of computers, wireless networks, sensors, and other modalities (such as mHealth devices) to create an environment to monitor, respond to, and assist in meeting the healthcare needs of individuals.[97,98] An example of uHealth is the development of smart home systems that provide persons with health concerns a safer environment in which to live more independently.[97] As the elderly population increases and people live longer with complex health conditions uHealth innovations can be used to detect changes in health status, communicate pertinent patient information, and alert healthcare providers to facilitate efficient interventions.[98]

Improve Healthcare Provider Shortages and Access to Care

As telehealth expands, further integration with informatics will continue. Telehealth encounters will be integrated within PHRs and EHRs. Self-care data will also be integrated into data repositories for individuals and populations. As the global population increases, the supply and distribution of healthcare providers can be optimized using telehealth to provide services regardless of the geographic location of those in need. Shortages in primary care providers and nurses, for example, can benefit from redistribution of portions of clinical expertise using telehealth as the export mechanism.[4,43]

Future migration of telehealth to uHealth will require practicing healthcare-provider licensure models that are not only interstate, but also international, enabling healthcare providers to practice in countries that have healthcare needs that can be met using telehealth technologies. This will require cooperation on the part of politicians, governments, and policy-makers on behalf of fully operationalized telehealth.[99,100]

REFERENCES

1. Health Resources and Services Administration (HRSA). *Telehealth.* HRSA; 2015. http://www.hrsa.gov/healthit/toolbox/RuralHealthITtoolbox/Telehealth/whatistelehealth.html.
2. American Telemedicine Association (ATA). *Telemedicine Defined.* ATA; 2015. http://www.americantelemed.org/about-telemedicine/what-is-telemedicine.
3. American Telemedicine Association (ATA). *What is Telemedicine?*; 2015. http://www.americantelemed.org/about-telemedicine/faqs.
4. Schlachta-Fairchild L. *International Competencies for Telenursing*; Geneva, Switzerland: International Council of Nurses; 2008.
5. Krupinski E, Nypaver M, Poropatich R, Ellis D, Safwat R, Sapci H. Clinical applications in telemedicine/telehealth. *Telemed J e-Health.* 2002;8(1):13–34.
6. University of Calgary, Health Telematics Unit. *State of the Science Report: Socioeconomic Impact of Telehealth Evidence Now for Health Care in the Future*; 2003. http://dspace.ucalgary.ca/bitstream/1880/43110/1/Socioeconomic%20Impact%20volume%20one.pdf.
7. Schlachta-Fairchild L, Elfrink V, Deickman A. Patient safety, telenursing, and telehealth. In: Hughes R, ed. *Patient Safety and Quality: An Evidence-Based Handbook for Nurses.* Rockville, MD: Agency for Health Care Research and Quality; 2008:1277–1316.
8. European Commission (EC). *Telemedicine for the Benefit of Patients, Health Care Systems and Society*; 2011. http://europa.eu/rapid/press-release_MEMO-11-282_en.htm?locale=en.
9. American Heart Association/American Stroke Association. AHA/ASA scientific statement: a review of the evidence for the use of telemedicine within stroke systems of care. *Stroke.* 2009;40:2616–2634.
10. European Coordination Committee of the Radiological, Electromedical and Healthcare IT Industry (COCIR). *COCIR Telemedicine Toolkit Supporting Effective Deployment of Telehealth and Mobile Health*; 2011. http://www.cocir.org/fileadmin/Publications_2011/telemedicine_toolkit_link2.pdf.
11. Medicaid CHIP Programs. *Telemedicine and Telehealth Overview*; 2015. https://www.medicaid.gov/Medicaid-CHIP-Program-Information/By-Topics/Delivery-Systems/Telemedicine.html.
12. HealthIT.gov. *What is Telehealth?*; 2014. https://www.healthit.gov/providers-professionals/faqs/what-telehealth-how-telehealth-different-telemedicine.
13. California Department of Healthcare Services. *Telehealth: Frequently Asked Questions*; 2015. http://www.dhcs.ca.gov/provgovpart/Pages/TelehealthFAQ.aspx.
14. Hall SC. *Army Telemedicine Programs Going Mobile*; 2013. http://www.fiercemobilehealthcare.com/story/army-telemedicine-programs-going-mobile/2013-05-13.
15. University of Miami Telehealth. *Teledermatology: University of Miami, Miller School of Medicine*; 2012. http://telehealth.med.miami.edu/services/teledermatology.
16. Darkins A, Cary M. *Telemedicine and Telehealth: Principles, Policies, Performance, and Pitfalls.* New York, NY: Springer Publishing Company; 2000.
17. House AM, Roberts JM. Telemedicine in Canada. *Can Med Assoc J.* 1977;117(4):386–388.
18. Johnston B, Wheeler L, Deuser J, Sousa K. Outcomes of the Kaiser Permanente tele-home research project. *Arch Fam Med.* 2000;9(1):40–45.

19. Darkins A, Ryan P, Kobb R, et al. Care coordination/home telehealth, and disease management to support the care of veteran patients with chronic conditions. *Telemed J e-Health*. 2008;14(10):1118–1126.

20. Department of Health (United Kingdom). *Whole System Demonstrator Programme: Headline Findings*. Department of Health; 2011. http://www.dh.gov.uk/en/ Publicationsandstatistics/Publications/ PublicationsPolicyAndGuidance/DH_131684.

21. AFHCAN Telemedicine Program Reaches Significant Milestone in Alaska. *Native American Times*; 2011. http://www. nativetimes.com/index.php/life/health/5615-afhcan-telemedicine-program-reaches-significant-milestone-in-alaska.

22. American Nurses Association. *Core Principles on Telehealth*. Washington, DC: American Nurses Publishing; 1998.

23. American Telemedicine Association (ATA). *About ATA*; 2015. http://www.americantelemed.org/about-ata/who-is-ata#. VndP7PkrJD8.

24. American Telemedicine Association. *Telemedicine Practice Guidelines*. http://www.americantelemed.org/resources/ telemedicine-practice-guidelines/telemedicine-practice-guidelines#.Vlz3bnarTIU. Accessed July 1, 2016.

25. Demiris G. Patient-centered applications: use of information technology to promote disease management and wellness. *J Am Med Inform Assoc*. 2008;15:8–13.

26. Continua Health Alliance. *Mission and purpose. Continua Health Alliance*; 2015. http://www.continuaalliance.org/about-the-alliance/mission-and-objectives.

27. *Personal Connected Health Alliance*. http://www.pchalliance. org/. Accessed June 30, 2016.

28. ZigBee Alliance. *Specifications*. ZigBee Alliance; 2015. http:// www.zigbee.org/what-is-zigbee/.

29. United States Department of Health and Human Services, Office of the National Coordinator for Health Information Technology. *Federal health IT strategic plan 2015-2020*. https://www.healthit. gov/sites/default/files/9-5-federalhealthitstratplanfinal_0.pdf. Accessed November 29, 2015.

30. Thielst C. *The Crossroads of Telehealth, Electronic Health Records & Health Information Exchange*; 2010. https://www.amia.org/ sites/amia.org/files/Crossroads-of-Telehealth-White-Paper.pdf.

31. World Health Organization (WHO). *Telehealth and Telemedicine will Henceforth be Part of the Strategy for Health for All [press release]*. Geneva, Switzerland: WHO; 1997.

32. Worley J. *Long Distance and Up Close: UK Telemedicine in the Vanguard of Patient Care*. Odyssey: University of Kentucky; 2010. http://www.research.uky.edu/odyssey/spring10/jicha.html.

33. Gagnon MP, Orruno E, Asua J, Abdeljelil AB, Emparanza J. Using a modified technology acceptance model to evaluate health care professionals' adoption of a new telemonitoring system. *Telemed J e-Health*. 2012;18(1):54–59.

34. American Nurses Association. *Competencies for Telehealth Technologies in Nursing*. Washington, DC: American Nurses Publishing; 1999.

35. American Nurses Association. *Developing Telehealth Protocols: A Blueprint for Success*. Washington, DC: American Nurses Publishing; 2001.

36. Canadian Society for Telehealth. *Canadian National Initiative for Telehealth Releases Framework of Guidelines for Telehealth*. Virtual Medical Worlds; 2003. https://www.isfteh.org/files/ work_groups/FrameworkofGuidelines2003eng.pdf.

37. College of Registered Nurses of Nova Scotia (CRNNS). *Telenursing Practice Guidelines*. CRNNS; 2008. https://crnns.ca/ wp-content/uploads/2015/02/Telenursing2014.pdf.

38. American Telemedicine Association (ATA). *Expert Consensus Recommendations for Videoconferencing-Based Telepresenting*. ATA; 2011. http://www.americantelemed.org/resources/ telemedicine-practice-guidelines/telemedicine-practice-guidelines/recommendations-for-videoconferencing-based-telepresenting#.VnddaPkrJD.

39. Hein MA. *Telemedicine: An Important Force in the Transformation of Health Care*. Washington, DC: International Trade Administration, US Department of Commerce; 2009.

40. Care WD, Gregory DM, Chermonas WM. Nursing, technology, and informatics: understanding the past and embracing the future. In: McIntyre M, McDonald C, eds. *Realities of Canadian Nursing: Professional, Practice, and Power Issues*. Philadelphia, PA: Wolters Kluwer, Lippincott Williams & Wilkins; 2010.

41. Jennett P, Yeo M, Pauls M, Graham J. Organizational readiness for telemedicine: implications for success and failure. *J Telemed Telecare*. 2003;9:27–30.

42. Duclos C, Hook J, Rodriquez M. *Telehealth in Community Clinics: Three Case Studies in Implementation*. California Health-Care Foundation; 2010. http://www.chcf.org/~/media/ MEDIA%20LIBRARY%20Files/PDF/PDF%20T/PDF% 20TelehealthClinicCaseStudies.pdf.

43. Schlachta-Fairchild L, Elfrink V. *International Telenursing Survey Report*. Frederick, MD: iTelehealth Inc; 2009.

44. Department of Health and Human Services. *Telemedicine Report to Congress*; 2001. http://armtelemed.org/resources/24-US_ DHHS_TM_report-to-congress_2001.pdf.

45. Pong RW, Hogenbirk JC. Licensing physicians for telehealth practice: issues and policy options; *Health Law Rev*. 2002;8 (1):3–14.

46. Robbings D. *Removing Barriers for the Advancement of Telemedicine*; 2011. http://cchpca.org/telehealth-advancement-ac.

47. Philipsen N, Haynes D. The multi-state nursing licensure compact: making nurses mobile. *J Nurse Pract*. 2007;3(1):36–40.

48. Telehealth Resource Center (TRC). *Licensure and Scope of Practice*; 2011. http://www.telehealthresourcecenter.org/ toolbox-module/licensure-and-scope-practice.

49. U.S. Government Printing Office. *Medicare and Medicaid programs: Changes Affecting Hospital and Critical Access Hospital Conditions of participation: Telemedicine and Privileging*; May 5, 2011. Washington, DC. Federal Register 76, no. 87.

50. Medicaid.gov. *Telemedicine.Medicaid.gov*; 2012. https://www. medicaid.gov/Medicaid-CHIP-Program-Information/By-Topics/Delivery-Systems/Telemedicine.html.

51. Chee J. *Tele-Medical Malpractice: Negligence in the Practice of Telemedicine and Related Issues*. The Center for Telehealth and E-Health Law; 2010. http://www.ctel.org/research/TeleMedical %20Malpractice%20Negligence%20in%20the%20Practice% 20of%20Telemedicine%20and%20Related%20Issues.pdf.

52. Manhattan Research Group. *Seven Percent of U.S. Physicians Use Video Chat to Communicate With Patients*. FierceHealthcare; 2012. http://www.fiercehealthcare.com/press-releases/seven-percent-us-physicians-use-video-chat-communicate-patients-1#ixzz1lGE7d5Ls.

53. American College of Emergency Physicians. *ER Visits Up Since Implementation of Affordable Care Act: Nearly 9 in 10 ER Docs Report Psych Patients Being Held in their ERs*; 2014. http:// newsroom.acep.org/2014-05-21-ER-Visits-Up-Since-Implementation-of-Affordable-Care-Act.

54. Jasper B. *Doctors' Virtual Consults With Patients to Double by 2020*. Forbes; 2015. http://www.forbes.com/sites/brucejapsen/ 2015/08/09/as-telehealth-booms-doctor-video-consults-to-double-by-2020/.

55. *Harris Logic Telehealth Solutions.* http://www.harrislogic.com/case-studies/telehealth-solutions. Accessed November 29, 2015.

56. *Secure Telehealth.* http://www.securetelehealth.com/telearticles-a-news.html. Accessed June 30, 2016.

57. *Teladoc.* http://www.teladoc.com. Accessed November 29, 2015.

58. *Online Care Anywhere.* https://www.onlinecareanywheremn.com/. Accessed November 29, 2015.

59. *Virtuwell.* https://www.virtuwell.com/. Accessed November 29, 2015.

60. *Relay Health.* http://www.relayhealth.com/solutions/clinical-solutions/medical-home-support. Accessed November 29, 2015.

61. Jordan-Marsh M. *Health Technology Literacy: A Transdisciplinary Framework for Consumer-Oriented Practice.* Sudbury, MA: Jones & Bartlett; 2011.

62. Lau C, Churchill S, Kim J, Matsen F, Yongmin K. Asynchronous web-based patient centered home telemedicine system. *IEEE T Bio-Med Eng.* 2002;49(12):1452–1462.

63. Agency for Healthcare Research and Quality. *Multiple Chronic Conditions*; 2015. http://www.ahrq.gov/professionals/prevention-chronic-care/decision/mcc/index.html.

64. *VA Telehealth Services.* http://www.telehealth.va.gov/ccht/; 2015.

65. Darkins A, Ryan P, Kobb R, et al. Care coordination/home telehealth, and disease management to support the care of veteran patients with chronic conditions. *Telemed J e-Health.* 2008;14(10):1118–1126.

66. *MyHealtheVet.* Welcome to MyHealtheVet. https://www.myhealth.va.gov/index.html. Accessed November 30, 2015.

67. *Garfield KM.* Telehealth and the homebound heart failure patient. http://www.telehealth.philips.com/customers_home_health_agencies.html. Accessed November 30, 2015.

68. Philips Telehealth Solutions. http://www.telehealth.philips.com/. Accessed November 30, 2015.

69. Wigmore I. *What is: Sensor*; 2012. http://whatis.techtarget.com/definition/sensor.

70. Kailas A, Chia-Chin C, Watanabe F. From mobile phones to personal wellness dashboards. *IEEE Pulse.* 2010;1(1). http://ieeexplore.ieee.org/xpl/login.jsp?tp=&arnumber=5506918&url=http%3A%2F%2Fieeexplore.ieee.org%2Fxpls%2Fabs_all.jsp%3Farnumber%3D5506918. Accessed November 30, 2015.

71. Sopher J. *Hot Health Care Trends for 2015: Eye Imaginations*; 2014. https://blog.eyemaginations.com/hot-health-care-technology-trends-2015/.

72. Szcaerba RJ. *Fashion 2.0 Complement Your Smart Phone with Smart Clothes forbes/tech*; 2014. http://www.forbes.com/sites/robertszczerba/2014/11/14/fashion-2-0-complement-your-smart-phone-with-smart-clothes/.

73. Soojung K. *New Memo: RFID: Smart Homes & Sociable Devices in Institute for the Future*; 2005. http://www.iftf.org/future-now/article-detail/new-memo-rfid-smart-homes-sociable-devices/.

74. The Learning Space. *An Overview of RFID in ICTS: Device to Device Communication.* Scotland: The Open University; 2012. http://openlearn.open.ac.uk/mod/oucontent/view.php?id=397529&section=7.2.

75. Center for Studying Health System Change. *Surprising Decline in Consumers Seeking Health Information.* Center for Studying Health System Change; 2011. http://www.hschange.com/CONTENT/1261/.

76. Fox S, Duggan M. *Pew Internet and American Life Project Health online 2013*; 2013. http://www.pewinternet.org/2013/01/15/health-online-2013/.

77. Healthy People 2020. *Health Communication and Health Information Technology*; 2010. http://healthypeople.gov/2020/topicsobjectives2020/overview.aspx?topicId=18.

78. Toner R. *Consumer Health Websites Accelerate Consumer-Driven Health Care Value Based Purchasing.* Thomas Jefferson University, Jefferson Digital Commons; 2009. http://jdc.jefferson.edu/cgi/viewcontent.cgi?article=1041&context=vbp&sei-redir=1&referer=http%3A%2F%2Fwww.google.com%2Furl%3Fsa%3Dt%26rct%3Dj%26q%3Dhistory%2520of%2520health%2520consumer%2520websites%26source%3Dweb%26cd%3D3%26sqi%3D2%26ved%3D0CEMQFjAC%26url%3Dhttp%253A%252F%252Fjdc.jefferson.edu%252Fcgi%252Fviewcontent.cgi%253Farticle%253D1041%2526context%253Dvbp%26ei%3DefYyT7iEOYLx0gGZ5o3kBw%26usg%3DAFQjCNGf0dlOmsTSJkvO6zj0cU8b6QY4Cg#search=%22history%20health%20consumer%20websites%22.

79. Health on the Net. *HONCode in Brief.* Health on the Net Foundation; 2008. http://www.hon.ch/HONcode/Patients/Visitor/visitor.html.

80. Lorence D, Abraham J. A study of undue pain and surfing: using hierarchical criteria to assess web site quality. *Health Inform J.* 2008;14(3):155–173.

81. Toms EG, Latter C. How consumers search for health information. *Health Inform J.* 2007;13(3):223–235.

82. Chan CV, Kaufman DR. A framework for characterizing eHealth literacy demands and barriers. *J Med Internet Res.* 2011;13(4).

83. Norman CD. Skinner HAeHealth literacy: essential skills for consumer health in a networked world. *J Med Internet Res.* 2006;8(2).

84. Nelson R, Joos IM, Wolf D. *Social Media for Nurses.* New York, NY: Springer; 2013.

85. Mechael PN. The case for mhealth in developing countries. *Innovations.* 2009;4(1):103–118.

86. Pare G, Jaana M, Sicotte C. Systematic review of home telemonitoring for chronic diseases: the evidence base. *J Am Med Inform Assoc.* 2007;14(3):269–277.

87. Polisena J, Coyle D, Coyle K, McGill S. Home telehealth for chronic disease management: a systematic review and analysis of economic evaluations. *Int J Technol Assess.* 2009;25(3):339–349.

88. Vinson MH, McCallum R, Thornlow DK, Champagne MT. Design, implementation, and evaluation of population-specific telehealth nursing services. *Nurs Econ.* 2011;29(5):265–277.

89. Miller EA. Solving the disjuncture between research and practice: telehealth trends in the 21st century. *Health Policy.* 2007;82(2):133–141.

90. Nkosi MT, Mekuria SM. Cloud computing for enhanced mobile applications. *Cloud Comput Technol Sci.* 2010;31:629–633. http://dx.doi.org/10.1109/CloudCom.2010.31:629-633.

91. Thuemmlar C, Fan L, Buchanan W, Lo O, Ekonomou E, Khedim S. E-health: chances and challenges of distributed, service oriented architectures. *J Cyber Security Mobil.* 2012;1(1):37–52.

92. Kalorama Information. *Remote Patient Monitoring Systems May Help Overstressed ICUs*; 2011. http://www.kaloramainformation.com/about/release.asp?id=2339.

93. European Commission (EC). *eHealth Benchmarking III: SMART 2009/0022*; 2011. https://ec.europa.eu/digital-agenda/sites/digital-agenda/files/ehealth_benchmarking_3_final_report.pdf.

94. Canada Health Infoway. *Telehealth Benefits and Adoption: Connecting People and Providers Across Canada.* Canada Health Infoway; 2010. https://www2.infoway-inforoute.ca/Documents/telehealth_report_2010_en.pdf.

95. Pew Research Center. *10 Facts About Technology Use in the Emerging World*; 2015. http://www.pewresearch.org/fact-tank/2015/03/20/10-facts-about-technology-use-emerging-world.

96. CNN. *Mobile Phone: Weapon Against Global Poverty*; 2011. http://www.cnn.com/2011/10/09/tech/mobile/mobile-phone-poverty/.

97. Agoulmine N, Deen MJ, Lee JS, Meyyappan M. U-Health smart home: innovative solutions for the management of the elderly and chronic diseases. *IEEE Nanotechnol Magazine*. 2011;5 (3):6–11.

98. Otto C, Milenkovic A, Sanders C, Jovanov E. System architecture of a wireless body area sensor network for ubiquitous health monitoring; *J Mobile Multimed*. 2006;1(4):307–326.

99. Miller EA. Solving the disjuncture between research and practice: telehealth trends in the 21st century. *Health Policy*. 2007;82(2):133–141.

100. Schlachta-Fairchild L, Castelli D, Pyke R. International telenursing: a strategic tool for nursing shortage and access to nursing care. In: Jordanova M, Lievens F, eds. *Proceedings of Medetel, the International Society of Telemedicine and eHealth Annual Conference*, Luxembourg: Luxexpo; 2008:399–405.

DISCUSSION QUESTIONS

1. What licensure model would be most useful to support telehealth clinical practice across international boundaries; for example, Canadian doctors or nurses (virtually) seeing and treating U.S. patients or U.S. pharmacists and occupational therapists (virtually) seeing and treating Australian patients?
2. How do the different models for delivering healthcare, including covering the cost of that healthcare, affect the telehealth programs in different countries?
3. What actions can individual healthcare providers take in the next 3 years to advance the benefits of telehealth for their profession?
4. Why has the telehealth adoption taken so long in the healthcare industry when Skype, cellphones, and other video conferencing applications have been used in personal and business interactions for decades?
5. How much does usability affect you and your friends when deciding to accept or reject the use of a new technology? Does this also apply in your role as healthcare provider?
6. What actions can individual healthcare providers take to improve their patients' eHealth literacy?
7. What needs to occur on an international basis for uHealth to be operationalized?
8. What are the first five steps you would take to start a telehealth program or application in the healthcare facility where you work?
9. What key success criteria for telehealth programs are "must have" and what criteria are "nice to have" when considering a new telehealth initiative?
10. What factor or factors will be most important in driving the exponential growth of telehealth in the future?

CASE STUDY

Mrs. Smith is 82 years old and is diagnosed with hypertension, diabetes, and congestive heart failure. Her two children live in California, whereas she lives in North Carolina in a small family home on 10 acres of land in the Blue Ridge Mountains. Mrs. Smith has been in the hospital four times in the last year because of congestive heart failure. As her eyesight and mobility get worse with age, she has found it a challenge to stay on her medical plan and to do her shopping for the right foods she knows she should be eating. Mrs. Smith's health plan, Purple Cross of North Carolina, assigned a nurse case manager to address her situation. Purple Cross provided a digital scale and a remote monitoring device that record Mrs. Smith's condition every day by uploading her weight and transmitting the answers to a series of questions on a touch screen kiosk. The case manager also coordinated delivery of Meals on Wheels, providing low-sodium, diabetic-compliant dinners to Mrs. Smith on an ongoing basis. The case manager calls Mrs. Smith twice a week, taking the time to educate her about her medications, her activities, and the disease-specific elements that will keep her healthy and out of the hospital. When the case manager identifies that Mrs. Smith can no longer organize her daily medications, a digital medication dispenser will be provided that will keep her on her medication regimen. The medication dispenser will be preloaded with Mrs. Smith's medications and will issue a subtle doorbell tone when it is time to take her medicines. With the combination of remote and real-time (telephonic) support persons and technologies, Mrs. Smith is able to remain in her home and avoid further inpatient admissions.

Discussion Questions
1. Which components are critical to Mrs. Smith staying safely in her home?
2. Describe whether Mrs. Smith's regimen might be augmented using telehealth applications.

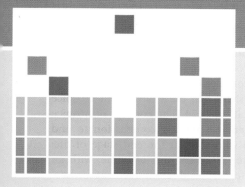

9

Home Health and Related Community-Based Systems

Karen S. Martin and Karen B. Utterback

No matter how dreary and gray our homes are, we people of flesh and blood would rather live there than in any other country, be it ever so beautiful. There is no place like home.

Baum LF. The Wonderful Wizard of Oz. Chicago, IL: George M. Hill Co.; 1900.

OBJECTIVES

At the completion of this chapter, the reader will be prepared to:

1. Describe home health, palliative care and hospice, public health, nurse-managed health centers, and other practice models.

2. Summarize the supporting electronic health records (EHRs) and information systems used at community and home-based practice sites.
3. Specify the value of the clinical data and information that can be generated by information systems used at practice sites.

KEY TERMS

home health, 154
hospice care, 155
Hospice Item Set (HIS), 157
Intervention Scheme, 161
nurse-managed health center, 155
Omaha System, 159

Outcome and Assessment Information Set (OASIS), 156
outcomes-based quality-improvement (OBQI), 158
palliative care, 155
Problem Classification Scheme, 160
Problem Rating Scale for Outcomes, 161
standardized datasets, 156

ABSTRACT ❖

Home care and related community-based systems located in the United States are changing rapidly. Information technology is accelerating those changes. This chapter will address (1) home health, palliative care and hospice, community based public health, nurse-managed health centers, and other community-based practice models; (2) the electronic health records (EHRs) and information systems used at community and home-based practice sites; and (3) the value of the clinical data and information that can be generated by these information systems. Core values of community-based clinicians include patient-centered care and services that are of high quality, efficient, and cost effective. Information systems began with billing systems and evolved to point-of-care solutions in the 1990s. The Outcome and Assessment Information Set (OASIS), Hospice Item Set (HIS), and patient-experience surveys are examples of home health and hospice standardized datasets. Using standardized terminologies is another strategy that complements community-based core values. The Omaha System, one of the standardized terminologies developed by home health nurses and recognized by the American Nurses Association, is described, and a clinical example illustrates how practice, documentation, and information management can enhance the quality of community-based care.

INTRODUCTION

Home care and related community-based systems located in the United States are changing rapidly and becoming increasingly linked to other providers in the healthcare community. Information technology (IT), related technological advances, the emphasis on big data, the transition to value-based care, and other national initiatives are accelerating these changes. Numerous references describe home health research, economics, and patient personal preference, suggesting that the home is the optimal location for diverse health and nursing services.[1a–6] Patient residences include houses, apartments, dormitories, trailers, boarding and care homes, hospice houses, assisted-living facilities, shelters, and cars. Although residences are the primary location where care is provided, many home care and related community-based organizations offer services at workplaces, schools, churches, community buildings, and other sites.

This chapter addresses home health, palliative care and hospice, community-based public health, nurse-managed health centers, and other community-based practice models; the supporting electronic health records (EHRs) and information systems used at the practice sites; and the value of the clinical data and information that can be generated by these information systems. The assessment, planning, intervention, and evaluation services that are part of these models range from promoting wellness and preventing disease to care of the sick and dying. Ideally, these services are captured in EHRs so that they can be quantified, analyzed, and used to measure the outcomes of care. Formal caregivers include nurses, social workers, physical and occupational therapists, speech-language pathologists, registered dietitians, home health aides, chaplains, physicians, and others. A team approach and interprofessional collaboration are required to address the intensity of the patient's and family's needs. Although the term *patient* is used consistently in this chapter, *client, customer, consumer,* and *member* are alternative terms often used in home health and community-based systems.

EVOLUTION AND MILESTONES

Home health and community-based systems have a long and distinguished history in this country. In the early years, care for those who were ill or dying was typically informal and provided by the women who lived in the household or neighborhood. Home health provided by formal caregivers originated in the 1800s and was based on the district nursing model developed by William Rathbone in England. In many communities, the initial programs evolved into visiting nurse associations (VNAs). The movement expanded rapidly in the United States, resulting in the formation of 71 agencies before 1900 and 600 by 1909.[7-9]

In 1893, Lillian Wald and Mary Brewster established the Henry Street Settlement House in New York City and developed a comprehensive program that was staffed by nurses and social workers. One of Wald's most impressive innovations was to convince the Metropolitan Life Insurance Company to include home visits as a benefit and to examine the cost effectiveness of care, a partnership that continued until 1952.[7-9]

Public health departments were established and expanded during the early years of the 20th century. Health department staff members were primarily nurses who focused on care of immigrants, milk banks for mothers and babies, communicable disease, and environmental issues. They were concerned about consistent practice standards, the patient record, and the collection of statistics.[10]

Home health services were included as a major benefit when Medicare legislation was enacted in 1965 and resulted in significant changes nationally. The benefit was designed to provide intermittent, shorter visits with temporary lengths of stay to persons age 65 and older; health promotion and long-term care services were not reimbursed. Nurses continued to represent the largest group of agency staff members; however, involvement of other professions was required. When a patient was admitted to service, the home health

agency was required to develop a plan of care, obtain the signature of a physician, and follow additional regulations.[11]

Hospice care was introduced in the 1970s. Florence Wald is acknowledged as the founder of the hospice movement in the United States; she established the Connecticut Hospice with interprofessional staff in 1974. The concept of hospice grew from a commitment to provide compassionate and dignified care to people who were at the end stage of life; the program offered care in the comfort of home, with an emphasis on quality of life. Medicaid reimbursement for hospice care began in 1980, and Medicare reimbursement began in 1983; reimbursement determines many aspects of the hospice programs.[10,12-14]

Nurses employed in home health and community-based settings were concerned about documentation, standardization, and accountability in addition to practice. Their concerns were similar to those of other healthcare professionals. Physicians advanced systems for nomenclature and classification beginning with the International Classification of Diseases (ICD) in 1893. In 1966, physician Avedis Donabedian described the well-known structure, process, and outcome framework for evaluating the quality of medical care.[15] Another physician, Lawrence Weed, developed a problem-oriented medical record in 1968 that was adaptable to computerization.[16] In 1986, Mary Elizabeth Tinetti developed and published a tool to measure mobility problems in elderly patients.[17] In 1990, Pamela Duncan developed a balance measure referred to as "functional reach" that is especially useful for her physical therapist colleagues who work in community settings. Functional reach can serve as a measure of frailty in elders to predict fall risk and help identify appropriate interventions.[18] Numerous studies have been conducted to confirm the value of Tinetti's and Duncan's tools and original research. During the last 25 years, many other respected and validated tools have been adopted into practice, including the use of required standardized data sets for home health and hospice. These tools ensure that objective data are captured as care is being delivered.

PRACTICE MODELS

Home Health

Home health is the delivery of intermittent health-related services in patients' places of residence with the goal of promoting self-care and independence rather than institutionalization. The intensity of services has increased dramatically as hospital stays have become shorter and patients are discharged with serious illnesses or soon after surgery and with complex treatment needs. The care delivered often focuses on supporting a safe transition back to the home following an episode of illness or exacerbation that required an inpatient or extended care facility stay.[4]

Home health interventions include medication reconciliation; teaching and coaching to improve the ability of patients, families, and caregivers to manage independently; coordination of care with other healthcare providers and community resources; and early detection of decline or exacerbation. Common treatments and procedures now include ventilators, renal hemodialysis, and intravenous therapy for antibiotics, chemotherapy, and analgesia, as well as delivery of total par-enteral nutrition and blood products.

An estimated 12,200 Medicare-certified home health agencies provide services across the country.[5,19–22] As the largest payer, Medicare accounts for 45% of total home health reimbursement. Medicaid, state and local governments, private pay, and private insurance are the other sources. Home health agencies provide services to approximately 12 million patients who ranged in age from infants to elders. More than 85% of all home health patients are over age 65. Recipients of home health services have diverse needs. Joint replacement with rehabilitation services and heart failure top the list for patients discharged from hospitals to home health. Diabetes, rehabilitation services, and heart failure are listed most often for all home health patients.[5,19–22]

Palliative Care and Hospice

Hospice care involves the delivery of services by teams of interprofessional clinicians for those who have exhausted curative treatment measures. Palliative care focuses on quality of life for patients and their families facing the problem associated with life-threatening illness. Whereas palliative care often begins once a cure is no longer possible and may be somewhat long term, hospice care is limited to patients with life expectancies of 6 months or less. Both palliative and hospice care involve holistic care, an emphasis on dignity, and being surrounded by the comforts of home and family. However, the programs have differences. Typically, palliative care services are focused on comfort, quality of life, and end-of-life or advanced care planning. Hospice involves symptom management with the goal of providing as much comfort and dignity as possible at the end of life. Hospice programs include bereavement follow-up for families after a patient's death. In this country, a stigma may be associated with end-of-life care. It is associated with giving up and the refusal to accept death as a natural process, although this is changing as evidenced by the growth in hospice programs.[6,23–25]

There were approximately 5800 hospice programs in 2013; about 3700 were Medicare-certified. More than 1.5 million patients received hospice services in 2013, with an average stay of 72 days. The average length of stay is increasing as hospice becomes more widely accepted. As the largest payer, Medicare accounted for 87% of hospice expenditures in 2013, with Medicaid and private insurance paying the rest.[6,13,24,25]

Community-Based Public Health

The basis of community-based public health practice is the individual, family, and community. Public health nurses and other clinicians provide services that address and include health education and wellness campaigns, immunization clinics, screening events, parent-child health and safety, communicable disease, family planning, environmental health, substance use, and sexually transmitted disease. Approximately 2800 city, county, metropolitan, district, and tribal health departments exist in the United States. Since 2008, local health departments have lost 51,700 of approximately 155,000 positions because of decreasing budgets, layoffs,

and attrition. Many public health nursing positions have been lost because of lack of funds.[26] In this chapter the emphasis is on computerization to support these types of public health services that are provided to individuals and families in the community.[27]

Public health services can also be directed toward the community with a focus on the whole population and primary prevention. Principles of public health and epidemiology or causality, as well as community assessment and public policy, are usually components of these types of public health programs. Chapter 11 focuses on public health informatics with an emphasis on population health of communities, countries, and global health.

Nurse-Managed Health Centers

Community health nurses, as well as advanced practice registered nurses, including clinical nurse specialists, nurse practitioners, and certified nurse midwives, provide care at urban and rural centers called nurse-managed health centers. These centers may have collaborative agreements with physicians and other interprofessional colleagues. Many centers are part of or associated with educational institutions. They provide clinical experiences for students and are located in underserved areas. Target populations include pregnant teens, fragile elders, low-income mothers and children, and others who may be underinsured or uninsured. Nurse-managed health centers offer primary care services, preventive care, chronic illness care, and care for specific conditions such as obesity. More than 250 centers exist in the United States; Philadelphia has more than any other city.[28]

Other Practice Sites

School, faith community, and occupational health nurses, as well as other clinicians, provide healthcare in noninstitutionalized settings. School nurses typically participate in classroom instruction, screen the school setting for safety hazards, provide medications in collaboration with parents and healthcare providers, work with children who have special needs, monitor immunization status, and provide and follow-up on screening procedures. Faith community nurses may function as case managers when they help their parishioners to obtain needed healthcare services, food, shelter, and supplies. Some provide educational and surveillance interventions for those who have chronic illnesses such as diabetes and cardiovascular disease. Occupational health nurses are often employed by businesses with a high risk of injury or with an emphasis on health promotion and wellness such as smoking cessation, weight loss, and regular exercise.

Similarities Among Practice Models

Because community-based clinicians have the opportunity to work with patients and their families over time, they embrace core values that influence their practice. Interprofessional collaboration and a seamless healthcare environment are essential. Practice is based on the consumer movement: people have rights and responsibilities, must be knowledgeable about their own healthcare, and must participate as partners in healthcare decisions. These values are linked to themes of access, cost, quality, and IT.

The power of the patient and family is an important core value. When a nurse or other healthcare professional enters a patient's home, the patient and family are in charge, not the clinician. Clinicians immediately observe indicators and collect data about patients' lifestyles, resources, and motivation. While providing care, clinicians identify patients' strengths and incorporate those strengths in the care process. The goal of community-based practice settings is to provide patient-centered care and include patients, their families, and their caregivers in care planning and delivery. In the hospital or long-term care facility, the nurse gives medications, changes dressings, and controls many aspects of care. In the home, nurses assist patients to provide their own care or assist family members or informal caregivers to provide that care.[10,29,30]

Clinicians who work in community settings need skills that demonstrate dedication, flexibility, and independence. Although they develop plans for their day and for each visit or encounter, those plans often need to be adapted and modified. It may not be possible to accomplish Plan A, so Plan B, C, or D may be substituted at a moment's notice. Colleagues, equipment, and references are not readily available to the extent that they are in hospitals and long-term care facilities. Selected help and supplies may be available in the trunk of a car or via cellphone, in the EHR, from the internet, or from a pager request. Clinicians always need to consider their safety. Environments may be difficult, dysfunctional, or even dangerous. Many patients and families welcome clinicians, although that does not always happen. Clinicians need to develop and rely on their basic education, ongoing education, life experiences, and common sense to function self-sufficiently and to enjoy their work responsibilities.

The Triple Aim model for healthcare was published in 2008 (Box 9.1). However, the primary concepts of the model have been the foundation and core values of home health and related community-based services from their inception: services that are patient centered, of high quality, efficient, and cost effective. Although the size, staffing, organization, board structure, and financial arrangements of the practice models summarized in this chapter vary markedly, all deal with limited financial resources. Clinicians who work in community settings must be very knowledgeable about costs and funding. Frequently they help patients and families understand and manage health-related financial issues. In many situations, Medicare and Medicaid funding regulations are the primary determinant of the type and length of home health and hospice services. Private insurance companies determine their own guidelines but typically follow Medicare's policies. Ever-changing regulations and reimbursement patterns, interest in private pay services, and the aging population contribute to altered services. Agencies that provide Medicare- and Medicaid-certified services must meet strict national regulations. Most states have additional licensing rules.[11]

STANDARDIZED DATASETS

Standardized datasets are required in Medicare-certified and hospice settings, and are found in other community-based settings. The concept of a standardized dataset in the community began more than 25 years ago with the Resident Assessment Instrument (RAI). This approach was adopted in response to a public outcry about the poor quality of care occurring in long-term or extended nursing facilities, and to the government's effort to bring visibility and transparency to care provided in these institutions. Over time, the use of standardized datasets has expanded from long-term care to home health, renal dialysis units, and other care settings. This approach provides a means to collect patient characteristics and measurements in a standardized manner that allows data aggregation for analysis. The aggregated data offer the opportunity for data-driven decision making related to care delivery and correlating payment systems to a predicted level of care needed by the patient.[31,32]

Standardized datasets have evolved largely without the adoption of standardized point-of-care and reference terminologies in practice settings. Although standardized terminologies in medicine have existed for centuries, the adoption of standardized terminologies in nursing and the other health professions began to take root about 45 years ago. However, adoption in practice has been limited and even more limited among the information systems commonly purchased by home health, hospice, and other community-based care settings. Although standardized datasets have served an important purpose, healthcare providers need additional strategies to achieve the care communication and coordination necessary to transform healthcare and achieve the Triple Aim for healthcare (see Box 9.1). Strategies need to include a focus on patient-centered care, best practices and evidence-based care, interprofessional care teams, and a value-based approach that can be quantified, analyzed, and used to measure the outcomes of care.[3,4,33,34]

Outcome and Assessment Information Set

The Outcome and Assessment Information Set (OASIS) is the standardized dataset that home health agency clinicians complete with their patients.[35] It is designed to determine payment and measure the quality and outcomes of practice. OASIS consists of 80-plus questions and response sets; collection requirements vary according to specific times during the

---

BOX 9.1 **The Triple Aim for Healthcare**

- Better care for individuals, described by the six dimensions of healthcare performance: safety, effectiveness, patient-centeredness, timeliness, efficiency, and equity.
- Better health for populations, through attacking "the upstream causes of so much of our ill health," such as poor nutrition, physical inactivity, and substance abuse.
- Reducing per-capita costs.

Adapted from Berwick DM, Nolan TW, Whittington J. The triple aim: care, health, and cost. *Health Aff.* 2008;27(3):759-769.

process of care (i.e., admission, transfer, resumption of care, follow-up, or discharge). An example of a question is M1240: Has the patient had a formal Pain Assessment using a standardized pain assessment tool? A second example is M1242: Frequency of Pain interfering with patient's activities or movement.

Public reporting, another benefit of the data and outcomes collected using the OASIS dataset, began in 2003. It allows the public to compare the outcomes of home health agencies in a local community to the state and national outcome averages.[36]

The OASIS dataset has undergone three major revisions. It is currently known as OASIS-C1/ICD-10.[35] Each major revision has involved modifications to the data collected, including exclusions, modifications, and additions. The latest iteration of the expanded dataset included reporting on key process measures and the transition from the use of ICD CM 9 to ICD CM 10 for diagnosis coding. These process measures will continue to evolve in support of the efforts to harmonize quality measures across care settings to improve data collection and analysis.

In 2014, the U.S. Congress passed the Improving Medicare Post-Acute Care Transitions Act (IMPACT). The new law requires that long-term care, skilled nursing, home health, and inpatient rehabilitation providers begin submitting standardized and interoperable data in 2019. The data collected will be used to evaluate and change payment methodologies between and among care settings to increase alignment with value-based purchasing initiatives.[37]

Hospice Item Set

The Affordable Care Act of 2010 required that the Secretary of Health and Human Services publish selected quality measures that must be reported by hospice programs. Those measures are referred to as the Hospice Item Set (HIS). The approach to develop a standardized dataset for hospice agencies has been industry driven rather than mandated by the CMS (Centers for Medicare & Medicaid Services). The Conditions of Participation for Hospice, effective in 2008, describe the expectation that the hospice industry determine the appropriate measures to collect and report nationally.[38] This approach reflects the fact that hospices had been collecting and reporting key quality measures through their associations and other data analysis partners for almost 20 years.[13,14,24] The CMS mandated that hospices begin their reporting processes with two measures: one that is patient related and one that is structural. It is expected that the number of measures will increase as the industry continues to identify, propose, and refine a dataset.[13,14,24]

Patient-Experience Surveys

Home health agencies, hospices, skilled nursing facilities, and dialysis centers are required to submit patient-experience surveys. These surveys, referred to as Consumer Assessment of Healthcare Providers and Systems (CAHPS), are designed to measure the interpersonal value of healthcare experienced by patients and contribute to their ability to make informed decisions about health plans and care providers.[39] Surveys provide an additional source of standardized data for aggregation and offer visibility and transparency about the care provided. It is expected that they will become increasingly important in the future because patient experience represents one of the key tenets of the Triple Aim for healthcare (see Box 9.1).

SUPPORTING HOME HEALTH WITH ELECTRONIC HEALTH RECORDS AND HEALTH INFORMATION TECHNOLOGY

Challenges related to distance, communication, productivity, and interprofessional practice are inherent in home health and related community-based services. Because of these challenges, agency providers are embracing national and global trends. Many trends focus on technology that facilitates communication and collaboration, such as cellular telephones, telehealth, remote patient monitoring, fall-detection device technology, sophisticated information systems, and point-of-care devices. The point-of-care devices are designed to make patient records available in the home when care is being provided and capture clinicians' documentation in real time, thereby supporting that care.[27,29,34,40–42]

The core values and practice models of community-based services have direct implications for technology and information systems. Systems must be designed to support the data, information, knowledge, and wisdom continuum as described in Chapter 2, and have interprofessional practice with the patient, family, and community as the central focus.[43–46]

Information systems used in community practice settings are evolving into next-generation systems. Software vendors are exploring the relationship of the design and function of their systems to improve their capabilities to support interprofessional practice, communication and collaboration, clinical decision support (CDS), and the ability to share information across care settings. Vendors and their healthcare provider customers are not only starting to share information with other providers but also encouraging patients to use personal health records to store their data in a longitudinal care record and plan.[42,45,47–49] In addition, information systems are viewed as a critical factor to achieving the Triple Aim for healthcare. Next-generation systems are expected to support the simplicity and connectivity that are essential to connecting caregivers across diverse locations and care settings. Interoperability and data exchange are required if all members of the healthcare team engage in a ubiquitous approach to care planning, collaboration, transparency, and efficiency in healthcare. Such developments are necessary for home health and community-based providers to have sharable and comparable data and participate in big data initiatives.[33,50–52]

Information systems were first adopted by home health agencies in the early 1980s. The development and use of these systems in home health, hospice, and other community-based settings have generally evolved in the following historical sequence to (1) support billing, (2) collect data at the point of patient care to support the financial needs of the business, (3) manage and support collection of standard clinical datasets, and (4) provide CDS. This evolution is analogous to the progression described in the data, information, knowledge, and wisdom continuum.

Billing Solutions

Initially, data within systems moved in one direction from the home health, hospice, or community-based agency to the third-party payer as an electronic claim. The payer, upon receiving the claim, reviewed and paid the claim. As financial systems and electronic capabilities advanced, bidirectional exchange of claims information management became commonplace. This allowed the payer to receive the electronic claim and return an acknowledgment of payment to the healthcare provider electronically.

Point-of-Care Solutions

The next milestone for information systems used by home health agencies and, to a lesser degree, by hospice services occurred as agencies recognized the value of capturing the clinicians' documentation that supported the interaction with the patient at the point of care. The principal value of these systems was to enable electronic capture of the service date and time for billing and payroll purposes.

In 1998, the value of point-of-care systems changed for home health agencies because of Medicare's transition from a cost-based reimbursement system to a prospective payment system. The prospective payment system was predicated on the use of a standardized assessment dataset designed to predict the patient's resource needs; the results of the dataset were associated with a payment rate. The standardized dataset OASIS was discussed earlier in this chapter.

Agencies that were computerized expected their software vendors to incorporate the OASIS dataset into their point-of-care systems to enable their clinicians to capture the information once, prepare, and then submit to their respective states for aggregation by the CMS. Home health agencies that had not adopted point-of-care solutions experienced a significant data-entry burden to remain in compliance with regulations. As a result, agencies accelerated their adoption of point-of-care information systems and EHRs as a strategy to reduce the regulatory burden and streamline their operations.

In addition to supporting the change in payment methodology, the collection of the OASIS dataset created an opportunity to introduce an **outcomes-based quality-improvement (OBQI)** process to home health. OBQI is a risk-adjusted and outcome-reporting tool used across time and viewed as a means to further move the risk from the payer to the healthcare provider by assigning a value-based purchasing facet to the model. OBQI represents the next step in evolving the payment system from fee for service to capitation or payment for care of a population. Fig. 9.1 depicts a continuum that illustrates the onset of CMS reimbursement through the transition of payment risk from the payer to the healthcare provider.

As adoption of OBQI grew, provider agency managers and administrators recognized the value of mining OASIS data and converting it to information to support business and operational decision making in their organizations. The information was transformed into knowledge involving the care their staff delivered, potential opportunities for improvement, and marketing their successes.[43,44]

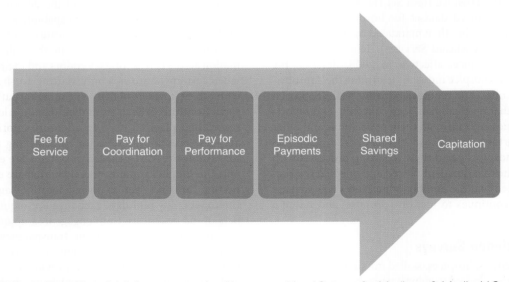

FIG 9.1 Transition of risk from payer to healthcare provider. (*Centers for Medicare & Medicaid Services [CMS]*. Oasis-C educational resources. CMS. http://www.cms.gov/Medicare/Quality-Initiatives-Patient-Assessment-Instruments/HomeHealthQualityInits/EducationalResources.html; 2010.)

An expected result of having information represented by OASIS and the HIS is the goal of understanding the following three questions:

- What is causing the outcomes?
- How can the outcomes be improved?
- How much improvement can realistically be expected?

Efforts to answer these questions have identified the need to know more about the processes being used to deliver care, specifically what care processes contributed to positive clinical outcomes. The knowledge of the outcomes has resulted in a need for increased predictability, visibility, and transparency in the use of best practices and evidence-based practice protocols.

In 2010, the OASIS dataset was revised to improve the quality of responses to outcome questions. Specifically, 16 process measures were added to the dataset. The data collected about these process measures are intended to clarify how best practices and evidence-based practice affect outcomes.[36,38,42,53] The CMS and other payers are using this knowledge to transition to payment methodologies that support value-based purchasing, bundled payments, and accountable care, each of which are contributing to the increasing need for payer and agency provider collaboration to ensure the best possible patient outcomes at the lowest possible costs.[34,53] This transition has already had an impact on practice and is predicted to have an even greater effect across the care continuum in the future.

Clinical Decision Support Systems

CDS systems are part of the next frontier for home health and other related community-based practice settings. Rouse described these systems as applications that analyze data and help healthcare providers make clinical decisions.[54] CDS systems generally use one of two approaches: (1) presenting best practices and evidence-based practice options to the clinician by finding and displaying what is known about the patient to a knowledge base using rule sets and an interface engine, or (2) using a process of machine learning that presents or displays best practices and evidence-based practice options to the clinician after analyzing the data entered and comparing them to similar patterns or scenarios that exist in the system. These systems have been challenging to implement because they are dependent on understanding the clinicians' workflow. Clinicians' workflow usually varies among patients and lacks structured clinical concepts, characteristics that are required to develop a knowledge base or machine learning.[54] In addition, standardized terminologies are required to develop effective CDS systems. The next goal for CDS systems is to achieve rapid learning systems that can support quick and widespread adoption of evidence-based practice. When these learning systems are used, the time needed to implement best practices and evidence-based practice will be significantly reduced. Reaching this goal will require health information networks that are capable of collecting and supporting analysis of large amounts of data in simple, clear terms and returning the findings to clinicians though CDS systems at the point of care.[33] See Chapter 10, for a more detailed discussion of CDS systems.

STANDARDIZED TERMINOLOGIES

The American Nurses Association (ANA) recognizes 12 reference and point-of-care or interface terminologies. These terminologies are described in detail in Chapter 22 and the references that accompany that chapter. Use of standardized terminologies is increasing in response to diverse factors. The national initiative to link reimbursement to value instead of volume serves as an important factor because providers will need quantitative data to confirm improved patient outcomes.[47,48,55–57] As noted by the Alliance for Nursing Informatics, the use of standardized nursing and other health terminologies:

> …is necessary and a prerequisite for decision support, discovery of disparities, outcomes reporting, improving performance, maintaining accurate lists of problems and medications, and the general use of and reuse of information needed for quality, safety, and efficiency.[55, p. 66]

It is critical that point-of-care terminologies are mapped to reference terminologies to the enable current and future interoperability and data sharing described in this chapter. The point-of-care terminologies recognized by the ANA have been or are being mapped.

Ideally, students are introduced to the 12 terminologies in their entry programs and clinical sites during their basic education, and they become somewhat familiar with them. In addition, students should understand the difference between reference terminologies, including Systematized Nomenclature of Medicine—Clinical Terms (SNOMED CT) and Logical Observation Identifier Names and Codes (LOINC), and point-of-care terminologies as discussed in Chapter 22.

Similarities and differences are evident when the terminologies are compared and contrasted.[56,58–60] Those that are especially pertinent to this chapter are summarized. Many authors note that whereas point-of-care terminologies were initially intended for use in specific settings (i.e., community, acute, or long-term care), healthcare delivery has changed dramatically, and boundaries have blurred. It is possible to implement most of the terminologies across the continuum of care. Developing a structure that is computer compatible was not the initial goal in the development of point-of-care terminologies. With the IT explosion and proliferation of software vendors, relationships are evolving between the terminologies and software developers of clinical information systems. When discussing point-of-care terminologies, it is important to remember the distinction between the terminologies and the individual software applications that may incorporate a terminology. Any one terminology can be used in the development of systems by multiple developers and vendors.

OMAHA SYSTEM

The Omaha System is an example of a point-of-care terminology recognized by the ANA that is mapped to SNOMED CT and LOINC, two of the reference terminologies. The Omaha System was initially developed (1) for home health and community-based use, (2) to operationalize the problem-solving process, (3) to provide a practical, easily understood, computer-compatible guide for daily use in community settings by interprofessional clinicians, and (4) to provide a tool to quantify, analyze, and use to improve the quality of care. From the early home health, hospice, public health, and school health focus, adoption began to expand in the 1990s, with both automated applications and paper-and-pen forms. Current use represents the continuum of care; it has extended far beyond the early community-based settings. More than 22,000 interprofessional clinicians, educators, and researchers use the Omaha System in the United States and a number of other countries with various types of software based on the Omaha System. Details about the application, users, clinical examples (case studies), inclusion in reference terminologies, research, best practices and evidence-based practice, and listserv are described in publications and on the website (www.omahasystem.org)[29,61,62]

Description

The Omaha System consists of the Problem Classification Scheme, the Intervention Scheme, and the Problem Rating Scale for Outcomes. Reliability, validity, and usability were established when the fourth federally funded research project was completed in 1993 (Box 9.2). The three components, designed to be used together, are comprehensive, relatively simple, hierarchical, multidimensional, and computer compatible. Since the first developmental research project in 1975, the Omaha System has existed in the public domain; thus the terms, definitions, and codes are not held under copyright. They are available for use without permission from the publisher or developers and without a licensing fee. However, the terms and structure must be used as published.[29,61]

The conceptual model is based on the dynamic, interactive nature of the problem-solving process, the clinician-client relationship, and concepts of diagnostic reasoning, clinical judgment, and quality improvement (Fig. 9.2). The patient as an individual, a family, or a community appears at the center of the model, reflecting a patient-centered approach. The central location suggests the many ways in which the system can be used, the importance of the patient, and the essential partnership between patients and clinicians.

The system was intended for use by nurses and all members of healthcare delivery teams. The goals of the research were to (1) develop a structured and comprehensive system that could be both understood and used by members of various disciplines, (2) foster collaborative practice, and (3) generate accurate and consistent aggregate data. Therefore the system was designed to guide practice decisions, sort and document pertinent patient data uniformly, and provide a framework for an agency-wide, interprofessional clinical information management system capable of meeting the daily needs of clinicians, managers, and administrators.[29,46,61–63]

Problem Classification Scheme

The **Problem Classification Scheme** is a comprehensive, orderly, nonexhaustive, mutually exclusive taxonomy designed to identify diverse patients' health-related concerns. Its simple and concrete terms are used to organize a comprehensive assessment, an important standard of interprofessional practice. The Problem Classification Scheme consists of four levels. Four domains appear at the first level and

---

BOX 9.2   Development of the Omaha System

As early as 1970, the clinicians and administrators of the Visiting Nurse Association (VNA) of Omaha, Nebraska, began addressing practice, documentation, and information-management concerns. Their goal was to identify a strategy that would translate theory into practice and share pertinent qualitative and quantitative data with healthcare professionals and the public. At that time, clinicians were not using computers, and there was no systematic nomenclature or classification of patient problems and concerns, interventions, or patient outcomes to quantify clinical data and integrate with a problem-oriented record system. These realities provided the incentive for initiating research and involving community test sites throughout the country. Between 1975 and 1993, the staff of VNA of Omaha conducted four extensive, federally funded development and refinement research studies that established reliability, validity, and usability. The work of Larry Weed was recognized. Avedis Donabedian, who developed the structure, process, and outcome approach to evaluation, was a valuable consultant.

Data from Donabedian A. Evaluating the quality of medical care. *Milbank Q.* 1966;44(2):166-206; Martin KS. *The Omaha System: A Key to Practice, Documentation, and Information Management.* Reprinted 2nd ed. Omaha, NE: Health Connections Press; 2005.

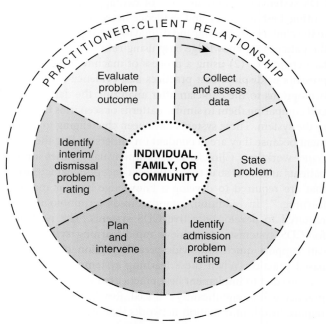

FIG 9.2 Omaha System model of the problem-solving process. (From Martin KS. *The Omaha System: A key to practice, documentation, and information management.* Reprinted 2nd ed. Omaha, NE: Health Connections Press; 2005.)

represent priority areas. Forty-two terms, referred to as client problems or areas of patient needs and strengths, appear at the second level. The third level consists of two sets of problem modifiers: health promotion, potential and actual, as well as individual, family, and community. Clusters of signs and symptoms describe actual problems at the fourth level. The content and relationship of the domain and problem levels are outlined in Box 9.3 and are further illustrated by the clinical example in Box 9.4. Understanding the meaning of and relationships among the terms is a prerequisite to using the scheme accurately and consistently to collect, sort, document, analyze, quantify, and communicate patient needs and strengths.

Intervention Scheme

The Intervention Scheme is a comprehensive, orderly, non-exhaustive, mutually exclusive taxonomy designed for use with specific problems. It consists of three levels of actions or activities that are the basis for care planning and services, providing the structure and terms to organize care plans and actual care. An important standard of interprofessional practice is providing interventions and leaving a data trail about the care that was provided. Four broad categories of interventions appear at the first level of the Intervention Scheme. An alphabetical list of 75 targets or objects of action and 1 "other" appear at the second level. Client-specific information generated by clinicians is at the third level. The contents of the category and target levels are outlined in Boxes 9.5 and 9.6, respectively, and are further illustrated by the clinical example in Box 9.4. The Intervention Scheme enables clinicians to describe, quantify, and communicate their practice, including improving or restoring health, describing deterioration, or preventing illness.

Problem Rating Scale for Outcomes

The Problem Rating Scale for Outcomes consists of three five-point, Likert-type scales used to measure the entire range of severity for the concepts of Knowledge, Behavior, and Status. Each of the subscales is a continuum that provides a framework for measuring and comparing problem-specific patient outcomes at regular or predictable times. Evaluation is an important interprofessional standard of practice. Suggested times include admission, specific interim points, and discharge. The ratings are a guide for the clinician as patient care is planned and provided. The ratings offer a method to monitor and quantify patient progress throughout the period of service. The content and relationships of the scale are outlined in Table 9.1 and are further illustrated by the clinical example in Box 9.4. Using the Problem Rating Scale for Outcomes with the other two schemes creates a comprehensive problem-solving model for practice, education, and research.

BOX 9.3 Domains and Problems of the Omaha System Problem Classification Scheme

Environmental Domain
Material resources and physical surroundings both inside and outside the living area, neighborhood, and broader community:
- Income
- Sanitation
- Residence
- Neighborhood/workplace safety

Psychosocial Domain
Patterns of behavior, emotion, communication, relationships, and development:
- Communication with community resources
- Social contact
- Role change
- Interpersonal relationship
- Spirituality
- Grief
- Mental health
- Sexuality
- Caretaking/parenting
- Neglect
- Abuse
- Growth and development

Physiological Domain
Functions and processes that maintain life:
- Hearing
- Vision
- Speech and language
- Oral health
- Cognition
- Pain
- Consciousness
- Skin
- Neuro-musculo-skeletal function
- Respiration
- Circulation
- Digestion-hydration
- Bowel function
- Urinary function
- Reproductive function
- Pregnancy
- Postpartum
- Communicable/infectious condition

Health-Related Behaviors Domain
Patterns of activity that maintain or promote wellness, promote recovery, and decrease the risk of disease:
- Nutrition
- Sleep and rest patterns
- Physical activity
- Personal care
- Substance use
- Family planning
- Health care supervision
- Medication regimen

From Martin KS. *The Omaha System: A Key to Practice, Documentation, and Information Management.* Reprinted 2nd ed. Omaha, NE: Health Connections Press; 2005.

BOX 9.4   John T. Little: A Man Who Received Home Health Services

Kelly S. Nelson, PT, DPT, PCS, CWS
*Assistant Professor, Department of Physical Therapy,
School of Pharmacy and Health Professions, Creighton University
Omaha, Nebraska*

Information Obtained during the First Visit/Encounter

John T. Little, age 79 years, had a fracture of his left femur that was surgically repaired with a pin 2 weeks ago. John spent 5 days in the acute care hospital followed by 9 days at the subacute rehabilitation facility. He was discharged to his home yesterday.

During the home health nurse's first visit, John's wife seemed relatively well informed. In John's presence she stated, "I am going to need help caring for him. It's a difficult time for us." The nurse summarized the agency's services including interprofessional providers, and the goals of care for both Mr. and Mrs. Little. The couple agreed when the nurse suggested that a home health aide visit to provide personal care.

John was resting in a hospital bed with an overhead trapeze and removable side rails. The equipment was set up before he came home. He moved in the bed with difficulty and needed assistance to roll or sit up. Mrs. Little could not find the mobility technique instructions that they were given yesterday. John, his wife, and the nurse discussed plans and goals for the physical therapist's visit later today and the occupational therapist's visit tomorrow.

The nurse indicated that the surgical site and John's skin were in excellent condition and offered evidence-based suggestions about bed mobility and prevention of skin shearing and breakdown. Mrs. Little reported that she could manage John's diet, fluid intake, and elimination. She said she would appreciate the use of a raised toilet seat and a shower chair.

Although John was reluctant to admit that he had pain, he rated it as a 4 on a 0-to-10 pain scale. Mrs. Little administered pain medication at least three times a day and as needed, indicating that she "would not wait for John to look miserable." She described how she evaluated John's pain and would use the pain scale as the nurse instructed. The nurse showed Mrs. Little a web site describing evidence-based pain management and gave her some printed instructional materials. Mrs. Little agreed to keep the nurse informed as John's need for pain medications changed and if other symptoms such as constipation occurred. The nurse mentioned several methods for achieving nonpharmacological pain relief and asked the couple to discuss their preferences before the nurse's next visit. They said they would do so.

Application of the Omaha System:
Domain: Physiological
Problem: Pain (High Priority Problem)
Problem Classification Scheme
Modifiers: Individual and Actual
- Signs/Symptoms of Actual: expresses discomfort/pain
- compensated movement/guarding

Intervention Scheme
Category: Teaching, Guidance, and Counseling
Targets and client-specific information:
- anatomy/physiology (diagnosis and surgery in relation to pain, joint, and pain management)
- relaxation/breathing techniques (consider options and decide)
Category: Surveillance

Targets and client-specific information:
- signs/symptoms—mental/emotional (attitude, emotions)
- signs/symptoms—physical (ability/willingness to move)

Problem Rating Scale for Outcomes
Knowledge: 3—basic knowledge (knows pain causes, need for medication, but not other options)
Behavior: 3—inconsistent knowledge (not tried additional options for pain relief, but willing)
Status: 3—moderate signs/symptoms (caused by injury and surgery)

Problem: Neuro-Musculo-Skeletal Function (High Priority Problem)
Problem Classification Scheme
Modifiers: Individual and Actual
Signs/Symptoms of Actual:
- limited range of motion
- gait/ambulation disturbance
- difficulty transferring
- fractures

Intervention Scheme
Category: Teaching, Guidance, and Counseling
Targets and client-specific information:
- occupational therapy care (plan of care)
- physical therapy care (plan of care)
Category: Surveillance
- durable medical equipment (bed set-up adequate, needs raised toilet seat and shower chair)
- mobility/transfers (bed mobility)
- signs/symptoms—physical (surgical site, skin condition)

Problem Rating Scale for Outcomes
Knowledge: 3—basic knowledge (recalls some instructions, can't find handout)
Behavior: 2—rarely appropriate behavior (limited mobility/activity)
Status: 2—severe signs/symptoms (minimal activity)

Domain: Health-Related Behaviors
Problem: Personal care (High Priority Problem)
Problem Classification Scheme
Modifiers: Individual and Actual
Signs/Symptoms of Actual:
- difficulty with bathing
- difficulty with toileting activities
- difficulty dressing lower body
- difficulty dressing upper body
- difficulty shampooing/combing hair

Intervention Scheme
Category: Case Management
Targets and client-specific information:
- paraprofessional/aide care (schedule 3 times/week)

Problem Rating Scale for Outcomes
Knowledge: 4—adequate knowledge (knows help needed)
Behavior: 4—usually appropriate behavior (requested assistance)
Status: 2—severe signs/symptoms (care is difficult because of John's physical condition)

BOX 9.4 John T. Little: A Man Who Received Home Health Services—cont'd

Problem: Medication Regimen
Problem Classification Scheme
Modifiers: Individual and Actual
Signs/Symptoms of Actual:
- unable to take medications without help

Intervention Scheme
Category: Teaching, Guidance, and Counseling
Targets and client-specific information:
- medication action/side effects (reports of pain, movement, non-verbal cues)
- medication administration (scheduling doses appropriately)

Category: Surveillance
Targets and client-specific information:
- signs/symptoms—physical (discussed effectiveness, constipation, other symptoms; will use pain scale)

Problem Rating Scale for Outcomes
Knowledge: 4—adequate knowledge (informed about pain medication, watch for changing needs)
Behavior: 4—usually appropriate behavior (good administration schedule)
Status: 3—moderate signs/symptoms (pain scale=4)

BOX 9.5 Categories of the Omaha System Intervention Scheme

Teaching, Guidance, and Counseling
Activities designed to provide information and materials, encourage action and responsibility for self-care and coping, and assist the individual, family, or community to make decisions and solve problems.

Treatments and Procedures
Technical activities such as wound care, specimen collection, resistive exercises, and medication prescriptions that are designed to prevent, decrease, or alleviate signs and symptoms for the individual, family, or community.

Case Management
Activities such as coordination, advocacy, and referral that facilitate service delivery; promote assertiveness; guide the individual, family, or community toward use of appropriate community resources; and improve communication among health and human service providers.

Surveillance
Activities such as detection, measurement, critical analysis, and monitoring intended to identify the individual, family, or community's status in relation to a given condition or phenomenon.

From Martin KS. *The Omaha System: A Key to Practice, Documentation, and Information Management.* Reprinted 2nd ed. Omaha, NE: Health Connections Press; 2005.

Clinical Example from Practice

The John T. Little clinical example (see Box 9.4) depicts the use of the Omaha System with a patient and his home health nurse. It describes evidence-based and community-based practice, introduces the system as a standardized terminology, summarizes interprofessional practice, and offers details about EHRs, standards, and other concepts. Many additional references describe the application and value of using point-of-care documentation.[29,46,61–63]

Interpretation of the Clinical Example

The clinical example illustrates the following:
1. *Patient-centered care and the power of the patient and the family:* These are core values of home health and other community-based services. The nurse asks for John and Mrs. Little to provide information about his status and asks them to share their preferences about pain relief during the next visit.
2. *Evidence-based practice:* The nurse follows the agency's evidence-based standards of practice in relation to skin care and medication management.
3. *Interprofessional practice:* The nurse, John, and Mrs. Little discuss plans for the home health aide, physical therapist, and occupational therapist.
4. *Practice and documentation using a standardized terminology:* The nurse uses the Omaha System to guide the assessment (Problem Classification Scheme), care plan (Intervention Scheme), and care delivery (Intervention Scheme). In addition, the nurse selects the baseline Knowledge, Behavior, and Status ratings (Problem Rating Scale for Outcomes) that will guide evaluation during future visits. Other members of the care team will also use the Omaha System. Although not described in the clinical example, the nurse would have completed the OASIS dataset and entered billing, supplies, and other data.
5. *Practice, documentation, and information management linkages:*
   a. All members of the care team use one integrated EHR for documentation and can follow the data trail about John's progress. They can revise the care plan and interventions as needed to improve the quality of care they provide.
   b. John's data will be analyzed and added to aggregate data. Outcome reports will be available to members of the care team, as well as to agency managers and administrators. As data are transformed to information and knowledge, quality of care can be monitored and improved as part of the agency's quality-improvement program.
   c. Requests for orders and regular reports will be sent to John's referring medical staff, who are external members of the care team.

BOX 9.6 Targets of the Omaha System Intervention Scheme

- anatomy/physiology
- anger management
- behavior modification
- bladder care
- bonding/attachment
- bowel care
- cardiac care
- caretaking/parenting skills
- cast care
- communication
- community outreach worker services
- continuity of care
- coping skills
- day care/respite
- dietary management
- discipline
- dressing change/wound care
- durable medical equipment
- education
- employment
- end-of-life care
- environment
- exercises
- family planning care
- feeding procedures
- finances
- gait training
- genetics
- growth/development care
- home
- homemaking/housekeeping
- infection precautions
- interaction
- interpreter/translator services
- laboratory findings
- legal system
- medical/dental care
- medication action/side effects

- medication administration
- medication coordination/ordering
- medication prescription
- medication set-up
- mobility/transfers
- nursing care
- nutritionist care
- occupational therapy care
- ostomy care
- other community resources
- paraprofessional/aide care
- personal hygiene
- physical therapy care
- positioning
- recreational therapy care
- relaxation/breathing techniques
- respiratory care
- respiratory therapy care
- rest/sleep
- safety
- screening procedures
- sickness/injury care
- signs/symptoms—mental/emotional
- signs/symptoms—physical
- skin care
- social work/counseling care
- specimen collection
- speech and language pathology care
- spiritual care
- stimulation/nurturance
- stress management
- substance use cessation
- supplies
- support group
- support system
- transportation
- wellness
- other

From Martin KS. *The Omaha System: A Key to Practice, Documentation, and Information Management.* Reprinted 2nd ed. Omaha, NE: Health Connections Press; 2005.

TABLE 9.1 Omaha System Problem Rating Scale for Outcomes

Concept	1	2	3	4	5
Knowledge: ability of client to remember and interpret information	No knowledge	Minimal knowledge	Basic knowledge	Adequate knowledge	Superior knowledge
Behavior: observable responses, actions, or activities of client fitting occasion or purpose	Not appropriate behavior	Rarely appropriate behavior	Inconsistently appropriate behavior	Usually appropriate behavior	Consistently appropriate behavior
Status: condition of client in relation to objective and subjective defining characteristics	Extreme signs/ symptoms	Severe signs/ symptoms	Moderate signs/ symptoms	Minimal signs/ symptoms	No signs/ symptoms

From Martin KS. *The Omaha System: A Key to Practice, Documentation, and Information Management.* Reprinted 2nd ed. Omaha, NE: Health Connections Press; 2005.

6. *External monitoring and quality control:*

a. Aggregate data about John and the home health agency's other patients will be submitted to CMS and other external third-party payers for reimbursement. In turn, they may select John's EHR for review, and a site visitor may accompany a team member on a home visit to observe John's care.

b. John's EHR may be selected for review by accreditation site visitors. They may also make a home visit to observe care. Many home health agencies are accredited by the Joint Commission, Community Health Accreditation Program (CHAP), or the Accreditation Commission for Health Care. The number of health departments that are accredited is increasing rapidly.

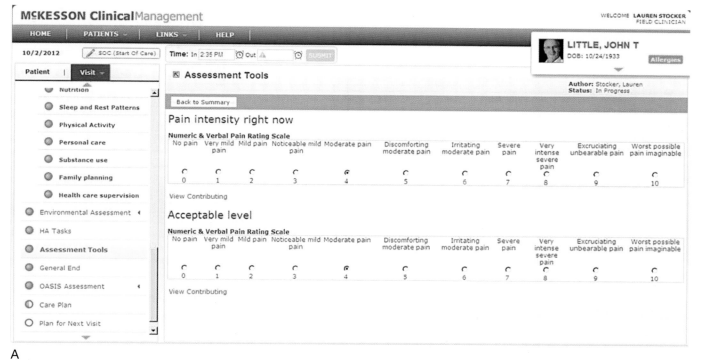

A

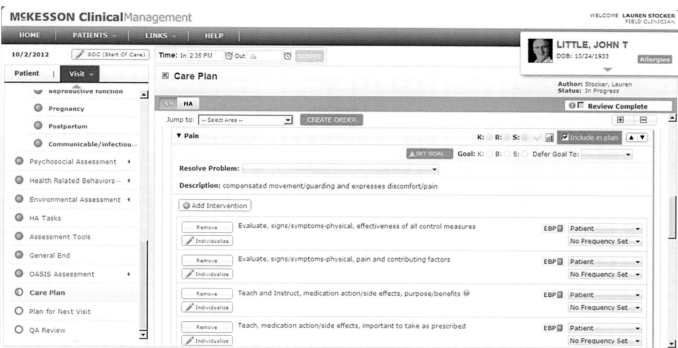

B

FIG 9.3 A, Pain assessment. B, Problem identification.

(Continued)

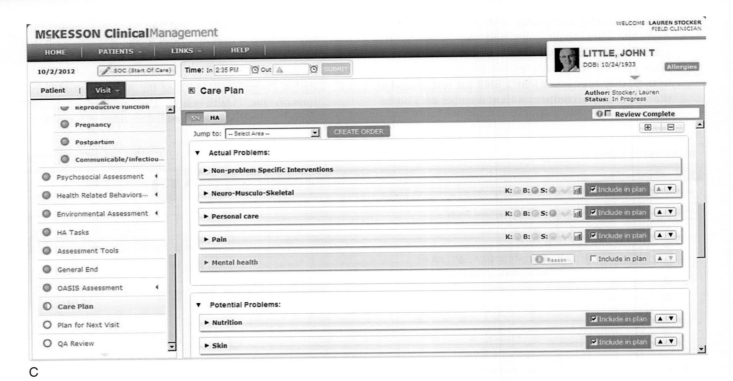

FIG 9.3, CONT'D C, Care planning. (Copyright McKesson Corporation.)

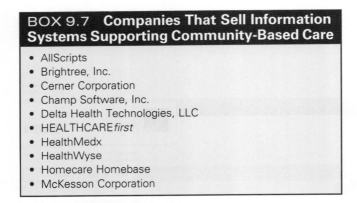

Examples of Electronic Health Record Screen Images

Three screen images are presented in Fig. 9.3 to illustrate a limited portion of John T. Little's EHR. Specifically, they depict pain assessment, problem identification, and care planning. The images are examples that enable the reader to visualize the application of concepts presented in this chapter. Note that the focus of the images varies but does not depict John's entire clinical record or other software modules that the home health agency would use. The images are part of McKesson Corporation's information system. McKesson Corporation and nine additional vendors are listed in Box 9.7 as examples of companies that sell information system solutions to diverse home health, hospice, and other community-based organizations in the United States. Note that these 10 companies are examples only; many additional companies sell information systems and niche software to similar organizations.

CONCLUSION AND FUTURE DIRECTIONS

The healthcare delivery system in the United States is under enormous pressure to change and create a more transparent, collaborative, efficient, and patient-centered system.[57] Adoption of EHRs and enabling the exchange of clinical information between members of the care team and across disparate systems are critical to achieving the goals of the U.S. Department of Health & Human Services, the Office of the National Coordinator for Health Information Technology, and the Triple Aim for healthcare.[33]

Home health, hospice, and other community-based care providers are actively engaged in envisioning and testing models of care. The evolving communication and collaboration models are designed to support safe transitions between care settings, effectively manage patient populations, and participate in accountable care organizations to achieve better clinical outcomes, better patient experiences, and lower costs. Accurate and consistent data generated by information system solutions and capable of being transformed into information, knowledge, and wisdom are key to each of these initiatives. The information system solutions should support patients across the care continuum and into their homes to ultimately enable them to successfully self-manage their care needs. It is critical to seamlessly share and update a common plan of care, including medications, allergies, problems, planned interventions, and goals and results.[29,33,47,48,61]

When considering the longer term, there is an opportunity to quantify and aggregate information about common patient populations, create knowledge of effective care teams and treatment approaches, and share the knowledge in real time or near real time with the care team. Rapid learning systems and delivering wisdom to the healthcare community represent the opportunity ahead.

REFERENCES

1. Buhler-Wilkerson K. Care of the chronically ill at home: an unresolved dilemma in health policy for the United States. *Milbank Q.* 2007;85(4):611–639.
2. Naylor MD, Van Cleave J. The transitional care model for older adults. In: Meleis AI, ed. *Transitions Theory: Middle Range and Situational Specific Theories in Research and Practice.* New York, NY: Springer; 2010:459–464.
3. Humphrey CJ, Utterback KB. The role of evidence-based clinical practice in emerging home care models. *Caring.* 2012;31 (10):26–30.
4. American Nurses Association (ANA). *Home Health Nursing: Scope and Standards of Practice*; 2nd ed. Silver Spring, MD: Nursebooks.org; 2014.
5. Avalere and the Alliance for Home Health Quality and Innovation. *Home Health Chartbook*; 2015. http://ahhqi.org/images/uploads/AHHQI_2015_Chartbook_FINAL_October.pdf.
6. Perry KM, Parente CA. Integrating palliative care into home care practice; In: Harris MD, ed. *Handbook of Home Health Care Administration.* 6th ed. Sudbury, MA: Jones and Bartlett; 2017:767–782.
7. Buhler-Wilkerson K. No place like home: a history of nursing and home care in the U.S. *Home Healthc Nurse.* 2002;20 (10):641–647.
8. Donahue MP. *Nursing: The Finest Art.* 3rd ed. St. Louis: Elsevier; 2011.
9. Dieckmann JL. Home health care: a historical perspective and overview; In: Harris MD, ed. *Handbook of Home Health Care Administration.* 6th ed. Sudbury, MA: Jones and Bartlett; 2017:9–25.
10. Stanhope M, Lancaster J. *Public Health Nursing: Population-Centered Health Care in the Community*; 9th ed. St. Louis, MO: Elsevier; 2016.
11. Centers for Medicare & Medicaid Services. *Home health conditions of participation.* Electronic Code of Federal Regulations; 2015. http://www.ecfr.gov/cgi-bin/text-idx?tpl=/ecfrbrowse/Title42/42cfr484_main_02.tpl.
12. Zerwekh JV, Warner KD. Clients receiving home health and hospice care; In: Allender JA, Rector C, Warner KD, eds. *Community and Public Health Nursing.* 8th ed. Philadelphia, PA: Wolters Kluwer; 2014:1041–1061.
13. National Hospice and Palliative Care Organization. *NHPCO's Facts and Figures: Hospice Care in America, 2014 edition.* Alexandria, VA: NHPCO; 2015. http://www.nhpco.org/sites/default/files/public/Statistics_Research/2014_Facts_Figures.pdf.
14. National Hospice Palliative Care Organization (NHPCO). *History of Hospice Care.* NHPCO; 2015. http://www.nhpco.org/history-hospice-care.
15. Donabedian A. Evaluating the quality of medical care; *Milbank Q.* 1966;44(2):166–206.
16. Weed L. Special article: medical records that guide and teach; *New Engl J Med.* 1968;278(12):593–600. 652–657.
17. Tinetti ME. Performance-oriented assessment of mobility problems in elderly patients; *J Am Geriatr Soc.* 1986;34(2):119–126.
18. Duncan PW. Functional reach: a new clinical measure of balance; *J Gerontol.* 1990;45(6):M192–M197.
19. National Association for Home Care & Hospice (NAHC). *Basic Statistics About Home care.* Washington, DC: NAHC; 2010. http://nahc.org/assets/1/7/10hc_stats.pdf 2015.
20. US Department of Health and Human Services Centers for Disease Control and Prevention. *Long-Term Care Services in the United States: 2013 Overview*; 2015. http://www.cdc.gov/nchs/data/nsltcp/long_term_care_services_2013.pdf.
21. California HealthCare Foundation. *U.S. Health Care Spending: Who Pays? 1960-2013*; 2015. http://www.chcf.org/publications/2015/11/data-viz.hcc-national.
22. Centers for Medicare & Medicaid Services (CMS). *National Health Expenditures 2014-2024 Forecast Summary.* CMS; 2015. http://www.cms.gov/Research-Statistics-Data-and-Systems/Statistics-Trends-and-Reports/NationalHealthExpendData/Downloads/proj2014.pdf.
23. Zerwekh JV. *Nursing Care at the End of Life: Palliative Care for Patients and Families*; Philadelphia, PA: F.A. Davis; 2006.
24. American Nurses Association (ANA) and Hospice and Palliative Nurses Association (HPNA). *Palliative Nursing—An Essential Resource for Hospice and Palliative Nurses: Scope and Standards of Practice*; Silver Spring, MD: Nursebooks.org; 2014.
25. Hurzeler RJ, Knight R, Hwu W-J, et al. Hospice care: pioneering the ultimate love connection about living, not dying; In: Harris MD, ed. *Handbook of Home Health Care Administration.* 6th ed. Sudbury, MA: Jones and Bartlett; 2017:783–798.
26. National Association of County & City Health Officials (NACCHO). *The Changing Public Health Landscape: Findings from the 2015 Forces of Change Survey.* NACCHO; 2015. http://nacchoprofilestudy.org/wp-content/uploads/2015/04/2015-Forces-of-Change-Slidedoc-Final.pdf.
27. Foldy S, Grannis S, Ross D, Smith T. A ride in the time machine: Information management capabilities health departments will need; *Am J Public Health.* 2014;104(9):1592–1600.
28. National Nursing Centers Consortium (NNCC); 2015. http://www.nncc.us.
29. Martin KS. *The Omaha System: A Key to Practice, Documentation, and Information Management*; Reprinted, 2nd ed. Omaha, NE: Health Connections Press; 2005.
30. Milone-Nuzzo P, Hollars ME. Transitioning nurses to home care; In: Harris MD, ed. *Handbook of Home Health Care Administration.* 6th ed. Sudbury, MA: Jones and Bartlett; 2017:455–466.
31. Anderson R, Leonard MA, Mansell J, et al. Brief history of resident assessment instrument/minimum data set; *American Health Information Management Association, Long-Term Care Insights*; 2015. https://newsletters.ahima.org/newsletters/LTC_Insights/2010/Summer/transition.html#history.
32. Centers for Medicare & Medicaid Services (CMS). *MDS 3.0 RAI Manual* CMS; 2015. https://www.cms.gov/Medicare/Quality-Initiatives-Patient-Assessment-Instruments/NursinghomeQualityInits?MDS30RAIManual.html.
33. Office of the National Coordinator for Health Information Technology. *Federal Health IT Strategic Plan 2015–2020*; 2015. https://www.healthit.gov.
34. Remington L. Value-based care solutions across the continuum; *The Remington Report.* 2015;23(5):3.
35. CGS. *Outcome and Assessment Information Set (OASIS).* CGS; 2015. http://www.cgsmedicare.com/hhh/coverage/oasis.html.

36. Centers for Medicare & Medicaid Services (CMS). *Home Health Quality Initiative*. CMS; 2015. https://www.cms.gov/Medicare/Quality-Initiatives-Patient-Assessment-Instruments/HomeHealthQualityInits/index.html?redirect=/HomeHealthQualityInits/14_HHQIOASISUserManual.asp.

37. United States Congress Public Law 113-185. *Improving Medicare Post-Acute Care Transitions Act of 2014 (IMPACT)*; 2015. http://www.gpo/gov/fdsys/pkg/PLAW-113publ185/pdf/PLAW-113publ185.pdf.

38. Centers for Medicare & Medicaid Services (CMS). *Hospice Quality Reporting*. CMS; 2015. https://www.cms.gov/Medicare/Quality-Initiatives-Patient-Assessment-Instruments/Hospice-Quality-reporting.

39. Centers for Medicare & Medicaid Services (CMS). *Consumer Assessment of Healthcare Providers and Systems*. CMS; 2015. https://www.cms.gov/Research-Statistics-Data-and-Systems/Research/CAHPS/index.html?redirect=/CAHPS/.

40. American Academy of Nursing. Putting "health" in the electronic health record: a call for collective action; *Nurs Outlook*. 2015;63(5):614–616.

41. Fazzi Associates. *2013-2014 National State of the Home Care Industry Study for Home Health and Hospice*; 2015. http://www.fazzi.com/tl_files/documents/Fazzi%20State%20of%20the%20Industry%20Study%20%20Report.pdf.

42. Robert Wood Johnson Foundation. *Data for Health: Learning What Works*; Princeton, NJ: Robert Wood Johnson Foundation; 2015.

43. Graves JR, Corcoran S. The study of nursing informatics; *Image J Nurs Sch*. 1989;21(4):227–230.

44. Nelson R, Joos I. On language in nursing: from data to wisdom; *Pennsylvania League for Nursing Visions*. 1989;1(5):6.

45. Martin KS, Monsen KA, Bowles KH. The Omaha System and Meaningful Use: Applications for practice, education, and research; *Comput Inform Nurs*. 2011;29(1):52–58.

46. Monsen KA, Finn RS, Fleming TE, Garner EJ, LaValla AJ, Riemer JG. Rigor in electronic health record knowledge representation: lessons learned from SNOMED CT clinical content encoding exercise; *Inform Health Soc Care*. 2015;21:1–15.

47. Minnesota Department of Health. *Recommendations Regarding the Use of Standard Nursing Terminology in Minnesota*. 2014; 2015. http://health.state.mn.us/e-health/standards/nursingterminology082114.pdf.

48. American Nurses Association (ANA). Standardization and Interoperability of Health Information Technology: Supporting Nursing and the National Quality Strategy for Better Patient outcomes. *Nurs World*; 2014. http://nursingworld.org/MainMenuCategories/Policy-Advocacy/Positions-and-Resolutions/ANAPositionStatements/Position-Statements-Alphabetically/Standardization-and-Interoperability-of-Health-Info-Technology.html.

49. Samuels JG, McGrath RJ, Fetzer SJ, Mittal P, Bourgoine D. Using the electronic health record in nursing research: challenges and opportunities; *West J Nurs Res*. 2015;37(10):1284–1294.

50. Bowles KH, Potashnik S, Ratcliffe SJ, et al. Conducting research using the electronic health record across multi-hospital systems; *J Nurs Adm*. 2013;43(6):355–360.

51. Westra BL, Choromanski L. Amazing news for sharable/comparable nursing data to support big data science; *Comput Inform Nurs*. 2014;32(6):255–256.

52. Westra BL, Latimer GE, Matney SA, et al. A national action plan for sharable and comparable nursing data to support practice and translational research for transforming healthcare; *J Am Med Assoc*. 2015;22(3):600–607.

53. Centers for Medicare & Medicaid Services (CMS). *OASIS User Manuals*. CMS; 2015. https://www.cms.gov/Medicare/Quality-Initiatives-Patient-Assessment-Instruments/HomeHealthQualityInits/HHQIOASISUserManual.html.

54. Rouse M. *Clinical Decision Support—Definition*. SearchHealthIT; 2015. http://searchhealthit.techtarget.com/definition/clinical-decision-support-system-CDSS.

55. Sensmeier J. Clinical transformation: blending people, process, and technology; *Nurs Manag (IT Solutions)*. 2011;42(10):2–4.

56. American Nurses Association (ANA). ANA recognized terminologies that support nursing practice. *Nurs World*; 2012. http://www.nursingworld.org/MainMenuCategories/ThePracticeofProfessionalNursing/NursingStandards/Recognized-Nursing-Practice-Terminologies.pdf.

57. Federal Register. *Patient Protection and Affordability Care Act: HHS Notice of Benefit and Payment Parameters for 2016*; Document number 2015-03751; 2015. https://www.federalregister.gov/articles/2015/02/27/2015-03751/patient-protection-and-affordable-care-act-hhs-notice-of-benefit-and-payment-parameters-for-2016.

58. Lundberg CB, Brokel JM, Bulechek GM, et al. Selecting a standardized language to increase collaboration between research and practice. *Online J Nurs Inform*. 2008;12(2):1–18. http://ojni.org/12_2/lundberg.pdf.

59. American Nurses Association (ANA). Inclusion of recognized terminologies within EHRs and other health information technology solutions. *Nurs World*; 2015. http://nursingworld.org/MainMenuCategories/Policy-Advocacy/Positions-and-Resolutions/ANAPositionStatements/Position-Statements-Alphabetically/Inclusion-of-Recognized-Terminologies-within-EHRs.html/.

60. Sewell J, Thede LQ. *Informatics and Nursing: Opportunities and Challenges*; 4th ed. Philadelphia, PA: Wolters Kluwer, Lippincott Williams & Wilkins; 2013.

61. Omaha System; 2015. http://www.omahasystem.org.

62. Monsen KA, Schenk E, Schleyer R, Schiavenato M. Applicability of the Omaha System in acute care nursing for information interoperability in the era of accountable care; *Am J Manag Care*. 2015;3(3):53–61.

63. Pruinelli L, Fu H, Monsen KA, Westra BL. Comparison of consumer derived evidence with an Omaha System evidence-based practice guideline for community dwelling older adults; *Stud Health Technol Inform*. 2014;201:18–24.

DISCUSSION QUESTIONS

1. The focus of this chapter is home health and related community-based systems. What are your experiences with such settings? Do you expect to have more contact with them in the future?

2. Patient-centered care is an important theme in this chapter. Think about your experiences in practice settings. Describe whether you consider your experiences to be patient centered.

3. Describe your interest in and experience with standardized terminologies. List at least three positive and three negative experiences with standardized terminologies. What can be done to transform the negative experiences to positive ones?

4. Describe your interest in and experience with point-of-care documentation. List at least three positive and three negative experiences with point-of-care documentation. What can be done to transform the negative experiences to positive ones?

CASE STUDY

The ABC Home Health Agency is a nonprofit, Medicare-certified organization established in the mid-1950s in a small Midwestern city. It is accredited by the Accreditation Commission for Health Care, Inc. The agency offers a continuum of preventive and therapeutic services that have an individual, family, and community focus. Clinicians provide services to patients ranging in age from infants to elders. The agency employs supervisory, administrative, IT, and support staff, as well as 45 clinicians: 25 nurses, 10 home care aides, 5 homemakers, 3 physical therapists, 1 occupational therapist, and 1 social worker. Staff members are on call 24 hours a day. ABC Home Health Agency services include (1) skilled home health and hospice; (2) home care aide and homemaker; (3) private duty, including nursing, personal care, and respite care; (4) wellness, flu, and immunization clinics; (5) school health; (6) jail health; and (7) durable medical equipment. There are two hospitals with about 100 beds and 15 physicians within the service area. The Agency has a good working relationship with both hospitals and the physicians. Many patients followed by the Agency have been referred from these services. Last year the Agency provided 20,345 home visits.

The Agency has used an automated billing, statistical, and financial management information system for 15 years. Clinicians enter all patient data using an unstructured, narrative, automated software system. The previous director, who has just retired, did not believe that the cost was justified to implement an EHR capable of capturing discreet clinical data to support tracking patient-specific assessment information, identifying the specifics of care, and generating outcome measures. You have just been hired as the new director. The board of directors asks you to investigate purchasing an EHR and submit your recommendations to them.

Discussion Questions

1. Should you introduce the clinicians to standardized terminologies and involve them in discussions about EHRs before contacting potential software vendors? Or should you contact vendors, select the best software, and tell the clinicians what you selected?
2. What steps would you need to complete before reporting to the board of directors?
3. What strategies will likely increase your chances of success? What strategies will increase your chances of failure?

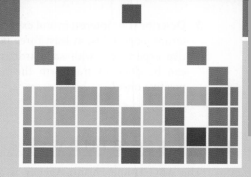

10

Clinical Decision Support Systems in Healthcare*

Kensaku Kawamoto and Guilherme Del Fiol

Since shortly after computers were first introduced into clinical settings in the 1960s and 1970s, clinical decision support (CDS) has been shown to be a powerful tool for positively affecting care delivery and patient outcomes.

OBJECTIVES

At the completion of this chapter, the reader will be prepared to:

1. Describe why clinical decision support is needed and its impact.
2. Explain the major types of clinical decision support.
3. Analyze best practices for clinical decision support.
4. Synthesize the current adoption status and the barriers to the wide adoption of clinical decision support.
5. Outline recent progress toward disseminating clinical decision support on a national level.

KEY TERMS

ABSTRACT ❖

Clinical decision support (CDS) is a key component of a variety of health information systems and a core component of electronic health record (EHR) systems. By providing the right information to the right person at the right time and at the right location, CDS systems can support effective clinical decision making and improve clinical care. CDS, encompassing various types of intervention modalities, has been shown to be effective for many decades. Important considerations in implementing CDS systems include the application of best practices and the incorporation of knowledge management capabilities. Despite its benefits, significant challenges limit the widespread adoption and impact of CDS. These challenges include a healthcare payment model that has traditionally rewarded volume over quality and the difficulty of scaling CDS capabilities across healthcare systems and their information systems. In recent years, several prominent efforts ensued to develop standards-based approaches to disseminating CDS on a national level. Moving forward, a need exists to capitalize on these ongoing initiatives to make advanced CDS available on a national scale.

*Acknowledgments: Kensaku Kawamoto (KK) has served as a consultant or paid speaker on CDS for the Office of the National Coordinator for Health IT, ARUP Laboratories, McKesson Health Solutions, ESAC, Inc., JBS International, Inc., Inflexxion, Inc., Intelligent Automation, Inc., Partners HealthCare, Hospital Sírio-Libanês, HL7 International, Massachusetts General Hospital, the RAND Corporation, and the Mayo Clinic. KK receives royalties for a Duke University-owned CDS technology for infectious disease management known as CustomID that he helped develop. KK was formerly a consultant for Religent, Inc. and a co-owner and consultant for Clinica Software, Inc., both of which provide commercial CDS services, including use of a CDS technology known as SEBASTIAN that KK developed. KK no longer has a financial relationship with either Religent or Clinica Software. Guillherme Del Fiol was supported by grant number K01HS018352 from the AHRQ. He has served as a paid speaker on CDS for HL7 International and Hospital Sírio-Libanês.

INTRODUCTION

Since the early days of health information technology (IT), the central goals of leveraging IT in medicine have been to help clinicians in their decision-making process to prevent errors, to maximize efficiency, to enable evidence-based care, and ultimately to improve health and healthcare. Over time, tools that support the clinical decision-making process have been generally designated as clinical decision support (CDS) systems.

According to the classic Institute of Medicine (IOM) report *To Err Is Human*, as many as 98,000 people die in hospitals in the United States every year due to preventable healthcare errors.[1] Many consider this a conservative number; more recent research has estimated that more than 400,000 people die prematurely every year due to preventable errors.[2] More than 15 years after the IOM report was issued, little has changed. *Consumer Reports*, addressing the same question, reported that "based on our review of the scant evidence, we believe that preventable medical harm still accounts for more than 100,000 deaths each year—a million lives over the past decade."[3, p. 2] Furthermore, a study by McGlynn et al. showed that, on average, patients in the United States receive only 54.9% of recommended medical care processes.[4] To a great extent, errors in healthcare are caused by process errors, information overload, and knowledge gaps.[1,5] Several factors further aggravate this problem, including rapidly evolving domain knowledge, an aging population having multiple comorbidities, and an increasingly complex healthcare delivery system. Ultimately this leads to a clinical information overload that significantly exceeds the human cognitive capacity.[6,7]

Many healthcare errors can be prevented, particularly through process improvement measures enabled by computerized information systems coupled with CDS tools. In fact, a large number of studies have shown that CDS tools help clinicians and patients adopt evidence-based care whenever applicable.[8] As a result, several relevant reports and regulations have called for the use of health IT to support healthcare decision making, such as the IOM's *Crossing the Quality Chasm*,[9] the National Quality Forum's (NQF's) *Driving Quality and Performance Measurement—A Foundation for Clinical Decision Support*,[10] the United States EHR Meaningful Use incentive program,[11] and the IOM's *The Future of Nursing: Leading Change, Advancing Health*.[12]

Definition of Clinical Decision Support

Multiple definitions of CDS have been proposed, but in general these definitions have evolved from a narrow scope, typically focused on alerts and reminders, to a broader scope that encompasses a much wider set of tools that provides patient-specific information to support clinical decision making. According to Osheroff, CDS comprises a variety of tools and interventions that "provide clinicians, staff, patients, or other individuals with knowledge and person-specific information, intelligently filtered or presented at appropriate times, to enhance health and health care."[13, p. 141] Similarly, the NQF defined CDS as "any tool or technique that enhances decision-making by clinicians, patients, or their surrogates in the delivery or management of health care."[10, p. 1] In light of these definitions, CDS can support several aspects of patient care decision making such as the following:

- Reminding about a specific care need (e.g., patient due for an immunization).
- Alerting about a specific care action that may impose risk to the patient (e.g., a drug interaction).
- Providing intelligent views of a patient's record that help cultivate a better understanding of the patient's status (e.g., intensive care reports, chronic disease management dashboards).
- Providing tools that assist in implementing and documenting decisions more efficiently and accurately

(e.g., documentation tools, order sets, medication reconciliation tools).
- Providing clinicians and patients with seamless access to patient-specific reference information available in online knowledge resources.
- Providing access to information about similar patients in the population along with their treatments and outcomes.
- Integrating information from nontraditional sources into the clinical workflow, such as patient self-reported outcomes, vital signs collected via wearable sensors, and patient dietary information, as well as relevant data about the patient's environment, such as air pollution and infectious disease rates.
- Applying advanced analytics to estimate risks for a specific individual, such as risk for hospital readmissions, risk for cardiovascular events, and risk for falls.

History

Since the early 1970s, when the first studies demonstrating the impact of CDS were published by groups at the Regenstrief Institute in Indiana and the Latter-Day Saints (LDS) Hospital in Salt Lake City, CDS has become one of the holy grails of health informatics. Although designed more than 3 to 4 decades ago, these examples of CDS are still relevant and some of them are still in use.

De Dombal Computer-Aided Diagnosis of Acute Abdominal Pain

According to a systematic review by Johnston et al.,[14] the first study to compare CDS with clinician performance was published in 1972 by de Dombal et al. on the diagnosis of acute abdominal pain.[15] The system comprised a Bayesian knowledge base and provided diagnostic probabilities as output.[16] An evaluation was conducted over an 11-month period at a general hospital in the United Kingdom, during which patient admissions due to acute abdominal pain were assessed independently by a physician and by the computer-aided diagnostic system.[15] The system's overall diagnostic accuracy was significantly higher than that of the most senior member of the clinical team (91.8% vs. 79.6%). The results of this seminal study demonstrated the strong potential of using computers to assist decision making for patient care.

Computer Reminders at Regenstrief Institute

One of the seminal randomized trials assessing the impact of a broad CDS intervention was published in 1976 by McDonald.[17] In this study, physicians at the Regenstrief Institute received patient-specific reminders about 390 patient management protocols on a myriad of clinical conditions. These reminders were automatically generated by the computer based on the patients' EHR and logic encoded in computable form. When a patient had a clinic visit, applicable reminders were printed and attached to the patient's chart. The study showed that physicians reacted to 51% of the events when exposed to reminders versus 21% when not exposed to reminders.

Clinical Decision Support Examples from the HELP System

A comprehensive set of CDS examples is provided by the HELP (Health Evaluation Through Logical Processing) System, a clinical information system developed in the late 1960s and used well into the 21st century at the LDS Hospital in Salt Lake City, Utah.[18] The HELP System includes a broad range of CDS tools that can be classified into the following four categories:

1. *Alerts* as a response to the presence of certain clinical data, such as life-threatening laboratory test results.
2. Tools that *critique* clinicians' decisions, such as the presence of drug interactions in medication orders.
3. Tools that provide on-demand diagnostic or therapeutic *suggestions*, such as computer protocols for ventilator management and antiinfective selection assistance.
4. *Retrospective* quality assurance tools.

Several of these CDS tools have demonstrated a significant impact on clinicians' decisions and patient outcomes, such as appropriate use of perioperative antibiotics, reduced postoperative wound infections, reduced hospital length of stay when clinicians received alerts for life-threatening conditions, and increased survival rate in patients with acute respiratory distress syndrome (ARDS) when computer protocols were utilized for ventilator management. A compendium of the HELP CDS tools and a summary of the effects of these tools on clinicians' decisions and patient outcomes are available in an article by Haug et al.[18]

CLINICAL DECISION SUPPORT TYPES AND EXAMPLES

Several taxonomies have been developed to classify CDS systems. A recent taxonomy was developed by the NQF as an extension of a functional taxonomy developed by researchers at Partners HealthCare.[19] The taxonomy is composed of four functional categories: triggers, input data, interventions, and action steps. *Triggers* are the events that initiate a CDS rule (e.g., a drug prescription). According to the NQF taxonomy, CDS can be triggered by an explicit request from a user, updates to a patient's data, user interactions with an EHR system, or a specific time. *Input data* are the additional data used in the background to constrain or modify the CDS, such as patient conditions, medications, diagnostic tests, and the care plan. *Interventions* are the possible actions that result from the CDS system, such as sending a message to a clinician, displaying relevant clinical knowledge or patient information, and logging that a particular event took place. *Action steps* are actionable alternatives offered to the CDS user, such as collecting or documenting information (e.g., reason to override an alert, completion of care recommended by CDS), requesting an order, and acknowledging a CDS recommendation. The complete NQF taxonomy is available in the NQF consensus report *Driving Quality and Performance Measurement—A Foundation for Clinical Decision Support.*[10]

One of the most current and comprehensive taxonomies was developed by Wright et al. using a Delphi method with 11 CDS experts.[20] The taxonomy classifies CDS types from the user ("front end") perspective into six overarching categories: medication dosing support, order facilitators, point-of-care alerts and reminders, relevant information display, expert systems, and workflow support. Each of these categories is broken down into subtypes, leading to a total of 53 CDS types. The following sections describe each of the six overarching categories and provide real-life examples.

Medication Dosing Support

This category includes tools that assist clinicians in finding and monitoring the most appropriate doses for medication orders. Tools vary from simple "pick lists" with allowed dose options to more complex dose calculation algorithms based on parameters such as patient weight, height, renal function, and hepatic function (Fig. 10.1). Researchers at the Brigham

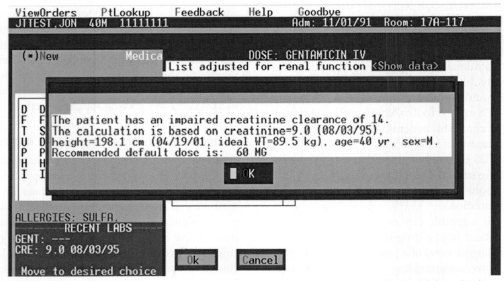

FIG 10.1 Dose adjustment recommendation for a gentamicin order in a patient with impaired renal function. The adjusted dose takes the patient's creatinine clearance and weight into account. (From the computerized provider order entry system at Brigham and Women's Hospital, Boston.)

and Women's Hospital designed several medication dosing support tools for a broad range of medications within their computerized provider order entry (CPOE) system.[21]

Order Facilitators

Broader than medication dosing support tools, order facilitators are tools that assist clinicians in the order entry process in general. Order sets are perhaps the most common example in this category.[22] They assist clinicians by providing a set of commonly used orders for a specific condition (e.g., community-acquired pneumonia) or service (e.g., internal medicine hospital admission orders, vascular surgery postoperative orders). In addition to expediting the order entry process, order sets may help to reduce errors and promote consistent care, reducing unnecessary variability, enabling more complete orders, and reducing the need for verbal orders. Most currently available CPOE systems provide order set capabilities.[19] Fig. 10.2 depicts a community-acquired pneumonia order set within the HELP2 system at Intermountain Healthcare.[22]

Point-of-Care Alerts and Reminders

Point-of-care alerts and reminders raise the clinician's or the patient's attention to important conditions or recommendations based on the patient's clinical data. One of the most common types of CDS, available in most CPOE and drug prescription systems, is an alert that notifies clinicians when a drug being prescribed interacts with other drugs the patient is already receiving. Similar examples include duplicate

therapy alerts, drug allergy alerts, and an alert when a patient's condition contraindicates the use of a particular drug. Similar to alerts, reminders are messages that aim to raise the clinician's attention to a particular patient's need to receive certain care, such as immunizations, cancer screening, fall prevention, and pain assessment. Fig. 10.3 shows a set of patient care reminders generated by the VistA EHR system at the Veterans Health Administration (VHA).

When designed appropriately, alerts have shown significant reduction in errors.[21] However, overuse of the alert mechanism may lead to a problem known as alert fatigue, where clinicians tend to ignore alerts because they are frequently false positives and not clinically significant.[23] Fig. 10.4 illustrates one way in which drug-drug interaction alerts may be presented without interrupting clinicians' workflow and therefore minimize alert fatigue. Other approaches to reducing alert fatigue include prioritizing alert display and improving the precision of the alert logic through contextual information about the patient, healthcare provider, and care setting to prevent false-positive alerts.[24]

Relevant Information Display

A different category of CDS addresses clinicians' information overload in the process of care in both patient information and domain knowledge. This broad category includes CDS tools that provide seamless access to relevant patient information or summarize prominent aspects of a patient's record to help clinicians understand the patient's condition and status. Intensive care daily reports that assist clinicians in patient

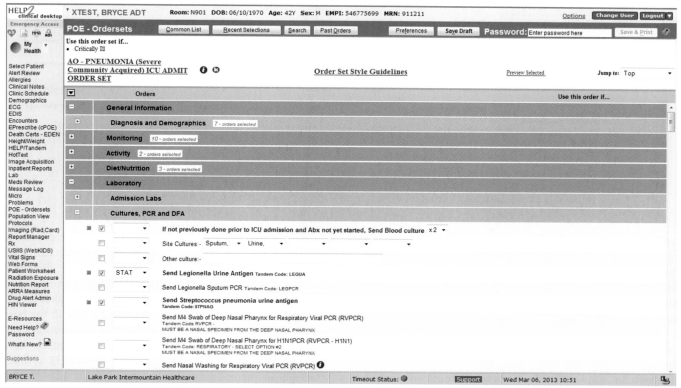

FIG 10.2 CPOE system with a community-acquired pneumonia order set. (From the HELP2 system at Intermountain Healthcare, Salt Lake City.)

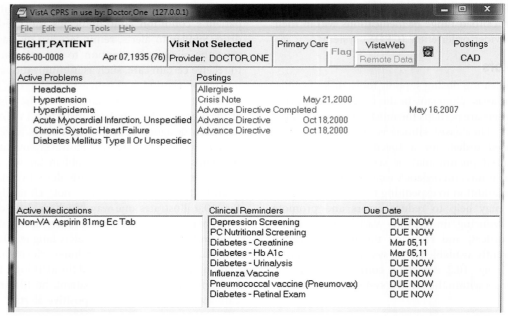

FIG 10.3 A set of care reminders (bottom right of screen) presented within the VHA's VistA Computerized Patient Record System. (Copyright Veterans Health Administration. All Rights Reserved.)

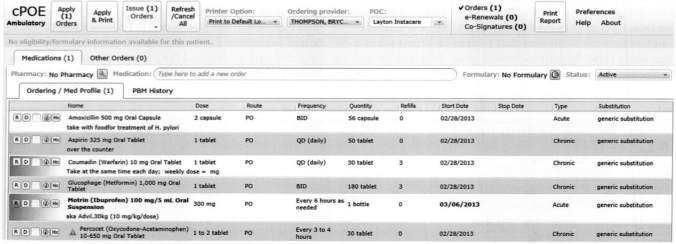

FIG 10.4 A medication prescription system coupled with noninterruptive drug interaction checking. Pairs of interacting drugs are color-highlighted. Different colors denote different levels of interaction severity. The figure also shows Infobutton links adjacent to each drug that clinicians can click to retrieve context-specific information. (From the HELP2 system at Intermountain Healthcare, Salt Lake City.)

rounds are one example of such tools. Another example is disease management dashboards that summarize relevant data for managing a specific condition. Fig. 10.5 shows a disease management dashboard developed at Duke University to assist the management of patients with chronic conditions such as diabetes, hypertension, and chronic kidney disease.[25]

In addition to the need for seamless access to relevant patient information, clinicians frequently raise domain knowledge questions when making patient care decisions. Research has shown that clinicians raise about two questions for every three patients seen and that more than half of these questions go unanswered.[26] With the advent of the World

Wide Web, several online health knowledge resources became accessible through desktop and mobile devices. Although these resources provide answers to most of the clinicians' questions, significant barriers limit their use at the point of care.[27] In essence, the amount of time it typically takes for clinicians to find their answers is not compatible with the busy clinical workflow.[28] To facilitate access to these resources and reduce barriers to their use in patient care, researchers have been enabling access to these resources within EHR systems through an increasingly popular approach to CDS known as "Infobuttons."[29] Leveraging contextual attributes about the patient, clinician, care setting, and clinical task at hand

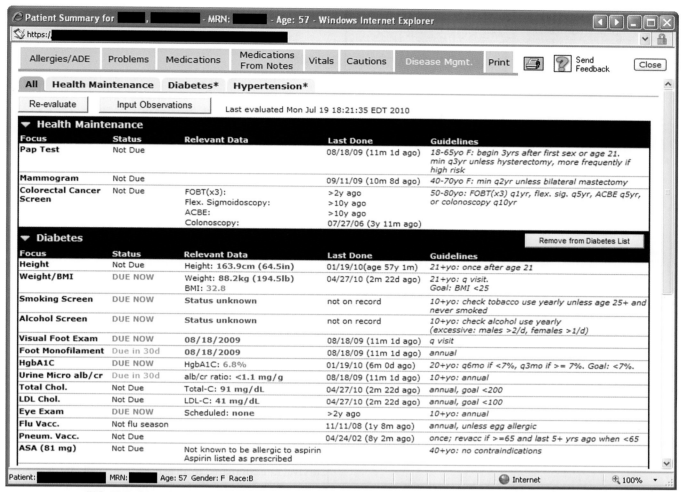

FIG 10.5 Chronic disease management module in use at the Duke University Health System. The system presents relevant data associated with evidence-based care recommendations. (Copyright Duke University Health System. All Rights Reserved.)

within an EHR, Infobuttons anticipate clinicians' information needs and provide automated links to relevant online knowledge resources. For example, a physician prescribing a medication for a patient who has chronic kidney disease might want to know if the medication is contraindicated or if its dose needs to be adjusted based on the patient's condition. An Infobutton positioned beside the drug name within the EHR would provide access to this kind of information from an external drug knowledge resource. Fig. 10.6 shows an example of Infobuttons within the HELP2 drug prescription module used at Intermountain Healthcare.[30]

Expert Systems

Expert systems provide diagnostic or therapeutic advice based on patient parameters. They typically contain more sophisticated computer logic than other forms of CDS and are less frequently found in commercial EHR systems.[20] Within informatics, the term *expert system* is also used to classify computerized systems that go beyond decision support and actually automate the decision-making process. This use of the term is described in Chapter 2.

The antibiotic assistant and ventilator management protocols described in the section titled CDS Examples from the HELP System are examples of this category of CDS. Another example is diagnostic decision support systems such as Iliad,[31] Quick Medical Reference (QMR),[32] and Dxplain.[33] These systems propose a list of candidate diagnoses based on a patient's signs and symptoms. Although diagnostic CDS tools have achieved a quite reasonable level of diagnostic accuracy, especially for differential diagnoses,[34] their use has been limited primarily to educational purposes.[35,36]

Workflow Support

The last category of CDS tools comprises tools that aid in important steps of the patient care workflow, such as care transitions, patient documentation, and orders. These workflow steps are susceptible to various types of errors and inefficiency that can be tackled with CDS. For example, medication errors in care transitions can be prevented with medication reconciliation tools[37]; structured documentation templates may facilitate consistent and efficient documentation[38]; and automatic steps in the ordering workflow, such

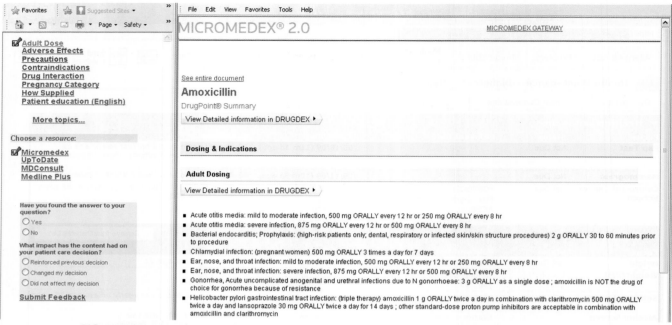

FIG 10.6 User interface presented to a physician who clicks an Infobutton beside the drug amoxicillin, when prescribed to an adult patient. The left side has a navigation panel with automated context-specific links to relevant resources. The right side contains the content itself, which was retrieved from external online resources. (Copyright 2012 Truven Health Analytics Inc. and Intermountain Healthcare. All Rights Reserved.)

as order approval, routing, and termination, may improve the overall efficiency and safety of the ordering process.[39,40]

CLINICAL DECISION SUPPORT IMPACT

Evidence of Effectiveness

Numerous research studies have evaluated the impact of CDS. In 2011, Jaspers et al. synthesized the findings from 17 high-quality systematic reviews of the impact of CDS on healthcare practitioner performance and patient outcomes.[8] Within these systematic reviews, 57% of 91 unique studies reported improved practitioner performance and 30% of 82 unique studies reported improved patient outcomes.[8] Improved practitioner performance was not always associated with a statistically significant improvement in patient outcomes, at least in part because studies of CDS interventions often lack large sample sizes and the associated statistical power required to reliably identify improvements in patient outcome metrics.

Examples of Clinical Decision Support Impact Studies

As one classic example of a CDS intervention resulting in positive outcomes, a study at Brigham and Women's Hospital in Boston found that a CPOE system with various CDS capabilities reduced nonintercepted serious medication errors by 86%, with increasing benefits seen with the introduction of additional CDS capabilities.[21] In another classic example, also described in the section titled CDS Examples from the HELP

System, the use of a rule-based CDS system for the mechanical ventilation of patients with ARDS resulted in a 60% survival rate compared to an expected survival rate of approximately 35%.[41] In another example, the impact of the antibiotic assistant developed by Evans et al. was assessed in a pre-post study. Compared to the preintervention period, use of the antibiotic assistant led to significant improvements in a variety of clinical measures, including antibiotic-susceptibility mismatches and adverse events caused by antiinfective agents.[42] Moreover, patients who received antiinfective therapy according to the regimens recommended by the CDS system had significantly reduced length of stay (10.0 days vs. 16.7 days, $p < 0.001$) and significantly lower total hospital costs ($26,315 vs. $44,865, $p < 0.001$) compared to patients who were not managed according to the CDS system's recommendations.[42]

Not all CDS interventions result in the desired outcomes, however. For example, in a randomized controlled trial involving 29 health centers, an external CDS system for diabetes management that was accessible through the EHR system did not result in any clinically significant changes in practitioner performance or patient outcomes.[43] In another example, a stand-alone CDS system designed to guide referrals for patients at increased risk for hereditary breast cancer was found to have limited impact in a randomized controlled trial involving 86 primary care practices, primarily due to the limited use of the tool by clinicians.[44] Last, a randomized controlled trial involving 60 primary care practices found no significant impact when a CDS system for asthma and angina management was made available to intervention clinicians as a separate path within their practices' EHR systems.[45]

Financial Impact of Clinical Decision Support

As with any investment, a healthcare institution should consider the expected financial impact when making decisions related to CDS investment. To the extent that CDS can facilitate desired changes in clinical practice patterns and patient outcomes, CDS can lead to positive returns on investment, for example, by reducing medical errors and lengths of stay. The VHA estimated that its health IT investments have resulted in more than $3 billion in net benefits, with CDS serving as an important catalyst for the return on investment.[46] In this analysis, CDS provided a financial return on investment to the VHA in reduced costs related to preventable adverse drug events, avoided admissions, and redundant or unnecessary laboratory and radiology tests.[47]

In assessing the financial impact of CDS, it is important to recognize that the financial benefits of CDS may accrue to stakeholders other than those investing in CDS. For instance, if a healthcare delivery organization invests in CDS to support influenza and pneumococcal vaccinations and the rate of hospitalizations for these conditions decreases, the organization may lose money because of the decrease in revenue-generating hospitalizations, whereas society, patients, and health insurers would likely benefit from the investment. In another example, if a healthcare delivery organization invests in CDS systems to ensure that low back pain results in expensive diagnostic imaging and surgical procedures only when clearly warranted, it may lose money because of the decrease in revenue-generating radiologic exams and surgeries; again, society, patients, and health insurers would likely benefit from the investment. Thus when assessing the financial impact of CDS, it is important to assess the impact in terms of the different stakeholders involved, particularly patients, healthcare delivery organizations, and health insurers.

In the case of organizations such as the VHA that serve as both a healthcare delivery organization and a health insurer, the financial incentives of the major stakeholder groups may align well. Other health organizations' incentives do not align as well but, as discussed later, healthcare payment models are beginning to change toward models in which the financial incentives of the key stakeholders are better aligned. Currently, however, because of the healthcare payment models in the United States, the issue of misaligned financial incentives will likely continue to be an important issue in the financial case for CDS.

Clinical Decision Support Adoption

Despite four decades of substantial evidence demonstrating the ability of well-implemented CDS to improve practitioner performance and patient outcomes, most commercial EHR systems and healthcare delivery organizations in the United States have implemented only basic CDS capabilities, such as alerts for drug-drug interactions and drug allergy contraindications.[13] According to a systematic review, 24% of all studies on the impact of health IT on patient care were

conducted at four healthcare organizations in the United States: the Regenstrief Institute, Brigham and Women's Hospital/Partners HealthCare, the U.S. Department of Veterans Affairs, and LDS Hospital/Intermountain Health Care.[47] Characteristics common to these four organizations are use of homegrown EHR systems that were developed and implemented gradually; a strong informatics culture; and strong clinician engagement in the system design, development, and implementation process. Unfortunately, the approach taken at these organizations with internally developed systems is unlikely to be feasible for disseminating CDS to most healthcare settings. Hence the broad dissemination of CDS remains one of the most significant challenges and prominent areas of research in healthcare informatics.

Challenges and Barriers to Clinical Decision Support Adoption

The dissemination of CDS is limited by a significant set of barriers, which collectively make CDS interventions not easily replicable. The most prominent barriers include the following:

- *Lack of incentives:* As discussed earlier, a key reason for the limited adoption of CDS is a healthcare payment model that often fails to reward the provision of higher-quality care and therefore investments in quality-enhancing technologies such as CDS. Within healthcare systems, CDS interventions often do not provide financial benefit to the individuals and organizations that must invest the resources to implement CDS.
- *Implementation challenges:* Successful CDS requires a well-designed implementation plan supported by a strong organizational culture and strategy. In fact, a recent meta-analysis identified local user involvement in the CDS development process as one of the key factors associated with successful CDS.[48] CDS implementations are an ongoing cycle requiring constant monitoring and updating of the underlying clinical logic to reflect changes in domain knowledge, local practices, workflow, and regulations. Ideally CDS should be seen as an integral component of a healthcare organization's quality and value improvement strategy that is operationalized as an organization-wide clinical knowledge management effort.[49,50]
- *Low EHR adoption:* Because CDS generally requires that a core information system such as an EHR or CPOE system be in place first, a barrier to CDS adoption has been the limited adoption of EHR and CPOE systems. However, this scenario is changing rather rapidly worldwide, partially due to incentives such as the Meaningful Use program in the United States. After the inception of this program, the rate of hospitals in the United States that have at least a basic EHR system increased from 9% in 2008 to 76% in 2014, with increasing use of advanced functionality.[51] Similarly, the adoption of EHR systems by office-based physicians increased from 17% in 2003 to 78% in 2013.[52]
- *Multiple data sources with little information exchange:* Most CDS logic requires data that are typically fragmented

across multiple data sources, such as laboratory; pharmacy; radiology; billing; admission, discharge, and transfer (ADT); and EHR systems. Moreover, a patient may have relevant data for CDS stored with many different healthcare organizations. These data sources are typically not shared with the EHR providing the CDS or not shared in a format that can be readily used by the CDS system. As a result, many implementations of CDS require additional data entry by users. In turn, little or no need for data entry is often suggested as a facilitator of successful CDS interventions.[48,53] Therefore a fundamental requirement for CDS adoption is the ability to exchange information with multiple data sources, ideally through a standards-based approach.

- *Lack of adequate CDS tools and capabilities in most EHR systems:* As mentioned earlier, most EHR systems offer only basic CDS capabilities and do not necessarily replicate successful CDS interventions developed and evaluated with "homegrown" or internally developed EHR systems. This limitation compromises the impact of CDS in most healthcare organizations that rely on commercial EHR systems.
- *"Cookbook medicine":* There is a belief among many physicians that the use of CDS reduces medicine from an art to a "cookbook" approach to patient care.[54] However, with the increased emphasis on evidence-based practice, standards of care, and best practices, this attitude is changing.
- *Lack of a framework for sharing CDS logic and capabilities:* As discussed later in this chapter, another important barrier to widespread CDS adoption has been the limited ability to scale most existing CDS logic and capabilities across healthcare organizations and health information systems.[13] This includes the lack of a business model for sharing CDS logic and capabilities, lack of a legal framework covering potential liability implications associated with CDS recommendations, lack of a widely adopted formalism for representing and sharing CDS knowledge, and lack of widely available, standards-based CDS tools and infrastructure.

CLINICAL DECISION SUPPORT BEST PRACTICES

While CDS interventions can profoundly impact clinical care, in a significant minority of cases they fail to result in meaningful improvements. Given the significant effort and cost that can be associated with implementing a CDS intervention, there has been major interest in identifying best practices for CDS to help maximize the likelihood that a CDS initiative will lead to the desired outcomes. In other words, substantial work has been done to make CDS more of a science than an art. These best practices also aim at contributing to the replicability and wide dissemination of CDS interventions.

As an important source of CDS best practices, seasoned experts have compiled guides for CDS best practices, two of which are discussed here. First, in 2003, Bates et al. published "Ten Commandments for Effective CDS: Making the Practice of Evidence-Based Medicine a Reality."[55] These 10 commandments are as follows:

1. Speed is everything.
2. Anticipate needs and deliver in real time.
3. Fit into the user's workflow.
4. Little things can make a big difference.
5. Recognize that physicians will strongly resist stopping.
6. Changing direction is easier than stopping.
7. Simple interventions work best.
8. Ask for additional information only when you really need it.
9. Monitor impact, get feedback, and respond.
10. Manage and maintain your knowledge-based systems.[55]

A second notable source of CDS best practices is *Improving Outcomes with CDS: An Implementer's Guide*, which was authored by experts in the field and published in 2011 by the Healthcare Information and Management Systems Society (HIMSS).[56] This book synthesizes best practices into worksheets to guide the reader through the CDS implementation and evaluation process. It also provides a practical framework for designing and implementing CDS interventions that follows the "CDS Five Rights," which refers to providing the right information to the right person using the right CDS intervention format, delivered through the right channel and at the right point in the workflow.

As a complement to these best practice guides, some researchers have attempted to quantitatively analyze the features of CDS interventions that are strongly associated with, and therefore potentially explain, the success or failure of those interventions. In particular, a systematic review led by Kawamoto analyzed 70 randomized controlled trials of clinician-directed CDS interventions to assess the degree to which the trial outcomes correlated with the presence or absence of CDS intervention features suggested as important by domain experts.[53] Through a multiple logistic regression analysis, this study found that a single feature was by far the most critical: the automatic provision of CDS as a part of clinician workflow (adjusted odds ratio 112.1, $p < 0.00001$). Although there were CDS interventions that included this feature but had no impact, the CDS interventions that were not automatically part of the clinician's workflow failed to result in a significant improvement in clinical practice. This finding suggests that unless a CDS intervention is provided automatically to end users as a part of their routine workflow, there is a high likelihood that the CDS intervention will remain unused and therefore will not have an opportunity to affect patient care positively. In addition, this study found that providing CDS along with a recommendation at the time and location of decision making, rather than just an assessment, were additional independent predictors of a positive outcome.

RECENT PROGRESS TOWARD DISSEMINATING CLINICAL DECISION SUPPORT ON A NATIONAL LEVEL

As noted throughout the chapter, CDS has the potential to significantly enhance the efficiency and effectiveness of healthcare delivery. Indeed, while CDS is not a silver bullet, it is a critical and largely underused resource for improving care and reducing costs, especially when implemented according to known best practices. Thus disseminating comprehensive CDS on a national level is a critical challenge. A number of initiatives are being developed to tackle the challenges and barriers to CDS adoption. The following sections review a series of relevant initiatives and progress that should contribute to overall CDS adoption.

Value-Based Payment Models

The recent trend with perhaps the most significant potential to spur nationwide adoption of advanced CDS is the current shift of healthcare payment from a fee-for-service model to approaches that reward the delivery of better quality and better outcomes at lower cost. Driven by the fundamental problem that the historical fee-for-service payment model leads to unsustainable and relentless increases in healthcare costs, health insurers are increasingly moving toward models of payment in which healthcare delivery organizations are reimbursed less for care volume and more for care value (outcomes relative to costs). For example, a RAND Corporation technical report from 2011 catalogs nearly 100 implemented and proposed payment reform programs and predicts accelerated payment reform moving forward.[57] Although it is difficult to predict how quickly and how deeply these changes will ultimately be adopted, this shift will likely have a profound impact on the degree to which healthcare delivery organizations are motivated to implement CDS-supported process changes to improve care quality and reduce care costs.

Meaningful Use Incentives for Electronic Health Record and Clinical Decision Support Adoption

In 2009 the U.S. federal government established a law providing approximately $30 billion in incentives for clinicians and hospitals to make "Meaningful Use" of EHR systems.[11] In 2012, the regulations related to this law were relatively limited with respect to CDS, requiring only that compliant EHR systems implement a handful of CDS interventions and support a standard approach for integrating context-relevant information resources, typically referred to as Infobuttons.[58] With the exception of the Health Level Seven (HL7) Context-Aware Knowledge Retrieval Standard (also known as the "Infobutton Standard"), the 2015 Meaningful Use EHR certification requirements do not specify standards for the implementation of CDS capabilities. Part of the problem is the low level of maturity and adoption of most CDS standards. Perhaps most important are the Meaningful Use program's powerful incentives for healthcare delivery organizations to adopt EHR systems. As EHR systems are critical enablers of robust and widely distributable CDS, this federal program significantly increases the prospect of a national base of EHR systems through which advanced CDS capabilities can be shared and widely used.

Statewide Health Information Exchanges

As noted in Chapter 5, health information exchanges (HIEs) enable the secure exchange of health information among healthcare providers in a defined region, often through secure web portals that enable authorized clinical access. Beyond EHR systems, HIEs can provide a platform to deliver CDS to clinicians on a large scale. The U.S. federal government has invested more than $500 million in recent years in support of statewide HIEs.[59] As such, this increase in the potential capabilities and reach of HIEs presents an additional opportunity for enabling CDS on a national scale.

Clinical Decision Support Standards

In general, there are two complementary approaches to sharing CDS across a large number of healthcare delivery organizations: (1) sharing structured CDS knowledge resources (e.g., order sets, alert definitions) and (2) sharing CDS capabilities over a secure internet connection (e.g., sending anonymous patient data to a secure web server, which returns evidence-based care recommendations).[60] In both approaches, a critical element is that common standards are used by the various interacting health information systems so that the approach can scale widely and be implemented at relatively low cost. In recognizing this need, a number of CDS standards that are required for a national approach to CDS have recently been developed and adopted by international standards development organizations such as HL7. Interested readers can obtain further details regarding the current state of CDS standards in a recent review article.[61]

National Clinical Decision Support and Knowledge Management Initiatives

To underscore the degree to which the national dissemination of advanced CDS has become an explicit priority for many relevant stakeholder groups, a number of efforts were initiated in recent years in which the nationwide dissemination of CDS is the explicit goal. The CDS Consortium, for example, is a public-private collaborative effort sponsored by the Agency for Healthcare Research and Quality (AHRQ) to assess, define, demonstrate, and evaluate best practices for knowledge management and CDS that can scale across multiple healthcare settings and EHR technology platforms.[62] This effort includes demonstrations of how the CDS interventions developed at one institution can be accessed over a secure internet connection and integrated with the different EHR systems of different healthcare delivery organizations. The CDS Consortium research contract began on March 5, 2008, with a 5-year grant that ended in July 2013 (www.partners.org/cird/cdsc/default.asp).[63]

Furthermore, the NQF, responsible for the development of the various quality measures required for EHR Meaningful Use compliance, has also placed significant focus on how CDS could improve healthcare provider performance with regard to the national quality measures developed by the group.[10] Also, the U.S. Office of the National Coordinator for Health Information Technology recently sponsored an effort known as Advancing CDS; one of the primary deliverables was a proposed national framework for CDS content sharing and an initial pilot implementation of that framework.[64] Finally, a multistakeholder effort known as Health eDecisions actively worked to identify, define, and harmonize standards that facilitate the emergence of systems and services whereby shareable CDS interventions can be implemented at scale,[65] and a follow-on effort known as Clinical Quality Framework is harmonizing these CDS interoperability standards with standards for electronic clinical quality measurement.[66] An important goal of these efforts is to develop and validate a standards-based approach to CDS scaling that can be incorporated into future federal regulations and programs.

Open Source, Freely Available Resources

As a practical matter, the implementation of a common standards-based approach to CDS can be facilitated by resources that are freely available in the public domain. In recognition of this potential enabling role of open source, freely available CDS resources, several CDS stakeholders have launched efforts to collaboratively develop such resources. One such initiative is known as OpenInfobutton (www.openinfobutton.org), which is sponsored by the VHA to develop an open source solution for supporting context-sensitive information retrieval in a standards-compliant manner.[67] An additional initiative in this area is OpenCDS (www.opencds.org), which is a multistakeholder collaborative effort to develop standards-based, open source resources to enable CDS at scale.[67]

RESEARCH CHALLENGES

Despite four decades of research, we are still in the infancy of CDS, and notable challenges must still be addressed to fully realize its benefits. To help focus effort toward achieving this goal, Sittig et al. compiled a list of the top 10 grand challenges in CDS through a consensus-building process (Box 10.1).[68]

One particular area of interest receiving significant attention is the desire to leverage large and heterogeneous data sources, also known as "big data," through advanced analytic and visualization methods.[69] To develop research on big data, the U.S. federal government has allocated a significant amount of research funding to the National Science Foundation (NSF) and the National Institutes of Health (NIH). Big data could advance CDS in several ways, including leveraging of free text data through natural language processing (NLP); the use of nontraditional data sources (e.g., patient self-reported data, wearable sensor data, environmental data); identification of similar patients in a population along with their treatments and outcomes; and the use of predictive analytics to identify patients at high risk of undesirable events such as hospital readmission,[70] who can then be targeted for appropriate management through CDS.

Population-based CDS is also another important area of research need. Historically, volume-based payment models provided healthcare systems with little or no incentive to improve the care of populations as a whole. With the increasing shift to value-based payment models, however, healthcare systems are starting to face much greater incentives for improving health at the population level. As such, the efficient and effective improvement of population health will likely represent a growing focus of CDS efforts moving forward.

BOX 10.1   Top 10 Grand Challenges in Clinical Decision Support

Improve the Effectiveness of Clinical Decision Support Interventions
1. Recognize the need for improvements in human-computer interfaces for delivering CDS.
2. Implement tools that automatically summarize the patient's clinical data, helping clinicians to understand the patient's condition and status.
3. Prioritize and personalize CDS recommendations to the user.
4. Account for patient's comorbidities.
5. Leverage the large amount of narrative text typically available in EHR systems.

Create New Clinical Decision Support Interventions
1. Help organizations prioritize CDS content development and implementation.
2. Leverage large clinical databases to create CDS.

The third category addresses some of the barriers to the wide adoption of CDS.

Disseminate Existing Clinical Decision Support Knowledge and Interventions
1. Disseminate CDS best practices.
2. Create a framework for sharing CDS knowledge and capabilities.
3. Create online CDS repositories.

Adapted from Sittig DF, Wright A, Osheroff JA, et al. Grand challenges in clinical decision support. J Biomed Inform. 2008;41(2):387-392. CDS, Clinical decision support; EHR, electronic health record.

Another area of growing interest is CDS interventions to promote patient-centered care (PCC), defined by the IOM as "care that is respectful of and responsive to individual patient preferences, needs and values, ensuring that patient values guide all clinical decisions."[9] Intelligent tools are needed to help patients understand their conditions and care alternatives, prioritize and carry out their care goals, and engage in shared decision making with their providers.[71-73] A systematic review reported by the AHRQ found an overall positive effect of PCC health IT interventions on healthcare processes, clinical outcomes, responsiveness to the needs and preferences of individual patients, promoting shared decision making, and improving patient-clinician communication.[74] However, studies reported a number of barriers for using these applications to enable PCC, such as lack of usability, low computer literacy in patients and clinicians, lack of standardization, workflow issues, and problems with reimbursement.

CONCLUSION AND FUTURE DIRECTIONS

Since shortly after computers were introduced into clinical settings in the 1960s and 1970s, CDS has been shown to be a powerful tool for positively affecting care delivery and patient outcomes. What has been lacking, however, is a business environment conducive to widespread CDS and technical approaches that enable large-scale CDS knowledge sharing. Today there are a number of changes taking place that address both of these critical challenges. Therefore there is a real opportunity for relevant healthcare stakeholders to come together and realize the vision of advanced CDS that is available ubiquitously and at low cost to support improved healthcare across the nation.

REFERENCES

1. Institute of Medicine (IOM). *To Err Is Human: Building a Safer Health System.* Washington, DC: IOM; 1999.
2. James J. A new, evidenced-based estimate for patient harms associated with hospital care. *J Patient Saf.* 2013;9(3):122–128.
3. Jewell K, McGiffert L. *Consumer Reports. To Err is Human—to Delay is Deadly*; 2009. http://safepatientproject.org/safepatient project.org/pdf/safepatientproject.org-ToDelayIsDeadly.pdf.
4. McGlynn EA, Asch SM, Adams J, et al. The quality of health care delivered to adults in the United States. *N Engl J Med.* 2003;348 (26):2635–2645.
5. Leape LL, Bates DW, Cullen DJ, et al. Systems analysis of adverse drug events: ADE prevention study group. *JAMA.* 1995;274 (1):35–43.
6. Stead WW, Searle JR, Fessler HE, Smith JW, Shortliffe EH. Biomedical informatics: changing what physicians need to know and how they learn. *Acad Med.* 2011;86(4):429–434.
7. Smith R. Strategies for coping with information overload. *BMJ.* 2010;341:c7126.
8. Jaspers MW, Smeulers M, Vermeulen H, Peute LW. Effects of clinical decision-support systems on practitioner performance and patient outcomes: a synthesis of high-quality systematic review findings. *J Am Med Inform Assoc.* 2011;18(3):327–334.
9. Institute of Medicine (IOM). *Crossing the Quality Chasm: A New Health System for the 21st Century.* Washington, DC: IOM; 2001.
10. National Quality Forum (NQF). *Driving Quality and Performance Measurement—A Foundation for Clinical Decision Support: A Consensus Report.* Washington, DC: NQF; 2010. http://www.qualityforum.org/WorkArea/linkit.aspx? LinkIdentifier=id&ItemID=52608.
11. Jha AK. Meaningful use of electronic health records: the road ahead. *JAMA.* 2010;304(15):1709–1710.
12. Institute of Medicine (IOM). *The Future of Nursing: Leading Change, Advancing Health.* Washington, DC: IOM; 2010.
13. Osheroff JA, Teich JM, Middleton B, Steen EB, Wright A, Detmer DE. A roadmap for national action on clinical decision support. *J Am Med Inform Assoc.* 2007;14(2):141–145.
14. Johnston ME, Langton KB, Haynes RB, Mathieu A. Effects of computer-based clinical decision support systems on clinician performance and patient outcome: a critical appraisal of research. *Ann Intern Med.* 1994;120(2):135–142.
15. de Dombal FT, Leaper DJ, Staniland JR, et al. Computer-aided diagnosis of acute abdominal pain. *Br Med J.* 1972;2(5804):9–13.
16. Horrocks JC, McCann AP, Staniland JR, Leaper DJ, de Dombal FT. Computer-aided diagnosis: description of an adaptable system, and operational experience with 2,034 cases. *Br Med J.* 1972;2(5804):5–9.
17. McDonald CJ. Protocol-based computer reminders, the quality of care and the non-perfectability of man. *N Engl J Med.* 1976;295(24):1351–1355.
18. Haug PJ, Gardner RM, Tate KE, et al. Decision support in medicine: examples from the HELP system. *Comput Biomed Res.* 1994;27(5):396–418.
19. Wright A, Goldberg H, Hongsermeier T, Middleton B. A description and functional taxonomy of rule-based decision support content at a large integrated delivery network. *J Am Med Inform Assoc.* 2007;14(4):489–496.
20. Wright A, Sittig DF, Ash JS, et al. Development and evaluation of a comprehensive clinical decision support taxonomy: comparison of front-end tools in commercial and internally developed electronic health record systems. *J Am Med Inform Assoc.* 2011;18(3):232–242.
21. Bates DW, Teich JM, Lee J, et al. The impact of computerized physician order entry on medication error prevention. *J Am Med Inform Assoc.* 1999;6(4):313–321.
22. Del Fiol G, Rocha RA, Bradshaw RL, Hulse NC, Roemer LK. An XML model that enables the development of complex order sets by clinical experts. *IEEE Trans Inf Technol Biomed.* 2005;9 (2):216–228.
23. Ash JS, Sittig DF, Campbell EM, Guappone KP, Dykstra RH. Some unintended consequences of clinical decision support systems. *AMIA Annu Symp Proc.* 2007;26–30.
24. Duke JD, Bolchini D. A successful model and visual design for creating context-aware drug-drug interaction alerts. *AMIA Annu Symp Proc.* 2011;339–348.
25. Lobach DF, Kawamoto K, Anstrom KJ, Russell ML, Woods P, Smith D. Development, deployment and usability of a point-of-care decision support system for chronic disease management using the recently-approved HL7 decision support service standard. *Stud Health Technol Inform.* 2007;129(Pt 2):861–865.
26. Covell DG, Uman GC, Manning PR. Information needs in office practice: are they being met? *Ann Intern Med.* 1985;103 (4):596–599.
27. Ely JW, Osheroff JA, Chambliss ML, Ebell MH, Rosenbaum ME. Answering physicians' clinical questions: obstacles and potential solutions. *J Am Med Inform Assoc.* 2005;12(2):217–224.
28. Hersh WR, Hickam DH. How well do physicians use electronic information retrieval systems? A framework for investigation and systematic review. *JAMA.* 1998;280(15):1347–1352.
29. Cimino JJ, Elhanan G, Zeng Q. Supporting Infobuttons with terminological knowledge. *Proc AMIA Annu Fall Symp.* 1997;528–532.
30. Del Fiol G, Haug PJ, Cimino JJ, Narus SP, Norlin C, Mitchell JA. Effectiveness of topic-specific Infobuttons: a randomized controlled trial. *J Am Med Inform Assoc.* 2008;15 (6):752–759.
31. Warner Jr. HR, Bouhaddou O. Innovation review: Iliad—a medical diagnostic support program. *Top Health Inf Manage.* 1994;14(4):51–58.
32. Bankowitz RA, McNeil MA, Challinor SM, Parker RC, Kapoor WN, Miller RA. A computer-assisted medical diagnostic consultation service: implementation and prospective evaluation of a prototype. *Ann Intern Med.* 1989;110 (10):824–832.
33. Barnett GO, Cimino JJ, Hupp JA, Hoffer EP. Dxplain: an evolving diagnostic decision-support system. *JAMA.* 1987;258 (1):67–74.
34. Berner ES, Webster GD, Shugerman AA, et al. Performance of four computer-based diagnostic systems. *N Engl J Med.* 1994;330 (25):1792–1796.

35. Lange LL, Haak SW, Lincoln MJ, et al. Use of Iliad to improve diagnostic performance of nurse practitioner students. *J Nurs Educ.* 1997;36(1):36–45.

36. Miller RA, Masarie Jr. FE. Use of the Quick Medical Reference (QMR) program as a tool for medical education. *Methods Inf Med.* 1989;28(4):340–345.

37. Bassi J, Lau F, Bardal S. Use of information technology in medication reconciliation: a scoping review. *Ann Pharmacother.* 2010;44(5):885–897.

38. Rosenbloom ST, Denny JC, Xu H, Lorenzi N, Stead WW, Johnson KB. Data from clinical notes: a perspective on the tension between structure and flexible documentation. *J Am Med Inform Assoc.* 2011;18(2):181–186.

39. Buising KL, Thursky KA, Robertson MB, et al. Electronic antibiotic stewardship—reduced consumption of broad-spectrum antibiotics using a computerized antimicrobial approval system in a hospital setting. *J Antimicrob Chemother.* 2008;62(3):608–616.

40. Topal J, Conklin S, Camp K, Morris V, Balcezak T, Herbert P. Prevention of nosocomial catheter-associated urinary tract infections through computerized feedback to physicians and a nurse-directed protocol. *Am J Med Qual.* 2005;20(3):121–126.

41. Thomsen GE, Pope D, East TD, et al. Clinical performance of a rule-based decision support system for mechanical ventilation of ARDS patients. *Proc Annu Symp Comput Appl Med Care.* 1993;339–343.

42. Evans RS, Pestotnik SL, Classen DC, et al. A computer-assisted management program for antibiotics and other antiinfective agents. *N Engl J Med.* 1998;338(4):232–238.

43. Hetlevik I, Holmen J, Krüger O, Kristensen P, Iverson H, Furuseth K. Implementing clinical guidelines in the treatment of diabetes mellitus in general practice: evaluation of effort, process, and patient outcome related to implementation of a computer-based decision support system. *Int J Technol Assess Health Care.* 2000;16(1):210–227.

44. Wilson BJ, Torrance N, Mollison J, et al. Cluster randomized trial of a multifaceted primary care decision-support intervention for inherited breast cancer risk. *Fam Pract.* 2006;23(5):537–544.

45. Eccles M, McColl E, Steen N, et al. Effect of computerised evidence-based guidelines on management of asthma and angina in adults in primary care: cluster randomized controlled trial. *BMJ.* 2002;325(7370):941.

46. Byrne CM, Mercincavage LM, Pan EC, Vincent AG, Johnston DS, Middleton B. The value from investments in health information technology at the U.S. Department of Veterans Affairs. *Health Aff.* 2010;29(4):629–638.

47. Chaudhry B, Wang J, Wu S, et al. Systematic review: impact of health information technology on quality, efficiency, and costs of medical care. *Ann Intern Med.* 2006;144(10):742–752.

48. Bright TJ, Wong A, Dhurjati R, et al. Effect of clinical decision-support systems: a systematic review. *Ann Intern Med.* 2012;157(1):29–43.

49. Rocha RA, Bradshaw RL, Hulse NC, Rocha BHSC. The clinical knowledge management infrastructure of Intermountain Healthcare. In: Greenes RA, ed. *Clinical Decision Support: The Road Ahead.* Burlington, VT: Academic Press; 2007:469–502.

50. Hongsermeier T, Kashyap V, Sordo M. Knowledge management infrastructure: evolution at partners healthcare system. In: Greenes RA, ed. *Clinical Decision Support: The Road Ahead.* Burlington, VT: Academic Press; 2007:447–467.

51. Charles D, Gabriel M, Searcy T. *Adoption of Electronic Health Record Systems among US Non-Federal Acute Care Hospitals: 2008-2014.* Washington, DC: Office of the National Coordinator for Health Information Technology; 2015. https://wwwhealthit.gov/sites/default/files/data-brief/2014HospitalAdoptionDataBrief.pdf.

52. Hsiao C-J, Hing E. *Use and Characteristics of Electronic Health Record Systems among Office-Based Physician Practices: United States, 2001–2013;* 2014. http://www.cdc.gov/nchs/data/databriefs/db143.pdf/.

53. Kawamoto K, Houlihan CA, Balas EA, Lobach DF. Improving clinical practice using clinical decision support systems: a systematic review of trials to identify features critical to success. *BMJ.* 2005;330(7494):765–768.

54. Cabana MD, Rand CS, Powe NR, et al. Why don't physicians follow clinical practice guidelines? A framework for improvement. *JAMA.* 1999;282(15):1458–1465.

55. Bates DW, Kuperman GJ, Wang S, et al. Ten commandments for effective clinical decision support: making the practice of evidence-based medicine a reality. *J Am Med Inform Assoc.* 2003;10(6):523–530.

56. Osheroff JA, Teich JM, Levick D, et al. *Improving Outcomes with Clinical Decision Support: An Implementer's Guide.* 2nd ed. Chicago, IL: Health Information Management and Systems Society; 2011.

57. Schneider EC, Hussey PS, Schnyer C. *Payment Reform: Analysis of Models and Performance Measurement Implications.* Arlington, VA: RAND Corporation; 2011.

58. Health Level Seven (HL7). *HL7 Context-Aware Information Retrieval (Infobutton) Standard.* HL7; 2010. http://wwwhl7.org/v3ballot2010may/html/domains/uvds/uvds_Context-awareKnowledgeRetrieval(Infobutton).htm.

59. US Office of the National Coordinator for Health Information Technology. State health information exchange cooperative agreement program. HealthIT.gov. http://healthit.hhs.gov/portal/server.pt?open=512&objID=1488&mode=2. Accessed July 6, 2016.

60. Kawamoto K. Integration of knowledge resources into applications to enable clinical decision support: architectural considerations. In: Greenes RA, ed. *Clinical Decision Support: The Road Ahead.* Boston, MA: Elsevier; 2007:503–538.

61. Kawamoto K, Del Fiol G, Lobach DF, Jenders RA. Standards for scalable clinical decision support: need, current and emerging standards, gaps, and proposal for progress. *Open Med Inform J.* 2010;4:235–244.

62. Middleton B. The clinical decision support consortium. *Stud Health Technol Inform.* 2009;150:26–30.

63. *Safe Patient Project.* www.SafePatientProject.org. Accessed July 6, 2016.

64. U.S. Office of the National Coordinator for Health Information Technology. CDS sharing. HealthIT.gov. http://healthit.hhs.gov/portal/server.pt/community/healthit_hhs_gov__cds_sharing/3789. Accessed July 6, 2016.

65. *Standards and Interoperability Framework.* Health eDecisions homepage. S&I Framework. http://wiki.siframework.org/Health+eDecisions+Homepage. Accessed July 6, 2016.

66. *Clinical Quality Framework Initiative.* S&I Framework. http://wiki.siframework.org/Clinical+Quality+Framework+Initiative. Accessed November 9, 2015.

67. Del Fiol G, Kawamoto K, Cimino JJ. Open-source, standards-based software to enable decision support. *AMIA Ann Fall Symp.* 2011;2127.

68. Sittig DF, Wright A, Osheroff JA, et al. Grand challenges in clinical decision support. *J Biomed Inform.* 2008;41 (2):387–392.

69. Ohno-Machado L. Big science, big data, and a big role for biomedical informatics. *J Am Med Inform Assoc.* 2012;19:e1.

70. AbdelRahman SE, Zhang M, Bray BE, Kawamoto K. A three-step approach for the derivation and validation of high-performing predictive models using an operational dataset: congestive heart failure readmission case study. *BMC Med Inform Decis Mak.* 2014;14–41.

71. Lenert L, Dunlea R, De Fiol G, Hall LK. A model to support shared decision making in electronic health records systems. *Med Decis Making.* 2014;34(8):987–995.

72. Flynn D, Knoedler MA, Hess EP, et al. Engaging patients in health care decision in the emergency department through shared decision making: a systematic review. *Acad Emerg Med.* 2012;19(8):959–968.

73. Legare F, Ratte S, Stacy D, et al. Interventions for improving the adoption of shared decision making by healthcare professionals. *Cochrane Database Syst Rev.* 2010;12(5):CD006732.

74. Agency for Healthcare Research and Quality. *Enabling Patient-Centered Care Through Health Information Technology;* 2012. http://www.ahrq.gov/clinic/tp/pcchittp.htm.

DISCUSSION QUESTIONS

1. Describe examples of CDS that are available within your organization.
2. Identify the most important barriers to CDS adoption at your organization.
3. Explain how healthcare reimbursement reform will affect healthcare organizations' use of CDS moving forward.
4. What recommendations do you have for the use of CDS to improve care value at your organization?
5. What opportunities do you see for CDS to facilitate the work of healthcare professionals?
6. When implementing a CDS system, what should the appropriate relationship be between local values and standards and national standards?

CASE STUDY

Imagine that you have been appointed Director of Clinical Decision Support at a healthcare delivery system. This healthcare system consists of several large hospitals and multiple outpatient clinics and uses the same EHR system across the enterprise. There has been limited CDS activity at the institution prior to your arrival. Now, with the increasing need to provide increased care value, the appropriate use of CDS is an institutional priority. The current CDS available at your institution consists primarily of off-the-shelf drug-drug interaction and drug allergy alerting, which is the source of significant clinician complaints due to the rate of false-positive alerts. There is a strong sense within the institution's administration that IT in general and CDS specifically should be leveraged to improve care value and to enable the institution to influence its clinical practice patterns more systematically and more rapidly. You have a reasonable budget and adequate staff to make meaningful changes and you do have support from key institutional stakeholders, including healthcare system executives, the nursing informatics officer, and the chief medical informatics officer. You have been asked to devise a strategic plan for CDS at your institution within 3 months of your arrival and to have concrete "wins" within 12 to 18 months.

Discussion Questions

1. Describe the approaches you would use to ensure that all aspects of patient care were considered when developing a CDS system. How would you prioritize the efforts of your CDS team? Potential areas on which to focus include areas in which payment rates are tied to national quality measures, CDS interventions that meet Meaningful Use requirements, readmissions for congestive heart failure and other care events for which payers are increasingly not reimbursing, and areas that have been identified as institutional priorities for clinical improvement.

2. How would you balance the need to deliver desired CDS capabilities quickly against the benefits of establishing robust infrastructure to enable future deliverables to be implemented more quickly?

3. Identify one area for quality and value improvement. Define the CDS interventions that you would implement to address this area of need. Describe how your approach aligns with the best practices discussed in this chapter, such as the CDS Five Rights, the CDS 10 commandments, and the desire to use standards-based, scalable approaches. How would you systematically measure the impact of these CDS interventions?

11

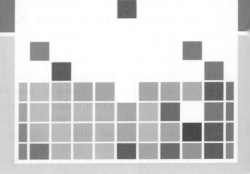

Public Health Informatics

Catherine Janes Staes

Public health informatics is the specialty where informatics methods and tools are used to solve public health problems or support population and public health goals.

OBJECTIVES

At the completion of this chapter, the reader will be prepared to:

1. Summarize critical public health functions and common workflows that may be supported by information technology.
2. Analyze the sociopolitical context for public health and other factors that influence the implementation of informatics solutions.
3. Critique key public health applications for infectious and chronic diseases.
4. Describe current efforts to improve the exchange of information between public health and clinical systems.
5. Explain why cloud computing is critical to the future of public health informatics.

KEY TERMS

immunization information systems (IISs), 193
information ecology, 198
information supply chain, 198

public health, 185
public health information, 190
public health surveillance, 191

ABSTRACT ❖

The chapter includes a description of the importance and unique features of public health practice and explores the differences between clinical and public health practice. It includes social and political challenges that affect public health informatics. A list of several major public health data systems is provided to help the reader understand the scope of information generated and used by public health, but these data systems alone are not informatics applications that transform data to knowledge. To illustrate public health informatics applications, the chapter includes a description of surveillance systems, immunization information systems, and the role of public health in a health information exchange. The chapter includes a description of the workflows associated with these systems and the value of information technology (IT), decision support, and standards. The next section describes the opportunities to leverage the electronic health record (EHR) to meet and promote public health goals. EHRs can be used to manage a population of patients in a single clinical practice or in a more complex medical home model. EHR data are used to generate and track quality performance measures important for preventing disease, reducing healthcare costs, and improving outcomes such as the Healthcare Effectiveness Data and Information Set (HEDIS) measures that concern antibiotic use, influenza vaccination, cancer screening, body mass index assessment, and other quality metrics. In addition, EHRs can be used to deliver patient-specific alerts for preventive or screening interventions. Finally, there is a discussion about the future of public health informatics and the need to leverage new technologies and paradigms to meet new challenges and resource constraints in the 21st century.

INTRODUCTION

The public health informatics specialty uses informatics methods and tools to solve public health problems or support population and public health goals. This definition transcends the walls of a public health department and recognizes that population and public health practice occurs in the community, in clinical sites, and in a variety of other settings outside the domain of a health department. Rapidly evolving technologies, standards, and partnerships have created new opportunities for monitoring and improving population health and preventing injury and disease. This chapter explains how informatics concepts can be applied to populations, with the goals of limiting health problems and promoting health.

PUBLIC HEALTH: A POPULATION PERSPECTIVE

Public health is the science, art, and practice of protecting and improving the health of populations. It has contributed substantially to improvements in health status throughout the world. For example, during the 20th century, life expectancy at birth among U.S. residents increased 62%, from 47.3 years in 1900 to 78.8 years in 2014.[1] Unprecedented improvements in population health status were observed at every stage of life across a variety of different metrics.[1a] While the average life span of persons in the United States increased by 30 years, 25 years of this gain were attributable to advances in public health.[2] Advances in medical diagnostic modalities, antibiotics, and other treatments and therapies are important, but prevention of death, illness, and disability can be attributed to public health strategies that reduce harmful exposures and promote health. For example, the Centers for Disease Control (CDC) and Prevention profiled 10 great public health achievements that affected health in the United States[3]:

- Vaccine-preventable diseases
- Prevention and control of infectious diseases
- Tobacco control
- Maternal and infant health
- Motor vehicle safety
- Cardiovascular disease prevention
- Occupational safety
- Cancer prevention
- Childhood lead poisoning prevention
- Public health preparedness and response

These achievements required multifaceted health policy, legal, taxation, and prevention program strategies applied in the community, the workplace, and the home. As an example, the recognition of tobacco use as a health hazard and the subsequent public health antismoking campaigns resulted in changes in social norms to prevent initiation of tobacco use, promote cessation of tobacco use, and reduce exposure to environmental tobacco smoke.[3] During the 30 years following the initial 1964 Surgeon General's report on the health risks of smoking, the prevalence of smoking among adults decreased from around 50% to 20%, and an estimated 1.6 million deaths from smoking were prevented.[4] Today, 50 years after the initial 1964 Surgeon General report, (1) research continues to newly identify diseases caused by smoking, including diabetes mellitus, rheumatoid arthritis, and colorectal cancer; (2) prevention efforts are still ongoing toward a goal of eliminating cigarette use; and (3) new health threats must be addressed concerning the emerging use of e-cigarettes.[5,6]

Despite the above achievements of the 20th century, the unprecedented improvements in sanitation and control of infectious diseases, and the fact that the United States spends more money on healthcare than any other nation in the world, the U.S. population still ranks near the bottom on most standard measures of health status when compared with other developed nations.[7] In a call to do better, Schroeder states that the pathways to better health do not generally depend on better healthcare and that even in those instances in which healthcare is important, too many Americans do not receive it, receive it too late, or receive poor-quality care.[7] In particular, though, Schroeder calls for improved efforts to address the behavioral patterns that affect health in the 21st century. Given that smoking and the constellation of poor diet and physical inactivity were the "actual cause" of about one-third of all deaths in the United States in 2000,[8] public health efforts in the 21st century need to tackle these and other modifiable behavioral risk factors to substantively affect population health. Going forward, public health priorities and activities will continue to evolve as the following occur:

- New problems arise, such as prescription drug abuse, organisms resistant to antimicrobial therapies, the spread of Ebola, or violent bioterrorism events seen on and after September 11, 2001.
- New priorities are recognized, such as the need to address the rising rates of obesity, gun violence, and behavioral risk factors, and the need to improve preparedness for natural and human-made disasters, and ensure food safety.
- A continued need exists to prevent and control infectious and chronic diseases, injuries, and behaviors (such as smoking) that cause high rates of morbidity and mortality.

To address these challenges, public health involves a diverse set of professionals and agencies that all have one common goal: to improve people's health and protect them from health risks. The professionals specialize in public health nursing, behavioral science and health education, epidemiology, environmental health, injury control, biostatistics, emergency medical services, health services, international health, maternal and child health, nutrition, public health laboratory practice, public health policy, and public health clinical practice. The agencies involved include local (city and county), state, and tribal health departments and federal agencies such as the CDC, the Food and Drug Administration (FDA), the Environmental Protection Agency (EPA), and the Census Bureau. The CDC includes the National Center for Health Statistics, the National Institute for Occupational Safety and Health, and other centers that focus on domains such as injuries, infectious disease, genomics, and global health. These governmental public health agencies partner with healthcare delivery systems and others to ensure the conditions for population health (Fig. 11.1).

When asked to define public health, people often mention service functions, such as "where you go to get your child immunized or to get a birth or death record," or job duties, such as "employing disease detectives that respond to outbreaks and inspectors who check restaurants." While correct, these responses are incomplete. Public health agencies provide direct clinical services similar to any health-care organization but also provide services, such as outbreak management and surveillance, that are not otherwise per-formed in a community.[9] A broad spectrum of public health practice is largely invisible to the general public because much of the goal of public health is to stop hazardous situations from arising.[10] When public health strategies function well, hazardous events do not occur, which creates a paradox: You often do not get grateful patients or communities when problems are prevented.[10] Some less visible examples of pub-lic health activities include monitoring of air and water, pre-vention and control of injuries, building of safe roadways, protection of the food supply, proper disposal of solid and

liquid waste and medications, rat control and mosquito abate-ment, surveillance of infectious and chronic diseases, and pre-vention and preparedness research (Fig. 11.2). This diverse set of activities can be summarized in the core functions and essential services for effective public health systems that were defined by the Institute of Medicine (IOM) Committee for the Study of the Future of Public Health. There are many oppor-tunities to use informatics strategies with these services.

The IOM framework developed in 1988 holds true today.[10] Public health agencies should perform three core functions: (1) assessment: "to regularly and systematically collect, assemble, analyze, and make available information on the health of the community, including statistics on health status, community health needs, and epidemiologic and other stud-ies of health problems"[10, p. 7]; (2) policy development: "to exercise its responsibility to serve the public interest in the development of comprehensive public health policies by promoting use of the scientific knowledge base in decision-making"[10, p. 8]; and (3) assurance: "to assure their constituents that the services necessary to achieve agreed upon goals are provided, either by encouraging actions by other entities (private or public sector), by requiring such action through regulation, or by providing services directly."[10, p. 8] "The committee recommends each public health agency involve key policy-makers and the general public in determin-ing a set of high-priority personal and communitywide health services that governments will guarantee to every member of the community. This guarantee should include subsidization or direct provision of high-priority personal health services for those unable to afford them."[10, p. 8] The essential services related to these functions are described in Box 11.1.

Public health practice differs from clinical practice in important ways that help illustrate core public health princi-ples. Most notably, public health is focused on prevention and maintaining the health of populations rather than treating individuals after they become injured or ill. The primary goal of clinical care is to obtain the best possible outcome for the individual receiving care. This paradigm leads to saving "one life at a time." In contrast, the primary goal of public health practice is to affect population health and ensure a healthy

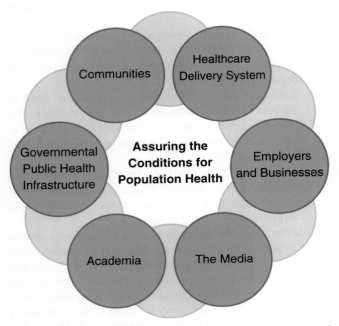

FIG 11.1 The public health system: government and some of its potential partners. (From Committee on Assuring the Health of the Public in the 21st Century. *The Future of the Public's Health in the 21st Century.* Washington, DC: The National Acad-emies Press; Copyright 2002, National Academy of Sciences.)

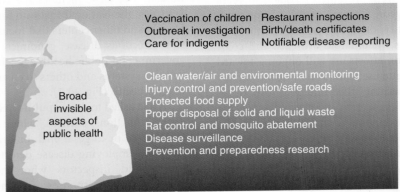

FIG 11.2 The visible and invisible work of public health. (Copyright 2010 Catherine States. Reprinted with permission.)

community. This is performed by encouraging healthy behaviors, focusing on prevention, and balancing individual autonomy with limitations on individuals that protect those individuals or others. For example, this balance is seen in smoking and helmet laws designed to limit exposures to known risks for injury and disease. The policies and strategies are designed to save "millions of lives at a time."

The diagnostic tools used in the two domains differ. Clinical providers measure the health of an individual using tools ranging from a stethoscope to sophisticated imaging or laboratory modalities. In contrast, epidemiologists and public health officers measure the vital status of a community using birth and death records, surveys, and surveillance data to understand the distribution and determinants of disease and health in their community. A list of the major surveys performed by the National Center for Health Statistics is available on its website.[11] Other important systems will be described later in the chapter.

The breadth of entities involved in medical and public health practice differs. A clinical provider primarily interacts with people and data associated with hospitals, laboratories, and other clinical care settings. In contrast, public health practitioners may perform work in a clinical setting but the assessment, policy development, and assurance functions often involve schools, the legislature, the workplace,

correctional facilities, food establishments, water systems, the community at large, and many other settings.

Public health interventions focus on events earlier in the causal pathway of disease (Fig. 11.3). While medical care addresses the diagnosis and treatment of disease, public health interventions focus on creating a safe environment to avoid or reduce exposure to hazards, promote healthy behaviors, and reduce the prevalence of risky behaviors and other risk factors. For example, public health practitioners focus on safely removing leaded paint in a child's community to avoid lead poisoning and advocate or require the use of helmets to prevent head injuries.

Public health practice differs from clinical practice in one additional significant way. The risk reduction strategies employed by public health are based on a population perspective to determine priorities and evaluate success. Three models for risk reduction are discussed extensively in *The Future of the Public's Health in the 21st Century*[12] and illustrated in Fig. 11.4. These models are based on three central realities in the development of effective population-based prevention strategies. First, disease risk is a continuum rather than a dichotomy. There is no clear division between risk for disease and no risk for disease regarding levels of blood pressure, cholesterol, alcohol consumption, tobacco consumption, physical activity, diet and weight, lead exposure, and other risk factors. Second, most often, only a small percentage of any population is at the extremes of high or low risk. The majority of people fall in

BOX 11.1 Core Functions and the Ten Essential Services for Effective Public Health Systems

Core Function: Assessment
Essential Services
- Monitor health status to identify community health problems.
- Diagnose and investigate health problems and health hazards in the community.

Core Function: Policy Development
Essential Services
- Inform, educate, and empower people about health issues.
- Mobilize community partnerships to identify and solve health problems.
- Develop policies and plans that support individual and community health efforts.

Core Function: Assurance
Essential Services
- Enforce laws and regulations that protect health and ensure safety.
- Link people to needed personal health services and assure the provision of healthcare when otherwise unavailable.
- Assure a competent public health and personal healthcare workforce.
- Evaluate effectiveness, accessibility, and quality of personal and population-based health services.
- Research for new insights and innovative solutions to health problems.

From Committee for the Study of the Future of Public Health. *The Future of Public Health*. Washington, DC: The National Academies Press; 1988.

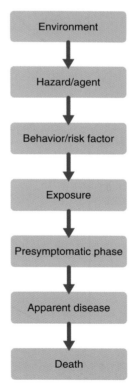

FIG 11.3 Causal pathway of disease. (Reproduced from Public health 101 for informaticians, Koo D, O'Carroll P, LaVenture M, 8, 585–97, 2001 with permission from BMJ Publishing Group Ltd.)

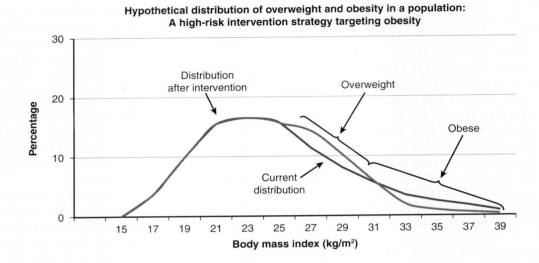

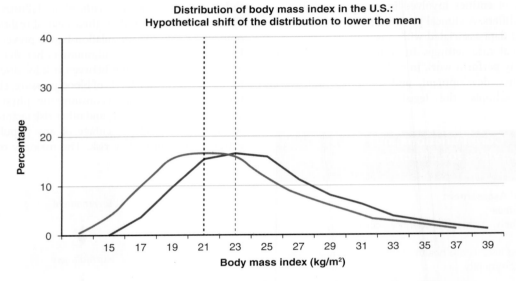

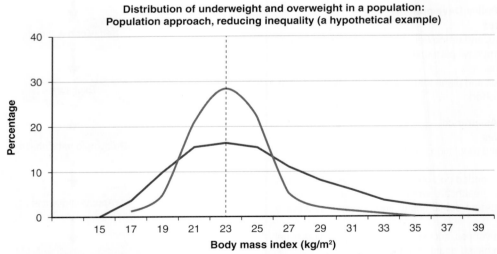

FIG 11.4 Models for risk reduction. (Printed with permission from Committee on Assuring the Health of the Public in the 21st Century. *The Future of the Public's Health in the 21st Century.* The National Academies Press; Copyright 2002, National Academy of Sciences.)

the middle of the risk distribution. Exposure of a large number of people to a small risk can yield a more absolute number of cases of a condition than exposure of a small number of people to a high risk. Third, an individual's risk of illness cannot be considered in isolation from the disease risk for the population to which he or she belongs.

Fig. 11.4 illustrates the hypothetical impact on the distribution of risk in a population when efforts are focused on only those at highest risk (see Fig. 11.4A), when strategies are employed to shift the mean level of risk for the entire population (see Fig. 11.4B), or when strategies attempt to limit variation in risk and tighten the distribution around the population mean (see Fig. 11.4C). American society experienced the second approach to disease prevention and health promotion when measures were taken to promote sanitation and food and water safety in the early 20th century and more recently when implementing policies about seat belt use, unleaded gasoline, and vaccination.[12] The second and third models (see Fig. 11.4B and C) are common strategies for evaluating quality improvement in the clinical setting. The clinical informatics strategies for assessing systems and process improvement are very useful in thinking about the application of informatics to population health.

Social and Political Challenges That Affect Public Health Informatics

Many aspects of public health are inherently governmental functions. As a result, the architecture of public health reflects the constitutional structure of the United States. The founding fathers of the United States did not envision a need for a national-level public health system. Such a vision was beyond the grasp of even our greatest thought leaders at the end of the 18th century. Further, the framers of the Bill of Rights saw the need to limit federal powers. The Tenth Amendment to the U.S. Constitution essentially states that any powers that are not reserved for the federal government or not prohibited for the states are in the realm of the states' authority. Because of the limits on federal authority and the relatively late development of a national public health infrastructure, public health laws and functions evolved primarily as state and local government functions.

The lead government agency for public health, the CDC, was not created until after World War II, long after the value of public health regulations for control of contagion were recognized. While the CDC evolved into its role as a national public health agency through its work in the 1950s and 1960s, its legislative authority is limited by the Tenth Amendment. Congress has not mandated, nor could it require, states to cooperate with the CDC except in situations where there is a threat to national security. So, how does the CDC get states and local governments to work with it toward national interests? It must use grants and contract vehicles to persuade states to work with the national government, including sharing of data. With respect to informatics, this means that the CDC cannot require states to maintain specific kinds of information systems or even to send data to the CDC. Data exchange with the federal government is voluntary and driven by obligations and incentives that are embedded in CDC-administered grants and contracts with the states.

An example of voluntary cooperation between the states and the federal government is the National Notifiable Disease Surveillance System (NNDSS). While states have all agreed to contribute data to the NNDSS to allow the country to track infectious diseases, integration of these data is difficult because each state is its own arbiter of the types of data it collects for each notifiable disease and even of the types of tests and findings considered relevant for reporting a condition. This immensely complicates the creation of a nationwide view of the impacts of disease.

In the same way that the national government has limitations on its authority in matters of public health, many state governments have similar challenges with municipal authorities. In states that provide for local Home Rule (Fig. 11.5), municipal governments have a broad delegation of authority, which may include authority for public health functions. In Home Rule states, state governments can regulate many aspects of health through the counties. However, state governments may have less control over city public health departments, which may adopt their own business practices for health investigations and use information systems that differ from those of state agencies. In general, it is large municipalities (such as New York, Baltimore, and Los Angeles) in which local public health officials may wield significant resources. In states without Home Rule, public health activities within the state tend to be more centralized and managed at the state level.

As a result of the history and structure of public health departments, public health authority and activity is largely a county function in the United States, but the responsibility for planning and policy is largely at the state and federal levels. This creates a continuing series of problems with data standardization, data ownership, lack of willingness to share data across levels of government, complexities with data integration, and system planning and development. In contrast, in countries with a strong national authority for public health issues, such as Canada, Great Britain, or China, a single information system can be used across the country to manage specific public health issues or even the entire public health enterprise. In the United States, informatics solutions must allow state and local governments to be the stewards of their own computational resources and data.

Sociological Context of Public Health

While public health, nursing, and medicine share a similar set of facts about disease, health, prevention, and treatment, each has a different approach to these problems and a different worldview. The worldview of a clinical practitioner is often patient-centric, which is reflected in the knowledge artifacts they produce and the computer systems developed to support their work. In contrast, public health software systems reflect the language and worldview of population health. Systems are developed to serve specific operational needs and, as a result,

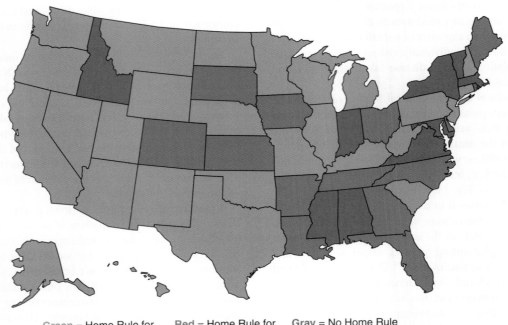

Green = Home Rule for   Red = Home Rule for   Gray = No Home Rule
selected municipalities   all municipalities

FIG 11.5 Distribution of U.S. states that allow Home Rule. (Data from American City County Exchange. *Federalism, Dillon Rule and Home Rule.* https://www.alec.org/app/uploads/2016/01/2016-ACCE-White-Paper-Dillon-House-Rule-Final.pdf; January 2016.)

focus on one type of public health activity or another. For example, public health departments might use one system to track patients with sexually transmitted diseases and another to track patients receiving immunizations.

In public health systems, data are typically captured about one event (disease, lead test result, immunization administered) at a time, often without the ability to directly link reports about an individual across different systems. The difference in the worldview of public health and the design of public health information systems complicates the tasks associated with sharing data across systems and, in particular, the task of integrating clinical systems with public health systems.

A second difference in worldview concerns the sharing of information. In many public health practice circumstances, clinical systems send data about an individual to a public health system without incurring any direct benefit for the patient or the healthcare provider. For example, information about patients is included in the hospital discharge datasets sent to the public health system, but this sharing of information does not benefit the patient or healthcare provider directly. In contrast, data movement in the clinical system occurs primarily for patient benefit or reimbursement. The Health Insurance Portability and Accountability Act (HIPAA) Privacy Rule recognizes and supports these differences, but sometimes clinicians are reluctant to share information because of their different worldview and training.

In 2003 the CDC published the following guidance:

The Privacy Rule permits covered entities to disclose protected health information (PHI), without authorization, to public health authorities or other entities who are legally authorized to receive such reports for the purpose of preventing or controlling disease, injury, or disability. This includes the reporting of disease or injury; reporting vital events (e.g., births or deaths); conducting public health surveillance, investigations, or interventions; reporting child abuse and neglect; and monitoring adverse outcomes related to food (including dietary supplements), drugs, biological products, and medical devices [45 CFR 164.512(b)]. Covered entities may report adverse events related to FDA-regulated products or activities to public agencies and private entities that are subject to FDA jurisdiction [45 CFR 164.512(b)(1)(iii)].

To protect the health of the public, public health authorities might need to obtain information related to the individuals affected by a disease. In certain cases, they might need to contact those affected to determine the cause of the disease to allow for actions to prevent further illness. Also, covered entities may, at the direction of a public health authority, disclose protected health information to a foreign government agency that is acting in collaboration with a public health authority [45 CFR 164.512(b)(1)(i)].[13]

It is the job of the public health informatician to develop tools or methods to translate the data representations generated by the public health and the clinical worldviews. This translation is necessary to enable interoperability and support the various uses of the information. For example, clinical records are usually patient centered whereas public health may request aggregated information such as the number of encounters for influenza-like illness during the week.

Two questions should be considered in the field of public health informatics:

- How can information and communication technologies improve the effectiveness of public health agencies?
- How can information and communication technologies improve the health of the American public?

It is important to understand that there is a difference between these questions. Improvements in population health will require addressing both of these questions and considering the goals, breadth of data quality, sources, needs, and the sociopolitical and governmental context in which informatics solutions are being applied. The Public Health Informatics Institute (PHII) has been instrumental in articulating the business processes within public health agencies to address the first question. A list of its resources is available at www.phii.org.

THE VALUE OF INFORMATICS FOR THE DOMAIN OF PUBLIC HEALTH

To demonstrate the value of informatics for the domain of public health, it is useful to explore current public health methods, applications, and processes. The descriptions will help the reader understand the value of informatics and the challenges encountered in the real world. A single chapter on the topic of public health informatics cannot begin to describe the breadth of public health systems, but examples will be instructive. The sections that follow describe surveillance as a public health method, immunization information systems as a public health application, and health information exchange and public health reporting as public health processes.

Surveillance

Public health surveillance is the ongoing collection, analysis, interpretation, and dissemination of data for a stated public health purpose.[14] The primary goal of surveillance is to provide actionable health information to public health staff, government leaders, and the public to guide public health policy and programs.[14] Hence surveillance activities and the information generated guide decisions and monitor progress. These are critical for meeting all three functions required of a public health system: assessment, policy development, and assurance. It is important to note that surveillance is an activity that often requires partnerships with private and public entities in the community and legislation to enforce it. Surveillance is difficult to delegate to others in the community, so it has generally been a public health department activity.

While new technologies, health reforms, and national security concerns affect surveillance efforts in the 21st century, the following specific goals of surveillance have not changed over time:

- Recognize cases or clusters of disease or injury to (1) trigger investigations, (2) trigger interventions to prevent disease transmission or to reduce morbidity, and (3) help ensure the adequacy of medical diagnosis, treatment, and infection control.
- Measure trends; characterize diseases, injuries, and risk factors; and identify high-risk population groups or geographic areas toward which needed interventions can be targeted.
- Monitor the effectiveness of public health programs, prevention and control measures, and intervention strategies, which includes providing information to determine when a public health program should be modified or discontinued.
- Develop hypotheses leading to analytic studies about risk factors for disease and injury and disease propagation or progression.
- Provide information to the public to enable individuals to make informed decisions regarding personal behaviors and to healthcare providers to ensure that they base their care of individual patients on the most current surveillance information available.[14]

Currently, surveillance of infectious diseases (through case reporting or sentinel surveillance) is performed at the local level where control efforts are localized and may be urgent. Surveillance of noninfectious events is typically managed by state health agencies because the interventions involved are often statewide and long term (such as cancer screening and prevention campaigns) and there are more resources to support electronic systems for vital records, immunization and cancer registries, newborn screening for heritable disorders, electronic laboratory reporting, and so forth. In addition, state agencies usually manage the hospital discharge datasets, claims data, and other administrative data that are generated from clinical encounters and shared with public health. State agencies conduct surveys for the Behavioral Risk Factor Surveillance System (BRFSS) and the Pregnancy Risk Assessment Monitoring System (PRAMS). Finally, the CDC and other federal agencies, such as the FDA, EPA, and the U.S. Department of Agriculture (USDA), monitor national trends and support state activities, conduct national surveys (e.g., National Health and Nutrition Examination Survey, National Health Interview Survey, Bureau of Labor Statistics' annual survey of work-related injuries and illnesses, federal tracking of coal workers' pneumoconiosis), interface with the World Health Organization (WHO) on global health concerns, and use data to generate research hypotheses.[14]

The range of events under surveillance span the causal pathway of disease (see Fig. 11.3), including environmental exposures (e.g., folate levels in fortified grains, fluoride levels in water, air and water quality, air lead levels in indoor firing ranges), hazards (e.g., leaded paint in older housing, toxic releases), behaviors and risk factors (e.g., prescription drug abuse, smoking, cancer screening, use of sunscreen, use of helmets when biking), exposure (e.g., needlestick injuries, newborns of mothers infected with hepatitis B, children in households with smokers), presymptomatic phase (e.g., blood lead levels in children), apparent disease or injury (e.g., persons diagnosed with hepatitis, tuberculosis, traumatic brain injury), and death. In their blueprint for surveillance in the 21st century, public health epidemiologists note that surveillance methods should match surveillance goals, data should be collected in the least expensive manner possible, and data should flow in an efficient, timely, and secure manner as defined by local, state, and federal laws.[14] High-quality data are needed if surveillance information is to be relied on, but data quality should match its use. Perfecting data can be costly and may not be necessary. With this in mind, the authors of the blueprint matched purposes for surveillance with methods commonly used (Table 11.1)[14] and noted that systems should be evaluated for efficiency and security as well as timeliness, sensitivity, positive predictive value, simplicity,

and flexibility of the system for the level of public health agency using the data.[15] In the 21st century, surveillance systems should also be evaluated on their sustainability and scalability to meet other needs and interoperate with existing systems.

To improve the timeliness with which outbreaks are detected (influenza outbreaks in particular), informatics researchers have been testing new signals for event detection, evaluating statistical models for finding significant events among normal variation, and devising new strategies for visualizing information and engaging a broader community. Table 11.2 illustrates the relationship between illness-related events and the variety of surveillance systems that may capture those events. The quest to identify early events must balance the potentially less predictive quality of the information with improved opportunities to identify infections and outbreaks

TABLE 11.1 Examples of Matching Surveillance Purposes With Methods

Purpose	Method
Provide case management; notify exposed partners; provide prophylaxis to contacts; detect outbreaks; quarantine exposed contacts; isolate cases; take regulatory actions to prevent exposures by others; target interventions to remediate hazards to exposed persons	Case reporting to local and state health departments by clinicians, healthcare facilities, and laboratories
Monitor common diseases for which detection of every case is not needed (e.g., influenza, Lyme disease)	Sentinel surveillance (collection of detailed information about a subset of cases) or sampling of suspected cases for full investigation
Monitor population vital statistics	Birth and death certificate reporting to states
Monitor population cancer incidence	Case reporting to state health department cancer registries by clinicians, healthcare facilities, and pathology laboratories
Monitor prevalence of childhood vaccination rates	Reporting of all childhood vaccinations by clinicians to state immunization information systems
Monitor population prevalence of risk factors and health-related conditions	Public health telephone, school-based, community, or other self-report surveys; public health examination surveys; analysis of de-identified electronic health record data, hospital data, claims data, and other clinical encounter data
Measure population levels of environmental and occupational risk factors	Public health or community and worker surveys; environmental monitoring and modeling; biomonitoring
Monitor antibiotic resistance in communities	Electronic laboratory reporting
Monitor characteristics and quality of care for health events and conditions (e.g., myocardial infarction, stroke, cardiac arrest, diabetes)	Quality improvement registries (e.g., Paul Coverdell National Acute Stroke Registry)
Detect evidence for an unreported change in community health or track situational awareness during public health emergencies	Analysis of de-identified clinical data by public health to detect changes in population health (syndromic surveillance)
Evaluate effectiveness of public health programs and interventions; monitor health trends in a population	Trend analysis of vital statistics reports, case reports, vaccination prevalence, clinical and billing data, population survey data, worksite injury and death reports, law enforcement records, special surveys
Characterize the epidemiology of specific diseases or injuries and develop hypotheses about and target interventions toward their risk factors	Analysis of population data or case-based data to describe disease or injury characteristics and risk factors

Adapted from Smith PF, Hadler JL, Stanbury M, et al. Blueprint version 2.0: updating public health surveillance for the 21st century. J Public Health Manag Pract 2012, http://dx.doi.org/10.1097/PHH.0b013e318262906e [Epub ahead of print].

TABLE 11.2 Relevant Surveillance Systems for Illness-Related Events

Illness-Related Event	Surveillance Systems That Capture the Event
Actions in the Home or Community	
Search for information about "flu" in Google	Google flu trends (www.google.org/flutrends/; http://www.healthmap.org/flutrends/)
Stay home from school	School absenteeism surveillance
Buy over-the-counter cough medicine	National Retail Data Monitor (https://www.rods.pitt.edu/site/content/blogsection/4/42/)
Read news article about possible outbreak in the community	HealthMap (www.healthmap.org/en)
Healthcare Surveillance	
Visit an urgent or emergency care setting and report chief complaint	Syndromic surveillance of chief complaints from all or sentinel clinics
Have a medically attended visit for influenza-like illness	U.S. outpatient influenza-like illness surveillance network (ILINet)
Be diagnosed with a reportable disease	National electronic disease surveillance system
Be hospitalized with influenza	Influenza hospitalizations CDC's flu activity & surveillance (www.cdc.gov/flu/weekly/fluactivitysurv.htm)
Get a laboratory test for a viral pathogen	Pathogen surveillance (GermWatch: https://intermountainhealthcare.org/health-information/germwatch/)
Receive positive lab result	Electronic laboratory reporting
Mortality Surveillance	
Succumb to illness and die	Death registration system (i.e., vital records)
Child less than 5 years	Influenza-associated pediatric mortality
Resident of a city included in the 122-city system	122 cities mortality reporting system

CDC, Centers for disease control and prevention.

and then implement control measures to prevent further spread. Events that occur earlier in the chain of illness-related events may be less specific and lead to false-positive signals. The quality of the detected signals must be evaluated before they are routinely used in public health practice.

Finally, there are new opportunities to use personal health records (PHRs) and social media to monitor indicators of health status and attitudes and beliefs in the community. For example, researchers at Harvard University have shown that online social networks may be an efficient platform for bidirectional communication with and data acquisition from populations with diseases, such as diabetes, that affect public health.[16] Unadjusted aggregate A1c levels reported by users from the United States closely resembled aggregate levels reported in the 2007–08 National Health and Nutrition Examination Survey (respectively, 6.9% and 6.9%, $p = 0.85$).[16]

In a second example, researchers archived and analyzed more than 2 million Twitter posts containing keywords such as "swine flu" and "H1N1" during the 2009 outbreak. These researchers found that user-generated content from the participatory web and social media tools has the potential to serve as a near-real-time source of data to trigger a public health response and serve as a vehicle for knowledge dissemination to the public.[17] These authors believe that "infodemiology" data can be collected and analyzed in near real time and have the potential for analysis of queries from internet search engines to predict disease outbreaks (e.g., influenza); monitor

people's status updates on microblogs, such as Twitter, for syndromic surveillance; detect and quantify disparities in health information availability; and identify and monitor public health–relevant publications on the internet (e.g., anti-vaccination sites, news articles, expert-curated outbreak reports). Such automated tools may be useful for measuring information diffusion and knowledge translation and for tracking the effectiveness of health marketing campaigns.[18]

Immunization Information Systems

Immunization information systems (IISs) are confidential, population-based, computerized databases that record all immunization doses administered by participating healthcare providers to persons residing within a given geopolitical area.[19] As one of the best examples of a public health informatics application, they interact with both clinical and public health systems, have successfully implemented vocabulary and messaging standards, can be used to deliver public health decision support in a clinical setting, and provide information useful for making public health policy and programmatic decisions. IISs are an important tool in achieving and maintaining effective vaccination coverage levels greater than 90% for universally recommended vaccines among young children (Box 11.2).[20] IISs represent the successful blending of multiple standards (including data, messaging, policy, interface, privacy, and so forth) managed by multiple governing bodies (Box 11.3).

IISs are in routine use throughout the United States. In 2008, 75% of children under 6 years of age had two or more immunizations recorded in a fully operational, population-based IIS (see Objective IID-18).[20] The Healthy People goal is to reach 95% by 2020 because vaccines are among the most cost-effective clinical preventive services.[20] Childhood immunization programs provide a very high return on investment. For example, for each birth cohort vaccinated with the routine immunization schedule[21] (this includes DTap, Td, Hib, polio, MMR, Hep B, and varicella vaccines), society saves 33,000 lives, prevents 14 million cases of disease, reduces direct healthcare costs by $9.9 billion, and saves $33.4 billion in indirect costs.[20]

At the point of clinical care, an IIS can provide consolidated immunization histories for use by a vaccination provider in determining appropriate client vaccinations.[19] When children receive vaccines in a variety of clinical settings, which is common, missing records can lead to repeated vaccinations (over-immunization) and added costs. In addition, an IIS can evaluate the consolidated record and provide recommendations based on the immunization schedules published and updated annually by the CDC.[19] Since the vaccine schedules are updated every year, analysts must access the CDC website to view the most current vaccine schedules and assess their structure and complexity for implementation in a decision support application. The schedules represent rule-based logic that may initially appear simple because it is primarily based on age. However, the schedule quickly becomes more complicated when one reads the footnotes, considers the required time lapse between vaccine doses, and determines whether a different schedule is required if a child or adult is overdue and needs "catch-up" vaccines. Embedded decision support can determine the vaccines due today and forecast the vaccines required in the future to help in scheduling appointments.

At the population level, an IIS provides aggregate data about vaccinations that are useful for surveillance and program operations and can guide public health actions to improve vaccination rates and reduce vaccine-preventable disease.[19] An IIS can also provide information for health plans and healthcare providers that need to track and report quality measures, such as the HEDIS measures.[22] Finally, IISs have provided previously unrealized critical functionality in public health emergencies. For example, only days after Hurricane Katrina in September 2005, the Houston-Harris County Immunization Registry was connected to the Louisiana Immunization Network for Kids Statewide, which provided immediate access to the immunization records of children forced to evacuate the New Orleans, Louisiana, area.[23] One year later, more than 18,900 immunization records were found by persons querying the system, representing avoided vaccinations.[23] The researchers estimated a cost savings of more than $1.6 million for vaccine alone and $3.04 million for vaccine plus administration fees.[23] Similarly, during a recent measles outbreak, the registry was instrumental in helping to prioritize contact tracing efforts. Named contacts with no measles vaccination information in the registry could be prioritized for intensive phone calling efforts to ensure that appropriate control measures were implemented.

Health Information Exchange

To succeed in its mission and carry out core functions, public health entities rely on data and partnerships with healthcare and other settings in a community. Health information exchange (HIE) initiatives and organizations provide an infrastructure to improve the required communication

BOX 11.4 Potential Health Information Exchange Applications for Use in Public Health

- Mandated reporting of lab findings
- Nonmandatory reporting of lab data
- Mandated reporting of physician diagnoses
- Nonmandatory reporting of clinical data
- Public health investigation
- Clinical care in public health clinics
- Population-level quality monitoring
- Mass casualty events
- Disaster medical response
- Public health alerting: patient level
- Public health alerting: population level

Adapted from Shapiro JS, Mostashari F, Hripcsak G, Soulakis N, Kuperman G. Using health information exchange to improve public health. *Am J Public Health*. 2011:101(4):616-623.

between public health and community partners. In the past, the primary aim of an HIE was to bring unavailable clinical data from patients' disparate health records to the point of care where clinicians and their patients need it most. The motivation for exchanging health data has been to create a complete health record to address safety and quality concerns, gain efficiencies, reduce duplication of effort and control costs, notify participants about problems and potential drug seekers, and perform research. Box 11.4 includes HIE applications for achieving these public health benefits. When public health agencies participate in an HIE, they can both provide and receive value from their participation. Public health benefits from participating in an HIE include the following additional benefits:

- More timely and complete receipt of disease reports.
- Faster transmission of better information to public health case managers (for communicable disease control, newborn screening follow-up).
- Easier identification and analysis of gaps in preventive health services (immunization, Papanicolaou smears) and of patterns that could improve performance.
- Easier identification and analysis of follow-up failures (treatment of sexually transmitted diseases, environmental evaluation of lead poisoning) and of patterns that could improve performance.
- Analysis and display of geographic distribution of illness or injury to focus public health interventions or services.
- Analysis and display of the temporal and geographic epidemic spread.
- Improved ability to communicate with selected healthcare provider and patient populations.[24]

Public health also provides value to HIE partners.[24,25] Public health can provide patient information (e.g., immunization records, newborn screening results, tuberculosis clinical findings, child health clinic records) and epidemiologic information to improve diagnosis (e.g., distribution and incidence of Lyme disease to improve a clinician's estimation of

pretest probability). A public health agency may serve as a trusted neutral party for confidential health information or may maintain a community master person index that can support the HIE using identifiers generated by healthcare organizations, birth records, and other sources.[26] Public health involvement in an HIE can reduce the cost and labor of reporting. Finally, public health can provide personalized patient care information available in the community and alert healthcare providers to urgent community health issues.

Public Health Reporting

In the United States, public health reporting to perform surveillance and implement control measures has been going on since the 18th century when tavern owners were asked to report persons with illness to a local board of health. Today, public health reporting to recognize and control communicable disease in a community is a quintessential public health activity. The rules concerning the diseases that should be reported and the actions to take if reporting is necessary vary among the 50 states, may vary among cities or counties within a state, may vary by disease, and sometimes vary by reporting entity (i.e., whether the reporter is a laboratory or a clinician) and other factors. As shown in Fig. 11.6, a local health department is often the agency responsible for (1) receiving reports from laboratories, clinicians, hospitals, and other reporters (e.g., schools, daycare centers); (2) investigating the situation; and (3) implementing control measures. Information gathered during the investigation informs the public health response and helps establish whether to count the event for surveillance purposes.

Local and state agencies may share a single web-based system or the two levels of governmental public health may have separate systems. Either way, more data are collected during an investigation than are needed for "notification" from the local to state health department. The information shared is often summary information ascertained after completing the investigation. Depending on the information available from the completed investigation, a disease report may be classified as a "confirmed" or a "probable" case, for example. This classification is used when summarizing surveillance data to consistently report similar events over time while still quantifying the unconfirmed but relevant events.

The information used by the state health department for surveillance is a subset of the information gathered during an investigation. When information is sent to the CDC as a "notifiable report," the record is de-identified and filtered again to include only the data needed for national surveillance. Finally, the set of conditions included in the NNDSS is not reported in every local and state jurisdiction and does not include all conditions reported everywhere.[27]

There are many complexities associated with the detailed processes of public health reporting but the high-level process shown in Fig. 11.7 illustrates a set of activities that is commonly carried out across the United States. Informatics solutions may be applied to each step in the process. For example, the first step in public health reporting concerns the

Selected examples from Utah:
>   Within 24 hours, report anthrax, measles, hepatitis A, tuberculosis
>   Within 3 days, report AIDS, influenza-associated hospitalization

Selected examples from Maryland:
>   Immediately report botulism, hepatitis A, rabies, pertussis
>   Within 1 working day, report AIDS, chlamydia, mumps, infectious meningitis

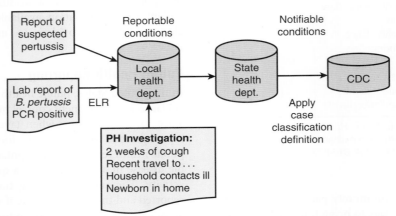

FIG 11.6 Overview of the current public health reporting process. (Copyright 2010 Catherine States. Reprinted with permission.)

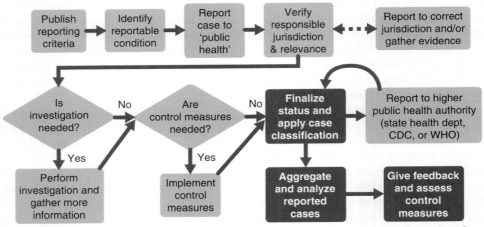

FIG 11.7 Process of public health case health reporting. (Copyright 2010 Catherine States. Reprinted with permission.)

publishing of reporting criteria (e.g., specifications). Currently, the guidance and regulations that laboratories and other reporters need to follow are described on websites and posters, and can often be found by using search terms such as "communicable disease reporting regulations for [state A or city B]." The information cannot be processed by electronic systems; it changes periodically, especially during an outbreak; and it differs among states and between states and the CDC. Case reporters must interpret the criteria expected and maintain the reporting criteria in their systems. This situation could be improved using knowledge management strategies that allow public health authorities to author structured content and disseminate the laboratory and clinical reporting specifications in both a human-readable format and a structured format for use by automated laboratory and

clinical systems. This strategy is being employed using the Reportable Condition Knowledge Management System (RCKMS), which is under development by the Council of State and Territorial Epidemiologists (CSTE).[28]

Several factors make it difficult for clinicians, laboratories, and others to identify reportable conditions. Underreporting is common when manual processes are involved and reporting relies on clinicians to remember to report.[29] Studies have shown a lack of knowledge among clinicians about reporting requirements.[30] In addition, even as the use of detection logic is becoming more common in laboratory and clinical systems, the sensitivity and specificity of logic can vary by reportable condition. For example, a single lab test result is sufficient for detecting chlamydia, a clinical diagnosis is required for identifying culture-negative tuberculosis or suspected measles, and a combination of laboratory and clinical findings is required to identify chronic hepatitis B infection.[31] There are informatics opportunities for defining and publishing detection logic (including codes such as International Classification of Diseases 10 [ICD-10], Logical Observation Identifiers Names and Codes [LOINC], and Systematized Nomenclature of Medicine-Clinical Terms [SNOMED-CT]) and using surrogate markers for reportable events, such as administration of hepatitis B immune globulin to a newborn as an indicator of an infected mother.

Challenges in the process of reporting a case or lab result to public health agencies result in delayed reporting, inefficient data gathering with incomplete reports, variable data collection, and nonstandard formats used to transfer the information (e.g., fax, phone, email, mail, web forms, electronic laboratory reports). Some of these challenges are being addressed by increased use of electronic health records (EHRs), Meaningful Use incentives, and Health Level Seven (HL7) standards.

While these factors improve the capabilities for the sender, there are also challenges on the receiving end of the transaction. Health departments must receive, sort, filter, deduplicate, and consolidate information that arrives "at their doorstep" via fax, phone, online web forms, and electronic messaging systems and from records routed from their state or other local health department colleagues using statewide electronic disease surveillance systems. Health departments often manage a large volume of reports using manual processes.

For example, in an observational study of workflow in a local health department, 3454 reportable conditions were manually entered into an electronic data system during an 18-month period of time.[32] In a prospective evaluation of the information being received, 18% of the reports were for other counties, 3% were not reportable, 16% were duplicates, and 18% were updates on previously reported cases.[32] Personnel resources are used to manage all of the paper arriving to find the new, relevant information among all incoming paper.

In an ideal world, a health department would receive complete information in a timely manner only once and updates and duplicates would be managed automatically. There are numerous informatics opportunities to do the following:

- Enable the use of specifications (computable logic) to define where and how reports should be sent, the urgency of reporting, and the information to include in a report.
- Automate information extraction of additional information in the EHR.
- Improve standardization of message structure and content.
- Enable secure information exchange.
- Create public health information systems to receive case reports and allow access by local and state public health entities.

Systems are being built to receive laboratory reports, but this is only part of the information required to manage persons with communicable diseases in municipalities, counties, and states.

The processes associated with performing an investigation and implementing control measures (such as excluding a person with salmonella from food service or daycare or vaccinating contacts of a person with meningitis) can be complex. Decisions must be made on incomplete and evolving information, and guidelines are often ambiguous. The situation could be improved by

- Automated linkage between clinical and electronic lab reports with information concerning updated or redundant reports
- Improved quality of the information in a report (e.g., include additional associated lab findings needed for investigation)
- Improved tools to explore the existing information[33]
- Decision support tools that improve the management of new information and apply guidelines

The processes associated with aggregating information across jurisdictions and sharing subsets of information with a higher authority could be addressed using new strategies. Currently, aggregation occurs by copying information and sending it up the chain. However, "central" aggregation is defined differently among different stakeholders and does not adequately support sudden unanticipated needs. Currently, ad hoc queries must be initiated or informal communication and data aggregation may be required. A goal for future systems should be the ability to perform dynamic aggregation across jurisdictions and to access complete data in their native environments, with appropriate permissions (Fig. 11.8). In addition, future systems should allow surveillance data to be more accessible to healthcare systems and the community for decision support in near real time.

In summary, case reporting and management will benefit from computable knowledge managed and served by public health authorities about what, how, where, and when to report; automated event detection; electronic, standardized information exchange; improved systems for receiving and integrating case reports; and the ability to access disparate systems with appropriate permissions to dynamically aggregate data across jurisdictions and respond to new situations, data, and priorities.

CONCLUSIONS AND FUTURE PUBLIC HEALTH INFORMATICS STRATEGIES

Transforming Practice With New Strategies

As discussed in this chapter, public health IT reflects the division of authority for population health between national, state, and local governments. In the past, this division was less important because records systems were largely paper based. Each department could have its own approach to information management and the departments to which it reported or with which it shared information had to manually convert information from one format to another. Given the complexities of data collection in the past, public health practitioners focused on information gathering to ensure the validity of the information supply chain for its own program. There was no

Goal:
• Dynamic aggregation across jurisdictions
• Access complete data in their native environments

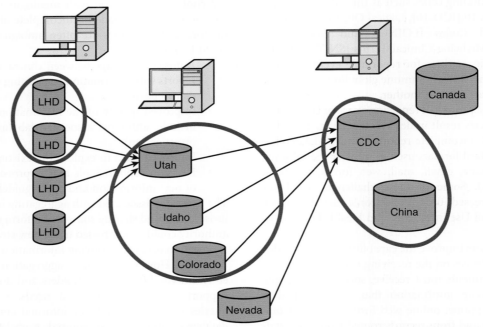

FIG 11.8 An example of dynamic aggregation across local health departments (LHDs) and state and national departments of health. (Copyright 2010 Catherine States. Reprinted with permission.)

way to reuse data across programs and it was not deemed highly important since the costs of reuse were almost as high as the costs of primary data collection and the validity of "reused" data could not be assured.

As public health practice moves into the future, the concept of the information supply chain needs to evolve toward an alternative model: an information ecology. Public health departments will receive, from a variety of sources, data that are repurposed for population health uses. Electronic data elements collected for one purpose (as part of one information supply chain) will be linked with other data to create an integrated environment. The old paradigm of public health programs setting up systems that measured specific factors, with primary data collection for surveillance, will be replaced by systems that generate healthcare, environmental, and commerce data that are relevant to public health. Perhaps the biggest change for public health is the idea that public health systems need to "give to get." In the past, federal, state, and local governments used legislative authority to mandate reporting to public health. Over the past few years, the government has increased efforts to implement syndromic surveillance by incentivizing healthcare providers to report emergency room data and other data to public health departments through the Meaningful Use regulatory process.[34] Efforts to require transmission of these data are controversial for both hospitals and provider organizations because of the cost involved and the lack of return for their efforts.

In the future, public health departments will need to partner with other data producers, add value to the data received, and republish those data to contribute to the local information ecology. An example of this approach concerns public health alerting in EHRs. Working with GE Healthcare, the CDC demonstrated an alternative approach based on a web services model that integrates syndromic surveillance in clinical workflows using decision support.[35] When a clinician sees a patient with a new complaint, he or she considers the following question: "Could this patient's symptoms be caused by an infectious disease?" Public health departments might answer this question by publishing "disease weather maps" for their local regions that clinicians could consult.[36] This type of decision support, whereby community-level information is summarized and displayed, is important but insufficient. Work can go further to create an interdependent system.

What would be most useful to clinicians is an individual specific interpretation of the current "epidemiologic weather." How could this be obtained? What if, instead of merely sending data to local public health departments when required, information systems could harness the power of computerized knowledge systems to highlight patterns of data indicative of the types of symptoms a patient might be experiencing to assist the practitioner in determining whether they match the pattern of a known public health problem? At the public health department, data would be stored to track the nature of symptoms in a community and the individual data would be matched to public health alerts in the region. If the symptoms are consistent with a known problem, the sending electronic records system might receive an alert from the public health system through secure messaging processes, informing the clinician that the patient may be part of a public health outbreak. This type of cycle defines information ecology: the public health department integrates with clinical care and provides interpretations of data generated by and sent from healthcare providers, which justifies the provider's costs of extraction and transmission of information.

In addition to increasing access to data from healthcare systems, the public health system has the opportunity to use data from an increasingly connected environment to measure and affect health in the community. Mobile devices with global positioning system (GPS) locators are tools for people to find their way, but could also be tools for governments to assess how active their citizens are in daily life. Do the regulations that try to make neighborhoods more walkable result in more people walking? In the past, observers would use clipboards and might sample streets or survey persons about how often they walk. But now a more efficient and accurate method for determining whether people are walking might be to see how many phones are moving around the community at walking speeds. Walkability might be defined by the patterns in which the phones move. Cellular phone companies have these data and they sell them for commercial use. Legislators and other policy makers need to consider how private business can be incentivized (or regulated) to provide this type of information to public health.

Similarly, in the past, understanding dietary patterns of a community has required extensive in-person or mail surveys to ascertain food consumption. These methods are expensive and time consuming and limit the use of such data for public health purposes. An alternative approach that uses existing sources of data to inform population dietary habits would be to analyze shoppers' purchasing habits. Many stores use shopper cards to track purchasing decisions and behaviors. These same data could be used by public health officials to monitor consumption of fresh fruits and vegetables, salt, and sodas and to identify other dietary needs and risks. The use of such data raises many privacy issues at an individual level.

However, public health operations may not always need individual-level data. Many policy issues could be addressed by geocoding the data and anonymizing data clustering at a home or work location. If one can understand that a particular neighborhood is a "hot spot" for sugary beverage use or salt intake, then targeted efforts can be made to work within the community to change the community's values and habits to promote health. As described earlier, the population perspective assumes that individuals have levels of risk that are reflected in their community. Disease prevention strategies focused on a community do not require that public health officials know that Mrs. Jones drinks too much soda. Public health officials need to know where to conduct an education campaign in schools to reverse trends of students who often prefer sugared beverages over healthier ones.

Advancing the Technical Infrastructure

The future of public health requires new advanced information technologies and infrastructures. However, public health departments, particularly local health departments, are resource-challenged environments. Departments often do not have the IT resources to take on new initiatives to connect themselves to clinical care systems or other sources of data, such as schools or occupational health entities that could provide the value-added capabilities discussed above. State governments may provide funding for IT, but it may be only for specific programs to capture very limited data. Likewise, federal public health programs provide their less-funded state colleagues with task-specific IT. While the availability of such technology might provide secondary benefits to local and state public health departments, the funding typically comes with contractual requirements that prevent technology resources from being used for other tasks. How can this problem be addressed and resolved? How can there be a future for public health informatics if resources are a continuing problem?

The CDC's first effort at helping the public health community to coordinate information management technologies was the Public Health Information Network (PHIN). This program proposed a set of communication and vocabulary standards for public health software designed to promote interoperability and support reuse of information. The PHIN program had a number of elements, including a standardized vocabulary based on the HL7 version 3.0 Reference Information Model (HL7 v3 RIM), solutions for composing value sets of standard codes for applications, an interoperability solution for transforming messages from one vocabulary to another, and a message transport solution called the Public Health Information Network Messaging System (PHIN-MS) for securely sending data from one public health department to another.[37] The success of the PHIN program was limited, except with regard to its transport solution, which was widely adopted. In general, the advantages of adopting one set of standards for vocabulary for public health systems were offset by the costs of implementation and the lack of fit between the HL7 v3 RIM vocabulary model and public health workflows. Public health departments found it easier and cheaper to continue to use their existing information management tools than to develop new tools based on the CDC standards or to convert existing tools to those specifications. PHIN continues to evolve as a program.[38] However, the question of whether a standards-based approach alone can achieve the ends of interoperability at a reduced cost remains open.

Standards are critical, but by themselves may not be adequate to provide the level of support needed to advance public health informatics. A flawed environment for acquiring systems results in agencies duplicating each other's efforts to develop and implement systems. Jurisdictions often implement proprietary, stand-alone systems that preclude data exchange, which is fundamentally important for surveillance and two-way communication. An alternative to individual jurisdictions creating the specifications for and purchasing software on their own, with inherent inefficiencies, may be the use of open source and collaborative development methods. Collaborative development can take many forms. In a project funded by the Robert Wood Johnson Foundation, a group of state laboratories at state public health departments collaborated to develop a set of shared business process specifications for a laboratory information system.[39] These shared specifications were then used to guide shared open source development of a laboratory information system, where different jurisdictions assumed responsibility for different modules of the final product. This same group went on to work collaboratively to develop its own information exchange solutions and worked as a group to modify the CDC's PHIN-MS software to support routing hubs (PHIN-MS was initially designed to support only point-to-point communications).

A service-oriented architecture (SOA), explained in Chapter 5, and open source methods may be useful in shared development. If a set of standard functions based on an enterprise architecture view can be developed to support public health applications, then these components could be reused to support a wide variety of additional public health applications. This concept is the foundation of the "service-oriented" systems approach. A critical issue is developing a set of modular programs designed to work together. These might include data transport tools like PHIN-MS, interoperability engines, standardized vocabularies, databases, master person indexes, and other critical components. Importantly, this set of components should be open source software that is available to potential developers at low or no cost. In an open source environment, public health departments with significant capabilities for developing software can work together to advance the field as a whole.

Currently the goal of many vendors of public health information systems (and other software systems as well) is to attempt to lock departments into proprietary systems, guaranteeing future revenue streams. Open source methodologies can help to prevent this situation. Some examples of successful open source software systems are[40]

- The community version of the TriSano case management application;
- OpenELIS, which is the public health laboratory information system described above; and
- OpenMRS, an enterprise-level medical records application that is widely used in Africa for public health applications.

Many public health departments, particularly local ones, have no significant capabilities to develop IT and typically lack the resources to hire vendors to support development or customization efforts. One approach to this lack of capability may be to move public health systems to the "cloud." As explained in Chapter 5, cloud computing systems migrate the location of software to a remote site where resources can be shared by different users. Examples of cloud-based software systems include Amazon.com, Facebook, and other web applications. These applications operate as software as a service (SaaS), where the developer attempts to present an integrated single application or a tightly integrated suite of applications.[41] BioSense 2.0[42] is an example of a SaaS application for public health. In this application, each state can receive, parse, store, and analyze data streams from the EHR systems in hospital emergency departments, as required by the government's

Meaningful Use program. Without this service, each state develops its own infrastructure to receive emergency department data. BioSense 2.0 allows states to rapidly develop procedures and use data sent in a prescribed format from the healthcare system, without the requirement to create their own infrastructure to manage the information. The system also allows states to share data across jurisdictions when necessary. For example, when a Super Bowl game draws large numbers of fans from cities in one region of the country to another, this creates a need to link emergency room data from those cities to detect outbreaks that may occur after the event, when people have returned home.

The approach to computing that may be the most relevant to public health is platform as a service (PaaS).[43] PaaS architecture is based on virtualization of an entire computer operating system. For example, a PaaS system might allow a user to access a functional "PC" (entire version of the latest version of Windows, for example) on a remote computer. This "PC" might have the entire library of relevant and most up-to-date public health programs on it. PaaS architecture would allow each public health department to select the applications it deems most relevant to its own workflows. These programs should draw on a public health SOA that would facilitate the creation of new public health applications. Applications could share databases and services for transforming and managing data. Because the operating system for each PC is identical, the task of configuring and managing software would be greatly simplified. A suite of applications could be created based on off-the-shelf components that work well together and public health departments could access and use this suite from any location with high-speed internet service. Moreover, the task of interoperability between users and jurisdictions would become greatly simplified as the network settings and application configurations would be known and standardized. Importantly, the degree of standardization afforded by PaaS architecture might help to create a market for public health applications that would rapidly foster improvement and expansion through competition among vendors. Lenert and Sundwall provide further discussion of issues related to the market and to SaaS versus PaaS systems for public health.[43]

Another future direction for public health informatics includes the integration of community-based information into EHRs or other aggregate databases. For example, Bazemore and colleagues recommend including community social, economic, occupational, and environmental factors that influence population health.[44] These factors are termed "community vital signs," and data are available from sources such as the U.S. Census surveys. Integrating these data would provide context-informed care in the future.

In conclusion, this chapter described the importance and unique features of public health practice and differentiated public health practice from clinical practice. The social, technical, and political challenges of public health and public health informatics were highlighted. The value of informatics tools in supporting public health's unique needs and mission was highlighted, and existing systems were reviewed. Current major public health informatics applications, such as surveillance and IIS, were described. The supporting workflows associated with these systems and the value of the IT, decision support, and standards that are necessary to make the systems work were reviewed along with the strengths and challenges associated with developing an information ecology. This chapter then reviewed the future strategies underpinning the public health information infrastructure. Increasing use of EHRs, standards to improve information exchange, social networking tools, and cloud-based and mobile computing methods will transform the way that public health accesses and uses information to improve the health of populations.

REFERENCES

1. National Center for Health Statistics. *Health, United States, 2015: with special feature on racial and ethnic health disparities.* Hyattsville, MD; 2016. http://www.cdc.gov/nchs/hus/index.htm.
1a. National Center for Health Statistics. *Health, United States, 2010: With Special Feature on Death and Dying.* Hyattsville, MD: Centers for Disease Control and Prevention; 2011.
2. Bunker JP, Frazier HS, Mosteller F. Improving health: measuring effects of medical care. *Milbank Q.* 1994;72:225–258.
3. Centers for Disease Control and Prevention. Ten great public health achievements—United States, 2001–2010; *MMWR Morb Mortal Wkly Rep.* 2011;60(19):619–623.
4. Centers for Disease Control and Prevention. Achievements in public health, 1900-1999. tobacco use—United States, 1900–1999. *MMWR Morb Mortal Wkly Rep.* 1999;48(43):986–993.
5. DHHS. *The Health Consequences of Smoking: 50 Years of Progress. A Report of the Surgeon General.* Atlanta, GA: U.S. Department of Health and Human Services, Centers for Disease Control and Prevention, National Center for Chronic Disease Prevention and Health Promotion, Office on Smoking and Health; 2014. Printed with corrections, January 2014. http://www.surgeongeneral.gov/library/reports/50-years-of-progress/50-years-of-progress-by-section.html
6. California Department of Public Health, California Tobacco Control Program. *State Health Officer's Report on E-Cigarettes: A Community Health Threat*; 2015. Sacramento, CA, https://www.cdph.ca.gov/programs/tobacco/Documents/Media/State%20Health-e-cig%20report.pdf.
7. Schroeder SA. We can do better: improving the health of the American people. *N Engl J Med.* 2007;357(12):1221–1228.
8. Mokdad AH, Marks JS, Stroup DF, Gerberding JL. Actual causes of death in the United States, 2000. *J Amer Med Assoc.* 2004;291(10):1238–1245.
9. *Public Health Data Standards Consortium.* White paper: building a roadmap for health information systems interoperability for public health; 2008. http://www.ihe.net/Technical_Framework/upload/IHE_PHDSC_Public_Health_White_Paper_2007_10_11.pdf/.
10. Committee for the Study of the Future of Public Health. *The Future of Public Health.* Washington, DC: National Academy Press; 1988.
11. National Center for Health Statistics. *Summary of NCHS Surveys and Data Collection Systems.* Centers for Disease Control and Prevention; 2015. http://www.cdc.gov/nchs/data/factsheets/factsheet_summary.htm.
12. Committee on Assuring the Health of the Public in the 21st Century. *The Future of the Public's Health in the 21st Century.* Washington, DC: The National Academies Press; 2002.
13. Centers for Disease Control and Prevention. HIPAA privacy rule and public health: guidance from CDC and the U.S. Department of Health and Human Services. *MMWR Morb Mortal Wkly Rep.* 2003;52:1–12.
14. Smith PF, Hadler JL, Stanbury M, Rolfs RT, Hopkins RS. "Blueprint version 2.0": updating public health surveillance for the 21st century. *J Public Health Manag Pract.* 2013;19(3):231–239. http://dx.doi.org/10.1097/PHH.0b013e318262906e.
15. Centers for Disease Control and Prevention. Updated guidelines for evaluating public health surveillance systems: recommendations from the Guidelines Working Group. *MMWR Recomm Rep.* 2001;50(RR-13):1–35.
16. Weitzman ER, Adida B, Kelemen S, Mandl KD. Sharing data for public health research by members of an international online diabetes social network. *PLoS One.* 2011;6(4):e19256.
17. Chew C, Eysenbach G. Pandemics in the age of Twitter: content analysis of tweets during the 2009 H1N1 outbreak. *PLoS One.* 2010;5(11):e14118.
18. Eysenbach G. Infodemiology and infoveillance: framework for an emerging set of public health informatics methods to analyze search, communication and publication behavior on the Internet. *J Med Internet Res.* 2009;11(1):e11.
19. Centers for Disease Control and Prevention (CDC). *Immunization information systems;* 2015. CDC; 2015. http://www.cdc.gov/vaccines/programs/iis/index.html.
20. Office of Disease Prevention and Health Promotion, National Center for Health Statistics. *Immunization and infectious diseases*; HealthyPeople.gov; 2015. http://www.healthypeople.gov/2020/topicsobjectives2020/default.aspx.
21. CDC (Centers for Disease Control). Immunization schedules CDC. http://www.cdc.gov/vaccines/schedules/index.html.
22. National Committee for Quality Assurance (NCQA). *HEDIS measures.* NCQA; 2015. http://www.ncqa.org/HEDISQualityMeasurement/QualityMeasurementProducts.aspx.
23. Boom JA, Dragsbaek AC, Nelson CS. The success of an immunization information system in the wake of Hurricane Katrina. *Pediatrics.* 2007;119(6):1213.
24. Foldy S, Ross DA. *Public Health Opportunities in Health Information Exchange.* Atlanta, GA: Public Health Informatics Institute; 2005.
25. Shapiro JS. Using health information exchange to improve public health. *Am J Public Health.* 2011;101:616–623.
26. Duncan J, Eilbeck K, Narus SP, Clyde S, Thornton S, Staes C. Building an ontology for identity resolution in healthcare and public health. *Online J Public Health Inform.* 2015;7(2). http://dx.doi.org/10.5210/ojphi.v7i2.6010. http://ojphi.org/ojs/index.php/ojphi/article/view/6010.
27. Centers for Disease Control and Prevention (CDC). *National Notifiable Diseases Surveillance System (NNDSS).* CDC; 2015. http://www.cdc.gov/nndss.
28. Council of State and Territorial Epidemiologists (CSTE). *Surveillance / Informatics: Reportable Condition Knowledge Management System.* CSTE; 2015. http://www.cste.org/group/RCKMS.
29. Overhage JM, Grannis S, McDonald CJ. Comparison of the completeness and timeliness of automated electronic laboratory reporting and spontaneous reporting of notifiable conditions. *Am J Public Health.* 2008;98(2):344–350.
30. Staes CJ, Gesteland P, Allison M, et al. Urgent care physician's knowledge and attitude about public health reporting and pertussis control measures: implications for informatics. *J Public Health Manag Pract.* 2009;15(6):1–8.

31. Klompas M, Haney G, Church D, Lazarus R, Hou X, Platt R. Automated identification of acute hepatitis B using electronic medical record data to facilitate public health surveillance. *PLoS One.* 2008;3(7):e2626.

32. Rajeev D, Staes C, Evans RS, et al. Evaluation of HL7 v2.5.1 electronic case reports transmitted from a healthcare enterprise to public health. *AMIA Annu Symp Proc.* 2001;2011:1144–1152.

33. Livnat Y, Gesteland P, Benuzillo J, et al. Epinome: a novel workbench for epidemic investigation and analysis of search strategies in public health practice. *AMIA Annu Symp Proc.* 2010;2010:647–651.

34. Federal Register. *Medicare and Medicaid Programs; Electronic Health Record Incentive Program-Stage 3 and Modifications to Meaningful Use in 2015 through 2017;* 2015. https://www.federalregister.gov/articles/2015/10/16/2015-25595/medicare-and-medicaid-programs-electronic-health-record-incentive-program-stage-3-and-modifications#t-11.

35. Garrett NY, Mishra N, Nichols B, Staes CJ, Akin C, Safran C. Characterization of public health alerts and their suitability for alerting in electronic health record systems. *J Public Health Manag Pract.* 2011;17(1):77–83.

36. Gesteland PH, Livnat Y, Galli N, Samore MH, Gundlapalli AV. The EpiCanvas infectious disease weather map: an interactive visual exploration of temporal and spatial correlations. *J Am Med Inform Assoc.* 2012;19(6):954–959.

37. Loonsk JW, McGarvey SR, Conn LA, Johnson J. The Public Health Information Network (PHIN) preparedness initiative. *J Am Med Inform Assoc.* 2006;13(1):1–4.

38. Centers for Disease Control and Prevention (CDC). *Public Health Information Network (PHIN) Tools and Resources;* 2015. http://www.cdc.gov/phin/index.html.

39. Public Health Informatics Institute (PHII). *The LIMS Project: Summary of Evaluation Findings.* PHII; 2007. http://www.phii.org/resources?search_api_views_fulltext=LIMS&sort=search_api_relevance%20DESC.

40. *Open Health News.* Software & Information Technology (IT); 2015. http://www.openhealthnews.com/resources/software-information-technology-it.

41. Badger L, Grance T, Patt-Corner R, Voas J. *Cloud Computing Synopsis and Recommendations of the National Institute of Standards and Technology;* 2013. Special Publication 800-146, http://csrc.nist.gov/publications/nistpubs/800-146/sp800-146.pdf.

42. Kass-Hout TA, Gallagher K, Foldy S, Buehler JW. A functional public health surveillance system. *Am J Public Health.* 2012;102 (9):e1–e2.

43. Lenert L, Sundwall DN. Public health surveillance and Meaningful Use regulations: a crisis of opportunity. *Am J Public Health.* 2012;102(3):e1–e7.

44. Bazemore AW, Cottrell EK, Gold R, et al. "Community vital signs": incorporating geocoded social determinants into electronic records to promote patient and population health. *J Am Med Inform Assoc.* 2016;23(2):407–412.

DISCUSSION QUESTIONS

1. How might you begin to develop a data and information exchange between acute care, subacute care, and home health settings that would support the work of public health? Do such systems already exist?

2. Monitoring population health status is a central public health activity. A variety of survey systems, such as the CDC's National Health and Nutrition Examination Survey (NHANES) and National Health Interview Survey (NHIS), as well as state and national reporting systems, such as the Behavioral Risk Factor Surveillance System (BRFSS), Pregnancy Risk Assessment Monitoring System (PRAMS), and National Electronic Disease Surveillance System (NEDSS), provide public health practitioners with the ability to assess health trends, identify and respond to emerging health hazards, and guide development of interventions and policies that address serious health conditions such as obesity, smoking, and diabetes. With the proliferation of EHRs within acute and ambulatory care systems, how much of this survey activity do you think can be folded in under routine data collection and exchange activities?

3. The primary goal of public health is to affect population health and ensure a healthy community. How might you see public health nurses using web-based tools to reach, manage, and educate populations of patients residing in targeted communities?

4. Part of the job of the public health informatician is to develop the tools required to translate between clinical and public health worldviews as they relate to information system development and data sharing across the specialties. As a clinical leader, by what means would you advocate to enable this sharing?

5. Personal health records are technological tools that are being implemented within the acute care setting to enable data exchange with EHRs and to encourage patient activation in healthcare. How might you foresee the use of patient-entered data from a PHR or patient portal as a public health surveillance tool?

CASE STUDY

You have been hired as an informatician at a state health department. The health department is developing systems to receive laboratory and clinical case reports from clinical settings, such as hospitals and doctor's offices. Your state has had an immunization registry in operation for several years and has been successful in getting cooperation from healthcare settings to send data to the system.

Discussion Questions

1. Why is the system for reporting immunizations and receiving results at the health department so successful, particularly in comparison to the struggles you are observing as the health department sets up its laboratory and case reporting systems?

2. What is the difference between the information required to report the administration of an immunization and the information required to report a person with a communicable disease?

3. What standard vocabulary is used to code a vaccine name and how is this vocabulary different from the LOINC or SNOMED-CT vocabularies required for laboratory and clinical case reporting?

4. What is the value proposition for a healthcare provider to participate in an immunization registry?

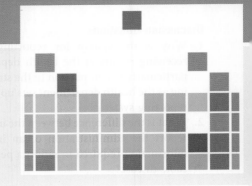

12

The Engaged ePatient

Sally Okun and Christine A. Caligtan

The ePatient is and will continue to be a pivotal force in accelerating the healthcare system's adaptation to the ever-evolving world of technology, information management, and communication.

OBJECTIVES

At the completion of this chapter, the reader will be prepared to:

1. List at least three "e" terms used to describe ePatients.
2. Explain the driving forces behind the emergence and continuing evolution of the ePatient movement.
3. Discuss the characteristics of digital healthcare consumers.
4. Describe how the quantified self uses health-related data.
5. Analyze the implications of ePatients for clinical practice.
6. Identify technological innovations likely to be used in routine practice by clinicians in the future when caring for patients.

KEY TERMS

ABSTRACT ❖

The term *ePatient* was coined long before the advent of the internet to describe patients who take an active role in their health and healthcare by being equipped, enabled, empowered, and engaged. Today, ePatients connect electronically to a vast array of digital health information and resources, such as traditional chat rooms, support sites, health-related social media, patient-to-patient research-based social networks, mobile devices, and wearable sensors. ePatients understand the value of engaging in a collaborative partnership with their healthcare providers and view the integration of participatory healthcare across the U.S. healthcare system as essential. The ePatient is and will continue to be a pivotal force in accelerating the healthcare system's adaptation to the ever-evolving world of technology, information management, and communication.

HISTORICAL BACKGROUND AND DRIVERS OF THE ePATIENT EVOLUTION

ePatient as a Pioneering Concept

As early as the 1960s clinical researchers[1] used emerging technology to test computer-based patient-driven medical interviews. Slack's philosophical view of "patient power" coupled with his belief that computers had a place in medical practice were controversial at the time. Often asked, "Will your computer replace the doctor?" Slack's response was as true then as it is today: "Any doctor who can be replaced by a computer deserves to be" (p. S135).[2] Empowering patients with innovative tools is about fostering effective partnerships with their healthcare providers that lead to better outcomes. Empowering consumers with innovative health and wellness tracking tools is about giving individuals the opportunity to lead more proactive and fulfilling lives.[3]

The use of the term *ePatient* predates the availability of online medical resources. In 1975 another pioneering physician, author, and researcher, Thomas Ferguson, was interested in the empowered health consumer. Ferguson coined the term *ePatient* and characterized ePatients as people who are equipped, enabled, empowered, and engaged in decisions about their health and healthcare.[4] By the early 1990s, with the rapid emergence of personal computers and the World Wide Web, Ferguson recognized the power and potential for consumer use of online health resources. In *Looking Ahead: Online Health & the Search for Sustainable Healthcare*, Ferguson wrote:

> The 21st Century will be the Age of the Net-empowered epatient, and … the health resources of today will evolve into even more robust and capable medical guidance systems which will allow growing numbers of epatients to play an increasingly important role in medical care. Online patients will increasingly manage their own healthcare and will contribute to the care of others. Medical professionals will increasingly be called upon to serve as coaches, supporters, and coordinators of self-managed care.[5]

Ferguson's work is largely seen as the impetus of the **ePatient movement** and his early observations, ideas, and recommendations continue to resonate. Today an **ePatient** is characterized as one who uses technology to actively partake in his or her healthcare and manages the responsibility for his or her own health and wellness.[6] ePatients are digitally enabled, seeking information, sharing their knowledge, and connecting with others. An ePatient manages health decisions on a daily basis and uses the internet and digital devices to supplement his or her health journey. The collection of data and knowledge from these sources helps to organize and support ePatients with contextual information and medical vocabulary necessary to converse with their healthcare providers.

The first evolutionary phase of the connected ePatient movement occurred as access to health information and health-related services became increasingly available through electronic means. By late 1999 the term **eHealth** emerged in the lexicon as a way to describe electronic communication and information technology (IT) related to health information and processes accessible through online means.[7]

In 2001, eHealth was described as "the use of emerging information and communication technology, especially the internet, to improve or enable health and health care" (p. 8).[8] Conceptually, the term *eHealth* was considered a bridge for both the clinical and the nonclinical sectors capable of supporting health-related tools for individuals and populations. For this potential to be fully realized, Eng believed that eHealth initiatives require integrated information systems that use common data elements and infrastructure standards that can serve multiple stakeholders, more commonly known now as interoperability. The implications of interoperability are more fully discussed in Chapters 5 and 22.

The term eHealth remains a broad concept used to describe internet or web-based activities that relate to healthcare, yet no consensus about the definition exists among researchers, policy-makers, clinicians, or patients.[9] Pagliaro et al. identified 36 different definitions of eHealth in publications and internet sources.[10] In the final analysis they felt that the definition put forth by Eng, augmented by Eysenbach's definition, appropriately represented eHealth and captured the fluid nature of emergence as a defining characteristic.[11] Eysenbach defined eHealth as:

> …an emerging field of medical informatics, referring to the organization and delivery of health services and information using the internet and related technologies. In a broader sense, the term characterizes not only a technical development, but also a new way of working, an attitude, and a commitment for networked global thinking, to improve healthcare locally, regionally, and worldwide by using information and communication technology.[11]

In addition to viewing eHealth as the delivery of health information to health professionals and consumers via the internet and telecommunications, the World Health Organization includes harnessing the power of the internet and e-commerce to improve public health services and business practices within healthcare.[12]

Our Connected World

This transformation must be considered in the context of the emergence of massive amounts of information on the World Wide Web, connected via the internet. Traversing the 20th and 21st centuries, the proliferation in the use of the internet has had an unprecedented impact on access to information, sharing, and connectedness; moreover, it has been a driving force in the emergence of the 21st-century consumer.

Just as growth in the number of individuals using online resources is assured, disparities between internet access "haves" and "have-nots" exist in large part due to cost, literacy, computer skills, language, and education. For some, the lack of access is intentional. It is a conscious decision not to use the internet. Nonetheless, the volume of internet users is staggering. In 1995 there were an estimated 16 million users. By 1998, when the search engine Google was launched, there were 147 million users. In 2001, only a decade after the graphic browser was conceived, 500 million users were online. By 2015 the number of global internet users surpassed 3 billion (Fig. 12.1).[13] A report by Ericsson, a global communications technology company, suggests that by 2021 there will be 6.3 billion people with smartphone subscriptions. The digital divide will continue to narrow as technology companies expand free and low-cost broadband access to those traditionally underserved.[14] A partnership led by Facebook and internet.org, is working to bring access to every person on earth, beginning with millions of people in sub-Saharan Africa via satellite.[15]

The emergence of the internet as a valuable tool for health and healthcare became better understood at the turn of the century. In *The Future of the Internet in Health Care: Five-Year Forecast*, Mittman and Cain declared, "Health care has discovered the internet and the internet has discovered health care!" (p. 1).[16] Between 1999 and 2001 the Institute

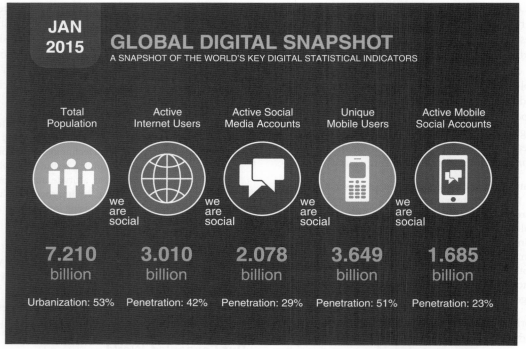

FIG 12.1 Global digital snapshot. (Data from We Are Social's Compendium of Global Digital Statistics. 2015. Copyright 2015, We Are Social.)

of Medicine (IOM) issued two reports published by the Committee on the Quality of Health Care in America that shed light on significant safety and quality issues related to health and healthcare in the United States. These reports continue to influence the emergence of a learning health system that is more patient-centric. Patients and those close to them are being included as integral members of the healthcare team, and technology is highlighted as a critical component for improving safety and quality. The IOM report, titled *Crossing the Quality Chasm: A New Health System for the 21st Century*, focused attention more broadly on the multiple dimensions of quality and safety concerns in need of fundamental change across the U.S. healthcare system.[17] To narrow the quality chasm, the report offered six specific areas that represent what healthcare ought to be for all Americans. Healthcare should be safe, effective, patient centered, timely, efficient, and equitable. In addition, the report provided "ten simple rules for the 21st century health care system" that describe what patients should expect from their healthcare (Box 12.1).

While the rules in the IOM report align well with the interests of ePatients, the report's most important contribution to the ePatient movement is the attention paid to using IT to improve the quality and safety of healthcare. This theme resonates throughout the report with recommendations that directly support the previously mentioned six aims. The report highlights the potential benefits of harnessing health-related applications for the internet that include consumer health, clinical care, public health, professional education, research, and administrative and financial transactions. Since the report, a number of health-related improvements have been initiated in both public and private sectors. The

Office of the National Coordinator (ONC) for health information technology released a report in 2015 that builds upon the messages in the IOM reports by providing an interoperability roadmap and long-term vision for connecting health and care across the United States.[18]

The recognition of safety and quality flaws in the U.S. healthcare system led many patients and those close to them to become vigilant advocates. Access to the internet, coupled with simplified search solutions offered by companies such as Alphabet Inc. (Google), made looking for health-related information online more feasible for an increasing number of people. Thus began the new generation of ePatients who started searching online for health information to learn more about their symptoms and conditions and to better understand the options available to treat and manage them.

An enduring source of rich data about the use of online resources is the Pew Research Center's Internet & American Life Project, which began to monitor basic online activities in 1999 to understand who was using the internet and what people were doing while online. Susannah Fox, named Chief Technology Officer for Health and Human Services in 2015, previously led the Pew Internet & American Life Project, which explored the impact of the internet on families, communities, work and home, daily life, education, healthcare, and civic and political life.[19] Findings from the Pew reports have shown that health information remains a popular online pursuit. In February 2011, the report found that 8 in 10 internet users look online for health information, making it the third most popular online activity, following e-mail and using a search engine.[20,21] In *Health Online 2013,* Pew researchers found that the internet is being used as a diagnostic tool by one third of U.S. adults.[22]

BOX 12.1   What Patients Should Expect From Their Healthcare

1. Beyond patient visits: You will have the care you need when you need it ... whenever you need it. You will find help in many forms, not just in face-to-face visits. You will find help on the Internet, on the telephone, from many sources, by many routes, in the form you want it.
2. Individualization: You will be known and respected as an individual. Your choices and preferences will be sought and honored. The usual system of care will meet most of your needs. When your needs are special, the care will adapt to meet you on your own terms.
3. Control: The care system will take control only if and when you freely give permission.
4. Information: You can know what you wish to know, when you wish to know it. Your medical record is yours to keep, to read, and to understand. The rule is: "Nothing about you without you."
5. Science: You will have care based on the best available scientific knowledge. The system promises you excellence as its standard. Your care will not vary illogically from doctor to doctor or from place to place. The system will promise you all

the care that can help you, and will help you avoid care that cannot help you.
6. Safety: Errors in care will not harm you. You will be safe in the care system.
7. Transparency: Your care will be confidential, but the care system will not keep secrets from you. You can know whatever you wish to know about the care that affects you and your loved ones.
8. Anticipation: Your care will anticipate your needs and will help you find the help you need. You will experience proactive help, not just reactions, to help you restore and maintain your health.
9. Value: Your care will not waste your time or money. You will benefit from constant innovations, which will increase the value of care to you.
10. Cooperation: Those who provide care will cooperate and coordinate their work fully with each other and with you. The walls between professions and institutions will crumble, so that your experiences will become seamless. You will never feel lost.

From National Research Council. *Crossing the Quality Chasm: A New Health System for the 21st Century.* Washington, DC: The National Academies Press, Copyright 2001, National Academy of Sciences.

For those interested in online health-related resources, the internet is much more than a unidirectional source of information. Web 1.0, as the early functionality is now known, provided information based on simplified search parameters; for healthcare resources it was known as Health 1.0. Since then, Web 2.0 has become available and is more sophisticated, with social engagement, interaction, and networking capabilities. Social media platforms such as Facebook, later followed by others such as Twitter, Instagram, Pinterest, and LinkedIn, demonstrate the power of the internet to support the formation of spontaneous social, commercial, and political groups rapidly and in real time.[23] For ePatients, Web 2.0 brought about Health 2.0, allowing previously unavailable interactive communication with other patients and healthcare resources across the country and around the world. Online patient communities range from traditional chat rooms and listservs to more formal social networking platforms. Patient-to-patient communities such as PatientsLikeMe, CureTogether, Inspire, and others have emerged as places where ePatients seek and find communities formed around common illnesses, treatments, or symptoms. Within these communities, patients connect with each other for various reasons, including emotional support, ongoing learning, and advocacy.

Google, Facebook, Amazon, and other online environments learn from user search behavior and other internet activity to serve up predictive content, confirming that Web 3.0 has arrived with Health 3.0 rapidly evolving along with Digital Health, Medicine 2.0, Connected Health, and mHealth. These terms and concepts represent the changing world of healthcare and its integration with current technology, making possible personalized health experiences through

the use of predictive search capabilities and more advanced cognitive computing.[24]

Health-related resources on the internet are constantly growing and becoming more innovative and complex. They provide ePatients with access to incredible resources and data previously unavailable, such as personal genetic information. To appreciate the power of technology, consider the Human Genome Project. It took 13 years and nearly $3 billion to complete the identification and sequencing of genes within human DNA.[25] In contrast, 23andMe, an internet company launched in 2007 offering direct-to-consumer kits, made it possible for anyone to access his or her personal genetic information quickly, simply, and for less than $500 (the price is now as low as $199).[26]

Another area of explosive growth has been in mobile technology or mHealth. Anyone with a smartphone can access thousands of health- and fitness-related applications. mHealth applications coupled with sensors and wearables are growing rapidly as technology becomes more sophisticated and increasingly connected to all aspects of fitness, wellness, and healthcare delivery. ResearchKit, introduced by Apple in 2015, allows consumers to participate in healthcare research from the palm of their hand. Within 24 hours of its launch, over 10,000 iPhone users signed up for the ResearchKit heart study.[27] With recent mobile technological advances, the collection and display of data are being presented in a more digestible format which helps inform decision making as well as the ability to share real-time updates within a social circle. Data visualization and infographics have become ever more mainstream and are used to enhance one's ability to view trends or patterns in health. The concept of mHealth is further explored in Chapter 15.

Policy and Legislative Influences

The economics of healthcare influenced the evolution of ePatients and their use of nontraditional and/or innovative sources for healthcare information. Patients with insurance have seen their out-of-pocket expenses, including deductibles and copayments, increase over the last decade, leading many to look for alternative ways to get answers and support for healthcare questions. The uninsured and underinsured are often left trying to manage their own and their family members' healthcare needs to avoid incurring expenses associated with various services. Additionally, with changes in the healthcare reimbursement structure shifting care from the hospital to home, patients and caregivers are assuming more responsibility for increasingly complex care needs. The responsibilities of self-managing health and navigating the healthcare system motivated many to become ePatients, to find, connect with, and learn from others who may share similar experiences.

Policy and legislative actions in the United States have been important drivers in the ePatient movement. In 2009 the American Recovery and Reinvestment Act was signed into law. A hallmark of this legislation destined to affect the next phase of the ePatient movement is the requirement known as Meaningful Use (MU), which sets specific objectives that eligible professionals and hospitals must achieve to qualify for incentive programs offered by the Centers for Medicare and Medicaid Services (CMS) for integrating electronic health records (EHRs) into their systems. Implementation of MU requirements is a multistage, multiyear endeavor with expectations that compliance will result in better clinical outcomes, improved population health outcomes, increased transparency and efficiency, empowered individuals, and more robust research data on health systems. MU requirements are not without controversy, which led CMS to propose modifications to certain requirements in April 2015. Stage 2 MU requirements for patient engagement were significantly reduced by making the requirement for patients to use technology for electronic download, view, and transmit of their medical records from 5% of eligible providers' patients to just one patient, prompting much criticism from ePatients and patient advocates.[28]

The focus on access to health information fueled the development of patient portals within EHR systems of large health systems, hospitals, physician practices, and other eligible healthcare providers. Another mechanism for ePatient health information access is personal health records (PHRs). PHR features vary from one system to another, but most support a menu of transactions including the ability to review test results, schedule appointments, refill prescriptions, and communicate via electronic messaging with healthcare providers. Estimates suggest that approximately 70 million people in the United States have access to PHRs, yet widespread adoption has been slow, and changes by CMS to the MU patient engagement requirements may impact prior expectations that the requirements would improve utilization. Other healthcare reform measures, including provisions in the Patient Protection and Affordable Care Act (PPACA) and the Health Care and Education Reconciliation Act of 2010, which amended the PPACA and became law on March 30, 2010, significantly affect healthcare coverage and care delivery. In 2015 Health and Human Services Secretary Sylvia M. Burwell set specific goals and a timeline for shifting Medicare reimbursements from volume-based care, commonly known as fee-for-service, to value-based care.[29] Patients and their healthcare providers will bear increasing responsibility for managing cost and care, leading to the need for more collaboration and engagement at the actual point of care.

Characteristics of Digital Healthcare Consumers

In a report titled *Health e-People: The Online Consumer Experience*, Cain, Sarasohn-Kahn, and Wayne introduced three categories of online healthcare consumers: those who are *well*, those who are *newly diagnosed* with an illness, and those who are *chronically ill* and their caregivers.[30] The report suggests that people in each group behave in certain ways on the internet and that their behavior is a reflection of their health status:

- *The well:* When the report was written, approximately 60% of consumers looking online for health and healthcare information were well. The online needs of the well are largely considered episodic and occasionally driven by the need to seek out specific information related to prevention and wellness. They tend to move across various resources both online and offline for information and they typically place value on convenience over loyalty.

- *The newly diagnosed:* This group represented only 5% of the total number of online health consumers in 2009. The newly diagnosed are driven by a sense of urgency to understand, manage, and mitigate a recent change in their health status. Their presence and behavior online depend largely on the nature of the condition and its usual trajectory. Most newly diagnosed individuals are expected to spend large amounts of time online in the weeks following the news of their diagnosis. Those diagnosed with a condition amenable to intervention and eventual resolution have different needs than those moving from a state of wellness to a state of chronic illness. For the latter, the need for online resources is expected to evolve and change to reflect changes in their health over time.

- *The chronically ill:* This group represented about 35% of online health consumers in 2009. Chronically ill patients who use online sites often align their loyalty to sites with resources, services, and support for their specific condition. According to the report, 51% of American adults living with chronic disease go online for health topics related to disease, medical procedures, medications, or health insurance information; 1 in 4 adults with a chronic illness have looked online for someone who shares the same condition.[31]

Caregivers and loved ones of those living with illness or disability often become active online. Contemporary ePatients are information seekers and data gatherers. They take personal responsibility for researching online and offline resources to improve their health and well-being. The *well* ePatient is inclined to peruse a host of digital resources episodically to prepare for medical appointments, investigate intermittent family health questions, or search just out of curiosity. *Active* ePatients (and their caregivers), including those newly diagnosed and those with chronic illnesses, are more invested in gathering important data points by tracking their health with the use of online self-management tools and biosensors, such as heart rate monitors, seizure trackers, mood maps, sleep diaries, and glucose monitors. Digital devices and wearables are becoming increasingly commonplace for monitoring mobility, medication adherence, and even for detecting behavioral changes.[32] Tracking their health data digitally in conjunction with online searches empowers ePatients to gain a sense of participation and ownership of their well-being, treatment options, and health.

As the evolution of the ePatient continues, more prominent examples of contemporary ePatients emerge. One emblematic ePatient is Dave deBronkart, who has dedicated himself to being a patient activist, blogger, international speaker at health and social media conferences, and health policy advocate for the ePatient movement.[33] His call to action came in 2007 when he received a diagnosis of Stage IV renal cell carcinoma that had spread to his muscles, bones, and lungs. He was told that his median survival time was about 24 weeks. With this prognosis, deBronkart was highly motivated to find an effective treatment and scoured the internet for viable options. With help from other patients on the Association of Cancer Online Resources (ACOR) website with a similar diagnosis, he learned about a promising clinical trial as well as tips on medications to avoid jeopardizing his trial eligibility. Armed with this information, he engaged in meaningful discussions with his clinician about his options. Fortunately, deBronkart had a favorable outcome and the treatment regimen from the clinical trial led to his successful recovery. One year after his treatment ended he began publicly sharing his story by blogging and participating in healthcare conferences and events. deBronkart believes that patients are the most underused resource within healthcare and champions the message of "Let Patients Help." His proactive research and engagement with his healthcare providers helped to provide a favorable outcome. However, he is always quick to state that what actually saved him was phenomenal medical science provided by experts in their field in an institution well grounded in patient-centered care. In recognition of his role in patient advocacy and the role of the patient in cooperative science, the Mayo Clinic Internal Medicine Chief Residents named deBronkart the 2015 Visiting Professor in Internal Medicine.[34]

Other ePatients are called to activism as a result of their experiences with the healthcare system. Regina Holliday chose art as the medium to express her family's difficult experiences during her husband's illness and untimely death.[35] Holliday shares her story in a powerful and provocative mural depicting the journey she and her family traveled through a fragmented and uncoordinated healthcare system. The journey was exemplified by her inability to access her husband's medical records in a timely way to ensure that he received needed care. The mural is titled *73 cents*, the price Holliday was told she would have to pay per page to make a copy of his medical record. Since completing the mural, Holliday has continued to bring a voice to the patient and family experience through art. Since 2010, Holliday has painted more than 372 poignant and thematic paintings while on-site at healthcare conferences, events, and policy meetings, using them as an opportunity for public advocacy. She founded a movement called the Walking Gallery where she and other artists depict patients' stories or elements of medical advocacy on the back of jackets or lab coats for government employees, technology gurus, medical professionals, social media activists, executives of companies, patients, and artists. Holliday and 43 other artists have painted 439 wearable images for the Walking Gallery. As of June 2016, 392 unique Walkers have joined the Gallery wearing 430 jackets. These jackets are often worn by their advocate owners at health-related conferences and events. When gathered together for a Walking Gallery exhibit, the images on each jacket convey powerful messages to the public about the importance of advocacy.

A new type of health consumer has emerged in the last decade. The **quantified self** (or quantified selfer) refers to a person invested in using tools and data to quantify and monitor daily experiences using personal metrics.[36] A quantified self measures a range of inputs such as food consumption, environmental factors, emotional and biophysical states, biometric data, and mental and physical performance. These data, collected at baseline and over time, can encourage and promote healthy behaviors and provide signals for early detection of illness or changes from the baseline state of health. The real-time feedback from the wearable sensors provides awareness of one's own physiologic response.[37]

Semantically, a quantified self may not consider himself or herself to be an ePatient but rather someone whose goals are to achieve and maintain good health and who has an innate interest in tracking personal metrics. This type of health consumer captures health-related data such as blood pressure, exercise, activity, sleep, and dietary intake using personal informatics tools for self-monitoring to track their progress toward his or her goals. This type of tracking has the potential to identify health changes more quickly and may affect outcomes favorably, especially in circumstances when a nuanced change leads to an early diagnosis. This potential is exemplified by the experience of Steven Keating; while a doctoral student at MIT's Media Lab, he collected and researched his own health data and symptoms, which led to the discovery of a brain tumor and successful timely treatment. Keating, relentless in the pursuit of his medical information, shares his journey on his website. In a *New York Times* article, Keating states, "there is a huge healing power to patients understanding and seeing the effects of treatments and medications."[38] The aggregation of personal metrics, lifestyle factors, and real-world experiences has the potential to expand healthcare providers' understanding of patient responses to wellness and illness, both behaviorally and physiologically.

Today a perfect, positive storm is brewing as technology, policy, legislation, patient-centered reform, and patients' interests in personal health data converge. Observing the evolution of ePatients from their earliest days to today is akin to watching a movie in slow motion. However, a shift to fast-forward is rapidly occurring; the impact of an increasing number of ePatients on health and healthcare will result in disruptive innovation for healthcare providers and healthcare delivery systems. More importantly, ePatients will continue to be a driving force in achieving improvements in the quality and safety of healthcare in the United States.

CONVERGENCE OF ePATIENTS, CLINICIANS, PATIENT-CENTERED MODELS OF CARE, AND INFORMATICS

Participatory Patient-Centered Healthcare

The maxim of "doctors know best" is a statement of the past. Until the early 21st century, the old paradigm was a paternalistic model in which the healthcare provider was the exclusive source of medical knowledge. Deeply rooted cultural assumptions in this old medical model view the patient as the uninformed layperson and the medical professional as the keeper of all health knowledge. In a clinician-controlled environment the patient is the outsider with little ability to gather and access data about his or her condition and is expected to play the "good patient" role. This is changing with patient-centered care models.

As patient-centered care models rapidly evolve in the United States, questions emerge about who should direct the care: the patient or the healthcare provider.[39] Patient-centeredness promulgates a model in which the patient is not only at the center of care but also a full member and partner of the healthcare team. Patients know best when it comes to having the most intimate understanding of their personal circumstances, their preferences, and their bodies. Yet in most healthcare organizations, including patient-centered medical homes and primary care practice settings, provider-directed care remains the norm, perhaps for political, legal, and reimbursement reasons.[40] Scherger suggests that the internet will test this paradigm of provider-directed care in much the same way that online banking, travel services, and other previously brokered services have given way to consumer control.[39]

The ePatient movement does not support replacing physicians and other healthcare providers. On the contrary, ePatients understand the value of collaborative patient-provider partnerships and seek healthcare providers who appreciate the value of allowing patients to participate. ePatients appreciate the need for provider-directed care for certain circumstances such as trauma, acute medical events, and surgical emergencies; however, the model of patient-centered care exists with the premise that patients are considered experts in their own care and self-management and must be allowed to exercise patient-driven controls. Patient-centered care is viewed as a critical component of achieving the Triple Aim of improving the experience of care, improving the health of populations, and reducing per capita costs of healthcare.[41] For patient-centered care to succeed, patients and their clinicians must have respectful partnerships within which patients and clinicians mutually determine how care will be directed and managed to meet needs.

An unprecedented opportunity exists to fundamentally change the experience of healthcare encounters for both patients and their clinicians. ePatients have the tools and skills to elevate discussions with their healthcare providers and use limited office visit time engaged in a more constructive dialog. This can result in greater satisfaction for both stakeholders. This meaningful collaboration between the ePatient and the healthcare provider, known as **participatory healthcare** or **participatory medicine**, is defined by the Society for Participatory Medicine as:

> …a cooperative model of healthcare that encourages and expects active involvement by all connected parties, including patients, caregivers, and healthcare professionals, as integral to the full continuum of care. The "participatory" concept may also be applied to fitness, nutrition, mental health, end-of-life care, and all issues broadly related to an individual's health.[42]

The Society for Participatory Medicine was founded as a movement in which networked patients shift from being mere passengers to responsible drivers of their health. Healthcare providers encourage and value them as full partners.

Participatory healthcare also requires ePatients and clinicians to use a variety of data sources to genuinely collaborate on shared goals and decision making for improved health and outcomes. Iverson, Howard, and Penney found that gathering information online fosters more patient engagement in health maintenance and care.[43] The movement toward participatory patient-centered care requires that ePatients, health professionals, and informatics systems align accordingly. Berwick offered three maxims that he finds useful when considering a participatory patient-centered model of care:

- The needs of the patient come first.
- Every patient is the only patient.
- Nothing about me without me.[44]

The last maxim is often associated with ePatients and calls for openness and transparency among all involved stakeholders, especially when it comes to their health data. deBronkart's notoriety flourished after his keynote presentation at the 2009 Medicine 2.0 conference titled "Gimme My Damn Data," which was picked up by Cable News Network (CNN) in a series on the empowered patient.[45] In response to the CMS decision to reduce the MU requirement for patient engagement, ePatients, advocates, leading consumer organizations, healthcare experts, policy-makers, and technology organizations launched a collaborative data liberation campaign on July 4, 2015, leading to the formation of "GetMyHealthData," an initiative promoting transparency and consumer access to digital health information.[46] In October 2015 the Alliance for Nursing Informatics (ANI) published a press release stating that it had joined the GetMyHealthData effort. "Encouraging nurses to get involved in the GetMyHealthData effort is a natural next step to the multi-year Consumer eHealth agenda of ANI," announced Judy Murphy, RN, FACMI, FHIMSS, FAAN, co-chair of ANI.[47]

While opportunities for health professionals' growth in participatory healthcare exist, it is equally important to acknowledge the challenges. Current care models may not be structured to support patient-centeredness and even well-intentioned clinicians may find it difficult to allocate sufficient time and resources to fully engage with ePatients who come with a well-prepared agenda. However, there is no doubt that ePatients will continue to push and advocate for their place in the healthcare system.

Many ePatients want to integrate empirical knowledge into their understanding of their health conditions. Therefore clinicians should engage these ePatients in developing a shared hypothesis based on data and patient-reported experiences to help explain symptoms and other findings. Developing a shared hypothesis and including the ePatient in creating a plan to manage care initiates a process known as guided discovery. Guided discovery includes integrating open-ended questions in the medical encounter, preidentifying data collection parameters that have meaning to the ePatient, planning time for analysis of collected information, completing an evaluation of outcomes, and recognizing that those results may require experimentation to achieve shared goals.[47] Clinicians must also take a proactive role in educating patients to safely and effectively use internet-based resources including social media sites. Examples of key points to consider in this education are included on Box 12.2.

The New Role of Clinicians and Informaticians in ePatient Care

Clinicians involved in informatics are uniquely positioned to participate in system changes that support ePatients' desire for data openness and transparency by helping to build data collection models that support connection, partnership, and guided discovery.[48] Patients and healthcare providers need the right tools at the right time to collect data to support their need to investigate and hypothesize health issues to create a shared plan. Clinicians may need to learn new skills and gain new knowledge to serve as a "guide" for ePatients as they integrate information and data from multiple sources while navigating their healthcare experience. It is within this culture of partnership that guided discovery of the ePatient's health and well-being can be fully realized.[49] Healthcare providers must be flexible and open to the possibility that patients may be more intimately adept at the experience of their own illness and that clinicians should not be expected to have all of the answers. However, ePatients expect their clinicians to use timely technology, including online and digital sources, to build their own knowledge and expertise.

ePatients have inherent knowledge of their sense of self and are encouraging the healthcare field to recognize and support this notion. As deBronkart has been known to say, "Patients have more skin in the game." ePatients look to

BOX 12.2 Key Points for Teaching Patients Safe and Effective Use of Social Media Sites

- Take the time to read the *Conditions of Use* and *Privacy Statement*. The website should be designed in such a way that you can read these documents before establishing an account.
- Read the *About* section to determine who has established the site and the mission or purpose of the site.
- Spend time learning how to navigate the site and set privacy/security setting before participating on the site.
- Lurk on the site until you learn the names and characteristics of frequent participants on the site as well as the personality of the social media group as a whole.
- If you are unclear about a comment that has been posted, ask questions. Other people in the group might have some of the same questions.
- Treat people with respect and kindness. If you think something that has been posted is incorrect, point out that it is different than your previous knowledge or experience and ask for more information or clarification.
- If you are feeling strong emotion such as angry, excitement and anxiety it is often helpful, to compose your comments and let them set for a bit of time before posting. Remember, once it is posted it is permanent.
- Carefully evaluate the information posted by others. Listen/read the whole conversation. Information may be accurate but not apply to your situation or case. The first answer to a question is not always the best answer and group consensus is not always correct.

Sources used include: Joos I, Nelson R, Smith M. *Introduction to Computers for Health Professionals*. Burlington, MA: Jones & Bartlett. 2014, box 12-1 and Nelson R, Joos I, Wolf DM. *Social Media for Nurses*. New York, NY: Springer Publishing Company. 2012, table 1.4.

clinicians not only for their clinical expertise but also for their willingness to support changing needs during the illness journey. Health professionals can demonstrate this willingness by understanding the value of online and digital technology resources to ePatients. Clinicians have the opportunity to research internet sites and digital devices that are relevant to their specialty, recommend those that provide value to them and their patients, and be open to learning about and exploring other resources and technology solutions favored by their ePatients.

The integration of patient-centered care models enabled by technology into the U.S. healthcare system will continue, and ePatients will be essential participants. As with any change, resistance should be expected. However, initial resistance will not stem the tide that is occurring across the country to create a partnership model of care that supports safety, efficiency, and health for all stakeholders.[50]

Health Informatics and ePatients

Disruptive communication technologies, such as the internet and digital devices, have drastically altered the way we communicate with one another. From electronic messaging, texting, and tweeting to updating social networks, posting pictures, and posting reviews, our experiences allow us to share knowledge, communicate, and connect in real time with others around the world. Online businesses are harnessing the power of communication and connection by researching buyer reviews and purchasing history data of customers to help drive sales. The idea of using buyer reviews can also be found within healthcare. One example is the Hospital Consumer Assessment of Healthcare Providers and Systems (HCAHPS), the first national, standardized, public report of patients' perspectives of their experiences with healthcare organizations and healthcare providers, which is now also in use in ambulatory and outpatient care settings.[51]

The aggregation of data across similar experiences is known as **crowdsourcing**. Crowdsourcing is useful in recognizing patterns within the population and can also help to expand our knowledge for public health. The idea of crowdsourcing information and participatory healthcare is growing; one example is PatientsLikeMe. This research-based online platform was created for patients to share and learn from real-world experiences and to produce outcome-based health data for advancing the current pace of research.[52] Imagine a patient who has recorded data about his or her symptoms over time; the historical data can lead to productive encounters with healthcare providers, but may also contribute to emerging knowledge about the experience of living with certain conditions. Crowdsourced data from real patients in real time expand and challenge how we view and study health.[53]

Despite the growing move toward participatory health and collaborative care, for most healthcare organizations the current health IT infrastructure does not foster interoperability for patients and healthcare providers so that they can interact and communicate effectively and efficiently. Immediate electronic access to one's health records and electronic messaging with healthcare providers is becoming more commonplace yet electronic transfer of information across systems remains a barrier to accessing information. Health informatics has been touted as one of the solutions in changing healthcare, which should improve quality, efficiency, and safety of care and decrease costs, but the delay in implementing systems is impeding the ability of healthcare to evolve more rapidly. An additional layer of data architecture is needed to support the integration of meaningful and relevant **patient-generated health data (PGHD)** at the point of care.[54] PGHD is defined as health-related data that is created, recorded, or gathered by patients, family members, and caregivers to address a health concern.[55] A pilot study using PGHD demonstrated significant improvement in epilepsy self-management and self-efficacy among veterans using online self-tracking tools in collaboration with their clinicians.[56]

Informatics alone cannot build the learning health system as described in the IOM's Learning Health System Series.[57] The vision of a learning health system aligns scientific knowledge, biomedical informatics, value-added incentives, and cultural norms to ensure that continuous improvement and innovation become natural by-products of the experience of healthcare. Consumer participation and collaboration are essential elements of a learning health system.

Transparency and Access to Data

Increasing transparency of medical documentation to patients offers new opportunities for patient engagement. The OpenNotes project, which began in 2010, evaluated the impact of sharing clinical encounter notes for primary care providers and patients online. Participating providers believed in transparency of medical documentation and the tangible benefits of sharing notes with patients. Nonparticipating providers indicated worry over the increased demand on their time and lengthier visits as well as an inability to record their thoughts candidly about sensitive issues regarding mental health, obesity, cancer, and substance abuse. In addition, nonparticipating providers noted that the transparency of the notes would negatively affect their current practices and have minimal positive effect on patients. In contrast, patients reported positive interest in reading clinical notes, and fewer than one in six patients expressed worry or confusion over reading the notes, regardless of demographic and health characteristics. Many patients in the study also indicated that they would consider sharing the notes with friends and family. Overall, the evidence suggests that giving patients access to their provider's notes may improve communication and efficiency of care and may lead to patients becoming more involved with their health and healthcare.[58] Since the initial study, many sites in the United States are participating in OpenNotes bringing access to more than 5 million patients.[59]

Many ePatient supporters are advocating transparency and challenging the question of who owns the data. Dave deBronkart has heavily advocated for transparency of data because of his experiences with inaccurate information in his health record and his family members' records that could have led to potentially fatal mistakes. For example, his mother's diagnosis of hyperthyroidism was transcribed incorrectly and treatment for hypothyroidism was prescribed. His wife's allergy to penicillin was not recorded and she was almost given the harmful medication. deBronkart reviewed his own health record and noted erroneous diagnoses.[60] Regina Holliday's advocacy work, mentioned earlier, is solidly in favor of access to the health record. She believes that no patient or family should ever have to struggle, as she did, to gain timely access to health records. Similar efforts in support of transparency and open access are occurring in the research realm. Interest has grown over the past several years and on June 4, 2012, a petition was signed by thousands of advocates urging the White House to make taxpayer-funded research available online to everyone. Due to public concerns, the Obama administration committed to giving public access to the results of federally funded research within one year of publication.[61]

ePatients attempt to access studies on their chronic illnesses, but closed access to research papers constrains their efforts. In addition, closed access prohibits patients who participated in studies from reviewing study outcomes. Not only are patients often limited in their access to research results from studies in which they participated, they are often denied access to their own health data collected as part of the research study. This practice within the research and publishing world creates a roadblock for patients and an imbalanced dissemination of knowledge. Progress has been made on sharing data from clinical trials with the release of an IOM report in 2015.[62] Groups such as Patient Centered Outcomes Research Institute and PatientsLikeMe have embraced open access as essential for all of their publications. Open access to research literature gives ePatients the ability to critically evaluate their best course of action.

HEALTH 3.0 EMERGES

Over the last decade, the internet has evolved from the static unidirectional experience of Web 1.0 to the dynamic and interactive environment of Web 2.0 within which collective intelligence is harnessed.[63] With this framework in mind, Van De Belt et al. identified definitions for the parallel evolution of Health 2.0 and Medicine 2.0, terms that are often used interchangeably.[9] They found 46 unique definitions from 44 articles, suggesting that the concept is continuing to develop. Seven recurrent themes indicated that a set of characteristics for Health 2.0 is emerging: (1) patients/consumers, (2) Web 2.0/technology, (3) professionals/caregivers, (4) social networking, (5) change of health care, (6) collaboration, and (7) health information or content.

ePatients participate across various health-related social media spaces: some blog; some tweet and retweet; some form patient-related pages on Facebook; some express their experiences through music and art; and some seek opportunities to communicate their messages at professional conferences, political gatherings, and citizen forums. ePatients influence the experiences of other patients on a global scale. As Health 2.0 gives way to Health 3.0, innovative environments continue to emerge in which collective intelligence and knowledge of multiple stakeholders is gathered, exchanged, and shared. The concept of Health 3.0 is built on Web 3.0, also referred to as the internet of things (IoT). With Web 3.0, a wide variety of monitors, such as those used to monitor one's home of health status, can be connected and managed from the internet, Health 3.0 provides new opportunities and raises new challenges. A fully connected home could make it possible for patients with limited cognitive abilities to remain in their home as opposed to a nursing home. However, while surfing the web can tell advertisers what websites a user frequently visits, things like biometric wearables collect and share much more personal data about a user's activities and overall health status. As U.S. Secretary of Homeland Security Michael Chertoff indicated, some caution is in order when it comes to IoT: "One shouldn't default to the position that connecting everything is perfect."[64]

However, the viral capability of social media provides ePatients with a powerful platform from which the experiences of even the most vulnerable can be collected, appreciated, and shared. Gaps exist in internet accessibility despite the proliferation of technology across all aspects of society. This digital divide has both individual and public health implications since those lacking access are unable to benefit from the

wisdom of collective knowledge to improve health outcomes, whether in real time or longitudinally. The gap between the internet "haves" and "have-nots" is beginning to narrow through collaborative efforts of countries and global technology companies working to bring access to anyone who wants it. While motivations for this movement may be commercially driven, engaging the global population in the digital world provides far-reaching opportunities to impact global health.

Virtual Patient Communities and Research Networks

In *Peer-to-Peer Healthcare*, Fox found that 18% of internet users were online to find others who may have similar health concerns.[65] Among those users living with chronic illnesses such as diabetes, heart, or lung conditions, 23% reported going online to look for others with similar experiences. The report also highlights that 71% of adults seek information, care, or support from a health professional during an acute moment of need. This important point reinforces the notion that ePatients want a partnership with healthcare providers to collaborate and share in decision making. Fox's *Health Online 2013* report indicates that the general public continues to use the internet for a variety of health-related needs with 72% of online users seeking health information in the previous 12 months.[22]

ePatients seeking health information and support are increasingly turning to a new generation of innovative tools and devices that include mHealth applications, comprehensive web-based content, interactive social networks, and wearable sensors that can seamlessly connect data to online sites. These digital environments provide the opportunity to reframe one's experience from "Why me?" to "Oh, you too? Tell me more." The interactions that occur provide support, validation, and a place to share ideas about how to live as well as possible with illness. This journey is depicted in Fig. 12.2.

One of the most transformative developments for ePatients has been the emergence of patient-focused virtual communities in which patients interact, sharing health-related data and learning from each other's experiences while being unbounded by geographic limitations, social stigma, or other limiting characteristics. Eysenbach et al. defined virtual community as follows:

…a group of individuals with similar or common health related interests and predominately non-professional backgrounds (patients, healthy consumers, or informal caregivers) who interact and communicate publicly through a computer communication such as the internet, or through any other computer based tool (including non-text based systems such as voice bulletin board systems), allowing social networks to build over a distance. (p. 1)[66]

In an online environment ePatients exchange information, compare notes, learn about treatment options, and engage in discussions that may seem superfluous and deemed not within the purview of the medical professional. For example, they can exchange tips on where to purchase wigs in preparation for chemotherapy, advice on raising children,

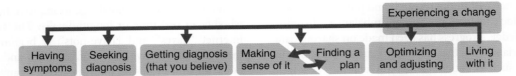

FIG 12.2 The patient and caregiver journey. (Copyright PatientsLikeMe. <http://www.pati entslikeme.com/patients/view/40?patient_page=1>; 2012.)

or advice on working while managing a chronic illness. Online communities can also function as a lifeline for those trying to manage the fear and uncertainty associated with illness. For many, including the uninsured, underinsured, and those with high-deductible plans, spending time online to explore ideas with others may be a reasonable first step in deciding what to do next about a health concern. Patients with rare diseases can search for specialists, researchers, and newly discovered information for their rare disease. Schweizer et al. found that among cancer patients, virtual communities play an important role in helping patients to cope with their situation.[67] Establishing social relationships with other cancer patients complements and supplements their offline social relationships. While emotional support is a benefit, evidence also exists that patients derive physical and quality-of-life benefits as well.[68]

The lines previously drawn between patients, care delivery, and health-related research are continually blurring. Studies show that Americans are increasingly willing to share their health data if it improves their outcomes or the outcomes of others like them.[69] Among veterans using the MyHealtheVet portal, 79% report interest in sharing access to their electronic health information with caregivers and non-VA providers.[70]

ePatients are looking for more than social support from their interactions with online communities. Nambisan found that patients participating in online health communities experienced enhanced perceived empathy when their information seeking was supported by relevant tools and data displays similar to those used by PatientsLikeMe (on this site ePatients have access to a variety of tools to share data about their health conditions, symptoms, treatments, and side effects).[71] In a user survey conducted in 2010, PatientsLikeMe members reported improved understanding of how their treatments worked, feeling more involved in decisions regarding their treatments, and better communication with members of the healthcare team.[72] Researchers identified a "dose effect" of connectedness among members of the site's epilepsy community.[73]

Health-related social networks and patient-powered research sites have become a rich resource for support, information, empowerment, and advocacy for ePatients and their caregivers. However, as with all activities on the internet, participants should review the terms of use and the privacy and data-sharing policies to ensure that they are well informed. Reputable sites display links to their privacy policies on every page of the site (Table 12.1).

Virtual communities share many of the characteristics of any social group and these characteristics may evolve and change as the community grows and matures. Most virtual communities can afford the user some degree of anonymity

TABLE 12.1 Patient Virtual Communities: User and Privacy Policies		
Patient Virtual Community	User Terms	Privacy Policy
Cure Together	http://curetogether.com/terms.php	http://curetogether.com/privacy.php
Patients Like Me	www.patientslikeme.com/about/user_agreement	www.patientslikeme.com/about/privacy www.patientslikeme.com/about/openness
Inspire	www.inspire.com/about/terms/	www.inspire.com/about/privacy/
Army of Women	www.armyofwomen.org/termsofuse	www.armyofwomen.org/privacypolicy
Association of Cancer Online Resources (ACOR)	http://www.acor.org/pages/termsAndConditions	http://www.acor.org/pages/privacyPolicy
Smart Patients	https://www.smartpatients.com/terms	https://www.smartpatients.com/privacy

since engagement is not typically face to face. This can be both a benefit and a risk. Patients may feel more comfortable sharing sensitive information anonymously than they would in person. Among 1267 polled members of PatientsLikeMe, 41% said that they have withheld information from their doctors about certain symptoms and 39% did not share information about lifestyle habits such as exercise, diet, and alcohol use. Reasons for withholding this information from their doctors included not wanting to be lectured, feeling too embarrassed, not thinking the information was important or the doctor's business, forgetting to bring it up, and fearing that the treatment they wanted would not be provided.

A survey conducted in 2011 by iVillage, an online community for women, found that women placed more trust in and value on information obtained from online women's communities than from other social networks.[74] The respondents believed that sites such as iVillage, CafeMom, and BabyCenter offered more expertise to understand and meet their needs.

Virtual communities may also carry risks, especially for novice ePatients who may feel uncertain or vulnerable in this environment. Many patient communities incorporate moderators as part of the experience, yet there is an inconsistent approach to how moderation is done in these communities. Research is emerging in this area but more is needed to characterize the effectiveness and quality of moderation in online communities.[75] Organizations that create and support online communities should measure user input to gauge the perceived benefits, risks, and social health of the community from the patient's perspective.

Online communities can be important sources of patient experience data that could be harnessed by researchers. Patient-reported outcome measures (PROMs) are gaining use among academic and clinical researchers, government and regulatory agencies, policy institutes, and patients themselves. Information collected within virtual patient communities offers a novel source of patient-reported outcome (PRO) data for meaningful measure development. Although of increasing interest, data generated by patients themselves, either actively reported or passively gathered from wearable or sensor devices, are not without challenges including the need to establish data standards and methodologies for data collection and analysis. The value of patient-generated health data is gaining favor across all sectors of health and healthcare, giving ePatients an unprecedented opportunity to impact care, policy, and payer decision making.[58]

CONCLUSION AND FUTURE DIRECTIONS

21st Century Health and Healthcare

As we look to the future for ePatients, consider the Google generation, a generation of computer users born after 1993. They have grown up with immediate access to information and knowledge sources that were previously unavailable. This generation is also called the Net generation, the Google generation, digital natives, and millennials. They are very skilled at navigating internet and digital resources and are accustomed to sharing data in real time in online environments.[76] Insight into this generation of users is important because they have little or no recollection of life without the internet. They are now adults, taking jobs, starting families, and will increasingly engage in decisions about their health and the health of their families. These are today's ePatients and their appetite for immediacy and responsiveness from online and digital tools will drive innovation across all consumer interactions including healthcare. Not far behind is Generation Z, also known as iGen or Digitarians. These future ePatients only know a world of access powered by the internet, having been raised with touch-enabled devices and the ability to connect to anyone globally.[77]

As these generations age and health technology continues to evolve, the term *ePatients* will make way for a more inclusive term, the eHealth consumer.

The evolution of the web might be summed up this way: Web 1.0 was akin to a library where you could access loads of information but you could not contribute anything. Web 2.0 has more of a community feel; it is a place where groups can gather, where you can exchange information, and where your contribution can be included and even judged by others for its value. So what does Web 3.0 enable? Browsers and devices are already acting more like a personal assistant, such as Apple's Siri. Search capabilities now harness user experience behavior to display content of interest including personally tailored advertising. Web 3.0 uses data from our online and digital exhaust to put current searches into context to deliver information that meets our needs and interests in the moment.

What does this mean for health and healthcare? In 2011, Topol described technological advances in medical devices and other diagnostic tools emerging in practice.[78] Just four years later he said that patients hold the future of medicine in their hands—literally, in the form of a smartphone. Topol suggests that the digitalization of medicine has now democratized it, calling this digitization medicine's "Guttenberg moment."[79] Research institutes like the P4 Medicine Institute are working to integrate systems biology, digital and information technology, clinicians, and patients to form **P4 Medicine**, medicine that is predictive, preventive, personalized, and participatory.[80] In April 2014, IBM Watson moved from being a Jeopardy champion to powering the IBM Watson Health Cloud of advanced cognitive and analytic technologies for health and healthcare.

As the vision of a learning health system is realized, patients and those close to them need opportunities to contribute. In May 2012 a summit was convened in Washington, DC, bringing together representatives from government, industry, nonprofits, and patients to build consensus on the core values and principles needed to support a person-centered, continuous learning health system on a national scale. Regina Holliday, the artist-in-residence for the 2-day summit, painted *Chaordic*, depicting powerful images of multiple stakeholders navigating the fine line between the chaos and order of our current healthcare environment as they converge to achieve the vision of a learning health system (Fig. 12.3).[81]

Since that time, attention to including patients as partners across all domains of health and healthcare has become commonplace. In 2012 an initiative called Patients Included created a charter to establish aspirations for patient participation in conferences and now provides a logo that is proudly displayed for those events that honor the charter's intentions.[82] Since 2013 the multiple centers across the National Institutes of Health (NIH) have engaged with external stakeholders, including patients, in workshops and events focused on the role of Citizen Science in biomedical research. President Obama used his 2015 State of the Union address to announce a bold initiative called Precision Medicine to recruit 1 million volunteers in a research effort aimed at understanding the

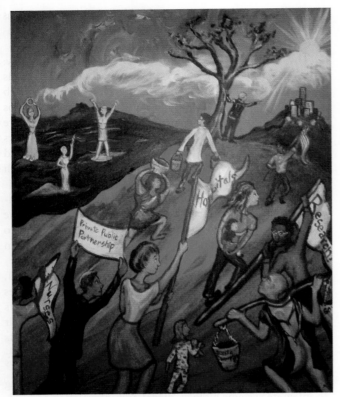

FIG 12.3 Chaordic. (Copyright Regina Holliday, 2012.)

individual differences in people's genes, environments, and lifestyles in hopes of developing more personalized and targeted therapies.[83] The 21st Century Cures Act, which passed the House of Representatives in July 2015 and is pending in the Senate, contains provisions that support patient engagement and participation in drug discovery and development processes including the use of patient experience data by the U.S. Food and Drug Administration in the benefit risk assessment of a new drug.[84]

We are nearing a time when the term *ePatient* may be irrelevant; a time when a person-centric health system welcomes equipped, enabled, empowered, and engaged people in creating health, together as partners in a peer relationship with their healthcare providers. A time when a continuously learning health system, supported by an ever-evolving technological infrastructure, can ensure personalized participatory medicine, preference-sensitive decision making, and shared accountability for achieving mutually agreed-upon value-based outcomes.

REFERENCES

1. Slack W, Hicks G, Reed C, Van Cura L. A computer-based medical-history system. *N Engl J Med*. 1966;274(4):194–198.
2. Slack W. The patient online. *Am J Prev Med*. 1999;16(1):43–45.
3. Patient empowerment—who empowers whom? *Lancet*. 2012;379(9827):1677. http://dx.doi.org/10.1016/S0140-6736(12)60699-1670.
4. Ferguson T. ePatients: how they can help us heal healthcare [white paper]. *e-patients.net*; 2007. http://e-patients.net/e-Patient_White_Paper_2015.pdf.
5. Ferguson T. Looking ahead: online health & the search for sustainable healthcare [online exclusive]. *Ferguson Report*. 2002;9. http://www.fergusonreport.com/articles/fr00901.htm.
6. Gee P, Greenwood D, Kim K, Perez S, Staggers N, Devon H. Exploration of the epatient phenomenon in nursing informatics. *Nurs Outlook*. 2012;60(4):e9–e16.
7. Della Mea V. What is ehealth (2): the death of telemedicine? *J Med Internet Res*. 2001;3(2):e22. http://www.jmir.org/2001/2/e22/.
8. Eng T. *The eHealth Landscape—A Terrain Map of Emerging Information and Communication Technologies in Health and Health Care*. Princeton, NJ: The Robert Wood Johnson Foundation; 2001. http://www.hetinitiative.org/media/pdf/eHealth.pdf.
9. Van De Belt T, Engelen L, Berben S, Schoonhoven L. Definition of Health 2.0 and Medicine 2.0: a systematic review. *J Med Internet Res*. 2010;12(2):e18. http://www.jmir.org/2010/2/e18/.
10. Pagliaro C, Sloan D, Gregor P, et al. What is ehealth (4): a scoping exercise to map the field. *J Med Internet Res*. 2005;7(1) http://dx.doi.org/10.2196/jmir.7.1.e9.
11. Eysenbach G. What is ehealth? *J Med Internet Res*. 2001;3(2). http://www.jmir.org/2001/2/e20.
12. World Health Organization. *Atlas of eHealth Country Profiles 2015: The Use of eHealth in Support of Universal Health Coverage Based on the Findings of the 2015 Global Survey on eHealth*; 2016. http://www.who.int/goe/publications/atlas_2015/en/.
13. We Are Social. *Digital, Social & Mobile in 2015*; 2015. http://wearesocial.net/blog/2015/01/digital-social-mobile-worldwide-2015.
14. Ericsson Mobility Report: On the pulse of the networked society; 2016. https://www.ericsson.com/res/docs/2016/ericsson-mobility-report-2016.pdf.
15. Internet.org by Facebook. https://internet.org Accessed 20.06.16.
16. Mittman R, Cain M. *The Future of the Internet in Health Care: Five-Year Forecast* [white paper]. California HealthCare Foundation; 1999. http://www.chcf.org/publications/1999/01/the-future-of-the-internet-in-health-care-fiveyear-forecast.
17. National Research Council. *Crossing the Quality Chasm: A New Health System for the 21st Century*. Washington, DC: The National Academies Press; 2001.
18. *Connecting Health and Care for the Nation: A Shared Nationwide Interoperability Roadmap Draft Version 1.0*; 2015. https://www.healthit.gov/sites/default/files/nationwide-interoperability-roadmap-draft-version-1.0.pdf.
19. Fox S, Jones S. *The Social Life of Health Information: Americans' Pursuit of Health Takes Place within a Widening Network of Both Online and Offline Sources*. Washington, DC: Pew Internet & American Life Project; 2009. http://www.pewinternet.org/Reports/2009/8-The-Social-Life-of-Health-Information.aspx.
20. Fox S. *The Social Life of Health Information*. Washington, DC: Pew Internet & American Life Project; 2011. http://www.pewinternet.org/Reports/2011/Social-Life-of-Health-Info.aspx.
21. Fox S. *Health Topics*; Washington, DC: Pew Internet & American Life Project; 2011. http://pewinternet.org/Reports/2011/HealthTopics.aspx.

22. Fox S. *Health Online 2013*. Washington, DC: Pew Internet & American Life Project; 2013. http://www.pewinternet.org/files/old-media//Files/Reports/PIP_HealthOnline.pdf.

23. Duggan M, Ellison N, Lampe C, Lenhart A, Madden M. *Social Media Update 2014*. Washington, DC: Pew Research Center; 2015. http://www.pewinternet.org/2015/01/09/social-media-update-2014/.

24. *IBM Watson Health*; 2015. http://www.ibm.com/smarterplanet/us/en/ibmwatson/health/.

25. National Human Genome Research Institute. *The Human Genome Project Completion: Frequently Asked Questions*. National Human Genome Research Institute; 2003 http://www.genome.gov/11006943.

26. 23andMe; 2016. https://www.23andme.com/.

27. Cortez M, Chen C. Thousands have already signed up for Apple Research Kit. *Bloomberg Bus*. 2015. http://www.bloomberg.com/news/articles/2015-03-11/apple-researchkit-sees-thousands-sign-up-amid-bias-criticism.

28. Federal Register. Medicare and Medicaid programs: electronic health record incentive program-modifications to meaningful use in 2015 through 2017. *A proposed rule by the Centers for Medicare & Medicaid Services*; 2015. https://federalregister.gov/a/2015-08514.

29. Burwell S. Setting value-based payment goals—HHS efforts to improve U.S. health care. *N Engl J Med*. 2015;372:897–899.

30. Cain M, Sarasohn-Kahn J, Wayne J. *Health e-people: the online consumer experience* [white paper]. California HealthCare Foundation; 2000. http://www.chcf.org/publications/2000/08/health-epeople-the-online-consumer-experience.

31. Fox S, Purcell K. *Chronic disease and the internet*. Pew Internet & American Life Project; 2010. http://pewinternet.org/Reports/2010/Chronic-Disease.aspx.

32. Reeder B, Chung J, Lazar A, Joe J, Demiris G, Thompson HJ. Testing a theory-based mobility monitoring protocol using in-home sensors: a feasibility study. *Res Gerontol Nurs*. 2013;6 (4):253–263.

33. deBronkart D. *About Dave*. e-Patient Dave; 2015. http://epatientdave.com/about-dave/.

34. deBronkart D. From patient centered to people powered: autonomy on the rise. *BMJ*. 2015;350:h148.

35. Holliday R. *The Walking Gallery. Regina Holliday's Medical Advocacy Blog*; 2015. http://reginaholliday.blogspot.com/2011/04/walking-gallery.html.

36. Technology Quarterly. The quantified self, counting every moment, technology and health: measuring your everyday activities can help improve your quality of life, according to aficionados of "self-tracking". *Economist*. 2012. http://www.economist.com/node/21548493.

37. Singer E. The measured life: do you know how much REM sleep you got last night? New types of devices that monitor activity, sleep, diet, and even mood could make us healthier and more productive [online exclusive]. *Technol Rev*. 2011. http://www.technologyreview.com/biomedicine/37784/.

38. Lohr S. The healing power of your own medical records. *The New York Times*. 2015. http://nyti.ms/1DmQsEj.

39. Scherger J. Future vision: is family medicine ready for patient-directed care? *Fam Med*. 2009;41(4):285–288.

40. Okun S, Schoenbaum S, Andrews D, et al. *Patients and Health Care Teams Forging Effective Partnerships*. Discussion Paper, Washington, DC: Institute of Medicine; 2014. https://nam.edu/perspectives-2014-patients-and-health-care-teams-forging-effective-partnerships/.

41. Berwick D, Nolan T, Whittington J. The triple aim: care, health and cost. *Health Aff*. 2008;27(3):759–769.

42. Society of Participatory Medicine. http://participatorymedicine.org; 2009.

43. Iverson S, Howard K, Penney B. Impact of internet use on health-related behaviors and the patient-physician relationship: a survey-based study and review. *J Am Osteopath Assoc*. 2008;108(12):699–711.

44. Berwick D. What "patient-centeredness" should mean: confessions of an extremist. *Health Aff*. 2009;28 (4):555–565.

45. deBronkart D. Gimme my damn data. *Keynote speech at: World Congress on Social Networking and Web 2.0 Applications in Medicine*. Toronto: Health, Health Care, and Biomedical Research; September 17, 2009. https://youtu.be/I9JBAuYvsng.

46. Get My Health Data. https://getmyhealthdata.org/; 2015.

47. ANI. *Press release: alliance for nursing informatics joins GetMyHealthRecord effort*; 2015.

48. Sarasohn-Kahn J. *The Wisdom of Patients: Health Care Meets Online Social Media*. California HealthCare Foundation; 2008. http://www.chcf.org/publications/2008/04/the-wisdom-of-patients-health-care-meets-online-social-media.

49. Dill D, Gumpert P. What is the heart of health care? Advocating for and defining the clinical relationship in patient-centered care [online exclusive]. *J Particip Med*. 2012;4:e10. http://www.jopm.org/evidence/reviews/2012/04/25/what-is-the-heart-of-health-care-advocating-for-and-defining-the-clinical-relationship-in-patient-centered-care/#footnote_82.

50. Sarasohn-Kahn J. *Participatory health: online and mobile tools help chronically ill manage their care*. California HealthCare Foundation; 2009. http://www.chcf.org/~/media/MEDIA%20LIBRARY%20Files/PDF/PDF%20P/PDF%20ParticipatoryHealthTools.pdf.

51. Hospital Consumer Assessment of Healthcare Providers and Systems (HCAHPS). HCAHPS fact sheet. *HCAHPS*; 2012. http://www.hcahpsonline.org/files/HCAHPS%20Fact%20Sheet%20May%202012.pdf.

52. PatientsLikeMe; 2012. http://www.patientslikeme.com/patients/view/40?patient_page=1.

53. Swan M. Crowdsourced health research studies: an important emerging complement to clinical trials in the public health research ecosystem. *J Med Internet Res*. 2012;14(2). http://www.jmir.org/2012/2/e46/.

54. Deering MJ. *Issue Brief: Patient Generated Health Data and Health IT*; Washington, DC: Office of the National Coordinator for Health Information Technology; 2013. https://www.healthit.gov/sites/default/files/pghd_brief_final122013.pdf.

55. HealthIT.Gov. *Consumer eHealth: patient-generated health data*. https://www.healthit.gov/policy-researchers-implementers/patient-generated-health-data; Accessed June 20, 2016.

56. Hixson J, Barnes D, Parko K, et al. Patients optimizing epilepsy management via an online community: the POEM Study. *Neurology*. 2015;85(2):129–136.

57. Institute of Medicine. *The Learning Health System Series*. Washington, DC: The National Academies Press; 2011.

58. Delbanco T, Walker J, Darer J, et al. Open notes: doctors and patients signing on. *Ann Intern Med*. 2010;153(2):121–125. http://annals.org/article.aspx?volume=153&issue=2&page=121.

59. Open Notes; 2015. http://www.myopennotes.org/who-is-sharing-notes/.

60. deBronkart D. The magic incantation (for rich products). *e-Patient Dave*; 2012. http://epatientdave.com/.

61. The White House: Expanding public access to the results of federally funded research; 2013. https://www.whitehouse.gov/blog/2013/02/22/expanding-public-access-results-federally-funded-research.

62. Institute of Medicine (IOM). *Sharing Clinical Trial Data: Maximizing Benefits, Minimizing Risk.* Washington, DC: The National Academies Press; 2015.

63. O'Reilly T. *What is Web 2.0: Design Patterns and Business Models for the Next Generation of Software.* O'Reilly; 2005. http://oreilly.com/web2/archive/what-is-web-20.html.

64. Meek A. What role should the government play in developing the internet of things? *Guardian.* 2015. http://www.theguardian.com/technology/2015/oct/14/government-regulation-internet-of-things.

65. Fox S. *Peer-to-Peer Healthcare.* Pew Internet & American Life Project; 2011. http://www.pewinternet.org/~/media//Files/Reports/2011/Pew_P2PHealthcare_2011.pdf.

66. Eysenbach G, Powell J, Englesakis M, Rizo C, Stern A. Health related virtual communities and electronic support groups: systematic review of the effects of online peer to peer interactions. *BMJ.* 2004;328(7449):1166.

67. Schweizer K, Leimeister J, Kremat H. The role of virtual communities for the social network of cancer patients. Paper presented at: 12th Americas Conference on Information Systems; August 4–6, 2006; Acapulco, Mexico.

68. Frost J, Massagli M. Social uses of personal health information within PatientsLikeMe, an online patient community: what can happen when patients have access to one another's data. *J Med Internet Res.* 2008;10(3):e15. http://dx.doi.org/10.2196/jmir.1053.

69. Grajales F, Clifford D, Loupos P, et al. *Social Networking Sites and the Continuously Learning Health System: A Survey.* Discussion Paper, Washington, DC: Institute of Medicine; 2014.

70. Zulman D, Nazi K, Turvey C, Wagner T, Woods S, An L. Patient interest in sharing personal health record information: a web-based survey. *Ann Intern Med.* 2011;155(12):805–810.

71. Nambisan P. Health information seeking and social support in online health communities: impact on patients' perceived empathy. *J Am Med Inform Assoc.* 2011;18(3):298–304.

72. Wicks P, Massagli M, Frost J, et al. Sharing health data for better outcomes on PatientsLikeME. *J Med Internet Res.* 2010;12(2). http://dx.doi.org/10.2196/jmir.1549.

73. Wicks P, Hixson JD. Blog: The Patient Engagement Pill—Lessons from Epilepsy. *Health Affairs Blog*; 2013. February 7, 2013.

74. Goudreau J. Online, women more likely to trust each other. *Forbes.* 2011. http://www.forbes.com/sites/jennagoudreau/2011/01/20/online-women-more-likely-to-trust-each-other-facebook-yahoo-twitter-myspace-marketing/.

75. Huh J, McDonald DW, Hartzler A, Pratt W. Patient moderator interaction in online health communities. *AMIA Annu Symp Proc.* 2013;2013:627–636.

76. British Library and the Joint Information Systems Committee. *Information behaviour of the researcher of the future*; 2008. http://discovery.ucl.ac.uk/177993/.

77. Levit A. Make way for generation Z. *The New York Times.* 2015. http://nyti.ms/1G2FPXD.

78. Topol E. *The Creative Destruction of Medicine: How the Digital Revolution Will Create Better Health Care.* New York, NY: Perseus Books Group; 2011.

79. Topol E. *The Patient Will See You Now: The Future of Medicine.* New York, NY: Perseus Books Group; 2015.

80. P4 Medicine Institute; 2012. http://p4mi.org/.

81. Holliday R. *The word of the day is "Chaordic". Regina Holliday's Health Advocacy Blog*; 2012. http://reginaholliday.blogspot.com/2012/05/word-of-day-is.html.

82. PatientsIncluded; 2015. http://patientsincluded.org/.

83. Precision Medicine Initiative; 2015. https://www.whitehouse.gov/precision-medicine.

84. 21st Century Cures Act. *H.R.6–114th Congress (2015–2016)*; 2015. https://www.congress.gov/bill/114th-congress/house-bill/6.

DISCUSSION QUESTIONS

1. Discuss reasons why clinicians may be reluctant to change their current practice to accommodate the principles of participatory medicine.

2. What ethical concerns do you have about the sharing of health data online?

3. Considering today's privacy rules, how can you be expected to maintain confidentiality when patients are sharing data so freely? How might privacy rules evolve?

4. Defend or refute the following: Patients should have real-time access to all information in their health records, including narrative notes.

5. How can we narrow the gap between technology "haves" and "have-nots"?

6. Develop strategies for working with ePatients and using patient-generated health data in your personal practice and consider if those strategies would be acceptable in your work setting.

7. Debate this statement: Employers who contribute to the cost of employee health insurance can require employees to monitor certain health parameters or pay a higher premium to maintain coverage.

8. If you believe that participatory healthcare should become the standard of care, what policy and legislative changes are needed to make that a reality?

9. Create a vision for the model of healthcare you want in place by 2020. What is the single most important characteristic of your vision on which you are unwilling to compromise?

10. In the interest of public health, shouldn't all capable patients be expected to monitor their health using accessible tools? What, if any, are the unintended consequences of that expectation?

CASE STUDY

A few weeks ago you were hired as Director of Patient Education for a regional medical center located in the Midwest. The medical center includes three community hospitals ranging from 175 to 321 beds, four outpatient clinics, and five centers of excellence. The five centers of excellence are located at two of the hospitals and focus on heart disease, cancer care, care of the aging, neuromuscular disorders, and women's health.

In your position you are responsible for coordinating patient education across the medical center, including all programs and print materials. Your staff includes three BSN-prepared nurses, one located at each of the hospitals. As one of your initial steps in this new position, you have completed an assessment of the current educational offerings and staff satisfaction with the quality of the current programs. One area of need stands out: The professional staff report that a growing number of patients have been joining online social networking sites. One staff member said, "I think they are all helping each other get online." These patients are now raising new and sometimes difficult questions about treatment options. None of the staff has explored any of the online sites, and they are afraid to join for fear that they could become involved in some sort of violation of the Health Insurance Portability and Accountability Act (HIPAA).

Discussion Questions

1. Describe how you would develop a staff education program and create an outline of key points that you would include.

2. Develop a patient handout that the staff can use to educate patients on the effective use of online social media materials.

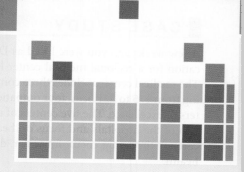

13

Social Media Tools for Practice and Education*

Heather Carter-Templeton

Peer-to-peer healthcare is a way for people to do what they have always done—lend a hand, lend an ear, lend advice—but at internet speed and at internet scale.

Susannah Fox

OBJECTIVES

At the completion of this chapter, the reader will be prepared to:

1. Describe social media tools and their benefits.
2. Explore the current and potential use of social media in healthcare and healthcare education.
3. Analyze the issues and challenges associated with the use of social media in healthcare and healthcare education.
4. Provide guidance for writing social media policies.

KEY TERMS

microblogging, 222
social media, 220

social networks, 221

ABSTRACT ❖

To better understand the concept of social media, this chapter starts with the definition of social media and describes the various tools included under this concept. Current and potential ways that both healthcare professionals and patients/consumers can use social media tools are explored. The challenges of social media in healthcare are examined within the context of privacy, confidentiality, inappropriate behavior, security, regulatory issues, and market pressure. To address these challenges, the chapter provides a comprehensive overview related to the development of social media policies in healthcare.

Acknowledgments: We would like to acknowledge and thank Diane J. Skiba, PhD, FACMI, ANEF, FAAN, Professor & Health Care Informatics Specialty Director, University of Colorado College of Nursing; Elizabeth Dickson, MS, RN, RN Clinical Applications Coordinator, U.S. Department of Veterans Affairs, Cheyenne, Wyoming; Paul Guillory, MS, RN-BC, Bar Code Medication Coordinator/Pharmacy Informaticist, Department of Veterans Affairs, Pacific Islands Health Care System, who wrote this chapter for the first edition of this book. We also wish to thank Heather Carter-Templeton, who revised this chapter and took on the role of author for this edition of the book.

WHAT IS SOCIAL MEDIA?

As noted by Kaplan and Haenlein, "Social media is a group of Internet-based applications that build on the ideological and technological foundations of Web 2.0, and that allow the creation and exchange of user generated content."[1, p. 61] Anthony Bradley of the Gartner Blog Network identified six core principles that differentiate social media from other forms of communication and collaboration:

1. Participation
2. Collective
3. Transparency
4. Independence
5. Persistence
6. Emergence[2]

These characteristics collectively define social media as "an on-line environment established for the purpose of mass collaboration."[3]

For many people in today's society, the most popular internet-based sites are those that allow the individual to make and maintain social connections with others. These sites offer user-friendly and easy ways to keep up with colleagues, family, and/or friends. Many relationships have been maintained or strengthened as a result of these platforms. Some relationships, including professional relationships, would not exist without these platforms. While social media sites and tools are easy to use in establishing and maintain relationships, the overall impact of social media on individuals, groups, and communities is often overlooked.[4]

Social media tools are undeniably transforming how groups and individuals acquire and disperse information, communicate with others, and connect to those with similar interests. It is of no surprise that consumers and businesses have gravitated toward these powerful tools. The healthcare field has not been isolated from this phenomenon and has recognized the potential of social media to increase awareness of healthcare services, disseminate health promotion and preventative education, recruit new clients, connect patients to others with similar experiences, and increase access to health services. Social media steps away from traditional print, radio, and one-way internet methods of mass communication and offers healthcare a new venue for fast, efficient means of sharing information concerning new services, health promotion programs, and advances in patient care.[5] For many, long gone are the days of waiting for a response from a physician to find the answer to a healthcare question.

The Healthcare Information and Management Systems Society (HIMSS) Social Media Work Group speculated that in the long term social media will become ubiquitous and be considered part of routine healthcare operations, in addition to being part of consumers' everyday lives. The group referred to the concept of "healthcare + social media = 'social health'."[6, p. 3] Several reports examining the future transformation of healthcare touted the use of social media as a viable method to meet the widespread needs of patient populations. The Bipartisan Policy Center,[7] in particular, asserted social media platforms can facilitate the promotion of health and wellness.

SOCIAL MEDIA TOOLS

Social media tools are web-based platforms that facilitate interaction and networking among their communities. Social media tools offer a form of communication that allows users to create diverse content for the purposes of sharing with others via online environments. Different types of social media platforms exist, including networking, media sharing, blogs, wikis, and microblogs. These different platforms form the foundation for an ever-growing list of applications. Table 13.1 demonstrates the evolving nature of social media applications using several well-recognized names.

There are various ways to classify social media tools. One method is a classification[1] system based on social theories (social presence[8] and media richness[9]) and two key social process elements (self-presentation and self-disclosure). This system is particularly useful for researchers examining the impact of social media tools. Assumptions that follow from this classification system include the following:

- The higher the social presence (awareness of the communication partners), the more communication partners can influence each other's behavior.[2]
- In terms of media richness, the more information that is shared, the less likelihood there is of ambiguity.
- Self-presentation focuses on how someone depicts his or her image.

TABLE 13.1 Development of Social Media Applications and/or Devices

Year	Device and/or Application
1978	Computerized bulletin board
1992	First smartphone released
1998	Blogger
2000	Friendstar
2002	MySpace
2003	LinkedIn and Facebook
2005	YouTube
2007	iPhone
2009	Twitter
2010	iPad and Pinterest
2010	Instagram
2011	Snapchat
2014	Learnist
The future	Interactions within an augmented virtual reality

Adapted from Nelson R, Joos I, Wolf D. *Social Media for Nurses*. New York, NY: Springer Publishing Company; 2013.

- Self-disclosure in the social media world involves the amount of personal information, including feelings and thoughts, that is shared.

Another way to categorize the use of social media tools is to understand that the structure of a social media site is dependent on its purpose and the exchange of information (Box 13.1).[6] A fairly simple method of organizing social media sites is to classify them by their types of tools. For example, these tools can commonly be divided into five categories:

- Social networking (Facebook)
- Blogging (http://thehealthcareblog.com) and wikis (http://wikidoc.org)
- Microblogging (Twitter, Vine)
- Social bookmarking or pinning (Pinterest) and social sharing news (Digg, reddit)
- Video or image sharing (YouTube, Vimeo, Instagram)

Social Networking

Social networks are online platforms that enable groups and individuals to connect with others who share similar interests. They transcend time and geographic restrictions, opening lines of communication and allowing users to share text, photographs, and videos. The notion is that social networks build on the wisdom of the crowd.[10] Social networks have changed the way individuals, businesses, and organizations experience and interact with the world of healthcare. Examples of health-related services provided by social networks include information sharing, social support, access to information on clinical trials, and processes for monitoring health status and data.[11]

Seemingly an infinite number of health-related social networking sites have been developed by both for-profit and not-for-profit groups, including healthcare institutions, companies' professional groups, voluntary associations, and health consumers. An example of a not-for-profit site is CaringBridge (www.caringbridge.org). This site allows users

---

BOX 13.1 **Social Media Structure**

- *Provider-consumer:* Information exchange between a medical provider or institution and patients or others in the healthcare community. A good example is the Mayo Clinic's Facebook page.
- *Consumer-consumer:* The use of social media by patients, families, or caregivers (consumers) to lend support or gather and share information relating to their diagnoses, treatments, or healthcare providers. A good example is the PatientsLikeMe community, where patients not only share information but their healthcare data on various outcomes.
- *Companies (life sciences)–consumers:* Pharmaceutical and medical device companies' use of social media to engage patients and providers, research use and side effects, market products, support or oppose legislation, and facilitate

notification of recalls. An example is AstraZeneca's use of Facebook and Twitter.
- *Advocacy group–consumer:* Engagement between consumers and advocacy organizations such as the American Heart Association or Autism Speaks.
- *Provider-provider:* Connection between medical providers for the purposes of clinical information and experience exchange. Good examples are Sermo for doctors and the American Nurses Association's NurseSpace.
- *Public health–provider/consumer:* Release of public health messages to promote safety and prevention. A good example is the Centers for Disease Control and Prevention's campaign for H1N1.

Adapted from Healthcare Information and Management Systems Society (HIMSS) Social Media Work Group. HIMSS white paper: Health care "friending" social media: what is it, how is it used, and what should I do? HIMSS. <http://s3.amazonaws.com/rdcms-himss/files/production/public/HIMSSorg/Content/files/HealthcareFriendingSocialMediav15%284%29.pdf>; 2012.

---

to create their own private and personal websites to facilitate health status information exchange and encourage support between friends and family members during health crises.

Examples of for-profit sites include PatientsLikeMe, CureTogether, and Inspire. These sites link patients with each other and facilitate data and information sharing among patients with similar diagnoses.

General social media sites also facilitate important aspects of health-related networking. A great example is Facebook, one of the more popular and well-known social networking sites. A wide range of individuals, businesses, healthcare institutions, companies, special interest groups, and health organizations have Facebook pages. Although not exclusively designed as a forum for healthcare, these Facebook pages are often accessed to gather healthcare information[12] and to market practices or institutions to patients.[13]

Blogging and Wikis

Blogs represent a web-based, chronological journal of an individual author's thoughts. They allow for asynchronous conversations and invite readers to comment and join the discussion.[14] Blogs contain a variety of media types beyond simple text, including links to other websites, video, and images. According to Sparks, O'Seaghdha, Sethi, and Jhaveri (2011), "The popularity of a blog hinges on its ability to draw together disparate individuals interested in a specialized topic, creating a community of ideas, interest, and expertise."[15, p. 512] Medical journals, healthcare facilities, nursing organizations, healthcare provider networks, and educational institutions commonly maintain blogs to relay the latest information and facilitate discussion.

Wikis are collaborative, web-based tools designed to compile information on a particular topic or group of topics. They provide a platform for the creation of a flexible document by allowing many authors to add and edit content. Wikis are often compared to an online encyclopedia. The best known wiki is Wikipedia. These sites usually provide search functionality and links to other articles. Examples of healthcare wikis include Wiki Project Med (https://meta.wikimedia.org/wiki/Wiki_Project_Med); Ganfyd (www.ganfyd.org), developed by medical providers and researchers to generate

healthcare-specific documents; and Clinfowiki (www.clinfowiki.org), focused specifically on clinical informatics.

Microblogging (Twitter)

Microblogging is a form of blogging in which entries are kept brief using character limitations. Twitter, the primary microblogging site, restricts blog threads known as "tweets" to 140 characters. These posts are delineated with a hashtag (#) symbol to organize "tweets" of a particular topic. Several examples of health-related hashtags used on Twitter can be seen at http://www.symplur.com/healthcare-hashtags/.

Twitter has emerged as an increasingly popular site for public health research and is used in many studies to track trends and behaviors related to illnesses and conditions.[16] It has also proved a useful tool for instant communication of vital information during crises or disasters.[14] Some authors have suggested that standard hashtags could be used to create a national conversation within and across disciplines. For example, Resling concluded a 2016 publication with a call for nursing leaders in Canada to consider the need for a national social media hashtag or series of hashtags that could be utilized to unify and extend professional messaging for registered nurses (RNs).[16a]

In 2009 Phil Baumann provided a multipurpose overview of different healthcare uses of Twitter, which continues to be a useful resource. See "140 Health Care Uses for Twitter" at http://philbaumann.com/140-health-care-uses-for-twitter/.

Social Bookmarking

Social bookmarking is a way to organize and store online resources. Unlike saving bookmarks to your individual computer browser, the bookmarks are tagged on a third-party website such as Delicious, Connotea, or Digg. Connotea allows users to bookmark websites as well as journals, a great advantage for researchers. There are three advantages to social bookmarking: "availability, tagging and collaboration."[17, p. 236] Availability means that users' bookmarks are accessible from any computer. The bookmarks are no longer tied to a particular computer; instead, the social bookmarking service allows users to connect and access all saved bookmarks. Second, tagging allows the creation of established tags that are meaningful to the user and not just those established by a computer algorithm. Users can share their tags with others in their network or join other networks to view their tags. In the spirit of social media, these tools facilitate collaboration within specific or general networks. The downsides of tagging are "no standardization with taxonomies such as MeSH [medical subject headings] terms, no hierarchical associations, and mis-tagging due to spelling errors and highly personalized tags."[17, p. 236]

Video and Image Sharing Content

Another method for sharing health information is through the video-sharing website YouTube. This social media channel allows visitors to view and share videos posted by individuals, businesses, and organizations. Content has been developed by both professional and amateur videographers and can be "liked" or "disliked." It can also be accurate or not so accurate. Because YouTube can present visual instruction for hands-on skills such as changing a tracheotomy dressing or giving an insulin injection, this site has a unique advantage for providing health education to patients and providers. Readily available content includes health-promoting exercise instructions, computer-generated depictions of how a condition such as diabetes affects internal organs, and general educational content on diseases. For example, during the Ebola epidemic in 2014, the Centers for Disease Control and Prevention (CDC) posted several videos to YouTube discussing the epidemic and how healthcare providers could protect themselves as well as others. Along with videos, there are podcasts, asynchronous recordings designed to provide healthcare information, and current events announcements.

Flickr is a public photo-sharing site that offers a forum for sharing photos and encouraging conversation and dialog. Medical facilities are actively using these social media tools to interact with clients, promote facility activities, and open alternate means of communication.

Foursquare, a social media tool designed specifically for mobile applications, allows users to "check in" at various venues, instantly communicating with friends and at times receiving discounts at "checked-in" locations (http://foursquare.com). Medical facilities that use mobile platforms are creating the opportunity for visitors to comment on their hospital experience.

Other healthcare sectors are turning to Second Life, a multiuser virtual environment (MUVE) or virtual world that allows users to create a three-dimensional arena with graphics and sound simulation for education and socialization purposes.[14] The disability community has embraced Second Life and has created the Virtual Ability Island[18]; several schools of nursing use this tool for educational purposes.[19]

SOCIAL MEDIA STATISTICS

As the use of social media platforms is becoming more widespread in today's society, social media statistics are constantly changing with a general upward trend. For example, as of 2015 nearly two-thirds of American adults (65%) use social networking sites, up from 7% social media usage in 2005.[20] This increased use is also seen in healthcare. For example, the number of social media–related articles indexed in healthcare library databases is increasing. The number of health-related institutions of with social media policies is also increasing. In addition, many scholarly journals and professional organizations are using social media to promote and share content, and healthcare organizations are creating and expanding social media pages. Many healthcare consumers turn to these resources to learn more about their conditions or to connect with others.

According to a recent report by PricewaterhouseCoopers Health Research Institute, one-third of healthcare consumers now use social media to find out more about their medical condition and symptoms and to share thoughts about their doctors, medications, and insurance companies with others.[20a] The following social medical–related statistics were also compiled by Referral MD:

- Greater than 40% of healthcare consumers are influenced by social media that inform them about health-related matters.
- People aged 18 to 24 are twice more likely than 45- to 54-year-olds to seek social media for discussions regarding health.
- Thirty-one percent of healthcare organizations have specific guidelines or policies for their staff pertaining to social media.
- Nineteen percent of smartphone users have at least one app focused on health. The most popular type of apps are related to diet, exercise, and weight loss.
- Many trust information found through crowdsourcing; 54% of patients are comfortable with their healthcare provider looking for information about their condition from online groups.
- Thirty-one percent of healthcare professionals use social media tools such as Facebook, Twitter, and LinkedIn to network.
- Forty-one percent of people surveyed said social media would influence their choice of healthcare provider and facility.
- Twenty-six percent of hospitals in the United States use some form of social media, with Facebook being the most popular platform used.
- Sixty percent of doctors believe social media improves the quality of care provided to patients.[21]

According to the International Telecommunication Union, "the number of active social media users surpassed the first billion in 2011, many of whom connect to social media using their mobile devices."[22, p. 5] In the United States, nearly four in five active internet users visit blogs and social networks daily, spending approximately 23% of their internet time at these sites.[23]

According to the National Research Corporation's Ticker survey,[11] one in five Americans use social media to obtain healthcare information. The Pew Research Center, in describing the social life of health information, revealed that 59% of U.S. adults have used the internet to obtain health information, while 46% of adults use social media.[24] Only 15% of those users (or 7% of all adults) have sought health information from a social media site.[24] Eleven percent of all adults have followed a friend's health experiences on social network sites and 17% of social network site users have used social networks to memorialize someone.[24] Twenty-four percent of internet users have sought drug reviews online.[24] Caregivers and those living with chronic conditions are most likely to seek information from social network sites.[24]

Health-related social network use is expanding rapidly. Specific social networks, such as PatientsLikeMe, MedHelp, and Inspire, present membership and daily usage statistics on their web pages and demonstrate an impressive number of members. Social media is also being used by hospitals throughout the United States. Results from a recent descriptive study found that there was variation among adoption of social media across hospitals. The majority (94.41%, 3351/3371) had a Facebook page, a Yelp page (99.14%, 3342/3371), and had the ability to check in via Foursquare (99.41%, 3351/3371); about half (50.82%, 1713/3371) had a Twitter account. Hospitals in large, urban areas classified as private nonprofit and teaching hospitals had higher utilization of these tools.[25] A majority of physicians have social media accounts for personal use,[12] including 28% using online professional physician communities, mainly for educational purposes but also to communicate with colleagues, socially and professionally. However, use by physicians to communicate with patients is rare.[12] Professional workforce sites such as LinkedIn allow healthcare professionals to connect with others in their field. Doc2doc, Sermo, and Student Doctor Network all offer forums designated specifically for physician collaboration and networking. Sermo is designed exclusively for physicians and can be used to hold "closed door" consultations with colleagues and access experts in the field.[14] Nurses and other healthcare specialists maintain their own profession-specific social networking sites to communicate field-relevant information, such as American Nurses Association's (ANA's) Nurse Space and NurseGroups.com.

Many major healthcare systems have realized the positive influence of social media and committed to the use of social networking tools to support the delivery of healthcare information, describe their services, recruit employees, and communicate their mission.[4] The U.S. Department of Veterans Affairs (VA) recognized the power of social media and is aggressively incorporating social media tools into its agenda. In December 2011 the VA announced Facebook pages for all of its 151 facilities, with more than 352,000 subscribers. While the Facebook sites restrict specific discussion of individual veterans, the staff members monitoring the site have at times intervened to lend support in mental health crisis situations.[26] The VA has its own YouTube channel, 64 Twitter feeds, a Flickr page for photos, and a veteran-run blog. The VA's *Directive 6515: Use of Web-Based Collaboration Technologies* not only highly encourages the use of social media but also "endorses the secure use of Web-based collaboration and social media tools to enhance communication, stakeholder outreach collaboration, and information exchange; streamline processes; and foster productivity improvements to achieve seamless access to information."[27, p. 1] The VA believes that the use of social media technologies will support

the organization's mission effectiveness through the benefits of speed, broad reach, targeted reach, collaboration, a medium for dialog, and expansion of real-time, sensitive communications.[27]

The Mayo Clinic has also embraced social media, pioneering a first-of-its-kind social media center. The Mayo Clinic Center for Social Media "exists to improve health globally by accelerating effective application of social media tools throughout Mayo Clinic and spurring broader and deeper engagement in social media by hospitals, medical professionals and patients."[28] The Mayo Clinic Center for Social Media's mission to "lead the social media revolution in health care"[28] is driven by a philosophy of improved health through patient empowerment and collaboration among healthcare providers. To facilitate the growth of social media in healthcare, the Mayo Clinic offers a residency training program that provides advanced intensive training in the use of social media.

Healthcare insurance companies are also joining the trend of using social media tools to promote well-being. Blue Cross and Blue Shield (BCBS) maintains a social media site for its members that allows individual profiles, blogs, discussion threads, and access to experts in nutrition, cooking, and health coaching. Pharmaceutical companies are using social media tools to provide customers and physicians with educational materials.[12] Input from physicians facilitates a relationship with pharmaceutical companies to "collaborate for adherence solutions" for improved patient outcomes.[12] These sites also offer customer and patient services, opening channels for medication users to discuss experiences and needs.[12]

BENEFITS OF SOCIAL MEDIA

There are several benefits associated with the use of social media. One of the most obvious benefits is the opportunity to improve provider-to-provider as well as patient-to-provider and provider-to-patient communication. Social media offers a means of communication between provider and patient that is more personable and can have the unintended consequences of an enhanced patient experience.[29] By improving communication and facilitating the swift transfer of information, the use of social media may correlate with a positive influence on patient outcomes.[30] These tools go beyond simple one-way communication, creating an engaging form of conversation between patient and provider.[31]

Another benefit is in the area of research. A growing number of studies describe potential benefits of social media. These studies can be divided into three general areas of research in social media: (1) description of the content on social media sites, (2) the use of social media, and (3) potential use of social networks for research. The first area examines the content of social media being disseminated through social networks and microblogging tools such as Twitter. Content analyses and text-mining techniques are used to assess the nature and quality of the content. Findings from this research include the following:

- The most common health conditions on social media are diabetes, cancer, pregnancy, mental health, and neurologic conditions.[32]

- Social networks are places where information, including personal experiences and personal stories, can be shared with the intended community.[33-36]
- The majority of the information is valid, although this can vary from network to network.[34,37-39]
- Twitter messages produce valuable public health information about the public's knowledge of antibiotics,[38] H1N1,[37,39] and seizures.[40] Researchers have validated Twitter as a real-time content, sentiment, and "public attention trend-tracking tool."[39, p. e14118]
- "Twitter might also be a promising platform for leveraging social support to motivate health behaviour change"[42, p. 1159] and promoting healthy behaviors.[41,43]

The second area of studies examined how specific patient populations used social media. PatientsLikeMe[44-46] is the most studied network to date. Other studies examined specific patient populations (oncology,[47-50] depression,[51] traumatic brain injury,[52] and asthma[53]). Highlighted findings are as follows:

- Benefits noted by patients included finding others with similar health conditions[44-48] and seeking information related to symptom management and treatments.[44-46]
- Patients used various techniques to search for other patients' video stories[47] and used them for encouragement[48] and social support.[49,51]
- Facebook had the largest number of social networks for breast cancer but most were for increasing public awareness and fundraising.[50]

The final area examined two major uses of social networks in the research process. First, researchers are recruiting potential clinical trial subjects from within disease-specific web and social networking sites that then provide this information to pharmaceutical companies, universities, and research labs.[10,13,54,55] Second, researchers are using social networks to accelerate clinical discoveries[10,56,57] and provide "a low-cost and scalable model of citizen science"[58, p. e19256] for data sharing and bidirectional communication within a disease population. According to Swan, "Self-run clinical trials and structured self-experimentation are emerging as patients no longer have to wait for formal research findings and pharmaceutical company-sponsored clinical trials. These efforts may fill the gap for orphan diseases and other conditions that do not make good business cases in the existing pharmaceutical model."[10, p. 500]

Additional benefits of social media include access to information and social support. Facebook, YouTube, and Twitter are the most common social media sites used by patients to obtain healthcare information or interact with other patients with similar diseases or health and wellness interests. "Social media platforms for online dialogue and support among individuals with common conditions, needs or interests support prevention, wellness, and healthy behaviors."[6, p. 14] Social media sites[59] not only foster social support but also enable patients to manage their own health conditions, typically at no direct cost to the patient. That is because many of for-profit sites make that profit by selling the data collected from patient postings as well as through targeted advertising to these patients.[4]

Two predominant forces are "driving online health conversation: (1) the availability of social tools and (2) the motivation, especially among people living with chronic conditions, to connect with each other."[22, p. 3] The most popular social media sites specifically geared toward patients (PatientsLikeMe, CureTogether, MedHelp, and Inspire) offer venues for dialog and also shift the power of achieving health and well-being into patients' own hands. As healthcare evolves from paternalistic to partnership models,[10] these two forces will continue to fuel the growth of social media in healthcare. The development of social media arenas has created a community of ePatients engaged in their health and healthcare decisions (http://e-patients.net/about-e-patientsnet). Many of these individuals will take part in quantified self-tracking (online data entry of condition, symptom, treatment, and other biological information to monitor personal progress) and search for "patients like me."[10]

CHALLENGES OF SOCIAL MEDIA

The world of social media is not free of challenges and opposition. Social media can enhance the consumer's and provider's healthcare experience but also has the potential to undermine the goals of healthcare.[60] Thus the strengths of social media's open platform and networking capabilities are also its greatest weaknesses. The uptake of new technology requires a careful appraisal and informed risk analysis. Unfortunately, many are not exploring the benefits of social media due to prolonged discussion and debate often stalled by skepticism and by those who are risk averse.[61]

While social media connections are facilitated through technology, the technology should not necessarily be the focal point, but it should serve as the medium used to connect with others. Many may be apprehensive about using social media platforms to communicate with others, offering reasons such as:

- It takes too much time to learn
- Participation may be seen as unprofessional by other healthcare providers
- It is too easy to make a mistake and post something that is prohibited by an employer's social media policy
- It is too easy to make a mistake and post something that compromises patient confidentiality

Social media has quickly developed into an acceptable form of mass communication.[62] However, managing the stakes associated with social media communication channels requires professionals that learn to effectively use these tools, work to share quality information, engage other stakeholders, and respond to feedback from others.

Health professionals should be aware of the dangers associated with social media use prior to engaging in its activities.[60,63] The primary principle influencing the use of social media in healthcare is the obligation to serve the best needs of the public; however, clinicians are bound by laws, practice ethics, and professional codes of conduct governing how and when to use social media applications. The digital environment is not isolated from the real world,[64] and professional standards that exist in one realm should carry over to the other. Moreover, naive and negligent social media practices bring about security vulnerabilities that can compromise

TABLE 13.2	Health Related Professional Guidelines and Social Media	
Professional Association	**Document Title**	**URL**
AMA	Professionalism in the use of Social Media	\<http://www.ama-assn.org/ama/pub/dab/9124a-abstract.page\>
ANA	ANA's Principles for Social Networking and the Nurse	\<http://www.nursingworld.org/MainMenuCategories/ThePracticeofProfessionalNursing/NursingStandards/ANAPrinciples.aspx\>
AMA; NZMSA AMSA	Social Media and the Medical Professions: A Guide to Online Professionalism for Medical Practitioners and Medical Students	\<Social_Media_and_the_Medical_Profession_FINAL_with_links.pdf\>
Federation of State Medical Boards	Model Policy Guidelines for the Appropriate Use of Social Media and Social Networking in Medical Practice	\<https://www.fsmb.org/Media/Default/PDF/FSMB/Advocacy/pub-social-media-guidelines.pdf\>
NCSBN	White Paper: A Nurse's Guide to the Use of Social Media	\<https://www.ncsbn.org/Social_Media.pdf\>
NMC	Guidance on Using Social Media responsibly	\<http://www.nmc.org.uk/standards/guidance/social-networking-guidance/\>
NMC	Social Networking Site Guidance	\<http://www.nmc-uk.org/Nurses-and-midwives/Advice-by-topic/A/Advice/Social-networking-sites/\>
RCN	Use of Digital Technology: Guidance for Nursing Staff Working With Children and Young People	\<http://www.rcn.org.uk/__data/assets/pdf_file/0008/586988/004_534_web.pdf\>
INRC	INRC Social Media Use: Common Expectations for Nurses	\<http://www.cno.org/globalassets/docs/prac/incr-social-media-use-common-expectations-for-nurses.pdf\>

AMA, American Medical Association; *ANA,* American Nurses Association; *NZMSA,* New Zealand Medical Student Associations; *AMSA,* Australian Medical Student Association; *NCSBN,* National Council of State Boards of Nursing; *NMC,* Nursing and Midwifery Council; *RCN,* Royal College of Nursing; *INRC,* The International Nurse Regulator Collaborative.

professional integrity and consumer confidence.[60] Fortunately private and professional organizations recognizing these issues have provided guidance regarding appropriate social media practices. Table 13.2 provides several examples. Each of these issues will be explored in more detail in the sections that follow.

Privacy and Confidentiality

The most significant challenge for healthcare providers who use social media is to maintain privacy and confidentiality. There is an innate relationship between privacy and sharing many aspects of a personal or professional situation. Digital social media tools have brought these challenges to the forefront. Prior to social media, with its open access, individuals and organizations had more control over what information was shared and who had access to that shared information. With online, real-time capabilities, that control is much more limited. This loss of control requires more attention and awareness with regard to personal information that can be quickly and easily shared within online social environments. Each social media application offers options, often referred to as settings, related to privacy. It is not always easy to find and determine how these options actually function. However, it is important to invest the time and effort necessary to understand these options. The advantages social media offers for professionals and scholars in terms of networking can be greater than the risks associated with privacy issues.[65]

Social media applications tout the ability for users to establish "many-to-many" relationships. As promising as that may sound, these open forums provide the opportunity for clinicians to inadvertently divulge consumer information to a vast number of people. A valuable mindset to have is to equate a social media application to the circumstances inside a hospital elevator;[66] any number of people can ride in an elevator and all can hear the conversations taking place within them. Further, healthcare providers are "dual citizens" in the social media arena[67] because they have professional and private uses for social media–generated content. This dual role increases the chance that professional boundaries may blur and may encourage clinicians to inadvertently communicate too openly.[68-74]

Healthcare providers are accountable to federal laws and professional standards that protect the privacy of patients' protected health information (PHI).[60,75] The Health Insurance Portability and Accountability Act (HIPAA) of 1996 defined the appropriate handling of PHI.[75] Government agencies and employees are further restricted by the Privacy Act passed in 1974.[76] Both require that a patient must provide authorization before healthcare professionals and organizations can release any part of the patient's record.[72,77] PHI refers to individually identifiable information that is related to the delivery of healthcare[78] and does not always indicate obvious identifiers such as name, social security number, and date of birth.[79] Additional information about the privacy and security rules within the HIPAA legislation is included in Chapter 26.

Even without explicit representation of such individually identifiable information, social media applications are rich with other details that could identify a particular consumer.[80] Social media profiles displaying a consumer's hometown, personal interests, and family photographs may be pieced together to reveal the consumer's identity. Consequently, healthcare providers may inadvertently reveal certain key facts that could lead others to recognize a specific patient.[79]

In addition to federal regulations, healthcare providers are bound by their professional codes of conduct, which regard privacy and confidentiality as compulsory. For example, the ANA's Code of Ethics states that the "nurse has a duty to maintain confidentiality of all patient information."[81, p. 6] Further, according to the ANA's Principles of Social Networking and the Nurse, "patient privacy is a fundamental ethical and legal obligation of nurses."[60, p. 4] Physicians are also committed to keeping patient information private. According to the American Medical Association's (AMA's) Code of Ethics,[82] physicians should not share confidential information without prior consent of the patient. In addition, the AMA has established a social media policy for physicians.[83] These standards apply even when healthcare providers are not physically in their clinical roles.[60]

Conscious awareness and diligent adherence to laws and professional standards may not be enough. Healthcare providers acting in good faith may still unwittingly expose consumers to privacy and confidentiality risks. The primary reason lies in the naive trust they may have in the privacy settings of the social media application itself.[72] Risks often arise because clinicians fail to invoke certain privacy settings in their social media accounts.[72] Further, social networking sites such as Facebook often push privacy barriers and wait until consumers complain before tightening privacy restrictions.[84] "Friending" is one example of a less conspicuous means of breaching privacy. A healthcare provider may "friend" a patient in hopes of keeping in better contact but fail to realize that the other "friends" on his or her account may also be able to view the patient's name and information.[70,85] Another critical point to consider is the consumers' own account settings, as they may not share the same level of social media literacy.[13] For instance, a patient may not realize that adding a healthcare provider as a friend may expose the patient to unwanted scrutiny from other friends. Although this is entirely the patient's choice, healthcare providers are responsible for advocating for the best interests of their patients.[81,82]

Another naive assumption about the use of social media is the belief that consumers are who they claim to be.[86] Healthcare providers unaware of identity impersonation or hacking may unknowingly be divulging private information to someone other than the intended consumer. Just because consumer social media pages may have images and some recognizable data do not quantifiably identify them as accurately representing those individuals. Unless clinicians have a means to authenticate the consumer's identity, there is no way to guarantee that any social media contact, no matter how secure or confidential, involves the intended individuals. The relative permanence of online activity[60] adds an even greater degree of harm when sharing information with consumers who are not validated.

Inappropriate Behaviors

In addition to the risk of jeopardizing patient privacy and confidentiality, healthcare providers are also in danger of openly engaging in inappropriate behaviors. The danger arises from a healthcare provider's "dual citizenship" in the social arena.[64] This dichotomous role can blur the personal and professional boundaries that exist more clearly in the physical world.[70,71,73,74,87] In some cases the information a healthcare provider shares with his family and friends may be inappropriate for the general public to see. Consequently, healthcare providers must maintain the same level of professionalism online as they would in a healthcare setting.[60,68,75]

Inappropriate behaviors can include questionable blog and photo postings, unprofessional commenting, and projecting attitudes unbecoming of respectable healthcare personnel.[88] Not only does such behavior tarnish the clinician's reputation; it can also result in disciplinary action. For example, physicians have been reprimanded for misrepresenting their credentials, improper internet prescribing, and sexual misconduct.[89] Moreover, news agencies from various countries around the world have reported incidences of clinician improprieties, including nursing students posting images of organs (e.g., displaying a photograph of a placenta), medical students being vulgar or sexually suggestive, and doctors engaging in unprofessional social "games" online.[90-92]

Although these behaviors reflect a lack of personal accountability,[87] other professional indiscretions can be even more profound. Healthcare providers may find themselves endorsing drug products or third-party businesses by joining their online groups or "friending" one of their employees.[93] Such activities, without the appropriate declaration of conflict of interest,[73] could give consumers false impressions.

Another indiscretion involves clinicians actively seeking out patient information online. In particular, behavioral healthcare providers face professional dilemmas when determining whether to view a client's social media site to gain further clinical insight.[94] Although intended to facilitate clinical evaluations, such actions could be viewed as a violation of the patient's trust.[94] Behavioral healthcare providers are also particularly challenged when gauging the appropriate amount of client contact: too much contact through social media could encourage client transference and too little could lead to patients feeling rejected or abandoned.[71] Further, nurses who are excessively passionate about social media use for consumer advocacy may also be vulnerable to crossing boundaries.[95] Patient advocacy is a professional obligation for nurses;[81] however, social media applications enable nurses to overstep their boundaries. In an effort to connect with patients and win patient approval, some nurses can end up disclosing too much of their own personal information and come across as flirtatious or self-centered and misrepresent their profession.[95] Healthcare providers can falter in attempts at appropriate online behavior if they do not keep the patients' best interests in mind and advocate for patient well-being.[68,95]

Healthcare providers who use social media must consider who might view their postings and what impact those postings could have on their individual careers as well as their profession.[60,96] They must always consider social media platforms to be public domain and open to others who are unintended participants.[68] Failure to recognize these truths can have untoward consequences. Organizations and academic programs have taken punitive steps to address inappropriate behaviors, including expulsion of students and suspension or termination of employees.[87,91,97,98] Licensing boards have held disciplinary hearings in response to member misconduct.[89] Employers have also passed over applicants that have questionable content on their social media sites. Insurance companies likewise use social media platforms to validate claims or check on beneficiaries.[99,100] Thus inappropriate behaviors could lead to loss of coverage or cancellation of insurance payments.[101]

Security

Social media applications reside on the internet, which is characteristically and notoriously unsecure.[102,103] This high-risk environment is one of the principal reasons why healthcare organizations often restrict employee access to social media sites.[87,104,105] Although there are few reports of social media–related security breaches in healthcare, organizations do not have to look far to comprehend the risk that social media use can bring. Even with strict security settings, healthcare information systems are still susceptible to viruses, spyware, phishing, and other internet threats.[102,105] The primary reasons for these vulnerabilities are the personnel themselves,[106,107] who succumb to social engineering deceptions and can inadvertently allow the social media site to be a vector for malicious behavior.[86,106] Social engineering is the use of tactics to lure or deceive people into doing something they would not normally do. Social media applications have made it easier for dishonest individuals to attack others by enabling contact with numerous people at relatively little or no cost and with virtually complete anonymity.[108] These deceptions can be carried out through the social media site's electronic mail, which can contain deleterious software or an infected link on someone's blog. The social media user's interaction with these malicious attacks enables harmful applications to bypass electronic defenses and enter an organization's previously secure network.[106]

Another avenue for perpetrators to infiltrate another computer network is by "malicious friending."[106] This occurs when a person who is accepted as a friend changes his or her profile to include malicious code or unwanted content.[106] Malicious friending can also happen through distal extensions, or friends of friends. Users who open up their privacy settings to friends may inadvertently allow extended friends into their personal sites and subsequently make themselves vulnerable to attack.[108] These vulnerabilities are considered a type of social engineering that thrives in the social media arena, where users are quick to assume trust in the social media platform as well as in other users.[107,109]

Even with sound judgment and scrupulous navigation, social media users may engender security vulnerabilities by placing too much trust in the social media platform they are using.[107] Hackers, or those who infiltrate websites for malicious purposes, can implant malicious code into the social media site itself.[107] This is often done through advertisements[107] or by deceiving users into accessing an alternate log-in screen.[110] There is also free software that allows anyone to access another's social media account when both are on an unsecured wireless network.[86] Further, sites like Twitter, which enable broadcasting of microblogs, can also promulgate the spread of malicious activity by disseminating abbreviated links to websites that appear safe but are in fact gateways that lead the recipient to a harmful internet location.[107,111]

The means by which users access social media platforms has also elevated security risks. In particular, more and more users engage in social media via mobile devices,[107,109,112] such as laptops, tablets, and smartphones. These devices increase social media use and have also made users more vulnerable.[113-115] The ease of social media use on these platforms can encourage users to divulge too much personal information.[116] Unwitting consumers who post their location and activity on their social networking site may, for instance, actually invite thieves to rob their homes.[114]

Social media use on a mobile device also opens the risk of additional threats from other third-party applications called remote access Trojans (RATs)[107,114] A RAT is a malware program that opens a backdoor to the user's computer, thereby opening up to a third-party administrative control over the user's computer. These RATs can appear harmless to the user while allowing third parties to access the user's personal information.[107,115,117] These apps can then share the information with others, destroy it outright, or use it to impersonate the content owner.[107,117] Moreover, apps often operate in the background, unnoticed by the user, and can steal passwords, personal account data, and other private information.[102] Finally, storing personal information, such as details of a social media profile, on a mobile device increases security vulnerabilities if the device is lost or stolen.[111,115]

Security breaches from any of these vulnerabilities can result in loss of data and varying degrees of criminal activity.[104] Hackers could obtain clinician passwords and gain access to a hospital's vast database of PHI, leading to privacy breaches and financial damages. While loss of financial data is damaging, access to PHI could lead to identity theft and cyberbullying or cyberstalking, and in turn significant emotional and mental turmoil. Identity theft has been labeled as one of the top five social networking scams.[110] Moreover, identity theft has been reported as one of the most frequent consumer complaints regarding internet use, second only to nondelivery of goods.[118] According to the Federal Trade Commission (FTC), identity theft is the number one consumer complaint category, and these grievances are continuing to grow.[119]

Social media application use can contribute to the threat of identity theft by expanding the user's digital footprint, described as lingering electronic information that can be linked back to the user who provided it.[120,121] The bits of information disseminated across the internet can be combined to form a more detailed profile of the individual.[121] Social media users' naive efforts to become visible to friends and relatives actually may make them "knowable" to others who may have malicious inclinations.[119] Thus the open and trusted sharing of personal information can turn on the user and be employed for purposes other than what the user intended.[122,123]

Cyberharassment and cyberstalking are also increasing.[118] These terms are synonymous with cyberbullying but refer to adult behavior, whereas cyberbullying generally refers to underage harassment.[124] Regardless of the terminology, these are all considered social threats and are described as the stigmatizing, bullying, and threatening of others. This intimidation can pose significant danger to the recipients and their affiliates or friends.[79] Cyberstalking is not limited to threats or intimidation directed at specific individuals; organizations can be targeted as well.[86] Discrimination can be directed toward an individual's or organization's religious affiliation, political views, sexual orientation, or group association;[80] it can even involve an individual's medical diagnosis or hospitalizations. Cyberharassment, sometimes called digital abuse, includes online threats or aggression toward individuals or groups with the objective of intimidating or coercing others who are perceived as being unable to retaliate.[125,126] Social media platforms, which enable anonymous activity, have propagated these behaviors in the internet environment.[126] In addition to practicing these behaviors in relative anonymity, cyberstalkers may also impersonate another individual, thus causing further harm while displacing the blame.[110] Healthcare providers are not immune to such behavior, as was seen when a British surgeon's identity was stolen and used to create a Facebook page that slandered an Olympic swimmer.[127]

Regulatory Issues

Many of the challenges and risks discussed here exist because social media sites and the internet as a whole are not effectively regulated.[60,128] The Federal Communications Commission (FCC)[129] is the U.S. government body responsible for regulating communication through various media, including those employed for internet use. In 2015 the FCC voted to maintain "net neutrality."[130] Net neutrality is the principle that internet service providers and governments regulating the internet should treat all data on the internet in the same manner, not discriminating or charging differentially by user, content, website, platform, application, type of attached equipment, or mode of communication.

One of the key agencies in healthcare, with legal authority to control who may contribute social media content, is the U.S. Food and Drug Administration (FDA).[131] The FDA regulates the distribution of drugs and medical devices.[131,132] Pharmaceutical companies often engage in social media to promote consumer interaction and adverse events reporting,[132] However, these companies must be cautious and avoid posting anything that could be interpreted as off-label promotion.[133] They must also be careful when using social media to respond to unsolicited requests for drug information, as this avenue reaches a broader audience and remains viewable for an indefinite period of time.[131] Consequently, pharmaceutical and device manufacturing companies must respond according to FDA guidance to not appear to be promoting their products for unapproved purposes.[131]

Further, as discussed earlier, healthcare provider behavior is governed by laws limiting the kinds of information to be disclosed and to whom. This is directly related to the appropriate use of consumers' PHI. In addition to patient content restrictions, healthcare providers must be aware of the medical information they post and the advice, if any, they provide. This information should be appropriate and reliable and avoid any copyright infringement.[134] Misinformation can be detrimental as well as dangerous to the individual and organization.[60,135] It is also critical that healthcare providers avoid engaging in behavior that might be regarded as fraudulent or an abuse of their position. Certain social media information exchanges could be construed as kickbacks or inappropriate in the medical-legal environment.[134,136] If healthcare providers use social media with the intention of providing care, they are using telehealth, allowing for the provision of care over a distance using telecommunication technology.[137] Accordingly, social media used as a form of telecommunication could be regulated by the clinician's state and local agencies overseeing telehealth licensing and scope of practice.[138] Additional information about these regulations can be found in Chapter 8.

In light of the absence of more definitive regulation of social media sites, some have pushed the need for the federal government to intervene.[139] The risk to the public regarding privacy, confidentiality, and information security would seem to endorse that sentiment. Still, others have suggested that social media sites engender crowd wisdom and can engage in their own self-regulation.[112]

Market Pressure

The myriad risks associated with social media use have caused some healthcare providers to avoid using these applications.[140] Yet consumer demand and in turn market pressure for social media applications in healthcare continue to grow. Healthcare providers who rely on advertising to increase clientele may have no other choice but to enter the social media arena.[140-142] Social media has become a driving force for corporate marketing as well as consumer ratings.[141,143] This is especially true as more and more social media resources are emerging to provide public opinion on goods and services.[144]

The fact is that consumers are the primary driving force for using social media in healthcare, and increasing numbers of consumers seek health information online.[145] The resource of choice for many consumers is a healthcare provider.[146] Consequently, consumers may search for and expect to learn more about their healthcare questions from clinicians using these sites.

As more and more private practice physicians join accountable care organizations (ACOs), marketing and consumer ratings will become more significant. The push to provide patient-centered care[147] in ACOs will add pressure to those organizations and physicians who are currently reluctant to use social media as one option to connect with their patients.

Many organizations and individual clinicians have recognized these trends and the value that social media tools can bring, such as ease of use, information sharing, and timely updates.[148,149] From a business perspective, healthcare institutions find the low cost of social media an economical means to market their resources,[150] educate patients, and engender client loyalty.[151] The increase in clientele gained from social media use[5,97] can counter the lack of financial reimbursement,[140,152] as well as the time and effort needed to stay involved in social media sites.[135,153] With this pressure, the number of participating organizations and clinicians is expected to grow, adding to the expanding use of social media to market healthcare goods and services. Nonparticipating individuals and groups may feel pressured to opt in, just so that they too may gain market exposure.

Within healthcare organizations, many often work tirelessly to make sure channels of communication are handled carefully. In most cases, healthcare organizations began to use social media for the purposes of marketing and public relations. These new and novel avenues of contact and dissemination offered healthcare organizations contemporary ways to reach those they served and potentially gain more consumers. Organizations often worked with those designated to maintain their websites and marketing materials to integrate their brand into the world of social media. Healthcare providers also began to use social media tools to discover how they might include them in their care and patient encounters. Social media platforms are becoming more and more intertwined into our daily lives and activities. Furthermore, many healthcare provider recruiters use social media to gain the attention of candidates and potential employees by direct contact or by publicizing a healthy work environment. Healthcare organizations will continue looking for innovative and relevant ways to use social media for consumer and provider engagement.[62]

Social media is clearly valuable in increasing organizations' visibility. Some organizations may question whether they can flourish and prosper without these tools. According to Allison, "It's the new coffee shop."[154, p 50] The two most likely platforms to connect with your patients are Twitter and Facebook. Prior to the advent of the internet, healthcare consumers used the advice of their friends and family when learning about health-related information and resources. That remains the same; however the amount of friends and contacts we can access easily is greater than before. Patients and healthcare consumers can now use these connections to broadcast their feelings about their care. In turn, this gives healthcare providers and organizations the opportunity to come in contact with consumers in real time.

A new source of healthcare-related information is now available in the form of rating sites that offer information from a patient perspective about quality of care. Consumers are more frequently posting their opinions online as to whether or not they like a particular service or experience.[144] Numerous websites allow patients to rate their physician or hospital experiences (e.g., Vitals.com, DoctorScorecard.com). General business websites such as Yelp also allow consumers to rate and post comments on various hospitals and healthcare service organizations. Consequently, consumers often seek ratings or rankings from others before making a decision about purchasing goods and services, including healthcare.[146]

One of the great risks of social media rating sites is not knowing what rating information, whether good or bad, is being shared.[143] For example, healthcare providers may be surprised to discover their services are being rated by a site they never heard of and by "patients" they have never seen. While one might challenge the authenticity of what is found on social media and the internet, this new source could potentially be useful as a complement to traditional methods of measuring quality of care. Some suggest future research exploring how suitable social media is in assisting to judge the quality of care offered by healthcare professionals and organizations.[155]

With the growing number of sites and consumer interest in them, healthcare organizations and clinicians may feel compelled to create a social media site to promote their strengths and perhaps counter any negative ratings.[141] Contributing to this urgency is the fact that organization rankings have been posted on hospital scoring websites such as Healthgrades, Hospital Compare (operated by the U.S. Department of Health & Human Services), and ConsumerReports.org.

Another compelling reason to enter the social media arena is to dispel misinformation and bridge the digital divide. Consumers have unprecedented access to health information on the internet but may encounter inaccurate data.[133,145,152,156] Social media enables the creation and propagation of inaccurate and misleading information.[60,96,128,157-159] Largely due to lack of oversight,[159] web-based information can be created by anyone[128] and be disseminated far too easily.[133] Just about anyone can enter, alter, edit, and even sabotage social media applications.[150] Moreover, authors of social media content do not need to identify themselves[158] or provide any credentials.[96] Site association can also perpetuate inaccuracies. Authors of blog content who are not members of the health profession may associate themselves with reputable sites in order to seem as though they are in the field.[96] Consumers may also be misled by inaccuracies or opinions that dominate a particular site.[153,160] For example, an overabundance of opposition to child vaccinations on certain sites[153,160] could dissuade parents from immunizing their children, even though vaccines are valuable and could even save a child's life.[161] Information, even when accurately presented, can be reviewed out of context in the social media arena,[162] and subjective healthcare material can be easily accessed, circumventing any disclaimers or warnings.[163]

Healthcare providers are in a position to counter inaccuracies by sponsoring a social media site themselves or guiding consumers to reputable sites.[157] By choosing the latter strategy, healthcare professionals can become apomediaries.[156] Apomediation involves standing by to direct consumers to high-quality information on the internet rather than standing between the consumer and the information, as has been the usual practice in the past.[156] Clinicians may do this in person by interpreting web-based healthcare information that patients bring to their office visits.[160,164] Clinicians could also perform outreach via social media applications to contact and guide consumers who post questions or concerns regarding health conditions or services. Caution in these situations is necessary, as clinicians do not control the content of the referred site and there is a chance that a healthcare provider could recommend an unreliable source.[156]

The final incentive to clinician adoption of social media use is to facilitate the bridging of the "digital divide." Since the inception of the internet there has been a disparate representation of tech-savvy users, who have the means and knowledge to use the web, and those who lack either the means or the wherewithal to navigate.[165,166] Social media emerged as a means to bridge this divide because there is relative uniformity of use of social media across cultural and economic groups.[145,166-168] More disabled consumers can be reached through social media use.[60] Consumers in the older age demographic are about the only ones that have been identified as underrepresented in the social media arena.[146,167-169] Nevertheless, clinicians could accommodate older consumers via the usual methods, including in-person visits, telephone calls, and written media, while expanding their impact to others via social media.

SOCIAL MEDIA IN EDUCATION

Although the use of social media is widespread and social media tools have the potential to play a pivotal role in facilitating the sharing of health information and knowledge among healthcare professionals, limited information exists to explain or demonstrate best practices for educating or preparing health providers for using this resource. Social media platforms can help facilitate the concept of crowdsourcing to expand knowledge among expert clinicians.[170] To stay current and relevant within society today, healthcare providers must learn how to employ the use of these technologies while confronting the obstacles and hurdles associated with the use of social media in healthcare. But to reach their full potential, providers must be prepared educationally to access evidence-based resources via social media tools.[171]

The use of social media to engage and facilitate discussions related to EBP among healthcare providers as students and professionals holds great potential.[172,173] Clinicians immersed in day-to-day practices can offer each other information about, for example, new diagnostic tests, using social media formats such as Twitter.[174] If healthcare providers can have their clinical questions answered on the fly, one might anticipate improved patient outcomes, retention, and satisfaction and reduced liability as potential benefits.

Many healthcare providers, including faculty, remain unaware of the potential Web 2.0 holds for connecting to other healthcare team members, despite evidence that concludes healthcare professionals and patients are empowered by information technology.[170] Furthermore, healthcare faculty must make an effort to engage in learning more about these tools in order to prepare a workforce that is ready to practice in a modern healthcare system. By understanding how social media, Web 2.0 tools, and applications operate, healthcare providers can effectively use these platforms and

tools to improve the health of individuals and communities they serve. However, much more research is necessary before best practice models can be established to use these tools to enhance our teaching and learning.

While social media platforms hold vast potential for augmenting professional networks and supplying valuable evidence-based information to healthcare providers and consumers, healthcare providers must be well aware of existing policies at the national, state, and organizational levels pertaining to the use of social media. A careful approach to using social media platforms can result in professional benefits without the violation of policies or rules regarding patient confidentiality.

POLICY

Healthcare organizations that use social media or permit the use of social media typically have policies that govern the use of such media. Most of the policies related to the use of social media address personal internet use by employees during work hours. The organization may specifically address what types of websites may be accessed during work hours or they may even maintain careful control of websites that may be accessed while in the facility. The policies typically do not address the use of social media outside of the workplace.[175,176]

Social media has the potential to enable healthcare providers to foster professional relationships while facilitating interpersonal communication and consumer education.[176] However, healthcare providers who use social media are subject to increased security vulnerabilities,[106,177] blurred professional boundaries,[67,69,73,168,178] and confidentiality breaches.[176,177] For these and other reasons, policies are needed to help guide organizations and clinicians through recommended social media practices.[179,180] In addition to risk avoidance, social media policies can also illuminate professional expectations and establish definitions for acceptable behavior. The three critical elements that a well-constructed social media policy could mitigate are information disclosure, professional integrity, and productivity.[87]

A social media policy should limit information disclosure. It must illuminate the behaviors that increase the potential for breaches of patient privacy and confidentiality as well as address how such violations conflict with privacy laws and professional ethical standards.[75,80,81] Social media policies should also engender professional integrity by discouraging clinicians from divulging too much of their own personal information in addition to discouraging them from creating or disseminating inaccurate or potentially harmful information.[60] Written guidelines could also require healthcare providers to create separate accounts for private and professional use when choosing to use social media for consumer engagement.[181] A social media policy should define acceptable limits for social media use and consequences for overuse.[180,182] It may further delineate the organization's definition of overuse, repercussions for loss in productivity, and ramifications if social media indulgence creates an impression among customers that clinicians are not paying attention to their work.[97]

Social media policies must also be congruent with federal, state, and local legislation and regulations. For example, social media policies must avoid regulating legally protected employee behavior. This issue is why the National Labor Relations Board (NLRB), an independent federal agency that enforces the National Labor Relations Act (NLRA), has taken an interest in social media policies that bar employees from discussing the terms and conditions of their employment on social media. The NLRA protects the rights of employees to speak about work conditions. This protection extends to certain work-related discussions carried out via social media platforms. In 2010, the NLRB began receiving charges related to employer social media policies and the disciplining of employees related to social media posts. The agency found reasonable cause to believe that some disciplinary actions violated federal labor law. This resulted in complaints being issued against employers for unlawful conduct. Additional information about this topic can be found in Chapter 25.

The final consideration regarding social media policy creation is to determine which level of development would best serve the needs of the public as well as the industry. Health-related public policies are created at the national or state level and establish authoritative oversight by the executive, judicial, or legislative branches of government.[183] These types of policies tend to protect the interests of certain groups of people, such as the elderly or underserved, or types of organizations, such as healthcare plans or employers.[183]

Organizational-level social media policies can be a primary means of mitigating risks associated with social media use.[184] They can also promote social media engagement by helping healthcare providers overcome knowledge barriers and issues of mistrust with social media applications.[133] Policies can establish appropriate boundaries between healthcare provider authority and consumer vulnerability,[95] foster user accountability,[185] and define appropriate consumer engagement.[186] Entering the realm of social media use without strategic planning, including sound policies, could result in unexpected consequences and security threats.[177,186] Healthcare providers have a responsibility to promote patient health and protect consumers.[81,187] Social policies can help healthcare providers positively affect the quality consumers' online and real-life social environment.[183]

Guidelines for Writing Policies

Policy development requires careful planning and implementation. Too lenient a policy would be ineffective; however, too stringent a policy becomes counterproductive and unenforceable.[67] It is also important to not enter the realm of social media policy too hastily[184] and to develop a strategy to make social media work for the organization.[184,188,189] There are no international standards guiding social media, so it is imperative that policies are carefully created to define appropriate social media behavior.[86] Healthcare organizations and providers should understand the reason they wish to engage in social media before attempting to create a policy.[188] Once this purpose has been clearly defined, guidelines can be crafted to

protect the organization and employees[190] and to circumvent draconian rules that might stymie social media use.[184,188]

Of equal importance to the content of a social media policy is the process used to create it.[182] The first step in constructing a sound policy is to form a project team. By bringing key stakeholders together, the organization can be sure that essential elements will be included in the policy.[86,148] The project team should consist of representatives from public relations, marketing, information technology (IT), legal, administration, representative healthcare and staff members, as well as the community.[186,190-192] These individuals should have a varying range of technological aptitude and experience with social media.[182] Invariably, staff member representation should include healthcare providers.[60,69] Not only do healthcare professionals advocate on behalf of patient interests, but they are able to help define and adhere to professional boundaries.[69] Healthcare professionals can also harness their commitment to ethics and scope of practice when providing recommendations for policy development.[60,193]

Subsequently, an assessment of the organization environment should be performed.[194] The outcomes of an assessment will enable the team to establish the intent and scope of the policy. It will also help the project team determine which social media platform to adopt: internally or externally hosted applications. Internally hosted applications are developed and operated by the organization using them.[86] Although more resource intensive, this type of application enables the organization to control the security of the site as well as the data generated from it.[86] Externally hosted platforms, such as Twitter and YouTube, have vendors that administer the application but also control the sites' security protocols.[86] Operating in the social media arena without complete control over site security can be an added risk for healthcare providers and organizations.

The outcomes of the environmental assessment and platform appraisal enable the project team to establish its objectives for the policy and to generate its content. Content will need to be concise, consistent, use simple vernacular,[182,184,190] be specific, and include the owner of the policy and responsibilities of the various departments involved,[86] the organization's attitude regarding social media, and the organization's view on acceptable behavior and consequences for misuse.[86,180,195] Content should also include relevant security, regulatory, and safety implications.[188]

Additionally, the policy should set a framework for appropriate social media etiquette.[190] As each application has different features, guidance should be written for each application (e.g., blogs, social networking, or content communities such as YouTube).[13] For instance, when posting blogs, employees may be able to state where they work but should never say that they speak on behalf of the organization unless they are in an official position to do so.[177,190] Also, when engaging in social networking, healthcare providers should not "friend" a current or former patient.[69,73] Further, regarding content communities, employees may not be allowed to "favorite" objectionable material that could be discovered by consumers and associated with the organization. Lastly, employees may be expected to

BOX 13.2 Sample Outline of a Social Media Policy

Introduction
- Define social media, including what is included under its umbrella (e.g., blogging, social networking, content sharing).
- State the intent of the policy, including how social media coincides with the organization's mission and values.

Purpose
- Define the purpose of the policy.
- Define the scope of the policy and whom it covers.
- Identify the policy's goals, including promotion of ethical and professional use of the various forms of social media.
- Link the policy to any other company policies that may have overlapping guidance, such as an information security policy.
- Link the policy to comply with any applicable regulations and laws, including Health Insurance Portability and Accountability Act, U.S. Food and Drug Administration regulations, and others.

Responsibility
- Identify the policy owners who created it and will do periodic updates.
- Identify the responsibilities of the organization's leadership, including their exemplary use of social media tools.
- Identify the responsibility of the information technology department and information security officer, including security and system monitoring issues (if any).
- Identify the responsibility of the marketing and public relations departments, including any monitoring of social media content.
- Identify the responsibility of all employees, including following company policy for employee conduct as well as the rules of behavior outlined within the policy.

Rules of Behavior (General)
Provide guidelines for acceptable and unacceptable use. Consider the following:
- Outline appropriate and inappropriate tone and content.
- Discuss content management—whether the organization has authority to remove or censor postings and other activity.
- Discuss company representation—employees may identify with the company but not speak on its behalf.
- Promote ethical behavior to coincide with professional standards organizations (e.g., American Nurses Association, American Medical Association).
- Promote legal behavior, such as avoidance of copyright infringement, defamation, conflicts of interest, and plagiarism.
- Expect privacy and confidentiality of patient and company information.

- Expect everyone to review each social media site's privacy policy.
- Expect a minimum level of privacy settings for each social media site used.
- Require that everyone create separate social media accounts for professional and personal activities.
- Describe reasonable usage amounts, including avoidance of excessive use.
- Consider having employees sign the "rules of behavior" and "etiquette" guidelines.
- Describe the consequences for violation of policy guidelines.
- Establish an environment of open communication, including reporting policy violations.

References
- Cite all sources for the content of the policy, including other company policies.
- Include any professional organization guidance.

Supplemental Guidelines on Social Media Etiquette
- Social networking
  - Define it and identify its uses or objectives for use.
  - Expect staff to create separate personal and professional accounts (to dissociate their "two lives").
  - Set guidelines for managing vendor contacts and "friending."
  - Provide guidelines for configuring site privacy settings.
  - Set guidelines for managing patient contact and "friending."
  - Set guidelines for managing negative comments.
- Blogging and microblogging
  - Define it and identify its uses or objectives for use.
  - Address the practice of link shortening.
  - Consider providing guidelines for user profile names.
  - Address the approval process (if any) for blogging on, or from, the company site.
- Content sharing
  - Define it and identify its uses or objectives for use.
  - Identify appropriate and inappropriate content.
  - Provide guidelines for configuring site privacy settings.
  - Describe the process when inappropriate content is discovered and how it will be retracted.
- Other—Add any other forms of social media within the organization's purview
  - Define it and include its uses or objectives for use.
  - Provide guidelines for configuring site privacy settings.
  - Set guidelines for managing etiquette according to the functionality of the application.

Adapted from Bahadur G, Inasi J, de Carvalho A. *Securing the Clicks: Network Security in the Age of Social Media.* OH: McGraw-Hill Osborne Media; 2011; Barton A, Skiba D. Creating social media policies for education and practice. In: Abbott PA, Hullin C, Ramirez C, Newbold C, Nagle L, eds. *Studies in Informatics: Advancing Global Health Through Informatics. Proceedings of the NI2012. The 11th International Congress of Nursing Informatics.* Bethesda, MD: AMIA 2012:16-20; Centers for Disease Control and Prevention (CDC). CDC social media tools, guidelines & best practices. CDC. <http://www.cdc.gov/SocialMedia/Tools/guidelines/?s_cid=tw_eh_78>; 2014; and Mayo Clinic. For Mayo Clinic employees. Version 2.9.7.1 Mayo Clinic. <http://sharing.mayoclinic.org/guidelines/for-mayo-clinic-employees>.

review each application's privacy policy and to enact specific privacy settings. Box 13.2 provides an example of the material covered in a social media policy.

A sound institutional policy can help address social media security needs,[190] but its mere creation should not be the end

of the process. Organizations are obligated to educate their employees about the policy.[86,190,196,197,199] Clinicians should understand that a primary objective of social media use is a positive consumer experience[200] and that the policy is designed to guide and protect everyone involved, from the consumers to the staff.[190] As the project team carries out the training, they will need to adjust their tactics according to the varying degree of social media experience among the staff.[190] One potentially successful method would be to train key individuals in each area of the organization and establish them as social media experts.[190] These individuals could be the resource for their respective areas, to help monitor for appropriate usage, train staff, and continuously update the ever-evolving nature of the social media landscape.

Resources for Policy Development

Creating policy does not have to be resource intensive or performed in isolation. Healthcare organizations may find internal and external resources to assist them with social media policy development. One resource is the institution's existing information security policy, which may be adapted to meet identified needs: it could provide foundational guidance to minimize threats, ensure privacy, and secure company data, and could be modified to include expected rules of behavior.[176,201] Healthcare organizations can also gain useful guidance from other institutions, government bodies, and professional organizations.[97,168,192,198,202] One valuable resource containing examples of existing healthcare policies was established by Chris Boudreaux and is located at http://socialmediagovernance.com/policies. The website contains examples of different policies from major healthcare providers across the country, including trendsetting organizations, such as the Mayo Clinic. The Mayo Clinic has established its own medical director[203] and created a Center for Social Media, dedicated to helping its clients connect with clinicians and make healthy choices.[28]

CONCLUSION AND FUTURE DIRECTIONS

If Healthcare + Social media = Social health (today)
Then Social health (today) = Health (future)[5, p. 3]

As discussed in this chapter, healthcare is discovering the opportunities and challenges offered by social media. By changing the media of communication, social media is changing the conversation and in turn the professional relationship between consumers and patients, healthcare providers, and healthcare institutions. The number and types of social media tools are expanding as the current tools are meshed and new tools are evolving. The use of social media by all ages and social and cultural groups is growing rapidly and can be expected to continue.

The use of social media is woven into the tapestry of healthcare; therefore the statement above by HIMSS Social Media Work Group[5] may in fact predict the future. Consumers and patients will lead the movement toward social health and healthcare professionals, and the healthcare delivery system will eventually join the social health movement. Federal initiatives such as the Health Information Technology Pledge (https://www.healthit.gov/patients-families/pledge-members) encourage healthcare professionals to educate consumers about being active participants in their healthcare and may increase the number of healthcare professionals and

consumers using social media. Rannie and Wellman[204] described the phenomenon of people connected to social media as networked individualism; it is the new "operating system" because it describes the ways in which people connect, communicate, and exchange information. The near-term future will likely determine the fate of this new operating system.

There is no doubt that the active role of the patients or consumers in their healthcare will continue to dramatically change the landscape of the healthcare arena over the next decade. The emergence of upcoming generations born into a world immersed in social media will result in consumers taking control of their personal health and will foster a community of both collaboration and independence to achieve an optimal state of well-being. The growing number of Baby Boomers already immersed in the social media space may also contribute to the changing healthcare landscape.[93] Despite the promise of social media in healthcare, this area is not without its challenges and risks.

REFERENCES

1. Fox S. *Medicine 2.0: Peer-to-Peer Health Care*. Paper presented at Medicine 2.0 Congress; September 11, 2011; Stanford, CA; 2011. http://www.pewinternet.org/2011/09/18/medicine-2-0-peer-to-peer-healthcare/.
2. Kaplan AJ, Haenlein M. Users of the world, unite! The challenges and opportunities of social media. *Bus Horiz*. 2010;53:59–68.
3. Bradley A. A new definition of social media. *Gartner Blog Network*; 2010. http://blogs.gartner.com/anthony_bradley/2010/01/07/a-new-definition-of-social-media/.
4. Nelson R, Joos I, Wolf D. *Social Media for Nurses*. New York: Springer Publishing Company; 2013.
5. Backman C, Dolack S, Dunyak D, Lutz L, Tegen A, Warner D. Social media + health care. *J Am Health Inf Manag Assoc*. 2011;82(3):20–25.
6. Healthcare Information and Management Systems Society (HIMSS) Social Media Work Group. *HIMSS White Paper: Health Care "Friending" Social Media: What is it, How is it Used, and What Should I Do?* HIMSS; 2012. http://www.himss.org/ASP/ContentRedirector.asp?ContentID=79496.
7. Bipartisan Policy Center. *Transforming Health Care: The Role of Health IT*. Bipartisan Policy Center; 2012. http://www.bipartisanpolicy.org/sites/default/files/Transforming%20Health%20Care.pdf.
8. Short J, Williams E, Christie B. *The Social Psychology of Telecommunications*. Hoboken, New Jersey: John Wiley & Sons; 1976.
9. Daft RL, Lengel RH. Organizational information requirements, media richness, and structural design. *Manag Sci*. 1986;32 (5):554–571.
10. Surowiecki J. *The Wisdom of Crowds*. New York: Anchor Books; 2005.
11. Swan M. Emerging patient-driven health care models: an examination of health social networks, consumer personalized medicine and quantified self-tracking. *Int J Environ Res Publ Health*. 2009;6:492–525. http://dx.doi.org/10.3390/jerph6020492.
12. National Research Corporation. *1 in 5 Americans Use Social Media for Health Care Information*. National Research

Corporation 2011. http://hcmg.nationalresearch.com/public/News.aspx?ID=9.

13. Modahl M, Tompsett L, Moorhead T. *Doctors, Patients, and Social Media.* QuantiaMD. Care Continuum Alliance; 2011. http://www.quantiamd.com/q-qcp/DoctorsPatientSocialMedia.pdf.

14. Bacigalupe G. Is there a role for social technologies in collaborative health care? *Fam Syst Health.* 2011;29(1):1–14. http://dx.doi.org/10.1037/a0022093.

15. Sparks MA, O'Seaghdha CM, Sethi SK, Jhaveri KD. Embracing the internet as a means of enhancing medial education in nephrology. *Am J Kidney Dis.* 2011;58(4):512–518.

16. Paul M, Dredze M. *You are What You Tweet: Analyzing Twitter for Public Health.* Johns Hopkins University, Department of Computer Science; 2011. http://www.cs.jhu.edu/~mdredze/publications/twitter_health_icwsm_11.pdf.

16a. Resling T. Social media and nursing leadership: unifying professional voice and presence. *Nurs Lead.* 2016;28(4):48–57. http://dx.doi.org/10.12927/cjnl.2016.24561. http://www.longwoods.com/content/24561.

17. Barton A. Social bookmarking: what every clinical nurse specialist should know. *Clin Nurse Spec.* 2009;23(5):236–237.

18. Skiba D. Nursing education 2.0: second life. *Nurs Educ Perspect.* 2007;28(3):156–157.

19. Skiba D. Nursing education 2.0: a second look at second life. *Nurs Educ Perspect.* 2009;30(2):129–131.

20. Pew Research Center. *Social Media Usage: 2005-2015;* 2015. http://www.pewinternet.org/2015/10/08/social-networking-usage-2005-2015/.

20a. PWC Health Research Institute. *Social Media "Likes" Healthcare: From Marketing to Social Business.* http://pwchealth.com/cgi-local/hregister.cgi/reg/health-care-social-media-report.pdf. Accesssed July 31, 2016.

21. Referral MD. *24 Outstanding Statistics and Figures on How Social Media Has Impacted the Health Care Industry;* 2013. https://getreferralmd.com/2013/09/healthcare-social-media-statistics/.

22. International Telecommunication Union. *Trends in Telecommunication Reform 2012: Smart Regulation for a Broadband World.* Geneva, Switzerland: International Telecommunication Union; 2012.

23. Nielson NM Incite. *State of the Media: the Social Media Report Q3;* 2011. http://blog.nielsen.com/nielsenwire/social/.

24. Fox S. *The Social Life of Health Information.* Pew Internet & American Life Project; 2011. http://pewinternet.org/Reports/2011/Social-Life-of-Health-Info.aspx.

25. Griffis HM, Kilaru AS, Werner RM, et al. Use of social media across US hospitals: descriptive analysis of adoption and utilization. *J Med Internet Res.* 2014;16(11).

26. Brewin B. *Looking for Friends in All the Right Places: VA Expands its Facebook Presence.* Nextgov-Technology and the Business of Government; 2011. http://www.nextgov.com/nextgov/ng_20111222_5947.php.

27. Department of Veterans Affairs (VA). *Use of Web-Based Collaborative Technologies: VA Directive 6515;* 2011. http://www.va.gov/vapubs/viewpublication.asp?pub_id=551.

28. *Mayo Clinic Center for Social Media.* About. Mayo Clinic. http://socialmedia.mayoclinic.org/. Accessed March 12, 2016.

29. Costa C. *The Perfect Storm of Social Media: Consumerization of Healthcare;* 2014. *Rescooped from,* http://www.scoop.it/t/mobile-technology-in-health-car/p/4029901277/2014/10/15/the-perfect-storm-of-social-media-consumerization-of-healthcare. Original source not available.

30. Piscotty R, Voepel-Lewis T, Lee S, Annis A, Lee E, Kalisch B. Hold the phone? Nurses, social media, and patient care. *Nursing.* 2015;45(5):65–67.

31. Ferguson C. It's time for the nursing profession to leverage social media. *J Adv Nurs.* 2013;69(4):745–747.

32. Orizio G, Schulz P, Gasparotti C, Caimi L, Gelatti U. The world of e-patients: a content analysis of online social networks focusing on diseases. *Telemed J E Health.* 2010;16(10):1060–1066.

33. Gallant LM, Irizarry C, Boone G, Kreps G. Promoting participatory medicine with social media: new media applications on hospital websites that enhance health education and e-patients' voices. *J Partic Med.* 2011;3.

34. Sajadi KP, Goldman HB. Social networks lack useful content for incontinence. *Uro.* 2011;78(4):764–767. http://dx.doi.org/10.1016/j.urology.2011.04.074.

35. Ahmed OH, Sullivan SJ, Schneiders AG, McCrory P. iSupport: do social networking sites have a role to play in concussion awareness? *Disabil Rehabil.* 2010;32(22):1877–1883. http://dx.doi.org/10.3109/09638281003734409.

36. Greene JA, Choudhry N, Kilabuk E, Shrank WH. Online social networking by patients with diabetes: a qualitative evaluation of communication with Facebook. *J Gen Intern Med.* 2011;26(3):287–292. http://dx.doi.org/10.1007/s11606-010-1526-3.

37. Kim S, Pinkerton T, Ganesh N. Assessment of H1N1 questions and answers posted on the web. *Am J Infect Control.* 2012;40(3):211–217. http://dx.doi.org/10.1016/j.ajic.2011.03.028.

38. Scanfeld D, Scanfeld V, Larson EL. Dissemination of health information through social networks: Twitter and antibiotics. *Am J Infect Control.* 2010;38(3):182–188. http://dx.doi.org/10.1016/j.ajic.2009.11.004.

39. Chew C, Eysenbach G. Pandemics in the age of Twitter: content analysis of tweets during the 2009 H1N1 outbreak. *PLoS One.* 2010;5(11). http://dx.doi.org/10.1371/journal.pone.0014118.

40. McNeil K, Brna PM, Gordon KE. Epilepsy in the Twitter era: a need to re-tweet the way we think about seizures. *Epilepsy Behav.* 2012;23(2):127–130. http://dx.doi.org/10.1016/j.yebeh.2011.10.

41. Keelan J, Pavri V, Balakrishnan R, Wilson K. An analysis of the human papilloma virus vaccine debate on MySpace blogs. *Vaccine.* 2010;28(6):1535–1540. http://dx.doi.org/10.1016/j.vaccine.2009.11.060/.

42. Kendall L, Hartzler A, Klasnja P, Pratt W. Descriptive analysis of physical activity conversation on Twitter. In: *Proceedings of the 2011 Annual Conference on Human Factors in Computing Systems* New York: Association of Computing Machinery; 2011. http://dx.doi.org/10.1145/1979742.1979807.

43. Gold J, Pedrana AE, Sacks-Davis R, et al. A systematic examination of the use of online social networking sites for sexual health promotion. *BMC Public Health.* 2011;11:583. http://www.biomedcentral.com/1471-2458/11/583.

44. Frost JH, Massagli MP. Social uses of personal health information within PatientsLikeMe, an online patient community: what can happen when patients have access to one another's data. *J Med Internet Res.* 2008;10(3). http://dx.doi.org/10.2196/jmir 1053.

45. Wicks P, Massagli M, Frost J, et al. Sharing health data for better outcomes on PatientsLikeMe. *J Med Internet Res.* 2010;12(2). http://dx.doi.org/10.2196/jmir.1549.

46. Wicks O, Keininger D, Massagli M, et al. Perceived benefits of sharing health data between people with epilepsy on an online platform. *Epilepsy Behav.* 2012;23:16–23. http://dx.doi.org/10.1016/j.yebeh.2011.09.026.

47. Overberg R, Otten W, de Man A, Toussaint P, Westenbrink J, Zwetsloot-Schonk B. How breast cancer patients want to search for and retrieve information from stories of other patients on the internet: an online randomized controlled experiment. *J Med Internet Res.* 2010;12(1). http://dx.doi.org/10.2196/jmir.1215.

48. Chou WYS, Hunt Y, Folkers A, Augustson E. Cancer survivorship in the age of YouTube and social media: a narrative analysis. *J Med Internet Res.* 2011;13(1). http://dx.doi.org/10.2196/jmir.1569.

49. McLaughlin M, Nam Y, Gould J, et al. A videosharing social networking intervention for young adult cancer survivors. *Comput Hum Behav.* 2012;28:631–641. http://dx.doi.org/10.1016/j.chb.2011.11.009.

50. Bender JL, Jimenez-Marroquin MC, Jadad AR. Seeking support on Facebook: a content analysis of breast cancer groups. *J Med Internet Res.* 2011;13(1). http://dx.doi.org/10.2196/jmir.1560.

51. Takahashi Y, Uchida C, Miyaki K, Sakai M, Shimbo T, Nakayama T. Potential benefits and harms of a peer support social network service on the internet for people with depressive tendencies: qualitative content analysis and social network analysis. *J Med Internet Res.* 2009;11(3). http://dx.doi.org/10.2196/jmir.1142.

52. Tsaousides T, Matsuzawa Y, Lebowitz M. Familiarity and prevalence of Facebook use for social networking among individuals with traumatic brain injury. *Brain Inj.* 2011;25 (12):1155–1162. http://dx.doi.org/10.3109/02699052.2011.613086.

53. Baptist AP, Thompson M, Grossman KS, Mohammed L, Sy A, Sanders GM. Social media, text messaging, and email-preferences of asthma patients between 12 and 40 years old. *J Asthma.* 2011;48(8):824–830. http://dx.doi.org/10.3109/02770903.2011.608460.

54. Atkinson NL, Saperstein SL, Massett HA, Leonard CR, Grama L, Manrow R. Using the internet to search for cancer clinical trials: a comparative audit of clinical trial search tools. *Contemp Clin Trials.* 2008;29(4):555–564.

55. Allison M. Can Web 2.0 reboot clinical trials? *Nat Biotech.* 2009;27 (10):895–902 [Erratum appears in Nat Biotech. 2010;28(2):178.].

56. Frost J, Okun S, Vaughan T, Heywood J, Wicks P. Patient-reported outcomes as a source of evidence in off-label prescribing: analysis of data from PatientsLikeMe. *J Med Internet Res.* 2011;13(1). http://dx.doi.org/10.2196/jmir.1643.

57. Wicks P, Vaughan TE, Massagli MP, Heywood J. Accelerated clinical discovery using self-reported patient data collected online and a patient-matching algorithm. *Nat Biotech.* 2011;29 (5):411–416. http://dx.doi.org/10.1038/nbt.1837.

58. Weitzman ER, Adida B, Kelemen S, Mandl KD. Sharing data for public health research by members of an international online diabetes social network. *PLoS One.* 2011;6(4). http://dx.doi.org/10.1371/journal.pone.0019256.

59. Fox S. *Medicine 2.0: peer-to-peer health care*; 2011. Paper presented at Medicine 2.0 Congress; September 11, 2011; Stanford, CA, http://pewinternet.org/Reports/2011/Medicine-20.aspx.

60. American Nurses Association. *Principles of Social Networking and the Nurse.* Silver Spring, MD: American Nurses Association; 2011.

61. Chretien KC, Kind T. Social media and clinical care: ethical, professional, and social implications. *Circulation.* 2013;127:1413–1421.

62. Thielst C. *Technologies in Healthcare Environments.* Chicago: HIMSS; 2014.

63. McNamara M, Kappel D. *ANA and NCSBN Unite to Provide Guidelines on Social Media and Networking for Nurses.* National Council of State Boards of Nursing; 2011. http://www.nursingworld.org/FunctionalMenuCategories/MediaResources/PressReleases/2011-PR/ANA-NCSBN-Guidelines-Social-Media-Networking-for-Nurses.pdf. https://www.ncsbn.org/2927.htm.

64. Baker SA. From the criminal crowd to the "mediated crowd": the impact of social media on the 2011 English riots. *Safer Commun.* 2012;11(1):40–49. http://dx.doi.org/10.1108/17578041211200 100.

65. Nicoll L, Chinn P. *Writing in the Digital Age: Savvy Publishing for Healthcare Professionals.* Philadelphia, PA: Wolters Kluwer; 2015.

66. Strategies for Nurse Managers. *Social Media: Patient Friend or Foe? Strategies for Nurse Managers*; 2012. http://www.strategiesfornursemanagers.com/ce_detail/272966.cfm.

67. Mostaghimi A, Crotty B. Professionalism in the digital age. *Ann Intern Med.* 2011;154:560–562.

68. Snyder L. American College of Physicians ethics manual sixth edition. *Ann Intern Med.* 2012;156(1):73–101.

69. Cole L. Professional boundaries and social media. *N Hampshire Nurs News.* 2012;6(1):7. http://nursingald.com/uploads/publication/pdf/106/NH1_12.pdf.

70. Jain SH. *Practicing medicine in the age of Facebook*; 2009. *N Engl J Med.* 2009;361:649–651. http://www.nejm.org/doi/full/10.1056/NEJMp0901277.

71. Luo J. *Social media link you in but raise thorny patient issues*; *Psychiatr News.* 2011;46(11):12–22. http://psychnews.psychiatryonline.org/doi/full/10.1176%2Fpn.46.11.psychnews_46_11_12.

72. MacDonald J, Sohn S, Ellis P. Privacy, professionalism and Facebook: a dilemma for young doctors. *Med Educ.* 2010;44:805–813. http://dx.doi.org/10.1111/j.1365-2923.2010.03720.x.

73. British Medical Association. *Using Social Media: Practical and Ethical Guidance for Doctors and Medical Students.* London, England: British Medical Association; 2011. http://www.medschools.ac.uk/SiteCollectionDocuments/social_media_guidance_may2011.pdf.

74. Davies M, Brannan S, Chrispin E, et al. New guidance on social media for medical professionals. *J Med Ethics.* 2011;37 (9):577–579.

75. Centers for Medicare & Medicaid Services (CMS). *HIPAA Security Series.* CMS; 2009. http://www.hhs.gov/ocr/privacy/hipaa/administrative/securityrule/securityruleguidance.html.

76. *Federal Trade Commission (FTC).* Privacy Act of 1974, as amended. FTC. https://it.ojp.gov/PrivacyLiberty/authorities/statutes/1279. Accessed June 7, 2016.

77. Department of Health and Human Services (HHS). *The Privacy Act.* HHS; 2007. http://www.hhs.gov/foia/privacy/index.html.

78. Department of Health and Human Services Office for Civil Rights. *OCR Privacy Brief: Summary of the HIPAA Privacy Rule.* Department of Health and Human Services; 2003. http://www.hhs.gov/sites/default/files/ocr/privacy/hipaa/understanding/summary/privacysummary.pdf.

79. Nosko A, Wood E, Molema S. All about me: disclosure in online social networking profiles: the case of Facebook. *Comput Hum Behav.* 2010;26:406–418.

80. Duffy M. Patient privacy and company policy in online life. *Am J Nurs.* 2011;111(9):65–69.

81. American Nurses Association. *Code of Ethics.* Silver Spring, MD: American Nurses Association; 2001.

82. American Medical Association (AMA). *AMA Code of Ethics.* AMA; 2011. http://www.ama-assn.org/ama/pub/physician-resources/medical-ethics/code-medical-ethics.page#.

83. American Medical Association (AMA). *AMA Policy: Professionalism in the Use of Social Media.* AMA; 2012. http://www.ama-assn.org/ama/pub/meeting/professionalism-social-media_print.html.

84. Terry K. *Why You Could—but Shouldn't—Use Facebook to Coordinate Care.* FierceHealthIT; 2011. http://www.fiercehealthit.com/story/why-facebook-shouldnt-be-used-care-coordination/2011-04-11.

85. Dimick C. Privacy policies for social media. *J Am Health Inf Manag Assoc*; 2010. http://journal.ahima.org/2010/01/06/social-media-policies/.

86. Bahadur G, Inasi J, de Carvalho A. *Securing the Clicks: Network Security in the Age of Social Media.* McGraw-Hill Osborne Media: OH; 2011.

87. Balog EK, Warwick AB, Randall VF, Kieling C. Medical professionalism and social media: the responsibility of military medical personnel. *Mil Med.* 2012;177(2):123–124.

88. Cain J. Social media in health care: the case for organizational policy and employee education. *Am J Health Syst Pharm.* 2011;68:1036–1040.

89. Greysen SR, Chretien KC, Kind T, Young A, Gross CP. Physician violations of online professionalism and disciplinary actions: a national survey of state medical boards. *J Am Med Assoc.* 2012;307(11):1141–1142.

90. Press Association. *Hospital Staff Suspended for Playing Facebook "Lying Down Game".* The Guardian; 2009. http://www.guardian.co.uk/uk/2009/sep/09/hospital-lying-down-game?INTCMP=SRCH.

91. Huckabee C. *Judge Orders College to Reinstate Student Who Posted a Placenta Photo Online.* Chronicle of Higher Education; 2011. http://chronicle.com/blogs/ticker/judge-orders-college-to-reinstate-student-who-posted-a-placenta-photo-online/29555.

92. Emery C. *Medical Students Using Facebook and Twitter Can Get Expelled.* KevinMD; 2009. http://www.kevinmd.com/blog/2009/09/medical-students-facebook-twitter-expelled.html.

93. Zickuhr K, Smith A. Digital differences report. *Pew Internet & American Life Study 2012*; 2012. http://pewinternet.org/Reports/2012/Digital-differences/Overview.aspx.

94. Tunick RA, Mednick L, Conroy C. A snapshot of child psychologists' social media activity: professional and ethical practice implications and recommendations. *Prof Psychol Res Pract.* 2011;42(6):440–447.

95. National Council of State Boards of Nursing. *A Nurse's Guide to Professional Boundaries.* Chicago, IL: National Council of State Boards of Nursing; 2011.

96. Lagu T, Kaufman EJ, Asch DA, Armstrong K. Content of weblogs written by health professionals. *J Gen Intern Med.* 2008;23(10):1642–1646. http://dx.doi.org/10.1007/s11606-008-0726-6.

97. Baldwin G. *Social Media: Friend or Foe?* Health Data Management; 2011. http://www.healthdatamanagement.com/issues/19_9/social-media-friend-or-foe-43067-1.html.

98. Doctors suspended after playing Facebook lying down game. *The Telegraph*; September 9, 2009. http://www.telegraph.co.uk/technology/facebook/6161853/Doctors-suspended-after-playing-Facebook-Lying-Down-Game.html.

99. Nance-Nash S. *What Insurers Could Do With Your "Social Media Score".* Daily Finance; 2011. http://www.dailyfinance.com/2011/12/12/what-insurers-could-do-with-your-social-media-score/.

100. National Insurance Commission. *The Use of Social Media in Insurance (draft).* National Association of Insurance Commissioners; 2012. http://www.naic.org/store/free/USM-OP.pdf.

101. Ewing SM. *Insurance Companies Using Social Media to Catch Fraud.* WUSA9.com; 2011. http://archive.wusa9.com/news/article/170054/373/Social-Media-Mining-By-Insurance-Companies.

102. Acoca B. *Scoping Paper on Online Identity Theft.* Organization for Economic Co-operation and Development; 2008. http://www.oecd.org/internet/consumer/40644196.pdf.

103. LaRose R, Rifon N. Your privacy is assured—of being invaded: websites with and without privacy seals. *N Media Soc.* 2006;8:1009–1029.

104. Fraser M, Dutta S. *Web 2.0: security threat to your company?* SC Magazine; February 17, 2009. http://www.scmagazine.com/web-20-security-threat-to-your-company/article/127417/.

105. Webroot. *New Webroot Survey Shows Web 2.0 is Top Security Threat to SMBs in 2010.* Webroot; 2010. http://www.webroot.com/us/en/company/press-room/releases/web-2-security-survey.

106. Centers for Disease Control and Prevention (CDC). *Social Media Security Mitigations.* CDC; 2009. http://www.cdc.gov/SocialMedia/Tools/guidelines/pdf/securitymitigations.pdf.

107. Nemey C. *Five Top Social Media Security Threats.* Network World; 2011. http://www.networkworld.com/news/2011/053111-social-media-security.html.

108. Investor.gov. *Investor Alert: Social Media and Investing—Avoiding Fraud.* U.S. Securities and Exchange Commission; 2014. http://investor.gov/news-alerts/investor-alerts/investor-alert-social-media-investing-avoiding-fraud.

109. Symantec. *Symantec Corporation Internet Security Threat Report 2014.* Vol. 19; 2009. http://www.symantec.com/content/en/us/enterprise/other_resources/b-istr_main_report_v19_21291018.en-us.pdf.

110. *Scambusters.org.* The 5 most common social networking scams. Scambusters.org. http://www.scambusters.org/socialnetworking.html. Accessed March 17, 2016.

111. Barwick H. *Virtualisation, Mobile Devices Pose Largest Security Risks: Symantec, Security Industry Leaders Weigh in on 2011 Security Trends.* Computerworld; 2011. http://www.computerworld.com.au/article/375028/virtualisation_mobile_devices_pose_largest_security_risks_symantec/.

112. Sarasohn-Kahn J. *The Wisdom of Patients: Health Care Meets Online Social Media.* Oakland, CA: California HealthCare Foundation; 2008. http://www.chcf.org/topics/chronicdisease/index.cfm?itemID=133631.

113. Hamada J. *Attempts to Spread Mobile Malware in Tweets.* Symantec; 2012. http://www.symantec.com/connect/blogs/attempts-spread-mobile-malware-tweets.

114. Symantec. *Symantec Report Finds Cyber Threats Skyrocket in Volume and Sophistication.* Symantec; 2011. http://wwwsymantec.com/about/news/release/article.jsp?prid=20110404_03.

115. Verizon. *Mobile Devices and Organizational Security Risk.* Verizon; 2010. http://www.verizonbusiness.com/resources/whitepapers/wp_mobile-devices-and-organizational-security-risk_en_xg.pdf.

116. Symantec. *Norton Study Reveals "Over-Sharing" of Holiday Cheer Puts Consumers at Risk.* Symantec; 2010. https://www.symantec.com/about/newsroom/press-releases/2010/symantec_1216_01.

117. SearchSecurity. *RAT (remote access Trojan)*; 2009. http://searchsecurity.techtarget.com/definition/RAT-remote-access-Trojan.

118. Internet Crime Complaint Center. *2010 Internet Crime Report.* National White Collar Crime Center; 2011. http://www.ic3.gov/media/annualreport/2010_IC3Report.pdf.

119. Federal Trade Commission (FTC). *Consumer Sentinel Network Databook for January–December 2011.* FTC; 2012. https://www.ftc.gov/reports/consumer-sentinel-network-data-book-january-december-2011.

120. Greysen SR, Kind T, Chretien KC. Online professionalism and the mirror of social media. *J Gen Intern Med.* 2010;25(11):1227–1229.

121. Madden M, Fox S, Smith A, Vitak J. *Digital Footprints: Online Identity Management and Search in the Age of Transparency.* Pew Internet & American Life Project; 2007. http://pewresearch.org/pubs/663/digital-footprints.

122. Lee DH, Im S, Taylor CR. Voluntary self-disclosure of information on the internet: a multi-method study of the motivations and consequences of disclosing information on blogs. *Psychol Market.* 2008;25:692–710.

123. Marx G. Ethics for the new surveillance. *Inf Soc.* 1998;14:171–185.

124. Aftab P. *Understanding Cyberbullying & Cyberharassment.* Wired Safety; 2015. http://wwwwiredsafety.org/index.php?option=com_content&view=article&id=193:cyberbullying-and-cyberstalking-and-harassment&catid=96:cyberbullying–stalking-a-harassment-&Itemid=41.

125. Dooley JJ, Pyzalski J, Cross D. Cyberbullying versus face-to-face bullying, a theoretical and conceptual review. *J Psychol.* 2009;217(4):182–188.

126. Spears B, Slee P, Owens L, Johnson B. Behind the scenes and screens: insights into the human dimension of covert and cyberbullying. *J Psychol.* 2009;217(4):189–196.

127. Daily Mail Reporter. *Brain Surgeon's Identity Stolen for Fake Facebook Slur on Olympic Gold Medalist.* MailOnline; 2008. http://www.dailymail.co.uk/news/article-1044714/Brain-surgeons-identity-stolen-fake-Facebook-slur-Olympic-gold-medallist.html.

128. Schmidt CW. Trending now, using social media to predict and track disease outbreaks. *Environ Health Perspect.* 2012;120(1):A30–A33.

129. Federal Communications Commission (FCC). *About the FCC.* FCC; 2011. http://transition.fcc.gov/aboutus.html.

130. Federal Communications Commission (FCC). *Press Release: FCC adopts strong, sustainable rules to protect the open internet*; 2015. https://www.fcc.gov/document/fcc-adopts-strong-sustainable-rules-protect-open-internet.

131. Food and Drug Administration (FDA). *Guidance for industry responding to unsolicited requests for off-label information about prescription drugs and medical devices.* FDA; 2011. http://wwwfda.gov/downloads/Drugs/GuidanceComplianceRegulatoryInformation/Guidances/UCM285145.pdf.

132. TNS Media. *Connecting with patients, overcoming uncertainty.* TNS Media; 2007. http://www.seyfarth.com/dir_docs/news_item/1d21aaf1-4ad5-4e22-af28-af3feea533e6_documentupload.pdf.

133. Baldwin M, Spong A, Doward L, Gnanasakthy A. Patient-reported outcomes, patient-reported information from randomized controlled trials to the social web and beyond. *Patient.* 2011;4(1):11–17. http://dx.doi.org/10.2165/11585530-000000000-00000.

134. Lawry TC. Recognizing and managing website risks. *Health Prog.* 2001;82(6):12–13. 74.

135. Sharp J. *Social Media in Health Care: Barriers and Future Trends.* iHealthBeat; 2010. http://www.iseek.org/news/fw/fw7580FutureWork.html.

136. Goldman D. *Legal Issues (part 2): Unique Issues in Health Care Social Media.* Mayo Clinic; 2010. http://socialmedia.mayoclinic.org/2010/08/02/legal-issues-part-2-unique-issues-in-healthcare-social-media/.

137. National Council of State Boards of Nursing (NCSBN). *Position Paper on Telenursing: A Challenge to Regulation.* NCSBN; 1997. https://www.ncsbn.org/TelenursingPaper.pdf.

138. American Telemedicine Association (ATA). *Telehealth Nursing: A White Paper Developed and Accepted by the Telehealth Nursing Special Interest Group.* ATA; 2008. http://www.americantelemed.org/docs/default-document-library/telenursingwhitepaper_4-7-2008.pdf?sfvrsn=2.

139. Noyes K. *Social Nets Need New Privacy Rule, Says Senator.* E-Commerce Times; 2010. http://www.ecommercetimes.com/story/Social-Nets-Need-New-Privacy-Rule-Book-Says-Senator-69862.html.

140. Hawn C. Take two aspirin and tweet me in the morning: how Twitter, Facebook, and other social media are reshaping health care. *Health Aff.* 2009;28(2):361–368.

141. Fluss D. Using social media for customer service is a strategic imperative: protect and enhance your company's image. *Cust Relationsh Manag*; December 2011. http://www.destinationcrm.com/Articles/Columns-Departments/Customer-Centricity/Using-Social-Media-for-Customer-Service-Is-a-Strategic-Imperative-78728.aspx.

142. Vartabedian B. *Are Physicians Obligated to Participate in Social Media? 33charts*; 2009. http://33charts.com/2009/10/are-physicians-obligated-to-participate-in-social-media.html.

143. Scott DM. *Be An Agent of Change.* EContent; 2011. http://www.econtentmag.com/Articles/Column/After-Thought/Be-an-Agent-of-Change-79113.htm.

144. O'Donnell O. DataContent 2011: Make Room for Data. *Inf Today.* 2012;18.

145. Powell JA, Darvell M, Gray JA. The doctor, the patient and the World Wide Web: how the internet is changing health care. *J Roy Soc Med.* 2003;96:74–76.

146. Fox S, Jones S. *The Social Life of Health Information.* Pew Internet & American Life Project; 2009. http://www.pewinternet.org/Reports/2009/8-The-Social-Life-of-Health-Information/01-Summary-of-Findings.aspx.

147. Centers for Medicare & Medicaid Services (CMS). *Accountable Care Organizations Overview.* CMS; 2012. https://www.cms.gov/ACO/.

148. Ajjan H, Hartshorne R. Investigating faculty decisions to adopt Web 2.0 technologies: theory and empirical tests. *Int Higher Educ.* 2008;11(2):71–80.

149. Mejias U. *Nomad's Guide to Learning and Social Software.* Australian Flexible Learning Framework; 2005. http://blog.ulisesmejias.com/2005/11/01/a-nomads-guide-to-learning-and-social-software/.

150. Boulos MNK, Maramba I, Wheeler S. Wikis, blogs and podcasts: a new generation of web-virtual collaborative clinical practice and education. *BMC Med Educ.* 2006;6:41. http://dx.doi.org/10.1186/1472-6920-6-41.

151. Chaiken BP. Social networking: a new tool to engage the clinical community. *Pat Saf Qual Healthc*. 2009;6(2):6–7.

152. Crampton K. *Social Networking and Health Information: an Emerging Consumer Health Resource? What Librarians Need to Know!* Gundersen Lutheran. Personal communication of PowerPoint slides: La Crosse, WI; 2016.

153. Robinson MA. Navigating the world of social media. *Alta RN*. 2012;67(6):42.

154. Allison JT. Using social media to engage communities. *Healthc Exec*. 2014;29(5):50–53.

155. Verhoef LM, Van de Belt TH, Engelen LJ, Schoonhoven L, Kool RB. Social media and rating sites as tools to understanding quality of care: a scoping review. *J Med Internet Res*. 2014;16(2).

156. Eysenbach G. Medicine 2.0: social networking, collaboration, participation, apomediation, and openness. *J Med Internet Res*. 2008;10(3):e22.

157. Young SD. Recommendations for using online social networking technologies to reduce inaccurate online health information. *J Health Allied Sci*. 2011;10(2):2.

158. Kaslow FW, Patterson T. Ethical dilemmas in psychologists accessing internet data: is it justified? *Prof Psychol*. 2011;42(2):105–112.

159. Myers SB, Endres MA, Ruddy ME, Zelikovsky N. Psychology graduate training in the era of online social networking. *Train Educ Prof Psychol*. 2012;6(1):28–36.

160. Keelan J, Pavri-Garcia V, Tomlinson G, Wilson K. YouTube as a source of information on immunization: a content analysis. *J Amer Med Assoc*. 2007;298(21):2482–2484.

161. Centers for Disease Control and Prevention (CDC). *Five important reasons to vaccinate your child*. CDC; 2011. http://www.cdc.gov/media/matte/2011/04_childvaccination.pdf.

162. Edwards IR, Lindquist M. Social media and networks in pharmacovigilance: boon or bane? *Drug Saf*. 2011;34(4):267–271. http://dx.doi.org/10.2165/11590720-000000000-00000.

163. Eysenbach G, Diepgen TL. Towards quality management of medical information on the internet: evaluation, labeling, and filtering of information. *BMJ*. 1998;317:1496–1500. http://dx.doi.org/10.1136/bmj. 317.7171.1496.

164. Rodrigues RJ. Ethical and legal issues in interactive health communication: a call for international cooperation. *J Med Internet Res*. 2000;2(1).

165. Baur C, Kanaan S. *Expanding the Reach and Impact of Consumer E-Health Tools*. Washington, DC: U.S. Department of Health and Human Services; 2006. http://www.health.gov/communication/ehealth/ehealthTools/default.htm.

166. Cashen MS, Dykes P, Gerber B. eHealth technology and internet resources: barriers for vulnerable populations. *J Cardiovasc Nurs*. 2004;19(3):209–214.

167. Mazman SG, Usluel YK. Modeling educational usage of Facebook. *Comput Educ*. 2010;55(2010):444–453.

168. Chou WS, Hunt YM, Beckjord EB, Moser RP, Hesse BW. Social media use in the United States: implications for health communication. *J Med Internet Res*. 2009;11(4). http://dx.doi.org/10.2196/jmir.1249.

169. Chu LF, Young C, Zamora A, Kurup V, Macario A. Anesthesia 2.0: internet-based information resources and Web 2.0 applications in anesthesia education. *Curr Opin Anaesthesiol*. 2010;23:218–227.

170. Okun S, Caligtan C. The evolving ePatient in health informatics: an interprofessional approach. In: Nelson R, Staggers N, eds. *Nursing Informatics: An Interdisciplinary Approach*. St. Louis: Elsevier; 2014.

171. Facchiano L, Snyder CH. Evidence-based practice for the busy nurse practitioner: part two: searching for the best evidence to clinical inquiries. *J Am Acad Nurse Pract*. 2012;24:640–648.

172. Archibald M, Clark A. Twitter and nursing research: how diffusion of innovation theory can help uptake. *J Adv Nursing*. 2014;7(3):e3–e5.

173. Ovadia S. Exploring the potential of Twitter as a research tool. *Behav Soc Sci Libr*. 2009;28(4):202–205.

174. Leung E, Tirlapur S, Siassakos D, Khan K. #BlueJC: BJOC and Katherine Twining Network collaborate to facilitate post-publication peer review and enhance research literacy via a Twitter journal club. *BJOG: An Int J Obstet Gynaecol*. 2013;120:657–660.

175. National Student Nurses' Association, Inc. *Recommendations for Social Media Usage and Maintaining Privacy, Confidentiality and Professionalism*; 2012. http://www.nsna.org/Portals/0/Skins/NSNA/pdf/NSNA_Social_Media_Recommendations.pdf.

176. National Council of State Boards of Nursing (NCSBN). *White Paper: A Nurse's Guide to the Use of Social Media*; 2011. https://www.ncsbn.org/Social_Media.pdf.

177. Chi M. *Security Policy and Social Media Use*. Sans Institute; 2011. http://www.sans.org/reading_room/whitepapers/policyissues/reducing-risks-social-media-organization_33749.

178. Goldman D. *Legal Issues (part 4): Specific Suggestions When Drafting Your Policies*. Mayo Clinic; 2010. http://socialmedia.mayoclinic.org/2010/08/09/legal-issues-part-4-specific-suggestions-when-drafting-your-policies/.

179. Boudreaux C. *Policy Database*. Social Media Governance; 2011. http://socialmediagovernance.com/policies.php#axzz1pjfBq4VE.

180. Shinder DL. 10 things You Should Cover in Your Social Networking Policy. *Tech Republic*; 2009. http://www.techrepublic.com/blog/10-things/10-things-you-should-cover-in-your-social-networking-policy/.

181. Lagu T, Greysen SR. Physician, monitor thyself: professionalism and accountability in the use of social media. *J Clin Ethics*. 2011;22(2):187–190.

182. Junco R. The need for student social media policies. *Educause Rev*. 2011;46(1).

183. Longest B. *Health Policy Making in the United States*. 5th ed. Washington, DC: Health Administration Press; 2010.

184. Dryer L, Grant M, White LT. *Social Media, Risk, and Policies for Associations*. Social Fish & Croydon Consulting; 2009. http://wwwsocialfish.org/wp-content/downloads/socialfish-policies-whitepaper.pdf.

185. Chretien KC, Azar J, Kind T. Physicians on Twitter. *JAMA*. 2011;305(6):566–568.

186. Scott PR, Jacka JM. *Auditing Social Media: A Governance and Risk Guide*. Hoboken, NJ: John Wiley & Sons; 2011.

187. American Nurses Association. *Social Policy Statement*. Silver Spring, MD: American Nurses Association; 2010.

188. Strom D. *Who Owns Your Followers? Time to Revise Your Social Media Policy*. Readwrite Web; 2011. http://readwrite.com/2011/12/27/time-to-revise-you-social-medi-/.

189. Wolfe I. *Before You Write that Social Media Policy…Stop, Look & Listen*; 2009. Toolbox.com; http://hr.toolbox.com/blogs/ira-wolfe/before-you-write-that-social-media-policystop-look-listen-45660.

190. Barger C. *The Social Media Strategist: Build a Successful Program from the Inside Out.* Ashland, OH: McGraw-Hill; 2011.

191. Ohio State Medical Association. *Social Networking and the Medical Practice.* Ohio State Medical Association; 2010. http://www.osma.org/files/documents/tools-and-resources/running-a-practice/social-media-policy.pdf.

192. Barton A, Skiba D. Creating social media policies for education and practice. In: Abbott PA, Hullin C, Ramirez C, Newbold C, Nagle L, eds. *Studies in Informatics: Advancing Global Health through Informatics. Proceedings of the NI2012. The 11th International Congress of Nursing Informatics,* Bethesda, MD: AMIA; 2012:16–20.

193. Bard R. *CEO outlook: embracing social media.* Can Nurse; 2012. https://canadian-nurse.com/en/articles/issues/2012/january-2012/embracing-social-media.

194. Malone RE. Assessing the policy environment. *Policy Politics Nurs Pract.* 2005;6(2):135–143.

195. Guiness A. *7 (More) Must-Haves for Your Social Media Policy.* Social Media Policy Templates; 2010. http://socialmediapolicytemplates.wordpress.com/.

196. Mayo Clinic. *For Mayo Clinic Employees.* Mayo Clinic; 2012. http://sharing.mayoclinic.org/guidelines/for-mayo-clinic-employees/.

197. American Council for Technology–Industry Advisory Council (ACT-IAC), Collaboration & Transformation (C&T) Shared Interest Group (SIG). *Best Practices Study of Social Media Records Policies.* Fairfax, VA: American Council for Technology; 2011.

198. Black T. *How to Write a Social Media Policy.* Inc; 2010. http://www.inc.com/guides/2010/05/writing-a-social-media-policy.html.

199. Goldman D. *Legal Issues (part 3): General thoughts on Developing your Social Media Policy.* Mayo Clinic; 2010. http://socialmedia.mayoclinic.org/2010/08/04/legal-issues-part-3-general-thoughts-on-developing-your-social-media-policy/.

200. AstraZeneca. *White Paper: Social Media in the Pharmaceutical Industry.* AstraZeneca; 2011. http://www.pharmaceutical-technology.com/downloads/whitepapers/category/social-media-in-the-pharmaceutical-industry/.

201. Photopoulos C. *Managing Catastrophic Loss of Sensitive Data: A Guide for IT and Security Professionals.* Rockland, MA: Syngress Publishing; 2008.

202. Goodchild J. *4 Tips for Writing a Great Social Media Security Policy;* 2009. http://www.csoonline.com/article/505593/4-tips-for-writing-a-great-social-media-security-policy.

203. Aase L. *Center Names New Medical Director.* Mayo Clinic Center for Social Media; 2011. http://socialmedia.mayoclinic.org/2011/12/19/center-names-new-medical-director/.

204. Rannie L, Wellman B. *Networked Individualism: What in the World is That?.* Pew Internet & American Life Project; 2012. http://networked.pewinternet.org/2012/05/24/networked-individualism-what-in-the-world-is-that-2/.

DISCUSSION QUESTIONS

1. What are the strengths of using social media in healthcare?
2. What are the challenges of using social media in healthcare?
3. Why are healthcare professionals slow to adopt social media as a tool in healthcare?
4. Is the use of social media in healthcare a fad?
5. In a hospital setting, what are the key questions that the C-suite (CEO, CFO, CNO, CIO) should ask about using social media?
6. How does social media affect the relationship between patients and their healthcare providers?
7. Is social media a part of patient-centric care?
8. How can health professional schools prepare future healthcare providers in the area of social media?
9. Describe the meaning of the following statement:
   If Healthcare + Social media = Social health (today)
   Then Social health (today) = Health (future)[7]
10. Describe networked individualism and the benefits for one's healthcare.

CASE STUDY

Social Media in Education and Healthcare

Grace Speak is a fourth-year student at Best University. She and her fellow classmates are working hard in their final courses and preparing for exams. Inspired by the teamwork that the healthcare profession espouses, Grace gets an idea for a study group. She thinks it will really help share case experiences, course notes, and study tips. Unfortunately, several members of her peer group live out of town, which makes it difficult for them to participate fully. Grace is torn, as she does not want to exclude them from the study group. When she voices her concerns to a classmate, her friend suggests using social media tools as the primary medium for sharing information.

Discussion Questions

1. What types of social media tools could Grace's study group use?
2. How would those tools facilitate the objectives of the study group?
3. What are some of the risks associated with using social media for such purposes?
4. What might Grace need to do from the outset when she forms the study group?

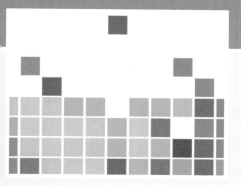

14

Personal Health Records

Bryan Gibson and Kathleen G. Charters

If trends in adoption and expansion of the functionality of personal health records (PHRs) persist, PHRs have the potential to become the platform for a more efficient, effective, and personalized healthcare system.

OBJECTIVES

At the completion of this chapter, the reader will be prepared to:

1. Describe trends and events leading to the development and adoption of electronic personal health records (PHRs).
2. Describe the history of Blue Button.
3. Describe the ideal PHR and its proposed benefits.
4. Explain the different types of PHRs and the pros and cons of each type.
5. Provide examples of existing PHRs, including their function and usage.
6. Evaluate current evidence regarding the effectiveness of PHRs as an approach to improve healthcare.
7. Explore issues affecting the adoption of current PHRs.
8. Discuss the future of PHRs.

KEY TERMS

ABSTRACT ❖

This chapter begins with a definition of the electronic personal health record (PHR) and a description of the historical trends contributing to the development and adoption of PHRs. This is followed by a discussion of the history of patient access to their electronic health records (EHRs) via Blue Button. Attributes of an ideal PHR and its proposed benefits are outlined along with types of PHRs, their pros and cons, as well as examples of current PHRs. The growing body of evidence supporting the benefits of PHRs is discussed in terms of the triple aim for healthcare (improving the patient's experience of care, improving health, and reducing costs). Issues in further improving the adoption of PHRs are outlined, and the chapter concludes with a discussion of the future of PHRs.

DEFINITIONS OF THE PERSONAL HEALTH RECORD

Although no single definition is universally agreed upon, several organizations have attempted to define the personal health record (PHR). A joint PHR Task Force of the Medical Library Association and the National Library of Medicine states the following:

> Electronic personal health record [is]: a private, secure application through which an individual may access, manage and share his or her health information. The PHR can include information that is entered by the consumer and/or data from other sources such as pharmacies, labs, and health care providers. The PHR may or may not include information from the electronic health record (EHR) that is maintained by the health care provider and is not synonymous with the EHR. PHR sponsors include vendors who may or may not charge a fee, health care organizations such as hospitals, health insurance companies, or employers.[1]

The Connecting for Health Personal Health Working Group of the Markle Foundation defined the PHR as

> An electronic tool that enables individuals or their authorized representatives to control personal health information, supports them in managing their health and ill-being, and enhances their interactions with health care professionals.[2]

These definitions emphasize two essential aspects of the PHR: The first is that the PHR serves as an information aggregator and storage system. The second is that the PHR is a tool, or suite of tools, that individuals or their delegates may use to manage their health.

THE DEVELOPMENT OF THE ELECTRONIC PERSONAL HEALTH RECORD

Individuals have long kept paper records of their healthcare as adjuncts to their medical records. Common examples include paper records of immunizations and lists of prescription medications or medical problems that people may keep in their personal files. A Harris Interactive poll found that most people thought it was a good idea to keep PHRs; 46% of those surveyed actually kept records, and 86% of those who did kept paper records.[3] Paper records serve several important functions: they minimize the need for individuals to remember the details of their medical history, they are portable, and they are shareable. There is some evidence that paper records may facilitate health behaviors.[4] While paper records likely remain the most common form of personal health information storage, the remainder of this chapter will refer to the electronic PHR.

The development and adoption of the PHR in the United States is the result of several converging historical trends:

- The rise of personal computing devices and the internet.
- The development of electronic health records (EHRs).
- Governmental policies related to health information technology (health IT).
- Consumer demands for the functions provided by a PHR.

The personal computing revolution began when desktop computers became affordable in the 1980s and continues today with the increasing adoption of mobile devices. Concurrent with the increase in adoption of personal computing devices was the development of the internet. In 2014, an estimated 84% of Americans had access to the internet,[5] thus paving the way for PHRs and other personal health technologies. With the internet the adoption of smartphones has exploded: in October 2014 it was estimated that 64% of

U.S. adults owned smartphones; this percentage is continuing to increase steadily.[6] (For detailed information on mHealth, see Chapter 15.) Fig. 14.1 presents the trends in the percentage of Americans owning common electronic devices from 2002 to 2014. As will be discussed later, mobile computing offers tremendous possibilities to expand the scope and functionality of PHRs.

While the widespread adoption and use of personal computing devices and the internet provide the infrastructure that makes PHRs possible, EHRs serve as the primary source of data populating the PHR. Large-scale implementation of EHRs began in the early 1990s at several integrated health systems, such as the Veterans Health Affairs (VHA),[7] Intermountain Healthcare in Utah, and the Regenstrief Institute in Indiana.[8]

In recent years, the U.S. government implemented policies specifically intended to increase the adoption of both EHRs and PHRs. In this chapter, we will only provide a brief overview of these polices and their relation to PHR adoption. See Chapters 25 and 27 for additional information on these policies.

The Health Information Portability and Accountability Act (HIPAA) of 1996 requires individuals to be granted access to their health records upon request. In addition, the law requires individuals to be provided with an audit trail describing who has accessed their health information and why.[9] HIPAA does not require this information to be provided or monitored electronically; however, since these provisions are most easily addressed with an electronic record, HIPAA could be seen as a first step in encouraging the adoption of PHRs.

Subsequent policy had a more direct effect on electronic records adoption. In April 2004, President George W. Bush set a goal that most Americans would have their medical

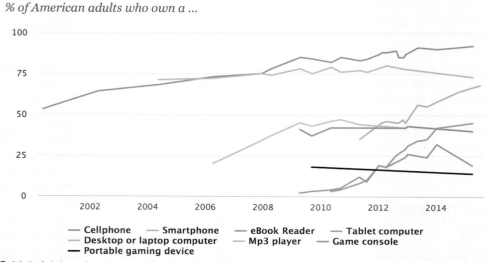

% of American adults who own a ...

Cellphone — Smartphone — eBook Reader — Tablet computer
Desktop or laptop computer — Mp3 player — Game console
Portable gaming device

FIG 14.1 Adult gadget ownership over time (2000–2014). As of July 2015, 68% of American adults have a smartphone. (From http://www.pewinternet.org/data-trend/mobile/device-ownership/)

information maintained in electronic records by 2014.[10] To facilitate this goal, the Office of the National Coordinator for Health Information Technology (ONC) was created and later funded by the Health Information Technology for Economic and Clinical Health Act (HITECH Act) of 2009. ONC is the "principal Federal entity charged with coordination of nationwide efforts to implement and use the most advanced health information technology and the electronic exchange of health information."[11]

In 2009, the American Reinvestment and Recovery Act of 2009 authorized the Centers for Medicare and Medicaid Services (CMS) to provide financial incentives for adoption and Meaningful Use of EHRs. As detailed in Chapter 27, the ONC proposed three stages of Meaningful Use, each characterized by a group of requirements necessary for certification. In 2010, CMS began to certify healthcare information system products for compliance with Stage 1 Meaningful Use. Eligible providers and eligible hospitals who used these products and met other specific criteria were and still are eligible for financial incentives.[12] The incentives are clearly driving adoption: the prevalence of hospitals in the United States with "basic" EHRs (as defined by Meaningful Use guidelines) increased from 9.4% in 2008 to 59.4% in 2013.[13] Similarly, outpatient clinics are increasingly adopting EHRs: in 2013, 48% of office-based physicians had a "basic" EHR system.[14]

In September 2012, the ONC finalized requirements that eligible providers who had met Stage 1 requirements would need to meet Stage 2 requirements in 2014 in order to be compliant. Some Stage 2 requirements directly tie the Meaningful Use of the EHR and PHR together. For example, Stage 2 states that patients visiting a certified healthcare provider must be able to access their EHR data electronically and that at least 5% of patients will actually use this function during a certification period. The rule also requires that patients discharged from the hospital must be able to view their information online and download and transmit that information within 36 hours of discharge from the hospital or, in the outpatient setting, within 4 days of the appointment. These requirements seem to be driving providers to offer their patients PHRs: in 2014 38% of patients reported being offered online access to the medical records.[15]

The final and possibly most important trend leading to adoption of PHRs is individuals' desire for the functions that PHRs provide. In 1998, Tang et al. conducted focus groups to explore patients' information needs and desires. The researchers found patients wanted to receive personalized, physician-endorsed health information and summaries of recent healthcare encounters as well as next steps in care. Participants thought being better informed would increase their understanding of their treatment plan, increase their motivation to comply with the plan, and improve their satisfaction with office visits.[16] A 2005 survey by the Markle Foundation found that 60% of those surveyed wanted a PHR that they could use for refilling prescriptions, communicating (e-mailing) with their doctor, and obtaining results over the

internet. In addition, over 70% supported the use of such a system to allow providers to review their medical records when needed.[17] A 2006 Harris Interactive poll reported similar findings; in addition, most people wanted the ability to schedule visits via the internet and wanted to be sent reminders for medical visits. About half of respondents wanted a system that could transfer self-monitoring data (such as blood pressures taken at home) to their doctors.[18] Recent surveys suggest that interest in PHRs continues to be strong: a national survey conducted in 2014 found that 57% of respondents who did not have a PHR would be interested in using one if it provided online access to their medical records.[19]

Blue Button for Patient Access to Electronic Health Records

The idea of patient access to EHRs has been discussed and debated since the 1990s.[20] However, early efforts to make EHRs available to patients resulted in wide variation in both content and presentation. The idea for Blue Button was developed during a meeting of the Markle Connecting for Health workgroup in 2010.[21] The vision was that by clicking on an image of a button, patients could access their records in either human-readable or machine-readable format. The symbol for Blue Button (Fig. **14.2**) and the slogan "Download My Data" are used to identify electronic access to health data views, downloads, and transmissions. Blue Button includes clinical, demographic, financial (explanation of benefits or invoices), and other information related to the health and medical care of patients.[22]

Initially pioneered by the CMS, Department of Defense, Department of Veterans Affairs (VA), and Social Security Administration, Blue Button was soon adopted by private health insurers, hospitals, and healthcare practices.[23,24] In 2011, the Department of Veterans Affairs held a prize competition called Blue Button for All Americans to encourage widespread use outside federal healthcare programs to benefit veterans who receive care from non-VA providers.[23] The same year, the ONC launched a pledge program to make it easier for patients to access their personal health information online and to encourage patients to use that information to improve their health.[24]

Blue Button challenges were designed to stimulate development of products by public and private organizations to make health information more usable and meaningful for patients. In 2012 and 2013, the ONC sponsored challenges to accelerate awareness of Blue Button and encourage developers to create apps that implement and use this functionality. The 2012 Blue Button Video Challenge asked participants to create inspiring and entertaining videos that introduce Blue Button and encourage viewers to learn more about it.[25] Eighteen videos were submitted, and they are now available online.[26] The 2012 Blue Button Mash Up Challenge built on this foundation, calling for development of an app that uses Blue Button–downloaded personal health data and

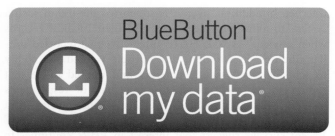

FIG 14.2 The Blue Button ® Logo. (From https://www.healthit. gov/patients-families/blue-button/blue-button-image)

combines it with other data to address the three-part aim of CMS: better healthcare, better health, and lower costs. Videos demonstrating the winning apps are available online.[27]

As awareness of Blue Button grew, the standards associated with Blue Button were also evolving. The ONC Standards and Interoperability Framework led to Blue Button + for data holders and receivers.[28] This combination of structure, transport mechanism (using a process called the direct protocol), and automation sets the stage for accelerated development of an ecosystem of tools and apps based on retrieving personal health data. Implementing Blue Button + Direct met the requirements of Meaningful Use Stage 2, requiring that patients be given the capability to view, download, and transmit their health data electronically.[29,30]

In 2013 a Blue Button Co-Design Challenge based on crowdsourced ideas was the foundation for apps to be developed using Blue Button + technical standards and to leverage policy drivers, such as rewarding efforts to engage patients in new ways. Use cases included combining data from a medical device with other health data; simplifying care for caregivers managing multiple chronic conditions; one-step patient-entered data about drugs, pharmacies, and preferred providers; and enabling a clear view of conditions a patient is at risk for and what preventive services are needed, as well as tracking preventive steps patients take on their own. The winning apps provide users with a variety of patient services and combine health information from multiple providers through Blue Button +.[31] GenieMD aggregates data from multiple providers so patients and their providers have a holistic view of all of the patient's medical conditions. ICEBlueButton provides immediate access to an In Case of Emergency (ICE) record, including allergies, medical conditions, and medications, by either nonmedical rescuers or emergency personnel using QR code scanning. CareTracker simplifies personal care among patients and their care teams and keeps everyone on the same page in real time.

The ONC provides an online tool, Blue Button Connector, to help patients find their health data so they can reference, check, share, and use apps.[32] Blue Button Connector users can select a source of their health information (health insurance, hospital or clinic, providers, pharmacy, lab, or immunization registry) and see what features are available for viewing, downloading, or securely sending records to an application. Blue Button Connector provides a list of health apps accepting information provided using nationally recognized standards, including but not limited to Blue Button + standards.[33] As of this writing, over 300 organizations pledged to provide patients with the information and tools they need to be partners in their own health.[34]

The question remains whether providing patients access to their health information makes any difference. Jika et al. conducted a systematic review of the effect of giving patients health record access and did an analysis of outcome measures based on eight reviews conducted between 2002 and 2014. They calculated the number of positive outcomes reported per every outcome measure investigated, finding mixed outcomes across both patient and providers, with approximately half of the reviews showing positive changes. They concluded there is:

> … a lack of empirical testing that separates the effect of record access from other existing disease management programs and there is currently insufficient evidence about the effect of patient accessible electronic health records on health outcomes for patients.[35]

PRINCIPLES OF AN IDEAL PERSONAL HEALTH RECORD

Aggregated from several publications and reports,[36] the following is a list of principles for an ideal PHR. No current system fully implements all of these principles; however, some current systems partially address them:

Comprehensive, longitudinal data storage. The PHR should serve as a persistent longitudinal record of individuals' health and healthcare over their life spans. Fully implementing this principle requires data integration from multiple sources (e.g., EHRs, pharmacies, and patient-entered data). Developing these kinds of interoperable records is one of the missions of the ONC and one of the primary reasons for the Meaningful Use criteria discussed above.

Data ownership, control, and privacy. Individual users (patients) should be considered the "owners" of data in PHRs. This principle has several corollaries: users should control access to their PHR, be able to annotate data created by others (e.g., data from EHRs), be able to create new data fields, and be able to assign a proxy who can control and use the system on their behalf. The Markle Foundation's report titled "Connecting for Health" focuses on this principle of users' ownership and control of the data in PHRs. Table **14.1** provides a summary of the core principles for PHR design delineated in their report. These core principles reflect the Federal Trade

Commission's Fair Information Practice Principles.[37] Additional information related to these principles is included in Chapter 26.

Portability. The system should be available to the user regardless of physical location. To this end, several PHRs are available as mobile phone applications.

Data sharing. The system should allow users to share all or parts of the PHR with others. The shared data should be provided in an electronic format that allows the receiver to manipulate the data (making the sender and receiver's records interoperable) rather than being available as read only.

Access. The system should provide a convenient means for users to access health-related information and services. This information or service may improve on or augment existing processes. Examples include the capability for secure messaging between patients and healthcare providers, the possibility of e-visits (e.g., web-based video or text consultations between patient and provider), online medication refills, and administrative functions such as scheduling of appointments.[38]

Unique and desired services. The system should provide users with unique services that are otherwise unavailable. Current PHRs provide functions that improve on existing healthcare processes. However, several authors[39] suggested that PHRs could provide a wider array of functions not currently available. For example, PHRs could provide decision aids to assist patients with complex therapeutic decisions, provide personalized motivational health promotion messages to facilitate healthy behaviors, and be used to elicit patients' goals and preferences and present those back to providers. These kinds of functions are needed if PHRs are to make a significant impact on users' behaviors and health.

Customization. PHRs should allow content customization to address individual users' needs. For example, the system might provide a translation service to help individuals understand clinical notes from EHRs.[40] Such information could be tailored to users' health literacy and numeracy. However, the ability to customize content in PHRs has yet to be implemented.

Proposed Benefits of an Ideal Personal Health Record

An ideal PHR has multiple proposed benefits. For example, by serving as a single comprehensive record, an ideal PHR could facilitate improved care coordination between healthcare providers, reduce repetitive tests and conflicting therapies, and improve patient safety.[41] Similarly, a function allowing users to assign a delegate or proxy to access and control their records might improve care delivered by informal caregivers

TABLE 14.1	Core Principles of Personal Health Record Design from Connecting for Health
1. Openness and transparency	Consumers should know what information has been collected about them, the purpose of its use, who can access and use it, and where it resides. They should also be informed about how they may obtain access to information collected about them and how they may control who has access to it.
2. Purpose specification	The purposes for which personal data are collected should be specified at the time of collection, and the subsequent use should be limited to those purposes, or others that are specified on each occasion of change of purpose.
3. Collection limitation and data minimization	Personal health information should only be collected for specified purposes and obtained by lawful and fair means. The collection and storage of personal health data should be limited to that information necessary to carry out the specified purpose. Where possible, consumers should have the knowledge of or provide consent for collection of their personal health information.
4. Use limitation	Personal data should not be disclosed, made available, or otherwise used for purposes other than those specified.
5. Individual participation and control	Consumers should be able to control access to their personal information. They should know who is storing what information on them, and how that information is being used. They should also be able to review the way their information is being used or stored.
6. Data quality and integrity	All personal data collected should be relevant to the purposes for which they are to be used and should be accurate, complete, and up to date.
7. Security safeguards and controls	Reasonable safeguards should protect personal data against such risks as loss or unauthorized access, use, destruction, modification, or disclosure.
8. Accountability and oversight	Entities in control of personal health information must be held accountable for implementing these principles.
9. Remedies	Remedies must exist to address security breaches or privacy violations.

(e.g., adults taking care of elderly parents).[42] Finally, a system like a PHR that is ubiquitously available and provides individuals with customized health promotion might improve individuals' self-management of health.[36,43]

Types of Personal Health Records

PHRs are often grouped into four main types: *stand-alone, untethered, tethered,*[44] and *networked.*[41,45,46] While the first three types do not provide all the desired functions of the ideal PHR described above, networked PHRs have the potential to address these deficits.[41]

Stand-alone personal health records store health information on an individual's computer or a USB device. These systems might be of use in particular cases (e.g., the capacity for emergency medical providers to access the person's USB stored data). These have not been widely adopted, likely because they require manual data entry by the user and the records are not interoperable with other systems such as EHRs.[44]

Untethered personal health records are web-based systems separate from an EHR. The advantage of these systems over stand-alone PHRs is that they are accessible anytime and can aggregate data from multiple sources. The drawback is that they do not link to healthcare providers; thus users cannot e-mail their doctors, request medication refills, view their medical records, or schedule appointments. Despite these deficits, proponents of untethered and stand-alone systems suggest that these formats offer users maximum control over the content included in their PHR.[47]

A tethered personal health record is linked to a single clinic or healthcare system. Because these systems allow the user to view EHR data via the PHR, they are sometimes called a *patient portal* (i.e., the system provides a portal into the person's medical information within the EHR). There are several advantages to these systems: they often provide direct access to functions such as secure messaging with healthcare providers, medication refills, and appointment scheduling, and because the PHR is usually automatically populated with EHR data, they require much less manual entry of data than untethered PHRs. The main disadvantage is that the information is linked only to one specific healthcare provider or system. This creates a problem for individuals with multiple healthcare providers in different healthcare systems because only the information from the linked system is represented in the PHR.

A *networked* PHR is proposed to address the limitations of a tethered PHR.[41] In a networked personal health record patients can integrate data from multiple sources, from different healthcare providers, health plans, or laboratories. The data are integrated through use of access services that conduct user authentication before allowing patient or proxy access to data. Ideally, users sign in once and gain access to comprehensive, integrated data. As with EHRs, the development of comprehensive, integrated PHRs is dependent on the wide implementation of data representation and data exchange standards that are still needed to create interoperable records. Fig. **14.3** depicts the differences in information flow between current processes and a networked PHR.

EXAMPLES OF EXISTING PERSONAL HEALTH RECORDS

Selected examples of existing PHRs are presented in this section. Additional examples of existing PHRs are available via recommended websites listed on the Evolve website.

One of the first electronic PHRs, the VHA's MyHealtheVet (MHV), was first piloted in 1999 and launched nationally in 2003.[48] MHV has two levels of use. The first level allows anyone to create an account online and use the system as an untethered, web-based PHR. The second level is for individuals receiving care through the VHA. These users can take full advantage of MHV's functionality by completing in-person authentication at their nearest VHA clinic or hospital. Once individuals are authenticated, they can use the system as a tethered PHR to exchange secure e-mails with their healthcare providers, view portions of their EHRs, view upcoming appointments, and receive wellness reminders.[49] As of August 2015, more than 1.9 million veterans were authenticated users of MHV, or greater than 30% of individuals who use the VHA for healthcare.[32] The majority of system adopters (75%) use the system to order prescription refills, with more than 70 million refills requested. In January 2010, the VHA began a rollout of secure messaging within MHV. Since then, secure messaging has been rapidly adopted. As of August 2015, 81% of authenticated MHV users have opted in to secure messaging with their healthcare team.[50]

Kaiser Permanente (KP) is an integrated nonprofit provider of both health insurance and healthcare in the United States. Between 2004 and 2010, KP implemented a system-wide EHR with a tethered PHR called My Health Manager.[33] The PHR provides secure messaging with healthcare providers, online appointment scheduling, and prescription refills. In 2013, 4.4 million of Kaiser's 9.1 million members were using the PHR (48.3% of all members). The PHR had over 131 million visits, with 34.4 million lab test results viewed online, 14.7 million secure e-mails sent, 3.6 million online appointment requests made, and 14.8 million online prescriptions refilled. A mobile phone PHR app was released by KP in 2012. It reached 1 million downloads in June 2014. Through the app, members can e-mail physicians, schedule or cancel appointments, get refills for a prescription, access lab results, and search for nearby KP medical facilities.[51]

Microsoft launched its web-based PHR platform, Health-Vault, in 2007. The system integrates data from multiple sources: individuals can upload documents and images, have their records added directly to HealthVault via fax from their healthcare providers, or pay a service to collect their records and digitize their medical information. HealthVault serves as an application platform. When an individual uses a Health-Vault application for the first time, he or she authorizes the application to access a specific set of data types from their record, and the application exchanges those data with the platform. One of the strengths of the platform is the ability to use compatible self-monitoring devices such as pedometers, glucometers, and blood pressure monitors to automatically capture

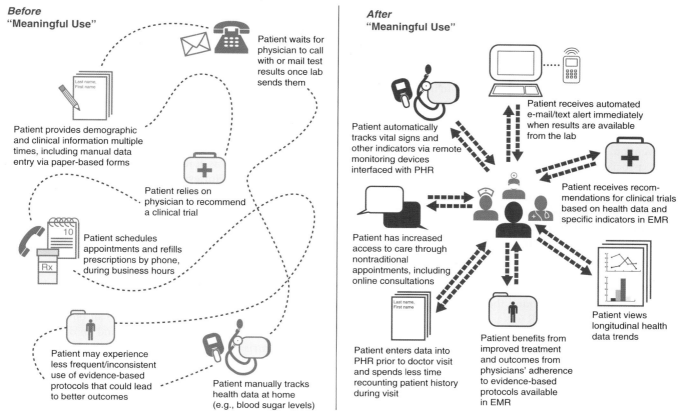

FIG 14.3 How Meaningful Use changes the healthcare experience for patients and families. *EMR,* Electronic medical record; *PHR,* personal health record. (From Health Research Institute. Putting patients into Meaningful Use. PricewaterhouseCoopers. <http://www.pwc.com/us/en/health-industries/publications/putting-patients-into-meaningful-use.jhtml> Page 2.)

data. A second strength of the platform is that app developers can leverage data in HealthVault when users allow access. As of August 2015, 251 devices can push data to HealthVault, and 120 apps make various uses of the data stored on the platform.[52] Depending on the number of data sources connected to the platform, HealthVault can function as an untethered, tethered, or networked PHR. For example, if all data sources for a specific patient were HealthVault partners, the patient's PHR would be a comprehensive, networked PHR.

CURRENT EVIDENCE OF BENEFITS OF PERSONAL HEALTH RECORDS

The Institute for Healthcare Improvement (IHI) first developed goals to improve individuals' experience of care, quality of care, and costs of care. These were later adopted by CMS and are referred to as the IHI triple aim for healthcare.[53] Each dimension should be considered when evaluating an intervention or healthcare process because these aims are interdependent and can at times be at odds with each other.[54] For example, an intervention that improves the quality of care might also increase costs. Similarly, a system that reduces costs might also degrade the person's experience of care. With

this in mind, evidence demonstrating the positive impact of PHRs across these three dimensions is increasing.[55,56]

Experience of Care

Evidence regarding the effect of a PHR on individuals' experience of healthcare is limited; however, user satisfaction surveys are generally very positive about the functions included in PHRs. For example, among individuals accessing their medical records online in 2013 or 2014, greater than 81% considered the information useful.[15] Similarly, most users of a tethered PHR reported high satisfaction (>86% were either satisfied or very satisfied) with functions such as online medication refills, secure messaging, and the ability to view lab test results.[57] Finally, patients from an academic medical system reported high satisfaction with secure messaging, as long as response times to their secure messages remained short.[58]

The flexibility offered by PHRs may also improve individuals' experience of care. This is suggested by the results of a survey of PHR users at the Geisinger Health System. Patients preferred e-mail communication for some interactions (e.g., requesting prescription renewals, obtaining general medical information) and preferred in-person communication for others (e.g., receiving treatment instructions).[59]

Quality of Care

Since PHRs are relatively new tools, evidence about the effects of PHR use on the quality of healthcare is limited and data on long-term outcomes are not yet available. The available evidence comes from two types of studies. The first are association studies that examined the relation between an individual's use of the PHR (usually secure messaging) and intermediate health outcomes. The second group of studies includes randomized controlled trials with the PHR as a component of a broader intervention.

In association studies, use of the PHR was related to improved intermediate health outcomes.[60] At KP Northwest, a positive association was found between patients' use of secure messaging and the likelihood of organizations meeting the recommended Healthcare Effectiveness Data and Information Set (HEDIS) performance measures for diabetes and blood pressure quality care.[61] This effect was significant, even after comparing users to nonusers, matched on age, gender, and healthcare provider. Similarly, a cross-sectional analysis of individuals with diabetes found the use of secure messaging in the MyGroupHealth PHR was associated with better glycemic control.[62] While the results of these studies are encouraging, these studies did not control for confounding factors such as the patient's self-efficacy, attitudes toward medical care, race, socioeconomic status, and health literacy.[62]

Several trials were conducted using a PHR as a component of a larger intervention. For example, two trials compared the effect of PHR use and an automated blood pressure cuff on subsequent blood pressure readings. In the first, the investigators compared three interventions: the PHR alone (UC); a home blood pressure monitor and the PHR (eBP); or a home blood pressure monitor, the PHR, and a pharmacist who engaged with the patient regularly via secure messaging (eBP-Pharm). The outcome of interest was the percentage of subjects whose blood pressure was controlled (<140/90 mm Hg) at a 1-year follow-up. Results were as follows: 56% of individuals in the eBP-Pharm group, 36% in the eBP group, and 31% in the UC group had controlled blood pressure at the end of the trial.[63] However, the eBP-Pharm group contains several variables, making conclusions less definitive about PHR effects. In a similar trial, Wagner et al. reported on a cluster randomized trial with either a PHR or none and automated blood pressure cuff or none for 1 year. Of 1686 patients approached, only 453 patients agreed to participate. The authors found no association between adoption of the PHR and blood pressure over 1 year. However, in a subgroup analysis, they found that patients who used the PHR more than twice a month reduced their blood pressure by 5 mm Hg. They also reported that increased PHR usage was associated with patients' perception of the usefulness of the system.[64]

Similar trials in individuals with diabetes showed that PHR-based care management modules are useful in affecting physiological outcomes[65] and reducing diabetes-related distress.[66] More recently a custom-built, untethered PHR with personalized messages about potentially inappropriate medication use had moderately positive effects on older adults' medication behaviors.[67]

While most work on PHRs affecting users' health focused on individuals with chronic disease, some studies addressed preventive health behaviors. For example, Lau et al. compared the effect of a PHR educational module on flu vaccination rates to a wait-list control among university students and found that the PHR module increased vaccinations rates and clinic visit rates.[68]

Cost/Utilization

Cost-benefit simulation of the effect PHR use and healthcare costs was estimated as quite positive (assuming >80% nationwide adoption).[69] However, actual data showing changes in healthcare costs are not yet available.[55] Several studies measured the association between PHR use and healthcare utilization. The assumption behind these studies is that shifting utilization away from in-person encounters will lead to decreased costs.

Zhou et al. compared 3201 users of KP's *My Health Manager* PHR with a nonuser group, matched for age and disease, and found PHR use was associated with reduced telephone calls to the clinic and a reduced number of outpatient visits per year.[70] Other investigators have found an opposite association. Harris et al. reported that increased use of secure messaging by individuals with diabetes in the My Group Health PHR was associated with increased outpatient visits.[62] Limitations of these two studies include that they are cross-sectional studies, and no determination was made as to whether the change in utilization was appropriate or not. For example, in the Harris study, use of the PHRs secure messaging function may help individuals realize they need to seek out care more regularly, and therefore increased utilization may have been appropriate.

In summary, the available evidence suggests that PHRs may improve patients' satisfaction with their quality of care, and PHRs also seem to change individuals' healthcare utilization patterns. The effects of this change on costs remain to be seen. Two facts qualify these statements. First, virtually all the evidence discussed above comes from studies of tethered PHRs used by integrated healthcare systems. More evidence from a more diverse sample is needed. Second, a common finding across these studies is that regular use of the PHR by patients is necessary to see improvements; therefore more research on engagement of patients with the PHR over time is needed.

CURRENT USE OF PERSONAL HEALTH RECORDS

Several studies found PHR users are more likely to have multiple medical problems than nonusers.[70,71] Even among individuals with the same disease, individuals with a higher disease burden may use PHRs more than those who are less ill. For example, Weppner et al. reported that among older individuals with diabetes, higher morbidity was associated with increased usage of secure messaging.[72] Similarly, a study of PHR use among individuals with chronic kidney disease found that about half of participants became frequent users of the systems and that this use occurred around the same time as clinic visits.[73]

Data on the frequency of logins to PHRs were reported for several systems. Among VA patients using MHV, approximately half report using the PHR monthly and 30% say they use it weekly.[74,75] Thirty percent of respondents in a California healthcare foundation survey about PHRs reported using PHRs monthly.[76] New enrollees logged in most frequently in the first month, but about half of respondents continued to access the portal at least monthly. Users most often examined laboratory and radiology results and sent secure messages to their healthcare providers.

Across settings the following PHR functions seem to be the most commonly used (in rough order of decreasing usage): laboratory results reviews, medication refills, patient provider secure messaging, after-visit summary review, medical condition review, appointment requests, immunization review, and allergy review.[48,77,78]

BARRIERS TO PERSONAL HEALTH RECORD ADOPTION

Self-reported PHR adoption as measured by at least one log-in to the system increased from 3% of the population in 2008[58] to approximately 20% in 2014.[15] As noted above, in some large integrated healthcare systems, adoption is even higher (i.e., >30% of VHA patients and >48% of KP members).

While this trend is encouraging, several barriers must be dealt with before PHRs will affect the majority of the population for a long enough time to influence long-term outcomes. These include awareness of PHRs, usability, interoperability of current systems, individuals' concerns over privacy, and the digital divide. In addition, providers' promotion of PHRs and integration of them into the clinical workflows will likely affect adoption and long-term use.

Awareness

A national survey by the California HealthCare Foundation in 2010 asked, "How much have you heard about websites where people can get, keep, and update their health information like test results and prescriptions?" More than half of respondents answered "not sure/not heard." A full 76% of respondents indicated that they had not heard about mobile phone programs to track their own health information.[76] In 2008 Fuji et al. examined rural physicians' awareness of PHRs and found that more than 25% of physicians had no awareness of PHR functions and 59% did not know whether their patients had or used PHRs.[79]

Weitzman et al. conducted interviews and focus groups with administrators, clinicians, and community members as a component of a formative evaluation of a PHR. They found that many individuals had limited awareness of PHRs yet held high expectations of what such a system should do. Common expectations were that the PHR would allow searching and linking within the record, that the system would include tailored communications, and that linkages would exist between self-reports and clinical data. The researchers commented

that these high expectations created a risk of disappointment when individuals encountered existing PHRs.[80]

These studies indicate the most significant barrier to widespread PHR adoption: the lack of awareness of PHRs.[15] To address this problem, several governmental and nongovernmental organizations recently launched websites to educate the public about PHRs. (See the appendix for a representative list.)

Usability

Poor PHR usability may also hinder adoption. For example, in a test of the usability of the MHV PHR, only 25% of users successfully completed registration with the system. In 2007, the National Health Service in the United Kingdom implemented a PHR called HealthSpace and found that adoption and use was much less than expected. Interviews with users suggested that users perceived it as neither useful nor easy to use.[81] Similarly, older adults with lower eHealth literacy were found to have significant difficulty in using a PHR to complete commons health management tasks.[82]

Schnipper et al. conducted usability testing of a medication management module embedded within a patient portal. The study highlighted the need for end user–specific interfaces and functionality in order to make the user experience easier and more efficient. For patients, this meant striking a balance between free-text, structured, and coded data fields to leverage the usefulness of patient-entered data without confusing or overwhelming patients. For example, drop-down menus and scrolls bars were found to be less confusing and more efficient than dynamic text boxes that would react to the word being typed when inputting data, such as medications and allergies.[83]

Privacy Concerns

A 2010 survey found that 63% of PHR users and 68% of PHR nonusers are "somewhat or very concerned" about the privacy of their health information.[84] Recent data suggest these concerns remain a serious barrier to PHR adoption.[15]

The Digital Divide

Research suggests that a "digital divide" exists in the United States. Individuals of lower socioeconomic status,[85] ethnic minorities,[86,87] those with low eHealth literacy,[88] and older individuals are less likely to adopt PHRs.[89] For example, Yamin et al. found that among 75,056 patients in the Partners Healthcare system, African Americans were half as likely as Caucasians to adopt a PHR, and individuals of lower income were about a third less likely to adopt the PHR as individuals of higher income.[85] Similarly, limited access to high-speed internet among veterans living in rural communities was identified as a barrier to adoption of the MHV PHR.[89] Despite this, a survey of Medicaid beneficiaries found most respondents were very interested in accessing personal health information online. Moreover, 90% of respondents reported they have access to the internet, and most use the internet once a week or more.[90]

Provider Engagement

Several recent studies showed clinician behaviors can markedly improve adoption of PHRs. For example, Krist et al.

found that implementing a clinic-based promotion of a patient portal increased adoption by 1% per month.[91]

In addition, other studies reported that aggressive marketing campaigns of tethered PHRs were successful in improving adoption of PHRs. In the first study, a total of 16 techniques were used, including automated greetings on the practice's telephone system, posters in waiting areas and examination rooms, postcard and letter mailings, staff speaking to the patients in the office or over the telephone, and on-site enrollment with a computer kiosk. Authors reported nearly a three-fold greater likelihood of PHR adoption among patients of practices employing five or more of these techniques.[85] At the Mayo clinic, North et al. compared the use of a promotional video to a paper instruction sheet and to a no-attention control group to promote PHR adoption and use. In the following 45 days, individuals' PHR adoption was 11.7% among individuals who saw the video, 7.1% among those who received the paper instructions, and 2.5% among the control group. The superiority of the video intervention persisted when the authors measured whether users went on to use the PHR to initiate secure messaging with their healthcare providers.[92]

Interoperability

As described earlier, PHR data and functions are constrained by the systems to which the PHR is linked. Current PHRs are integrated with a limited number of systems and therefore represent only a subset of the data and services that an ideal PHR should include. It is likely that a comprehensive, ideal PHR would be more attractive than current PHRs and would be adopted at a higher rate.

In principle, all that is required to address the data requirements of an ideal PHR is for all healthcare data systems in the United States to agree to use the same data representation and exchange standards. Several data representation and exchange standards have been developed and proposed, including Continuity of Care Record (CCR), Clinical Document Architecture (CDA), and Continuity of Care Document (CCD). For additional information about standards, see Chapter 22. As an example standard, CCR was developed by a consortium of medical societies and adopted by the American Society for Testing and Materials (ASTM).[93] By describing the exact format of the information to be exchanged, this and other standards provide the possibility for portable and syntactically interoperable PHRs. Recent laws and policies, such as the promotion of Nationwide Health Information Exchange by the ONC[94] and the development of accountable care organizations created in the recent Patient Protection and Affordable Care Act, are intended to promote and use interoperable records and should facilitate PHR adoption.

Summary of Adoption

While the Federal Communications Commission estimates that 90% of Americans will have internet access by 2020[95] and the adoption of mobile devices appears to be decreasing the digital divide (at least in terms of ownership),[7] adoption and usage of PHRs remains limited. Further work is needed to increase awareness of PHRs, address patients' concerns about privacy, and improve usability and functionality of existing PHRs. Finally, the interoperability and functionality of PHRs, while steadily improving, are limited by nationwide adoption of relevant standards and policies.

THE FUTURE OF PERSONAL HEALTH RECORDS

Though early in their evolution, currently available PHRs have positive effects on patients' experience of care, healthcare outcomes, and healthcare use. If the patients' desire for PHR functions persists and trends in adoption continue, PHRs have the potential to become the platform for a more efficient, effective, and personalized healthcare system. To achieve this promise, improvements in current systems as well an expansion of the scope and functionality of PHRs are needed.

The available evidence for current PHRs is generally positive. However, most PHR evaluations have been limited to primary care settings in a small number of integrated healthcare systems. Evidence is needed regarding the adoption, use, and efficacy of current systems in larger and more diverse groups of healthcare settings and among users of varying age, ethnicity, race, socioeconomic level, and disease status. Similarly, current efforts to promote adoption of PHRs (e.g., marketing campaigns to increase awareness) and governmental policy changes to promote adoption need to be evaluated and may need to be refined for specific subpopulations.

As pointed out at the beginning of this chapter, PHRs serve two main functions: as data storage systems and as a suite of tools intended to improve care. Both of these functions need to be expanded in future PHRs. In terms of data storage, the ultimate goal is to develop PHRs that are comprehensive, longitudinal records of individuals' health. To migrate toward this goal, systems will need to become more interoperable and networked.[41] The barriers to interoperability are not technical but rather political and economic. Recent governmental policy regarding the development of accountable care organizations to shift incentives in the U.S. healthcare system may also drive the promotion and adoption of PHRs.

In terms of functionality, Krist et al. have argued that current PHRs are just the beginning and that the functionality of these systems should evolve to become more personalized and effective over time.[39] The first step in making PHRs more patient-centered is to include services that only a few tethered PHRs currently include, such as allowing proxies to access PHRs, granting PHR access to minors, viewing EHR notes, viewing a full list of diagnoses, patient control over information access, inclusion of a "break the glass" function that would allow access for emergent service providers, and clinician response to e-mails in less than 24 hours.[96] PHRs could also be used to collect patient-reported behaviors and outcomes.[97] This type of patient-generated data could then be integrated into care. For example, EHRs are commonly missing information on individuals' occupational and family medical history.[98] These data could be captured via the PHR. Similarly, mobile systems could be used to capture observations of daily living, such as measures of dietary behaviors or self-report of symptoms, and present them back to patients as personalized real-time feedback.[99] Finally, research on

PHRs as "persuasive technologies" (technologies intended to change people's attitudes and behaviors)[100,101] is in its infancy but holds great promise.

In summary, PHRs are evolving tools with great potential to facilitate improvement in the health of individuals and the efficiency of healthcare. While current trends are encouraging and substantial progress has been made in recent years, significant work remains to be done if PHRs are to reach their full potential.

REFERENCES

1. Jones DA, Shipman JP, Plaut DA, Selden CR. Characteristics of personal health records: findings of the Medical Library Association National Library of Medicine Joint Electronic Personal Health Record Task Force. *J Med Libr Assoc.* 2010;98(3):243–249.
2. *Markle Foundation.* Connecting for Health Common Framework for Networked Personal Health Information; 2008. http://www.markle.org/health/markle-common-framework/connecting-consumers.
3. Harris Interactive. Two in five adults keep personal or family health records and almost everybody thinks this is a good idea. *Harris Interact Healthc News.* 2004;13(4):1–5.
4. Jerden L, Weinehall L. Does a patient-held health record give rise to lifestyle changes? A study in clinical practice. *Fam Pract.* 2004;21(6):651–653.
5. *Americans' Internet Access: 2000–2015*; 2015. http://www.pewinternet.org/2015/06/26/americans-internet-access-2000-2015/.
6. *Cell Phone and Smartphone Ownership Demographics*; 2014. http://www.pewinternet.org/data-trend/mobile/cell-phone-and-smartphone-ownership-demographics/.
7. Timson G. *The History of the Hard Hats.* http://www.hardhats.org/history/hardhats.html. Accessed March 24, 2012.
8. McDonald C. The Regenstrief Medical Record System: a quarter century experience. *Int J Med Inf.* 1999;54:225–253.
9. Nielsen J. Heuristic evaluation. In: Nielsen J, Mack RL, eds. *Usability Inspection Methods.* New York, NY: John Wiley & Sons; 1994:25–62.
10. *The Office of the President.* Executive Order 13335. Federal Register 30 April; 2004.
11. *Office of the National Coordinator for Health Information Technology.* Electronic Health Records and Meaningful Use. https://www.cms.gov/Regulations-and-Guidance/Legislation/EHRIncentivePrograms/2016ProgramRequirements.html. Accessed June 27, 2016.
12. *Office of the National Coordinator for Health Information Technology.* Electronic Health Records and Meaningful Use. http://healthit.hhs.gov/portal/server.pt?open=512&objID=2996&mode=2. Accessed July 1, 2016.
13. ONC. Adoption of Electronic Health Record Systems among U.S. Non-federal Acute Care Hospitals: 2008–2013; 2015. https://www.healthit.gov/sites/default/files/data-brief/2014HospitalAdoptionDataBrief.pdf.
14. Furukawa MF, King J, Patel V, Hsiao C-J, Adler-Milstein J, Jha AK. Despite substantial progress in EHR adoption, health information exchange and patient engagement remain low in office settings. *Health Aff.* 2014;33(9):1672–1679.
15. Patel V, Barker W, Siminero E. *Trends in Consumer Access and Use of Electronic Health Information;* 2015. https://www.healthit.gov/sites/default/files/briefs/oncdatabrief30_accesstrends_.pdf.
16. Tang P, Newcomb C. Informing patients: a guide for providing patient health information. *J Am Inform Assoc.* 1998;5(6):563–570.
17. Markle Foundation. *Attitudes of Americans Regarding Personal Health Records and Nationwide Electronic health Information Exchange;* 2005. http://www.markle.org/publications/951-attitudes-americans-regarding-personal-health-records-and-nationwide-electronic-hea.
18. Harris Interactive. Few patients use or have access to online services for communicating with their doctors, but most would like to. *Wall Street J Online.* 2006;5(16).
19. *Annual Xerox EHR Survey: Americans Open to Viewing Test Results.* Handling Healthcare Online. http://news.xerox.com/news/Xerox-EHR-survey-finds-Americans-open-to-online-records. Accessed June 27, 2016.
20. McLaren P. The right to know. *BMJ (Clinical Research Ed).* 1991;303(6808):937–938.
21. *Markle Foundation.* Shaping the future of health care: Improving health and health care, while protecting privacy for all.
22. *HealthIT.gov DoHaHS.* Your records: logo and usage. https://www.healthit.gov/patients-families/blue-button/blue-button-image. Accessed November 27, 2015.
23. *Affairs DoV.* Investing in innovation: Blue Button provider contest. http://bluebutton.devpost.com/rules. Accessed June 27, 2016.
24. *HealthIT.gov DoHaHS.* The Blue Button Pledge. https://www.healthit.gov/patients-families/pledge-info. Accessed June 27, 2016.
25. *Services DoHaH.* Blue Button video challenge rules. http://bluebuttonvideo.devpost.com/rules. Accessed November 27, 2015.
26. *Services DoHaH.* Blue Button video challenge submissions. http://bluebuttonvideo.devpost.com/submissions. Accessed November 27, 2015.
27. *Challenge HD.* Blue Button mash up challenge. http://www.health2con.com/devchallenge/blue-button-mash-up-challenge/#description. Accessed November 27, 2015.
28. *Services DoHaH.* Blue Button + Implementation Guide. http://bluebuttonplus.org/index.html. Accessed November 27, 2015.
29. *HealthIT.gov DoHaHS.* Will using Blue Button satisfy the "patient and family" requirements of Meaningful Use? https://www.healthit.gov/providers-professionals/faqs/will-using-blue-button-satisfy-patient-and-family-requirements-meaningf. Accessed November 27, 2015.
30. *Services DoHaH.* V/D/T and Blue Button+. http://bluebuttonplus.org/mu2.html. Accessed November 27, 2015.
31. *Services DoHaH.* Blue Button co-design challenge. http://www.health2con.com/devchallenge/blue-button-co-design-challenge/#background. Accessed November 27, 2015.
32. HealthIT.gov DoHaHS. Blue Button connector. http://bluebuttonconnector.healthit.gov/. Accessed June 27, 2016.
33. *HealthIT.gov DoHaHS.* Blue Button connector apps. http://bluebuttonconnector.healthit.gov/apps/. Accessed November 27, 2015.
34. *HealthIT.gov DoHaHS.* Who is pledging IT? https://www.healthit.gov/patients-families/pledge-members. Accessed November 27, 2015.
35. Jilka S, Callahan R, Sevdalis N, Mayer E, Darzi A. Nothing about me without me: an interpretative review of patient accessible electronic health records. *J Med Internet Res.* 2015;17(6).
36. Krist A, Woolf S. A vision for patient-centered health information systems. *JAMA.* 2011;305(3):300–301.

37. Commission FT. *Fair Information Practice Principles*. September 23; 2012.

38. Ahern D, Woods S, Lightowler M, Finley S, Houston T. Promise of and potential for patient-facing technologies to enable meaningful use. *Am J Prev Med*. 2011;40(5S2):s162–s172.

39. Krist A, Woolf S. A vision for patient-centered health information systems. *JAMA*. 2011;305(3):300–301.

40. Zeng-Treitler Q, Goryachev S, Kim H, Keselman A, Rosendale D. Making texts in electronic health records comprehensible to consumers: a prototype translator. *AMIA Annu Symp Proc*. 2007;846–850.

41. Detmer D, Bloomrosen M, Raymond B, Tang P. Integrated personal health records: transformative tools for consumer-centric care. *BMC Med Inform Decis Mak*. 2008;8:45.

42. Zulman D, Nazi K, Turvey C, Wagner T, Woods SS, An L. Patient interest in sharing personal health record information: a web-based survey. *Ann Intern Med*. 2011;155:805–810.

43. Archer N, Fevrier-Thomas U, Lokker C, McKibbon K, Straus S. Personal health records: a scoping review. *J Am Med Inform Assoc*. 2011;18:515–522.

44. Endsley S, Kibbe D, Linares A, Colorafi K. An introduction to personal health records. *Fam Pract Manag*. 2006;13(5):58–62.

45. Woods S, Weppner W, McInnes D. Personal health records. In: Hebda T, Czar P, eds. *Handbook of Informatics for Nurses and Healthcare Professionals*. Upper Saddle River, NJ: Prentice Hall; 2012.

46. Vincent A, Kaelber D, Pan E, Shah S, Johnston D, Middleton B. A patient-centric taxonomy for personal health records (PHRs). *Am Inform Assoc Proc*. 2008;2008:763–767.

47. Simons W, Mandl K, Kohane I. Model formulation: the PING personally controlled electronic medical record system: technical architecture. *J Am Inform Assoc*. 2005;12:47–54.

48. Nazi K, Woods S. My HealtheVet PHR: a description of users and patient portal use. *Am Inform Assoc Proc*. 2008;6:1162.

49. *Veterans Health Administration*. MyHealtheVet. https://www.myhealth.va.gov/index.html. Accessed June 7, 2016.

50. *MyHealtheVet product intranet website*: statistics. vaww.va.gov/MYHEALTHEVET/statistics; 2011.

51. *Kaiser Permanente 2014 Annual Report*. Oakland, CA, Kaiser Permanente; 2014. https://share.kaiserpermanente.org/static/kp_annualreport_2014/.

52. *HealthVault*. https://www.healthvault.com/us/en. Accessed November 27, 2015.

53. *Institute for Healthcare Improvement*. The IHI triple aim. http://www.ihi.org/offerings/Initiatives/TripleAim/Pages/default.aspx. Accessed March 24, 2012.

54. Berwick D, Nolan T, Whittngton J. The triple aim: care, health, and cost. *Health Aff*. 2008;27(3):759–769.

55. California Healthcare Foundation. *Measuring the Impact of Patient Portals;* 2011. http://www.chcf.org/publications/2011/05/measuring-impact-patient-portals.

56. Osborn C, Maybery L, Mulvaney S, Hess R. Patient web portals to improve diabetes outcomes: a systematic review. *Curr Diab Rep*. 2009;10(6):422–435.

57. Ralston J, Carell D, Reid R, Anderson M, Moran M, Hereford J. Patient web services integrated with a shared medical record: patient use and satisfaction. *J Am Med Inform Assoc*. 2007;14:798–806.

58. Liederman E, Lee J, Baquero V, Seites P. Patient-physician web messaging the impact on message volume and satisfaction. *J Gen Intern Med*. 2005;20:52–57.

59. Hassol A, Walker J, Kidder D, et al. Patient experiences and attitudes about access to a patient electronic health care record and linked web messaging. *J Am Med Inform Assoc*. 2004;11(6):505–513.

60. Shaw R, Ferranti J. Patient-provider internet portals—patient outcomes and use. *Comput Inform Nurs*. 2011;29(12):714–718.

61. Zhou Y, Kanter M, Wang J, Garrido T. Improved quality at Kaiser Permanente through e-mail between physicians and patients. *Health Aff*. 2010;29(7):1370–1375.

62. Harris LT, Haneuse SJ, Martin DP, Ralston JD. Diabetes quality of care and outpatient utilization associated with electronic patient-provider messaging: a cross-sectional analysis. *Diabetes Care*. 2009;32:1182–1187.

63. Green BB, Cook AJ, Ralston JD, et al. Effectiveness of home blood pressure monitoring, web communication, and pharmacist care on hypertension control. *JAMA*. 2008;299(24):2857–2867.

64. Wagner PJ, Dias J, Howard S, et al. Personal health records and hypertension control: a randomized trial. *J Am Med Inform Assoc*. 2012;19(4):626–634.

65. McMahon GT, Gomes HE, Hohne HS, Hu TM, Levine BA, Conlin PR. Web-based care management in patients with poorly controlled diabetes. *Diabetes Care*. 2005;28(7):1624–1629.

66. Fonda SJ, McMahon GT, Gomes HE, Hickson S, Conlin C. Changes in diabetes related distress related to participation in an internet-based diabetes care management program and glycemic control. *J Diabetes Sci Technol*. 2009;3(1):117–124.

67. Chrischilles EA, Hourcade JP, Doucette W, et al. Personal health records: a randomized trial of effects on elder medication safety. *J Am Med Inform Assoc*. 2014;21(4):679–686.

68. Lau A, Sintchenko V, Crimmins J, Magrabi F, Gallego B, Coiera E. Impact of a web based personally controlled health management system on influenza vaccination and health services utilization rates: a randomized controlled trial. *J Am Med Inform Assoc*. 2012;19(5):719–727.

69. *The Value of Personal Health Records Center for Information Technology Leadership*; 2008. http://tigerphr.pbworks.com/f/CITL_PHR_Report.pdf.

70. Zhou Y, Garrido T, Chin H, Wiesenthal A, Liang L. Patient access to an electronic health record with secure messaging: impact on primary care utilization. *Am J Manag Care*. 2007;13:418–424.

71. Ralston J, Rutter C, Carrell D, Hecht J, Rubanowice D, Simon G. Patient use of secure electronic messaging within a shared medical record: a cross-sectional study. *J Gen Intern Med*. 2009;24(3):349–355.

72. Wepner WG, Ralston JD, Koepsell TD, et al. Use of a shared medical record with secure messaging by older patients with diabetes. *Diabetes Care*. 2010;33(11):2314–2319.

73. Phelps RG, Taylor J, Simpson K, Samuel J, Turner AN. Patients' continuing use of an online health record: a quantitative evaluation of 14,000 patient years of access data. *J Med Internet Res*. 2014;16(10).

74. Nazi K, Woods S. My HealtheVet PHR: a description of users and patient portal use. *Am Med Inform Assoc Ann Symp Proc*. 2008;6:1162.

75. Nazi K. Veterans' voices: use of the American Customer Satisfaction Index (ACSI) Survey to identify MyHealtheVet personal health record users' characteristics, needs, and preferences. *J Am Med Inform Assoc*. 2010;17:203–211.

76. California Healthcare Foundation. *Consumers and Health Information Technology: A National Survey;* 2010. http://www.chcf.org/publications/2010/04/consumers-and-health-information-technology-a-national-survey#ixzz1razHRCuv.

77. Ralston J, Hereford J, Carrell D. Use and satisfaction of a patient Web portal with a shared medical record between patients and providers. *AMIA Annu Symp Proc.* 2006;1070.

78. Gerber DE, Laccetti AL, Chen B, et al. Predictors and intensity of online access to electronic medical records among patients with cancer. *J Oncol Pract/Am Soc Clin Oncol.* 2014;10(5): e307–e312.

79. Fuji KT, Galt KA, Serocca AB. Personal health record use by patients as perceived by ambulatory care physicians in Nebraska and South Dakota: a cross-sectional study. *Perspect Health Inf Manag.* 2008;5:15.

80. Weitzman E, Kaci L, Mandl K. Acceptability of a personally controlled health record in a community-based setting: implications for policy and design. *J Med Internet Res.* 2009;11(2).

81. Greenhalgh T, Hinder S, Stramer K, Bratan T, Russell J. Adoption, non-adoption, and abandonment of a personal electronic health record: case study of HealthSpace. *BMJ.* 2010;341:5814–5825.

82. Taha J, Czaja SJ, Sharit J, Morrow DG. Factors affecting usage of a personal health record (PHR) to manage health. *Psychol Aging.* 2013;28(4):1124–1139.

83. Schnipper JL, Gandhi TK, Wald JS, et al. Design and implementation of a web-based patient portal linked to an electronic health record designed to improve medication safety: the Patient Gateway medications module. *Inform Prim Care.* 2008;16:147–155.

84. *California Healthcare Foundation Consumers and Health Information Technology: A National Survey*; 2010. http://www.chcf.org/publications/2010/04/consumers-and-health-information-technology-a-national-survey#ixzz1razHRCuv.

85. Yamin C, Emani S, Williams D, et al. The digital divide in adoption and use of a personal health record. *Arch Int Med.* 2011;171(6):568–574.

86. Roblin DW, Houston 2nd TK, Allison JJ, Joski PJ, Becker ER. Disparities in use of a personal health record in a managed care organization. *J Am Med Inform Assoc.* 2009;16(5):683–690.

87. Goel MS, Brown TL, Willimas A, Cooper AJ, Hasnain-Wynia R, Baker DW. Patient reported barriers to enrolling in a patient portal. *J Am Med Inform Assoc.* 2011;18(suppl 1):i8–i12.

88. Noblin AM, Wan TT, Fottler M. The impact of health literacy on a patient's decision to adopt a personal health record. *Perspect Health Inf Manag/AHIMA, Am Health Inf Manag Assoc.* 2012;9:1–13.

89. Schooley BL, Horan TA, Lee PW, West PA. Rural veteran access to healthcare services: investigating the role of information and communication technologies in overcoming spatial barriers. *Perspect Health Inf Manag.* 2010;7(Spring). 1f.

90. Willis JM, Macri JM, Simo J, Anstrom KJ, Lobach DF. Perceptions about use of a patient internet portal among Medicaid beneficiaries. *Am Med Inform Assoc Proc.* 2006;1145.

91. Krist AH, Woolf SH, Bello GA, et al. Engaging primary care patients to use a patient-centered personal health record. *Ann Fam Med.* 2014;12(5):418–426.

92. North F, Hanna BK, Crane SJ, Smith SA, Tulledge-Scheitel SM, Stroebel RJ. Patient portal doldrums: does an exam room promotional video during an office visit increase patient portal registrations and portal use? *J Am Med Inform Assoc.* 2012;18: i24–i27.

93. eASTM 2369-05e2 Standard Specification for Continuity of Care Record. http://enterprise.astm.org/filtrexx40.cgi?+REDLINE_PAGES/E2369.htm. Accessed April 1, 2012.

94. Borycki E, Kushniruk A. Identifying and preventing technology-induced error using simulations: application of usability engineering techniques. *Healthc Quart.* 2005;8. Spec No:99-105.

95. Federal Communications Commission. *National Broadband Plan*; 2010. http://www.broadband.gov/download-plan/.

96. Reti S, Feldman H, Ross S, Safran C. Improving personal health records for patient centered care. *J Am Med Inform Assoc.* 2010;17:192–195.

97. Glasgow RE, Kaplan RM, Ockene JK, Fisher EB, Emmons KM. Patient-reported measures of psychosocial issues and health behavior should be added to electronic health records. *Health Aff.* 2012;31(3):497–504.

98. Institute of Medicine. Committee on Patient Safety and Health Information Technology. *Health IT and Patient Safety: Building Safer Systems for Better Care.* 2011.

99. *Robert Wood Johnson Foundation.* Project Health Design. http://www.projecthealthdesign.org/. Accessed March 15, 2012.

100. Fogg B. *Persuasive technology: using computers to change what we think and do*, vol. 1. San Francisco: Morgan Kaufmann; 2003.

101. Chatterjee S, Price A. Healthy living with persuasive technologies: framework, issues, and challenges. *J Am Med Inform Assoc.* 2009;16(2):171–179.

DISCUSSION QUESTIONS

1. In addition to those trends discussed in the chapter, what societal and technological trends do you see that might promote increased adoption and use of PHRs?

2. What specific types of data or functions do you think would draw people who are not current PHR users to adopt and use the PHR? How do you think this might vary by user attributes (e.g., age, disease status, health literacy)?

3. Examine information on the web about PHRs and current health policies. What new information did you discover and how will this information affect the adoption and use of PHRs?

4. In your health organization, what are the main barriers to PHR adoption and use?

5. What is the nurse's role in engaging populations to understand information about their health and understand how to access health information resources?

6. In thinking about a PHR that patients can use to annotate their EHR data (e.g., comment on the problem list), what steps do you think patients will likely take to correct their data? What do you think the advantages and disadvantages of such a system would be?

7. Examine the PHRs that are available to you: what are their relative benefits and disadvantages?

CASE STUDY

An academic medical center in the western United States recently adopted a commercial EHR and plans to adopt and integrate a PHR with its EHR. The hospital CEO drafts a vision statement that states, "By using the latest technology, University Hospital will improve how our patients experience healthcare. Instead of patients coming to us for help, we will be there wherever and whenever they need us, asking, 'How can we help you?' This initiative will make healthcare easier to access and more convenient to use, improve patients' health, and reduce the rising cost of healthcare in our area."

Discussion Questions

1. What is your role in engaging populations to understand information about their health and how to access health information resources?
2. What steps would patients take to correct their data?
3. What barriers should this facility anticipate in rolling out the PHR, and what tactics should the organization take to overcome them?

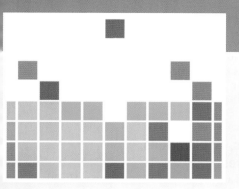

mHealth: The Intersection of Mobile Technology and Health

Sarah J. Iribarren and Rebecca Schnall

Of the world's seven billion people, six billion have mobile phones. However, only 4.5 billion have access to toilets or latrines.

United Nations Deputy Secretary-General Jan Eliasson[1]

OBJECTIVES

At the completion of this chapter, the reader will be prepared to:

1. Define mHealth and what makes it unique from other health information technology applications.
2. Describe driving forces behind the mHealth movement.
3. List mHealth application domains and describe examples of mHealth uses in healthcare settings in the United States and in developing countries.
4. Explore the current state of mHealth research evidence.
5. Discuss benefits and challenges to mHealth implementation.
6. Discuss implications for mHealth research.
7. Describe potential future directions and gaps in mHealth development and uses.

KEY TERMS

connected health, 255
eHealth, 255
mHealth, 255

mHealth tools, 256
mobile applications, 257
sensors, 257

ABSTRACT ❖

This chapter analyzes mobile health (mHealth) technologies and their potential to transform the access, management, and delivery of healthcare services as well as to restructure patient-provider relationships across the globe. Topics discussed include the emergence and driving forces leading to vast mHealth activities, examples of the range of ecosystems where an array of mHealth technologies are used, and benefits and barriers to its implementation. Potential directions and emerging trends are described.

INTRODUCTION

What Is Mobile Health?

Mobile health, commonly referred to as mHealth, m-Health, and more recently as "connected health," is described as a catalyst for healthcare change.[2,3] Widespread recognition exists for mHealth technologies' potential to address and overcome disparities in health services access, health inequities, shortage of healthcare providers, and high costs for healthcare.[4] mHealth falls under the umbrella of eHealth or the broad use of information and communication technologies (ICT) to support health and health-related fields. The World Health Organization's (WHO's) Global Observatory for eHealth (GOe) defines mHealth as "medical and public health practice supported by mobile devices, such as mobile phones, patient monitoring devices, personal digital assistants (PDAs), and other wireless devices."[5] Simply put, it is the use of mobile devices or wireless technology to achieve health objectives.[6] Before discussing examples from the nascent field of mHealth, this chapter explores what makes it unique from other health ICT.

mHealth was initially a term used interchangeably with telehealth (healthcare at a distance), but by the turn of the 21st century, mHealth was emerging as its own field with distinct characteristics different from telehealth. In 2000, the movement toward mobile and wireless was defined as "unwired e-med."[7] Later, Istepanian et al.[8] indicated m-Health "represents the evolution of e-health systems from traditional desktop 'telemedicine' platforms to wireless and mobile configurations." mHealth is redefining the original definition and concept of telemedicine as medicine practiced at a distance to include the new mobility and invisible communication technologies.

With this definition, the term mHealth was recognized as a new field of study. Within the Federal Health Information Technology (IT) Strategic Plan 2015–20, produced by the U.S. Office of the National Coordinator for Health Information Technology (ONC), telehealth and mHealth are noted as separate technologies and services.[9] Unlike telehealth, which often requires more advanced tools, mHealth uses consumer-grade hardware and allows for use of the technology with greater mobility. In a review of technologies and strategies to improve patient care with telemedicine and telehealth, Kvedar et al.[2] stated that mHealth has increased consumer access to telehealth services and suggests the term "connected health" be used to encompass the entire family of technologies and services. Although the delineation between mHealth and telehealth may be more nuanced within the larger umbrella of eHealth, mHealth tools, such as mobile phones with video capability, can be used for telehealth to deliver care at a distance. One example is the use of video conferencing on mobile devices rather than desktop computers. One thing is clear—the focus of mHealth is on taking advantage of a ubiquitous tool carried and used by most people in their daily lives. The

rapid proliferation of mobile technologies and recognition of their inherent potential for improving health has resulted in major reports and global surveys, dedicated conferences and journals, and centers of expertise focused on the field of mHealth.

Mobile Health Tools, Applications, and Examples of Uses

Labrique et al. developed a taxonomy of 12 common mHealth applications/domains and recommended mHealth strategies be viewed as integratable systems fitting into existing health systems rather than standalone solutions.[10] Table 15.1 lists the 12 common mHealth application domains, describes the functions of mobile devices used within each domain, and provides examples of applications in healthcare settings.

mHealth technologies comprise a wide range of tools with various technical capabilities and functionalities to support health-related programs. For example, short messaging service (SMS), or texting, is a core mobile phone function enabling one- and/or two-way communication commonly employed in mHealth initiatives. Globally over 350 billion text messages are sent monthly, exemplifying its extensive

TABLE 15.1 **Examples of Common Mobile Health Application Domains, Functions Used Within Each Domain, and Examples in Healthcare Settings**

Common Application Domains	Examples of Functions	Examples in Healthcare Settings
1. Client education and behavior change	• SMS • MMS • IVR • Voice communication/audio clips • Images	• Smoking cessation programs • Medication adherence support • Appointment reminders
2. Sensors and point of care diagnostics	• Mobile phone camera • Devices and sensors with connectivity • Built-in activity tracking sensors	• Physical activity tracking (weight loss) • Location, travel near disease outbreaks • Dongle—test HIV and syphilis
3. Registries and vital events tracking	• SMS • Voice communication • Digital forms	• Disease surveillance/ Contact tracking • Real-time reporting (e.g., potential Ebola patient) • Tracking and monitoring patients • Momentary ecological assessment
4. Data collection and reporting	• SMS • Voice communication • Digital forms	• Health surveys • Disease registration
5. Electronic health records	• Digital forms • Mobile web (WAP/GPRS)	• Personal and healthcare facility based
6. Electronic decision support: information, protocols, algorithms, checklists	• Mobile web (WAP/GPRS) • Apps assisting with storing information • IVR	• Treatment algorithms

Continued

TABLE 15.1   Examples of Common Mobile Health Application Domains, Functions Used Within Each Domain, and Examples in Healthcare Settings—cont'd

Common Application Domains	Examples of Functions	Examples in Healthcare Settings
[a]7. Communication (Provider-provider, patient-provider): User groups, consultation	• SMS • MMS • Mobile phone camera	• Connecting providers to expert consultation (e.g., sharing video, images) • Connecting patients to providers (e.g., sharing physiological data collected using an app)
8. Provider work planning and scheduling	• SMS alerts • Interactive electronic client list • Mobile phone calendar	• Healthcare visit alerts, reminders for post-procedures follow up
9. Provider training and education	• SMS • MMS • IVR • Voice communication • Audio/video clips, images	• Guidelines (e.g., treatment for cholera) at fingertips
10. Human resource management	• Web-based performance dashboards • Global positioning Service (GPS) • Voice communication • SMS	• Frontline healthcare worker support
11. Supply chain management	• Web-based supply dashboards • GPS • Digital forms • SMS	• Vaccine campaigns • Drug authentication
12. Financial transactions and incentives	• Apps • Transfer of airtime minutes	• Mobile money transfer and banking apps

Modified from Labrique AB, Vasudevan L, Kochi E, Fabricant R, Mehl G. mHealth innovations as health system strengthening tools: 12 common applications and a visual framework. *Glob Health Sci Pract.* 2013;1(2):160–171. http://dx.doi.org/10.9745/GHSP-D-13-00031.
[a]Domain 7 was modified from the original Provider-Provider Communication domain to Communication to include communication strategies applied with mHealth tools to increase communication between patients and providers.
GPRS, General packet radio service; *IVR*, interactive voice response; *MMS*, mobile message service (text messaging with photo or video capability); SMS, short message service.
WAP, Wireless Application Protocol.

use.[11] Its frequent use in mHealth programs is due to a number of reasons: (1) it is more economical than a phone call; (2) SMS is versatile, as it can be sent, stored, or answered; (3) it is retrieved at the user's convenience; and (4) SMS is available on all phone types.[12]

On a more functionally advanced level, smartphones combine features of a personal computer operating system with other features useful for mobile or handheld use. More complex functionalities include general packet radio service (GPRS), third- and fourth-generation mobile telecommunications (3G and 4G systems), global positioning systems (GPS), and Bluetooth technology.[5] Additional smartphone tools include cameras, calendars, mobile applications (apps), multimedia messaging with pictures or video, gaming, educational tools, mobile internet access, and wearable devices and sensors. Before describing examples of mHealth programs, it is helpful to understand the features offered by various mobile

devices. Table 15.2 provides a list of the main characteristics/features for common mHealth devices.

Mobile apps are important mHealth tools for smartphone and tablet mobile devices. In the past few years, the number of health-related apps based on the two leading platforms, iOS and Android, that are available to consumers has more than doubled.[13] In fact, a 2015 study by the IMS Institute for Healthcare Informatics identified over 165,000 health-related apps,[14] compared to about 40,000 in their 2013 report.[15] Fig. 15.1 provides the categories of apps available to consumers based on the IMS study. Of the 26,864 downloaded apps selected for their evaluation, two-thirds targeted wellness management (e.g., fitness, lifestyle and stress, and diet and nutrition), and one quarter were for disease treatment and management, medication reminders and information, women's health and pregnancy, and disease specific.[14] For the disease-specific apps, 29% focused on mental health.

TABLE 15.2 Device Type and Characteristics/Features

Device Type	Characteristics/Features
Basic phone	2G GSM. Services include: SMS; USSD; calling, alarm clock, calculator, flashlight.
Feature phone	Same as above with added internet-enabled services (usually limited, e.g., downloading music), often with camera (still pictures), internet on EDGE or 2.5G networks (if enabled) and removable memory cards (some).
Smart phone	Same features as basic and feature phones typically with graphical interfaces and touchscreen capability, built-in Wi-Fi and GPS, 3G + internet access, video camera, ability to install and use apps, Voice Over Internet Protocol (VoIP) or phone calls over internet rather than cellular service with internet service.
Tablet	Same as smartphone with larger screen size and memory, faster processor (enabling playback), touchscreen with virtual keyboard.

2G, Second-generation; *GPS*, global positioning system; *GSM*, global systems for mobile communication; *SMS*, short message service; *USSD*, Unstructured Supplementary Service Data; *VoIP*, Voice Over Internet Protocol.
Adapted from World Bank. *Information and Communications for Development 2012: Maximizing Mobile.* Washington, DC: World Bank; 2012; and Global Health eLearning Center. *mHealth Basics: Introduction to Mobile Technology for Health.* In: Lee CK, Raney L, L'Engle K, eds. 2014.

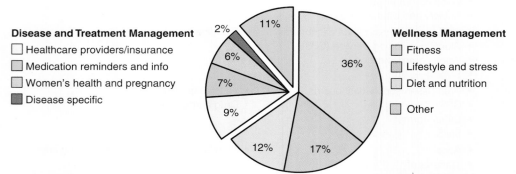

FIG 15.1 Categories of apps available to consumers. (From IMS Institute for Healthcare Informatics. *Patient Adoption of mHealth. Use, Evidence and Remaining Barriers to Mainstream Acceptance.* Copyright © 2015 IMS Health Incorporated and its affiliates.)

However, the majority of the apps had simple functionality, with over half only providing information, thereby limiting their role in healthcare. About 10% included the capacity to link to a sensor or a device.[14]

Client Education and Behavior Change

The mHealth domain of client education and behavior change largely focuses on the client to improve knowledge, modify attitudes, and support behavior change.[10] Many examples of mHealth interventions exist in this domain. MomConnect, an initiative in South Africa, is an example of a program providing pregnant women with tailored information through text messages about pregnancy, birth, and care of an infant.[4] Registrants also have access to the health system through help desk tools and feedback services. In England, Florence is an SMS-based intervention for any health condition, allowing patients to engage in their healthcare and linking client data directly into clinician software.[16]

Numerous healthcare-related apps have been designed to promote behavior change, support self-management of chronic diseases, and offer healthcare providers easy access to healthcare information at the point of care.[17] Apps are a useful tool for behavior change because of their popularity, connectivity, and increased sophistication.[18] Apps can support added functionalities beyond, for example, text messaging. They have the potential for real-time data collection, graphic feedback, interactivity, and links to social networking. Twine-Health is an example of an app integrated into healthcare systems that was a finalist in the 2014–15 Health Acceleration Challenge sponsored by Harvard Business School and Harvard Medical School. TwinHealth is a cloud-based platform together with a synchronized patient app that empowers patients in managing their chronic diseases and establishes personalized plans using a model of collaboration. In a randomized controlled trial (RCT), the team found hypertension was significantly reduced in an intervention group using a model of continuous care with technology support, including coaching. This was in contrast to the control group of standard face-to-face office visits. Costs were approximately $75 per patient year for the intervention group, compared to $250 for the control group.[19] Other examples of apps supporting behavior change targeted diseases such as schizophrenia[20] and depression.[21]

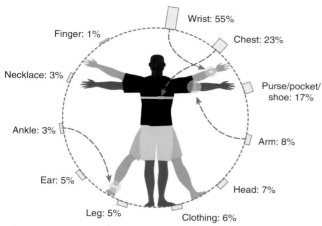

Wrist: 55%
Finger: 1%
Chest: 23%
Necklace: 3%
Purse/pocket/shoe: 17%
Ankle: 3%
Arm: 8%
Ear: 5%
Head: 7%
Leg: 5%
Clothing: 6%

FIG 15.2 Sensor types and location. (From IMS Institute for Healthcare Informatics. *Patient Adoption of mHealth. Use, Evidence and Remaining Barriers to Mainstream Acceptance.* Copyright © 2015 IMS Health Incorporated and its affiliates.)

Sensors and Point-of-Care Diagnostics

Sensors provide links from mobile phones to an external device for longitudinal data collection or patient monitoring and point-of-care diagnostics. Fig. 15.2 highlights types and locations of sensors or wearable technology for collecting physiological information. The data can be synced to mobile devices for monitoring. For example, AliveCor is a U.S. Food and Drug Administration (FDA) approved heart monitor that attaches to the back of an iPhone. It produces a single lead electrocardiogram that is storable and can be shared with a healthcare provider.[22] Researchers found the device to be feasible, suggesting the technology could become an important tool for clinical use.[22]

Registries and Vital Events Tracking

This domain encompasses the identification, recording, and tracking of individuals for a specific disease or event. For example, EbolaTXT was launched in five West African countries to raise awareness about important Ebola information and provided a convenient way community members could report potential new cases using SMS.[23] Fig. 15.3 provides a graphical overview of the EbolaTXT program and campaign. The program was advertised, and participants could opt in by texting a key word to initiate an interactive educational quiz covering, for example, important hygiene steps. Over 30,000 unique participants interacted with the program in Malawi, Ghana, and Mali and Sierra Leone.

Data Collection and Reporting

Mobile devices are replacing paper-based documentation as well as office-based devices such as computers by allowing data to be directly deposited into central servers from a mobile device. Potentially this will result in fewer errors by moving data collection closer to the actual event, using built-in checks to ensure data accuracy, completion, and quicker program evaluation. After pilot testing, Uganda rolled out a national data collection and reporting system using mobile devices to strengthen health reporting. The District Health Management Information Software System version 2 (DHIS 2) is used for the recording of routine health data by various healthcare personnel (e.g., records assistants, district health officers, and other health workers).[24] Using this approach, researchers found increased completeness and timeliness for outpatient reporting.

mPower is an app to help collect patient-reported symptoms related to Parkinson's disease for a research study using questionnaires (e.g., tremors and movement), memory games, phone collected sensor data (e.g., continuous location data feeds that provide position without divulging exact locations), and wearable device data using AppleHealth.[25] This app gives patients an option to work with researchers to understand their evolving health.

Electronic Health Records

Through the use of mobile-adapted electronic health records (EHRs), patients' health records can be accessed or updated in settings outside traditional hospitals or clinics. For example, Fazen et al.[26] developed an Android application, AccessMRS, that interfaced with an EHR to support community health volunteers providing maternal and child health services in Kenya.

Electronic Decision Support

Algorithms and protocols provide the information source for the development of electronic decision support tools for healthcare professionals. mHealth programs using point-of-care decision support tools and automated algorithms fall into this domain. In Tanzania, an electronic version of Integrated Management of Childhood Illness protocol (eIMCI) demonstrated greater adherence to protocols using the mobile phone–based support app than the usual paper-based approach.[27]

Decision support on a mobile platform is also available to patients and consumers. The app SnapDx is a free diagnostic tool downloadable from the AppStore that does not require the use of Wi-Fi. Symptoms are entered and the results show a list of diagnoses and the percent probability of a disease. Another decision support–related app, AllergyCast (Zyrtec), claims to help identify sources of allergies by triangulating consumer/patient symptoms, live pollen data, and live weather data (wind speed and humidity).[28]

Communication (Provider-Provider, Patient-Provider)

mHealth apps can be used to support direct voice exchange, images, or sound for immediate remote consultation. A provider-provider example is ePartogram, an electronic, tablet-based tool used in Kenya to provide decision support tools along with real-time, expert consultation to prevent and manage complications of labor.[23,29] A patient-provider example, WelTel, was one of the first large-scale mHealth interventions evaluating outcome measures for antiretroviral therapy adherence.[30] Patients were sent an e-mail asking

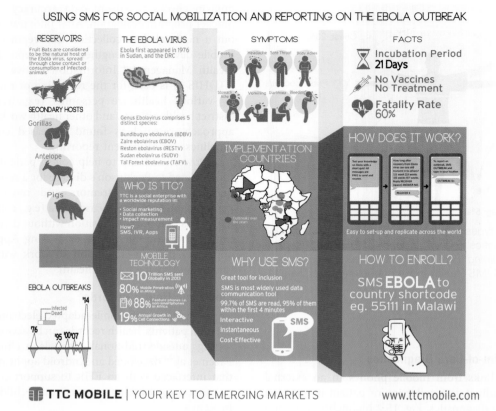

FIG 15.3 Graphical overview of EbolaTXT campaign. (Used with permission of TTC Mobile, Copyright © 2016.)

how they were doing with their treatment. If they responded positively, there was no action. If participants responded they had issues or did not respond, a nurse would directly contact the patient to identify needs and provide appropriate support. In the study on 538 participants, results indicated those receiving text messages had significantly improved adherence to antiretroviral therapy and lower rates of viral suppression compared to those receiving usual care. One example of a service patients can sign up for to communicate with a healthcare provider is HealthTap, an app allowing patients to ask their providers questions directly.[31]

Provider Work Planning and Scheduling

This domain includes alerts for healthcare visits, adherence to treatment regimens, or reminders for follow-up for postcare procedures.[10] For example, the Mobile Technology for Community Health (MoTeCH) initiative in northern Ghana supports work planning and scheduling by calculating upcoming care schedules for each client and, when care is due, notifies the client and community health workers.[32]

Provider Training and Education

Training and education is being provided using a number of mobile technology features (e.g., video, interactive exercises, quizzes, informational messages). A number of mobile apps provide access to continued health and medical education

guidelines and protocols, particularly useful to frontline health workers and providers in remote areas.

Human Resource Management

mHealth can assist with human resource management by helping healthcare workers to triage patient needs and focus on patients in need of extra support during treatment. This is particularly important in settings in which attention from healthcare workers is largely unavailable, costly, or difficult to access due to geographic distances.

Supply Chain Management

mHealth tools are being used to track and manage medication and other healthcare-related commodities. For example, cStock is a program implemented in Malawi to support supply chains for community management of diseases.[23]

Financial Transactions and Incentives

Mobile money applications facilitate payment for healthcare services, provide incentives to providers complying with protocols, and allow users to transfer money to others.[23] In rural Kenya, the feasibility of a mobile money-transferring platform (mPESA) was evaluated using SMS and conditional cash transfers for vaccine coverage.[33] Of the 72 mothers enrolled in the study, 90% of their children received their first vaccinations on time, and 86% received the second vaccination within 4 weeks of their scheduled dose.

DRIVING FORCES OF MOBILE HEALTH

mHealth has grown from an emerging field to a mainstream component of eHealth activities. Some of the driving forces fueling the mHealth movement include (1) technology (access, reduced cost, and its increasing functionality), (2) the consumer/patient engagement movement, (3) global health or connected health (expanding healthcare services to remote and marginalized populations), and (4) research, policy, and business (both cost savings and earning potential).[5,34]

Technology

Near ubiquitous access to mobile devices, along with their range of functionality and increased capabilities, are some of the driving forces of the rapid growth of mHealth.

Access

Mobile phone subscribers have grown from less than 1 billion in 2000 to more than 7 billion in 2015, equating to a penetration rate of 97% worldwide.[35] Indeed, the mobile phone was cited as the most rapidly adopted technology on the planet.[36] For example, many countries in Africa have leaped to mobile as a first telecommunication service infrastructure, bypassing landlines. A working paper by the Center for Global Development published in February 2015 examined trends in the infrastructure services in Africa and identified mobile phone service as the most widely available type of infrastructure across Africa.[37] Of the 33 countries examined, only 4 had mobile phone service coverage available for less than 80% of the area, while the remainder had mobile phone networks available for between 80% and 100%. In contrast, wide disparities exist for the availability of other services. Electricity was between 18% to universal availability in only five countries, piped water ranged from 11% to 89%, and sewer service was available for less than 10% in five countries, while only seven countries had over 50%.

While mobile phone connectivity is available in the overwhelming majority of Africa, inconsistent access to electricity often requires that phones are charged using alternative methods such as a solar energy source, a car battery, or a central charging station.[38] In another study, commissioned by the World Bank, one in five living at the base of the economic pyramid ($2.50 per day income) in Kenya sacrificed usual expenses, such as food, in order to reload mobile phone airtime. The most widely used app in this country was for mobile money transferring.[39]

While the United States has been a leader in traditional telecommunications, mobile phones are replacing landline connections. More than half of Americans aged 18 to 44 (44.1% of all adults) and of children under 18 (54.1% of all children) lived in wireless-only households according to a report released in June 2015.[40] Furthermore, in the United States, with the advent of the mobile phone, the gaps in the "digital divide," or those who have access to digital technology and those who don't, have narrowed.[41] As of January 2014, 90% of Americans owned a cell phone. Ownership was similar across racial and ethnic groups and community type (urban, suburban, and rural) and only slightly more for higher-income families (84% for those with household incomes less than $30,000/year and 98% for those with a household income of $75,000/year or more). The differences among age groups ranged from 74% for those 65 and older to 98% for ages 18 to 29.

Although smartphones are becoming more accessible globally, the majority of people worldwide are using basic phones.[42] In 2014, smartphone penetration was 37% globally, 33% in Latin America, and 63% in the United States.[42] Since 2011, China has been the world's leading smartphone market. A report by Mobile Futures, a diverse group of nonprofit organizations, found more mobile devices than personal computers are bought in China.[43]

Access to the internet determines the range and capabilities for mobile devices. Globally, 34% of households in developing countries have access to the internet in comparison to 80% in developed countries.[35] Although mobile phone ownership in the United States is similar across ethnicities and community type, there are noted differences in how access to the internet is obtained. U.S. minorities rely more on their phone for internet access. In contrast to only 4% of white smartphone owners, 13% of Hispanics and 12% of blacks must depend on their smartphone for internet access. That is, they do not have broadband access at home and have few options for going online other than with their cell phone.[44]

Range and Capabilities

The range of tools and capabilities of mobile devices has expanded along with availability. As outlined above, mHealth tools range from basic to more sophisticated mobile phone features. The functional capacity of mobile devices has increased exponentially with each smartphone generation. According to a 2015 report, 5G is in the very near future and will allow even faster speeds, help enable simultaneous use of different wireless pathways, and connect "virtually any and every thing."[43]

Consumer/Patient Engagement and Empowerment

The impact of the mHealth evolution goes well beyond the introduction of this technology. The use of mobile devices is transforming peoples' lives by changing the way people work and interact. With penetration into nearly all sectors of society and with these devices almost always turned on and near their users, smartphones and web-enabled devices are arguably considered by most people essential to everyday life.

In addition, healthcare models are changing through patient engagement and empowerment,[45] thereby increasing collaborative care, and changing the roles of both consumers and providers.[46] mHealth is implicated as the basis for the consumer-led, data-driven healthcare revolution.[34] Patient empowerment is being driven by consumers (1) having increased access to health information and basic medical knowledge as well as (2) being able to capture their own data.[3] mHealth is a catalyst for moving the locus of control from provider to patient and toward a more collaborative care approach.[47]

As described in Chapter 12, provider-determined care is shifting to participatory healthcare delivery models and changing how health knowledge and personal data are accessed and shared. Mobile devices have greatly impacted how communication and information access occurs. For example, communication by brief mobile messaging (e.g., text messaging or multimedia messaging through apps) is common and continues to increase. In fact, mobile messaging traffic is forecasted to be upwards of 27.7 trillion messages per year by the end of 2016.[48]

A major contributor to the mHealth evolution is the development, proliferation, and use of apps and sensors. The 100 billion mobile app downloads from the Apple store alone speaks loudly to consumer interest in mobile features.[49] Such mHealth tools support consumer/patient engagement by providing easy access to health information and personal data and also by enabling them to collect their own health data.[34] A 2014 report estimated mHealth-centric wearable devices will account for over 150 million unit shipments by the end of 2020.[50] The data collected by these devices can be used to individually modify behaviors and can also be shared with healthcare providers, family, or friends. Wireless devices and apps are making activities such as data collection, analysis, and sharing simple. With apps, patients can track and share upwards of 60 health indicators (e.g., respiratory rate, body temperature, activity, nutrition); they can self-diagnose and proactively manage their health and wellness.

Global Health and Connected Healthcare

Access to healthcare systems in rural, isolated, and resource-limited settings is a major driver of global mHealth implementation and research. The WHO recognized mHealth as a tool for strengthening health systems and improving health outcomes across the globe, especially in low- and middle-income countries (LMICs).[5] In response, global key stakeholders, such as governments, national healthcare institutes, and healthcare professionals, expressed interest or invested in mHealth initiatives.[51]

Research, Policy, and Business

Research, policy, and the growing business potential are stimulating mHealth growth.

Research

Two important guides providing principles for mHealth intervention development, implementation, and evaluation are the *Guide for mHealth Development, Design and Testing*[52] and the *Principles for Digital Development*.[53] These guides have been endorsed by major donor organizations and outline best practices into technology-enabled programs for sustainability in mHealth projects. A common purpose for both these guidelines is to build a common strategy to mitigate overlap and waste and improve collaboration among various healthcare key stakeholders at local, regional, or national levels.

There are three main phases described in the *Guide for mHealth Development, Design and Testing*, with accompanying documents and tools to guide the iterative process. These phases include (1) concept development, (2) solution design and testing, and (3) planning for implementation. The first two phases guide potential mHealth implementers in identifying the needs and technological literacy of the target population and in becoming familiar with the context within which the program will be implemented. The planning-for-implementation phase highlights iterative steps of incorporating feedback from users and partners and revising the content and system as needed before scale and sustainability can be achieved. Examples of this same principle using the *Principles for Digital Development* include "reuse and improve" (e.g., use, modify, and extend existing tools and platforms rather than build new ones) and "use open standards, open data, open source, and open innovation."[53]

The ONC's Federal Health IT Strategic Plan 2015–20 on how health IT can improve health goals includes mHealth technologies and services in three of the four goals.[9] For example, Goal 2 concerns transforming healthcare delivery and community health using person-centered care and self-management supported by health IT and specifically mentions mHealth as a strategy.[9] This report recommends improving mHealth research by using (1) sound intervention development principles, (2) guidance from established theoretical framework/underpinning, and (3) rigorous research methodologies (Goal 3C).[9] Research on the impact of mHealth technologies is growing but remains scarce.[54] As of July 2016, 256 mHealth trials were registered at https://clinicaltrials.gov/ with the term mHealth in their title or abstract. Funding calls related to mHealth initiatives have encouraged research. The state of the evidence is described the sections below.

Policy

After the rapid surge in the number of mobile apps available to the public, the FDA released guidance on mobile medical apps in 2013.[55] The agency indicated it will oversee a targeted risk-based subset of apps to focus on patient safety for cure, mitigation, treatment, or prevention of disease.[55,56] For example, apps considered high risk and those that act as medical devices, such as electrocardiogram machines, will require premarket approval. With other mHealth apps, the FDA will exercise only regulatory discretion.[57] That means apps with functionality to track health information like blood pressure and transfer the data to healthcare providers or generate health advice from patient-specific information might be considered of moderate risk but will not require premarket oversight.

A 2015 report including mHealth policy was produced in collaboration across leading organizations (e.g., United Nations, Microsoft, NetHope) highlights the United Nations Sustainable Development Goals (SDGs) as the next stage of commitment by world leaders to reduce extreme poverty in all forms by 2030.[58] The report is the *SDG ICT Playbook:*

From Innovation to Impact. It addresses technological areas such as mHealth to assist the SDGs achievements.

Business: Economic Potential and Cost Savings

mHealth is a lucrative business. Estimates indicate the mHealth market will account for nearly $13 billion in 2015 alone.[50] Further growth is anticipated at nearly 40% over the next 6 years despite barriers on regulation, patient acceptance, and privacy concerns.[50] Goldman Sachs analysts forecast an opportunity in savings from digital healthcare of $305 billion for the United States.[59] For healthcare systems, globally and particularly in low-resource settings, mHealth has the potential to increase healthcare quality, decrease costs, and create additional capacity for healthcare systems.[5,60] For example, in Latin America, estimates of mHealth services in Brazil and Mexico will extend medical attention to 28.4 million and 15.5 million new patients, respectively, at an estimated cost reduction of $17.9 billion.[61]

Service costs, such as traditional provider visits, are projected to significantly decrease with health digitalization. For example, Armstrong et al.[62] modeled the cost-effectiveness of replacing ambulatory surgical follow-up visits with mobile app home monitoring. Taking into account the total of healthcare system, patient, and external borne costs, they found the total cost difference between mobile app and in-person follow-up care was the equivalent of $223, with in-person follow-up being more expensive than mobile app follow-up care. However, research on mHealth intervention cost-effectiveness or cost-savings remains limited.

MOBILE HEALTH BENEFITS AND CHALLENGES
Mobile Health Evolution and Evidence

mHealth has evolved from early clinical decision support at the bedside using PDAs to the use of personal supercomputers.[34,63,64] Over the last decade, increased research and literature on mobile technologies reflect the mHealth's evolution.[54] While a number of research studies were conducted, a review of these studies demonstrate that research is still in the early stages with limited scope and mixed results.

Labrique et al. describes the first era of mHealth as experimental proliferation or what was criticized as "pilititis"—that is, a large number (piles) of pilot studies conducted within a short time frame and not extending past the pilot phase. This is a natural state of disruptive technology or innovation introduction.[51] Early, proof-of-concept projects often focus on evaluating technology feasibility and acceptability versus impact assessment. With the rapid increase in peer-reviewed literature and larger-scale research projects, we may now be transitioning into a second phase, an empirical era.[54]

The evidence base for mHealth continues to grow with an increase in outcomes research.[23] For example, authors of Cochrane Reviews assessed mobile messaging's impact on self-management of long-term illness,[65] promotion of preventive healthcare,[66] adherence to antiretroviral therapy in patients with HIV infection,[67] attendance at healthcare appointments,[68] and the effects of apps for asthma outcomes.[69] Other systematic reviews evaluated how mHealth can be used to improve adherence to any medication regimen[70] or usage of antenatal/postnatal care and childhood immunization.[71] High-quality evidence was identified for interventions using mobile messaging to support smoking cessation[66] and to improve adherence to antiretroviral therapy.[67] Some evidence of effectiveness or studies with positive outcomes were identified for mHealth interventions to improve adherence to any medication and to improve antenatal/postnatal care attendance and childhood immunization.[70,71]

Limited, low-to-moderate quality, or insufficient evidence was found for mobile messaging to improve self-management of long-term illnesses[65] or rate of appointment attendance,[68] and for asthma apps.[69] Overall, authors indicated a need for further high-quality evidence, particularly for understanding long-term mHealth effects, cost-effectiveness, a broader variety of settings, and risks and limitations of such interventions.[65,66,68,70,71]

Similarly, two systematic reviews conducted by Free et al.[72] found modest improvements in care delivery and mixed results for outcomes using mHealth technology-based health behavior change or disease management interventions.[73] Among 59 trials of mHealth interventions to improve disease management and 26 for health behavior change, findings indicate improved adherence for antiretroviral medication, smoking cessation, and increased physical activity in diabetics, but not lower body weight.[73]

A number of reviews assessed market availability of health-related apps for specific health topics, their functionalities, and content quality. For example, reviews were conducted to identify and evaluate apps to support chronic diseases such as diabetes[74] and chronic pain,[75,76] as well as for the prevention, detection, and management of cancer,[77] depression,[78] and bipolar disorder,[79] and medication self-management.[80]

Reviews also are available on apps for the prevention and support of infectious diseases such as healthcare-associated infection prevention,[81] HIV,[82] and tuberculosis.[83] Little is known about the length of app use. Although no health outcome was reported, Becker et al[84] found 29% (3406/11,688) of users of an app to support medication adherence used it at least once a week for at least 4 weeks and 27% (3209/11,688) continued to use it for at least 84 days.

Benefits

Many actual and potential benefits of mHealth were already discussed throughout this chapter and have been identified by experts in the field.[3] mHealth tools have the potential to support consumers/patients in being better informed and more involved in their healthcare. Beyond access to healthcare knowledge, mobile phones can support patients to participate proactively in their care and be aware of their health through active self-monitoring.[14] Sensors have the potential to provide real-time measures with highlights of day-to-day variations, and they may be as ubiquitous as phones themselves in the future. In summary, actual and potential benefits include the following:

- Increasing the reach and access to healthcare services (e.g., routine or emergency) and information (e.g., diagnostic, specialty services).
- Improving efficiencies and lowering healthcare systems expenses (e.g., increased data collection accuracy and completeness, rapid collection)
- Empowering individuals or populations for health behavior modifications and disease prevention
- Greater patient access to medical information to improve health outcomes
- Greater access to personal data
- Decrease in operational stresses on healthcare organizations

Challenges

The actual and potential value of mHealth is highly agreed upon, but challenges and barriers still exist.[14,47] Chapters 5, 8, and 22 discuss a number of challenges related to interoperability; these also apply to mHealth-based interventions. Equally challenging are the issues of human resources, funding, infrastructure, privacy (which is discussed in greater detail in Chapter 26), and legal and regulatory issues (discussed further in Chapter 25 and described from a global perspective in Chapter 34).

Issues for developing and low-income areas include the following:

- Patients frequently changing phones or numbers or phones getting lost or stolen
- Use of pay-as-you go plans, running out of credit, cost of texting
- Inconsistency of a reliable power source to charge devices
- Projects relying on smartphones where access to smartphones remain too expensive to be sustainable (globally, basic-feature phones are more common)
- Gender inequities
- Need to accommodate many languages
- Basic literacy, digital literacy, and health literacy
- Scale-up and integration into existing systems

The three biggest mHealth challenges identified by experts in the United States, according to the Economist Intelligence Report, were:

- Patient misinterpretation of data
- Poor health decisions
- Data privacy risks and legal risks[3]

Patient Misinterpretation of Data

Concern exists that mHealth consumers may misinterpret their data or rely on information from apps or devices without consulting a healthcare professional.[57] For instance, 25% of Americans surveyed indicated they trusted symptom checker apps, websites, or home-based vital sign monitors as much as they did their healthcare provider, and 26% reported using these resources instead of going to a healthcare provider.[85] Tripp et al.[86] identified pregnancy-related apps and reviewed their purposes and popularity. They concluded the reduced reliance on healthcare professionals was concerning due the

popularity and availability of interactive, personalized information from these apps.

Data Privacy Risks

Data security, privacy, confidentiality, and human subjects' protection are major concerns for mHealth adoption and expansion.[14,47,57] Large amounts of data are being collected on multiple devices and transferred elsewhere for central collection and analysis. Confidence in security and privacy of patient information is a major concern everywhere; the potential exists for information to be intercepted by third parties.[87] Similar to other areas in informatics, legal questions exist such as to whom the data belongs as well as licensing issues for treatment across state lines. Legal risks impact the roles and accountability of data, particularly continuous remote monitoring. Information handling requirements have increased due to the vast amounts of data and information generated from mobile devices. As a result, greater storage capabilities and data integration into large data sets are needed.[34] No protocol exists for the interpretation of the intensity of data.[47] With the massive amounts of data and information, one of the big questions is who will monitor and be responsible for all the data.[46]

Legal Risks: Safety, Regulation, and Oversight of Data

With over 165,000 health-related apps available to consumers/patients and millions of downloads, little evidence exists about their effectiveness, risks, safety, or even if or how long they are used after they are downloaded.[14] In addition, the development and consumer demand for health apps and sensors are outpacing regulation and policy.[57,76] Currently no medical-specific regulations are available to assure reliability and validity of app content, and only a small number of apps are FDA approved.[57] In fact, many apps are not current with clinical guidelines, and the functionalities and quality of apps are limited.[79]

Given the growing numbers of apps and little scientific evidence, it is understandable consumers and healthcare providers are challenged to become "app literate" or able to identify and recommend efficacious, credible, and reliable apps.[78] Although many apps likely could cause little harm, those supporting diagnostic decisions could have serious repercussions.[57] Misinformation is also a concern. For example, Acne App claimed its mobile app could cure acne by emitting colored light from a cell phone. The Federal Trade Commission sued the marketer of this app, claiming unfair and deceptive practice. The app information was not verified and information was potentially harmful (as well as not efficacious) to patients.

To help healthcare providers determine which apps to recommend to patients, a number of third-party organizations are providing tools to rate, evaluate, or curate certified apps, such as Happtique, HealthTap, Wellocracy, and Health AppScript.[88] For example, the Health AppScript uses a proprietary algorithm to rank apps based on six weighted areas[14]:

1. Licensed healthcare professional input
2. Endorsement by recognized associations (e.g., professional and hospital associations)

3. Consumer ratings (e.g., download and rating volume, retention)
4. Development quality (e.g., data management privacy and security)
5. Functionality (e.g., data management and control, clinical sensor compatibility)
6. Clinical outcomes

However, no evidence was found for how the validity of the tool was established. Readers can also consult the FDA's website for information on approved apps.[89]

Manual methods to evaluate apps are proposed. The Institute for Healthcare Informatics used seven functionality criteria and four functional subcategories for app assessment.[15] Another tool to classify and assess the quality of mobile apps uses five measures and is called the mobile app rating scale (MARS): [90]

1. Engagement (e.g., interest, interactivity, customization)
2. Functionality (e.g., performance, ease of use)
3. Aesthetics (e.g., layout, graphics, visual appeal)
4. Information (e.g., quality and quantity of information, credibility, evidence base)
5. Subjective quality (e.g., if recommended, willingness to pay, star rating)

MARS was used to review and rate existing apps to support heart failure symptom monitoring and self-management.[91] For reporting findings of a targeted app evaluation, recommendations are provided by the Quality and Risk of Bias Checklist for Studies That Review Smartphone Applications.[92]

Finding a viable business model to maintain an intervention is another challenge. Suggestions for remedies include selling mHealth services or creating subscriptions to premium content and advice for the collected data.[3] For example, the BlueStar app for type-2 diabetes management is only available by prescription and was the first app to receive approval to be prescribed for disease therapy and to be eligible for insurance reimbursement.[93] Once better evidence is available about the effectiveness of mHealth measures and how to classify them, reimbursements through insurance companies may be less of an issue.

Leading mHealth Organizations, Key Resources, and Information Repositories

To address a number of the challenges identified in this chapter, leading organizations have established repositories and helpful guides for mHealth development, implementation, and evaluation. Table 15.3 provides a list of several of these resources.

FUTURE DIRECTIONS OF MOBILE HEALTH AND CONCLUSIONS

An unprecedented opportunity exists to leverage humanity's most pervasive global technology platform into revolutionizing healthcare. Currently the use of technology is shifting from networks and hardware to software and

services.[94] The next generation of mHealth apps using 5G is likely to revolutionize and transform healthcare, with its projected speeds 100 times faster than today that can support billions of simultaneously connected devices. This level of connectivity will enable reaction times that can support the precise control of autonomous vehicles, improve network reliability, and reduce energy use by a factor of 1000.[43]

The future points to the connectivity of anything and everything. Multiple forms of sensors monitoring physiological responses will capture tremendous amounts of data over extended periods and will likely change what we know about our bodies. By 2020, over 78.5 million consumers globally are estimated to use home health technologies and remote monitoring tools, up from 14.3 million in 2014.[95] This revolution of data-gathering sensors monitoring everything is called the Internet of Things (IoT) and is mobile, virtual, and instantaneous.[96]

Wearable technology such as the Apple Watch (an "intelligent health and fitness companion"), Jawbone, and Smart Scale (monitoring body fat) is already here and widely used. Smartphones are being fitted for testing blood, saliva, and sweat, and breath tests.[3] The challenge will be how to analyze and respond to the growing databases of information. The fields of big data and personalized medicine will likely integrate to allow better understanding of the impacts and capacities of mHealth data.

Major players in the sphere of data and technology integration include Apple's HealthKit and GoogleFit, which were both released in 2014. These are central platforms to aggregate healthcare information, collect fitness and health data, access personal medical information (diagnoses, lab tests), develop tools such as apps or integrate ones existing or in use by healthcare facilities, and allow users to choose what will be shared with healthcare teams. According to a Reuters poll, 14 of 23 top hospitals in the United States have rolled out programs using Apple's HealthKit service.[97] In addition, the Apple ResearchKit, an open-source software framework, will likely transform how individuals or patients become involved to advance medical research.

mHealth is changing the delivery of healthcare, though its continued role in the future of global healthcare delivery seems certain. It is uncertain how mHealth will evolve in response to the challenges outlined above. mHealth has the potential to empower patients, allowing them to take control of their health; healthcare may become more personalized and responsive to individual needs. The ideal would be for integrated systems to shift from the current reactive, disease treatment focus to a proactive, disease prevention focus, including problem detection at early stages outside healthcare structures. A tighter integration of mHealth into health systems will allow even greater results than today. The future focus on mHealth and its health impacts is assured in part because the National Institutes of Health (NIH) included mHealth as one of its main goals in its NIH-wide 2016–20 strategic plan.[98]

TABLE 15.3   Leading Mobile Health Organizations, Key Resources, and Databases

Resource/Report	Aim	Link
K4health	Key considerations, planning, and evaluation of mHealth interventions	https://www.k4health.org/toolkits/mhealth-planning-guide
Nine Principles of Digital Development	Established to support integration of best practices into technology-enabled programs	http://digitalprinciples.org/
mHealth Compendium	Focuses on mHealth strategies, best practices, and technical capacities for health in Africa	https://www.msh.org/sites/msh.org/files/mhealth_compendium_volume_3_a4_small.pdf
Healthcare Information and Management Systems Society (HIMSS)	mHealth Roadmap	http://www.himss.org/ResourceLibrary/mHimssRoadmapLanding.aspx?ItemNumber=30480&navItemNumber=30479
John's Hopkins Global mHealth Initiative	Resources, mHealth news, webinars	http://www.jhumhealth.org/
mHealth Evidence, mHealth Knowledge,	Database of literature demonstrating the feasibility, usability, and efficacy of mobile technologies in healthcare	https://www.mhealthevidence.org/
mHealth Registry	Register projects with the WHO to synergize the added advantage in the space	Mregistry.org
NIH	mHealth information from the National Institutes of Health	https://obssr.od.nih.gov/scientific_areas/methodology/mhealth/
Global Health Learning Center	mHealth Basics: Introduction to Mobile Technology for Health. United States Agency for International Development (USAID).	http://www.globalhealthlearning.org/course/mhealth-basics-introduction-mobile-technology-health
Apple research kit	An open-source framework for developing health apps	http://www.apple.com/researchkit/
mHealth working group	Community to share resources and ideas on mHealth challenges and successes and project inventory	https://www.mhealthworkinggroup.org/project
The Groupe Speciale Mobile Association (GSMA) mHealth Tracker	Database of programs	http://www.m4dimpact.com/data/products-services
Center for Health Market Innovations	Learn about and connect with programs to improve the health of the world's poor	http://healthmarketinnovations.org/programs
Federal Health IT Strategic Plan 2015-2020[9]	U.S.-based health IT plan that includes mHealth as a tactic	https://www.healthit.gov/sites/default/files/federal-healthIT-strategic-plan-2014.pdf
SDG ICT Playbook: From Innovation to Impact[58]	Recommendations for investments in e-health. Produced in collaboration across leading organizations, e.g., United Nations, Microsoft, NetHope	http://www.knowledgefordevelopmentwithoutborders.org/2016/01/07/sdg-ict-playbook-from-innovation-to-impact/
Health Organization's Global Observatory for eHealth (GOe)	Report on a 64-country survey on broad applications of information and communications technology	http://www.who.int/goe/en/

NIH, National Institutes of Health; *ICT,* information and communication technologies, *SDG,* sustainable development goals.

REFERENCES

1. U.N. Centre. *Deputy UN, Chief Calls for Urgent Action to Tackle Global Sanitation Crisis;* 2013.
2. Kvedar J, Coye MJ, Everett W. Connected health: a review of technologies and strategies to improve patient care with telemedicine and telehealth. *Health Aff (Millwood).* 2014;33 (2):194–199.
3. The Economist Intelligence Unit Ltd. *How Mobile Is Transforming Healthcare: Power to the Patient;* 2015.
4. Mendoza G, Okoko L, Konopka S, Jonas E. Arlington, VA: African Strategies for Health project, Management Sciences for Health; 2013. mHealth Compendium. Vol. 3.
5. World Health Organization. *mHealth: New Horizons for Health Through Mobile Technologies.* Geneva, Switzerland; 2011. http://www.who.int/goe/publications/goe_mhealth_web.pdf/.
6. Global Health eLearning Center. mHealth Basics: Introduction to Mobile Technology for Health. In: Lee CK, Raney L, L'Engle K, eds. 2014. https://www.globalhealthlearning.org/course/mhealth-basics-introduction-mobile-technology-health.

7. Laxminarayan S, Istepanian RS. UNWIRED E-MED: the next generation of wireless and internet telemedicine systems. *IEEE Trans Inform Technol Biomed.* 2000;4(3):189–193.

8. Istepanian R, Laxminarayan S, Pattichis CE. *M-Health: Emerging Mobile Health Systems.* New York, NY: Springer; 2006.

9. The Office of the National Coordinator for Health Information Technology (ONC). *Federal Health IT Strategic Plan 2015–2020.* Office of the Secretary, United States Department of Health and Human Services; 2015. https://www.globalhealthlearning.org/course/mhealth-basics-introduction-mobile-technology-health.

10. Labrique AB, Vasudevan L, Kochi E, Fabricant R, Mehl G. mHealth innovations as health system strengthening tools: 12 common applications and a visual framework. *Glob Health Sci Pract.* 2013;1(2):160–171.

11. Mobile Marketing Association. *Industry Overview*; 2014. http://www.mmaglobal.com/about/industry-overview/.

12. International Telecommunication Union. *The World in 2013: ICT Facts and Figures*; 2013. http://www.itu.int/en/ITU-D/Statistics/Pages/facts/default.aspx/.

13. Research2guidance. *mHealth App Developer Economics 2014: The State of the Art of mHealth App Publishing.* Berlin, Germany: research2guidance; 2014.

14. IMS Institute for Healthcare Informatics. *Patient Adoption of mHealth. Use, Evidence and Remaining Barriers to Mainstream Acceptance.* Parsippany, NJ: IMS Institute for Healthcare Informatics; 2015.

15. IMS Institute for Healthcare Informatics. *Patient Apps for Improved Healthcare: From Novelty to Mainstream.* Parsippany, NJ: IMS Institute for Healthcare Informatics; 2013.

16. England NHS. *NHS England—TECS CASE STUDY 002: Florence text messaging to monitor a range of conditions*; 2014.

17. Boulos MN, Wheeler S, Tavares C, Jones R. How smartphones are changing the face of mobile and participatory healthcare: an overview, with example from eCAALYX. *Biomed Eng Online.* 2011;10:24.

18. Hale K, Capra S, Bauer J. A framework to assist health professionals in recommending high-quality apps for supporting chronic disease self-management: illustrative assessment of type 2 diabetes apps. *JMIR Mhealth Uhealth.* 2015;3(3).

19. Moore J, Marshall M, Judge M, et al. Technology-supported apprenticeship in the management of hypertension: a randomized controlled trial. *JCOM.* 2014;21(3).

20. Ben-Zeev D, Kaiser SM, Brenner CJ, Begale M, Duffecy J, Mohr DC. Development and usability testing of FOCUS: a smartphone system for self-management of schizophrenia. *Psychiatr Rehabil J.* 2013;36(4):289–296.

21. Burns MN, Montague E, Mohr DC. Initial design of culturally informed behavioral intervention technologies: developing an mHealth intervention for young sexual minority men with generalized anxiety disorder and major depression. *J Med Internet Res.* 2013;15(12).

22. Baquero GA, Banchs JE, Ahmed S, Naccarelli GV, Luck JC. Surface 12 lead electrocardiogram recordings using smart phone technology. *J Electrocardiol.* 2014;48(1):1–7.

23. Levine R, Corbacio A, Konopka S, et al. Arlington, VA: African Strategies for Health, Management Sciences for Health; 2015. mHealth Compendium. Vol. 5.

24. Kiberu VM, Matovu JK, Makumbi F, Kyozira C, Mukooyo E, Wanyenze RK. Strengthening district-based health reporting through the district health management information software

25. Sage Bionetworks. *mPower: Mobile Parkinson Disease Study*; 2015. parkinsonmpower.org/.

26. Fazen LE, Chemwolo BT, Songok JJ, et al. AccessMRS: integrating OpenMRS with smart forms on Android. *Stud Health Technol Inform.* 2013;192:866–870.

27. Mitchell M, Hedt-Gauthier BL, Msellemu D, Nkaka M, Lesh N. Using electronic technology to improve clinical care—results from a before-after cluster trial to evaluate assessment and classification of sick children according to Integrated Management of Childhood Illness (IMCI) protocol in Tanzania. *BMC Med Inform Decis Mak.* 2013;13:95.

28. McNEIl-PPC Inc. *Allergy Forcast Tools and Apps*; 2015. https://www.zyrtec.com/allergy-forecast-tools-apps/.

29. Paper-Based and Electronic Partogram Systems to Safe Lives at Birth (PartoMa). *ClinicalTrials.gov*; 2014. https://clinicaltrials.gov/ct2/show/NCT02318420/.

30. Lester RT, Ritvo P, Mills EJ, et al. Effects of a mobile phone short message service on antiretroviral treatment adherence in Kenya (WelTel Kenya1): a randomised trial. *Lancet.* 2010;376(9755):1838–1845.

31. HealthTap. *Doctors Are Making House Calls Again*; 2015. https://www.healthtap.com/.

32. Macleod B, Phillips J, Stone AE, Walji A, Awoonor-Williams JK. The architecture of a software system for supporting community-based primary health care with mobile technology: the mobile technology for community health (MoTeCH) initiative in Ghana. *Online J Public Health Inform.* 2012;4(1). http://dx.doi.org/10.5210/ojphi.v4i1.3910.

33. Wakadha H, Chandir S, Were EV, et al. The feasibility of using mobile-phone based SMS reminders and conditional cash transfers to improve timely immunization in rural Kenya. *Vaccine.* 2012;31(6):987–993.

34. Patrick J. How mHealth will spur consumer-led healthcare. *mHealth.* 2015;1(14):1–9.

35. International Telecommunication Union. *The World in 2015: ICT Facts & Figures.* Geneva: Author; 2015. http://www.itu.int/en/ITU-D/Statistics/Documents/facts/ICTFactsFigures2015.pdf.

36. International Telecommunication Union. *The World in 2009: ICT Facts and Figures*; 2009. http://www.itu.int/net/pressoffice/backgrounders/general/pdf/3.pdf/.

37. Leo B, Morello R, Ramachandran V. *The Face of African Infrastructure: Service Availability and Citizens' Demands.* CGD Working Paper 393, Washington, DC: Center for Global Development; 2015.

38. Mungai C. The mobile phone comes first in Africa; before electricity, water, toilets or even food. *Mail Guardian Africa.* 2015;17(10). http://mgafrica.com/article/2015-03-03-mobile-come-first-in-africa-before-electricity-water-toilets-or-even-food.

39. infoDev. *Mobile Usage at the Base of the Pyramid: Research Findings from Kenya and South Africa.* Washington, DC: World Bank; 2013.

40. Blumberg S, Luke J. *Wireless Substitution: Early Release of Estimates from the National Health Interview Survey, July-December 2014 (Released 06/2015).* US Department of Health and Human Services, Centers for Disease Control and Prevention, National Center for Health Statistics; 2015.

41. Pew Research Center. *Mobile Technology Fact Sheet*; 2014. http://www.pewinternet.org/fact-sheets/mobile-technology-fact-sheet/.

42. Statista. *Global Smartphone Penetration from 2008 to 2014 (in percent of new handset sales).* http://www.statista.com/statistics/218532/global-smartphone-penetration-since-2008/; 2015.

43. Kohlenberger J. Mobilizing America: Accelerating Next Generation Wireless Opportunities Everywhere. *Mobile Future*; 2015. http://mobilefuture.org/wp-content/uploads/2015/09/5G-Paper-.pdf.

44. Anderson M. *Racial and Ethnic Differences in How People Use Mobile Technology.* Washington, DC: Pew Research Center; 2015.

45. Patel V, Barker W, Siminerio E. *Individuals' Access and Use of Their Online Medical Record Nationwide. ONC Data Brief, No. 20.* Washington, DC: Office of the National Coordinator for Health Information Technology; 2014.

46. Staggers N, McCasky T, Brazelton N, Kennedy R. Nanotechnology: the coming revolution and its implications for consumers, clinicians, and informatics. *Nurs Outlook.* 2008;56 (5):268–274.

47. Whittaker R. Issues in mHealth: findings from key informant interviews. *J Medl Internet Res.* 2012;14(5).

48. Crocker P. *Converged-Mobile-Messaging Analysis and Forecasts.* Tyntec; 2013. http://www.smithspointanalytics.com/Converged_Mobile_Messaging.pdf.

49. Statista. *The Statistics Portal. Cumulative Number of Apps Downloaded from the Apple App Store from July 2008 to June 2015 (in billions)*; 2015. http://www.statista.com/statistics/263794/number-of-downloads-from-the-apple-app-store/.

50. Research SNS. *The Mobile Healthcare (mHealth) Bible: 2015-2020.* SNS Research Marketing Intelligence & Consultancy Solutions; 2014.

51. Labrique A, Vasudevan L, Chang LW, Mehl G. H_pe for mHealth: more "y" or "o" on the horizon? *Int J Med Inform.* 2013;82(5):467–469.

52. United States Agency for International Development (USAID). *The mHealth Planning Guide: Key Considerations for Integrating Mobile Technology into Health Programs*; 2015. https://www.k4health.org/toolkits/mhealth-planning-guide/.

53. Digital Development Principles Working Group. *Principles for Digital Development*; 2015. http://digitalprinciples.org/about/.

54. Fiordelli M, Diviani N, Schulz PJ. Mapping mHealth research: a decade of evolution. *J of Med Internet Res.* 2013;15(5).

55. US Food and Drug Administration. *FDA Issues Final Guidance on Mobile Medical Apps*; 2013. http://www.fda.gov/NewsEvents/Newsroom/PressAnnouncements/ucm369431.htm/.

56. US Food and Drug Administration. *Mobile Medical Applications. Guidance for Industry and Food and Drug Administration Staff.* Rockville, MD: US Department of Health and Human Services Food and Drug Administration; February 9, 2015.

57. Kuehn BM. Is there an app to solve app overload? *JAMA.* 2015;313(14):1405–1407.

58. NetHope. SDG ICT Playbook. *From Innovation to Impact.* 2015.

59. Stern C. Goldman Sachs says a digital healthcare revolution is coming—and it could save America $300 billion. *Business Insider.* 2015. http://www.businessinsider.com/goldman-digital-healthcare-is-coming-2015-6.

60. GSMA. *Socio-Economic Impact of mHealth: An Assessment Report for the European Union*; 2013. http://www.gsma.com/connectedliving/wp-content/uploads/2013/06/Socio-economic_impact-of-mHealth_EU_14062013V2.pdf.

61. GSMA. *Socio-Economic Impact of mHealth: An Assessment Report for Brazil and Mexico*; 2013. http://www.gsma.com/connectedliving/wp-content/uploads/2013/06/Socio-economic_impact-of-mHealth_EU_14062013V2.pdf.

62. Armstrong KA, Semple JL, Coyte PC. Replacing ambulatory surgical follow-up visits with mobile app home monitoring: modeling cost-effective scenarios. *J Med Internet Res.* 2014;16(9).

63. Lee NJ, Chen ES, Currie LM, et al. The effect of a mobile clinical decision support system on the diagnosis of obesity and overweight in acute and primary care encounters. *ANS Adv Nurs Sci.* 2009;32(3):211–221.

64. Sheehan B, Nigrovic LE, Dayan PS, et al. Informing the design of clinical decision support services for evaluation of children with minor blunt head trauma in the emergency department: a sociotechnical analysis. *J Biomed Inform.* 2013;46(5):905–913.

65. de Jongh T, Gurol-Urganci I, Vodopivec-Jamsek V, Car J, Atun R. Mobile phone messaging for facilitating self-management of long-term illnesses. *Cochrane Database Syst Rev.* 2012;12.

66. Vodopivec-Jamsek V, de Jongh T, Gurol-Urganci I, Atun R, Car J. Mobile phone messaging for preventive health care. *Cochrane Database Syst Rev.* 2012;12.

67. Horvath T, Azman H, Kennedy GE, Rutherford GW. Mobile phone text messaging for promoting adherence to antiretroviral therapy in patients with HIV infection. *Cochrane Database Syst Rev.* 2012;3.

68. Car J, Gurol-Urganci I, de Jongh T, Vodopivec-Jamsek V, Atun R. Mobile phone messaging reminders for attendance at healthcare appointments. *Cochrane Database Syst Rev.* 2012;11(7):CD007458.

69. Belisario MJS, Huckvale K, Greenfield G, Car J, Gunn LH. Smartphone and tablet self management apps for asthma. *Cochrane Database Syst Rev.* 2013;11.

70. Anglada-Martinez H, Riu-Viladoms G, Martin-Conde M, Rovira-Illamola M, Sotoca-Momblona JM, Codina-Jane C. Does mHealth increase adherence to medication? Results of a systematic review. *Int J Clin Pract.* 2015;69(1):9–32.

71. Watterson JL, Walsh J, Madeka I. Using mHealth to improve usage of antenatal care, postnatal care, and immunization: a systematic review of the literature. *BioMed Res Int.* 2015;2015:153402.

72. Free C, Phillips G, Watson L, et al. The effectiveness of mobile-health technologies to improve health care service delivery processes: a systematic review and meta-analysis. *PLoS Med.* 2013;10(1).

73. Free C, Phillips G, Galli L, et al. The effectiveness of mobile-health technology-based health behaviour change or disease management interventions for health care consumers: a systematic review. *PLoS Med.* 2013;10(1).

74. Martinez-Perez B, de la Torre-Diez I, Lopez-Coronado M, Sainz-De-Abajo B. Comparison of mobile apps for the leading causes of death among different income zones: a review of the literature and app stores. *JMIR Mhealth Uhealth.* 2014;2(1).

75. Wallace LS, Dhingra LK. A systematic review of smartphone applications for chronic pain available for download in the United States. *J Opioid Manag.* 2014;10(1):63–68.

76. de la Vega R, Miro J. mHealth: a strategic field without a solid scientific soul. A systematic review of pain-related apps. *PLoS One.* 2014;9(7):e101312.

77. Bender JL, Yue RY, To MJ, Deacken L, Jadad AR. A lot of action, but not in the right direction: systematic review and content

analysis of smartphone applications for the prevention, detection, and management of cancer. *J Med Internet Res.* 2013;15(12).

78. Shen N, Levitan MJ, Johnson A, et al. Finding a depression app: a review and content analysis of the depression app marketplace. *JMIR Mhealth Uhealth.* 2015;3(1).

79. Nicholas J, Larsen ME, Proudfoot J, Christensen H. Mobile apps for bipolar disorder: a systematic review of features and content quality. *J Med Internet Res.* 2015;17(8).

80. Bailey SC, Belter LT, Pandit AU, Carpenter DM, Carlos E, Wolf MS. The availability, functionality, and quality of mobile applications supporting medication self-management. *J Am Med Inform Assoc.* 2014;21(3):542–546.

81. Schnall R, Iribarren SJ. Review and analysis of existing mobile phone applications for health care-associated infection prevention. *Am J Infect Control.* 2015;43(6):572–576.

82. Schnall R, Bakken S, Rojas M, Travers J, Carballo-Dieguez A. mHealth technology as a persuasive tool for treatment, care and management of persons living with HIV. *AIDS Behav.* 2015;19 (Suppl 2):81–89.

83. Iribarren S, Schnall R, Stone P, Carballo-Diéguez A. Smartphone applications to support tuberculosis prevention and treatment: Review and evaluation. *JMIR Mhealth Uhealth.* 2016;4(2).

84. Becker S, Kribben A, Meister S, Diamantidis CJ, Unger N, Mitchell A. User profiles of a smartphone application to support drug adherence—experiences from the iNephro project. *PLoS One.* 2013;8(10).

85. Philips Survey. *Consumer Attitudes Towards Healthcare Technology;* 2012. http://www.newscenter.philips.com/pwc_nc/us_en/standard/resources/corporate/press/2012/Philips_Health_Infographic_12.12_F.jpg/.

86. Tripp N, Hainey K, Liu A, et al. An emerging model of maternity care: smartphone, midwife, doctor? *Women Birth J Aust Coll Midwives.* 2014;27(1):64–67.

87. Schnall R, Higgins T, Brown W, Carballo-Dieguez A, Bakken S. Trust, perceived risk, perceived ease of use and perceived usefulness as factors related to mhealth technology use. *Stud Health Technol Inform.* 2015;216:467–471.

88. Dan L. *The Rise of Third Party mHealth App Stores;* 2013. http://histalkmobile.com/the-riseof-third-party-mhealth-app-stores/.

89. US Food and Drug Administration. *Device Approvals, Denials and Clearances;* 2014. http://www.fda.gov/medicaldevices/productsandmedicalprocedures/deviceapprovalsandclearances/default.htm.

90. Stoyanov SR, Hides L, Kavanagh DJ, Zelenko O, Tjondronegoro D, Mani M. Mobile app rating scale: a new tool for assessing the quality of health mobile apps. *JMIR Mhealth Uhealth.* 2015;3(1).

91. Masterson Creber RM[1], Maurer MS, Reading M, Hiraldo G, Hickey KT, Iribarren S. Review and analysis of existing mobile phone apps to support heart failure symptom monitoring and self-care management using the Mobile Application Rat5ing Scale (MARS). *JMIR Mhealth Uhealth.* 14;4(2):e74. doi: http://dx.doi.org/10.2196/mhealth.5882.

92. BinDhim NF, Hawkey A, Trevena L. A systematic review of quality assessment methods for smartphone health apps. *Telemed J E Health.* 2014;21(2):97–104.

93. *BlueStar, the first prescription-only app.* Doctors start prescribing the BlueStar app for diabetes management. http://spectrum.ieee.org/biomedical/devices/bluestar-the-first-prescriptiononly-app/. Accessed September 20, 2015.

94. World Bank. *Information and Communications for Development 2012: Maximizing Mobile.* Washington, DC: World Bank; 2012.

95. Tractica. Home Health Technologies. *Medical Monitoring and Management, Remote Consultations, Eldercare, and Health and Wellness Applications: Global Market Analysis and Forecasts.* Boulder, CO: Tractica; 2015.

96. Burrus D. The internet of things is far bigger than anyone realizes. *Wired.* 2015. http://www.wired.com/insights/2014/11/the-internet-of-things-bigger/. Accessed November 9, 2015.

97. Farr C. Apple's health tech takes early lead among top hospitals. *Science;* 2015. http://recode.net/2015/02/05/apples-health-tech-takes-early-lead-among-top-hospitals/. Accessed October 15, 2015.

98. *NIH.* NIH-wide strategic plan fiscal years 2016-2020: turning discovery into health. National Institutes of Health. http://www.nih.gov/sites/default/files/about-nih/strategic-plan-fy2016-2020-508.pdf/. Accessed January 29, 2016.

DISCUSSION QUESTIONS

1. Describe the components of an mHealth intervention to support a patient with a chronic condition.

2. What are the strengths of using mHealth technologies in clinical practice?

3. What are the barriers to using mHealth technologies in clinical practice?

4. Explain some of the risks involved in using mHealth technology.

5. How can mHealth technologies be used to support patient care?

6. How might mHealth change the patient-provider relationship?

CASE STUDY

Henry Brown is a 67-year-old American living in the rural central United States. He is prescribed multiple medications for hypertension, depression, diabetes mellitus type 2, and a recent bacterial infection. Henry is not alone. In fact, estimates suggest at least 70% of the U.S. aging population is prescribed multiple medications due to the rapid increase in the prevalence of chronic diseases. This presents a major challenge for our healthcare system. Most medications require consistent adherence to the prescribed regimen for them to achieve therapeutic effect. Yet it is known that adherence rates remain suboptimal across populations and disease states. Because Henry uses a smartphone, his primary healthcare provider might recommend a mobile app called the Medication Tracker to help him manage his complicated medication regimen. Henry's primary healthcare provider recognizes apps have the potential to address the specific needs of patients in a manner that is timely, cost-effective, informative, and engaging. This app can be configured to deliver automated, personalized messaging to remind Henry to take his medication; can help Henry reinforce good self-management behaviors; can provide education on his chronic diseases; and can provide information about his medications, such as black box warnings, side effects, and contra-indications for use.

Discussion Questions

1. Describe the factors that Henry's primary healthcare provider should consider when selecting an app for him.
2. Identify the features most important to facilitate the primary treatment goals of Henry and his primary provider.
3. Describe how Henry should communicate his activities with the app to his primary healthcare provider.
4. List some risks for Henry associated with using this app.

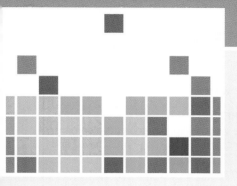

16

Strategic Planning and Selecting an Information System

Cynthia M. Mascara and Mical Debrow

The pace of change in healthcare is anticipated to only accelerate, and both the organization and the vendor must be able to adapt quickly.

OBJECTIVES

At the completion of this chapter, the reader will be prepared to:

1. Use an institution's vision and strategic plan as a guide in selecting a new or upgraded healthcare information system.

2. Organize and implement a system selection process using the initial phases of the systems life cycle.

3. Prepare a request for information (RFI) and a request for proposal (RFP).

KEY TERMS

request for information (RFI), 278
request for proposal (RFP), 278
requirements definition, 274
strategic alignment, 271

strategic vision, 271
systems life cycle (SLC), 273
vendor, 279

ABSTRACT ❖

This chapter provides direction and guidance for the utilization of a systematic process in the identification and selection of a healthcare information system. The most critical factor in a selection process is strategic alignment with both the organization and the information technology department. Understanding the systems life cycle and performing an assessment of an organization's requirements are essential to a successful selection process. The chapter describes the requirements of both a request for information and a request for proposal. Evaluation criteria for system selection are also explored. Appraisal of vendors and their capabilities to meet current and future needs are outlined.

INTRODUCTION

This chapter provides an overview of the system selection process within a healthcare environment. Box 16.1 lists steps that are usually part of the process. However, it is important to realize that the specific steps used for each purchase of a healthcare information system will vary depending on the size and mission of the institution, the significance of the purchase to the institution, the governance model of the institution, and a number of external factors. In addition, a systematic process should be used when selecting a new system; however, the process is not linear but rather somewhat reiterative as new information and insights develop during the process.

When the decision has been made to identify and select a new or first healthcare information system, an initial search will quickly identify that although some vendors have exited the health information technology (IT) (or health information systems [IS]) market, more than 200 companies remain marketing health IT. This large number of choices must be narrowed to a reasonable number of systems that can meet the organization's unique needs by considering factors such as the size, type, complexity, and unique cultural aspects of the organization. Although the natural inclination of an organization is to reach out to well-known companies or those used in the local community in selecting a system, a systematic process involving a thorough review of available information systems is recommended. However, selecting a new system or upgrading a current system is doomed to failure if that process is not based on a careful analysis of the institution's current status and desired future. This chapter provides the framework for that process.

STRATEGIC VISION AND ALIGNMENT

A **strategic vision** is the desired future state. **Strategic alignment** involves matching two or more organizational strategies to ensure that they synergistically support the organization's goals and vision. Before beginning the system selection process for any new or updated system, the institution must develop and implement a strategic vision and plan. In addition, the information technology (IT) department

BOX 16.1   Steps in the System Selection Process

Identify the Project as a Formal Organizational Priority
- Have the organization executives endorse the project as a priority, define its initial scope, and provide start-up resources.

Identify Responsible Groups/Individuals
- Establish the interdisciplinary selection committee, outline scope of responsibilities, and provide release time for individuals.
- Establish reporting relationships for the selection committee.

Perform Initial Internal and External Data Collection
- Review the mission and goals of the institution and how this project relates to them.
- Review resources, both internet-based and available literature, on real installations of the new project. If available, work with a formal project manager to formulate project steps.
- Attend trade shows and major conferences related to the project.
- Obtain related guidelines/regulations.
- Develop initial system specifications.
- Develop a list of vendors that offer the planned new system.
- Review computerized, manual, and/or paper processes and forms in use.
- Identify information systems that could interface with the project.
- Identify all current projects that might interface or conflict with the project.
- Develop lists of institutions/contacts with project experience.

Develop Goals, Benefits, and Scope of Project
- Prepare a statement outlining the goals, benefits, and scope of the project.
- Develop feasibility statement and refine system specifications.

- Send RFI to potential vendors (optional).
- Review the responses to the RFI (optional).
- Create a list of potential vendors for RFP distribution.

Develop and Distribute RFP
- Conduct preliminary site visits for specification development.
- Define and prioritize system requirements—"must have" and "nice to have."
- Create an RFP, including a standardized response format and weighted evaluation criteria (best value across clinical, technical, vendor, pricing).
- Develop and include criteria and mechanisms for vendor responses and committee evaluation.
- Finalize the list of potential vendors.
- Finalize and distribute RFP to potential vendors.

Analyze Vendor Proposals and Make Recommendation(s)
- Evaluate responses to RFP across at least these factors: clinical functionality, technical capability/feasibility, financial aspects, project timeline, and vendor attributes, including projected company stability.
- Have vendors conduct demonstrations using scenarios the committee devises. Use formal evaluation criteria to rate them.
- Conduct site visits and use formal evaluation criteria to rate the vendors.
- Combine findings and develop decision recommendations.

Conduct Contract Negotiations
- Include the RFP as part of the contract, including vendor responses to issues or questions.
- Review and iterate the agreement (see Chapter 18).
- Sign the agreement and begin the installation process.

RFI, Requests for information; *RFP*, request for proposal.

must develop its own strategic vision and plan in alignment with and guided by the organization's strategic vision and plan. It is essential that these plans consider the multiple internal and external stakeholders, including users of the patient's healthcare information such as physicians, nurses, ancillary healthcare staff, payers, regulatory groups and, finally, the patient.

The strategic vision and plan for an organization provides a long-term road map for the organization and is critical in light of economic, regulatory, and market pressures. Strategic planning in healthcare is used to determine the desired future of the organization. It involves a variety of organizational processes, including, for example, external and internal scans. The strategic plan sets the goals, objectives, assignments, and measures based on the community's needs and provides the direction for the organization when planning how it will achieve its clinical and financial goals and objectives. The plan will provide guidance in selecting the information systems that most closely align with the desired future of the organization, stakeholder buy-in, engagement, productivity, and efficiency. The strategic vision and plan should also create a

sense of urgency that begins with the vision of the organization. Strategic plans typically do not address issues or problems but rather chart the direction of the organization.

The IT plan should align with the organization's mission, vision, and overall strategic plan. Strategic planning for both the organization and the IT department is not a linear process; rather, it is iterative in nature and requires consideration of multiple variables, including future goals and directions.

Key factors in identifying and selecting information systems are the business plans for the organization and the IT department. It makes little sense to consider $20 million systems when the business plan states a maximum of $10 million. However, cost is not the only consideration. System selection teams must review key objectives of the organization and the IT department to ensure that the objectives of the selection team are in alignment with the institution and the IT department before proceeding with selection of potential information systems. Once objectives are aligned, the team is ready to begin the process of identifying and selecting the systems that will most closely align with the economic, operational, and clinical objectives of the organization. The stakeholders in each of those three areas must be heard, considered, and educated about what systems can and cannot do to support the objectives of different stakeholders within the organization. No system in isolation supports the practices of medicine or nursing, improves financial reporting of outcomes, and changes the operation of the organization. Rather, systems support the decision makers and stimulate process changes in these areas in order to realize institutional objectives. A thorough review and understanding of the clinical objectives as well as the financial and operational objectives of the organization and the IT department are essential, as these should guide the ongoing evaluation and system selection process.

Once the alignment of objectives has been completed, the IT department should review and update the inventory of existing systems. All of the current systems in place in the organization should be identified, including independent departmental systems as well as large integrated systems and those buried in areas outside IT. A review of the inventory allows the organization to identify overlapping functionality as well as gaps among systems. It is not unusual for multiple systems that accomplish the same task or goal to be in place. This happens when individual departments have implemented systems they need without addressing the organization's overall plan. Within the objectives of the IT department, clinical, financial, and operational goals of the organization are considered in identifying which systems are to be replaced and why.[1]

Answering a series of questions provides a straightforward approach for the institution to determine which systems may be replaced or updated:

1. *Need for the system.* What are the functions that the system addresses, and how frequently do those functions occur? In addition, are there some tasks or functions that are not addressed by the system? Is current staff using the system? Have work processes been developed to accomplish tasks or functions that the system does not address or that the staff find difficult to accomplish using the system?
2. *Development process.* Which information systems are in development and what is the nature of the development team and its methodology? New is not always better, but neither is what is familiar and comfortable. Are the requirements of the stakeholders being met, including management, financial, clinical, and operational stakeholders as well as the largest group of stakeholders, patients and their families?
3. *Basic structure.* What parts or functions can be observed? Are these items working to meet today's requirements or tomorrow's desired function? Does the current system work as designed and to meet future needs?
4. *Functionality.* What are the system response times, accuracy, reliability, and ease of use for end users? What are the plans to continue development of the system to meet new and ongoing requirements? How are the new and ongoing requirements determined?
5. *Impact.* How does the system affect providers, patients, processes, and the organization's users in nonpatient

care areas? Does the system support data collection and reporting?
6. *Integration.* How does this system interface with other systems in the institution from a technical perspective as well as from a workflow perspective?

The following key areas are important in detailing and documenting this institutional analysis:

1. Mission-critical requirements
2. Regulatory and accreditation requirements
3. Financial and increased net revenue requirements
4. End user demands and functionality requirements that are "must have"
5. End user demands and functionality requirements that are "nice to have"

This assessment of the institution's current status and needs will form the basis for future documentation and specifications. The systems analysis is an internal document and is best presented in comparative format (such as a spreadsheet) that is easy for technical and nontechnical readers to evaluate. An additional approach is to document the strengths and weaknesses of each system. Using the data and information from this assessment, the institution should carefully document system requirements from both an institutional and a department perspective. These requirements will then be used to develop key criteria to use during the system identification and selection process.[2]

SYSTEMS LIFE CYCLE

Knowledge about the life cycle of an information system will help in understanding the importance of a carefully designed system selection process in obtaining overall success in meeting an organization's needs. The systems life cycle (SLC) is a framework for understanding the process of developing or configuring, implementing, and using an information system. This process is described in a series of sequential logical steps or phases, listed as follows. These phases are based on the Staggers and Nelson SLC model discussed in Chapter 2 and depicted in Fig. 2.8:

1. Analyze
2. Plan
3. Develop or purchase
4. Test
5. Implement or go-live
6. Maintain and evolve
7. Evaluate
8. Return to analyze

System selection, the focus of this chapter, involves the first three phases of the SLC model: analyze, plan, and develop or purchase. The remaining phases of the SLC model are discussed in Chapter 19.

Analysis and Requirements Definition

The project planning and analysis phases often occur concomitantly in a recursive process. In this section, for the purposes of discussion, analysis is presented first, although others may decide that the planning step is first. The decision to purchase and implement a new information system usually begins with the realization that the systems currently in place do not meet the needs of the organization and its users. At this point the selection team should identify specifically which type of information system needs to be replaced or added by the organization by completing the analysis described in the previous section. However, this initial understanding of needs does not provide enough information to begin a formal search process, as one cannot determine if a system meets the organization's needs without a thorough evaluation and understanding of those needs or requirements.

Requirements definition is the process of determining the specific needs that the organization has for an information system and the specific functionality that is desired. This analysis is built upon the institutional inventory and analysis discussed in the previous section. However, at this point in the system selection process the analysis is focused on the specific system being selected, and the specifications are much more detailed. Therefore a detailed plan for data gathering is essential to effectively determine system requirements. Components of the requirements definition plan include the following:

1. *Review and, if necessary, update the inventory of current information systems and functionality.* The focus at this point is on those systems that will interface with or be directly affected by the new system. This evaluation should include a list of the components and functions of each system, listing the tasks that can be performed as well as any supporting information to better describe the functionality. An understanding of the general data flow between systems is also important in determining system requirements.

2. *Inventory paper documents and forms.* It is also important to obtain samples of all paper forms currently in use as well as reports from current information systems. Including paper forms in the inventory as opportunities for additional automation may drive the development of additional requirements for a new information system. Importantly, the paper process should not be replicated; forms are used to understand requirements, especially for subspecialties and linkages between departments. In addition, the selection committee will benefit from reviewing forms and templates that are commonly part of the system selection process. Examples of these types of documents can be seen in Box 16.2. The preferred sources for these documents are ones that the institution has used in the past with previous system selection committees, however; examples of these types of forms can be obtained from professional organizations such as Healthcare Information and Management Systems Society (HIMSS) or downloaded from the internet. While each selection committee will need to design their own forms, the opportunity to review several examples can be very insightful.

3. *Interview and observe staff.* The selection team should plan to interview hospital staff in various departments and roles regarding their work. One goal of the interviews is a determination of which functions are currently supported by an

---

BOX 16.2 Documents and Forms Commonly Used in Systems Selection

- RFI and/or RFP template
- RFI and/or RFP cover letter
- Proposal cover letter
- Disqualification or rejection letter
- Nonbinding letter of intent
- Scoring or decision matrix

RFI, Requests for information; *RFP,* request for proposal.

BOX 16.3 Sample Interview Questions

Strengths
- Which features and functions of the current system do you find useful?
- How does the current system support you in providing safe patient care?
- Is the current system easy to navigate and use? If so, which features support this?

Weaknesses
- Which features of the current system do you dislike, and why?
- Is the system difficult to use? If so, why?

Opportunities
- Are there any features or functionality that you feel are missing from the current system?

Threats
- Are there any shortcomings or issues with the current system that may create a risk to patients that you are caring for?

---

information system as well as functions and documentation that are not yet supported by an information system. Interview questions should also be used to gain an understanding of the decisions that staff will need to make as they perform their job functions and to determine which data are needed for these decisions. Management and frontline staff can provide valuable information about the work that is actually performed and how data are collected and used, while observations of the staff at work may uncover additional requirements and provide an increased understanding of the use of data. Members of the selection team should include interview questions for key stakeholders and frontline staff to elicit their opinions and experience with the current information system. The SWOT strategic analysis tool is useful in guiding these questions. SWOT is an acronym that represents the identification of strengths, weaknesses, opportunities, and threats.[3] Box 16.3 contains several sample interview questions to consider. Additional insights can be obtained if the users can demonstrate their answers on the current system as well as describe their experiences.

4. *Collect samples of system and manual reports.* The selection team should collect samples of reports that are provided by existing information systems as well as reports that are

generated manually. In addition, frontline staff, management, and hospital administration should provide information about their specific data needs, including other desired reports that are not currently available. Consideration should be given to data and reports that would support the hospital in determining how well they are meeting regulatory and accreditation requirements defined by organizations such as The Joint Commission (TJC) and Centers for Medicare & Medicaid Services (CMS).

5. *Develop process and dataflow maps.* Developing process and dataflow maps for each function or role will also clearly document the data needs of various groups of users.[4] Process maps illustrate an organization's workflow, which is a series of steps representing work activities and resources that follow a path to produce desired outcomes or outputs.[5] A thorough analysis of the workflow of future users of the new information system will help identify system requirements that may not have been identified during the interview process. Dataflow diagrams are often used to document this type of information. See Figs. 16.1

and 16.2 for examples of how this type of information may be documented.

6. *Identify hospital standards and policies and regulatory and accreditation requirements.* Hospital standards of care and policies as well as evidence-based practice must be supported by the information system that is selected. In addition, regulations established by state and federal governments and requirements of accreditation groups such as TJC must be considered. An example of legislation that has had a great impact on clinical information system functionality is the Health Information Technology for Economic and Clinical Health (HITECH) Act, signed in 2009. The goal of this legislation is to promote the adoption and Meaningful Use of health IT. Specific information about the HITECH Act and Meaningful Use can be found at www.healthit.gov/policy-researchers-implementers/health-it-legislation-and-regulations and in Chapter 27. The selection team should identify precise and clear system requirements related to how the information system might support the organization in meeting these

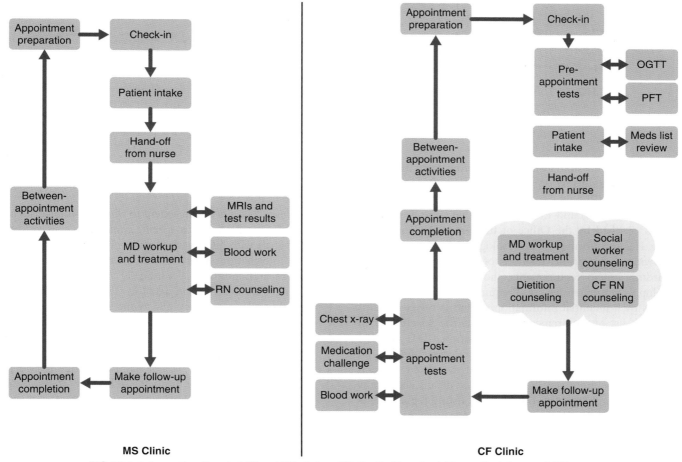

MS Clinic   **CF Clinic**

FIG 16.1 Information flow in MS and CF clinics. *CF,* Cystic fibrosis; *MD,* medical doctor; *MRI,* magnetic resonance imaging; *MS,* multiple sclerosis; *OGTT,* oral glucose tolerance test; *PFT,* pulmonary function test; *RN,* registered nurse. (Modified from Unertl KM, Weinger MB, Johnson KB, Lorenzi NM. Describing and modeling workflow and information flow in chronic disease care. *J Am Med Inform Assoc.* 2009;16:830. With permission from BMJ Publishing Group Ltd.)

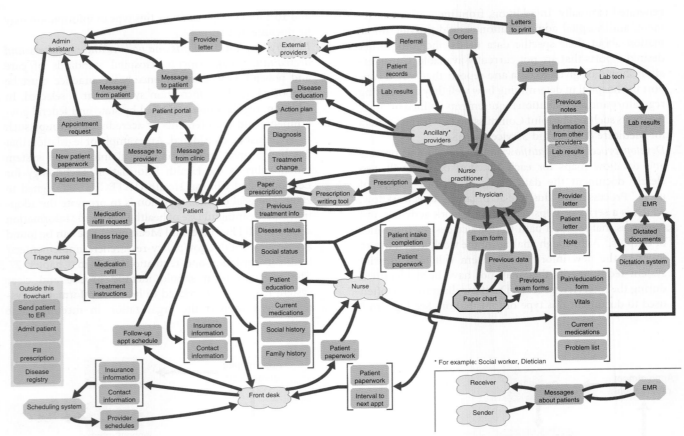

FIG 16.2 Information flow in chronic disease care. *Admin*, Administration; *appt*, appointment; *EMR*, electronic medical record; *ER*, emergency room. (From Unertl KM, Weinger MB, Johnson KB, Lorenzi NM. Describing and modeling workflow and information flow in chronic disease care. *J Am Med Inform Assoc.* 2009;16:832. With permission from BMJ Publishing Group Ltd.)

standards. One strategy may be to narrow down the field of potential vendors by starting with the Certified HIT Product List (CHPL), which provides a list of electronic health records (EHRs) and EHR modules that have been tested and certified by the Office of the National Coordinator for Health Information Technology (ONC).[6]

Following these various methods of information collection regarding system requirements, the selection team should develop a comprehensive list of requirements that it will evaluate as each potential information system is reviewed. This thorough list of requirements will guide the selection team as it develops the request for information (RFI) and the request for proposal (RFP). When developing the list, an effective strategy is to list the objectives related to each requirement without specific decisions or details about how the software will meet this objective. By listing requirements as objectives instead of specific descriptions of how these objectives are to be met, the team will not limit potential vendor solutions before it has had a chance to evaluate them.

Objectives can be logically grouped into several categories that will facilitate organization of the requirements list:

1. *Patient care objectives.* Determine the types of patient data that should be entered as well as any specific patient care areas that may require special processes, such as the emergency department, critical care units, or labor and delivery areas. Examples of patient care objectives are listed in Box 16.4.

2. *Usability.* Usability is the extent to which a product can be used by specific users in specific contexts to achieve specific goals with effectiveness, efficiency, and satisfaction.[7] The information system that is selected should be easy to use and intuitive. A variety of methods for testing usability are described in detail in Chapter 21. Improved usability improves safety and reduces user frustration as well as the time needed for educating users to effectively and efficiently use the system. For example, the user should be able to easily find a patient in the system and then proceed to view or enter patient data. Efficiency considerations should not be limited to bedside users only. System reports providing summarized patient data for management and administration can also greatly improve efficiency. See Box 16.5 for examples of efficiency objectives.

3. *IT department objectives.* The IT department will also be able to identify key requirements for a new information system. These may be related to the degree of customization allowed as well as the ease of customization. These factors will affect the IT resources needed to implement and maintain the

BOX 16.4 Example Requirements for a Hospital Information System: Patient Care Objectives

1. Patient care documentation (assessments and notes) by clinical users
   - Nursing
   - Physician
   - Social work and case managers
   - Nutrition
   - Wound care
   - Respiratory therapy
   - Pharmacy
   - Occupational therapy and physical therapy
   - Other ancillary users
2. Orders management
   - Order entry, including order sets by stakeholder groups
   - Order selection menu based on physician clinician specialty
3. Care plan and problem list
4. Patient data displays
   - Summary view of patient data
   - View longitudinal data across visits
5. Clinical decision support and alerts
6. Medication reconciliation
7. Patient discharge processes
   - Instructions and prescriptions
   - Continuity of care document, summary of care
8. Requirements for special care areas
   - Medical and surgical units
   - Critical care units
   - Step-down units
   - Ambulatory services
   - Psychiatry
   - Rehabilitation
   - Long-term care
   - Labor and delivery
   - Oncology

BOX 16.5 Example Requirements for a Hospital Information System: Efficiency Objectives

Data Collection
- Ease of data entry by end users
- Does the orders management system support customization for different categories of users?
- How long does it take for an end user (pharmacy, nurses, physicians) to enter a complex medication order?
- Does the system support difficult orders such as total parenteral nutrition, chemotherapy, and future orders?

Integration
- Is integration or interface with other systems supported, allowing bidirectional communication of data and information?
- Does the system support point-of-care data collection device integration, such as vital sign monitors?

Data Retrieval
- Ease of data retrieval by end users
- Is the process for viewing results easy to use while providing flexibility for the end user to choose what is needed?

Reports
- Are reports available to supply data needed to users at various levels, including the frontline staff, management, and administration?
- Is the creation of customized reports possible, and does the skill set needed for this exist within the organization?

system. Information regarding hardware and third-party software requirements should also be included in the IT objectives, as this will affect both the initial cost of implementation and the cost of maintenance. Another key objective is the ability of the information system to support data security and protection of patient confidentiality. The importance of this factor is highlighted as an objective of Meaningful Use certification as outlined by the HITECH Act.

4. *Organization objectives.* The organization will have additional objectives for the information system. Some of these may be related to how the organization can meet regulatory and payer requirements such as those of the American Recovery and Reinvestment Act (ARRA) and the Patient Protection and Affordable Care Act (PPACA).

Project Planning

Effective project planning requires the use of formal project planning tools, processes, and principles. Because of the importance of solid project planning, project management

has emerged as a formal specialty within and outside health and is the focus of Chapter 17 in this book. During the project planning phase, the high-level project goals are identified and established. The goals for the system should be in alignment with the strategic vision of the organization. Any change or improvement in an information system should directly support the ability of the organization to meets its goals. Goals may be directly related to the information system, such as ease of data entry and data retrieval. Systems that support accurate and easy data access support improved decisions during care. In addition, systems that allow easy and accurate data entry support improved patient care and can be designed to provide information about patient outcomes.[8]

When selecting an information system, it is also important to consider whether the system functionality is appropriate for the type of patients cared for by the facility, including inpatients, outpatients, and patients of the emergency department and specialty areas such as psychiatry. Goals may also be related to the ability of the system to facilitate the achievement of regulatory goals such as compliance with CMS measures and successful Meaningful Use attestation. Financial goals might include the budget guidelines for purchase, implementation, and ongoing maintenance related to the information system. Finally, the selection team must understand the goals related to system implementation, including the ease of implementation, the degree to which the software can be customized to meet specific needs, and the resources required to implement and maintain the system.

Another important aspect of project planning is the creation of the information system selection team and development of their roles and responsibilities. System selection is best accomplished by a multidisciplinary team representing the departments and roles that will be affected by the system to be purchased by the organization. This team should include representation from nursing; physicians; ancillary departments such as pharmacy, occupational and physical therapy, respiratory therapy, nutrition, social work and case management, infection control, and quality and risk management; IT technical specialists; and hospital administration. Clinical representatives must be involved in every step of the system selection process. Their input is key to the identification of requirements and system selection, as technology can support clinicians in providing better patient care. However, some of the department representatives on the team may not have previous experience with the system selection process. The system selection process will be more effective if the initial meetings of the team include a clear statement of the scope of the project and an orientation to the system selection process. The IT department must also be included in the system selection team. Ideally there are clinical and IT representatives who have had previous experience with the system selection process. The organization should carefully consider the goals of this group as well as the leadership. Requirements of users as well as the IT staff who will be supporting the system are important to consider. For more information about informatics governance and its role in the system selection process, see Chapter 28.

Develop or Purchase

Once analysis and planning are completed, the institution must decide if it will (1) develop a new system, (2) reconfigure or upgrade the current system, or (3) select a new system. For the purposes of discussion, this chapter is presented with the assumption that a decision has been made to select a new system. Reconfiguring or upgrading a current system is discussed in Chapter 19.

Developing, Obtaining, and Evaluating Requests for Information and Requests for Proposals

Once the selection team has been established and oriented to the system selection process, its first job is to develop a request for information (RFI). The RFI will determine who should be encouraged to submit a request for proposal (RFP). Understanding the essentials of RFIs and RFPs facilitates decision making and selection processes. Basically, the RFI is an information step in vendor evaluation. The organization prepares a list of system goals and high-level requirements and asks vendors to respond to them with specific information such as projected costs. Larger institutions often have a template with sections, such as a description of the institution already provided. Common sections often found in an RFI can be seen in Box 16.6.

BOX 16.6   Sections of a Request for Information

Purpose of Request
A brief statement describing the type of information system that the institution is planning to select. For example, is it searching for an electronic health record for use in physician offices or a classification and staffing system for use in the outpatient clinics?

Background
The description of the institution, including mission size and number and type of patients treated.

Qualifications
Any specific qualifications required by the vendor. For example, does it need to have been in business for 5 or more years?

Information Requested
A list of specific elements that should be answered. For example:
- Size, history, and financial status of the company
- Basic system architecture and software configuration
- Number of installations and selected names of customers

Time and Type of Response
This section includes the due date for the response, where the response should be sent, and who the vendor should contact if the vendor has any questions. The vendor should be discouraged from contacting anyone else at the institution.

The response to an RFI describes the vendor's experience and product and how it communicates with clients. Any vendor that cannot meet the RFI expectations or omits requested information may not remain on the evaluation list. An RFI is requested from potential vendors to determine which of their products and services are potentially available in the marketplace to meet the institution's needs. The response also lets organizations know the capability of the vendor in terms of strengths and offerings. For example, if the vendor has consistently installed in small community hospitals and the institution is a large academic medical center, this may not be a vendor worth further investigation.

RFIs are commonly used on major procurements, such as hospital information systems, but they are not an invitation to bid, so some vendors will not respond, even if they have systems that meet requirements. An RFI is not binding on either party and may or may not lead to an RFP. An RFI should inform the vendor of the organization's goals and how they will be achieved. An RFI should be specific enough to foster clear collection and evaluation of responses that enable a comparison of vendors to determine from whom more detailed responses (e.g., including price, quality of delivery, guarantees, and other considerations) to an RFP should be requested. This is not an insignificant step, as the organization will be investing large dollar amounts and committing resources to a new information system.

For financial considerations (actual bids for a health IT product), organizations should submit an RFP. Common

BOX 16.7 Major Components of a Request for Proposal

- Overview of the institution and its mission
- Project overview—purpose, goals, rationale for the project
- Project overview—teams, locations, services/specialties, proposed schedule
- System specifications—e.g., functional, technical, interfaces, data integration, current installed systems related to the new project or projected Agile development for specific areas
- Services requested (what is needed from the vendor)—e.g., training, installation, maintenance and support, equipment, required uptime, response to issues
- Vendor requirements and information—e.g., number of installed sites, qualifications of vendor team personnel, projected company stability
- Projected pricing and payment provisions (high level)
- RFP evaluation criteria
- Submission guidelines (a standardized format for responses)
- Any exclusions—e.g., timelines for responses, company size, or lack of monolithic system capabilities

sections of a RFP are provided in Box 16.7. An RFP is an invitation for vendors to submit back to an organization a formal proposal that clearly spells out what system (including functionality and capability) can be delivered and at what price. The RFP gives the vendor a very clear and detailed understanding of what the organization is looking for in a system and starts the negotiation process based on price and quality of delivery. An RFP requires much more effort and is done at the stage where the organization clarifies its expectations and receives assurances from the vendor that it can deliver the system on the organization's timetable and terms. The RFP is a more complete and formal step, with the vendor response often translating directly into the formal contract.

The RFP is the organization's way of soliciting competitive bids to supply a specific information system. An RFP should include detailed information about the organization as well as questions that elicit differences among competing vendors. An RFP should solicit cost quotes for installation and implementation and security standards, as well as delivery time (and estimated completion time) and resource requirements. Resource requirements should be spelled out for both the organization and the vendor in the response. The best RFP also seeks information on total cost of ownership (TCO) over the expected lifetime of the system. The RFP should require information such as corporate information on the vendor as well as its history with this kind of system. Customer references that can and should be validated must be part of the response from the vendor.

Prior to issuing an RFP, an organization should establish certain items:

1. The organization's needs as outlined in the organizational and IT vision and strategic plan, and the specific needs.

2. The organization's evaluation criteria. These should include vendor experience, vendor staff strength, market and industry understanding, and differential advantages such as usability or available functionality and cost.

When responses are received, they should be evaluated in total—not just on cost or any other single criteria. Following that, the organization should interview the vendors that have live, working systems and distinguish between available functions and future capability or functionality. Healthcare systems or hospitals will be using this information system for years, even decades, to come. Organizations want to ensure that available functionality is real today and will continue to grow with the needs of the health system or hospital.[9]

As much as everyone dislikes deadlines, organizations need to set a time limit for responses to both RFIs and RFPs; 6 to 8 weeks should be the outside limit of the timeline, although very complex organizations such as the Department of Defense may allow 60 to 90 days. Also, allow a sufficient time for the organization to evaluate responses adequately; healthcare today moves at a very fast pace, but ensure that the organization has carefully measured the responses and interviewed those who can deliver.

Evaluating Vendors

There are some basic characteristics to look for when finding an information system vendor. A fundamental element is the fit between the organization and the vendor. For example, is the organization small and more informal? Is the vendor large and bureaucratic? Does the organization make change rapidly? Can the vendor do the same? Does the vendor come across as professional? Also, a vendor should be expected to have a great deal of experience in the same type of facility or organization that is seeking an information system.[10] Information system support (24/7) and the help desk, as well as education and training, are key areas to examine when deciding on the vendor for a product. New or replacement systems without proper installation and implementation can be doomed from the start. For additional information on vendors, check the data available from the major IT research groups: Forrester, Gartner, HIMSS Analytics, and KLAS. These major research firms provide clear, unambiguous analysis of vendors and systems. Table 16.1 gives additional information about these research groups.

Additionally, valuable information is available from the HIMSS at www.himss.org. A detailed analysis of vendor research should include visiting the vendor's website. Also, a number of internet blogs have comments, both positive and negative, about vendors. An example is HIStalk at http://histalk2.com. Organizations should also validate information with peers in other hospitals and health systems.

Selecting the System

Now that the selection team has defined objectives and requirements for the new system, developed an RFI and RFP, and completed research about various vendors, the team must have a plan for how it will select an information system.

TABLE 16.1   Major Healthcare Information Technology Research Firms in the United States

Firm and Location	Overview
Forrester Research, Inc. Cambridge, Mass. www.forrester.com	Forrester is a global research and advisory group. Forrester serves clients as they face increasingly complex business and technology decisions on a daily basis. To help them understand, strategize, and act on opportunities brought about by change, Forrester provides proprietary research, consumer and business data, custom consulting, events and online communities, and peer-to-peer executive programs. Forrester guides leaders in IT, marketing, and strategy and the technology industry through independent, fact-based insight, ensuring their business success today and tomorrow.
Gartner, Inc. Stamford, Conn. www.gartner.com	Gartner is an IT research and advisory company. Gartner delivers the technology-related insight necessary for its clients to make the right decisions every day. From CIOs and senior IT leaders in corporations and government agencies, to business leaders in high-tech and telecom enterprises and professional services firms, to technology investors, Gartner is a partner to clients in 12,000 distinct organizations. Through the resources of Gartner Research, Gartner Executive Programs, Gartner Consulting, and Gartner Events, it works with every client to research, analyze, and interpret the business of IT within the context of its individual role. Gartner is headquartered in Stamford, Conn., and has 5000 associates, including 1280 research analysts and consultants, and clients in 85 countries.
KLAS Research Orem, Utah www.klasresearch.com	KLAS conducts over 1900 healthcare provider interviews per month, working with over 4500 hospitals and over 3000 doctor's offices and clinics. KLAS is independently owned and operated. KLAS has ratings on over 250 healthcare technology vendors and over 900 products and services. KLAS publishes approximately 40 performance and perception reports per year. KLAS is headquartered in Orem, Utah, with independent researchers working throughout North America. The name KLAS is an acronym comprising a letter from each of the founders' names.

CIO, Chief information officer; *IT,* information technology.
Information is adapted from the appropriate company's website.
Adapted from Forrester Research Inc. at www.forrester.com, Gartner Inc. at www.gartner.com, and KLAS Enterprises LLC at www.klasresearch.com.

The team must take steps to develop specific system evaluation criteria and a process for recording its individual and group decisions. This should be done before actually reviewing the RFI and RFP responses so that each team member can begin to evaluate and score the various information systems as soon as information is obtained. One effective approach is to develop a scoring system, where all of the system requirements are listed and each requirement is given a numeric score or weighted numeric score based on the degree to which it meets each objective. By using numeric ratings, organizations are able to obtain an overall score for each vendor's system. It may help to classify the requirements as "must have" or "nice to have," because this information will be useful as findings are evaluated. As team members complete the scoring document for systems, it is essential that they be open-minded and broadly explore all options presented by various vendors. The software that vendors present may meet the requirements but in a manner that is different from what was anticipated.

During the evaluation process, it is important to evaluate potential software products very rigorously since the amount of time and money invested in purchasing and implementing an information system is quite large. The impact of a new health information system on an organization's users cannot be minimized, so the task of evaluating and selecting a system should be given adequate attention and resources. Vendors responding to an RFP will provide presentations and demonstrations aimed at showing how the system can meet or exceed the requirements. In the past, organizations have found it helpful to script scenarios for the vendors to follow during the demonstrations. In this way, the organization can tailor the scenarios to its own patient populations and highlight the patient flow across modules. For example, a script may be developed following a patient from outpatient to the operating room, post–anesthesia recovery, intensive care, and surgical unit, then back to outpatient.

During this process, clinicians, IT, and hospital leaders should remember to focus on deployed, working systems only, as these are what will be delivered once the system is purchased. Vendors will spend some time explaining what their plans are for future development, but it is important for all to know what can actually be configured and implemented when receiving the software. Plans for future development by the vendor can be considered. However, there is no guarantee when new functions will be available or how they will actually work if delivered.

After initial presentations by various vendors, the selection team will have good ideas about the top contenders for the organization. Once the group has narrowed down the list to a handful of vendors, it should arrange for site visits to actual customers using the information systems. Working with the vendor in planning the site visit can be helpful, but there are important reasons to not give a vendor complete control in selecting the site or planning the details of the visit. Often, a vendor will select a site that is most successful and innovative. It may be more advantageous for the selection team to find a site themselves that is more representative of their institutional goals and objectives. The selection team should also determine if the site selected for the visit will receive direct or indirect remuneration from the vendor for providing a site visit.

The site visit team should be interdisciplinary and use specific evaluation criteria to guide the visit. This will allow the team to see how this organization has configured the system to work at its site. The biggest advantage of a site visit is the opportunity to talk with people at various levels to obtain their opinions and information about their experiences with the system. In planning for the visit, ask for sessions or opportunities where all can talk with various clinical users of the system, such as nurses, physicians, and ancillary users. IT staff will also want to talk with IT representatives to get their opinions and perspective. Some of these frank discussions will be most effective if the vendor representative is not present, allowing the staff at the hospital site to be more open and honest. After the visit, there are often additional questions. The selection team should obtain the names and contact information for individuals they may want to contact after the site visit with follow-up questions.

As the group evaluates various information systems, keep in mind the TCO. This is a financial estimate of the cost of implementing and maintaining the information system over the life of the project, also known as life-cycle costing.[11] This estimate should include all hardware, software, and resource costs associated with all phases of the project, including design, implementation, testing, and ongoing support over the entire life span of the system. Typical life cycles are about 11 years but can run much longer. During the evaluation phase make sure that the group obtains this type of information from the vendor. Include discussions about the frequency of software updates and upgrades and the IT resources needed to test and implement these changes. Ask how specific change requests from one organization are prioritized and what the average time lapse is from request to delivery. Include discussions about the frequency and duration of planned downtimes to accomplish updates.

Once the information systems have been reviewed and the vendors offering these systems have been evaluated, the selection task force makes a recommendation. If possible, the recommendation should include two or three potential options with a ranking and rationale statement for each option. The rationale should include the pros and cons of each option. Usually the decision on which product to recommend is made at the next-to-last meeting of the task force. The meeting should start with a general summary of the findings for each vendor and its product. Plenty of time should be given for discussion. If there are any major disagreements on which product to select, it is helpful if key administrative personnel such as the chief information officer (CIO) and the vice-president for the department most affected by the new system join the discussion.

At the final meeting of the task force, members should agree on the items to be placed in the contract including the scope of the implementation. This might include plans such as implementation in a pilot unit or units only versus the entire hospital. The final job of the IT staff for this product selection task force is to summarize the process and findings in a report for senior management. The final report includes the recommended products and vendors as well as the rationale for each recommendation. The report should also include any recommendations for the contract and implementation process.

Preparing for Contract Negotiations

For major purchases, contract negotiations are usually performed by a negotiating team. The composition of this team will vary depending of the organization, the specific anticipated purchase, and the governance model of the organization. In many organizations, especially large ones, the negotiations will occur at the executive level. These may be a team consisting of the contracts lawyer, the CFO, and/or the CIO, although in other organizations, the composition may be at a lower organizational level and include a project leader and key technical IT representation. In any case, the chair and members of the selection committee should be available for questions from the negotiating term once the formal negotiations begin. The vendor should be informed about the specific personnel performing contract development and negotiations and adhere to any communication restrictions.

Contracts or licensing agreements are described in detail in Chapter 18; however, the selection team should play a key role in planning for these negotiations and supporting the negotiating team during the process. The final report of the selection committee should include specific recommendations for items to be placed in the contract. Examples of such items are specific training programs and training supplies to be offered by the vendor or the stipulation that the hospital or clinic will be a test site for new functionality that is very important to the hospital or clinic.

During the negotiation process, the negotiating team may also call on the selection committee to review sections of the contract that could be misinterpreted. Examples include the following:

- The vendor should be asked to provide a definition of all vendor-specific terms and concepts referred to in the contract. These definitions can be reviewed by the selection team to ensure these definitions are consistent with the institutions understanding of these terms or concepts.[12]
- The contract should include a detailed explanation of line items in the pricing schedule. The selection term can review these explanations describing the line items, especially those items that might be misinterpreted and raise questions or concerns.
- The contract should include clear definitions of data ownership, especially when discussing aggregate data. Again the selection terms can help determine if these definitions are consistent with other institutional projects and goals.
- The contract should include the experience level of vendor staff who will provide project assistance for implementation, training, and support.[5] Again the selection committee can assist in reviewing these qualifications, especially vendor staff who are not providing technical type support.

Establishing a Working Relationship with the Vendor

From the day the RFI is mailed, the institution will begin managing its vendor relationship. The tone and nature of these relationships can be expected to change through the life cycle. However, an effective open and professional relationship can be key to success throughout the total project. Managing a vendor relationship requires skilled and careful leadership and a level of personal finesse. Vendor managers are usually experts in their own subject matter area. In many cases, they also have project management and business skills. But not every vendor manager has leadership expertise. Therefore communicating with the vendor is as important as communicating with an organization's stakeholders. Establishing communication channels and information flow between local clinicians, IT, and leaders and the vendor can lead to increased efficiency, reduced costs, and better service. The vendor will play a key role in local success. Building mutually strong relationships with a chosen vendor is critical and can ultimately strengthen overall performance. Vendor management is more than getting a lower price or better service. Properly managed vendor relationships can give the vendor and institution a significant competitive advantage. A successful vendor relationship shares local priorities and mutually agrees upon factors such as the following:

- Definition of a quality implementation
- Metrics for successful adoption of the system
- Elements of the vendor's quality assurance program, including measurable outcome metrics—not just response times and limits to unplanned downtime and upgrades but the real outcome to end users

A good vendor must understand and share priorities, but the organization must first communicate those priorities. If a vendor cannot help with stated priorities, a good vendor will disclose this limitation or weakness up front. Thus it is absolutely essential that the chosen vendor becomes a partner in the implementation, optimization, and ongoing use and upgrades of the organization's information system. There is a concrete need to drive contract terms and obligations, but in the end, no contract will adequately cover all long-term goals and expectations. A solid, true collaborative partnership with a vendor will provide for such needs. When some things go bad, as they most assuredly will at some point, the organization will be better served to have a partner at the table, not just a vendor. Early on, demand proof of concept. If an organization is seeking value, then the group needs to see it first-hand. A good vendor will prove it can be done.

The International Organization for Standardization (ISO) has developed a set of minimum standards, practices, terminologies, and requirements that, when adopted, demonstrates a vendor's products and services have achieved a minimum level of quality. ISO certification demonstrates a vendor's commitment to quality and service. These standards are outlined on the ISO website (www.iso.org). It is important to note the ISO does not perform certification but does provide the standards for certification. Actual ISO certification must be performed by an outside certification body. In reviewing the ISO standards, note that clinical practice varies around the world, and students will need to adapt minimum standards to their country's requirements.

CONCLUSION AND FUTURE DIRECTIONS

When selecting an information system, clinicians, IT, and leaders need to understand the vendor's plan for responding to changes in the market and regulatory environments. The pace of change in healthcare is anticipated to only accelerate, and both the organization and the vendor must be able to adapt quickly. The group may wish to review the selected vendor's history with response to changes such as these, including the timeliness of software changes and compliance. In the future, the vendor model may erode from full-service or monolithic health IT products such as EHR to commodity or component providers. For example, organizations may choose their pharmacy applications from one vendor and clinical documentation from another. The interoperability requirements being promulgated today would then allow organizations to compile functions using off-site cloud computing versus installing huge systems on-site. However, with this more futuristic notion, the phases and concepts listed in this chapter are still needed.

REFERENCES

1. Sittig D, Hazelhurst BL, Palen T, Hsu J, Jimison H, Hornbrook MC. A clinical information system research landscape. *Permanente J*. 2002;2(6):1–6.
2. *How to Implement EHRs*; 2014. https://www.healthit.gov/providers-professionals/ehr-implementation-steps/step-3-select-or-upgrade-certified-ehr/.
3. Helms MM, Moore R, Ahmadi M. Information technology (IT) and the healthcare industry: a SWOT analysis. *Int J Healthc Inform Syst Informat*. 2008;3(1):75–92. http://dx.doi.org/10.4018/jhisi.2008010105.
4. Staccini PM, Joubert M, Quaranta JF, Fieschi M. Towards elicitation of users requirements for hospital information system: from a care process modeling technique to a web based collaborative tool. *Proc AMIA Symp*. 2002;732–736.
5. Damelio R. *Basics of Process Mapping*. 2nd ed. Boca Raton, FL: CRC Press; 2011.
6. *How do I select a vendor?*; 2013. https://www.healthit.gov/providers-professionals/faqs/how-do-i-select-vendor/.
7. *International Organization of Standards (ISO)*; 2008. http://www.usabilitynet.org/tools/r_international.htm.
8. Nurse leaders discuss the nurse's role in driving technology decisions. *Am Nurse Today*. 2010;1(5):16-19. http://www.americannursetoday.com/Article.aspx?id=6142&fid=6116/.
9. Adler KG. How to select an electronic health record system. *Fam Pract Manag*. 2005;12(2):55–62.
10. Gortzis LG. Selecting healthcare information systems provided by third-party vendors: a mind map beyond the manuals. *Inform Health Soc Care*. 2010;35(1):1–9.
11. Cellucci F. What is the true TCO for information technology projects? *ConnectivITy*; 2011. http://www.docutech.com/blog/bid/54338/What-Is-The-True-TCO-For-Information-Technology-Projects/.
12. Craig JB. Life cycle of a health care information system. In: Englebardt S, Nelson R, eds. *Health Care Informatics: An Interdisciplinary Approach*. St. Louis: Mosby; 2002:181–208.

DISCUSSION QUESTIONS

1. How do strategic vision and alignment affect decisions made in your organization?
2. What is the role of healthcare providers in the identification and selection of a healthcare information system?
3. The selection team should be an interdisciplinary team, but how should the chair of the committee be selected?
4. What is the impact of a well-defined and complete RFI and RFP process on identification and selection of a healthcare information system?
5. What are the key roles and functions in identification of system requirements?
6. Why are vendor relationships with management essential? Brainstorm ideas for maintaining good site–vendor relationships.

CASE STUDY

You have been chosen to participate in the selection team for a new clinical information system to be purchased and implemented at the community hospital where you are a staff nurse. The selection team has been asked to develop an initial list of requirements that they would like to use for the evaluation of potential systems in relation to documentation of assessments for interprofessional use, including nursing, physicians, and some other departments such as physical therapy and occupational therapy. The selection team has decided to group the requirements that they identify into the following categories:

- Patient care objectives
- Usability
- IT department objectives
- Organization objectives

Your task for this case study is to use the key considerations listed below to develop a list of system requirements for electronic documentation in a clinical information system, grouping the requirements into the four categories listed above. The key considerations include information that the selection team has gathered in anticipation of developing system requirements.

Key Considerations for System Selection

Findings from Inventory of Current Systems and Functionality
- Electronic laboratory and radiology report results are produced by ancillary information systems.
- The intensive care units (ICUs) have an ICU information system where some documentation is done electronically, including vital signs, intake and output, and some interfaced data from monitoring systems.

Findings from Inventory of Paper Documents and Forms
- Nursing notes and care planning currently are documented only in the paper chart on medical/surgical units.

- Physician progress notes and orders currently are documented only in the paper chart.
- There are numerous paper forms and various versions of forms in use with no consistency across the organization.
- Paper order sets are in use. Some order sets are physician specific, with multiple versions for the same diagnosis or procedure. None appear to be evidence based.

Findings from Staff Interviews and Observations
Direct observation studies were conducted in the ICU, medical/surgical units, and pediatric unit. Observations and interviews also were conducted in various other clinical departments including Physical Therapy (PT), Occupational Therapy (OT), and wound care. The study revealed that there are similarities in the types and needs of data collection in all of these areas. Key findings included the following:
- Need to be able to document using structured data such as predefined drop-down boxes.
- Need to be able to enter free-text comments.
- Entry of an electronic assessment must include the user's electronic signature and the current date and time.
- All entries must have the capability to be edited, and changes to the document must be tracked by the system.

SWOT Analysis
A SWOT analysis of the current documentation was conducted with the following findings:
- *Strengths.* Structured electronic data in the ICU facilitates accurate and timely data collection.
- *Weaknesses.* Lack of standardization may result in inconsistent patient care.
- *Opportunities.* An electronic order management and documentation system could support evidence-based practice methodology.
- *Threats.* Paper documentation is difficult to read and could result in patient safety issues.

17

Project Management Principles for Health Informatics

Michele Mills

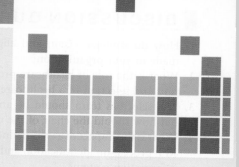

As costs continue to increase and more government regulations are mandated, healthcare professionals need to approach strategic initiatives and projects in a proven, methodical way by using formal project management principles.

OBJECTIVES

At the completion of this chapter, the reader will be prepared to:

1. Distinguish between the terms project, program, and portfolio in a healthcare setting.
2. Describe the need for formal project management in contemporary organizations.
3. Understand general project management processes and procedures and knowledge areas.
4. Describe the skills required for successful project management discipline.

KEY TERMS

portfolio management, 285
program management, 285

project management, 285

ABSTRACT ❖

Because of the increased demand for effectiveness and efficiency in healthcare delivery, leaders at all levels are forced to determine the best way to use available resources, whether these are human, physical, or monetary. Project management, a systematic approach to planning and guiding project processes from start to finish, is a proven way to improve outcomes that can directly and positively impact costs through the efficient and effective use of limited resources for health information technology (IT). Fundamental project management practices allow organizations to reach strategic goals within a planned timeline within cost parameters. A strong project management discipline includes high degrees of communication, organization, interpersonal leadership, cross-functional team coordination and negotiations, problem solving, attentiveness to detail, technical and business domain knowledge, and the ability to methodically guide the project processes through organizational governance parameters using these formal steps:

- Initiation or preplanning
- Formal planning with the creation of a project plan
- Implementation and execution of that project plan with measurement of progress and performance
- Project closure through delivery of value through project objectives

INTRODUCTION

Dr. Armstrong started a small ear, nose, and throat (ENT) clinical practice that was recently acquired by a large local hospital network. Each morning he meets with his clinic nurses and staff to review a list of patients treated the day before to ensure information in their files is complete and correct. Up to now, he has not been able to fully expand his office capabilities to include a full electronic health record system. Instead, he and his office staff spend time reviewing paper patient forms. He was just informed that hospital administration found his clinic to be losing revenue because they are not accurately capturing all the patient data required for efficient billing. He understands the importance of optimization for the patient experience and efficiency of cost, which a streamlined electronic patient documentation process would likely provide. He and the hospital would like a health IT solution within 3 months. He has proposed they select a few key patient paper forms they could convert into electronic forms that would integrate into the hospital system.

Later that week, Dr. Armstrong had conversations with hospital administration and the information technology department about making his forms electronic. He found a larger hospital initiative already underway for an enterprise document management system that would integrate departmental documentation into the larger hospital electronic health record (EHR) system. That initiative had an expected timeline of 18 months. Under his current timeline constraints, Dr. Armstrong negotiated a small capital budget to get a temporary electronic solution in place for a few of his critical ENT patient forms until the larger solution was available. The biggest question on his mind at this point was, "How in the world am I going to get this all done in 3 months?!"

In a complex organization like a hospital, where many clinics and physicians have competing priorities and demands, healthcare providers are often responsible for ensuring that tools, processes, infrastructure, and capabilities are in place to meet the demand for excellent patient care. A structured process called project management is an essential technique for clinicians and informaticians to know. Project management is defined by the Project Management Institute (PMI) as "a temporary endeavor undertaken to create a unique product, service, or result. The temporary nature of projects indicates a definite beginning and end. The end is reached when the project's objectives have been achieved or when the project is terminated because its objectives will not or cannot be met, or when the need for the project no longer exists."[1]

Project management is indispensable in health IT, as it is a structured approach to help ensure effective implementations of healthcare initiatives. A strong project management process includes initiation or preplanning, formal planning, creation and implementation of a project plan, and measurement of progress and performance.[2] A health IT project might focus on the implementation of a single application or initiative within a short timeline, such as providing a temporary electronic documentation solution for Dr. Armstrong's clinic.

Program management, on the other hand, involves larger implementations, like a large-scale hospital document management application or an organization-wide EHR system. With program management, there are multiple, aligned projects affecting many teams or departments that are coordinated and managed in concert.

Portfolio management is even more complex and involves the creation of common programs and projects that are not necessarily related but are important to combine and view as a whole. One example would be a clinical portfolio where all projects and programs that directly affect patient care are managed or aligned in a common category. Other portfolios might be a financial or a technology infrastructure portfolio. Effective management of portfolios is essential for a healthcare organization to adequately prioritize and approve new project requests and to work strategically on projects throughout the years. Portfolio management provides an essential foundation for decisions and discussions in governance committees as projects are prioritized and funded.[3]

THE NEED FOR PROJECT MANAGEMENT IN HEALTHCARE ORGANIZATIONS

Project management can improve the quality of health IT project outcomes, provide accountability of expenses, and reduce inefficiencies through structured change control processes. The Project Management Institute (PMI), an association created to improve organizational success and mature the profession of project management, has conducted a number of studies related to the impact of project management. These studies reveal that nearly 80% of all projects fail to meet their objectives if they do not have some type of structured project methodology.[4]

Applying appropriate processes, methodologies, and tools within a hospital setting can have multidimensional benefits by reducing variability across processes, providing standardization across projects, and increasing the overall project success rate. This is important in any industry but even more critical in a healthcare environment where multiple stakeholders, departments, clinics, and providers functioning under a single hospital umbrella must coordinate between competing priorities, budgets, capital expenses, and large enterprise initiatives. Many healthcare projects across departments can overlap or even clash. This is because departments are frequently regarded as separate entities or "silos" where clinical projects and initiatives are often carried out independently at the discretion of a leader and at times without aligning project goals with the larger organizational objectives. In the case of Dr. Armstrong, without a coordinated and structured project management approach at the hospital, his ENT clinic might implement a software solution for his particular electronic patient forms that may be incompatible with the hospital document management system. This could result in rework for interoperability/integration and a waste of valuable resources in the longer term, although it may provide a short-term solution for his area.

Projects implemented by healthcare practitioners themselves are often done with the best intent, but practitioners are seldom trained in formal project management methodologies. They may lack the skill set and knowledge base to properly mitigate project risks, define the scope of the project, develop realistic schedules, or manage resource issues throughout a given project timeline. Without these requisite skills, organizations may have projects with inconsistent outcomes, including cost overruns, time delays, and/or poor quality deliverables. At the macro level of hospital administration, this can often create conflicts where differences in project implementations from department to department result in an inability to estimate annual costs and departmental performance. Without a standardized approach, it is difficult to gather and measure organizational performance metrics, prepare performance reports, forecast financial data, and understand financial impacts and human capital costs of organizational initiatives. Standardized and consistent project management is needed throughout the organization at all levels to optimize process and project outcomes across all entities. The most effective organizations have formal strategic plans showing what they can and will do, so there is a clear understanding of what is expected across organizational departments and levels. Project management best practices can help create transparency and visibility within the organization and helps eliminate many of these issues.[5]

Good use of project management techniques can help align key areas and ensure skills and tools are consistently applied to health IT. This is important because healthcare must generate revenue while in a competitive landscape, control costs, operate within government regulations, and not compromise quality, patient care, or satisfaction. Project management can help ensure delivery of initiatives and projects on time and within budget and provide well-defined value requirements that positively affect the organization's financial performance, productivity, and delivery of patient services. It can also enhance patient satisfaction either directly or indirectly.[5]

Project management serves as an effective way to bring all of these concepts together to more efficiently appropriate resources in support of an organization's goals (Fig. 17.1). Fig. 17.1 shows project management areas surrounded by typical stakeholders. A PMI "Pulse of the Profession" study showed that projects within high-performing organizations are able to meet planned goals two-and-a-half times more frequently than those in low-performing organizations.[3] Additionally, high-performing organizations waste about 13 times less money than low performers. The need for strong project management skills and a solid understanding of the process has never been more important in healthcare.[6]

PROJECT, PROGRAM, AND PORTFOLIO MANAGEMENT

As defined earlier project, program and portfolio management are three levels of focus in formal project management. The following section explores each level and their interrelationships.

Project Management

A **project** refers to an undertaking that is time bound and delivers a particular product or service. It is a temporary undertaking ending after a set of goals are achieved, involving the application of knowledge, ideas, and skills to execute a plan of action.[2] More specifically, a project consists of goals, activities, a timeline, projected risks, and mitigation plans. Each project has an appointed manager who leads the effort. An example of a project is the purchase of a perinatal clinical system that needs to be integrated with the current EHR.

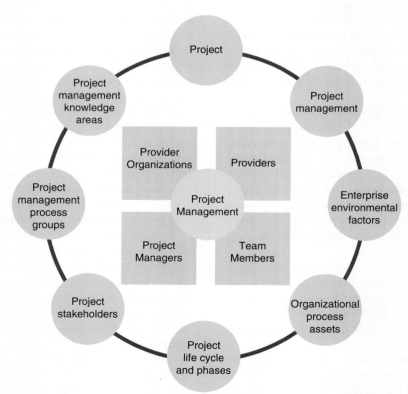

FIG 17.1 Coordination areas of project management. (Adapted from Bhide, D. Patient care—a project management perspective. <http://www.projectmanagement.com>; 2011.)

To comply with project management best practices, project processes, documentation, and procedures must follow a methodical approach through a series of defined phases that each have a specific set of deliverables and steps that must be completed before the next phase should begin. These project phases include initiation, planning, execution, and closure. Monitoring and control formally takes place during the planning and executing phases when most activities are moving at a fast pace. Monitoring and controlling and are not necessary during two phases—initiating and closing—because the work has not been defined (initiating) or it is completed (closing). See Fig. 17.2 for a graphic depiction of these concepts.

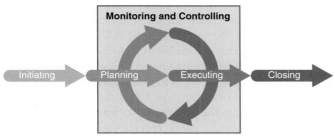

FIG 17.2 Project management phases. (Copyright Michele Mills, 2015.)

Project Process Groups

The PMI provides various process groups (or steps) and knowledge areas critical to the success of a project or program.[3] These process groups and associated activities form the primary foundation for the life cycle of a project (Table 17.1):

- *Initiating activities* are generally the most important activities and yet often the most rushed or undervalued. The initiation phase of a project requires a project manager (PM) to gather initial information and resource estimates so that project viability can be assessed. This includes activities like submission of a formal project proposal or business case for approval from leadership teams, prioritization of competing projects at the program or portfolio governance levels, and approvals for capital funding and operational budget from hospital administration. Initial project scope and timelines should be established so leaders can balance the impact on resources and existing workloads. Projects should have organization visibility so larger risks and impacts on architecture and existing initiatives can be mitigated across efforts. This can help mitigate unnecessary spending and ensure solid alignment organization strategic goals and objectives. Once projects are approved, funded, and resourced, formal project planning can begin.
- *Planning activities* lay the foundation for the project life cycle and are used to track future project performance.

TABLE 17.1   Project Management Process Groups (Steps)

Process Group	Description	Activities and Steps
Initiation	Project managers collect sufficient data to make a determination about the viability of a project and to assess what is needed.	• Define objectives • Define scope • Define purpose • Define deliverables • Provide financial and human capital estimates • Obtain necessary approvals and funding • Create project proposals
Planning	Project managers collaborate with domain and subject matter experts to create a detailed plan to guide the project team throughout project execution and closure.	• Create project charters • Break down deliverables into workable tasks • Create project plan • Identify critical work path and schedule • Assign resources • Create communication plan • Identify risks and create risk mitigation plans • Create testing plans • Create quality assurance plans • Create release management plans • Create education and training plans
Execution	Staff and vendors begin building the project deliverables and providing them to customers for testing and sign-off. Monitoring and control of the project are significant to ensure the executed plan does not deviate from the original purpose or scope.	• Complete project tasks • Monitor and control time, cost, quality, change, risks, issues, procurements, customer acceptance, communications, etc. • Adhere to plans established in planning phase
Closure	The project is delivered (includes communication with and handoff to operations and maintenance teams).	• Create ongoing support models for operations and maintenance • Document lessons learned

Planning is where projects are formally defined by project teams and subject matter experts who decompose project deliverables into workable tasks as part of the overall project plan. The plan will assist project leaders with time management, cost estimation, quality, change, risk, and issues throughout the life of a project. Often this step is where healthcare project advocates struggle, because there is a constant need to deliver "quicker, better, faster" and rush to implement a product or solution. Key risks may not be fully planned for or even considered, and tasks greatly affecting the scope or timeline may not be identified early enough to mitigate them. Steps may be left out completely. Defining the project through planning helps team members achieve defined goals and objectives and serves as a basis for good communication and evaluation for managing project staff and external vendors about timelines and budgets. Skipping this step or even inadequately completing this step typically hinders progress throughout the life of a project and affects the long-term results stakeholders seek. Once a formal project plan has been completed, resourced, and scheduled, the project is ready for execution.

- *Executing activities* often take the most time and resources to complete. The execution phase ultimately defines the success of a project. This is where the build of project deliverables and customer testing and approval occurs. Use of solid management processes, including effective monitoring and control of all elements of a project—time, cost, quality, change, management of risk, issues, procurement, customer acceptance, and communications—can help ensure success at the execution phase.[7] PMs monitor challenges encountered during development, and risks should be mitigated through well-thought-out risk plans. Risk management should include requisite changes to project scope. Any issues should be well controlled to keep the project on schedule and avoid project derailment. Once goals are met, project closure can begin.

  Project management theory often assumes a "best-case scenario" view. All project types can be managed based on these best case methodologies, but healthcare tends to have more uncontrollable variables. For example, compare healthcare with manufacturing, which is an industry with embedded processes. In manufacturing, every process step builds on the next in sequential order. Healthcare projects rarely follow precise processes because of variables that are out of a PM's control (e.g., regulatory change), so project management methodologies in a healthcare environment must take these kinds of unexpected events into account. Successful project management in healthcare is absolutely attainable, but it requires a strong understanding of the culture and limitations to "perfect" project management.

- *Closing activities* include release management, project delivery, documentation of lessons learned, and formal handoffs to operational and maintenance teams.[2] These steps are critical to define and complete in a healthcare setting because some of the same people (resources) who worked on a project are often the ones who maintain that project's outcomes. Equally important is the fact that a project, by definition, has a beginning and an end. Therefore a clear delineation of the end of every project is needed to understand when maintenance and operational phases begin. Also, PMs should conduct a postimplementation review to gather and share lessons learned and define next steps. Typical deliverables in this phase include documentation for support and specific communications to inform stakeholders the project has ended.

For instance, Dr. Armstrong's initiative to capture accurate and complete billing data through electronic patient forms for his ENT clinic is an example of a project in healthcare. His project should have a formal PM and a clear definition of project goals, objectives, and deliverables. Paper forms included in the project scope should be discussed, selected, and approved. Required data elements need to be identified, and resources need to be allocated to the project. A well-defined plan for execution should be formulated, so a solid understanding of the work required is communicated to the project team. This will enable them to meet the aggressive 3-month timeline. Monitoring project progress and controlling changes to scope is critical to ensure accurate patient data is captured on the new electronic forms and issues and risks are resolved to keep the project within budget and timeline constraints. A formal closing process can then effectively deliver a production-ready system for his clinic without affecting patient care, cost, or quality of service.

Key Knowledge Components

PMI knowledge areas or components of formal project management align directly with the project management process groups, activities, and steps and are vital to successful delivery. These include project integration, scope management, time and cost management, quality management, human resource management, communication management, risk management, and procurement management[2]:

- **Project integration** includes the development of a project charter. A project charter or management plan outlines the direction and management of overall project execution, monitoring and control processes for scope, schedule and resource management, performance of change control procedures, and project closure and release management steps. This area focuses on how project issues will be managed, tracks changes to the original plan, and coordinates replanning, if necessary.
- **Scope management** focuses on work of the project and clarifies boundaries and areas to include or exclude. Scope management involves collecting project requirements (desired functions) and defines the scope in more detail. This includes creating a work breakdown structure, scope verification, and validation process with stakeholders and key project sponsors and outlines scope change control. Without a well-defined scope document, there is no way to know if a project is in or out of scope at any particular phase.
- **Time management** includes estimations of task effort (by complexity), determines the project schedule, and records actual completion dates. This knowledge area includes

monitoring and control of schedule and resources, ensuring project teams are empowered to be productive, and reporting accurate time spent on activities (effort) throughout the project. This is closely aligned with cost management, especially for estimating resources required for tasks and task durations, as these directly align with project costs.

- **Cost management** involves the cost of resources such as materials, equipment, facilities, labor, and other related services. Determining cost estimates, budget, and financial controls all fall into this category.
- **Quality management** includes creating deliverables that meet an acceptable quality level and the quality of the project management process itself, focusing on quality assurance and quality control. Quality assurance consists of auditing and comparing initial quality requirements against quality control measurements. Quality control involves monitoring results of quality activities, which include project deliverables and project management results. An example of this would be tracking a project budget or schedule during the project life cycle.
- **Human resource management** is the management of people and includes aspects like team acquisition, team development, and processes for project resource issue resolution. PMs work closely with RMs to ensure they are in sync throughout a project.
- **Communication management** includes meeting management, risk actions and assessments, project plans, project reviews, stakeholder identification, and project information distribution. Stakeholder communication should be frequent and include project status, issues, risks, and successes to adequately manage expectations.
- **Risk management** includes both project threats and opportunities. These are plausible scenarios that may or may not impact the scope, timeline, or resources of a project, given a set of circumstances. Both have uncertainty so must be managed to avoid delays or project failure. The focus is on planned risk management, identification of

risks, performance of qualitative and quantitative risk analysis, and monitoring and control of risks. Risk identification is most effective if done during the planning phase and should include outcomes and possible solutions to threats if the given scenario materializes.

- **Procurement management** includes acquiring products or services from outside the project team. This includes working with vendors, contractors, and service groups.

Benefits of Improved Project Performance

Organizations realize increased efficiency in service delivery and enhanced customer satisfaction when following formal project management process areas and using key knowledge components. In healthcare, project management can provide benefits listed in Box 17.1.[5] Finally, fundamental project management practices allow organizations to reach strategic goals within a planned timeline within cost parameters.[2]

Program Management

A program refers to a group of related projects managed together. Program management is the art of cohesive coordination of various interrelated projects such as those for an EHR (imaging, documentation, barcode medication administration, etc.). The logic behind program management is that it is less complicated, less costly, and more operationally efficient to control similar projects together than separately. Resource sharing can then occur, as projects might be able to be managed by the same person or with shared resources, leading to significant efficiencies, financial savings, and coordination across projects. Program management ensures goals, project steps, and resource needs are in sync.[8] Ultimately, projects in a program are more likely to achieve the agreed-upon set of objectives when managed together rather than separately. An example would be an enterprise-wide document management system where multiple departments and clinics have competing requirements and workflows that must be managed under the umbrella of a single software installation that requires well-managed

---

BOX 17.1 Project Management Benefits

1. *Provide a guide for project teams to follow.* This helps the team as a whole stay on task and avoid issues that could delay the project or overrun the budget.
2. *Impact patient outcomes.* Projects can affect patient safety outcomes. Those with quality deliverables may include improved patient safety (e.g., computerized physician order entry alerts for medication interactions).
3. *Potentially enhance patient satisfaction.* Projects that are delivered on time and under budget and those including quality measures could impact patient satisfaction.
4. *Provide better team performance on future projects.* With positive project outcomes, project teams will likely be inspired to perform more effectively on future projects. Likewise, with negative project outcomes, teams can learn from a project "postmortem" or as a "lessons learned" exercise and not repeat the same mistakes twice.

5. *Improve the organizational standing and competitive edge.* With continued successful project outcomes, an opportunity exists for more positive standing in the organization and community with a stronger competitive edge. Superior performance is marketable.[12]
6. *Improve organizational efficiency and effectiveness.* Project management can allow for more flexibility in how work is prioritized by portfolio committees. Teams are able to work efficiently and effectively.
7. *Anticipate risks.* Project management techniques help organizations plan for risks. Managers can see risks in future projects before they become problematic.
8. *Increase project quality.* Techniques can result in achieving quality project outcomes more consistently.

CPOE, Computerized physician order entry.

coordination, phased implementation, or various subprojects to run in parallel (Fig 17.3).

Portfolio Management

Portfolio management centralizes the management of processes, methodologies, and technologies used by PMs, program managers, and project management offices (PMOs). This allows collective management of the entire suite of current and proposed projects, such as all projects supporting patient care (pharmacy, laboratory, EHRs, imaging, etc.). The purpose of portfolio management is to determine an optimal resource mix for project implementation and scheduling that is most effective in achieving an organization's operational and financial goals. In healthcare, these goals include patient care, quality, and cost goals.

A portfolio includes projects that are combined together as a logical group, but they are not necessarily linked directly together as in program management.[3] This might include aligning projects, programs, and operations with strategic objectives and investing resources in the right work to deliver the expected value.[4] All projects within the portfolio do, however, have similar strategic goals or initiatives. Like program management, portfolio management allows for better prioritization and optimization of projects as well as creating the opportunity for efficiencies (Fig. 17.4).[9] According to research, many organizations find mature portfolio management provides invaluable tools to sync projects and programs with strategic business goals. For organizations describing themselves as highly effective at portfolio management, 62% met or exceeded expected return on investment (ROI)

targets. Among this group, 89% said senior managers had an understanding of what portfolio management meant and how it is used. This helped mitigate individual departments expending monies and labor on single department initiatives. It also assisted in collaborative decision making for organization priorities. Organizations rated highly effective at portfolio management were twice as likely to adopt portfolio management to help them innovate within their sectors. Over half of minimally effective organizations did not take portfolio management as seriously,[5] resulting in less favorable outcomes.

Portfolio management can remove a portion of organizational politics and deliver clarity across project goals and processes. With structured evaluation of projects and selection, there is more visibility to organizational politics and political maneuvering. Projects are either viable or not, based on the more objective criteria put in place for each portfolio. This does not mean politics will be completely eliminated, but they are made visible, not hidden, with project management processes. Portfolio management is also likely to result in greater organizational stability and realization of projected benefits. For those reasons, it is not surprising that, according to the PMI research, leaders of highly effective organizations are three times more likely to understand portfolio management principles than minimally effective ones.[3]

Despite the benefits, initiating a portfolio management process can be difficult because portfolio managers must sometimes convince leaders these processes are best for their business. Strong leadership skills are essential for portfolio management. Without it, particularly in large healthcare organizations, projects across entities are disconnected, invisible project lists exist, and hidden agendas are common.[6]

Benefits of Portfolio Management

In the past, estimating and managing resources, using formal project management, and fostering alignment with strategic goals was said to be important, but it was not recognized as a critical aspect of organizational success. Project management provides a way to do this, bringing great value to organizations.

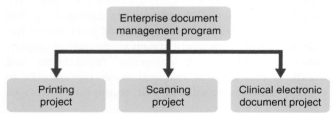

FIG. 17.3 Sample healthcare program. (Copyright Michele Mills, 2015.)

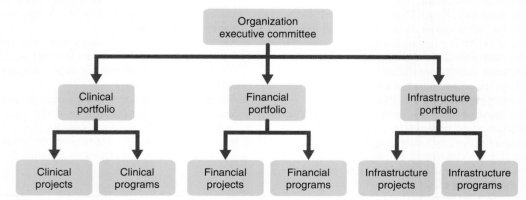

FIG. 17.4 Sample healthcare portfolio management structure. (Copyright Michele Mills, 2015.)

Portfolio management is a way to improve implementation of myriad organizational initiatives. In a healthcare environment, portfolio management can mitigate uncoordinated, decentralized efforts. This allows for an efficient sharing of resources, where feasible, and a better appraisal of what needs to be accomplished. Additionally, it provides an avenue for measuring ROI at the highest organizational level.[4]

While portfolio management requires organizational discipline and maturity, it is well worth the effort. It helps clarify organization-wide priorities and project and resource expectations upfront. Staff will appreciate the stability of being able to predict their efforts day to day, and they will likely work more effectively on approved tasks throughout the year. Organizations reap benefits by working strategically, targeting investments, gaining advantage against competitors, reducing or avoiding costs, and having the ability to comply more effectively and quickly with government regulations as well as effecting risk reduction through mitigation or elimination.

Portfolio Governance

Portfolio governance plays a significant role in a healthcare organization and its strategy. It is difficult to be successful if no clear plan is available on existing and proposed projects or about how resources are allocated. No matter how an organization's portfolio governance is structured, articulating it clearly provides guidance to the organization.

In most organizations with formal governance process, separate portfolio governance committees determine priorities and funding. They also decide if, when, and how any reprioritizations occur within the respective portfolios, based on resource availability. Projects and programs are categorized as a portfolio of investments and are meant to deliver maximum value. Cost is a factor, because it is important to stay in business, but money alone will not bring long-term success. To accomplish a strong ROI from each project or program, outcomes need to be measurable, weighted, and reviewed by a governance committee. Projects and programs of little value can be eliminated during prioritization or yearly reprioritization in portfolio governance meetings. It is most effective for any industry, but particularly healthcare, to prioritize at the beginning of the year (fiscal or calendar) and not continuously reprioritize throughout the year unless urgent issues occur. This allows staff to focus on planned efforts, rather than deal with the chaos of shifting priorities every day, week, or month. All portfolios should roll up to an organization's executive level committee for prioritization of projects and programs for the entire organization.[7] Once that is completed, individual portfolio prioritization can be done more effectively (see Fig. 17.4).

Strong portfolio governance committees manage ongoing and projected initiatives to determine if a set of projects can or should be implemented. Alignment of this decision-making process, new project selection for capital investments, and strategic planning is critical. The 2014 PMI *Pulse of the Profession: Portfolio Management* states that "alignment of projects to organizational strategy most likely contributes to

the surprising result that nearly one half of strategic initiatives (44%) are reported as unsuccessful."[2] Thus each committee needs a good understanding of resource management, project risks, and financial management, as these are key to the success of any project management governance model.[9] Utilizing project management practices will strengthen deployment of organization resources so they are working on the "right projects at the right time."[4]

Inherent risk exists in any project or program implemented in a healthcare environment. Integrating cost, schedules, contingencies, and risk response plans in a group with portfolios allows committees to review projects and programs holistically to mitigate issues before projects are funded or implemented. This enables organizations to have more visibility and less uncertainty about upcoming efforts.[9]

ROLES AND RESPONSIBILITIES: PROJECT, PROGRAM, AND PORTFOLIO MANAGERS

Project, program, and portfolio managers need to have a variety of skills in order to bring people, tools, and processes together in successfully delivering project objectives and value. Each of these roles requires strong leadership. Leaders are typically visionaries, collaborators, committed to organizational goals, excellent communicators, good problem solvers, and results oriented. They are accountable team players and can see the "big picture" of a project or program holistically. Project and program managers must be able to effectively communicate the project or program purpose, direction, and desired results to the project team and stakeholders so they can motivate people to deliver their best effort.[10]

The most effective leaders are collaborative in nature and include their project team(s) in the project strategy, risk assessment, planning, and decision making. Leaders must have strong, visible, and consistent commitment to their project, positively impacting the outcome. Without that, a team will likely not have confidence in their activities, or they may not understand expectations for a successful outcome. Leaders must be able to identify and react quickly to urgent issues. They work with the end goal in mind to help guide them through the project management process journey, basing their decisions and actions on outcomes they want to achieve. A solid project management discipline includes PMs who possess skills with high degrees of communication, organization, interpersonal leadership, cross-functional team coordination, negotiation, problem solving, attentiveness to detail, and knowledge about technical and business domains. Specific responsibilities and activities for each managerial level are outlined in the following sections.

Project Manager

PM roles and responsibilities span the beginning to the end of a project. PMs are responsible for controlling any project changes that occur, ensuring progress is monitored continuously and that performance is measured periodically.

PM activities include a major focus on project planning, budget allocations, and resource allocations. They bring structure to a healthcare environment to ensure projects and programs are delivered on time and on budget and within the set scope and requirements.[7]

Project planning is a significant role of PMs. They manage project overall planning and project deliverables. Their key role is to bring people and processes together to keep a project moving at an optimal pace and to ensure project deliverables are completed accurately and efficiently within the project deadline. Moving too quickly and rushing a project under pressure can often lead to missed details, so PMs have a responsibility to help stakeholders and staff manage the pace of delivery.

PMs monitor and continuously assess the project as well as record and manage issues throughout the course of the project execution. Issues are sometimes urgent and may impact scheduled implementation deadlines. If a team member working on a project reports that a current task or deliverable is not feasible because of a given environmental or hardware issue discovered in the process, this can delay or stop the project. These obviously need to be resolved immediately to avoid a negative impact on a project.

A PM is obliged to control the project scope so it does not diverge from what has been planned. Sometimes stakeholders who are highly engaged in the project may want more than can realistically be achieved within a given timeline and can add additional, unplanned requirements during the execution phase. This increase of original scope, or "scope creep," should be avoided or managed to avoid delays to project schedules. Most IT projects and programs tend to grow in scale and complexity as they progress, especially as more people get involved. One reason for this is that as more stakeholders see details of the project, they think of additional ideas. This is not always a negative situation, but adding more functions during scope creep still needs to be managed and/or mitigated. The most important aspect of scope creep is the creation of a scope document. Without such a document, how can you really assess your "scope creep"? It is essential to have a full understanding of what is in and out of scope so projects can be effectively managed.

An example of how scope creep can impact a project or program negatively is the delivery of an EHR in a large hospital. Hospital ABC planned to link 10,000 physicians with 200 hospitals around the world. The organization felt this project was an imperative for its future competitiveness and the project was worth the effort and cost to implement it. However, the organization had an immature internal project management process. Organizational leaders scheduled project implementation with the vendor without any requirements or input from the PM who would be managing the program for budget and timeline. The PM was given a gross project outcome—18 months and a budget of $25 million—but additional project functions were not defined as part of the implementation. As a result, the program ended 5 years later with a budget that doubled from the original estimate. The major lesson learned for the organization was that the lack of documentation of requirements from the beginning created project failure for the budgeting aspect. Not having that initial information about the project created a situation where the PM was not adequately prepared or able to manage scope creep.

To manage a project's potential scope creep, a PM should begin with a strong scope document. Project scope documentation should include information about project time, cost, and resources. It provides an overview of what the project team is expecting to achieve and how the work will be accomplished. It can be used to clarify what stakeholders can expect and what the parameters are for any changes that may be requested (scope creep).

This situation is not unusual in low-maturity organizations, unfortunately. Without documentation to help manage scope creep, leaders are forced to repeatedly push out go-live dates to accommodate critically needed changes. There is no way to show stakeholders what was originally agreed to. How can they effectively determine which changes are appropriate? For an IT PM, this type of situation can be a career killer. Managing scope creep well can help ensure project success and a PM's long career in healthcare project management.

At each performance measurement stage, the PM must update the sponsor and other stakeholders and solicit their help when necessary. Budget allocations for projects and programs are typically estimated to make certain the allocated funds are adequate for the effort to be successful. This is an area where a strong PM with excellent leadership skills can excel. In particular, successful PMs will be able to indicate what the requirements are and make them realistic. PMs provide vital information to leaders so the latter can make decisions based on solid data.

Resource allocation is another significant role for a PM. PMs need to understand the depth of resource requirements throughout a project or program. Thus a proper analysis of requirements is essential to determine the amount of resources needed at each stage. A PM may be responsible for hiring staff or consultants for a project or provide enough detail to directors or resource managers (RMs) who do the hiring. The PM is ultimately responsible for providing the most comprehensive information possible for adequate resources to be secured.

To avoid conflicts with resource allocation, PMs and RMs should determine at the beginning of a project or program what the parameters will be. The following are a few basic questions PMs can ask before activities begin:

1. Who is responsible for allocation of team members' time for the project or program?
2. What role will the RM play on the project, if any?
3. How will the RM and PM coordinate the work? What is the frequency of this coordination?

Some organizations have managers serve a dual role of both RM and PM simultaneously. This is not a recommended way to manage projects or programs because of the conflicting needs and goals of each role. Operationally, RMs must ensure their operational area continues to run in parallel with whatever projects or programs are in progress. Likewise, PMs must fulfill their duties to make certain nothing gets off track. When an RM is expected to do both, project management suffers. RMs can have an understandable bias toward their own teams, which can impact health IT project outcomes negatively.

Program Manager

Program managers are tasked with similar roles and responsibilities as PMs. They guide organization leaders and multiple projects, so their efforts need to be especially well coordinated. Like a PM, they are responsible for planning, executing, and delivering a program or collection of related projects within the defined program scope and schedule. Monitoring progress of individual projects, they coordinate activities across the group of projects in their program, which adds a level of complexity.

A program like the implementation of an EHR requires someone like a program manager to oversee the entire overarching implementation of the system among many clinics and departmental areas. Each area has requirements that may be managed as individual projects with their own individual, respective PMs. Projects and team members within a program cooperate to allow resources to be streamlined and synchronized to meet overall program objectives. Some elements of project management, like reporting to stakeholders, are typically more frequent in a program to prevent overlooking a small but critical element. Program managers' skills are typically at a higher level of strategic leadership, cross-functional team coordination, organizational resource negotiation, and communication due to the increased complexity of their responsibilities.

Portfolio Manager

A portfolio manager is responsible for centralized management of portfolio processes, methods, and structures to ensure successful flow of projects within a portfolio. The portfolio manager provides information about projects, programs, and resources within a portfolio to governance committees who will evaluate new requests based on strategic alignment. In a healthcare setting, portfolio management involves organizing projects to focus, for example, on patients, quality outcomes, and financial goals. Portfolio managers can help committees determine which projects should be given priority in terms of resource allocation, availability, realistic completion timelines, and project overlap because they should be aware of stakeholder demand and have high-level insight to requirements and deadlines of the projects within the portfolio.

Portfolio managers play a key role in ensuring project and program risks are known to committees and controlled to avoid poor project selection or delays. The ultimate success of a portfolio is dependent on the performance of individual projects. Portfolio managers should perform a value assessment for each completed project to provide information to leadership about long-term value. This requires comparing initial definitions of benefits against actual results.

PROJECT MANAGEMENT TOOLS

Some PMs use productivity software like Microsoft Word and Excel to perform project management functions. Microsoft Office has various free templates in Excel, Word, and PowerPoint of use for program evaluation review technique (PERT) and Gantt charts that outline project tasks and their interrelationships, as explained in the following section. These are low-cost options for a department or organization that is small to medium sized or those working on small projects limited to a low number of users and activities. Aspects to track are project scope determination, timelines, budget, resource assignment, and project documentation. There are also many project management software tools on the market that provide the same functionality but are built into the system.

PERT charts are used to schedule, organize, and coordinate tasks in a project. Using the foundation of an "activity list" (Fig. 17.5), these charts provide a graphical view of a project as a network diagram consisting of numbered "nodes" (Fig. 17.6). These nodes can be either circles or rectangles that represent events or milestones. They are linked by labeled vectors or directional lines that represent tasks. The direction of an arrow on a line indicates a task sequence. These are dependent or serial tasks. Tasks between nodes that are not dependent on the completion of one node to start the other

Activity	Description	Predecessor(s)	Optimistic time (0)	Pessimistic time (P)	Most likely time (M)	Expected time (0+4M+P)/6
A	Project team selection	—	10	16	14	12
B	Do site assessment; Select pilot site	—	5	13	9	8
C	Equipment selection	A	8	12	10	8
D	Network design and installation	B	9	17	9	9
E	Equipment installs	B, D	17	24	23	16

FIG. 17.5 PERT activities list. (Copyright Michele Mills, 2015.)

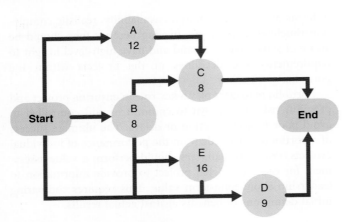

FIG. 17.6 PERT chart (activities in days).

node and can be undertaken simultaneously are called parallel or concurrent tasks.

Gantt Charts

A Gantt chart is a graphical view of the duration of tasks and activities shown as a progression in a timeline. A simplified view of the schedule and milestones is provided in Fig. 17.7. After that, managers would add task relationships and predecessors of each and put them into a graphical template (Figs. 17.8 and 17.9).

Task	Duration
Workflow analysis and redesign	12 months
Equipment selection	1 month
Hardware installation	1 month
Software configuration	2 months
Evaluate backup system	3 months
Determine how old data will be converted	3 months
Go-live planning	3 months

FIG. 17.7 Key tasks and durations in a Gantt chart. (Copyright Michele Mills, 2015.)

PERT charts are preferred by some PMs, rather than Gantt charts, because they clearly show task dependencies. They can, however, be more difficult to interpret, particularly in a complex project. PMs often use both tools to ensure they can interpret all the details effectively.

More scalable tools can be found in the market, but which one to select is dependent on the organization's strategy. Does the PM need to report only basic information (e.g., how much time project team members are spending on each task)? Does the PM need to go further and link project time to cost? Does the organization require the PM to be able to provide information about a large volume of projects and nonproject work? As with any software purchase, it is important to fully understand what is required before purchasing a product. Selection of a project tool is the ultimate project for an organization looking to reduce costs, meet mandated government regulations, and focus on strategic initiatives more methodically. More complicated medium- to large-sized organizations would be well served if they select a more formalized tool.

PROJECT AND PORTFOLIO MANAGEMENT SOFTWARE SELECTION

For complex or medium to large organizations, purchasing a formal project management tool can be justified. Depending on an organization's needs, a wide variety of options exist. In Gartner's Project and Portfolio Management (PPM) Magic Quadrant report, information is provided about various project management software (Fig. 17.10).[11] Gartner's review included both on-site and cloud-hosted options. Their report emphasizes that the current demand for IT PPM software will continue to gain traction due to increased speed and types of organizational change. Today PMs are more focused on digitalization and having cloud-based options. Most tools will have what an organization needs to be successful, but they must be prepared to do some work to get what they need.[9]

"Selling" a complex PPM system and discipline to your own organization can be difficult. Having a senior-level executive sponsor is critical. To do this, the PM should resist the temptation to speak about PM theoretical concepts. Leaders will focus on how new software will help the organization's bottom

Task	Duration	Predecessors
Workflow analysis and redesign	12 months	4
Equipment selection	1 month	4
Hardware installation	1 month	2
Software configuration	2 months	
Evaluate backup system	3 months	
Determine how old data will be converted	3 months	1
Go-live planning	3 months	1

FIG. 17.8 Task relationships and predecessors in a Gantt chart. (Copyright Michele Mills, 2015.)

#	EHR Implementation	Jul	Aug	Sep	Oct	Nov	Dec	Jan	Feb	Mar	April	May	June
1	**Workflow analysis and redesign**												
1.1	Office layout and patient scheduling	▓	▓	▓	▓	▓	▓	▓	▓	▓	▓	▓	▓
1.2	Evaluate transition from batch to queue system					▓	▓	▓	▓	▓	▓	▓	
2	**Equipment selection**												
2.1	Determine type of equipment					▓							
2.2	Determine equipment vendors						▓						
3	**Hardware installation**												
3.1	Installation team member selection						▓						
3.2	Installation plan						▓						
4	**Software configuration**												
4.1	Customize Patient Data Collection					▓							
4.2	System Testing									▓			
5	**Evaluate backup system**												
5.1	Create initial system backup for review							▓	▓				
5.2	Set up a scheduled backup of the system										▓		
6	**Determine how old data will be converted**												
6.1	Decide data to be converted									▓	▓	▓	
6.2	Perform data conversion test									▓	▓	▓	
7	**Go-Live Planning**												
7.1	Determine your roll out strategy									▓	▓	▓	
7.2	Create go-live schedule for staff									▓	▓	▓	

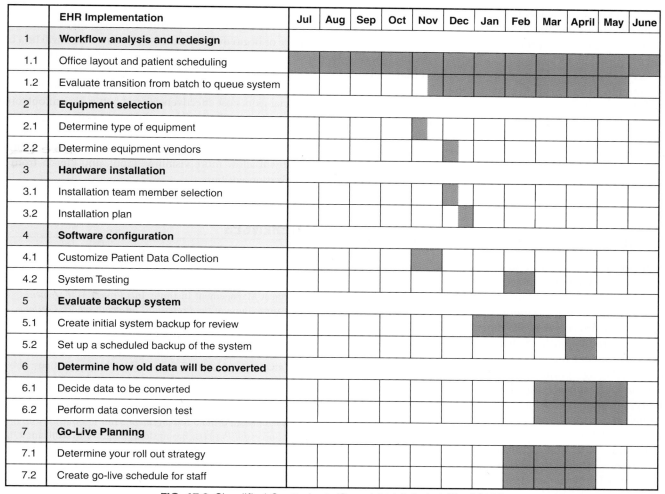

FIG. 17.9 Simplified Gantt chart. (Copyright Michele Mills, 2015.)

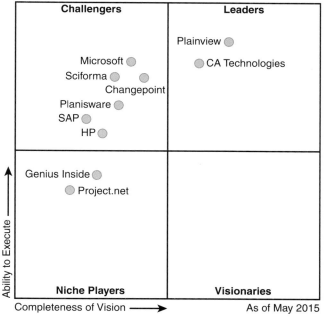

FIG. 17.10 Gartner Magic Quadrant 2015. (Copyright © 2016 Gartner, Inc. and/or its Affiliates. All rights reserved.)

line. What kind of data does the PM have to show them? How are projects being compromised today, and how can an effective tool help correct the problems? PMs can answer questions either by providing leaders with information about a specific project or by a process that demonstrates value. PMs could use, for example, two projects to show a comparison—one managed using project management software and one without. Measuring projects before and after they started will allow empirical data to emerge. In healthcare IT, it would be useful for PMs to show links with improvement(s) to monetary, patient care, or quality data. Once PMs have a senior leader in their corner, they should be well on their way to finding the right tool for the organization.

CONCLUSIONS AND FUTURE DIRECTIONS

High-performing organizations use project management processes to maximize project success and organizational value. Through consistent use of project management practices, healthcare organizations can deliver value through high-quality projects that are more cost effective to implement. The result can be better patient care, higher quality, and financial and human resources leading to higher profit margins. Though profit maximization is not always the primary aim of healthcare organizations, it is needed for sustainability. Integration of project management in healthcare is a significant step toward achieving overall cost-effective, quality healthcare delivery for patients by aligning all levels of the organization with strategic objectives.

Currently, healthcare organizations are only beginning to adopt formal project management techniques, tools, and process groups. As healthcare organizations mature in their processes, more will adopt these systematic, formal techniques to ensure more favorable project outcomes.

The future of project management in health IT is a positive one. As more and more organizations work to cut costs, they are seeing advantages in the use of project management principles, processes, and tools. The cost of purchasing an effective, scalable project management system pales in comparison to the cost of unnecessary waste. Expansion

beyond basic project management into the more complex areas of program and portfolio management will either mature or begin over the next 3 to 5 years. There will be a better understanding of the importance of effective prioritization techniques to gain competitive advantage, focusing efforts on appropriate projects and programs with substantial ROIs of financial gain, cost effectiveness, and better patient outcomes and satisfaction. These all have the purpose of meeting overall organization objectives, rather than only the individual, personal desires of a stakeholder. The project management of the future will allow more visibility, input, and buy-in from all organization entities.

REFERENCES

1. Project Management Institute, Inc. *A Guide to the Project Management Book of Knowledge: PMBOK.* 5th ed. Newtown Square, PA: PMI Publications; 2013: 417.
2. Project Management Institute, Inc. *Project Management Institute Pulse of the Profession® in-depth report: Portfolio Management.* Project Management Institute; 2014. http://www.pmi.org.
3. Project Management Institute, Inc. *The Standard for Portfolio Management.* Newtown Square, PA: PMI Publications; 2006.
4. Mulcahy R. *Top Reasons Projects Fail*; 1999. http://www.pmi.org.
5. Bhide D. *Patient Care—A Project Management Perspective*; 2011. http://www.projectmanagement.com.
6. Rajegopal S. *Portfolio Management: How to Innovate and Invest in Successful Projects*; Basingstoke: Palgrave Macmillan; 2012.
7. Harrison FL, Lock D. *Advanced Project Management: A Structured Approach.* 4th ed. Aldershot: Gower; 2004.
8. Thiry M. *Program Management.* Burlington: Gower; 2010.
9. Reiss G. *Project Management Demystified: Today's Tools and Techniques*; London, UK: E&FN SPON; 1995.
10. Matthews D, Cooke-Davies T. *HSI: Portfolio Management Optimizes Your Strategic Position*; 2013. http://www.pmi.org.
11. Stang D, Handler R, Jones T. *Gartner Magic Quadrant. Magic Quadrant for IT Project and Portfolio Management Software Applications, Worldwide.* Gartner, Inc.; 2015.
12. Berkun S. *Making Things Happen: Mastering Project Management.* Revised ed. Sebastopo: O'Reilly Media; 2008.

■ DISCUSSION QUESTIONS

1. Discuss why some healthcare organizations continue to underutilize formal project management practices.
2. What effects will a fully implemented project management methodology have on an organization? How might it impact the budget?
3. What are additional benefits for healthcare organizations that utilize project management?
4. How can project management enhance healthcare quality or patient care?
5. Project management can help mitigate unrealistic or even made-up deadlines imposed by managers or leaders. Explain the relevance of this benefit in healthcare.
6. Discuss how healthcare project management can be optimized to be different from other industries.
7. Hospitals are separated in many individual and specialized departments that respond differently to project management. Discuss different aspects of an ideal healthcare organization that could be enhanced through project management.
8. Discuss the various challenges limiting actualization of project management in a healthcare environment. How can these challenges be resolved?

9. How can project management help reduce negativity about healthcare organizations that patients might hear about in the news media?

10. What are the advantages portfolio management in a healthcare environment?

CASE STUDY

A PM's ability to achieve a successful outcome can be impacted by the lack of standardization of project management processes. This case study is designed to help you understand the importance of the standardization of project management practices and identify ways you can influence the use of standard processes to determine what the potential problems and solutions might be.

You are a program manager who has been asked to implement a new electronic health record (EHR) to help meet new regulatory guidelines. You are enthusiastic about your role but have concerns about the lack of project management processes in your organization. You fully understand the ramifications of failure with the implementation, and so you are looking for ways to mitigate issues with a large number of departments involved.

You know that an EHR needs to be focused on patient care, quality, and business and clinical workflows. A multidisciplinary implementation team needs to be assembled and must include clinicians and IT and operational staff. Training for staff at all levels is required. IT will need to be engaged to customize templates and workflows.

The organization is unsure what value having one EHR will provide, so communication about benefits of such a system is important. You have a good relationship with external organizations who have implemented their own EHRs. You are planning a meeting with some of them to see what you can glean from what they learned, during implementation.

You need to effectively define the scope of work your project teams are expected to deliver. You are constrained by availability of clinical resources and related funding. You are told that both of these are not flexible, and your sponsor emphasizes the political nature of the situation. She asks for your input on how to best deal with these constraints from a project management perspective.

Discussion Questions

1. What do you propose to your stakeholder as possible solutions to the resource constraint issue? What might be project risks if resources are constrained?
2. How would you implement project management processes in your project even if they are not yet systemwide?
3. What would your first steps be to implement project management in this EHR initiative?
4. If there is resistance to the use of project management techniques, how might you influence stakeholders on adopting these processes?
5. Discuss why some healthcare organizations continue to underutilize formal project management practices.
6. What effects will a fully implemented project management methodology likely have on an organization? How might this impact the budget?
7. Hospitals are separated into many specialized departments that respond differently to project management. Discuss different aspects of an ideal healthcare organization that could be enhanced through project management.

18

Contract Negotiations and Software Licensing*

Jon C. Christiansen

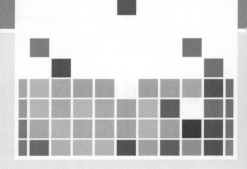

Never underestimate the leverage that a healthcare organization has to contractually protect itself.

OBJECTIVES

At the completion of this chapter, the reader will be prepared to:

1. Understand the implications of contract provisions commonly included in an agreement (contract) for software licensed to a healthcare organization (HCO).
2. Learn how to participate in the process of negotiating an agreement for software by understanding key elements,

compromises, and additional essentials to incorporate into the agreement.

3. Understand who should be involved in the negotiation process and roles these persons play.

KEY TERMS

cloud licensing, 300
derivative works, 300
limitations and exclusions of liability, 313
open source software, 300
service level agreement (SLA), 305

software as a service (SaaS), 300
software escrow, 305
software license agreements, 298
software warranty, 305

ABSTRACT ❖

Healthcare organizations (HCOs) need a negotiating team with the expertise and knowledge to properly assess and negotiate software license agreements with vendors. This team will need to represent different interests, including user, technical, finance, and legal interests of the HCO. The agreements provided by software vendors tend to be very one-sided and do not adequately protect HCOs or address all HCO needs. "Legalese," the legal terms and language of contracts, is not harmless and in many respects affects technical, business, and financial issues, including business continuity, data protection, return on investment, and other value propositions. HCOs should not underestimate their leverage to negotiate for better terms

in their software license agreement with vendors. This chapter describes a process for health information technology (IT) contract negotiation and provides a description of contract terms, related issues, and negotiation compromises.

INTRODUCTION

Healthcare organizations (HCOs) depend on computer software for the delivery of healthcare services to patients and for most, if not all, of their business operations. It is unimaginable today that an HCO could function without the use of software for a wide variety of applications and purposes, including clinical care, billing, security, compliance, research, and operations. Software vendors who provide the software are diverse in size, expertise, resources, ability, and the solutions they offer, but one practice they have in common is their insistence on software license agreements (also referred to as contracts) as a prerequisite to using their software. The term "vendor" refers to the licensor, service provider, or other company that licenses or provides the software to the HCO. The term *HCO* is used generically in this chapter to mean not only the HCO itself but also, when the context allows, the HCO's leadership or the designated representatives on a team doing the contract negotiations.

A negotiating team for a software agreement may be at the executive level or comprised of other designated team members

---

*The author of this chapter is a founder and managing attorney of TechLaw Ventures, PLLC, a law firm that focuses on transactions and disputes relating to technology and innovation. He has three decades of experience in representing licensors and licensees of software and information technology assets, including large healthcare organizations. He is also a founder and owner of EscrowTech International, Inc., a software and SaaS escrow company. The views expressed in this chapter reflect the bias, knowledge, and experience of the author, especially with respect to the types of software escrows discussed in this chapter.

who first work with the vendor on the terms and conditions of the agreement. Then, the agreement is signed by an executive such as the chief executive officer (CEO), chief financial officer (CFO), or the chief information officer (CIO) who is authorized to sign purchases or contracts and make financial commitments. A negotiating team's typical composition is listed in Box 18.1.

Although this chapter does not address Stark, anti-kickback, Health Information Portability and Accountability Act (HIPAA), and other regulatory issues, those issues must always be carefully considered and accounted for by the HCO. Details about legal issues may be found in Chapter 25, HIPAA is discussed in Chapter 26, and regulatory issues such as Health Information Technology for Economic Clinical Health (HITECH) and Meaningful Use are in Chapter 27.

This chapter focuses on commercial software license agreements rather than open source software licenses. It is written primarily to address traditional "on-premises" software licenses, but much of what is said about "on-premises" licenses also applies to cloud-based services. The chapter does include a discussion of cloud-based services (e.g., software as a service [SaaS] licenses) and is written from the perspective of informing healthcare professionals and informaticians who are expected to take a leadership role in understanding the

implications of these types of agreements. It is not written for attorneys but rather for others responsible for understanding and approving software license agreements and ensuring that the HCO complies with those agreements. By necessity, the chapter is not completely comprehensive (i.e., any given software license agreement is likely to include additional provisions not mentioned here and may not include some provisions that are mentioned). However, the chapter does provide a description of the topics and contractual provisions deemed the most relevant to the intended reader.

When purchasing a license for software that is "mission critical" or highly important, the HCO should be sure to understand what it is agreeing to and should make sure that the agreement makes sense in the context of the "real world" in which the HCO will use the software. Software license agreements can be relatively simple, but more often they are lengthy and complex and even confusing. They include provisions that address significant business and technical issues. They may also include provisions that are referred to as "legalese" or "boilerplate." These legalese or boilerplate provisions should never be dismissed or overlooked as "routine" or "harmless." These provisions, if enforced, can create some very unpleasant surprises with business, technical, financial, and/or patient care consequences.

In dealing with these types of agreements, there are three key points to always remember (Box 18.2).

OVERVIEW OF LICENSING AGREEMENTS

Intellectual Property Concepts Relevant to Software

Software is a "work of authorship" under the copyright laws. There is always a copyright to any software that is original (i.e., not copied from someone else). Copyrights only protect "expression" and not ideas, methods, facts, concepts, inventions, or systems. Writing computer software is analogous to writing a book. Both are expressions protected by copyright, but the concepts and ideas in them are not. Therefore copyrights can protect software against copying and even

---

BOX 18.1 Contract Negotiating Team Composition

- **The CFO.** This person or designed representative represents the financial interests of the HCO.
- **An attorney.** This attorney should generally understand relevant healthcare technology, intellectual property rights, and contract law. Experience in software license agreements is essential for proper representation.
- **The CIO** or designated representative. This team member understands the relevant technology, including the information systems of the HCO and the licensed software.
- **Key users.** One or more key stakeholders represent the software users and know what functionality and features are needed or expected by those users. These stakeholders may include a chief medical informatics officer or chief nursing informatics officer for a clinical system and/or clinical executive such as the chief medical or nursing executive.
- **Contract administrators.** If the HCO has contract administrators, then one of them may also be on the negotiating team.
- **Compliance officer.** This officer is needed to make sure that the agreement adequately and properly addresses HIPAA, Stark, anti-kickback, and other regulatory issues and does not include any provisions that could be construed as violating applicable law or patient privacy.
- **Security expert.** Software licenses and related services and data storage often trigger security concerns. A member of the HCO's security team should be involved not only to identify security risks in the agreement but to make sure that the agreement proactively address security risks as needed in a manner consistent with the HCO's security policies and practices.

CFO, Chief financial officer; *CIO,* chief information officer; *HCO,* healthcare organization.

BOX 18.2 Key Points About Agreements

- A vendor's form of agreement is not written to protect the HCO (i.e., the agreement is almost always very one-sided and written to protect the vendor).
- The HCO leadership should take the time and make the effort to clearly understand what the agreement says and what that means to the institution.
- The HCO leadership should negotiate these agreements to ensure the agreement meets the HCO's needs. Of course, the HCO leadership may not always have sufficient leverage to require the vendor to make the desired changes or to even negotiate the agreement, but in the author's experience, HCOs are more likely to underestimate their leverage than to overestimate it. Vendors need and want sales and can be reasonable. In the end, they want customers who are willing to sign up for software and services.

HCO, Healthcare organization.

against derivative works based on the software (a derivative work copies or includes at least some of the original expression). Infringement of a copyright requires that the original work be copied. Independent creation, even independent creation that was inspired by ideas and concepts in the original work, is not copyright infringement.

It is important to understand that copyright and patent are two different concepts. Copyright is a form of protection provided to the authors of "original" works. A patent protects the "invention" of an inventor. Sometimes, software includes or represents a patentable invention or the use of the software may be or involve a patentable method. If patented, the invention or method is protected by the patent, and to that extent the software is protected by the patent. Patent protection applies to inventions.[1] Therefore, patent protection is potentially much broader than copyright protection but is more difficult and expensive to obtain. A software vendor might have one or more patents applicable to its software. It is also possible that another person owns a patent that is infringed by the HCO's use of the software. A patent can be "innocently" infringed. Being unaware of the patent does not excuse infringement and is not a defense, but can be a mitigating factor when it comes to damages payable to the owner of the patent. If software is licensed to an HCO and if the vendor (licensor) owns a patent applicable to the software, then there is no infringement of the vendor's patent by the HCO because of the license. But the license is no defense if another person owns a patent that is infringed.

Trade secrets are a third form of intellectual property applicable to software. A trade secret is information that is not generally known to others and not readily ascertainable by others.[2] Trade secrets are protected against misappropriation (e.g., taking by improper means). Software can include trade secrets. The source code to commercial software is often held by the owner of the software as a trade secret. Open source software is not a trade secret, as the software and its source code are typically made available to the public and therefore are generally known to the public. Typically, when commercial software is distributed, it is the object code or executable code version of the software that is distributed and the source code is withheld from distribution. In such cases, the source code may be a trade secret.

Why Are Contracts Used for Software Licensing?

Vendors will insist on using a binding contract, such as a software license agreement, when licensing commercial software to an HCO. License agreements provide the vendor with contractual protection of its software in addition to intellectual property protection. They create binding obligations such as payment obligations and restrictions on use as well as limitations of liability and disclaimers that protect the vendor. However, a license agreement can also protect HCOs by including obligations and warranties binding on the vendor that give the HCO assurance as to the software and its functionality, performance, and compatibility, as well as other protections (e.g., indemnification against claims that the software infringes another person's intellectual property).

The Concept of Licensing Versus Sale

Software is "licensed," not sold, when distributed to customers. If the software itself were sold, this would give ownership to the customer, which is unacceptable to a vendor wanting to license the software to others. A license is, in effect, permission to use the software. A license to use software is sold, but the software itself is not sold. If the software were sold, it presumably means that the copyrights and other intellectual property in and to the software were also sold. Then the vendor would no longer have any rights to license the software to others without the permission of the new owner.

The media (e.g., DVDs) on which the software resides and is distributed to an HCO (1) may be owned by the HCO as a purchaser, or (2) may be leased or loaned to the HCO (i.e., the vendor owns the media). Ownership of the media is not an issue when software is downloaded by the HCO via the internet from the vendor or is remotely accessed and used by the HCO via the internet as in a software as a service (SaaS) agreement. Software as a service (SaaS) is a software distribution model where applications are hosted by a vendor and made available to customers over a network, typically the internet.

"On-Premises" Licensing Versus Licensing Through the "Cloud"

Traditionally, software licenses have been "on-premises" licenses, meaning that the software (usually the executable code but not the source code) is installed and runs on a computer or network located at the facility of the licensee (e.g., the HCO). (See Table 18.1 for definitions of the terms source code, executable code, and interpretive code.) Cloud licensing takes a different approach. The software resides and runs on the vendor's server(s), and the licensee (e.g., the HCO) remotely accesses and uses the software through the internet (e.g., via a web browser).

An example of cloud licensing is SaaS licensing. "True" SaaS can be characterized by a single instance of the software running on the vendor's server(s) that is accessed and used by multiple licensees (i.e., "multitenant"). This maximizes some of the benefits of a SaaS solution (e.g., the cost of hosting, running, maintaining, and supporting a single instance of the same version of

TABLE 18.1	Definition of Terms
Term	**Definition**
Source code	Software written in a programming language such as C++. The source code is understandable to the human programmer.
Executable code (machine code or object code)	Source code compiled into a format understandable by computers (machine code).
Interpretive code	Source code written in a specific language that is "interpreted" on the fly when the software is run to produce code that the computer can execute.

the software reduces costs when those costs can be shared by multiple licensees). The term *SaaS* can also apply to solutions that are not single instance or multitenant, although some persons may not consider such solutions as "true SaaS."

Other cloud services and licenses (and terms that are used to identify them) include hosting, managed services, on-demand services, and application service provider (ASP) services. Some agreements are structured as a hybrid between or combination of an "on-premises" license and a "cloud" license. For example, some vendors will license the software through an "on-premises" license but then offer hosting services through a services agreement (e.g., a hosting or managed services agreement). In such cases, the HCO is licensed to use the software under the license but engages the vendor through a services agreement to host and run the software for the HCO on the vendor's servers. If the services agreement were to terminate, it remains possible for the HCO to run and use the software on its own computers or network under the terms of the "on-premises" license agreement.

The Vendor's Contract: Healthcare Organizations, Beware!

Typically, the vendor has a standard template for a license agreement. However, it is often possible to negotiate the terms of any software license, as the vendor's version should be viewed by the HCO as only a starting point. The vendor's form of agreement is mostly designed to protect the vendor as opposed to protecting the HCO. The agreement usually includes legalese that can mislead, surprise an HCO, or in some cases offend basic concepts of fairness. It often fails to include many protections and assurances important to the HCO. Health providers and informaticians involved in contract negotiations should not be distracted by the "friendliness" of a vendor or with the developing informatics–vendor relationship, but rather they should focus on gaining a clear and objective understanding of what is in the agreement. HCOs should not hesitate to negotiate aggressively for the needs of the healthcare institution. Vendors can be persuaded to change their agreements, but they will not do so if no demand or request for change is clearly made. *HCOs should not underestimate their leverage.* While HCOs should negotiate firmly and aggressively for the need of the institution, a collegial, professional manner is always the most effective way to reach an acceptable agreement. The HCO and its representatives should have and maintain an amicable and professional relationship with the vendor at all times, and contract negotiations are no exception.

The Mechanics and Process of Contract Negotiation for a Software License

Although situations will vary, the progression of a negotiated agreement is likely to include a process similar to the one outlined in Box 18.3. As is illustrated, the process involves numerous "back and forth" steps.

The reason for having the vendor prepare a second draft is that this allows the agreement to move closer to what the HCO needs and wants in an agreement before the HCO starts to change the agreement. Assuming that the vendor accommodates some of the changes requested by the HCO in the first teleconference or meeting, there will be fewer changes that the HCO needs to make in its final draft (i.e., third draft). In the process, there should be shared control of the agreement document, by taking turns in preparing response drafts that are redlined to show changes to the prior draft. Two major tips for version control are listed in Box 18.4.

Before the Agreement Is Signed: Due Diligence

Even the best agreement is not a substitute for due diligence (see also Chapter 16 on system selection processes). The HCO should check with other users and even visit their sites.

BOX 18.3 Typical Negotiating Process for an Agreement

1. Vendor's standard form of agreement—Draft #1.
2. HCO reviews Draft #1.
3. Telephone conference or meeting with the vendor to discuss Draft #1.
4. Vendor prepares Draft #2.
5. HCO reviews Draft #2.
6. HCO prepares Draft #3.
7. Vendor reviews Draft #3.
8. Telephone conference or meeting with the vendor.
9. Vendor prepares Draft #4.
10. Repeat as necessary to reach final agreement.

HCO, Healthcare organization.

BOX 18.4 Tips on How to Control the Versions of a Draft Contract

Tip #1: If a vendor insists that it must control all drafting and refuses to provide an editable draft that is not locked or protected, simply inform the vendor (especially its salespeople) that this will greatly delay the negotiating process, as the HCO must then "type up" (or convert from a locked PDF) the entire agreement from the uneditable draft provided by the vendor to create an editable draft so that changes can be "tracked" and then sent to the vendor in an editable form. Given the complexity and length of license agreements, this is not a trivial issue, as the HCO's representatives responsible for the agreement and negotiating process will incur much more review time if they cannot rely on "document comparison" and "tracking" functionality in word processing software that can be used on editable documents. Also, manual typing, text readers, and other conversions can introduce errors. In any event, a careful reading of the final version of the agreement is critical before it is signed. This will ensure no provisions in the contract were changed during the numerous steps without the HCO knowing the changes.

Tip #2: Whenever there is a teleconference or meeting to negotiate the agreement, it is always advantageous to the HCO if the then-most-recent draft on the negotiating table (other than the first draft) is a draft provided by the HCO, even if that means reducing the frequency of the calls or meetings to negotiate.

HCO, Healthcare organization.

Although somewhat uncomfortable for both the vendor and the HCO, the HCO can ask who has recently discontinued use of the vendor's software and why. References provided by the vendor are not likely to include customers with bad experiences or complaints that the HCO might need to know about. Sometimes vendors are asked to provide financial statements so that the financial stability of the vendor can be assessed. Suddenly losing support and maintenance services (not to mention hosting or SaaS services) from a vendor in bankruptcy or buyouts can be a huge problem.

Always conduct due diligence on alternative vendors to get the best value. This also strengthens negotiating leverage with the first vendor and puts the HCO in position, should the need arise, to terminate negotiations with the first vendor and more rapidly move to negotiations with a second. The HCO needs to know its requirements and must clearly communicate those requirements to the vendor. Document the responses from the vendor to these requirements, including those presented during demonstrations of the software. Outside consultants/experts engaged by the HCO may be useful to it in the due diligence and negotiating process.

Use the Request for Proposal Process

Request for proposal (RFP) or request for information (RFI) or similar mechanisms are worth the effort, time, and expense if the software is mission critical or of high importance or high cost to the HCO. The RFP process, outlined in Chapter 16, sets forth the HCO's requirements and expectations for the software, including its functionality, performance, compatibility, etc. Do not overlook data, data migration, and data warehousing issues, if relevant. The RFP should also be used to ask relevant questions of prospective vendors, including costs. The more comprehensive the RFP, then the more comprehensive the response should be from the vendor. This will reduce the likelihood of misunderstandings and surprises later. Traditionally, an RFP is used with multiple vendors and is the basis for a bidding, comparison, and selection process, but even if there is only one vendor in the running, the RFP process is extremely valuable and very important in successfully negotiating a good license agreement.

The vendor's response to the RFP should be made a part of the license agreement. For example, the license agreement can reference the vendor's response and state that the vendor stands behind its response (i.e., that the response is accurate and that any promise or assurance in the response will be met by the vendor). Because of the nature of "Entire Agreement" clauses (see the next section), the response will be of no effect if not incorporated into the license agreement.

If the vendor objects to the inclusion of its response to the RFP in the license agreement, then the HCO should insist that the HCO relied on the vendor's response in the selection of the vendor. If the vendor still objects, the HCO should offer to allow the vendor to correct or clarify its response, and then the corrected or clarified response should be added to the agreement. If the corrections reveal some unpleasant surprises, it is better for the HCO to know before rather than after signing the agreement.

Although it is not common to do so, the RFP should be used to address the tough contract issues (including legal issues) that inevitably arise in contract negotiations (e.g., limitations of liability, termination, and scope of use). Negotiating these is much more difficult after the vendor knows that it has been selected, so now is the time. This approach can reduce the amount of time spent negotiating the agreement and can lead to a better result for the HCO.

The "Entire Agreement" Clause: Know What This Means!

An "Entire Agreement" clause also known to attorneys as an integration clause might read as follows:

> Entire Agreement. This Agreement is the entire agreement between the parties with regard to the subject matter of this Agreement and supersedes and incorporates all prior or contemporaneous representations, understandings or agreements, and may not be modified or amended except by an agreement in writing signed by the parties hereto.

What does this mean? Since no competent attorney for the vendor will allow you to negotiate this out of the agreement, the HCO must put everything it is relying on in the agreement. Exhibits, addendums, appendices, and documents that are incorporated by reference into the agreement can be used for this purpose. Statements made by salespersons, demonstrations, marketing materials, and other peripheral statements and documents do not count unless they are incorporated into the agreement. The agreement should identify what the HCO is paying for (Box 18.5).

MAJOR STEPS OR STAGES IN THE PERFORMANCE OF A LICENSE AGREEMENT

Although there is significant variation, a mission-critical license agreement might include the steps and stages listed in Box 18.6.

BOX 18.5   Elements in an Agreement Typically Paid for by HCOs

- Licensed software/databases
- Hardware
- Third-party software
- Technical and end user documentation
- Customizations

- Interfaces
- Implementation services
- Support
- Maintenance
- Other services (e.g., data migration)

HCO, Healthcare organization.

SPECIFIC COMPONENTS OF THE LICENSING AGREEMENT

Major components of a licensing agreement are located in Box 18.7. Specifics are discussed in the following sections.

Definitions of Terms

The agreement should include definitions of all vendor-specific terms and concepts, as mentioned in Chapter 16. The system selection team, negotiating team, or designated representatives should review these to ensure they are consistent with the HCOs use of the terms and for clarity.

Time Schedule

The license agreement should include a time schedule to keep the vendor on time (e.g., a project timeline for purchasing hardware, installing initial software, customizing the software, building interfaces, training, testing, acceptance, and go-live events). The contract should contain a good estimate of the initial project from start to go-live and acceptance testing. For example, a community hospital may project an 18-month timeline that is broken into discrete events. The time schedule should address most major stages, objectives, or milestones of the project, not just delivery of the software. The time schedule can be tied in whole or in part to an implementation plan (project plan). (For more information about project management, see Chapter 17.) Generally, vendors resist contractual time commitments, but usually an HCO can get some meaningful time commitments or at least good faith estimates. Even if the estimates are nonbinding, they create expectations and increase the probability that the project will be completed within an expected time frame. Furthermore, payment milestones or monetary incentives can be tied to milestones, even if the dates associated with the milestones are nonbinding estimates. For example, the vendor would not be in breach of the agreement for failing to meet an estimated time schedule date for a given milestone, but if that milestone is also a payment milestone, then payment may be delayed until the milestone is met.

Assuming that the vendor is committed to a time schedule, the agreement should indicate the consequences of a failure to meet the schedule. Such consequences may include liquidated damages, credits, discounts, or delay in payments. For example, if a go-live date is missed by more than a week, the contract may specify that the license fee might be reduced by a specified amount. In response, some vendors may seek financial incentives for early or timely performance of the schedule. In our previous example, a vendor might receive a bonus payment for an early go-live date. Assuming the vendor accepts the concept of a binding time schedule, the HCO should expect the vendor to insist on exceptions for delay or nonperformance caused by the HCO, another supplier, or a *force majeure* (disruptions caused by causes beyond the control of the vendor such as natural disasters or other unforeseeable circumstances beyond the control of a group). The vendor may also insist on building a margin for error into the time schedule.

Scope of the License
Who Are the Users?

Fundamentally, the license is permission from the vendor for the HCO to use the software. The license agreement needs to define who may use and access the software. Obviously, this includes the HCO and its employees, but a broader scope may be needed. Do others (nonemployees) need to use or access the software? Often, the answer is yes! Affiliated corporations, companies, and organizations (e.g., a subsidiary or sister corporation) may need to be included as users of the software. Other examples are (1) independent physicians having admitting privileges at the HCO's hospitals; (2) independent healthcare providers and clinics (e.g., to share medical records or perform billing); (3) patients or their family members who will see screen displays or output generated by the software;

BOX 18.6 Steps in the Performance of a Mission Critical License Agreement

- Create specifications (before or after signing of the agreement).
- Develop customized components and interfaces, if needed.
- Deliver the defined software and documentation (the "deliverables").
- Install and implement the software.
- Train HCO's personnel.
- Conduct acceptance testing of the software and then accept the software if it passes the testing.
- Determine when the warranty period begins.
- Determine when the maintenance and support phases begin.
- Conduct future phases and projects, if applicable.

HCO, Healthcare organization.

BOX 18.7 Main Components of a Licensing Agreement

- Definition of terms
- Time schedule
- Scope of the license
- Scope of use
- Derivation works
- Software and SaaS escrow
- Specifications
- Software warranties
- Service level agreements
- Acceptance
- Maintenance and support, other services (e.g., implementation support)
- Revenue recognition and payments
- Dispute resolution
- Termination
- Limitations and exclusions of liability
- Special clauses—confidentiality, intellectual property infringement

SaaS, Software as a service.

(4) consultants, other independent contractors (e.g., programmers), and volunteers; and (5) in some cases affiliated foundations or staff and students from affiliated institutions of higher learning. For example, the emergency department may contract with an outside billing agency. This outside agency needs to be mentioned as a user. Otherwise, billing and reimbursements will be negatively affected. The HCO needs to anticipate who the users will be and then make sure that the license agreement allows for those users.

Rights

The basic rights to software under a license are permissions to
- Use the software
- Copy the software as needed for licensed use
- Generate and use the output of the software (e.g., screen displays and reports)

Sometimes, but not often, other rights are included in a software license:
- Disclose the software or its output or screen displays to others
- Distribute the software to others—special cases
- Modify the software and create derivative works based on it

Restrictions and License Metrics

The scope of the license will often be subject to "internal use" or "permitted use" restrictions. The language may vary, but the HCO should be comfortable that these types of restrictions do not prohibit the intended use of the software. For example, a simple restriction that the software may only be used for internal purposes might prohibit a use of the software that benefits or involves others outside of the HCO. The scope of a software license is often defined or limited by various license metrics, such as those listed in Box 18.8.

HCOs should anticipate that applicable license metrics might be exceeded at some time in the future and to provide for the same discounted pricing originally negotiated to cover the excess. An annual "true up" of the license is a good approach. In other words, the agreement should allow for a review of the situation annually and for the payment of additional license fees if needed to cover the excess. With this approach, the HCO will not be in breach of the agreement

for exceeding a license metric provided that the HCO does a "true up" at the end of each year.

Scope of Use
Number of Copies

The license might include limits on the number of copies of the software. An extreme example might be the following clause: *Vendor grants to HCO a license to use one copy of the software and to have and maintain one back-up copy of the software.* This is a problem because multiple copies of the software can be found in the areas listed in Box 18.9.

An HCO will certainly exceed a one copy limit just by virtue of the fact that software held in the computer's memory (e.g., random access memory, or RAM) is legally considered under the copyright laws as a copy of the software and that there will be a copy of the software on the hard drive. Any limitation on the number of copies should reflect the reality of the technology and the use.

Environments and Instances

Sometimes a license is limited to certain number and types of environments and instances. If so, and at the very least, the HCO will need to be licensed to use the software in a "production environment" or to use one "production instance" of the software. The HCO's technical advisors should review this wording carefully to be sure that it is adequate in the context of expected use. Often the HCO will want the right to use the software in more than one production environment or in other environments, such as testing, training, development, and recovery environments. The same is true if this concept is expressed in terms of "instances" or some other technical terminology.

Derivative Works

Normally, a software license will prohibit the HCO from modifying the software or creating derivative works based on the software. But if the HCO needs to maintain, customize, or enhance the software, then the HCO will need to expand the license to include permission to modify and create derivative works. In such case and at a minimum, the agreement needs to require the vendor to provide the materials listed in Box 18.10 to the HCO.

The HCO will also need programmers, employees, or contractors with the necessary abilities to use the source code to maintain, customize, and enhance the software. More may be needed, depending on the particulars of the software and

---

BOX 18.8   Typical License Metrics in a Software License

- Number of "named" users (either by specific name or by category such as physician, nurse or pharmacist)
- Number of "concurrent" users
- Number of computers, servers, or workstations
- Number of processors or other measure of processing power
- Number of users or seats
- Number of procedures, images, reports, etc.
- Specific site or facilities
- Entire enterprise, etc.

BOX 18.9   Where Copies of Software Might Exist

- The master copy provided by the vendor
- Updates of the software
- Memory (e.g., RAM)
- Storage devices (e.g., hard drives)
- Backups (and other archive and disaster recovery storage)
- Nonproduction (non-live) environments used for testing, training, development, etc.

> **BOX 18.10   Materials to Be Provided to the Healthcare Organization If Derivative Work Rights Are Granted**
>
> - Source code and comments (if not already delivered as part of the software)
> - Development environment (to the extent not commercially available)
> - Programming documentation (e.g., compilation and build instructions)
> - Updates to the foregoing to keep current with the software used by the HCO
> - Anything needed by developers to understand the source code

HCO, Healthcare organization.

> **BOX 18.11   Types of Specifications in Agreements**
>
> - Features and functionality
> - Reports, forms, screen displays, output, input
> - Compatibility with hardware, operating system, third-party software, etc.
> - Communications and networking
> - Minimum system requirements
>   - System software (e.g., operating system)
>   - Other third-party software
>   - Hardware and peripheral devices
>   - Communications, networking, interfaces, etc.
> - Performance (e.g., response time; and latency in the case of a SaaS solution)
> - Interfaces, etc.

SaaS, software as a service.

environments in which it is developed and used. Also, third-party software may be needed.

Software and Software as a Service Escrows

For mission-critical or highly important software, an escrow may be included with the license agreement for business continuity purposes. For instance, if the vendor goes out of business or otherwise ceases to provide maintenance of the software (e.g., to fix programming errors or to update the software), the HCO may be left in an untenable position. A software escrow is a means to provide protection of the HCO if such event arises. For a software escrow, a neutral third-party escrow company holds the source code, programming documentation, and other items needed for maintenance and modification of the software. The escrow agreement includes release conditions and release procedures and legalese addressing intellectual property and bankruptcy law issues. A release condition is typically the bankruptcy or insolvency of the vendor, the vendor's breach of maintenance or other obligations, the discontinuation of maintenance and support by the vendor, the vendor going out of business, or in any other manner the vendor discontinuing support and maintenance of the software. The occurrence of a release condition entitles the HCO to receive the escrowed materials from the escrow company.

A SaaS escrow is an escrow for a SaaS or other cloud-based software solution. It is similar to the typical software escrow described previously, but also includes having the escrow company maintain a mirror or very similar solution on its own server in a condition that can be brought live and online for the HCO's use in the event that a release condition occurs or the HCO's access to the software is terminated by the vendor. The frequency of data updates to the escrow's server is just one of many details to be addressed in the escrow agreement. How "hot," "warm," or "cold" the escrowed solution (at the escrow company's data center) is affects cost and how quickly the escrowed solution can be brought live for the HCO.

Specifications

The HCO should not shortchange the required specifications, as these define the software that the HCO expects to receive. Specifications may apply to warranties, acceptance, payment

milestones, and maintenance obligations of the vendor. The initial draft of the license agreement from the vendor will likely include few or no specifications. The HCO should negotiate for meaningful specifications and preferably create and negotiate them prior to the signing of the agreement. Sometimes, the specifications need to be created after signing. If so, then stage 1 of the agreement can focus on the creation of the specifications. If parties agree on the specifications (which is almost always the case), then they proceed to subsequent stages of the agreement. If they do not agree, then the agreement is terminated.

Many types of specifications can be included in the agreement, such as those in Box 18.11. If the agreement includes custom development and if the development is "agile," then few if any specifications may exist. Agile software development[3] has its advantages that may outweigh the protections that we try to achieve for the HCO in an agreement.

Software Warranties

Sometimes the vendor offers no warranty (i.e., software is provided "as is" without any guarantee). The HCO should refuse to accept such an agreement. A good software warranty addresses most or all of the components in Box 18.12. The vendor is likely to have in its draft of the license agreement disclaimers or protections listed in Box 18.13.

There may be other disclaimers or limitations. For example, a clause may state that the software is not intended or licensed for high-risk uses or applications. The HCO should seek clarification that those high-risk uses or applications do not apply to healthcare or the specific purposes the HCO intends for its use of the software.

Service Level Agreements

When the license agreement is a SaaS agreement, a service level agreement (SLA) is often included as part of, or in addition to, the SaaS agreement. The SLA is intended to define certain service levels and the consequences of a failure to meet those levels. Typically, the service levels are not commitments of the vendor. The vendor is not in breach of contract for

---

BOX 18.12 Components of a Software Warranty

A good software warranty addresses most or all of the following:

- Programming errors (a "No Error" warranty is not realistic)
- Compliance with specifications
- Compliance with documentation
- Performance problems
- Output or input problems or errors
- Interface, network, or communications problems
- Compatibility
- Minimum system configuration

Other warranties may address:

- No self-help code or termination triggers
- No viruses or harmful code
- Compliance of the software with applicable laws and government regulations (e.g., HIPAA)
- Meaningful Use certification
- Vendor owns software or has right to license
- No conflict with other contracts or rights of others
- Non-infringement of intellectual property
- Compliance with privacy, security, and IT policies

BOX 18.13 License Agreement Disclaimers or Protections

- No warranties clause or "as is" approach (you get only what you get)
- A clause requiring the HCO to agree that there are no warranties that are not expressly included in agreement
- A clause disclaiming all implied warranties, including the following implied warranties:
  - Merchantability
  - Fitness for a particular purpose
  - Non-infringement

HCO, Healthcare organization.

---

failure to meet those levels but is only obligated to provide the specified remedy (e.g., credits as explained later on if the levels are not achieved).

Uptime

The most common service levels address uptime versus downtime (i.e., availability of the software to the HCO), response time, resolution time, latency, and performance. When calculating uptime (or downtime), scheduled downtime for maintenance and updates is commonly not considered downtime. Also, health professionals and informaticians need to understand that 100% uptime is typically not feasible. For each increment toward 100% uptime, expenses can increase dramatically and be unaffordable. However, redundant systems can be designed and implemented to support critical areas. Leaders will want to weigh the areas supported by the software (mission critical, patient safety) with their tolerance for downtime. Some may need 100% (intensive care,

operating rooms), while business offices could have less stringent requirements.

Obviously, scheduled maintenance should not include emergency fixes. Adjustments are also made for downtime caused by the HCO (e.g., connectivity issues or failure to meet the vendor's requirements). Force majeure events (i.e., disruptions beyond the control of the vendor such as natural disasters like floods, war, or lightning strikes) are also often excluded from uptime calculations. The HCO should ensure that the vendor is obligated to maintain disaster recovery solutions sufficient to overcome many force majeure events (see Chapter 20 on downtime and disaster recovery). Because of these adjustments to uptime calculations, an uptime service level of 99.999% is not likely to reflect true uptime and availability of the software. The appropriate uptime percentage should be based on a number of factors, including the criticality of the software and impact that downtime would have on the HCO. An uptime of 99.999% is generally considered the gold standard, but lesser uptimes may be appropriate and less costly (i.e., the HCO would likely have to pay more for the gold standard). Even if an uptime percentage of near 100% is achieved, there can still be other issues, such as network bottlenecks, poor latency, and other performance problems.

There can be disagreement about what "uptime" means. Does it simply mean that the HCO is able to access the software? What if some critical functionality of the software is producing errors or is not functioning but 90% of the functionality is available? The agreement should be clear. *A very favorable clause for the HCO would define "uptime" as the time during which the software, including all of its functionality and without material error, is available for access and use by the HCO.*

Performance

In the context of a SaaS agreement, users will not tolerate a painfully slow performing solution, and the SLA should be drafted to address this. Sometimes this type of performance is described as response time (i.e., the time for the computer running the software to respond to the user's input of a command). These performance issues can be very complex and difficult to precisely define in an SLA, and slow performance is not necessarily the fault of the vendor or the software. A simpler solution, but often unacceptable to the vendor, is to use general wording to define a service level in terms of reasonableness (e.g., response time will not be unreasonable).

Response Time and Resolution Time

A different type of response time is the time it takes for the vendor to respond to a notice of a problem. It is easy to draft this type of response time in an SLA. Resolution time is much more difficult. Without knowing what the problem is, the vendor will be hesitant to commit to a resolution time or even to guarantee that the problem will be resolved. Nonetheless, the HCO should attempt to build these concepts into the SLA or into warranties elsewhere in the agreement. One compromise is to have good response times coupled with an assurance by the HCO that diagnosis or troubleshooting of the problem will begin within the response time period and that efforts to resolve the problem will be diligently pursued to completion as soon as reasonably possible. This should also include a promise to provide a workaround solution, if practicable, while the permanent resolution is being worked on. This compromise may be better expressed as a warranty or contractual promise outside of the SLA and in some other part of the agreement instead.

Problem Severity

An SLA commonly defines the problem in terms of different categories of severity. Simplistically, categories will range from critical to nothing more than a minor fix or a change request. The HCO should carefully review the actual wording used by the vendor to define severity categories, because a lesser category may result in a long and unacceptable resolution time. For example, the resolution time for a low-severity category might be nothing more than a promise by the vendor to include a fix in the next release of the software without any assurance as to if and when the next release will take place. The HCO should insist that a patient safety issue is critical and should be addressed within a few hours.

The agreement may spell out response times and severity levels in simple terms or very complex details. The HCO should note that a "response" is not a solution. A response time of 30 minutes may only mean that the vendor's support personnel will acknowledge receipt of a support ticket. The agreement should at least require diligence in diagnosing and troubleshooting the problem and then solving it. Temporary workaround solutions should be provided, if practicable, by the vendor while the HCO is waiting for a permanent fix.

Vendors vary on their contractual commitments to fix a problem. The range of commitments include those listed in Box 18.14.

Remedies

The usual remedy for a failure to meet an SLA level is a credit to be applied against future payments to the vendor. For uptime, the credit may be defined as a percentage of the SaaS fee for the time period measured based on the level of uptime achieved for that same period. As the level of uptime decreases, the credit increases. Remedies other than credits can be used in an SLA, but vendors are typically reluctant to use anything other than credits. The HCO should make sure that the SLA allows for use of the credit to pay for any obligation to the vendor, not just as a credit against future payments of a SaaS fee. For example, the HCO should be allowed to apply credits toward additional services (e.g.,

training, consulting, custom development, data migration, and additional software products). It should also allow for the HCO to collect cash for the credit if the credit still exists at the time the agreement terminates.

Vendors usually include a clause in SLAs to the effect that the credit or other remedy is the sole and exclusive remedy for a failure to meet an SLA level. The HCO should be leery about this. For example, this should never apply to a breach by the vendor of an obligation to provide maintenance of the software. As a more extreme example, if the credit for uptime is capped at 25% of the SaaS fee, then literally the SLA would still require the HCO to pay the remaining 75% of the SaaS fee even if uptime were 0%. Of course that would be outrageous, but the literal wording of many SLAs actually mean this. As ultimate protection, the HCO should insist on the right to terminate the SaaS agreement if the SLA levels are significantly or continuously not met. This termination right is in addition to other remedies.

Acceptance of the Software

After implementation, the HCO should have the right to test and then accept (or reject) the software. Acceptance should be based on conformance of the software to the acceptance criteria. Acceptance criteria can include those listed in Box 18.15.

If a problem (i.e., nonconformance with any acceptance criterion) is discovered through the testing, then the HCO should reject the software and the vendor should be required to fix the problem and redeliver the software for retesting. If and when no problem is discovered, then the HCO should accept the software. The process may be repeated as necessary.

In some situations, it may be important to first do pre-live (preproduction) testing of the software before it is used and tested in a "live" ("production") environment. With this approach, the HCO does not risk using the software in a live environment (on live data and at the risk of patients' well-being) until after it is accepted through pre-live testing. But testing based on live data in a live environment is still important because live testing can reveal problems not discovered in a pre-live environment. In effect, the testing and acceptance (or rejection) process is repeated for the live environment.

Sometimes vendors want separate acceptance testing of software components, applications, and interfaces. If done

---

BOX 18.14 The Range of Vendor Commitments to Fix Problems

- Absolute commitment that errors will be fixed!
- Best efforts to fix
- Commercially reasonable efforts to fix
- "You get what you get"—which may be a late fix or no fix

BOX 18.15 Typical Acceptance Criteria in an Agreement

- Relevant provisions in the agreement (such as functionality or software performance once installed)
- Warranties
- Response to RFP or RFI issues
- Specifications exhibit
- Free of known errors
- End user documentation and other documentation
- Specifications published by the vendor

RFP, Request for proposal; *RFI*, request for information.

separately, this might not reveal problems that arise when the whole system (all components, applications, and interfaces) is used and should not be acceptable to the HCO. A possible compromise is to have a preliminary acceptance of each component, application, or interface, followed later by final acceptance testing of the complete system.

For a multisite solution, testing of the software at one site may not reveal all problems when the software goes live for all sites, especially if there is transmission or sharing of data between sites or other interactions between sites. Final testing and acceptance for all sites is advisable.

Software acceptance should be one of the payment milestones on which a portion of the license fee is conditioned. But vendors may resist this for revenue recognition reasons.

Remedies for Rejection

The HCO's right to reject the software if acceptance criteria are not met should be expressly stated in agreement. The vendor should be obligated to fix problems and redeliver for a repeat of acceptance testing. The entire software should be retested, not just the corrected portion of the software because correcting one problem may lead to a new one.

Often a difficult issue to negotiate with the vendor is the concept of an absolute obligation to fix versus an effort to use "best efforts" or "commercially reasonable efforts" to try to fix. This is just one more issue to negotiate. There may be time limits on the time to complete a fix or to provide a workaround solution. What happens if acceptance testing still fails after repeated attempts to correct the problem? How many tries and how long will the vendor have to correct problems? This needs to be negotiated and addressed in the agreement.

In the event of ultimate failure, vendors will usually say that the HCO will get a refund of the license fee but only for the software components or applications that fail. There is no refund for other software components and applications that pass and are accepted and no refund for services (e.g., installation, implementation, training). This should be unacceptable to the HCO. For example, if some of the accepted software components require an unaccepted component, then the HCO should be able to reject everything. (As a reminder, for more detail on downtime and disaster recovery, see Chapter 20.)

The HCO should have the option to elect one of the following remedies in Box 18.16 if the software ultimately fails to pass acceptance testing.

Maintenance and Support

Maintenance and support by the vendor of the software are essential in most license agreements. An HCO should not rely on continued use of software that is not adequately maintained and supported by the vendor. Maintenance and support include some or all of the components listed in Box 18.17.

HCOs may employ various tactics to reduce maintenance and support costs, which involve high costs to the organization. The HCO may create its own help desk to discount or

---

> **BOX 18.16 Possible Remedies If Software Fails Acceptance Testing**
>
> 1. Final rejection of the software by the HCO
>   - Software is de-installed and erased or destroyed or, if this is a SaaS solution, access to the software is terminated.
>   - The HCO receives a complete refund.
>   - Of what? Some or all of the license fees, hardware payments, third-party software fees, fees for customization, implementation and development, other fees, etc.?
>   - This would need to be negotiated.
> 2. Acceptance of the software "as is" with compensation for the nonconformance with the acceptance criteria.
>   - Compensation can be a partial refund, credit, some free services, or additional software licenses.
>   - This acceptance should not excuse the vendor's obligation to maintain the software.
> 3. Some other solution that the vendor and HCO agree to.

HCO, Healthcare organization; *SaaS,* software as a service.

> **BOX 18.17 Maintenance and Support Components in an Agreement**
>
> Maintenance components include the following:
> - Fix programming errors
> - Fix failure to conform to documentation
> - Fix failure to comply with specifications
> - Fix performance problems (e.g., response time, latency issues)
> - Fix anything that's a breach of warranty after warranty period
> - Keep software current with laws, regulations, etc.
> - Provide workaround solutions
> - Provide updates, upgrades, new versions, and future releases.
>
> Support includes some or all of the following:
> - Telephone calls and access to help desk
> - E-mail support
> - Answering questions but not training
> - Website support
> - Access to other support resources
> - Consultation
> - Diagnosis and troubleshooting of software problems
> - Solve software problems
> - Site visits if necessary

---

reduce fees payable for support. Through the HCO's help desk, support personnel provide frontline or first-tier support to HCO users of the software. Then the vendor's support personnel provide backup or second tier support to the HCO's support personnel as needed, not to other HCO users.

The agreement should clearly indicate the support hours of the vendor. Will support only be available during business hours (in which time zone?) or is 24/7 support needed? This depends on the nature of the software and the HCO's reliance on it. The HCO or its attorney should not automatically demand 24/7 support, because it is likely going to cost much more. If 24/7 support is needed, then it should be included.

Maintenance Fees

Fees for maintenance and support are typically 12% to 24% and more typically 15% to 22% of the license fee per year. If the license agreement is a SaaS agreement, the maintenance and support is typically included in the annual or other recurring SaaS fees.

The HCO should seek to cap increases on these fees. The cap may be based on a percentage or CPI (a specified customer price index) or other limit. The HCO should also consider negotiating for multiyear fixed prices to facilitate budget planning and to preserve discounts.

A significant issue is how long the vendor will commit to provide support and maintenance. This should be at least 5 years and preferably for a longer period sufficient to cover the expected return on the investment. HCOs should not be locked into the same number of years. They should be able to terminate support and maintenance after any year, because a reason for discontinuing use of the software may arise. No one wants to explain why the HCO is paying for support and maintenance of software no longer being used. Although this approach is not reciprocal, many provisions exist in a license agreement that are not reciprocal. Moreover, vendors should not sell licenses if they cannot assure long-term support.

Payment for support and maintenance should also entitle the HCO to updates and new releases of the software. The fine print in the agreement may make exceptions to this obligation or charge extra fees in some cases. Scrutiny of the agreement is needed.

The agreement should indicate how far back versions of the software will be supported and maintained. For example, an agreement may indicate that only the most current version of the software will be supported and maintained, but the HCO may want to continue to use prior versions. Upgrading to a new version may be costly, time consuming, and inconvenient. Security issues may arise when a new version is implemented. At some point, upgrading becomes necessary, as the HCO cannot reasonably expect the vendor to continue to support and maintain versions that are long outdated. Compromises on this issue often include support and maintenance for one or two of the most recent prior versions or giving the HCO a period of time to upgrade. After that is resolved, another good idea is to require the vendor to support and maintain old versions if the HCO is willing to pay a premium, a "just in case" precaution.

If the overall software solution includes third-party software, then support of the third-party software may not be covered by the support and maintenance obligations in the agreement and may instead depend on the support and maintenance provided by the third party. Make sure this is understood prior to signing the agreement and is adequately addressed.

Other Services

The license agreement should include other vendor services that the HCO needs or may want (e.g., those listed in Box 18.18).

BOX 18.18 Other Services to Include in a License Agreement

- Installation and implementation
- Training
- Data conversion
- Interfaces
- Development, customizations

BOX 18.19 Services to Include for Implementation Efforts

- Implementation approaches, such as "big bang" or incremental
- Vendor personnel and their qualifications
- Initial training for HCO functional and technical teams with specified approaches such as "train the trainer"
- Vendor "go-live" implementation support team as adjuncts to site super-users
- Consultation services (e.g., experts to act as implementation teams or experts who assess a site's implementation plans)

HCO, Healthcare organization.

System Implementation or Installation Support

Agreements often include services in support of system implementation, as listed in Box 18.19.

A significant issue can be "hours vs. results" when purchasing additional services. Is the HCO just buying "hours and effort" or "results"? For example, paying by the hour or day is no assurance as to how many hours or days it may take to complete a project or task. Or is the HCO buying results and basing payment on results (e.g., paying a fixed fee for completion of a project or task)? These are different approaches, each with pros and cons. If the HCO insists on a fixed-fee approach, the quote from the vendor is likely to build in a healthy margin for error, possibly resulting in a higher cost to the HCO. This approach gives certainty in budgeting and a greater chance that the results will be obtained without cost overruns. If the "buying hours and efforts" approach is used, the HCO should also include in the agreement the number of hours that the vendor estimates in good faith is needed for completion. The estimate can help the HCO negotiate if the vendor exceeds the estimated hours and asks for more.

The HCO should include in the agreement an open-ended obligation for the vendor to provide other or additional services at the option of the HCO, if they are needed by the HCO, as not everything can be anticipated at the time the agreement is signed. Needs may occur for additional assistance on installation, implementation, and data conversion; for more training; for more customization and interfaces; or for more consultation. Although additional fees (plus expenses) will have to be paid, it is worth having the option, if needed.

Outsourcing to Data Centers for Hosting and Software Management Services

If the software license is an "on-premises" license, the HCO should include the right to have a third-party data center host the software for the HCO and even to provide software management and other data center services. A typical license agreement includes restrictions that prohibit transferring or disclosing the software to any third party, and these restrictions would prohibit the HCO's use of third-party data centers to host the software for the HCO. Here is a sample clause that gives the HCO the right to use a third-party data center and other vendors for other purposes:

> HCO may outsource to other vendors any of HCO's needs or requirements for information technology equipment, resources, or services, including, without limitation, hosting, co-location, application management, and data center services. If and to the extent that any such outsourcing is applicable to any of the licensed software licensed to HCO under this Agreement, then this Agreement and the licenses granted to HCO will be reasonably expanded, if and as necessary, to allow such outsourcing, including, without limitation, the right for the licensed software to be run on servers, computers or processors of such vendors, or at their data centers for HCO. Any such vendor must agree in writing that it will not store, run, or use the licensed software for any purpose other than services for HCO and to protect the licensed software from any unauthorized copying, use, or access by others.

Revenue Recognition and Payments

From the vendor's perspective, revenue recognition issues drive or affect many key provisions in the agreement. These issues may arise from:

- Conditions on payment
- Delivery of software not existing at the time the agreement is signed
- Payment milestones (e.g., acceptance)
- Possible refunds or other elements

Do not be caught by surprise—this is a huge issue to many vendors, especially those that are public companies. The HCO should expect pressure to commit or finalize the agreement by the end of the quarter or end of the year, but the negotiating team should work together to avoid being affected by this pressure! There is always the next quarter or next year, and the urgency felt by the vendor will return. Often discounts are conditioned by the vendor on a signing of the agreement by a certain deadline, with the expectation that the HCO will concede on points of negotiation to meet the deadline. This is pressure on the vendor, not the HCO.

Payments

Is the HCO getting the best price? Generally, an HCO should not have to pay list price for a software license, and any discounts should have a long-term life for future purchases. Sometimes HCOs and other customers ask for "most favored nations" pricing and terms, but this is extremely hard to get from an established vendor for good reasons from its perspective.

When negotiating the agreement, look for opportunities to lock in prices or discounts on optional software, expansions,

or future projects. *The HCO has the most leverage before signing the agreement, not after.* The HCO should negotiate for a payment schedule that ties some payments to milestones and acceptance. This is a good way to motivate a vendor to stay on schedule. The agreement will often provide that the HCO pay for the vendor's expenses and other charges, especially with respect to some services. This should not apply to support and maintenance services. For other services, expenses should be reasonable, capped, and documented.

The HCO should consider credits, refunds, or other financial consequences for delays, breaches, or other failures by the vendor. If custom development or lengthy and complicated implementations and rollouts are involved, this can be important. For legal reasons, these credits, refunds, and other financial consequences should not be characterized as "penalties," even though non-attorneys tend to do so. In some cases, it may be appropriate to characterize them as "liquidated damages." When faced with the prospect of credits, refunds, or other financial consequences, a vendor may respond by asking for incentives (e.g., additional payment) if time schedules or other performances are overachieved by the vendor. The HCO should be prepared for this response by the vendor and probably should reject it.

The HCO should make sure that everything is covered. The vendor should provide line-by-line pricing for the system selection and/or the negotiating team to review. This is the "no unpleasant surprises" approach to payment obligations. Open-ended obligations to pay for services (e.g., implementation) may lead to unexpected budget overruns.

Overview of Termination

If things go wrong, the termination provisions may be the most important part of the license agreement. The agreement may be terminated simply because its term expires or because both parties agree to an early termination. Sometimes the agreement includes a clause giving the HCO the right to terminate for convenience or dissatisfaction or something other than a breach of the agreement by the vendor. For example, a failure of the vendor to meet a nonbinding time schedule or an SLA performance level might not be a breach of the agreement but could be expressed in the agreement as triggering a right on the part of the HCO to terminate the agreement. It would be a mistake for the HCO to give a similar right to the vendor. Other termination rights may include termination for bankruptcy, insolvency, or breach.

It should be noted that a license agreement usually includes a survival clause that indicates that certain provisions of the agreement will continue in effect after termination of the agreement. Confidentiality provisions are one such example. Although rarely the case in a vendor's form of agreement, the license itself can survive, but other provisions, such as maintenance and support, will terminate.

Termination for Breach

Nearly every license agreement includes a clause giving each party the right to terminate the agreement in the event that the other party breaches the agreement. Sometimes, one-sided license agreements only give the vendor this right, but in such cases, it is typically easy for the HCO to successfully negotiate for reciprocity.

From the perspective of the HCO, termination, even if for a breach by the HCO, can be much more dangerous and unreasonable than meets the casual eye. If the software is mission critical, it is not practical or realistic to expect the HCO to suddenly stop using the software being relied upon. For example, if the electronic health record of the HCO is reliant on the software, the HCO could not possibly stop use of it without terrible consequences to patients and operations. With a typical "termination for breach" clause, that is exactly what the HCO is agreeing to. Without a license, continued use of the software would be an infringement of the copyright and other intellectual property of the vendor. Typically, provisions are included that obligate the HCO to stop using the software upon termination.

An agreement includes many provisions that can potentially be breached by the HCO. For example, confidentiality provisions could be inadvertently or carelessly breached. Other restrictions, such as a prohibition against benchmark testing, may be breached without realizing that the agreement includes this prohibition. Exceeding the scope of the license is also a breach and can be done unintentionally. What if there is a dispute about the timing or amount of a payment? The vendor would likely claim a breach and threaten termination if the HCO does not concede and pay the disputed amount. Examining the agreement will reveal many provisions that might be breached.

In the case of an "on-premises" license, the HCO might out of necessity, for the sake of patients, ignore a notice of termination by the vendor and continue to use the software running on the HCO's computers, even though the HCO would be without support and maintenance. The vendor would then be forced to seek an injunction from a court to order the HCO to stop use. Hopefully, a court would not issue such an order if patient safety were jeopardized, but it may be hard to explain to the court why the HCO agreed that it would stop use upon termination for breach and now refuses to do so. The situation is riskier in the case of a SaaS license because all the SaaS vendor needs to do is terminate access by the HCO to the software running on servers at the vendor's data center. Hopefully, the vendor would not do this, but it is unwise for the HCO to agree to this provision. In any event, the vendor is likely to use the threat of termination to extract concessions to its advantage.

At the very least, the HCO should insist that the agreement include provisions that require (1) the breach be "material" in order to justify termination and (2) the vendor give the HCO notice of the breach and a 30-day opportunity to cure the breach before termination. If the breach is timely cured, then no right exists for the vendor to terminate. Sometimes more than 30 days is needed to complete a cure, so the HCO should request a clause that allows for an extension of the 30 days if the cure begins within the 30-day period and is diligently pursued to completion.

Is the Breach Curable?

A troubling issue is whether or not a given breach is curable. For example, is a breach of confidentiality curable once a disclosure of confidential information has been made? If the breach is not curable, then no cure is available in a timely manner and the right to terminate will be triggered. Some vendors specifically state in their agreements that the right to cure does not apply to noncurable breaches. Also, it is often not clear as to what it takes to cure a breach. The HCO should seek to include a provision to the effect that the breach will be deemed cured if the HCO discontinues the breach and takes reasonable steps to prevent a repeat of the breach.

Sometimes the HCO may dispute that an alleged breach has occurred. For example, the vendor may claim that the HCO has failed to make a maintenance fee payment in full and is in breach. The HCO may believe that the maintenance fee is less than what the vendor claims (e.g., there might be a dispute about a cap on maintenance fee increases). The vendor may then send a notice of breach and threaten termination of the license, a draconian consequence for the HCO and unfairly disproportionate to the amount in dispute. The HCO, faced with this "termination blackmail," may need to concede on the payment. It cannot risk that a court might conclude that the vendor's interpretation of the agreement is correct or that the vendor may stop support and maintenance or, in the case of a SaaS license, "flip a switch" and terminate the HCO's access to and use of the software running on the vendor's servers. Even if termination by the vendor is wrong, the vendor may have little or no monetary liability because of limitation and exclusion of liability provisions in the agreement. Limitation and exclusion of liability provisions are discussed later in the chapter.

The ultimate protection for an HCO is to include in the agreement a provision to the effect that the license will survive termination of the agreement even if there is a breach of the agreement. This does not excuse the breach, as the HCO remains liable for damages caused by the breach. The vendor can still obtain injunctive relief to stop the breach, but it is very difficult to get vendors to agree to this. Their attorneys are often adamant that termination of the license is essential for protection of the vendor's software and intellectual property. This concern is somewhat overstated because (1) the HCO is only seeking the right to continue to use the software within the scope of a license that the HCO has already paid for, and (2) the vendor can always obtain injunctive relief against any use, disclosure, distribution, or copying beyond the scope of that license.

Assuming that the HCO cannot get the ultimate protection described previously, the following clause or a variation is reasonable despite the vendor's dislike for it. It will as often as not be accepted by the vendor:

> In view of the "mission critical" nature of the Licensed Software to HCO and HCO's reliance on it and of the responsibility of HCO to protect the safety, health, and wellbeing of patients, Vendor may not suspend or terminate the License

[or any services or rights of HCO under this Agreement or any access to or use of the Licensed Software by HCO or its users] unless this Agreement is terminated in accordance with this Section. The vendor may terminate this Agreement only upon a material breach of this Agreement by HCO that is not cured by HCO within 30 days after receiving written notice from the vendor of such breach. The notice must specifically identify the provisions of this Agreement that are breached and must state the actions that the vendor believes are necessary for HCO to cure the breach and must give notice of the vendor's intention to terminate the Agreement if the breach is not cured. If more than 30 days are needed to cure the breach, then HCO will be allowed such additional time as is reasonably required for the cure, provided that HCO gives notice of the need and begins the cure within the 30-day period and that HCO is thereafter diligent in pursuing the cure to completion. If the breach is not curable, then for the purposes of this Section, the breach will be deemed cured if HCO takes reasonable steps to prevent a repeat of the breach. HCO remains liable for damages caused by its breach and nothing in this Section excuses monetary liability for those damages, but damages are subject to the agreed upon limitations of liability. If HCO disputes in good faith that a material breach has occurred, then the issue must first be decided through the dispute resolution provisions and, if necessary, litigation in accordance with governing law and forum provisions of this Agreement. If a court holds that a material breach occurred, then HCO shall have an opportunity to cure the breach as described above (or to address an incurable breach as described above) in order to preserve its license and rights and to avoid termination of the Agreement by the vendor. The 30-day cure period will begin when HCO receives notice of the final decision of the court in writing and such 30-day cure period is subject to extension as described above. Nothing herein permits HCO to use, distribute, or copy the Licensed Software outside the scope of the License and rights granted to HCO. Nothing prohibits or delays Vendor from obtaining an injunction to stop HCO from using, distributing, or copying the Licensed Software outside of such license and rights or from otherwise infringing or misappropriating any intellectual property or confidentiality information of Vendor.

Do not think that the nightmare of termination cannot happen. It does and can happen, although rarely. Even if a vendor is very unlikely to abuse termination rights in the agreement if the HCO acts in good faith and is repentant, the HCO is still exposed to the "termination blackmail" threat when the HCO disputes the existence of a breach or disputes what the remedy should be for the breach.

As a final comment on the issue of termination, the importance of this issue is proportional to the significance of the HCO's reliance on the software and the ease of transitioning to a substitute solution in the event of termination. Many situations exist where the HCO can, with relative safety, ignore the issue because the risk or downside of termination is so low that negotiating with the vendor is not justified. If the software is mission critical to the HCO, then the risk can be summed up as follows: (1) the probability of a serious termination issue occurring is very low, but (2) in the unlikely event

that it does occur, the consequences can be very serious. In a worst-case scenario, it may be difficult for the HCO's representatives responsible for approving the agreement to explain to management why the HCO agreed to allow the vendor to terminate or threaten to terminate the use of mission critical software.

Transition and Transition Period

As an additional protection in the event of termination, the HCO may want to add a clause entitling it to transition rights and a transition period. A clause of this nature might read as follows:

> In the event that the Agreement is terminated for any reason or expires and if the safety, health, or wellbeing of any patients or healthcare or business operations of the HCO are jeopardized or compromised by such termination or expiration, then the HCO will be entitled to a reasonable transition period to transition to computer programs, products, services, and solutions from another vendor that are a substitute for the Licensed Software, Services, and Solution of this Agreement. During this transition period, HCO may continue to use and exercise the License and rights with respect to the Licensed Software, Services, and Solution pursuant to this Agreement and subject to this Agreement. In effect, the transition period is an extension of the term of this Agreement and delays termination or expiration until the end of the transition period. The transition period must be sufficient in duration to allow for an orderly transition to substitute computer programs, products, services, and solutions, but HCO may not extend the transition period beyond one year. HCO will give notice to Vendor after the transition period ends.

Sometimes, especially for a SaaS license, the transition clause will require the vendor to provide transition services at the vendor's current standard fees plus expenses.

Exclusive Remedy Clauses

License agreements frequently include exclusive remedy clauses that state that the HCO's sole and exclusive remedy for a breach is limited to one specific remedy and not others. For example, a section may state that if the services are not performed in accordance with the warranties, then the exclusive remedy is that the services will be re-performed. What if the re-performed services continue to be in noncompliance? Even if performed properly later, there is no compensation to the HCO for the delay. The agreement may even include a provision stating the exclusive remedy still applies even if the remedy "fails of its essential purpose." The provision then leaves the HCO without a meaningful remedy.

No other damages or remedies can be recovered if the exclusive remedy clause is enforced! Usually an exclusive remedy clause is applied to warranties, but they can be applied to any obligation in the agreement. Sometimes vendors are overly aggressive and broad in the language of an exclusive remedy clause and incorrectly (or unfairly or illogically) apply it to any breach of the agreement! For example, an exclusive remedy may mention having a vendor re-perform an activity as the sole remedy for any breach of the agreement. However, this action would be illogical for a security or confidentiality breach by a vendor. The exclusive remedy should make sense in the context of the specific breach to which it applies and should only apply to specific breach of contract claims, not to other claims such as negligence or damage to property.

Limitations and Exclusions of Liability

A license agreement will almost always include clauses on limitations and exclusions of liability. These clauses are not harmless "legalese." The HCO should understand these clauses from a business point of view and not expect to be able to totally negotiate these clauses out of the agreement, but details may be negotiable.

Limitation of Liability

A limitation of liability clause limits the HCO's liability to an amount or cap that cannot be exceeded. For example, "In no event shall Vendor's aggregate liability exceed an amount equal to the license fee paid to Vendor under this Agreement." For the HCO, it may be better to increase the cap to all amounts paid under the Agreement (e.g., to further include amounts paid for support, maintenance, training, implementation, and other services). If the agreement is a SaaS agreement, then the cap may be an amount equal to 1 year of the SaaS fee or some other very limited amount much less than the total fees under the agreement. The consequence of an HCO agreeing that the vendor's liability is limited means that the HCO cannot recover damages from the vendor in excess of the cap, even if the HCO can prove a higher amount of damages.

Exclusion of Liability

An exclusion of liability clause totally excludes certain types of damages from recovery. For example, "In no event shall Vendor be liable for any consequential, indirect, special, punitive, or incidental damages, or for any loss of business, opportunity, profits, revenue, data, or programs." The consequence of the HCO agreeing to this means that the HCO recovers nothing for these types of damages, even if the HCO can prove that it suffered the damages. Only direct damages remain recoverable, subject to the limitation of liability cap described previously.

Reciprocity and Exceptions

The HCO should insist these clauses are reciprocal so they benefit the HCO, not just the vendor. When these clauses are made reciprocal, the vendor will often insist on exceptions for infringement of its intellectual property, breach of confidentiality, indemnification, and possibly some other clauses. The HCO should negotiate for other exceptions, such as breach of a business associate agreement or data security agreement, intentional breaches, willful misconduct, and wrongful suspension or termination. For example, if the

vendor wrongfully suspends or terminates a SaaS license and access to the software, the HCO would have little or no monetary recourse against the vendor because the limitation and exclusion of liabilities would prevent recovery of the most significant damages, including loss of revenue and disruption of business. This would be a terrible surprise to the HCO. Having these exceptions in the agreement will make a SaaS vendor leery about being too quick to suspend or terminate services for fear of being exposed to unlimited liability for doing so wrongfully.

Insurance

The vendor should agree to maintain adequate liability insurance, including cyber-liability insurance governing data privacy, security breaches, and business continuity. The HCO may need recourse against the insurance for negligence and other covered fault of the vendor, or the HCO may need to be additionally protected. The HCO should carefully consider whether it should be named as an additional insured party in the vendor's insurance policy, because existing insurance policies may not cover claims against another insured (e.g., the HCO). The limitations and exclusions of liability should not limit or exclude any losses and liabilities covered by the vendor's insurance policies. The HCO insurance advisor or risk management officer should work with the HCO's negotiating team in deciding on adequate insurance requirements expected of the vendor.

Dispute Resolution

Some license agreements require a dispute resolution process before litigation or arbitration. For example, a requirement may exist for a meeting to discuss and attempt to resolve the dispute. If that meeting is unsuccessful, the dispute must be escalated to a higher level of management of both parties for discussion and resolution. Only if this process has been followed without success may a party proceed with litigation or arbitration. This is generally a good approach for HCOs, especially if the dispute resolution process is a prerequisite to termination or suspension of a license or the agreement.

Special Clauses
Confidentiality

The license agreement typically includes confidentiality protections for the parties and their confidential information. The HCO's confidential information may include RFPs, plans, financial information, and anything that can be learned by the vendor's access to any networks or computer systems of the HCO. The party receiving the other party's confidential information should agree not only to keep the information confidential but also to not use it for any purpose other than performing obligations or exercising rights under the agreement. The HCO should expect to see some or all of the following exceptions in Box 18.20 to the confidentially provisions.

BOX 18.20 Exceptions to Confidentiality Provisions

- Information that is or becomes (through no fault of the receiving party) publicly known or generally known in the industry or profession of either party
- Information known to the receiving party prior to first disclosure by the other party
- Information that is lawfully disclosed on a nonconfidential basis by third parties to the receiving party
- Information that is independently created by or for the receiving party

---

The HCO should make sure that these exceptions do not apply to protected health information or other personally identifiable information, or to any obligation under a business associate agreement or data security agreement. The confidentially provisions should not prohibit a disclosure required by law, regulation, or court or government order, but a protective order or similar protection should be sought.

An important issue is the duration of the confidentiality obligations. The confidentiality obligations may expire after a certain number of years after the date of the agreement or after the date of first disclosure. Or they may never expire unless and until one of the previously given exceptions applies.

The vendor will include provisions that specifically protect the software and documentation against disclosure or transfer to others. It is not always clear if and to what extent protections apply to screen displays and output (e.g., reports). Because of the broad and restrictive nature of confidentiality provisions, the HCO may want to include an exception for incidental disclosures:

> Nothing in this Confidentiality Section or any other confidentiality provisions of this Agreement prohibits any disclosure that reasonably or inherently occurs as part of the licensed use of the Licensed Software or the servicing by contractors of hardware or systems for the HCO. By way of non-limiting examples, screen displays, interfaces and reports generated by the Licensed Software may be visible to visitors to HCO's facilities and reports and other output generated by the Licensed Software may be given to others in the ordinary course of business.

The HCO may want to go beyond the protections of a business associate agreement when it comes to patient data. The agreement should include provisions that protect patient data even if the data are de-identified and aggregated. Some vendors are eager to extract and use patient-related data and other data of the HCO for commercial or analytic purposes. This should be prohibited by more than just a business associate agreement, and careful attention should be given to any permission or license relating to data. If the vendor, especially a SaaS vendor, is to hold or store any of the HCO's data, then data security provisions will be needed in addition to the confidentiality provisions of the agreement.

Intellectual Property Infringement

The license agreement should include a warranty of non-infringement and a clause indemnifying (providing compensation for a particular loss) the HCO and its users of the software against claims that the software or its licensed use infringes or misappropriates any patent, copyright, trade secret, or other intellectual property. Often the vendor will not offer a warranty of non-infringement, saying instead that it only offers an indemnification clause that can be complex and include exceptions that need to be carefully considered. The clause might indemnify against monetary judgments payable to the owner of the intellectual property, but often not against the HCO's own losses or damages if it must suddenly cease use of the software because of an infringement claim. The HCO will want the broader indemnification protection.

Indemnification by the Healthcare Organization and Disclaimers by the Vendor of Responsibility

The vendor may seek to have the HCO indemnify the vendor against claims by others arising from the HCO's use of or reliance on the software or its use, results, and output. It is not uncommon to see vendors disclaim responsibility for the results and output of the software and to require HCOs to examine and verify those results and output, such as accuracy of medication calculations. How practical is it for the HCO to verify? Some will say, "Isn't this the purpose of the software?" The best approach is to delete these types of provisions, especially indemnification by the HCO, and simply make each party responsible for its own fault in the event of any claims by a third party.

Restrictive Covenants and Feedback Clauses

The HCO should take careful note of restrictive covenants and feedback clauses and should only agree to them if they are reasonable and understood by the HCO. Restrictive covenants include noncompetition clauses and other restrictions on doing business or conducting certain activities with others and clauses that prohibit the hiring or solicitation of the other party's personnel.

Feedback clauses may require the HCO to assign ownership of feedback and its intellectual property to the vendor. Feedback is typically defined as suggestions, ideas, recommendations, improvements, and enhancements relating to the software or a service of the vendor. This can become a serious problem if the HCO wants to use or commercialize the feedback independent of the vendor or to share the feedback with other vendors. At most, a feedback clause should only grant to the vendor a nonexclusive license to use the feedback in the vendor's software and services. The license should be granted on an "as is" basis without any warranty. Any feedback clause requires careful consideration and possible exceptions (e.g., for copyrights and patents).

Governing Law and Forum Clauses

These clauses indicate which jurisdiction's (e.g., state's) law will govern the agreement. The forum clause indicates the jurisdiction and venue for any litigation between the parties (i.e., where a lawsuit will take place). It may seem odd, but a court in one state may apply the law of another state to the agreement and dispute. With respect to jurisdiction and venue, one compromise is to say that a party may only bring an action in the state (or more specific venue) of the other party. This may discourage litigation.

Right to Assign the Agreement and License

License agreements generally prohibit an assignment (of license and other rights and delegation or transfer of duties and obligations) or transfer of the agreement to a third party. Given the possibility that the HCO may merge with or be acquired by another entity someday, it is a good idea to at least allow the HCO to assign or transfer the agreement in the event that the HCO or its assets or business is acquired by sale, merger, or otherwise. A change of HCO control should not be deemed as a prohibited assignment or transfer.

Use of the Healthcare Organization's Name, Marks, and Logos

The license agreement should prohibit the vendor from using the HCO's name, trademark, service mark, or logo in any marketing, sales, or promotional materials; on a website; or in any other public communication without the written consent of the HCO in each case, including the right of prior review. Use of the HCO's name in a list of customers or a press release may be permitted by the agreement without that consent. Vendors should not be allowed to use these materials to imply any HCO affiliation, endorsement, or sponsorship of the vendor or its software, product, or service. Similar restrictions should be considered for the name of any officer, researcher, developer, clinical informatician, physician, or other healthcare professional employed by the HCO.

Data Usage and Data Ownership

The agreement should specify data ownership, especially for aggregated data generated through use of the vendor's software. The HCO will want to consider carefully how population health data will be managed, define who owns those resulting data, and include these aspects in the agreement.

CONCLUSIONS AND FUTURE DIRECTIONS

License agreements are an essential part of an HCO's software procurement process. An understanding of those agreements and a willingness to negotiate for reasonable terms and conditions can reduce risk, save money, and protect the HCO against unpleasant surprises. An agreement, no matter how favorable to the HCO, is never an acceptable substitute for due diligence prior to the signing of the agreement or for a careful and systematic vendor selection process. After the agreement is signed, the HCO should have a process for ensuring and monitoring compliance with the agreement and for utilizing the protections and advantages successfully negotiated into the agreement. Although it may seem obvious, the HCO should have an organized archive of agreements and an index and summary of the important agreements that can be consulted when needed. Finally, never underestimate the leverage that an HCO may have to contractually protect itself. The future of license agreements will only grow more complex as technology and data become more distributed over time. As data are merged from different sources, data ownership and security breaches will continue to be issues in the future.

REFERENCES

1. *Section 101 of the U.S. Patent Laws (35 U.S.C. 101)*, 2016.
2. *Uniform Trade Secrets Act Definition*. https://www.law.cornell.edu/wex/trade_secret. Accessed July 20, 2016.
3. *Agile Software Development Processes*, 2016. https://en.wikipedia.org/wiki/Agile_software_development.

DISCUSSION QUESTIONS

1. Thinking about your own organization, outline the composition of a team to assist with a generating a licensing agreement to integrate all imaging services in your facility across ultrasound, radiology, and cardiology. Give the rationale for each team member.
2. Discuss what steps organizations might take for due diligence. How might these protect the organization beyond having a good contract in place?
3. In this chapter, the author recommends numerous sections to a licensing agreement. Which ones surprised you?
4. Your electronic health record (EHR) vendor was sold to another company. What provisions in the agreement will be the ones you will look for to ensure patient care is not compromised as a transition occurs?

CASE STUDY

Best Bet Hospital is a tertiary care medical center with 500 acute care beds, 35 ambulatory clinics, a Level-1 emergency department, a 75-bed skilled nursing facility, and telehealth services for both stroke and dermatology services. The leadership decided to change its EHR after a 10-year life cycle and shift to a SaaS agreement. You are the long-term care representative on the selection committee. Due to your expertise in health care, leadership has asked you to assist with the licensing agreement for this purchase.

Discussion Questions

1. Give an overview of the particular needs (functional aspects) of long-term care that should be included in a licensing agreement.

2. Glancing over the sections in this chapter, create an outline of the most important areas to consider in the licensing agreement.

3. Best Bet wants to reduce maintenance and support costs. What are some ways this might be accomplished? What areas should be included in the licensing agreement to support these?

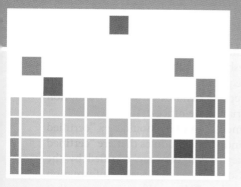

19

Implementing and Upgrading an Information System

Christine D. Meyer

No matter whether the health information system is new or an upgrade, the ultimate goal in implementations is to provide the highest level of care at the lowest cost with the least risk.

OBJECTIVES

At the completion of this chapter, the reader will be prepared to:

1. Discuss regulatory and nonregulatory reasons for implementing or upgrading an electronic information system.
2. Compare the advantages and disadvantages of "best of breed" and integrated system approaches in selecting healthcare information system architecture.
3. Explain each step in developing an implementation plan for a healthcare information system.
4. Develop strategies for the successful management of each step in the implementation of a healthcare information system.
5. Analyze the benefits of an electronic information system with an integrated clinical decision support system.
6. Explain the implications of unintended consequences or e-iatrogenesis as they relate to implementing an electronic health record (EHR).

KEY TERMS

best of breed, 323
big bang, 330
e-iatrogenesis, 321
phased go-live, 330

scope creep, 322
Tall Man lettering, 321
workarounds, 325

ABSTRACT ❖

This chapter analyzes the processes for implementing a health information system with a specific emphasis on an electronic health record (EHR). The decision to implement a new health information system or to upgrade a current system is based on several factors, including (1) providing safe and up-to-date patient care, (2) meeting federal mandates such as Meaningful Use (MU) and Medicare Access and CHIP Reauthorization Act of 2015 (MACRA) requirements, and (3) leveraging advanced levels of clinical decision support. Implementing EHRs entails multilayered decisions at each stage of the implementation. Major decisions include vendor and system selection, determining go-live options, redesigning workflows and processes, and developing procedures and policies. The timeline and scope of the project is primarily dictated by expenses, staff, resources, and the drop-dead date for go-live. Success depends on a well-thought-out and detailed project plan with regular review and updating of the critical milestones, unwavering support from the organization's leadership, input from users during the design and build phases, thorough testing, end user education, mitigation of identified risk factors, and control of scope creep. The implementation of an EHR is never finished. Medication orders, nonmedication orders, and documentation screens or fields will continuously need to be added, modified, or inactivated; patches will be installed and tweaks to workflows and functionality will be ongoing.

INTRODUCTION

This chapter focuses on the implementation of healthcare information systems. Of course, many different types of applications are used within a healthcare information system. The general principles for implementing different applications are the same; however, to demonstrate these general principles, this chapter will focus mainly on the implementation of an EHR. In 2004, President George W. Bush promoted the idea of a fully functional electronic medical record (EMR) for Americans within 10 years.[1] This proposal officially initiated the massive changes that we continue to witness in health informatics. Healthcare information systems are widely used today in many diverse settings. Small hospitals, ambulatory clinics, and small physician practices generally implement a simple and streamlined system with limited features and are tailored for a quicker implementation and easier long-term maintenance. Large medical centers, multifacility enterprises, and multiphysician practices with more complex needs typically opt to install a more robust system that allows for customizations. However, there are still hospitals and physician practices without an EHR or that have an outdated system that cannot accommodate recent regulatory mandates. An outdated system may be one reason to implement or upgrade a health information technology (health IT) solution, but there are others.

REASONS TO IMPLEMENT OR UPGRADE A HEALTHCARE INFORMATION SYSTEM

There are several reasons why a health organization (hospital organization, physician office, or clinic) may decide that a major change is needed. A careful review of the reasons for the change will start the process of deciding whether to install a new information system or upgrade the current system. One of the primary reasons for making such a major change is changing government regulations.

Changing Government Regulations
The American Recovery and Reinvestment Act

The American Recovery and Reinvestment Act (ARRA), enacted in 2009, spawned the Health Information Technology for Economic and Clinical Health (HITECH) Act. One of its primary goals was that each person in the United States would have a certified digital medical record by 2014, including the electronic exchange of health information across healthcare institutions to improve quality of healthcare. As discussed in detail in Chapter 27, the HITECH Act created a $27 billion federally funded incentive program providing Medicare and Medicaid payments over 5 to 10 years to three groups: (1) eligible providers (EP), (2) eligible hospitals (EH), and (3) Critical Access Hospitals (CAH). CAH are defined as rural hospitals certified to receive cost-based reimbursement from Medicare. Within the HITECH Act, there are two EHR incentive programs: the Medicare EHR Incentive Program administered by the Centers for Medicare and Medicaid Services (CMS) and the Medicaid EHR Incentive Program, which is governed by individual states and territories.

It is important to note that these government incentive programs were not established to cover the total cost of implementing an EHR system but to encourage or "incentivize" healthcare organizations and healthcare providers to use an EHR in a meaningful way, called Meaningful Use (MU), and to foster faster rates of adoption across the nation.[2] Other terms often used for this incentive program are "stimulus funds," "stimulus package," or simply "ARRA funds."[3]

CMS established the criteria for MU, which included minimal thresholds for select objectives. There are three stages in the EHR Incentive Program. Stage 1, which began in 2011, emphasized capturing patient data that was expected to be shared with other healthcare professionals and the patient. Stage 2 began in 2014 and focused on advanced clinical practices and providing patient portals where patients could

access their medical records. Stage 3, slated to begin in 2017, accentuates data interoperability and patient outcomes while increasing the thresholds for the objectives and clinical measures.[4] Additional requirements include the submission of detailed and timely reports demonstrating MU adoption to CMS and the appropriate state offices.

To meet MU requirements, an EHR should be a "certified complete EHR" or have individual modules that are "certified EHR modules." This means that they are certified by the Office of the National Coordinator for Health Information Technology (ONC). Complete EHR certification means that the system has the functionality, required data elements, and logic to support ambulatory, emergency room, outpatient, and inpatient MU requirements. EHR module certification means that the ancillary application meets one or more requirements. Most hospitals and physician offices purchase a commercial system that is deemed certified, meaning that the vendor incorporated these essential capabilities. A list of certified products can be found at http://oncchpl.force.com/ehrcert?q=chpl.

The Certification Commission for Health Information Technology (CCHIT) tested and certified new software applications beginning in 2006. However, in 2015 it ceased testing and certifying EHRs for financial reasons and changed its role to advising healthcare providers on how to comply with the government's regulations and providing guidance to health IT developers on how to meet the government's requirements for a certified EHR. The CCHIT works with the Health Information and Management Systems Society (HIMSS) to advance programs and policies that strongly promote interoperability and to advocate using IT between patients and providers as another tool to transform healthcare.[5]

The newly defined recertification program is structured so that the ONC now serves to manage or oversee the program, which involves several agencies or organizations that are responsible for the actual testing and certification of the products.[6] The flowchart shown in Fig. 19.1 illustrates the organization and flow for testing and certifying new EHR products.

However, the MU criteria do not require purchasing a commercial, certified product. A few hospitals and eligible providers have developed their own "homegrown" EHRs that may or may not include commercial components. CMS welcomes organizations to certify their systems using the EHR Alternative Certification for Healthcare Providers (EACH) program. The EACH program is a three-step program to certify homegrown systems or existing EHR technology not already covered by a vendor certification. The program provides a mechanism to obtain certification by demonstrating that the system meets the U.S. Department of Health & Human Services (HHS) MU requirements.[7] For example, the Regenstrief Medical Record System (RMRS) in Indiana is an EMR system that began in 1972 and expanded to several additional major hospitals.[8] Other medical centers that successfully opted for this alternative include Geisinger Health System, Marshfield Clinic Health System, Landmark Hospitals (Chartpad), and Brigham and Women's Hospital.[9,10]

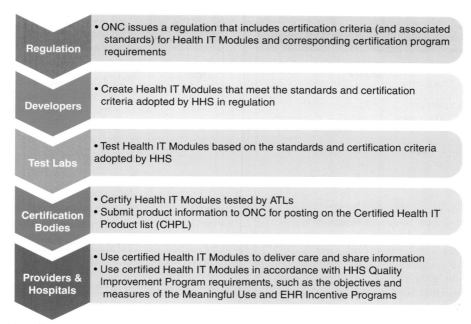

FIG 19.1 The certification process at a glance. (Source: *US DHHS Office of the National Coordinator. ONC. About the ONC Health IT Certification Program.* <https://www.healthit.gov/policy-researchers-implementers/about-onc-health-it-certification-program>; September 20, 2016.)

U.S. hospitals were initially slow to adopt an EHR system. However, the impact of HITECH can be clearly demonstrated. A 2011 survey conducted by the American Hospital Association found that the percentage of U.S. hospitals that had adopted EHRs doubled from 16% to 35% between 2009 and 2011. However, in 2014 the ONC reported that 76% of hospitals implemented at least a basic EHR system, and almost 97% of those implemented a certified EHR technology.[11]

The Transition from ICD-9-CM to ICD-10-CM Codes and from HIPAA Version 4010 to HIPAA Version 5010

In 2015 the CMS issued a mandatory transition from the International Classification of Diseases (ICD)-9-CM codes to ICD-10-CM codes. The requirement has also served as a major impetus for providers and healthcare facilities to upgrade their current EHR or to implement a new one. ICD-10-CM codes are used to classify all inpatient and outpatient diagnoses, report medical care and cause of deaths, process payments, calculate trends, and perform statistical analyses. Early versions of healthcare information systems could not adopt the new ICD-10-CM codes because they were configured to accept three to five numeric-only characters. The ICD-10-CM codes have three to seven characters in which the first and third characters are always alpha characters, the second character is always numeric, and characters four through seven are either alpha or numeric.[12] The ICD-9-CM system had 13,000 codes to define diagnoses and procedures. In contrast, the ICD-10-CM version contains over 68,000 diagnostics codes, which allows for a more detailed definition and better reporting for reimbursement and biosurveillance. Another difference between the two systems is that ICD-10-CM does not include procedure classifications, so there is a separate ICD-10-PCS (procedure coding system) with over 71,000 procedure codes that are used by hospitals for inpatient procedures (Table 19.1).[13] During the migration to ICD-10, the Centers for Disease Control and Prevention (CDC) suspended new additions or modifications to the ICD-10-CM and the ICD-10-PCS codes. However, in 2016 the CDC added nearly 1900 new diagnosis codes to the ICD-10-CM codes and 2651 new inpatient procedure codes to the ICD-10-PCS starting in fiscal year 2017.[13] A complete list of all ICD-10 codes is available at www.cdc.gov. and www.cms.gov.

The United States has lagged behind other countries in the implementation of ICD-10 codes. When the conversion occurred in the United States, 138 other countries were already using ICD-10 codes to track mortality, and 99 countries were using these codes to track morbidity (Table 19.2).[12]

In addition to the ICD-10 conversion, in 2012 all health plans, healthcare providers, and clearinghouses that conduct business electronically were required to convert the Health Insurance Portability and Accountability Act (HIPAA) standard for electronic transactions from Version 4010 to Version 5010. Version 5010 was important because it accommodated the move to ICD-10-CM and ICD-10-PCS code sets. While the conversion to ICD-10 and HIPAA Version 5010 were major challenges, what is important for the informatician to understand is that these types of requirement changes can be expected to occur on a regular basis as legislation and technology continue to change.

TABLE 19.1 Comparison of ICD-9-CM and ICD-10-CM Codes

Characteristic	ICD-9-CM	ICD-10-CM
Field length	3-5 characters	3-7 characters
Available codes	Approximately 13,000 codes	Approximately 68,000 diagnostic codes
Code composition (i.e., Numeric, alpha)	Digit 1 = alpha or numeric Digits 2-5 = numeric	Digit 1 = alpha Digits 2-3 = numeric Digits 4-7 = alpha or numeric
Character position within code	Characters 1-3 = category Characters 4-5 = anatomic site, etiology, manifestation[a]	Characters 1-3 = category Characters 4-6 = anatomic site, etiology, severity, or clinical detail[b] Character 7 = extension
Available space for new codes	Limited	Flexible
Overall detail embedded within codes	Ambiguous	Very specific
Laterality	Does not identify right versus left	Often identifies right versus left
Sample code	438.11, late effect of cerebrovascular disease, speech and language deficits, aphasia	I69.320, speech and language deficits following cerebral infarction, aphasia following cerebral infarction

From ICD-10 State Medicaid Readiness Medicaid ICD10 Implementation Handbook.docx. <http://www.medicaid.gov/Medicaid-CHIP-Program-Information/By-Topics/Data-and-Systems/ICD-Coding/Downloads/icd-10-implementation-assistance-handbook.pdf>; 2016.
ICD, International Classification of Diseases.
[a]Not always the case for ICD-9-CM.
[b]Not always the case for ICD-10.

TABLE 19.2 Examples of Countries That Use ICD-10 Codes

Year Adopted	Country
1994 to 1997	Scandinavian countries (Denmark, Finland, Iceland, Norway, Sweden)
1995	United Kingdom
1997	France
1998	Australia
1999	Belgium
2000	Germany
2001	Canada
2015	United States (original compliance date—October 1, 2013)

Adapted from Brooks P. ICD-10 Overview. <http://www.cms.gov/Medicare/Medicare-Contracting/ContractorLearningResources/downloads/ICD-10_Overview_Presentation.pdf>; 2010 (slide 15).

Best Practices: Incorporating Evidence-Based Content and Clinical Decision Support Systems

With each new release, information systems become more complex and robust, enabling them to incorporate evidence-based content (called evidenced-based practice [EBP]) and to use clinical decision support (CDS) features in the system. Detailed information on EBP and CDS is included in Chapter 3 and Chapter 10; however, one of the most frequently quoted definitions for EBP is one proposed by Sackett et al.: EBP is "the conscientious, explicit, and judicious use of current best evidence in making decisions about the care of individual patients. The practice of evidence based medicine means integrating individual clinical expertise with the best available external clinical evidence from systematic research."[14, p. 71] EBP involves making decisions

for clinical care based on the most current recommended treatments for specific diagnoses. These recommendations are derived from an ongoing review and analysis of high-caliber, peer-reviewed scientific studies in the literature. While entering orders from an EBP order set, the practitioner may override any of the recommended diagnostic or treatment options based on the individual needs of the patient. Some healthcare providers strongly object to a preconfigured EBP order set, referring to it as "cookbook medicine," and resist incorporating it into practice. Berner offers an analogy of CDS including EBP similar to the nursing process of the traditional "five rights" for medication administration: "The clinical delivery system should provide the *Right* information to the *Right* person in the *Right* format through the *Right* channel at the *Right* time."[15, p. 7]

A major challenge to EBP is remaining current due to the continuous discovery of new knowledge and the resulting changes to recommended best practices guidelines that are embedded in EHRs. Commercial products can assist organizations in updating protocols by providing current EBP clinical solutions, such as order sets and care plans. Most major EHRs have been upgraded with common CDS features that help meet some of the specific MU mandates, such as alerts for critical lab results or a history of methicillin-resistant *Staphylococcus aureus* (MRSA) on new admissions, pregnancy warnings on select medications and diagnostic tests, drug allergies, drug–drug interactions, drug–diagnosis warnings, dosage range limits, the capture of specific data such as smoking status and advance directives, and immunization reminders.

The advantages of using a system that incorporates evidence-based content and CDS include the following:
- Defines standardized, appropriate care and reduces variability of care for common diagnoses.
- Defines local or facility-owned orderables (elements that can be ordered using computerized provider order entry [CPOE] available at that facility.

- Triggers alerts and other CDS features based on locally built logic (rules). For instance, an alert may be triggered if (1) blood products are ordered on patients who request no blood products be administered, (2) pregnancy category teratogenic medications are ordered on patients of childbearing age with an unknown pregnancy status, or (3) the potassium level is below a preset level on patients receiving digitalis medications.
- Collects detailed metrics for specific reports required to meet MU criteria. These reports address a variety of MU requirements such as patient education, smoking status assessment, native language, discharge instructions, deep vein thrombosis prophylaxis in select patient populations, and the use of thrombolytic and antithrombotic medications in stroke patients.
- Enables a more timely update of treatment plans based on best practices. The study Translating Research into Practice (TRIP), conducted by researchers sponsored by the Agency for Healthcare Research and Quality (AHRQ) in 1999, concluded that it took an average of 10 to 20 years to incorporate new clinical findings into general clinical practice.[16] This time lag between the discovery of new treatment options and the use of this new knowledge at the point of care is sometimes called the "lethal lag" or "fatal lag." CDS and EBP are likely to accelerate the incorporation of new findings into clinical practice.

Patient Safety and Improved Quality of Care

Before MU rules were initiated, most healthcare leadership and professionals cited patient safety as the primary reason for implementing an EHR; however, with the rapid adoption of EHRs it may appear to some healthcare professionals that the sole reason for implementing an EHR is to qualify for the incentive package. In response to this concern, leadership needs to communicate to staff that the primary deciding factors for implementing or upgrading an EHR include patient safety, improved quality of patient care, and efficiency. ARRA is not the reason for the implementation or upgrade but rather is the match that has ignited the process. Reinforcing this message on a regular basis through all the stages of the implementation cycle helps counteract resistance to using the system.

For example, EHRs help decrease medication errors, especially if closed-loop bedside barcoding medication administration is an integral piece of the system. Quality of care and outcomes improve when decision support mechanisms, standardized order sets, and care plans based on best practices are incorporated in the EHR. Besides being aware of all the positive functionalities and advantages of the EHR, staff also need to be well informed on what the EHR cannot do.

Major implementations can elicit strong pushbacks from hospital staff for a variety of reasons. A primary reason is that a major implementation often involves changes in well-established workflows and processes, resulting in a temporary decrease in productivity, particularly in the early stages when clinicians are still learning the system. In addition, while the new system may offer significant advantages to the institution

(e.g., a decrease in medication errors, reduced time between order entry and delivery of services, or a dramatic decrease in telephone calls from nursing and pharmacy to physicians about illegible or questionable orders), individual practitioners may focus on the disadvantages that personally affect them, such as an increase in time to enter admission orders or immediate post-op orders.

In a paper world, some healthcare providers created their own personal order sets for their practice and titled them using their name, such as Dr. Smith's Routine Admission Orders for Surgery. Once records become electronic, personalized order sets are discouraged. Each specialty should collaborate to create a single order set for each of its common procedures, diagnoses, surgeries, and admissions, incorporating EBP. This approach minimizes wide variances in care and avoids an IT maintenance nightmare to keep individual physicians' order sets up to date. One of the most important success factors in the implementation of an electronic health system is to involve as many users as possible in the design and planning of that system and discuss the inevitable changes to workflows, processes, policies, and procedures.[17]

The number of unnecessary verbal or telephone orders has long been a major patient safety issue, even though certifying organizations voice strong warnings against using them for simple convenience. The Joint Commission (TJC) has a standard requiring that all verbal and telephone orders be recorded and "read back" to the ordering healthcare provider.[18] This scenario exemplifies another source of clinician frustration because the clinician must remain on the telephone while the person recording the verbal order retrieves the electronic record, enters it into the system, goes through all prompts, and reads the order back to the ordering practitioner. One study examined the number of verbal and telephone orders pre-CPOE and post-CPOE and reported a 12% reduction in the number of verbal orders and a 34% decrease in unsigned verbal orders after implementation.[19]

Using the EHR to perform a task for which it is not designed or using a poorly designed system may produce poor results or outcomes. Published studies report a variety of unintended consequences for EHRs. Ash et al. identified nine types of unintended consequences and corresponding interventions to minimize each of these risks.[20] A few of the unintended consequences are associated with human error, such as selecting the wrong patient or the wrong medication from a list. They refer to this type of error as a juxtaposition error. Recommended strategies to decrease unintended consequences are very similar to the best practices for a successful implementation discussed later in this chapter.[21] Weiner et al. coined a new term, e-iatrogenesis, to describe the most critical of the new type of errors seen in EHRs.[22] Other types of errors include users who fail to validate or read the list of all orders entered during a session before final acceptance or who accept the defaults for select orders without review.

The EHR may use **Tall Man lettering** (i.e., the use of mixed-case lettering) for look-alike names of medications recommended by the Institute for Safe Medication Practices (ISMP). Studies indicate that using mixed-case lettering in similar drug names helps decrease medication errors during order entry, medication dispensing, and medication administration by highlighting the differences in the drug names. A few examples of medication names using Tall Man lettering are NiFEDipine versus niCARdipine, DOBUTamine versus DOPamine, and CISplatin versus CARBOplatin.[23]

Another safety benefit associated with the implementation of an EHR is that it can enforce the use of CMS-approved abbreviations. In addition, EHRs can incorporate real-time updates or revisions to the order item master (a master list of orderable items) and electronic order sets. For example, Darvon and Darvocet were recalled in 2010 because of serious cardiac arrhythmias. Institutions with EHRs were able to quickly remove these medications from the pharmacy formulary, automatically inactivating Darvon and Darvon equivalents on all electronic order sets.

HIPAA legislation that was originally drafted in 1996 mandated unique national patient identifiers to ensure patient safety and promote interoperability. However, privacy advocates voiced strong opposition, and Congress passed laws preventing the development of unique national patient identifiers. HIMSS has recently reintroduced a strong argument for a National Patient Identifier (NPI) and Patient Matching strategy using demographic attributes that are considered relatively stable and unlikely to change. Many proponents believe that we cannot achieve true interoperability until it is in place.[24] Examples of attributes include first name, middle name, last name, maiden name, date of birth, gender, driver's license number, street address, city, state, ZIP code, and phone number.[26] Both proponents and opponents can cite scenarios in which data attributes may prove unstable and the algorithms that are used do not address enough data elements. An ONC report found that patient matching accuracy oftentimes depended on whether it was matching patients internally or externally across organizations. The error rate varied widely from 10% in IT sophisticated organizations to an alarming 40% to 50% rate when matching across enterprises.[25] Keith Fraidenburg, vice-president of the Education and Communications College of Healthcare Information Management Executives, who strongly supports an NPI, believes that an NPI (which must be encrypted) should not be the sole source of patient authentication. He wants to see a multidimensional strategy using NPI with retinal or thumb scans.

NEW IMPLEMENTATION VERSUS AN UPGRADE

Once the decision has been made that a major change is needed in the current information system, the next question is whether to upgrade or implement a new system. Answering the question "Do we need to make a change?" leads to the follow-up question, "What specific changes are needed?" The institution or healthcare provider should begin by determining what level or degree of change is needed to achieve

their goals, including meeting MU requirements. If there already is a well-established homegrown system, it is often wiser to upgrade. Making this decision can be supported by using the EHR Alternative Certification for Healthcare Providers (EACH) process to consider the level of scope needed.

Many competing factors must be evaluated in deciding whether to implement a new system or upgrade the current system. In Chapter 16, which explains the process for selecting a health information system, the assumption is made that the institution is planning to purchase a new system. However, a formal implementation process is used whether an institution selects a new system or upgrades a current system. Once that decision is made, the institution will move forward to the implementation phase of the systems life cycle.

Sufficient Resources

The three major resources that will have the most impact on whether to implement a new system or to upgrade an existing one are staff, budget, and physical or environmental constraints. Having a sufficient number of available and knowledgeable staff with the specific skill sets needed for each step in the process is imperative to the success of the project. The needed skill sets relate to the following:

- Installing and testing new hardware, software, and wireless networks
- Designing, building, and modifying applications
- Testing new applications and interfaces
- Providing staff education and support
- Maintaining hardware, software, and wireless networks

The project manager will usually create a grid of all resource assignments for easy tracking and reference. Regardless of the type of project, informatics projects are expensive and often incur unexpected costs for items such as adding computer memory, upgrading wireless systems, and developing new interfaces. Funds must be allocated for staff, servers, hardware such as new computers, scanners, printers, wiring, antennas, training rooms, software, and post-live vendor support. Physical requirements may include creating additional space in the clinical units, patient rooms, dictation areas, doctor lounges, etc.

Risk Factors

A good project plan identifies all probable and possible risk factors that may interfere with achieving a successful project completed on time, with sufficient quality, and within budget. A risk management plan lists corresponding reasonable strategies to mitigate the identified risks. Some risk factors can be anticipated with plans to minimize their effect, such as an upcoming accreditation inspection, the possibility of a strike by workers, new construction, and remodeling. Unexpected risk factors may be a loss of key project players, a publicized sentinel event, or a natural disaster in the area.

Scope Creep

Scope creep is one of the most frequent causes of project delays. Scope creep is defined as changes in the scope of the project during the implementation that frequently

reviewed in all end user training classes. Student reactions to this information in these classes can be an important alert concerning workflow processes that need additional discussion and/or design.

Building or Tailoring the Product

Once the current workflow is understood and redesigned, teams work to build or tailor the EHR to match the new workflow. Typically, clinical analysts work with vendor analysts to tailor a product for the current environment. Actual end-users are often involved in the process. At a minimum, once a module is initially tailored, analysts have end users assess the module in an iterative fashion. The following tips can be useful in this design process:

- Design and build the system to keep the number of clicks and amount of scrolling to an absolute minimum. Employees, such as physicians and others whose income can depend on their ability to manage more patients in less time, in particular will calculate the time it takes to perform common tasks. Excess clicking can be a huge user dissatisfier and can discourage users. To avoid excessive clicks, implementation analysts often use what is commonly referred to as the 80/20 rule. The term *80/20* refers to a mathematical formula proposed by an Italian economist in 1906 that states that 80% of our results or outcomes are derived from 20% of our efforts or causes.[31] An example of applying the 80/20 rule in health informatics is to assign default responses when a specific response is selected 80% of the time. For instance, builders will prefill as many of the fields as possible in order entry, with prompts such as "Routine" for the priority and "Once" for the frequency for all laboratory and radiology orders to facilitate faster order entry. The underlying rule is to minimize all keystrokes and excessive scrolling whenever possible. Default settings can be especially useful in saving time, but they also need to be evaluated carefully to ensure that they do not increase safety issues.

- Do not ask clinicians to respond to prompts that they cannot answer. For example, most radiology systems have a mandatory prompt for "Method of Transportation." Physicians most likely do not know if the patient requires a gurney or a wheelchair and will typically select the first option to place the order. Some organizations now use a default of "Wheelchair" or a term such as "Call Unit" for the "Method of Transportation." Avoid the overuse of alerts in order to minimize alert fatigue. Alert fatigue occurs when a user becomes desensitized to pop-ups or alerts if too many are triggered during an average session. Set the level of sensitivity so that only critical medical alerts fire and those with marginal clinical significance are suppressed.

- Maintain a consistent look and feel to the screens so the same information is always found in the same place on the screen and color-coding is consistent on every screen. Ideally this consistency should extend across vendors and institutional departments.

Testing

Implementing or upgrading an electronic health system involves extensive testing. The different types of testing must be carefully planned and conducted throughout the project. These include hardware, software, and functional testing. Functional testing is used to determine whether the system functions as designed and works effectively with the newly structured work processes. All testing should be done first within a module. Once all modules are functioning correctly, integrated testing across modules is performed using patient flow scenarios. Table 19.3 outlines several different types of testing that are often part of the testing protocol.

A test plan is often created in a spreadsheet format. The plan should include fields for the name of the test, date of the test, name of the tester, log-in used for the test, role of the tester (e.g., medical doctor [MD], nurse practitioner [NP], registered nurse [RN], respiratory therapist [RT], unit secretary [US]), test objective, and test instructions. An example of such a test plan is shown in Fig. 19.3.

TABLE 19.3	Different Types of Testing During an Implementation and Post Go-Live	
Testing Type	**Description**	**Examples**
ADT testing (see Fig. 19.3)	ADT testing involves testing for every possible type of ADT transaction used in the organization for inpatients, outpatients, serial patients, and preadmits. These transactions include admit; discharge; transfer; cancel admit; cancel discharge; cancel transfer; change beds, rooms, or departments; merge accounts; etc.	The tester will ask registration to admit several new patients. Tester will verify that patient is in correct department, room, and bed, and all data entered during admission are correct. Admissions then will cycle through the various transactions, with the tester validating each change.
Unit testing and functional testing	Unit testing is a very basic type of testing where the tester runs through the basic functionalities and features of an application. It is a high-level cursory walk-through of the application. The goal is to identify deviations from the expectations and to correct these unexpected results. The tester will not test every order or documentation field but will need to test every possible scenario.	For a CPOE application, the tester will enter interfaced and noninterfaced orders in the application and follow them through. The tester will verify that order details display appropriately and that orders are received in the ancillary system.

Continued

TABLE 19.3 Different Types of Testing During an Implementation and Post Go-Live—cont'd

Testing Type	Description	Examples
Integrated testing	Integrated testing tests the transmission of messages between all systems such as the healthcare information system, laboratory, radiology, pharmacy, dietary, cardiology, etc. This test includes testing all bidirectional order messages and results going across the interface(s).	The tester will enter different kinds of orders in the CPOE system to interfaced ancillary applications like laboratory, radiology, pharmacy, dietary, and cardiology, and then cycle through all actions that are permitted per user role, including canceling the order, discontinuing the order, modifying the order, holding the order, etc. This also includes testing "unsolicited" orders, orders that originate in an ancillary system. An example of an unsolicited order is when the laboratory system initiates an order in response to the result of a previous order such as performing an HIV Western blot if HIV antibody is positive.
Hardware testing	Hardware testing includes the capability of hardware interfacing with the EHR such as computers, printers, label printers, barcode printers, tablets, scanners, modems, etc.	The IT team will test that diet requisitions print in the dietary department, but dietitian consults print to the dietitian's office at the specific times based on table settings. Another example is that lab labels print in the patient departments for specimens that are collected by the nurse but print in the lab for specimens that are collected by lab personnel.
Volume testing	Volume testing is sometimes called "stress testing." Systems are built to accommodate the largest number of users accessing the system at the same time with no or minimal reduction in overall performance.	Early morning physician rounding and early afternoons are typically peak times for accessing the EHR. This type of testing may include asking a large group of students to log on and perform a variety of tasks simultaneously.
Security testing	Different staff members will have different reasons to access an EHR, and their roles will define what they can and cannot do in the system. Security testing checks that each provider type is able to perform functionalities specific to the role (entering orders, vital signs, nursing documentation, viewing results, medication reconciliation, etc.) but is prohibited from unauthorized actions, viewing, or access.	The IT department will validate that nursing assistants have the security to document vital signs, height, weight, I&O, and percentage of meals consumed but not be able to review the chart or enter orders. Another example is that a physician or RN can perform medication reconciliation with a change in the level of care but a nursing assistant cannot.
ARRA-related Meaningful Use testing	With the introduction of Meaningful Use, eligible providers, hospital organizations, and CAH must test their ability to collect required information and demonstrate that they meet Meaningful Use criteria.	A few of the CMS requirements for MU Stage 1 include • Assessing all patients for VTE prophylaxis • Recording smoking status on more than 50% of patients 13 years and older • Recording advance directives for more than 50% of patients 65 years and older • Providing more than 50% of patients with an electronic copy of their discharge instructions at time of discharge, upon request • Reporting hospital clinical quality measures to CMS or the states

ADT, Admission, discharge, and transfer; *ARRA*, American Recovery and Reinvestment Act; *CAH*, Critical Access Hospitals; *CMS*, Centers for Medicare and Medicaid Services; *CPOE*, computerized provider order entry; *EHR*, electronic health record; *I&O*, intake and output; *IT*, information technology; *RN*, registered nurse; *VTE*, venous thromboembolism.

The testing process requires that a testing environment be created within the organization's electronic system. Box 19.2 lists the different environments that are usually created in order to install and maintain a healthcare information system. These environments can be conceptualized as copies of the live environment. Testing is best done in an environment as close to reality as possible. Using the test environment to execute test plans, the implementation team will develop detailed test plans for each staff group such as healthcare providers (physicians, physician assistants, and advanced practice registered nurses), staff nurses, pharmacists, unit secretaries, and ancillary personnel for each application. Test plans evaluate information and data flow throughout the application, including, for example, messages, allergies,

Date: Tester Ext:

Tester
Name: Tester Dept.

Application:
ABC Clinical System
Test Title:
ADT Test PLAN
Test Objective:
To test each inbound and outbound ADT interface planned for the system
Test Conditions:
Only test message types relevant to customer site

Test Instructions:
1. Review the test steps defined below and execute the steps as they are written. Please attempt to execute all steps of the test.
2. Review the expected results for each step.
3. If the result is achieved, select PASS in the Status column.
4. If a different result is achieved, select FAIL in the Status column.
5. If the result is Fail, describe the actual outcome in the Actual Outcome/Exception Description column.
6. If you are unable to execute a step because of a defect or an error, try to navigate to a point where you can resume the steps and indicate what you did in the Actual Outcome column.
7. If it is not possible to continue with the test, indicate what happens in the Actual Outcome column.

Test Execution & Results:

Step #	Step Description	Test Data	Expected Results	Date Executed	Status	Actual Outcome/ Exception Description	Issue ID	Pass	Fail
1			**ADT** **(A01) Admit Pt**						
1.01	Admit a patient in the HIS system. Assign a station, room, and bed.		Interface receives an ADT A01 message. Message posts successfully. Patient visit accessible in HealthView.					0	0
1.02								0	0
1.03								0	0
2			**(A02) Transfer Pt**						
2.01	Transfer a patient in the HIS system to a different station, room, or bed.		Interface receives an ADT A02 message. Message posts successfully. Patient visit accessible in Healthview, with correct location.					0	0
2.02								0	0
2.03								0	0
3			**(A03) Discharge Pt**						
3.01	Discharge a patient in the HIS system.		Interface receives an ADT A03 message. Message posts successfully. Patient visit accessible in Healthview with discharge date.					0	0
3.02								0	0
3.03								0	0
4			**(A04) Register Pt**						
4.01	Register a patient in the HIS system.		Interface receives an ADT A04 message. Message posts successfully. Patient visit accessible in Healthview.					0	0
4.02								0	0
4.03								0	0
5			**(A05) Pre-Admit Pt**						
5.01	Pre-admit a patient in the HIS system.		Interface receives an ADT A05 message. Message posts successfully. Pre-admit patient visit accessible in Healthview.					0	0
5.02								0	0
5.03								0	0
6			**(A06) Transfer O/P to I/P**						
6.01	Transfer an outpatient visit to inpatient status. Assign to a station.		Interface receives an ADT A06 message. Message posts successfully. Patient visit accessible in Healthview in correct location.					0	0
6.02								0	0
6.03								0	0
7			**(A07) Transfer I/P to O/P**						
7.01	Transfer an inpatient visit to outpatient status.		Interface receives an ADT A07 message. Message posts successfully. Outpatient visit accessible in Healthview.					0	0
7.02								0	0
7.03								0	0
8			**(A08) Update Pt Info**						

FIG 19.3 Sample test plan. *ADT,* admission, discharge, and transfer; *HIS,* healthcare information system; *Pt,* patient. (Copyright McKesson Corporation.)

BOX 19.2 Healthcare Information System Online Environments

- *Live or production* environment refers to the healthcare information system application's actual use with patient and hospital data. Testing and teaching should not be done using this environment since changes are very likely to affect patient care.
- *Build* environment refers to a copy of a healthcare information system application that is used to configure and customize an application. Building usually occurs at the module level. Once a module is designed, it is moved to the test environment.
- *Test* environment refers to a copy of the healthcare information system application that is used to test the application. It should be a complete copy of the most recent version of the actual application. The test version of the software should not be an empty shell but should reflect the actual type and

amount of data one would expect to see in the live environment.
- *Teaching* environment refers to a copy of the healthcare information system application that is used for teaching users. Like the test version of the software, this version should not be an empty shell but should reflect the actual type and amount of data one would expect to see in the live environment.
- *Teaching/testing* environment refers to the combined use of a healthcare information system application for both testing and teaching activities. This does require careful scheduling since testing should not occur at the same time that a class is using the environment for teaching. However, the advantages are that this approach saves resources, and using the test environment for teaching provides additional testing for the application.

orders, test and other diagnostic results, automatic and manually demanded reports, and archiving of the patient's record post discharge. If this is an upgrade implementation, medical facilities often have ready-made test plans that they use with each upgrade but modify to accommodate changed or new functionalities, improved features, and fixes to previous defects. An upgrade test plan differs from a new implementation test plan in that the upgrade test plan typically has a short list of test items or orders for each department versus a new implementation that involves testing every item in the order item dictionary, as well as every prompt and combination of prompt responses on each order. Testing includes all devices such as computers, printers, handheld devices, barcode scanners, etc.

PREPARING FOR GO-LIVE

Preparing for go-live involves deciding on the go-live approach; developing the go-live plan, support, and schedule; and preparing the end users.

Big Bang or Incremental Go-Lives

There are two approaches to a go-live: big bang or incremental (also called a phased or a staged approach). The **big bang** approach occurs when all applications or modules are implemented at once. This approach is favored by vendors and facilities conducting large upgrades. With a **phased go-live** approach, both paper and electronic environments exist at the same time within the healthcare institution; however, the existence of both paper and electronic environments forces the clinician to use different workflows in patient units that have implemented the system than in units that have not, potentially creating safety concerns. The advantages of the big bang approach are that it is usually less expensive and implementation time is shorter, allowing staff to return to a new normal and see early improvements in the project metrics more quickly. The negatives associated with the big bang approach are the significant reductions in productivity seen immediately at go-live and for a short time afterwards due

to users' unfamiliarity with the new system and a large influx of requests to tweak the system (Box 19.3).

The incremental approach is usually selected when a facility has limited resources that cannot support a house-wide implementation or when the facility has a low tolerance for or ability to respond to institutional changes. There are a variety of ways to employ this method. Some facilities may decide to go-live with specific staff groups such as nurses, unit secretaries, and ancillary staff, including laboratory, pharmacy, radiology, respiratory therapy, physical therapy, occupational therapy, speech therapy, and dietary, followed by physicians and other clinicians a short time later. Others may choose to go-live with select clinical departments or product lines (e.g., patient flow within a specialty such as surgery). Reasons for selecting the first units to go-live may be based on their perceived support and enthusiasm for the project or their low number of admissions, transfers, and discharges. Advantages of the incremental approach are that it allows time to make changes to the build or the workflows and does not decrease productivity house wide while creating constant change for end users. The early adopters or the new users of the initial departments normally will share their experiences, perceptions, and satisfaction with others. However, this communication can either support or speak against the project. The disadvantages include the potential for errors due to multiple systems and the possibility that the project can be protracted and workflow disruptions will occur over a longer period, although on a smaller scale. Another factor to consider with the incremental approach is the availability of support for each successive unit. Most vendors typically like to transition from their implementation or services team to the support team 2 to 4 weeks after initial go-live. Continued support can be expensive for organizations. This also means that the organization will be calling vendor employees who may not be familiar with the build, workflows, and customizations when issues arise with each new mini go-live. Repetitive go-lives also tax the IT department and the superusers and delay the deployment of fixes and physician requests from the initial go-live departments. Sometimes the rollout is more

---

BOX 19.3   Advantages and Disadvantages of the Big Bang Approach

Advantages

- Eliminates staff having to use two systems or processes in different departments, which decreases the number of errors
- Total cost of entire implementation is lower
- Project is less likely to stall and is more likely to fully implement the system
- Shorter implementation cycle and shorter implementation pain
- Quicker improvements in EHR-related metrics (decreased use of nonformulary medications, decreased pharmacy callbacks)
- Immediate compliance with American Recovery and Reinvestment Act–mandated requirements for Meaningful Use to receive "stimulus" funds
- On-site and remote support personnel and implementation consultants from the vendor are available for the initial days of the go-live

Disadvantages

- Significant decrease in productivity in the initial days and immediately after go-live, with a gradual return to baseline
- Less time to make changes to the build or workflows
- Changes in workflows and processes are turned on house-wide with everyone on same learning curve, making implementation pain and anxiety greater
- Must plan for large number of support personnel in the information technology department and roaming superusers to all departments

---

BOX 19.4   Advantages and Disadvantages of the Incremental Approach

Advantages

- Allows time to make changes to build and workflows with each new batch of users
- Early reports of success breed enthusiastic support for the upcoming departments
- Less impact on productivity
- Restricts implementation pain to a smaller number of select users or departments

Disadvantages

- Staff that circulate through the organization must use two workflows, which can increase the number of errors
- Project may stall due to users' dislike of using different processes or workflows in different departments and changes that are made after each mini go-live
- Total cost of entire implementation is higher due to extended support and training
- Longer implementation time that will leave staff with the feeling that the system is "not ready for prime time."
- Delays compliance with American Recovery and Reinvestment Act–mandated requirements for Meaningful Use to receive "stimulus" funds
- Most vendors transition customers to their support division within 2 to 4 weeks post go-live
- Early reports of dissatisfaction may dissuade others from embracing the system

---

prolonged than originally planned or it may even stall indefinitely due to user dissatisfaction. The early go-live users who do not see quick resolution of easily fixed issues will complain because the support staff is too busy with the next go-live unit (Box 19.4).

Detailed Go-Live Plan

A detailed go-live plan includes each planned activity as a line item assigned to a specific individual or team with a completion date for each task. The go-live plan should include critical tasks that are scheduled to be completed a few days to a few weeks before the go-live date. Some project managers may break down the immediate days before go-live to the number of hours before go-live, marking tasks that must precede other tasks. Some of these may include cross-checking the patient census between the new and old systems, backloading a specific number of days of diagnostic tests results and medications into the new EHR, and confirming that all active and future orders on all patients are in the new HER.

Education and Training

A common mistake in an implementation or upgrade is not planning sufficient time to thoroughly train end users or failure to allot a sufficient budget to conduct training.[32] Education of all end users is a mini project and is best assigned to a person or facility education department that can coordinate or oversee all of its components. In fact, training is complex enough that software support in the form of a learning management system (LMS) is often used. An LMS includes planning and tracking the end users trained and the results of any competency tests. A training plan must address the development of teaching plans, training manuals, and job aids that provide instructions on common tasks and can be used during training and on the job. Different types of training must be developed for the different groups of end users, including physicians, students and/or outside faculty, nurses, pharmacists, unit secretaries, and ancillary personnel such as respiratory therapy, rehabilitative services, clergy, quality control, etc. For example, physicians will need instruction on using CPOE, viewing test results, viewing charting, and performing medication reconciliation, while nurses will need education related to order review, order entry, nursing documentation, and medication administration.

Policy and procedures for dealing with the consequences for not attending and/or passing the training should be developed as part of the training plan. For example, should providers with order-entry privileges be suspended if they have not demonstrated that they are competent to use the system for order entry? If yes, how should this policy be implemented if there are patients who are dependent on this provider for the management of their care?

Questions to consider in planning education hours are the number of users to be educated, education methodology including online or traditional classroom, the timing and length of the classes for each user group, the number of training rooms and training devices available, the training schedule, and trainers for each group. The content of the course should reflect the scope and standards for practice with role-specific processes, decisions, tasks, workflow and policy changes, and supportive EHR functions for each group of users. During training, common user errors or system quirks should be highlighted to help users avoid them. MU-related tasks such as assessing smoking status, advance directives, and immunization status should also be addressed so that users understand the importance of completing those data fields. Privacy and security policies, including not sharing one's log-in and password and accessing only those medical records the user needs to review, should be emphasized in every class. The consequences for violating privacy and security policies and practices should also be clearly stated.

Trainers

Depending on the organization's structure, the trainers might be in-house staff, vendor educators, temporary consultants, superusers or power users, or a mix of these. Organizations need to identify how professional students such as nursing or medical students will be educated on the new EHR. Some have regularly scheduled classes where students can register to attend while others take a "train the trainer" approach using the school's educators to provide the education. If the organization is using a big bang approach, it will often need to bring in temporary trainers in order to get all users trained and then

revert to in-house educators or superusers following go-live for new hires, system upgrades, and remediation training. The advantages of using in-house educators are that they are familiar with the organization's policies and usually have a background in adult education. Vendor educators and consultants frequently know the application very well but are not familiar with the organization's future workflows and policies. Superusers who can spend time with students who are having difficulties are valuable as assistants in the classroom. Training is an ongoing process that will continue after go-live to orient new hires and to address new responsibilities or changes in staff roles that consequently cause changing workflows.

Training Methodology

Most organizations use a combination of different training methods. One of the most popular methods is an instructor-led class in a classroom that contains all of the equipment needed to demonstrate essential functionalities, including printers, barcode scanners, identification bands, medication labels, etc. The advantages of instructor-led training are the ability for end users to ask questions, quick clarification of complex concepts, and easy identification of users who may need additional help. The primary disadvantages are the expense and resources needed to have multiple instructor-led classes. In addition, the number of students per session is limited, and no-shows are common among nurses and physicians since training competes with patient care needs. Another common training method includes a blended approach in which end users complete an "anytime/anywhere" online module about EHR basics and then attend a brief instructor-led session. These are also used as mini-refreshers or primers during upgrades.[33] A major drawback to using a variety of approaches is the constant need to update all of the training materials with the introduction of new functionalities. No matter the approach, the use of competency tests to assess proficiency is recommended.

With a CPOE implementation, most organizations create a new position for CPOE liaisons who are dedicated to clinician training 24 hours a day, 7 days a week. Physicians may be unable or unwilling to attend scheduled classes and prefer just-in-time or one-on-one education.[34] Some organizations employ physician liaisons who are dedicated exclusively to assisting physicians. Even though this is a labor-intensive strategy, physicians quickly become adept at their new workflows, report greater user satisfaction, and have a greater likelihood of using and being satisfied with the new system.

Length of Class and Class Schedule

Depending on the EHR functions needed, class time will vary. For example, CPOE classes for unit secretaries in an organization where prescribers will be expected to use CPOE may be 2 to 3 hours, whereas the same classes for healthcare providers may require 6 to 8 hours. Once the total number of users and the number of hours for each learning module are determined, a training schedule is developed, often using the LMS mentioned earlier. With a house-wide go-live, training will need to be provided around the clock. If users must attend class during their off-duty time, organizations will have to consider paying overtime. Alternately, if user education is incorporated into the 40-hour workweek, replacement staff may be required. End users should not be expected to attend class immediately after a shift when they are most likely tired and may not be able to leave their department when planned. Education should be conducted as close to the go-live date as possible to facilitate retention of the new knowledge and skills, with a goal of no more than 4 weeks pre-live. It is recommended that users have access to a device that points to the train environment to practice and become more familiar with the system. Some hospitals dedicate one device on each clinical unit that is in a remote location like the break room, while others reserve a readily accessible classroom with several devices. Once a significant majority of employees has completed the training, the institution is ready for go-live.

GO-LIVE

During the initial weeks of the go-live, organizations must plan to provide close support ("elbow-to-elbow" support) for end users. Many institutions will provide 24/7 support for a week or two and a few may offer it for several weeks. Assigning superusers wearing easily identifiable apparel to roam departments offering assistance to users is an excellent tactic that is well received by the end users. Issues, questions, and misunderstandings should be reported to the project team, which then catalogs, prioritizes, and tracks them for resolution and future reference. Additional tips include the following:

- Avoid a go-live date that falls on a weekend, a Monday or Friday, or close to a major holiday when vendor support personnel may be less available. Two exceptions to this guideline are the implementation of a new financial system, which must start at midnight on the first day of the month for billing purposes, and a big bang implementation, which is typically scheduled to start on a weekend to minimally affect surgery and procedure services.
- Set up an organized and well-equipped command center for the go-live that includes the following:
  - A highly publicized hotline number for assistance; incoming calls need to roll over to a bank of well-staffed phones.
  - A system for reporting, cataloging, assigning criticality, and assigning skilled resources to identified issues and problems.
  - A hotline number is one communication method, but urgent issues need to be addressed and, if necessary, escalated immediately to the vendor or IT department for resolution. Stock the command center with supplies such as whiteboards, poster boards, phones with outside access, preprinted "Issue Reporting" forms, printers, office supplies, meals, snacks, and water. Devices must be loaded with new software and integrated with upstream ADT and downstream (laboratory, radiology, pharmacy, dietary, electrocardiography, etc.) systems for immediate troubleshooting.

- Devise several different mechanisms to obtain and give user feedback in a timely manner.
- Include clearly identified people associated with the command center and project. For example, roaming superusers could wear an identifying T-shirt, vest, or large easy-to-read badge in the project "color."

Other go-live tactics include the following:

- Give small gifts to units (donuts or bakery items, boxes of candy, popcorn tins, balloons for desks).
- Use posters or banners in main lobbies, atriums, and waiting rooms.
- Provide a well-publicized process for end users to communicate with the implementation team and change-control committee (which collects and prioritizes system changes).
- Provide a generic e-mail address for users to ask questions, request a change or new item, or make suggestions, with prompt feedback to users' questions and requests.
- Create a suggestion box that allows anonymous input and has scheduled collections.
- Place notebooks in staff lounges with scheduled pickups and returns.
- Send e-mails to all users that include FAQs and "Tips and Tricks."

POST-LIVE MAINTENANCE

A vendor-supported implementation is officially over when the system formally transitions from the vendor's services team to its support division. With in-house development, the project leader announces when the go-live is over. Maintenance is an ongoing process that involves a variety of tasks such as applications updates, patches for identified defects, and a continuous revision of the system in response to users' requests. This includes revising documentation screens, adding new content, creating new orders such as new medications, and deactivating obsolete content such as outdated interventions and medications that are no longer in the hospital formulary. While outdated content is deactivated from user access, a record of the content must be maintained. For example, if a drug is removed from the formulary, a record of when this drug was in the formulary must be maintained. The change control committee receives input for new content, such as newly defined order sets, as well as requests for revisions to current order sets so that they align with updated best practices. Users may discover system flaws that were not detected during testing, and these need to be submitted to the change control committee and vendor. In addition, the IT departments should conduct regularly scheduled rounds to the clinical units to solicit input from the users.

As mentioned earlier, major reasons to implement EHRs are patient safety, improved patient care, and clinical outcomes. One of the final tasks in the implementation plan is to evaluate whether and how the system made a difference according to the metrics identified and collected during the preimplementation phase. This collection of data is typically performed approximately 3 to 6 months after the go-live to allow users to become more proficient with the EHR.

Implementing a new EHR or upgrading an older version is a process without a definitive end point. After installation, an EHR will require software upgrades, new hardware, ongoing training of staff, and education of IT staff.[32]

CONCLUSION AND FUTURE DIRECTIONS

Meeting MU criteria as well as future criteria developed to support the Medicare Access and CHIP Reauthorization Act of 2015 (MACRA) and the Merit-Based Incentive Payment System (MIPS) will continue to spur growth of EHRs. In the future, increasing numbers of patients will interact with their healthcare providers via electronic means to set up appointments, send questions, request prescription refills, and retrieve their health record, including test results. There will be rapid movement away from stand-alone outpatient EHR systems toward integrated systems. Mobile devices such as smartphones and iPads will play a larger role in patient–clinician relationships and nurse–patient–family relationships in the home. Health-related apps that allow for home monitoring of vital signs, blood glucose levels, electrocardiography monitoring, and fetal monitoring will become commonplace.

In the future, the United States may develop a registry to track EHR-related safety issues. The registry could be used to monitor safety and adverse issues and initiate timely notifications to medical providers and patients.[35] In a similar vein, the Institute of Medicine advocates the creation of a new federal agency or National EHR Safety Board under the auspices of HHS to oversee EHR safety. Presently there is no formal national or global process through which organizations or individual users can report possible EHR-related safety issues. The IOM also recommends that the federal agency have the authority to (1) require IT vendors to register their products and communicate negative events associated with their applications, (2) establish mandatory IT safety criteria, and (3) publish an annual report on identified safety issues and strategies in an effort to minimize or eliminate them.[36–38] No matter whether the EHR is new or an upgrade, the ultimate goal in implementations now and in the future is to provide the highest level of care at the lowest cost with the least risk.

REFERENCES

1. The White House. *Promoting Innovation and Competitiveness: President Bush's Technology Agenda.* The White House; 2004. http://www.whitehouse.gov/infocus/technology/economicpolicy200404/innovation.pdf.
2. One Hundred Eleventh Congress of the United States of America. *The American Recovery and Reinvestment Act of 2009, Title XIII.* Heath Information Technology; 2009. http://www.gpo.gov/fdsys/pkg/BILLS-111hr1enr/pdf/BILLS-111hr1enr.pdf.
3. *Healthcare Information Technology Standards Panel (HITSP).* HITSP Quality Measures Technical Note ED, VTE, and Stroke Examples for Implementation of the HITSP Quality Interoperability Specification: HITSP/TN906.
4. Centers for Medicare & Medicare Services (CMS). *CMS Fact Sheet: EHR Incentive Programs in 2015 and Beyond*; 2015.
   https://www.cms.gov/Newsroom/MediaReleaseDatabase/Fact-sheets/2015-Fact-sheets-items/2015-10-06-2.html.
5. Terry K. *CCHIT Exits EHR Certification Business.* Information Week; 2014. http://wwwinformationweek.com/healthcare/policy-and-regulation/cchit-exits-ehr-certification-business/d/d-id/1113632.
6. *Health IT.gov.* ONC Health it Certification Program FAQs. https://www.healthit.gov/policy-researchers-implementers/permanent-certification-program-faqs. Accessed July 10, 2016.
7. US DHHS Office of the National Coordinator ONC. *About the ONC Health IT Certification Program*; November 3, 2015. https://www.healthit.gov/policy-researchers-implementers/about-onc-health-it-certification-program.
8. Duke JD, Morea J, Mamlin B, et al. Regenstrief Institute's Medical Gopher: a next-generation homegrown electronic medical record system. *Int J Med Inform.* 2014;83(3):170–179.
9. Braunstein M. *How a Healthcare Clinic Plans to Become a Software Company.* InformationWeek; 2015. http://wwwinformationweek.com/software/enterprise-applications/how-a-healthcare-clinic-plans-to-become-a-software-company/a/d-id/1320339?.
10. Mace S. *Tech Tactics for the Long-Term.* HealthLeaders Media; 2016. http://wwwhealthleadersmedia.com/technology/tech-tactics-long-term?page=0%2C1.
11. Charles D, Gabriel M, Searcy T. *Adoption of Electronic Health Record Systems among U.S. Nonfederal Acute Care Hospitals: 2008–2014*; April 2015. ONC Data Brief No. 23. https://www.healthit.gov/sites/default/files/data-brief/2014HospitalAdoptionDataBrief.pdf.
12. Centers for Medicare & Medicaid Services (CMS). *ICD-10 Overview*; 2012. https://www.cms.gov/Medicare/Medicare-Contracting/ContractorLearningResources/downloads/ICD-10_Overview_Presentation.pdf.
13. AHA News Now. *New ICD-10 Diagnosis Codes Released*; 2016. http://news.aha.org/article/160322-new-icd10-diagnosis-codes-released.
14. Sackett DL, Rosenberg WM, Gray JA, Haynes RB, Richardson WS. Evidence based medicine: what it is and what it isn't. *Br Med J.* 1996;312(7023):71–72.
15. Berner ES. *Clinical Decision Support Systems: State of the Art.* Agency for Healthcare Research and Quality; 2009. http://healthitahrq.gov/images/jun09cdsreview/090069ef.html.
16. Agency for Healthcare Research and Quality (AHRQ). *Translating Research into Practice (TRIP)-II: Fact Sheet*; 2001. http://www.ahrq.gov/research/trip2fac.htm.
17. Menachemi N, Collum T. Benefits and drawbacks of electronic health record systems. *Risk Manag Healthc Pol.* 2011;4:47–55. http://dx.doi.org/10.2147/RMHP.S12985.
18. Joint Commission of Accreditation of Healthcare Organizations. *Hospitals' National Patient Safety Goals.* The Joint Commission. 2004. http://wwwjointcommission.org/PatientSafety/NationalPatientSafetyGoals/04npsgs.htm.
19. Kaplan JM, Ancheta R, Jacobs BR. Clinical informatics outcomes research group: inpatient verbal orders and the impact of computerized provider order entry; *J Pediatr.* 2006;149:461–467.
20. Ash JA, Sittig DF, Dykstra R, Campbell E, Guappone K. The unintended consequences of computerized provider order entry: findings from a mixed methods exploration. *Int J Med Inform.* 2009;78:S69–S76. http://dx.doi.org/10.1016/j.ijminf2008.07.15.

21. Ash JA, Stavri Z, Kuperman GJ. A consensus statement on considerations for a successful CPOE implementation. *J Am Med Inform Assoc.* 2003;10:229–234. http://dx.doi.org/10.1197/jamia.M1204.

22. Weiner JP, Kfuri T, Chan K, Fowles JB. e-Iatrogenesis: the most critical unintended consequence of CPOE and other HIT. *J Am Med Inform Assoc.* 2007;14:387–388. http://dx.doi.org/10.1197/jamia.M2338.

23. Institute for Safe Medication Practices (ISMP). *FDA and ISMP Lists of Look-alike Drug Names with Recommended Tall Man Letters*; 2011. http://www.ismp.org/tools/tallmanletters.pdf.

24. Ritz D. *Opinion: It's Time for a National Patient Identifier*; 2013. http://www.himss.org/News/NewsDetail.aspx?ItemNumber=21464.

25. Office of the National Coordinator for Health Information Technology. *Patient Identification and Matching Final Report*; 2014. https://www.healthit.gov/sites/default/files/patient_identification_matching_final_report.pdf.

26. Terry K. *National Patient Identifier Struggles for Life* CIO; 2015. http://www.cio.com/article/2972266/healthcare/national-patient-identifier-struggles-for-life.html.

27. Agency for Healthcare Research and Quality (AHRQ). *Percentage of Verbal Orders*; 2009. https://healthit.ahrq.gov/sites/default/files/docs/page/percentage-of-verbal-orders-quick-reference-guide.pdf.

28. Ash JA, Fournier L, Zoë Stavri P, Dykstra R. Principles for a successful computerized physician order entry implementation. *AMIA Annu Symp Proc.* 2003;36–40. http://www.ncbi.nlm.nih.gov/pmc/articles/PMC1480169/pdf/amia2003_0036.pdf.

29. Sklardin NT, Granovsky SJ, Hagerty-Paglia J. *Electronic Health Record Implementation at an Academic Cancer Center: Lessons Learned and Strategies for Success.* American Society of Clinical Oncology; 2011. Educational Book, http://www.asco.org/ASCOv2/Home/Education%20&%20Training/Educational%20Book/PDF%20Files/2011/zd900111000411.PDF.

30. McGonigle D, Mastrain K. *Nursing Informatics and the Foundation of Knowledge.* Sudbury, MA: Jones and Bartlett Publishers; 2009.

31. Hafner AW. *Pareto's Principle: The 80-20 Rule.* Ball State University; 2003. http://www.bsu.edu/libraries/ahafner/awh-th-math-pareto.html.

32. Grant JT. Allow time to implement EHR. *Ophthalmol Times.* 2010;35(7):54–56.

33. Jain V. Evaluating EHR, systems. *Health Manag Technol.* 2010;31(8):22–24.

34. Classen DC. Leading patient safety expert speaks on CPOE implementation strategy and success factors. *J Healthc Inf Manag.* 2004;18:15–17.

35. Consumer Reports. Dangerous devices. *Consum Rep.* 2012;77(5):24–28.

36. Goedert J. New report echoes call for national EHR safety board. *Health Data Manag.* 2011.

37. Institute of Medicine (IOM). *Health IT and Patient Safety: Building Safer Systems for Better Care*; 2011. http://www.iom.edu/hitsafety.

38. Sittig DF. Safe electronic health record use requires a comprehensive monitoring and evaluation framework. *J Am Med Assoc.* 2010;303(5):450–451. http://dx.doi.org/10.1001/jama.2010.61.

DISCUSSION QUESTIONS

1. Discuss the reasons why some institutions experience significantly more satisfaction or dissatisfaction during an implementation than do others.

2. What are some of the approaches that can be used to coordinate care during an incremental go-live as patients are transferred from units that have gone live to units still waiting to go live?

3. When developing new workflow processes using a systems approach, the work of patient care or specific tasks often shift from one department to another. While the new workflow can make the care provided to patients more efficient and effective for the institution as a whole, certain departments may experience more rather than less work. What are some approaches that can help users accept the new workflow?

4. Workarounds develop when employees find a quicker and/or easier way to complete a task. However, workarounds can create new and dangerous situations. Given the motivation for developing a workaround and the danger these can create, what are some of the guidelines or principles that should be used in managing workarounds?

5. Should insurers offer incentives to patients to select healthcare providers who are using EHRs to engage patients in managing their own care?

6. Review the EMR Adoption Model (EMRAM), an eight-step scale developed by the HIMSS to monitor hospitals' and health systems' EHR progress toward a paperless or near paperless system, at http://www.himssanalytics.eu/emram. What are the characteristics of the organizations who have successfully achieved Stage 7 status?

7. What are the advantages and disadvantages of a Healthcare Information Technology Standards Panel (HITSP)–certified health IT system versus a homegrown IT system that meets certification standards?

8. Should employees who have repeatedly failed to attend go-live classes be subjected to discipline measures?

9. Identify creative strategies to encourage physicians and other clinicians to participate in the implementation of a new health IT system.

10. Discuss ramifications and causes regarding interoperability issues among electronic health systems and applications.

CASE STUDY

Middleville Hospital, located in a small rural town, is a 58-bed acute care facility with both inpatient and outpatient services. The hospital consists of more than 600 employees and more than 300 volunteers. It is a community-owned, not-for-profit hospital dedicated to providing compassionate, accessible healthcare close to home. The facility primarily serves one major county and nine surrounding counties. The hospital has a homegrown EHR system, but its functionality just barely meets Meaningful Use Stage 2 criteria. The hospital's primary goal is to implement a certified EHR, but the leaders are weighing the benefits of two options: recruiting a skilled professional to rebuild the current system or purchasing a commercial system. There is pressure to make a decision as soon as possible.

What are the musts, constraints, and barriers?

- The new system must be fully implemented and operational no later than June 2017.
- The EHR must be able to meet MU Stage 3 criteria.
- The hospital has a very small IT department and a modest budget.
- The new EHR requires larger servers, new devices, central monitors, printers, and tablets.
- The wireless infrastructure must be upgraded to eliminate known dead spots in areas of the facility.
- The hospital wants to more effectively take advantage of select features such as clinical decision support and incorporate best practices or evidence-based medicine.

Discussion Questions

1. Based on what you read in this chapter and the case study, compile an initial list of functional requirements (functions needed) for the new EHR.
2. Create a brief evaluation plan by developing five or six criteria for evaluating vendors' products.

Case Study Follow-Up

The hospital made a list of all pros and cons of rebuilding a homegrown system or buying a commercial product. Realizing that regulations governing healthcare and reimbursement will only become more complicated, the hospital decided to go with a vendor-supplied EHR. Ultimately, it decided to purchase a fully integrated electronic health system that shares a common database to eliminate the issues often seen with interfaces.

Fourteen months later, the EHR went live house-wide for all staff, including housekeeping and pastoral services. The implementation included the functionality to meet MU and the installation of new servers and hardware in addition to an upgrade of the wireless network. All staff can even view a large monitor showing occupied, clean, and dirty beds that is updated by housekeeping.

The new EHR benefits are many. Initially the physicians grumbled about having to do "secretaries' work" in CPOE, but they gradually came to realize the benefits for their patients. Pharmacy reports a 55% decrease in nonformulary medications and a 73% reduction in physician callbacks. The time between a "stat" medication order and administration of the medication and the time between a "stat" lab test order and posting of the lab results have also decreased significantly. Due to the introduction of order sets based on best practices and evidence-based medicine, the hospital has seen a dramatic decrease in its 30-day readmission rates for heart attack, heart failure, and pneumonia patients compared to the U.S. national average and now has the lowest rates in the county.

Discussion Questions

1. Brainstorm two additional factors you would evaluate for this installation.

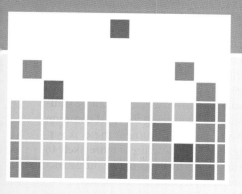

20

Downtime and Disaster Recovery for Health Information Systems

Nancy C. Brazelton and Ann M. Lyons

The primary objectives for downtime and disaster planning are to protect the organization and the patients served by minimizing operational disruptions.

OBJECTIVES

At the completion of this chapter, the reader will be prepared to:
1. Explain downtime risk assessment.
2. Analyze considerations for a health system inventory.
3. Describe an assessment tool for evaluating a downtime event.
4. Summarize the clinician's role in system downtime planning.
5. Summarize information technology's role in system downtime planning.
6. Establish key components of a business continuity plan for an organization.
7. Formulate communication strategies for downtime in an organization.

KEY TERMS

application, 338
bolt-on system, 341
business continuity, 348
clinical application, 340
cold site, 345
configuration management database (CMDB), 341
data center, 338
disaster recovery, 348
downtime, 337
electronic data interchange (EDI), 340
electronic health record (EHR), 341

enterprise resource planning (ERP), 340
high availability, 351
hot site, 345
human-made disaster, 338
incident response team (IRT), 347
information systems, 337
natural disaster, 338
picture archiving and communication system (PACS), 338
revenue cycle, 349
service level agreement (SLA), 345

ABSTRACT ❖

Healthcare entities are complex operations that are increasingly dependent on computerization. This chapter identifies tactics related to planning for and responding to computer downtime events and disasters. Focus areas include the clinical impact, the information technology (IT) impact, business continuity, and communications. A model for assessing the level of downtime response is provided.

INTRODUCTION

Healthcare entities, no matter how small or large, are extremely complex businesses that are increasingly dependent on computerization in their quest to provide exceptional healthcare. The employees of these healthcare organizations move through a unique labyrinth of systems, machines, workflows, regulatory requirements, business rules, and tools to provide the best care for patients and their families and to keep the business intact. Healthcare organizations select from a variety of vendors, adopt information systems at different rates, and implement systems in the order that works best for them.

Given the importance of information systems within any healthcare entity, institutions and their employees must be prepared for the many variations of downtime, including those caused by human errors, software and hardware failures, severed power cables, software viruses that invade the firewall, and disruptions caused by Mother Nature. The bulk of literature around the topic of downtime is in white papers, blogs, and industry group publications found via internet searches. The very few research articles discuss current trends and strategies.[1,2] The impetus to publish is often spurred by a downtime event experienced by the authors, who encourage readers to get plans in place.[3–5] Anderson reports a study conducted by AC Group that determined that each hour of downtime can cost $488 per physician per hour.[6] In their time and motion study, the authors determined that a physician spends 2.15 minutes during recovery for each minute the system was unavailable. A report estimates the average cost of a downtime is $8000 per minute.[7] The costs are staggering when translated to a large healthcare enterprise. Given the cost and the risk to patient care, the priorities for every healthcare institution are working to prevent downtime and recovering quickly if an incident occurs.

This chapter focuses on practical, tactical ways to put plans in place for managing health system downtime and disaster recovery. Tips and tools for downtime risk assessments, downtime and disaster response planning, clinical and information technology (IT) system recovery, and business continuity are provided. The chapter also provides information on developing a communication strategy and ideas for keeping patients safe and the business functioning, because downtime does happen.

DOWNTIME RISK ASSESSMENT

Planning for downtime can and should occur from project inception through system support, and maintenance and must include all existing systems and infrastructure. The complexity and criticality of the organization will determine how extensive an exercise this must be. Potential types of downtime and their impacts on the systems should be anticipated, and mitigation plans must be put in place.

Downtimes can be classified by the root cause and the degree of impact. A general network related incident or outage is different from a power outage or a planned software upgrade. A single noncritical software application may be unavailable, which will have a much lower impact than a total outage of the admission, discharge, and transfer (ADT) system. It is important to also consider the users or processes that are impacted.

Determining the root cause of a downtime is not always straightforward. The first step is to determine what is and what is not functioning; however, this first determination may not be the final answer. For example, a network downtime may be diagnosed easily by asking the following questions: Can you access the internet *and* the intranet? How about the computer next to you? What about the computer on the unit downstairs? If the answer to these questions is "no," suspect an entire network downtime. However, networks in many healthcare enterprises are now segmented for security purposes and include a series of switches, firewalls with coded rules, as well as the actual fiber network, cable pulls, and other components. This makes diagnosis of the specific network problem or the location of the problem more complex, potentially increasing the length of the network downtime. Also, external factors may exist, such as telecommunication fiber vendors that may be having problems as well as the millions of miles of fiber infrastructures vulnerable to physical damage, commonly referred to as "backhoe outage."

Thus the first step in preventing or managing a downtime is to determine what might cause a downtime and then to perform a risk assessment of the impact for each potential downtime. This step can be iterative with step three discussed below, which is compiling an inventory of existing applications and systems. Classifying all potential downtimes and putting them into mutually exclusive categories can be difficult. It is usually best to start by identifying the most common technology source of downtimes and document these. A systematic approach starting with infrastructure is more likely to ensure a comprehensive list. Begin by dividing the infrastructure into IT infrastructure and physical infrastructure.

IT infrastructure includes the network and application delivery systems, such as those listed in Box 20.1. Examples of physical structures include those listed in Box 20.2. Some overlap exists between the IT infrastructure and the physical infrastructure, and partial versus complete downtimes must be considered. Box 20.3 includes examples of both IT infrastructure and physical infrastructure. The order of the elements does not reflect their priority. Networks include both hardware and software components and therefore need to be examined from both aspects.

The second step is to identify the most common potential causes of a downtime in the facility, areas of vulnerability, and the most likely scenarios of natural disasters or human-made disasters in the geographic area. Is the facility or data center on an old or outdated power grid? Is the building only rated to withstand a 6.5 magnitude earthquake in an area where experts predict one much stronger? Is the facility's generator located in an area that is vulnerable to flooding? Common disasters are noted in Table 20.1; these lists are not

---

BOX 20.1   Sample Elements of Information Technology Infrastructure

- Electronic health record software
- Clinical and ancillary system software (e.g., physiologic monitoring, endoscopy, registry databases)
- **Picture archiving and communication system (PACS)**
- Laboratory applications
- Cardiology applications
- Radiology applications
- Anesthesia systems
- Surgical processing systems
- Revenue cycle software
- Interfaces or the interface engine
- Enterprise data warehouse

BOX 20.2   Examples of Information Technology Physical Structure

- Hardware related to the chillers that keep the data center cool
- Storage (physical hardware that stores the electronic health record, e-mail, and other third-party systems)
- Electrical power
- Network switches and hubs
- Biomedical devices
- Any component of the buildings themselves

BOX 20.3   Information Technology and Physical Infrastructure

Information Technology Infrastructure

- Application delivery system (e.g., Citrix)
- Asset management
- Biomedical devices with software components and network requirements
- Databases
- E-mail, other communications
- Enterprise data warehouse
- Help desk and computer support
- Identity management (e.g., active directory)
- Interface engine
- Interfaces
- Keyless entry systems or other security software
- Middleware servers
- Network
- Scanning software
- Security systems
- Software applications list with interdependencies identified (will be unique to each organization)
- Telecommunication systems (hospital operators, paging, cellphone, analog, Voice Over Internet Protocol)
- Web services

Physical Infrastructure

- Batteries
- Biomedical devices
- Buildings and facilities (list most likely maintained by an environment of care committee per requirements of accreditation and regulatory agencies)
- Cabling
- Chillers for data center
- Electrical power
- Emergency power outlets (red plugs)
- Generators and fuel supply
- Help desk and computer support
- Inventory (think broadly; replacement computer hardware to patient care supplies and paper forms)
- Medical record (paper) storage
- Medical gasses
- Network cables and other physical components
- Operator switchboard
- Pneumatic tube systems
- Physical security of buildings
- Printers (include printers for patient ID labels/wristbands)
- Reports
- Storage area network; other storage
- Scanners
- Servers
- Switches and hubs
- UPS (uninterruptible power supply)
- Utilities: power, heating, cooling, water

IT, Information technology; UPS, uninterruptible power supply.

TABLE 20.1   Downtime Vulnerabilities and Common Human-Made and Natural Disasters

Most Significant Downtime Vulnerabilities	Human-Made Disasters	Natural Disasters
Buildings or data center not to current code or vulnerable to natural or human-made disasters	Biologic: Intentional	Biologic
Cyber attack	Cyber attack	Dam failure
Lack of recovery site	Explosion: Intentional (bomb)	Drought
Lack of disaster planning or business continuity planning	Explosion: Unintentional (natural gas line rupture)	Earthquake
Lack of backups or inability to recover from backups	Fire	Fires, wildfires,[14] smoke
Lack of high availability or failover for critical systems or applications	Hazmat incident	Flood Heatwave
Lack of downtime planning	Nuclear incident	Hurricane
Outdated or aging physical infrastructure	Pandemic	Landslide, mudslide, debris flow
Outdated or aging technology (i.e., not on current or supported level of code or servers that are no longer supported)	Terrorist attack	Pandemic
Power grid and supply	Workforce violence, shootings, loss of life of key personnel	Snowstorm, blizzard
System resources at or near capacity (disk space, database, storage, etc.)		Space weather, geomagnetic storm Tornado Tsunami

TABLE 20.2 System Inventory Considerations

Type of System	Examples
Core clinical applications	Electronic medical record (EMR), electronic health record (EHR), emergency department, computerized provider order entry (CPOE), clinical documentation, medication administration record (MAR), surgical services, and anesthesia information system
Ancillary service and procedure area information services	Pharmacy, radiology and imaging, laboratory, arterial blood gas, cardiology, endoscopy, respiratory, neurology, nutrition care, dictation, health information management, biomedical devices (physiologic monitors, vital sign machines, intravenous pumps, ventilators, pneumatic tube systems, etc.)
Online reference databases	Drug information references; patient education; policies and procedures; disease, diagnosis, and interventional protocol databases; formulas or health-related calculators
Revenue cycle	Admission, discharge, and transfer; enterprise scheduling; preauthorization; facility and technical billing; health information (HIM), document management (scanning), coding; professional and physician billing; claim scrubbers; print vendors; address verification; electronic data interchange (EDI) transactions; benefit checking
Business, finance, and personnel	E-mail, office software, cash collections, credit card transactions, banking, business intelligence, reports and reporting, supply chain and enterprise resource planning (ERP), budgeting, human resources, payroll, staff scheduling, keyless entry, facilities and engineering, telephone systems and wiring, telephone operators, paging systems, wireless communication devices
Miscellaneous	Printers, Bluetooth devices (scanners, label printers), reports, data warehouse, barcode scanning, print vendor, internet-based public web pages, intranet and related internal web sites, wikis, clinical health information exchanges, retail outlets (retail pharmacies, gift shops, food service)

Note: This is not a complete list.

TABLE 20.3 Special Considerations by Area for Acute Care Setting

Area	Specialty Requirements
Anesthesia	Ventilators, anesthetic gases, frequent vital signs
Automated charge capture	Can be from many systems
Cardiac catheterization lab	Hemodynamic monitors, image capture, documentation for registries
Emergency department	Tracking patients in the waiting room and through the department
Endoscopy	Image capture and specific discreet documentation for registries or billing
Health information	Coding, release of information, maintenance of the legal medical record, legal cases, insurance queries, scanning solutions
Physicians, advanced practice clinicians	CPOE, clinical decision support systems, diagnostic test results, dictation
Newborn intensive care	Bedside monitoring and extracorporeal membrane oxygenation devices, ventilators, intravenous pumps
Nursing	Care planning, CPOE, Bar Code Medication Administration or electronic medication administration record, telemetry, patient communication systems with nurses, clinical decision support reminders, nursing databases (e.g., patient education resources)
Nutrition care	Assessments, nutrition care system, consultation notes, CPOE
Obstetrics	Fetal monitoring, mother and baby monitoring and documentation during the labor period, preterm wave forms, information from mother's record that needs to be available on newborn's record for continuity of care
Outpatient procedure areas	Point of care systems, registration and scheduling, medication-dispensing machines (i.e., Pyxis and Omnicell)
Pharmacy	Medication dispensing machines (Pyxis and Omnicell), robots, inpatient versus retail pharmacy ordering systems, intravenous pumps that contain drug-specific information (Alaris, etc.), pharmacy ordering system often interfaces with the medication supplier
Physical, occupational, and speech therapies	Therapy systems have specific patient education content
Physiologic monitoring	Often supported by biomedical engineering and has vendor-specific content
Radiology, imaging, and picture archiving and communication system	Image and procedure capture, multiple modalities, questionnaires
Respiratory therapy	Contains respiratory measures like ventilator settings, ventilator weaning parameters, respiratory treatments and measurements

CPOE, Computerized provider order entry.

mutually exclusive but instead provide a starting point for planning at a specific organization.

The third step is to complete an inventory of all systems and document them. All systems in use at the organization should be inventoried, because each is important to some aspect of the business. A sample inventory is located in Table 20.2.

An inventory list can be surprisingly difficult to compile and may involve doing walk-throughs of departments and units to observe systems and devices that end users are actually using in their day-to-day workflow. This is especially critical if the institution has a hybrid system (i.e., a system using multiple vendors for specific functionality). For instance, the ancillary systems within a hospital often have a limited amount of data requirements but highly specific ones. For example, the pharmacy may have homegrown applications perhaps to assist in adjudicating pharmaceutical costs in addition to major modules in an electronic health record (EHR). These unique systems are added on to the main EHR because of the need for specific functionality or perhaps because the ancillary application was built and implemented prior to the EHR. Table 20.3 lists areas that may have special considerations within an acute care setting. In addition, readers should remember to bear in mind the outpatient and ambulatory settings that may have unique requirements as well as specialty populations such as pediatrics[8] or geriatrics.

To locate applications, consider functional operations, type of personnel, data and information being processed or consumed, how and where vital records are housed, and policies and procedures that guide the business or practice.[9] This compilation will involve persistently reaching out to all members of the IT team or others who host applications or provide some component of infrastructure for input. The more specific and complete the inventory, the more useful and helpful it will be in the event of an actual planned or unplanned downtime. Due to the difficulty of getting a very complete inventory, it is best to start with the most critical applications and work on less critical ones later. Minimally, the inventory should include the items listed in Box 20.4.

Other data useful for general system support and downtime planning should be carefully documented as well. These items may be part of the application inventory, or they may be housed in a separate document, including those listed in Box 20.5.

System dependencies, configuration diagrams, and interface data should also be documented and stored in a place that is easily accessible and backed up on a routine basis as the final step. Best practices for maintaining this inventory and documentation from an Information Technology Infrastructure Library (ITIL) perspective is a configuration management database (CMDB) that has configuration items unique to the organization. However, many tools or combinations of tools are available for this purpose, such as shared drives and folders, spreadsheets, databases, vendor-supplied tools, wiki sites, collaboration software, document management systems repositories, or even simple paper notebooks.

With the appropriate data collected, IT should work very closely with the organization's emergency preparedness and disaster planning groups in planning for disasters. Having some component of IT downtime as a part of disaster drills is a very effective way for IT and staff to practice disaster response and hone plans. The federal government has published many helpful articles and websites to assist in institutional and personal planning and in case of an actual disaster.

BOX 20.4 Inventory Items

- Vendor name
  - If developed in-house, where is the source code and other documentation?
  - Date of contract and its current location
- Application or module name
  - Date of original go-live
- Current version
  - Date of upgrade
- Categorization (site defined): major/minor, Tier I/II/III, other
- Host model (where the application or service is located): in-house or remote
  - If remote, supported by whom?
- Interfaces, both inbound and outbound
- Third-party bolt-on systems
- Other key dependencies
- Primary use
- Primary users and number of users
- Business owners
- Information technology contacts
- Notes and comments

BOX 20.5 Elements for General Systems Support

- A checklist for the IT team to follow when a planned or unplanned downtime occurs
- Checklists and role definition cards for the clinicians, caregivers, and registration staff
- Known system vulnerabilities
- Documentation of frequent error messages
- Patterns of error messages indicating known problems or pending system failure
- Knowledge objects used in supporting or maintaining system
- Contact information with phone numbers for vendors and the teams supporting the application
- Service level agreements with key users of the application
- Preferred user communication plan for planned and unplanned downtimes
- Plan to deploy nonclinical staff to support clinicians or perform duties assigned by the command center
- Unit- or department-based workflow diagrams
- Unit or department blueprints that document all electronic devices connected to the wired or wireless network
- Agreed-upon time for planned changes and maintenance work, also known as a change window
- Policies, procedures, rules, or standards from information technology or the broader organization applying to the particular application

These include the Federal Emergency Management Agency (FEMA) website at www.ready.gov and several others, including the National Incident Management System (NIMS), Public Health Emergency and the U.S. Department of Health and Human Services, and an educational curriculum developed the Veterans Health Administration (VHA).[10–13]

DOWNTIME AND RESPONSE PLANNING

Once the system documentation is developed and the risks are understood, the healthcare institution is ready to define the different types of potential downtimes. These can be depicted on a continuum indicating the degree of significance for each potential downtime. The significance of the different downtimes will depend on the level of complexity and the installed base of the institution. For example, if the organization has results review implemented and a single results feed is down, the response will be very different than if the organizations has a mature EHR and the network is unavailable. Context makes a difference. For instance, is this a physician's office with a single provider and a very experienced staff or a huge integrated delivery network (IDN) spread across multiple states or geographic regions?

Consider both planned and unplanned downtimes. If a downtime is scheduled, there should be ample time to plan; however, if the downtime is unexpected, no contingency plans may be in place. A worst-case scenario of an unplanned downtime is a total loss of the network occurring midweek at the start of the business day when the hospital and clinic schedules are full, all operating rooms are in use, and the emergency department is busy and expecting two traumas (one via flight service) on a snowy winter day when 20% of staff is late due to road conditions.

Table 20.4 identifies a number of elements that will influence the impact of an individual downtime. The list in Table 20.4 is not intended to be followed linearly. Different scenarios or error messages will lead down different paths, just as different symptoms might lead to different diagnoses in patient care. In direct patient care, readers would take different actions if a patient's temperature increased by a half-degree Celsius and the heart rate increased by 10 beats per minute over the last 45 minutes, as opposed to if a patient had a sudden decrease in heart rate to 30 beats per minute. Some events allow for a measured response, whereas others require immediate attention. The same process occurs when managing EHRs or other systems. Being able to quickly translate error messages and recognize patterns are keys to reducing the length of the downtime and restoring clinician and staff workflow.

Once the organization has clear definitions for downtimes and has methods of assessing the significance of potential events,[4] the emergency preparedness and disaster planning

TABLE 20.4 Impact Considerations

Attribute	Continuum
Expected or actual duration	≤1 h to >4 h; should also plan for catastrophic events in which network or systems may take weeks to months to rebuild
Time of day	The slowest night of the week to about the busiest day of the week (think OR scheduling pattern)
Number of users affected and scope of outage	Single user or department to the entire facility; partial to full; single system or infrastructure component to complete loss of application, network, or building
IT infrastructure	Intact to completely damaged and replacement parts need to be ordered
Impact on workflow	Users are able to carry on activities with minimal disruption to complete change in workflow reverting to paper/manual systems
Complexity of IT installs and criticality of applications	Single system with review-only functionality to an organization that is >90% electronic and paperless with multiple systems for all business and healthcare requirements
Planned or unplanned	Downtime scheduled during agreed-upon service level agreement and system comes back up as promised to an unexpected system-wide downtime with no estimated time to recovery
Complexity of health system or complexity and criticality of unit or department affected	Single office to multistate integrated delivery network; office that still keeps paper records to a fully electronic ICU with patients on multiple assistive devices
Communication methods and mechanisms	Communicate in person or via two-way radios or satellite phones until communications systems are back online (analog phones, VOIP phones, paging, cellphones, internet, intranet, faxing)
Redundancy of infrastructure and the ability to recover	No redundant systems or infrastructure to fully redundant, highly available system in a co-located data center
Maturity of downtime plans, policies, and procedures and availability of backup supplies	No plans or supplies to mature and tested policy, procedure, and plans with stocked supplies and staff aware of them

ICU, Intensive care unit; IT, information technology; VOIP, Voice Over Internet Protocol.

team can develop the response, communication, and recovery plans. A comprehensive and accurate assessment will provide a reliable starting point for the team responding to the downtime, thereby decreasing chaos and saving critical time at the start of an event. The downtime plan will include different levels of interventions for various events. For example, a downtime event with a simple application may be managed with a decision tool. An example of a simple decision tree is shown in Fig. 20.1. However, this same approach may become too cumbersome when dealing with multiple systems. In these cases, an organization may use a "level" system such as the one shown in Table 20.5.

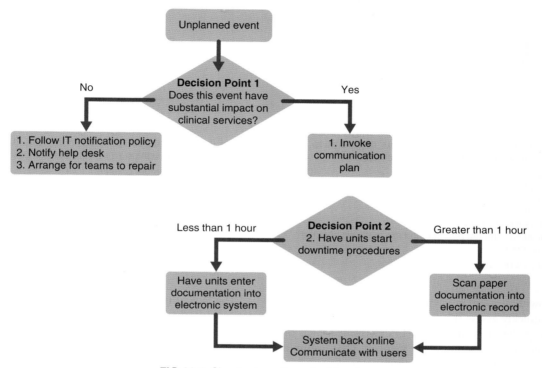

FIG 20.1 Simple downtime decision tree.

TABLE 20.5 Downtime Levels

	Definition	Response Examples
Level 1	Part of a system down or unavailable but minimal impact and no loss of content or data integrity. Expected time to recovery less than 1 hour.	IT team and targeted users only are involved per standard SLA. Service desk agent communicates with user.
Level 2	Complete system unavailable, data may be unavailable, and data will have to be entered into the system to maintain integrity. Expected time to recovery up to 4 hours.	IT team and targeted users are involved per standard SLA. Unit-based downtime plans invoked. May require additional communication to stakeholders and plans for reentry of data.
Level 3	Multiple systems unavailable, big impact on workflow, and content may be unavailable and will have to be entered into the system to maintain integrity. Expected time to recovery greater than 4 hours.	IT incident response team involved along with multiple teams. Downtime plans invoked. Broad communication to the organization. Notification to key stakeholders and administration. Plan for reentry of data.
Level 4	All systems and network unavailable but root cause is known and recovery is possible. Users must complete downtime plans. Estimated time to recovery greater than 4 hours.	IT incident response team involved, along with multiple teams. Downtime plans invoked. Broad communication to the organization. Notification to key stakeholders and administration. Plan for reentry of data. May involve emergency response team and opening of command center.
Level 5	All systems and network unavailable. Major catastrophic event and facility structure may be compromised. Systems and infrastructure need to be rebuilt. System-wide emergency plans and response invoked.	All hands on deck and event directed per emergency response team or administration. May require communication to the wider community.

IT, Information technology; SLA, service level agreement.

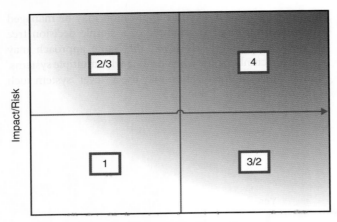

Plot each component in one of the four quadrants to determine where the items cluster

1. Time of day/number of users
2. IT infrastructure affected
3. System criticality
4. Planned versus unplanned
5. Health system complexity
6. Communication: Amount required and are methods affected?
7. Ability to recover

FIG 20.2 Downtime Determinator Model.

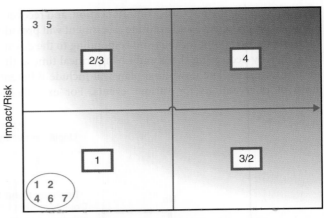

Plot each component in one of the four quadrants to determine where the items cluster

1. Time of day/number of users
2. IT infrastructure affected
3. System criticality
4. Planned versus unplanned
5. Health system complexity
6. Communication: Amount required and are methods affected?
7. Ability to recover

FIG 20.3 Downtime determinator Quadrant 1 example.

With a downtime event involving multiple systems, the use of a tool to quickly assess the significance of the downtime event will help the IT team and users determine which of the predefined responses should be invoked. One example of such a tool is the Downtime Determinator depicted in Fig. 20.2, a tool developed by the authors. The x-axis is the length of downtime (or time to recovery) and the y-axis is the impact and risk. Each of the seven risk attributes is plotted on the Downtime Determinator tool in one of the four quadrants, and a pattern or cluster of numbers will start to emerge. The pattern of numbers becomes the basis for evaluating the event.

Using the risk attributes described previously, quadrant responses would be defined by the organization and might be similar to the earlier examples provided with the levels. For example, when the majority of numbers cluster in the lower left quadrant, this should invoke a quadrant 1 response; numbers clustered in the upper right quadrant should invoke a quadrant 4 response. The lower left quadrant represents the least critical events, and the upper right quadrant represents the most critical events. The Downtime Determinator displays the numbers 2/3 and 3/2 in the upper left and lower right quadrants, respectively. Each organization will need to assign quadrants 2 and 3 based on its assessment of each individual downtime event, after considering the impact and risk versus time. There may be times when the length of the downtime is so long that the event warrants a quadrant 3 (more intense) response. There may be other times when the event is so massive that even though the downtime is scheduled for 30 minutes, the impact to the organization is so great that it warrants a quadrant 3 response.

The Downtime Determinator is similar to the "level" system mentioned earlier, as both have four categories. However, the Downtime Determinator allows for more specificity and nuances in responses because each of the attributes can be considered separately and responded to in relation to other attributes. When using a tool such as the Downtime Determinator, each organization would customize the tool by defining each attribute and delineating time along the x-axis that is significant to the organization. Four scenarios are outlined below using the Downtime Determinator, ranging from least to most impact:

- **Scenario 1:** Level I trauma center and teaching hospital. Planned EHR downtime from 02:00 to 05:00 on a Wednesday night. IT infrastructure and communications intact (Fig. 20.3).
- **Scenario 2:** Community hospital. Unplanned downtime of the hospital billing system at 15:30 on a Monday. Multiple staff unable to do work, but patient care is not affected. Recovery expected in 3 hours. System requires replacement of a hard drive; the hard drive is available locally, and it should be delivered to the data center by the vendor shortly. Communications intact (Fig. 20.4).
- **Scenario 3:** Acute care hospital with multiple intensive care units (ICUs) with a physiologic monitoring system interfaced to the EHR via bedside medical device integration (BMDI). The vendor-specific server is damaged due to a water spill in the communication closet, and the BMDI unexpectedly quits working at 08:00 on a Saturday morning. The vendor indicates a 2-week lag until a replacement server will be available (Fig. 20.5).

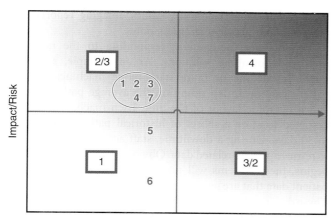

Plot each component in one of the four quadrants to determine where the items cluster

1. Time of day/number of users
2. IT infrastructure affected
3. System criticality
4. Planned versus unplanned
5. Health system complexity
6. Communication: Amount required and are methods affected?
7. Ability to recover

FIG 20.4 Downtime determinator Quadrant 2 example.

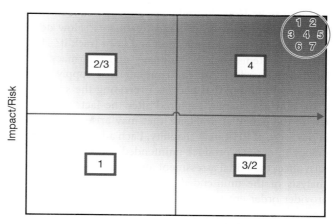

Plot each component in one of the four quadrants to determine where the items cluster

1. Time of day/number of users
2. IT infrastructure affected
3. System criticality
4. Planned versus unplanned
5. Health system complexity
6. Communication: Amount required and are methods affected?
7. Ability to recover

FIG 20.6 Downtime determinator Quadrant 4 example.

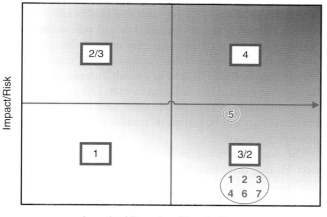

Plot each component in one of the four quadrants to determine where the items cluster

1. Time of day/number of users
2. IT infrastructure affected
3. System criticality
4. Planned versus unplanned
5. Health system complexity
6. Communication: Amount required and are methods affected?
7. Ability to recover

FIG 20.5 Downtime determinator Quadrant 3 example.

- **Scenario 4:** An F-16 military airplane crashes into the data center of an academic medical center at 19:00 on a Friday night during training exercises. The data center is destroyed physically, a large fuel spill covers the area, and there is complete IT system downtime. The

hospital and campus are otherwise intact. The academic medical center has a hot site that can host approximately 30% of critical systems and a cold site that has capacity to host the remainder of the systems. The critical hot site applications can be available in 24 hours, but the remaining 70% of applications to be built in the cold site will take 30 days for complete recovery (Fig. 20.6).

As seen with these scenarios, the clustering of numbers helps guide the response of the organization in managing the event or disaster. A quadrant 1 event (scenario 1) should be a routine event that is managed with standard processes, communications, and service level agreements (SLAs) that are already in place. With a quadrant 4 major disaster (scenario 4), the response should be massive and system- and organization-wide. Such a disaster would have a significant impact on the ability of the organization to carry on the business of healthcare. Taking time to plan and put realistic processes into place before the event will determine whether the organization will continue to care for patients safely and have the business remain intact.

Clinical Impact and Planning: Acute Care Focus

With the increased use of technology at the point of care and in the clinical environment, healthcare organizations must now precisely determine their response when technology is unavailable. How do clinicians find historical data, including recent vital signs, the first of three troponin results, the history and physical prior to surgery, and the last time the PRN (as needed) pain medication was given, with the patient's response to it? How do healthcare providers document new events, medications, orders, and treatments? How does the pharmacy dispense a medication and keep track it? How do ancillary systems such as radiology and pharmacy receive handwritten orders? Do the computerized supply cabinets have programming that permits overriding the system and, if so, how are charges captured after the fact? These are a few of the potential problems that may arise at institutions in the event of EHR unavailability. Each addition to the technology in use can produce unintended consequences and in turn affect the initial assessment and resulting plan. A 4-year analysis of the unintended consequences of computerized provider order entry (CPOE) identified nine types of unintended consequences.[15] A list of these unintended consequences is included in Box 20.6.

Logically, the more electronic components in the organization, the more complex troubleshooting becomes. The elements that need to be considered include inpatient and outpatient venues, networks, intranets, printers, databases, interfaces, storage hardware, published applications, and layering software used to manage the myriad devices in an institution. Failure at any of these points may result in some sort of downtime for clinicians. Reducing the risk of a downtime can be accomplished by using the approaches outlined in the following sections.

Redundant Systems

Redundant systems, also known as backup systems, provide clinicians the ability to access some if not all patient data during an electronic downtime. If clinicians can recover just enough information to carry on with patient care from the point at which the downtime begins, care can proceed safely.[16] Therefore a subset of critical data must always be available, even during downtime. Each individual organization should define the required subset of data according to applications and services. Suggestions are basic demographics, orders, medication administration records (MARs),

---

BOX 20.6   Unintended Consequences of the Impact of Computerized Provider Order Entry

- More/new work issues
- Workflow issues with mismatch of order entry and related activities
- Never-ending demands
- Paper persistence
- Communication issues with changes in communication patterns
- Emotions
- New types of errors introduced by use of a computer
- Changes in the power structure
- Overdependence on technology

Modified from Ash JS, Sittig DF, Poon EG, Guappone K, Campbell E, Dykstra RH. The extent and importance of unintended consequences related to computerized provider order entry. *J Am Med Inform Assoc.* 2007;14(4):415-423.

---

most recent vitals, laboratory values, imaging reports, and physician and provider progress notes.

Vendors are increasingly responding to the need for improved downtime solutions. As an example, a vendor might install one or more stand-alone machines in each patient care area, depending on the average patient census and geographic layout of the unit. Each machine might be designed to store a subset of historical patient data for up to 30 days. During a downtime, staff access these machines to retrieve patient-related data. Obviously, once the downtime begins, these systems will no longer be updated, and new patient data that are generated must be maintained manually. These data must be entered back into the EHR by keying them into the system or scanning them in after the system is up again. Because healthcare providers may need printed data during the downtime event, each machine should be directly connected by cable to a printer so it is not dependent on the down network connection for printing services. Another benefit of these machines is that they can be portable. In the event of a hospital evacuation, these machines can be removed from the premises and data from these machines can be used until a recovery plan is in place.

However, this particular redundant downtime solution has limitations. One concept that is difficult for clinical and IT staff to understand is that once the network becomes unavailable, these downtime machines are no longer updated with patient information. This requires the healthcare providers to check the new manually recorded data as well as the historical data maintained in the temporary system when providing care. Another limitation is that the data may be organized differently than in the EHR, and as a result, information may be displayed or printed in a different format. This can cause confusion and even errors in patient care. Also, data entry for the downtime may not be complete, resulting in a fragmented or incomplete record.

The downtime solution using temporary machines must meet Health Insurance Portability and Accountability Act (HIPAA) requirements for security, privacy, and confidentiality. As a result, these machines require an extra layer of encryption to prevent information theft in the event that the machine is removed from the hospital. However, these encryption systems typically are add-ons that slow down the response time of patient care applications running on the machines.

Other terms used to describe redundant systems are *shadow*, *mirror*, or *read-only systems*. The downtime system described previously is a shadow or mirror system that is only able to be read by clinicians. Clinicians cannot add any patient data to this type of system. Some shadow or mirror systems duplicate the EHR. In the event that the primary system crashes, the secondary system automatically, and hopefully seamlessly, transitions the clinician to the secondary system. The clinician continues to document orders, medications, or care. Generally, these systems reside on separate hardware that "mirrors" the configuration of the primary system. These systems are generally more robust than the redundant downtime solution described previously, encompassing a similar look and feel and often read and write capability. These systems are beneficial because clinicians use their current log-in and password to access the system, the look and feel of the system are almost identical to the EHR, and printing can be available.

Redundant systems often resemble the configuration of the existing EHR, requiring a substantial financial investment with the vendor. The financial investment can be an obstacle; therefore a business case should be made with and for the clinicians on behalf of patients. The more mature the EHR, the more dependent the clinicians are on the system to get information to provide patient care. Investing in a backup system of this caliber is arguably a necessity after institutions have reached a certain level of EHR maturity, and organizations should assess this requirement frequently.

In addition to the previously discussed solutions, home-grown, web-based solutions are available for use by clinicians prior to a planned downtime. For example, a web-based solution may be configured so that clinicians can print an MAR or all current patient orders. These have proven helpful during planned upgrades because they provide clinicians with enough information to weather the upgrade as well as provide a place to begin manual documentation of patient care during the downtime.

DOWNTIME POLICIES AND PROCEDURES

Approved downtime policies and procedures are needed to guide the clinical team. These policies should be prescriptive, include roles and responsibilities, and define workarounds or manual procedures that allow for the continuity of critical functions. They should include specific instructions about required data entry to the legal and permanent EHR record at the conclusion of the downtime. Examples of downtime policies are available in the literature and on the internet.[16–19]

A best practice is for patient units to have up-to-date, physical "downtime" boxes.[21] Each box contains documentation forms specific to the patient care area, instructions for paper form completion, and a plan for managing the paper documents on the unit. For example, ICUs may revert to traditional six-panel paper flow sheets. Other patient care areas have screenshots of the electronic "patient admission" form or other forms directly from the EHR. When no preprinted forms are available, blank or lined pieces of paper are used and work as long as healthcare providers are aware of documentation requirements. Each downtime box should be stocked to last at least 24 hours and have instructions for restocking the forms. Each patient care area is expected to maintain and customize the contents of its "downtime" box.[20] Informaticians can partner closely with clinicians to create downtime policies and procedures to ensure that clinical requirements are matched with available IT solutions.

INFORMATION TECHNOLOGY IMPACT AND PLANNING

The IT impact and downtime risk can be reduced by following a systematic process when changes are applied to the "production" or "live" system. One approach is to organize a

service management program to organize a risk assessment and downtime planning document. Service management is a discipline for managing IT systems that focuses on the customer and the business and its operations, as opposed to simply being technology-centric. The service life cycle includes service strategy, service design, service transition, service operation, and continual service improvement.[21] Interestingly, this life cycle is similar to both the system development life cycle used to implement computer systems[22] and the nursing process.[23] Various process-based systems exist to assist the IT team in instituting a service management program, including ITIL,[21,24] Six Sigma, and total quality management (TQM). These systems require the use of standardized terminology, problem identification and management, change control measures, and communication patterns. The benefits of using these systems are agreed-upon, realistic service levels; predictable and consistent processes; metrics; and alignment with business needs.

Implementing a service management program requires financial and time commitments from the organization, the IT executives, and all members of the IT team, but is well worth the investment. Commitments are needed from the IT staff to fill roles on committees such as the change advisory board, incident response team (IRT), and IT service management. The benefits of a service management program include having a framework with clear rules and processes to structure IT activities so fewer unplanned events occur. One of the disadvantages of a service management program is that the program will invariably increase the time to implement new code or new functionality. This additional time might turn into an advantage, as waiting may reduce knee-jerk reactions from users. It also gives the IT team more time to test the new functionality and discover any dependencies. Waiting also benefits clinicians because they can negotiate a standard change time and reduce unnecessary downtimes.

DISASTER PLANNING

Organizations are obligated to maintain contingency and disaster plans in order to be compliant with the HIPAA security rule of 1996, the U.S. Department of Health and Human Services, and accreditation bodies. A separate set of IT policies should exist to supplement the organization's overall disaster plan and include security and privacy components. Senior leadership of the IT department, the security and privacy office, the emergency preparedness group, and senior leadership from the broader organization should review and approve the plans.[9] These plans should be frequently reviewed, tested, and revised as needed. Staff need to be updated on a consistent basis so they are prepared to implement contingency and disasters plan with minimum effort. Considerations for the IT components of an IT disaster plan are listed in Table 20.6.

Once contingency and disaster plans are implemented and at the point when the institution is converting back to its standard systems, the organization needs to be prepared to test the

TABLE 20.6 Information Technology Contingency and Disaster Recovery Plan Considerations

Element	Activities
Staff competencies	• Identify and agree on roles and responsibilities. • Create comprehensive system documentation and make it widely available. • Demand "knowledge transfers"; all members to avoid SPOFs. • Develop stakeholder relationships. • Update emergency contacts for vendors and IT staff.
Data backups	• Preserve all critical data associated with the patient, the business, finances, payroll, and personnel. • Be knowledgeable about retention policies of medical records and business documents for the organization and state. • Schedule backups on duplicate data on tapes, disks, and optical disks. • Store data in one of the clouds and/or across multiple servers.
Off-site storage of removable media	• Include a secure plan for transporting the media to an offsite location. • Encrypt data.
Adequate storage	• Evaluate storage capacity and procedures proactively.
Development and test domains for all systems	• Test all changes to production prior to promoting the code to production using a formal process.
System monitoring and notifications	• Keep a spreadsheet of common errors to help speed up diagnostics. • Introduce various types of downtimes to a test (nonproduction) system and evaluate the error messages or system issues; for example, in the nonproduction system, turn off the interfaces to see what types of errors or alerts you receive in the monitoring. • Work with the database team to mimic at-capacity database tables and carefully monitor system errors that are displayed.
Continuity plans	• Design systems that are highly available and redundant. • Archive source code with a reputable third-party company. • Complete negotiations up front for replacement hardware with commitments on days to ship and configure. • Arrange colocation sites with adequate network bandwidth and dual network pathways. • Develop reciprocal agreements or consortium arrangements. • Consider hot sites, warm sites, and cold sites.
Postevent review and revision	• Have formal process for the review that is inclusive of stakeholders. • Complete and document event review as near to the event as possible.

Data from Hoong LL, Marthandan G. Factors influencing the success of the disaster recovery planning process: a conceptual paper. *Research and Innovation in Information Systems (ICRIIS), 2011 International Conference.* 2011;1-6:23-24. doi:10.1109/ICRIIS.2011.6125683; Federal Emergency Management Agency (FEMA). IT disaster recovery plan. <http://www.ready.gov/business/implementation/IT>; 2012.
IT, Information technology; *SPOF,* single point of failure.

clinical system rapidly to ensure that all aspects of the system are functioning as planned. Therefore having up-to-date test plans for all clinical systems is an integral part of turning around a downtime quickly once hardware and database issues have been resolved. Software upgrades can and do occur frequently. If the test plans are not current, the testing process may not be reliable. In addition, without systematic preplanned processes in place, it is difficult to enlist the help of non-IT people. Keeping test plans up to date ensures that people external to the recovery team can assist with testing and getting the system online sooner.

Disaster Recovery

Preparedness and planning are the keys to **disaster recovery** following either a simple incident or a catastrophic event. In fact, the process of planning can be as beneficial to an organization as the final written plan. Recovery should include all components identified as crucial: network, servers, connectivity, data, telecommunications, hardware, software, desktops, security, wireless, and any other specific items.

The goal of disaster recovery is to recover the business fully and completely. Depending on the severity of the event or disaster, it may be necessary to do an incremental recovery. Key administrative leaders, with input from the staff, should be involved in the decisions about the sequence of recovery of systems or applications. All employees in an organization will likely have changed workflows during the disaster, and it is important that they understand their roles during the disaster or downtime and during the recovery period. The steps to actual recovery will be different for each event and for each organization. Because of this complexity and the time involved to develop a comprehensive disaster recovery plan, an organization may choose to hire outside consultants instead of using internal resources.[25,26]

Business Continuity

Business continuity management is a complementary process to disaster recovery. **Business continuity** has a larger scope than recovering only IT systems. It also includes determining which administrative and healthcare services must be available using a defined timeline and identifying which systems can be excluded from initial recovery. Business continuity management outlines the functions, processes, and systems needed to allow the core business of providing health services to continue.

A tier system works well for this purpose, and each organization will have unique requirements. For example, Tier I applications would be identified as critical and are recovered first. The organization defines the expected time to recovery based on the requirement for service and available resources. As a general rule, the faster the recovery must occur, the more expensive the recovery process will be. The cost should also be evaluated in comparison with the cost of the downtime. For a Tier I application to be recovered in 24 hours or less, it is likely that a hot site would be required with hardware standing by. Tier II applications would come next and may be identified as needing to be available within 72 hours. Finally, Tier III and Tier IV may be identified as requiring recovery within 1 week and 1 month, respectively. For healthcare, business continuity includes providing care of both patients and the revenue cycle. Defining business continuity should be a formal process that includes the following:

- A business impact analysis that takes into consideration the institution's business needs and the needs of the community for healthcare services
- Definition of recovery strategies
- Development of a formal plan
- Exercises to test the plan

As with other elements discussed previously, this process will need resources (both human and financial) from the organization's senior leadership.[27,28]

Part of business continuity includes the downtime boxes mentioned earlier in this chapter. Every business unit needs to have a downtime box that includes items such as registration forms, charge sheets, fax forms, and other commonly used forms for that business area. Consider keeping paper instructions about how to fill out and use paper forms in a downtime box. This is important because some of the newer clinicians have never written paper orders or documented a clinical assessment on paper. In addition, it is a good idea to have these documents stored on a portable media device to be kept in the downtime box. In the event of a disaster, these forms can be stored on a second portable device and kept in a secure location. Organizations should make specific assignments to ensure that these are kept up to date and staff review the downtime box procedures periodically.

Communication

Communication is an integral part of any downtime. Five components of communication plans are needed to determine the following:

- Who needs to know the details?
- What details are needed?
- What media or modes of communication will be used?
- Who will communicate what information?
- What systems or workflow processes are affected?

Of course, the more complex the downtime is, the more people need to be notified and the more information needs to be communicated. For example, if the bedside monitoring device is not transmitting data to the EHR, only the ICU staff need to be notified. If the EHR database becomes corrupt, then all clinicians who use the system will need to be notified, as well as all IT teams and possibly hospital administration and the risk management department.

Fahrenholz et al.[18] compiled a downtime communication template useful to readers. Their questions are as follows:

- What system will be down?
- When will the downtime begin?
- How long will the system be unavailable?
- Why will the system be down?
- What changes are being made to the system?
- Who will be affected and what can the end user expect?
- What procedures should be followed during the downtime?

These guidelines can be adapted for any facility's use during both planned and unexpected downtimes.

If the facility uses a tool for IT service management such as ITIL, the procedures discussed here will be used. If people in the facility do not use one of these systems, they should use other sources[29,30] to develop policies and procedures to ensure that communication is managed properly. Communication occurs most predictably and reliably when the responsibility belongs to one consistent team or group of people. A service management or equivalent team works well to manage the communications. Whoever is designated as the primary communication team must work very closely with the IRT and the help desk. Communications are coordinated, and the help desk is kept informed of the event and of the information it should supply to end users as inquiries are made about the event. The help desk is critical to communication, as in most cases, staff experiencing technical problems will contact the help desk first. Plus, in most healthcare institutions, the help desk staff are on-site and have on-call agents available 24 hours a day. Training the help desk staff to manage these communications allows the infrastructure and application teams to work on resolving the problems. Some tools that might be used in addition to managing the trouble ticket queue are continuous or intermittent conference calls, individual and group paging for the IT department, individual and group instant messaging, webcasts, updated web pages, group e-mail updates, recorded phone messages, and coordination with hospital operators. Multiple means of communication need to be considered when planning for an event. The technical problems causing the downtime or the disaster event may also eliminate certain communication modes. For example, if the network is down, an e-mail cannot be sent with information about managing the event to the clinical units and Voice Over Internet Protocol (VOIP) phones will not work.

The hospital telecommunications operators can manage many aspects of the communication plan, including individual and group pagers, cellphones, tablets, and other communication devices for clinicians and the operational areas. Sending information to these communication devices may help manage information distribution during sudden or extended downtimes. A best practice in the age of internet-based phone systems is to have some analog phones available in key hospital areas because they function during network and electrical downtimes. These phones can be identified by using a different color of phone, such as red. Hospital telecommunications operators can also use the overhead paging system in the hospital to distribute information. The point is to be sure to include these hospital operators in the downtime communication plans.

In the event of a major disaster, satellite radios and phones can be used. Satellite phones and radios are network independent but require electricity to recharge their batteries. The local emergency management office in the organization will have more information about these capabilities.

Responsibilities

The IT staff is responsible for communicating the necessary information to the help desk agents. In addition, some electronic systems contain notification alert capability. For example, planned downtimes can be communicated using the notification system in the facility's EHR. Obviously this method would not be available during an EHR downtime, but it can be used to announce a planned downtime or when any of the ancillary systems are offline.

IT leaders are responsible for communicating with the organization's senior leadership and the public relations department so they can manage media relations with the community. Social media applications can also be used to manage information with the media and to distribute information to staff in the event of a downtime (assuming that staff members have subscribed to the service and the service can provide the appropriate level of security and privacy).

Other mechanisms may be in place, depending on the institution and the setting. For example, if the institution is affiliated with a university, a "campus alert" system may be available. Using this system, notifications can be sent via e-mail, cellphone, work phone, home phone, or a combination of these. This communication strategy can be very helpful during disaster drills as well as unexpected events. Numerous ways exist to communicate with hospital employees and leadership, IT staff, news media, and the public. Finding the right combination for the facility's budget and staff and formalizing the ownership of specific communication will facilitate the workflow transitions during EHR downtimes at the facility.

CONCLUSION AND FUTURE DIRECTIONS

This chapter identifies tactics for health system downtime planning and disaster recovery. It challenges clinicians and informaticians to assess, plan for, respond to, recover from, communicate about, continue business during, and prevent downtimes and disasters when possible. The primary objective for downtime and disaster planning is to protect the organization and the patients who are served by that organization by minimizing disruption to the operations. This includes minimizing economic loss; ensuring organizational stability; protecting critical assets of the organization; ensuring safety for personnel, patients, and other customers; reducing variability in decision making during a disaster; and hopefully

minimizing legal liability.[5] In healthcare and health IT, the single most important reason to carry out the activities described in the chapter carefully and methodically is the ability to provide uninterrupted, exceptional service and safe care to all patients.

In the future, the potential impact of downtimes and disasters will continue to grow as healthcare entities become more dependent on technology and as individual healthcare institutions continue to become part of a larger network. This should drive administrators to invest additional human and material resources in assessing and planning to minimize the impact of potential threats. Advances in technology can be expected to offer better solutions than currently exist. These solutions may be less costly as new and improved technology eventually reduces the potential for downtimes. Additional research is very much needed to help clinicians and health systems understand the experience of downtime workflow interruptions, the patient safety implications, and the operational impacts. In addition, research should be initiated to drive a standard approach to downtime planning for health systems, disaster recovery, and business continuity efforts. Many focus areas might be addressed along the continuum of disaster planning to business continuity, where research could have a very positive impact for the health system and its clients.

REFERENCES

1. Menon S, Singh H, Meyer A, Belmont E, Sittig DF. Electronic health record-related safety concerns: a cross-sectional survey. *J Healthc Risk Manag.* 2014;24(1):14–26.
2. Sittig DF, Gonzalez D, Singh H. Contingency planning for electronic health record-based care continuity: a survey of recommended practices. *Int J Med Informat.* 2014;83:797–804.
3. Polaneczky M. *When the Electronic Medical Record Goes Down. The Blog That Ate Manhattan;* 2007. http://www.tbtam.com/2007/03/when-the-electronic-medical-record-goes-down.html.
4. Getz L. Dealing with downtime: how to survive if your EHR system fails. *For the Record.* 2009;21(21):16. http://www.fortherecordmag.com/archives/110909p16.shtml.
5. Capital One. *Business Continuity and Disaster Recovery Checklist for Small Business Owners.* Continuity central; 2011. http://www.continuitycentral.com/feature0501.htm.
6. Anderson M. *The Costs and Implications of EMR System Downtime on Physician Practices.* XML Journal; 2011. http://xml.sys-con.com/node/1900855.
7. Ponemenon Institute. *2013 Cost of Data Center Outages;* 2013. http://www.emersonnetworkpower.com/documentation/en-us/brands/liebert/documents/white%20papers/2013_emerson_data_center_cost_downtime_sl-24680.pdf.
8. Durry A. Are we ready? Pediatric disaster planning. *Nurs Made Incredibly Easy.* 2015;13(5):30–37. http://dx.doi.org/10.1097/01.NME.0000470082.48212.01.
9. Wold GH. Disaster recovery planning process. *Disaster Recovery J;* 2011. http://c.ymcdn.com/sites/www.rfmaonline.com/resource/resmgr/crfp/disasterrecoveryplanningproc.pdf.
10. FEMA. *National Incident Management System;* 2015. https://www.fema.gov/national-incident-management-system.
11. FEMA. *NIMS Implementation Activities for Hospitals and Healthcare Systems;* 2006. https://www.fema.gov/pdf/emergency/nims/imp_hos.pdf.

12. Office of the Assistant Secretary for Preparedness and Response Hospital Preparedness Program. *National Guidance for Healthcare System Preparedness;* 2012. http://www.phe.gov/Preparedness/planning/hpp/reports/Documents/capabilities.pdf.

13. Office of the Assistant Secretary for Preparedness and Response Hospital Preparedness Program. *Hospital Preparedness Program Overview;* 2014. http://www.phe.gov/Preparedness/planning/hpp/Pages/overview.aspx.

14. Morse S. *California Hospitals Prepared as Wildfires Rage, Association Says;* 2015. http://www.healthcarefinancenews.com/news/california-hospitals-prepared-wildfires-rage-association-says.

15. Ash JS, Sittig DF, Poon EG, Guappone K, Campbell E, Dykstra RH. The extent and importance of unintended consequences related to computerized provider order entry. *J Am Med Inform Assoc.* 2007;14(4):415–423.

16. Nelson N. Downtime procedures for a clinical information system: a critical issue. *J Crit Care.* 2007;22:45–50.

17. University of Texas Health Science Center at Houston. *Emergency Management Plan;* 2015. https://www.uthealthemergency.org/UTHealth-Emergency-Management-Plan.pdf.

18. Fahrenholz CG, Smith LJ, Tucker K, Warner D. *A Practical Approach to Downtime Planning in Medical Practices.* American Health Information Management Association; 2009. http://library.ahima.org/xpedio/groups/public/documents/ahima/bok1_045486.hcsp?dDocN.

19. Williams College: Office of Information Technology. *Downtime Policy.* http://oit.williams.edu/policies/downtime/. Accessed June 13, 2016.

20. Vaughn S. Planning for system downtimes. *Comput Inform NU.* 2011;29(4):201–203.

21. Arraj V. ITIL: the basics. *Best Management Practice.* White Paper; 2010. http://www.best-management-practice.com/gempdf/itil_the_basics.pdf.

22. Whitten J, Bentley L. *System Analysis and Design Methods.* 7th ed. McGraw-Hill Higher Education: New York, NY; 2007.

23. American Nurses Association. *The Nursing Process.* Nursing World; 2012. http://nursingworld.org/EspeciallyForYou/What-is-Nursing/Tools-You-Need/Thenursingprocess.html.

24. Hoerbst A, Hackl WO, Blomer R, Ammenwerth E. The status of IT service management in health care: ITIL in selected European countries. *BMC Med Inform Decis Mak.* 2011;11:76.

25. Hoong LL, Marthandan G. Factors influencing the success of the disaster recovery planning process: a conceptual paper. In: *Research and Innovation in Information Systems (ICRIIS), 2011 International Conference;* 2011:23–24. http://dx.doi.org/10.1109/ICRIIS.2011.6125683.

26. Federal Emergency Management Agency (FEMA). *IT Disaster Recovery Plan;* 2012. http://www.ready.gov/business/implementation/IT.

27. Federal Emergency Management Agency (FEMA). *Business Continuity Plan;* 2012. http://ready.gov/business/implementation/continuity.

28. Nickolette C. *Business Continuity Planning Description and Framework.* Comprehensive Consulting Solutions, Inc; 2001. http://www.comp-soln.com/BCP_whitepaper.pdf.

29. Healthcare and Public Health Sector. *Working without technology: how hospitals and healthcare organizations can manage communication failure.* n.d. http://www.phe.gov/Preparedness/planning/cip/Documents/workingwithouttechnology.pdf. Accessed June 13, 2016.

30. (x)matters. *Proactive Communications During Major Incidents. Best Practices Beyond Incident Resolution (whitepaper);* 2015. http://www.xmatters.com/resource/proactive-communications-during-major-incidents/.

DISCUSSION QUESTIONS

1. Explain the importance of an organization-specific downtime risk assessment.
2. Describe the pros and cons of different assessment tools for evaluating downtime events and discuss scenarios in which they might be used to their best advantage.
3. Compare and contrast the roles of the informatician, the clinician, and IT personnel in system downtime planning.
4. Describe key components of a business continuity plan and (a) how they might differ for different types of organizations and (b) how they might differ depending on EHR maturity level.
5. Contrast different communication methods for system downtime events and summarize the pros and cons of each.

CASE STUDY

At your Level 2 trauma center, an unplanned EHR downtime occurs at 17:00 on a Tuesday. After 1 hour of troubleshooting and working with the vendor's help desk, the IT team attempts a system reboot, which is unsuccessful. The vendor is in a different time zone, so specialists have to be called in from home to respond to this incident. The initial assessment is that the downtime is due to database corruption and the system will have to be recovered from backup systems. Unfortunately, the system is not configured with high availability techniques, nor is it redundant. The IT department estimates that it will take 8 hours to recover the system, for a total downtime of 10 hours.

Discussion Questions

1. Plot each component on the Downtime Determinator for both part 1 and part 2 of the scenario as it unfolded, and document your IT response, end user response, and communication plans.
2. Make changes to the assessment and plans to account for changes to the scenario.

21

Improving the User Experience for Health Information Technology

Nancy Staggers

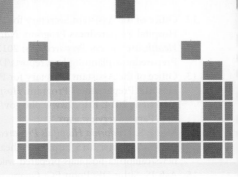

Usability has a strong, often direct relationship with clinical productivity, error rates, user fatigue, and user satisfaction[1]

OBJECTIVES

At the completion of this chapter, the reader will be prepared to:

1. Compare and contrast the terms *user experience, human factors, ergonomics, human-computer interaction, usability,* and *design thinking*.
2. Discuss the potential benefits of incorporating usability into organizational processes.
3. Describe the goals of usability and user-centered design.
4. Identify the major components to consider in human-computer interaction and usability studies.
5. Analyze methods for conducting usability studies and relate them to a specific purpose of a usability study.
6. Outline components of four different usability tests related to their position in the systems life cycle.
7. Explain the basic steps in conducting a usability test on a healthcare IT product.

KEY TERMS

contextual inquiry, 362
design thinking, 355
discount usability methods, 359
ergonomics, 353
focused ethnographies, 361
heuristic evaluations, 359
human factors, 353
human-computer interaction (HCI), 354

joint cognitive systems, 357
sociotechnical system, 352
task analysis, 361
think-aloud protocol, 361
usability, 354
user interface, 356
user-centered design, 354

ABSTRACT ❖

The usability of health information technology (IT) products is a worldwide concern. U.S. federal agencies are responding to this challenge by developing regulations and reports to guide improved user experiences (UXs) for health IT products. Health professionals and informaticians require a suite of skills to understand concepts about the UX and to conduct usability tests. This chapter provides the knowledge and skills to meet those needs. First, the chapter outlines the need for attention to the UX. Terms are defined, the concepts of usability goals are presented, and user-centered design precepts are discussed. Potential benefits for improved UX are outlined. Available human-computer interaction (HCI) frameworks are listed; one framework is explained in detail, and selected methods particular to UX evaluations are explained. Then types of usability tests are discussed and linked to the systems life cycle. Examples of actual usability studies in health settings are provided. These techniques will allow readers to design and conduct usability tests to determine the effectiveness and efficiency of and satisfaction with health IT products.

INTRODUCTION TO IMPROVING THE USER EXPERIENCE

Readers can easily describe their frustrations with today's poorly designed health information technology (IT) products. Solutions to these health IT issues involve the systematic study of the user experience (UX) that incorporates a wide variety of available resources. This section of the chapter outlines users' current experiences with health IT. After terms are defined, potential benefits are discussed for improved UX to health IT product users and health organizations.

The Current User Experience With Health Information Technology Products

UX issues with health IT products are a worldwide concern. The expansion of mobile health (mHealth) and electronic health records (EHRs) in particular has resulted in complex interactions among multiple users, IT products, and environments, all with varying characteristics. These complex interactions, known as a sociotechnical system, coupled with complex health systems, are magnified as users interact with health IT.

Convincing evidence exists that UX issues in health IT can result in patient safety problem and errors.[1-3] In the United States, The Joint Commission (TJC) issued an alert in mid-2015 concerning sentinel events related to health IT. TJC evaluated 3375 previous adverse event reports, identifying 120 health IT-related sentinel events.[4] One third of these stemmed from factors related to the human-computer interface, while 24% stemmed from workflow and communication issues. Lack of interoperability and difficulties in extracting relevant data from vast quantities of information can result in omissions and errors in care continuity mechanisms such as handoffs.[5,6] Moreover, providers have difficulty finding critical information and developing the "big picture" of the patient.[7,8] In the federal sector, an ambulatory EHR application serving more than nine million patients failed to support providers during patient encounters, did not allow them to obtain situation awareness of the patient (the "big picture" of the patient), promoted work-arounds for the existing nonintegrated systems, and greatly increased frustrations because of required structured documentation.[9] Last, potential patient safety issues occurred with two different Electronic Medication Administration Records (eMARs) because nurses could not easily view patients' medications to determine those missed and those due.[10,11]

Physicians are currently very vocal about their dissatisfaction and productivity issues with EHRs. Their perceptions about EHR usability were increasingly negative between 2010 and 2013, according to a national survey.[12] In a letter signed by 30 physician organizations in 2015, the American Medical Association (AMA) issued a call for solutions to poorly designed EHRs.[13]

Other healthcare professions are similarly affected but less outspoken. However, a recent call to action was issued to improve nurses' UXs, especially for EHRs.[14] Nurses are particularly affected by excessive documentation requirements. For example, admission assessments in acute care can take from 30 to 60 minutes and involve 532 clicks, structured documentation does not reflect the nuances of care (a pick list cannot capture how a patient feels about dying, for example), and nurses indicated that EHRs are a hindrance to care because they take time away from patients.[8] These issues could be ameliorated by incorporating known UX principles and processes to improve the UX with health IT.

DEFINITIONS OF TERMS AND THEIR RELATIONSHIPS

Despite discussion in the literature for more than 30 years, precise definitions for UX terms are a source of debate and overlapping concepts. The relationship of terms is depicted in Fig. 21.1. As demonstrated in the figure, UX is the most inclusive of these terms, with human factors, ergonomics, human-computer interaction (HCI), and usability embedded within it. Usability and ergonomics overlap and intersect human factors and HCI. These terms overlap in conceptual definitions and also because the physical attributes of ergonomics may be combined with software, which is more the purview of usability and HCI.

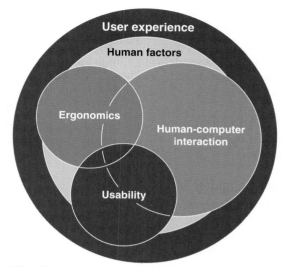

FIG 21.1 Terms and Their Relationships. (Adapted and expanded from Staggers N. Human factors: imperative concepts for information systems in critical care. *AACN Clin Issues.* 2003;14(3):310-319; quiz 397-318.)

User Experience

The term *user experience* encompasses all aspects of users' interactions.[15] The International Organization for Standardization (ISO) 9241-11 defines the term as "a person's perceptions and responses that result from the use or anticipated use of a product, system or service."[16,17] Schaffer indicates that UX is concerned with a range of experiences, from walking into a bank to designs that fit into complex ecosystems with many users interacting.[18] To achieve a high-quality UX, a seamless merging must occur from the talents of multiple disciplines, such as engineering, graphic and industrial design, interface design, psychology, and domain experts in the discipline at hand.[19,20] ISO 9241-11 is being revised at the time of this writing. Readers are encouraged to search ISO for new revisions beginning in mid to late 2017.

Human Factors

According to the Human Factors and Ergonomics Society (HFES), human factors is "the scientific discipline concerned with the understanding of interactions among humans and other elements of a system, and the profession that applies theory, principles, data and methods to design in order to optimize human well-being and overall system performance."[17] Simple examples include a design for opening a door efficiently, how to turn on the lighting for one area of a room from a bank of light switches, and how to safely and efficiently operate the controls to drive a car. In healthcare, human factors might concern the design of a new operating room to better support workflow, teamwork, and patient flow, or identifying obstacles to intensive care nurses in their task performance.[21] See Donald Norman's classic book about the design of everyday objects such as lighting and even teapots.[22]

Ergonomics

The term ergonomics is used interchangeably with human factors by the HFES in Europe, but in the United States and other countries, its focus is on human performance with physical characteristics of tools, systems, and machines.[23] For example, ergonomics issues might address the design of a power drill to fit a human hand or the design of chairs to promote comfort and safety. In healthcare, ergonomics can be the number, types, and locations of computer workstations or the physical design of a mobile device to support care. Ergonomics also deals with the design of a surgical instrument to fit the human hand to perform desired functions effectively and efficiently.

Human-Computer Interaction

Human-computer interaction (HCI) is the study of how people design, implement, and evaluate interactive computer systems in the context of users' tasks and work.[24] As with human factors, HCI draws on the disciplines of psychology and cognitive science, computer science, sociology, and information science and on the discipline of the user at hand. HCI can be addressed throughout the systems life cycle to include the design, development, purchase, implementation, and evaluation of applications. HCI topics can include the following:

- The design and use of devices such as an intravenous pump or a touchpad on a computer
- User satisfaction with computerized provider order entry (CPOE)
- Patient usage rates of mHealth apps or personal health records
- Users' perceptions of eMARs
- The standardization (or not) and meaning of icons on a patient portal
- Principles of effective screen design, including mobile application design
- Analysis of the capabilities and limitations of users and matching these to mHealth designs

Usability

The term usability is often used interchangeably with HCI when the product is a computer, but usability also concerns products beyond computers. Usability is also more focused on interactions within a specific context or environment for a specific product. Formally, the ISO defines usability as the extent to which a product can be used by specific users in a specific context to achieve specific goals with effectiveness, efficiency, and satisfaction.[16] A product with good usability allows users in a particular context to achieve their goals when interacting with a product.[24] Usability is, however, fundamentally concerned with human performance, and in the case of healthcare, interactions that promote safety rather than only subjective data. Usability can include the following dimensions:

- Speed and errors in interactions with a health IT product
- Ease of learning and remembering interactions after time has elapsed
- User satisfaction or perceptions about the interactions with health IT
- Efficiency and accuracy of interactions

- Designs to promote error-free or error-forgiving products
- Seamless fit of an information system to the tasks and goals of users

THE GOALS OF USABILITY

The overall goals of usability are established by the ISO. Fig. 21.2 depicts the ISO usability goals[19]:

- *Effectiveness* is the accuracy and completeness with which specified users achieve specified goals in particular environments, including worker and consumer or patient safety.
- *Efficiency* includes the resources expended in relation to the accuracy and completeness of goals achieved.
- *Satisfaction* is the level of comfort and acceptability that users and other people associate with the product or work system and deals with users' perceptions.[19]

Dimensions of usability correlate to potential benefits of UX depicted in Fig. 21.3, and (as discussed in detail in the next section) include improvements for individuals or groups of individuals in the following areas: productivity and efficiency, effectiveness in product use, safety, and cognitive support (an aspect of effectiveness).

USER-CENTERED DESIGN

UX experts employ a process of user-centered design composed of the following three axioms:

- An early and central focus on users in the design and development of products
- Iterative design
- Systematic measures of the interactions between users and products[23,24]

These principles were derived nearly 30 years ago by Gould and Lewis and are more salient than ever because contemporary environments are filled with an array of complex tools. An early and central focus on users means understanding users in depth—that is, their characteristics, environment,

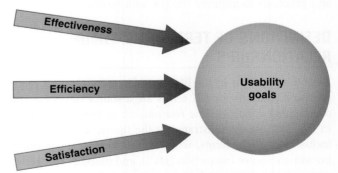

FIG 21.2 Usability goals. (From HIMSS Usability Task Force. *Promoting Usability in Health Organizations: Initial Steps and Progress Toward a Healthcare Usability Maturity Model.* Chicago, IL: Healthcare Information and Management Systems Society; 2011. Reprinted with permission from HIMSS.)

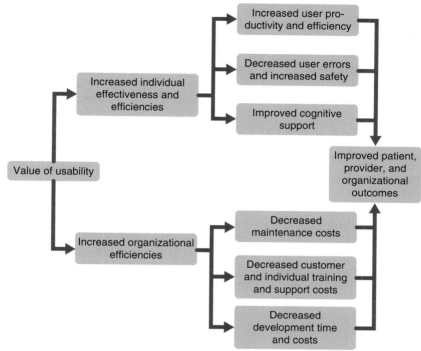

FIG 21.3 The value of usability to health organizations. (From HIMSS Usability Task Force. *Promoting Usability in Health Organizations: Initial Steps and Progress Toward a Healthcare Usability Maturity Model.* Chicago, IL. Copyright © Healthcare Information and Management Systems Society; 2011.)

and tasks.[24] Direct contact with actual users is needed early and often throughout a design or redesign process. Iterative design means having rounds of design and having key users evaluate product prototypes to determine their effectiveness and efficiency in the care process and health decisions. One design is never adequate, and typically at least three rounds are necessary. Once a design is available, even on paper or in PowerPoint, designers or informaticians work with users to determine any issues by having them systematically interact with and respond to the design. Specific methods to accomplish this are explained in subsequent sections. The important point is that major usability issues are identified and corrected early in the process. Design and evaluation then occur in a cycle until major usability issues are corrected. This dynamic, iterative process, which includes the three axioms listed above, is known as user-centered design. Importantly, structured and systematic observations, including identified measures, are necessary. Usability goals and axioms apply not only to developing products but also to the selection, purchase, customization, and redesign of products.

This kind of design allows us to integrate health data, information, and knowledge into health IT products. For example, a well-designed eMAR would filter medication routes to match the particular medication, eliminating inappropriate options (e.g., being able to chart an antacid as an intravenous medication or administer a tablet in the left arm). Although this sounds like common sense, current designs in major EHRs often do not accommodate this kind of filtering.

Design Thinking

Many UX professionals embrace a creative process called "Design Thinking." The process is complementary to User-Centered Design (UCD) discussed previously because it focuses on understanding problems from a user's perspective but the process concentrates on innovative solutions. Design thinking began in earnest in 1987 with Peter Rowe's book titled *Design Thinking.* Stanford University expanded this work for business, calling it a process for creative solutions. Essentially design thinking is a formal process of addressing ill-defined problems through creative design, using an iterative process of creating and testing multiple designs, as in UCD, to evaluate their fit as an appropriate solution.[25]

Potential Benefits of Improving the User Experience

A white paper from the Healthcare Information Management and Systems Society (HIMSS) describes how to incorporate UX or usability in health organizations.[19] This publicly available white paper includes a section on the benefits of usability to healthcare summarized here.

Usability can add value to organizations across a range of areas. Usability ROI material is available from (1) nonhealthcare projects such as Bias and Mayhew[26] and Nielsen,[27] (2) the User Experience Professionals Association website, and (3) Dey Alexander Consulting.[28] To the author's knowledge, no research is yet available about large-scale ROI or cost savings for UX efforts in healthcare projects. Thus material is cited from non-healthcare applications. However, findings from non-healthcare IT projects are very likely to extend to healthcare because of the often dramatic changes that usability can create. Fig. 21.3 outlines potential areas of value when UX is improved in health organizations.

Increased Individual Effectiveness

Usability can positively affect at least three areas of particular interest in health IT:

1. Increased user productivity and efficiency
2. Decreased user errors and increased safety
3. Improved cognitive support

Increased User Productivity and Efficiency. One of the most prevalent complaints about health IT in general and EHRs specifically is that the technology impedes users' productivity. For example, outpatient visits were reduced from four to three per hour after an ambulatory EHR was fielded.[29] A cognitive work analysis of the same system in a laboratory setting showed a large number of average steps to complete common tasks, a high average execution time, and a large percentage of required mental operators.[30]

Employing usability processes helps improve productivity and efficiency. The Nielsen Norman Group estimated that "productivity gains from redesigning an intranet to improve usability are eight times larger than costs for a company with 1,000 employees; 20 times larger for a company with 10,000 employees; and 50 times larger for a company with 100,000 employees."[27, p. 5] Website redesign statistics for the 42 cases collected by Nielsen Norman yielded an average increase in user productivity of 161%. After testing intranets for low and high usability, these authors projected a savings of 48 hours per employee if intranets were redesigned for high usability. Souza et al. cited usability research showing that two-thirds of buyers failed in shopping attempts on well-known sites.[31] Thus poor usability on intranets can mean poor employee productivity.

Decreased User Errors and Increased Safety. One of the major reasons why health IT is installed is to reduce errors in healthcare.[32] While clearly some classes of errors such as medication errors can be reduced with health IT, technology can create unintended consequences and new errors due to poor usability.[33,34] For example, Kushniruk et al. were able to identify how certain types of usability problems were related to errors as physicians entered prescriptions into hand-held devices.[35]

Nielsen and Levy collected case studies and found a decrease in user error rates in 46 redesign projects measuring user error.[36] Another study showed a 25% decrease in user errors after screen redesign.[37] Users found needed information only 42% of the time on 15 large commercial websites, even when they were directed to the correct home page; 62% gave up looking for desired items on websites.[27] Redesigns could prevent errors in these types of interactions; thus incorporating usability can potentially decrease errors in health IT products.

Improved Cognitive Support. Stead and Lin concluded that the premier EHRs in the United States in 2009 did not provide the required cognitive support for clinicians (i.e., tools for thinking about and solving health problems).[7] This is still true today. Cognitive support may include designs to provide an overview or summary of the patient, information "at a glance," intuitive designs, and tailored support for clinicians in specific contexts. An example of how usability can provide cognitive support is the work on novel physiologic monitoring designs. Researchers employed UCD and usability testing techniques to create novel designs integrating physiologic data in a graphic object.[38–40] The new design provided integrated, "at a glance" pictorial data to show changes to clinicians. These graphic objects are now being incorporated in vendors' products as an adjunct to numeric data displays. Another example is the design and testing of new displays for ICU nurses after researchers performed a comprehensive study of their tasks and cognitive requirements.[41]

Increased Organizational Efficiencies

Well-designed user interfaces and systems translate into organizational efficiencies, including the following:

- Decreased maintenance costs
- Decreased customer and individual training and support costs
- Decreased development time and costs

Decreased Maintenance Costs. Eighty percent of software life cycle costs occur in the maintenance phase and are related to unmet user requirements and similar usability problems.[42] Usability experts estimated that by correcting usability problems early in the design phase of a project, two different U.S. airline projects reduced the cost of those fixes by 60% and 90%.[43] At IBM, researchers concluded that it is more economical to consider users' needs early in the design cycle than to solve them later.[44]

Decreased Customer and Individual Training and Support Costs. A study by Microsoft showed that time for support calls "dropped dramatically" after a redesign of the print merge function in Word.[43] Business analysts found that a well-designed user interface had an internal rate of return of 32%, realized through a 35% reduction in training, a 30% reduction in supervisory time, and improved productivity.[37] Logically, a well-designed user interface would require fewer resources to support, less time and effort in training, and decreased time on support calls. Souza also cited a web redesign at Lucy.com that resulted in a 20% reduction in support calls.[31]

Decreased Development Time and Costs. According to Marcus, the rule of thumb in many usability-aware organizations is that the cost-benefit ratio for usability is $1:$10:$100.[45] Once a system is in development, correcting a problem costs 10 times as much as fixing the same problem during design. If the system has been released, it costs 100 times as much relative to fixing the problem in design. This estimate is frequently quoted, and while it may be overly optimistic, its main point is clear: It is far more expensive in time, costs, and effort to correct issues later in the development life cycle than to complete an informed design at the beginning of a project.

Best practices in usability engineering could alleviate major reasons for inaccurate cost estimates by managers in these areas: frequent requests for changes by users, overlooked tasks, users' lack of understanding of their own tasks, and insufficient communication and understanding between users and analysts.[43] By including usability techniques, two companies reduced time spent on development, one by 40%[43] and another by 33% to 50%.[46] An ROI analysis by Karat indicated a $10 return on each dollar invested in usability.[47] According to Landauer, when usability is factored in at the beginning of a project, efficiency improvements can be greater than 700%.[48] On a national level Landauer estimated in 1995 that the inadequate use of usability engineering methods in software development projects cost the U.S. economy about $30 billion per year in lost productivity. Of course, the cost would be even more substantial now.

Incorporating usability into health IT provides significant value to all such projects; therefore it is essential that healthcare team members, informaticians, and IT staff understand and apply usability principles and processes in their work. This chapter provides readers with an understanding of the knowledge and skills to conduct usability tests.

HUMAN-COMPUTER INTERACTION FRAMEWORKS FOR HEALTH INFORMATICS

Frameworks provide guidance for understanding essential components that improve the UX. They are helpful in completing UCD processes, usability tests, IT adoption evaluations, and usability research. This section of the chapter provides an overview of existing frameworks and describes in detail the Health Human–Computer Interaction Framework (HHCI).

Human Factors and Human–Computer Interaction Frameworks

Various HCI frameworks and models with different foci are available[49-58]:

- Fit Between Individuals, Task, and Technology (FITT), with the elements connected by interactions and influences[49]
- User, Function, Representation, and Task Analyses (UFuRT, or TURF). System knowledge is distributed across multiple users who have differences in expertise and cognitive characteristics. It includes a task analysis portion to describe steps in tasks and interactions.[58] More recently, this framework was renamed TURF.[59]
- A framework for employing usability methods to redesign a fielded system[54]
- A framework for technology-induced error[51]
- A combined health IT adoption and HCI model[52]
- Joint cognitive systems[53]
- Systems Engineering Initiative for Patient Safety (SEIPS) 2.0, which incorporates human factors

concepts of configuration, engagement, and adaptation, a model at a higher level of abstraction for systems[60] The last two models bear more discussion. Hollnagel and Woods coined the term *cognitive systems engineering*, acknowledging that sociotechnical systems, or complex technologies embedded within social systems, are increasingly prevalent yet have frequent system failures.[53] The authors devised a cyclic model called contextual control model, or CoCom, with the following elements: event, modifies, constructs, determines, acts, and produces. Users and context are major components of the model. Importantly, joint cognitive systems imply that information is shared or distributed among humans and technology. This framework is useful for examining teamwork in healthcare, such as those for patient care.

SEIPS 2.0 is a model centered on work systems. Work performance results in a sociotechnical system with people as one component. People (or a person) are central to work systems, and support for the design of work is necessary. Support includes the design of work structures and processes using human factors science. Often work systems include technology, but SEIPS may also be used to examine work without technology.[60]

An analysis of the existing frameworks found each helpful but inadequate for health usability studies. Missing elements across frameworks included (1) interactions among disparate users, including patients, although SEIPS acknowledges groups of people and CoCom and TURF mention information distribution, (2) characteristics and actions of products and users, (3) a focus on context, and (4) a developmental timeline. Context is critical in particular because it defines the kinds of users, tasks, and work design.[58,59] A developmental time element is also necessary because it accounts for users changing (maturing) in their interactions over time.[52,55] Therefore a new framework was created.

The Health Human–Computer Interaction Framework

The HHCI Framework is described here. The current framework builds on early work by Staggers and Parks describing nurse-computer interaction.[61] It was expanded to include groups of healthcare providers and interactions with patients.[55] The framework is adapted further here to acknowledge that IT may be only one example of an available health IT product (e.g., others might be physiologic monitors or intravenous pumps).

The elements of the framework are outlined in Fig. 21.4. Information (e.g., patient care, administrative, or educational information) is the exchange mechanism. Interactions occur in a system of mutual influences where elements (e.g., individuals, health IT) act and respond based on specific characteristics. Context is paramount with all interactions embedded within a context. This means that any outcomes of interactions are distinct, as they are defined by a context. The developmental timeline indicates that interactions change over time. Thus the outcomes of interactions are different based on when an interaction occurs in time.

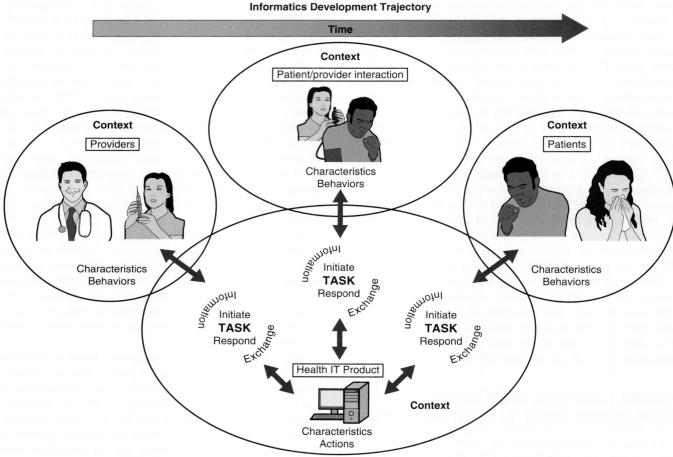

FIG 21.4 Health human–computer interaction framework. (Copyright Nancy Staggers. Reprinted with permission.)

Humans or products can initiate interactions. The information is processed through either the product or the humans, according to characteristics. The recipient then reacts to the information; for example, a healthcare provider could read and respond to an e-mail from a patient, or a product might process interactions after the Enter key is pressed. Iterative cycles continue as humans behave and products act according to defined characteristics. Goals and planning are implicit within the tasks displayed in the framework.

Essential Components for Improving the User Experience

The important point in this section is that using a framework or model can greatly assist readers to think comprehensively about UX for health IT and the conduct of usability studies. Readers may choose a framework to match the need at hand. Methods can then be applied as appropriate, while ensuring that critical elements are under consideration. This idea is expanded in later sections to illustrate how the framework assists usability testing. In summary, product interactions are a complex part of a sociotechnical system. Critical elements to consider are as follows:

- Users and their characteristics
- Interactions
- Tasks (goals of tasks)

- Information
- Products and their characteristics
- Context
- Interactions mature over time (developmental timeline)

SELECTING METHODS TO IMPROVE THE USER EXPERIENCE

UX methods can be at a more strategic level or project-based. For instance, strategic UX methods were outlined by the American Medical Informatics Association (AMIA) in 10 recommendations to improve patient safety and quality of care by improving the usability of EHRs (Box 21.1).[62]

To effect these recommendations and also apply concepts to health IT in local projects, readers will want to know some specific methods for analyzing UX in health IT systems. Techniques to improve the UX can be informal or formal, simple or complex, and employ a few individuals or a wide range of users. Readers or researchers can design small projects or sophisticated studies by combining usability precepts with usability-specific or traditional research designs and methods such as quantitative, qualitative, or mixed methods. The type of usability study is dependent on the purpose of the project; when the assessment is targeted within the systems life cycle; the desired outcome of the project; and available resources, including time, people, and

---

BOX 21.1   American Medical Informatics Association Recommendations for Improving Electronic Health Records Usability

- Accelerate a research agenda for usability a human factors in health IT.
  - Prioritize standard use cases.
  - Develop a core set of measures for adverse events related to health IT use.
  - Research and promote best practice for safe implementations of EHRs.
- Create new policies.
  - Include usability concerns as a part of the standardization and interoperability across EHRs.
  - Establish an adverse event reporting system for health IT and voluntary health IT event reporting.
  - Develop and disseminate an education campaign on the safe and effective use of EHRs.
- Develop industry guidelines.
  - Develop a common user interface style guide for select EHR functionalities.
  - Perform actual usability assessment on patient-safety sensitive EHR functionalities.
- Create clinical end-user recommendations.
  - Adopt best practices for EHR system implementations and ongoing management.
  - Monitor how IT systems are used and report IT-related adverse events.

AMIA, American Medical Informatics Association; *EHR,* electronic health records; *IT,* information technology.

BOX 21.2   User Experience Methods and Techniques

An excellent resource for UX methods and techniques is the Usability.gov website. This resource includes content such as the basics about usability, project management, and visual design. For our purposes here, the most relevant content is the section on "how to and tools."

Usability projects can be done at any point in the systems life cycle from initial work (to identify usability issues; clarify requirements; and assess initial designs, technical prototypes, or simple computerized applications) to iterative development of solutions, product selection, product customization, or evaluation of a system after installation.[63] The important point is that UX experts recommend usability tests early and often.

UX, User experience.

---

money. However, any study can use the elements from the HHCI framework as a guide (Box 21.2).

UX methods were developed over decades and are robust. This section of the chapter concentrates on unique, proven UX methods to choose and apply. These include discount usability methods and other UX methods described later.

Discount Usability Methods

Nielsen developed techniques he called discount usability methods to reduce the number of required users in usability projects and to use early design prototypes. Meant for UX experts, this method has proven useful for others involved in designing projects.[64,65] A discount usability method offers economies of time, effort, and cost and can be completed at any point in the systems life cycle. The most common technique is heuristic evaluation.

Heuristic Evaluation

The definition of a heuristic is a "rule of thumb" or guideline. Heuristic evaluations (HEs) compare products against accepted usability guidelines to reveal issues. Nielsen recommends that three to five experts complete independent evaluations and then combine issues into a master list after discussion and consolidation. HE violations of guidelines are made and severity scores are then assigned to the identified issues.[65] Importantly, dual domain experts (experts in both UX and the field to which the application is geared)

can find 81% to 90% of existing usability problems and increased numbers of major issues with the application.[66] HE is a commonly employed technique, and readers can complete an HE after only a modest amount of training.

A number of usability heuristics are available to evaluate applications:

- Nielsen's 10 heuristics[67]
- Zhang et al.'s 14 heuristics[68]
- Dix et al.'s 10 heuristics[23]
- Shneiderman's 8 golden rules[69]
- HIMSS's 9 usability principles[1]

Zhang et al.'s guidelines have been used extensively in health applications and devices. These authors combined Nielsen's and Shneiderman's heuristics and applied them to a project evaluating two infusion pumps, finding 192 and 121 heuristic violations, respectively, categorized into 89 and 52 usability problems. Using this technique, they concluded that the pump with the higher violations might contribute to more medical errors than the other one.[68] Zhang et al.'s 14 adapted heuristics and definitions are outlined in Table 21.1. Once readers develop a basic understanding of the meaning of each heuristic, they can evaluate a health IT product against the heuristics as in the following examples.

Examples of a Heuristic Evaluation Project. Guo et al. used Zhang's heuristics to evaluate a vendor's eMAR installed at a tertiary care center.[11] The authors received training on the eMAR, defined typical tasks that nurses complete using the product, and also modified Zhang's heuristics to include concepts about patient safety. The authors independently completed the defined tasks and compared their interactions to the heuristics, synthesized results, and found 233 violations for 60 usability problems. Problems included having to manually update the screen by clicking an "as of" button to refresh the screen and ensure that the most current medication orders were being viewed. Nurses had great difficulty in determining medications given "at a glance." These results have implications across all three usability goals of effectiveness, efficiency, and satisfaction, and also raise potential patient safety issues.

Researchers evaluated the Veterans' Administration's eMAR using a similar process to the one listed above; however, they

TABLE 21.1   Zhang Heuristics and Nielsen Severity Rating Scheme

Heuristic Category	Definition
Consistency and standards	Consistency across all aspects of the product: methods of navigation, messages and actions, meaning of buttons, and terms and icons. Congruence with known screen design principles for color and screen layout. Consistency with ISO (International Organization for Standardization) usability guidelines.
Visibility of system state	Users understand what the system is doing and what they can do with the product from the system messages, information, and displays.
Match between system and world	The technology matches the way users think and do work, uses appropriate information flow, has typical options that users need, and includes expected actions by the system.
Minimalist	No superfluous information. System and screen design targeted to primary information users' needs. Use of progressive disclosure to display details of a category of information only when needed. The exception can be designs for expert users where screen density is preferred.
Minimize memory load	Minimizing the amount of information and tasks users have to memorize to adequately use the technology. Product makes use of sample formats for data input, such as a calendar for date format.
Informative feedback	The technology provides prompt and useful feedback about users' interactions and actions (e.g., feedback that orders were placed).
Flexibility and efficiency	The ability to tailor and customize to suit individuals' needs. Includes novice and expert capabilities (e.g., string searches).
Good error messages	Tell users what error occurred and how users can recover from the error. Not abstract or general such as "Forbidden!" Need to be precise and polite and not blame the user.
Prevent errors	Catastrophic errors must be prevented (e.g., mixing pediatric medication order dosing between kilograms and pounds or delivering a radiation dose with the device left wide open instead of being tailored to tumor size).
Clear closure	Users should know when a task is completed and all information is accepted. Displays should include progress toward 100% completion versus using a series of bars.
Reversible actions	Whenever possible, actions and interactions should be able to be undone within legal limits in electronic health records. If actions cannot be reversed, there is a consistent procedure for documenting the correction of any misinformation in the system.
Use the users' language	The technology uses language and terms the targeted users can comprehend and expect. Health terms are used appropriately.
Users in control	Users initiate actions versus having the perception that the technology is in control. Avoid surprising actions, ending up in unexpected places, and loud sounds with errors.
Help and documentation	Provide help for users within the context the actions occur (context sensitive). Embed help functions throughout the application.

Severity Scale Rating Element	Definition
0—No usability problem	No need to correct the issue.
1—Cosmetic problem	Correct the issue only if extra time and fiscal resources allow. Lowest priority.
2—Minor problem	Annoying issue with minor impact. Low priority to fix.
3—Major usability problem	Issue with major impact to use or training or both. Important to fix. Considerations are the numbers and kinds of users affected by a persistent problem.
4—Usability catastrophe	Severe issue that must be corrected before product release, especially those related to patient safety.

Data from Zhang J, Johnson TR, Patel VL, Paige DL, Kubose T. Using usability heuristics to evaluate patient safety of medical devices. *J Biomed Inform.* 2003;36(1,2):23-30; Nielsen, J. Severity ratings for usability problems. http://www.useit.com/papers/heursitic/severityrating.html/; 1993.

also validated UX findings with the site barcode medication administration nurse coordinators.[10] Findings included 90 usability problems and 440 heuristic evaluation violations. Fifteen issues were rated as catastrophic, with nurses particularly impaired in situation awareness or having the ability to develop a "big picture" of what was happening with patients and their medications. An example was medication preparation for a group of patients. The application allowed nurses to access only one patient's medication list at a time even though they cared for groups of patients, so they developed workarounds such as using paper 4 × 6 index cards to organize medications for times throughout a shift. HE provided insights about how this application needed to be improved to support nurses' cognitive processes and medication activities.

Traditional Usability Methods

A large suite of methods is available to conduct UX examinations of health products and processes. Three of these methods—think-aloud protocol, task analysis, and contextual inquiry/focused ethnographies—are presented here.

Think-Aloud Protocol

Think-aloud protocol involves a small number of actual application users (vs. experts). Even as few as five users can offer rich data about UX issues. Users talk aloud while they interact with a product and observers record their experienced usability problems. As users voice what they are trying to do, they indicate where interactions are confusing and provide other thoughts about the product. This allows a detailed examination of the specified tasks, in particular to uncover major effectiveness issues. This method may be used in the design, redesign, development, or evaluation of applications at any time in the systems life cycle. Think-aloud methods are often used in conjunction with other techniques.

With this technique, researchers first determine a specific set of tasks for users to complete, such as tasks to operate an infusion pump or use an mHealth app. Defining tasks ahead of time provides structure and consistency across participants and guides users through the procedure. Participants are asked to complete the tasks and talk aloud during the session. Methods to capture the session can include observing and taking notes, audio- or video-recording using software such as Morae or even a smartphone, and handwritten diaries or issue logs.[23] The resulting material is then analyzed by grouping issues or using a schema such as HE categories to label findings. The analysis portion of this method can be time consuming, depending on the complexity of the product, the number of users tested, and the number of tasks. However, the information gained by using this method is robust and helpful in pinpointing areas needing redesign.

Task Analysis

Task analysis is a generic term for a set of more than 100 techniques that range from a focus on cognitive tasks and processes (called cognitive task analysis) to observable user interactions with an application (e.g., a systematic mapping of team interactions during a patient code). Task analyses are systematic methods used to understand what users are doing or required to do with a health IT product. They focus on tasks and behavioral actions of the users interacting with products. These methods provide a process for learning about and documenting how ordinary users complete actions in a specific context.[33,70,71] Task analyses are helpful to identify task completeness, the correct or incorrect sequencing of tasks (especially their fit to cognitive tasks), accuracy of actions, error recovery, and task allocation between humans and products. Task analysis is typically used early in the systems life cycle to determine user requirements for design or to determine redesign when rich data are needed. This technique may be used to analyze areas for redesign. One type of analysis, cognitive task analysis, is particularly useful for understanding users' goals while interacting with products.[72] A task analysis can be used, for example, to determine who is attending to patients' preventive health alerts in a clinic because alerts are seen by a variety of healthcare providers.

Sample methods of task analysis include the following:
- Interviews
- Observations
- Shadowing users at their actual work sites
- Observing users doing tasks
- Conducting ethnographic studies or interviews[71]

A critique of cognitive task techniques is available for readers who want to find the right method for their project.[73] References on the specifics of performing task analyses are available.[70–72]

Sample output from a task analysis is listed in Table 21.2. After observations and interviews, evaluators record user actions (e.g., a flow chart with task descriptions). Evaluators might video-record users as they interact with an mHealth application, asking users to perform specific tasks and use a think-aloud protocol to uncover tasks (especially cognitive tasks) and requirements.

Example of a Task Analysis. Researchers video-recorded nurses as they interacted with an existing eMAR in an inpatient application.[74] They also observed nurses' medication management tasks in the actual setting in a variety of acute care units. The researchers created a task flow diagram of medication tasks that included cognitive tasks and delineated deficiencies with the current application. By using task analysis to define requirements, the researchers could then develop a novel and more effective eMAR.

Contextual Inquiry or Focused Ethnographies

Ethnography methods are borrowed from anthropology and sociology, where fieldwork and analyses of people in cultural and social settings are completed. Focused ethnographies

TABLE 21.2 Sample Output From Task Analyses

Type of Task Analysis Output	Description
Profiles of users or personas	Short narrative, visual descriptions, and/or summaries about the characteristics of users
Workflow diagrams	A flow diagram of tasks or cognitive processes performed by users
Task sequences or hierarchies	Lists of tasks order by sequence or arranged to show interrelationships
Task scenarios	Detailed descriptions of events or incidents, including how users handle situations
Usability issues	A list and classification of usability problems with a product
Affinity diagrams	Bottom-up groupings of facts and issues about users, tasks, and environments to generate design ideas
Video and audiotape highlights	Clips that illustrate particular observations about users and tasks in a context

Adapted from Staggers N. Human-computer interaction. In: Englebardt S, Nelson R, eds. *Information Technology in Health Care: An Interdisciplinary Approach.* Philadelphia, PA: Harcourt Health Science Company; 2001:321-345.

and contextual inquiry involve interacting with users in their actual sites or "field settings." They concentrate on individuals' points of view and their experiences and interactions in social settings, rather than on just the actions of those individuals.[75,76] However, researchers are observers rather than a part of the society. During observations, detailed descriptions are generated with an emphasis on social relationships, interactions with IT, and their impact on work. Ethnographies have become important in understanding the UX and describing the impact of complex products.

Example of a Focused Ethnography or Contextual Inquiry

Ash et al. used this method to research the impact of CPOE on users in acute care facilities in the United States.[34,77,78] They completed interviews, focus groups, and observations and outlined unintended consequences for CPOE: new and more work, workflow issues, unusual system demands, disruptions in routine communications, extreme user emotions, and overdependence on the technology. Their studies are considered seminal works in informatics.

FORMAL USER TESTING

"Usability measurements are to user interface design what physical exams are to patient care."[79]

User tests may be done at any point in the systems life cycle, but they are often completed as summative tests—that is, after a product is nearly or completely developed and/or fielded. At that point, more objective methods are employed. A critical aspect of conducting a usability test is measuring human performance and having a larger sample of users. To assist readers, a taxonomy of usability measures is presented in Table 21.3. This table is adapted from Sweeney et al. and from Staggers and expanded here.[55,80,81] The taxonomy includes measures from three perspectives: users, experts, and organizations. Researchers recommend at least 15 users for summative testing.[82] The important points are that usability is measurable and that a suite of measures is available. In addition to the objective measures in the table, questionnaires are available to measure users' perceptions of or satisfaction with their product interactions.

Usability Questionnaires

At least four questionnaires are available to measure user interaction or user interface satisfaction:
- System Usability Scale (SUS)[83,84]
- Questionnaire for User Interaction Satisfaction (QUIS)[85]
- Purdue Usability Testing Questionnaire[86]
- Software Usability Measurement Inventory (SUMI)[87]

The SUS is considered an industry standard among UX professionals and has been used widely on a variety of products outside of and internal to healthcare.[83,84] The SUS is a publicly available, 10-item scale developed in 1986 by John Brooke at Digital Equipment Corporation.[83]

Developed in the late 1990s, QUIS addresses users' overall perceptions of a product, including overall reaction, terminology, screen layout, learning, system capabilities, and other subscales such as multimedia applications.[85] QUIS subscales can be mixed and matched to fit the application at hand. Participants can complete the QUIS in about 5 to 10 minutes. Reliability and validity assessments are available for this tool.

The Purdue Usability Testing Questionnaire has 100 open-ended questions about how features adhere to accepted guidelines. Students would need to be familiar with design guidelines before using this questionnaire.[86] However, reliability and validity assessments of the questionnaire are not reported.

Less information is available about the SUMI, including its assessed reliability and validity. The instrument has three components: an overall assessment, a usability profile, and an item consensus analysis.[87] The usability profile examines areas such as efficiency, helpfulness, control, and learnability. The consensus component addresses adherence to well-known design alternatives such as categorical ordering of data in a simple search task.

SELECTING A TYPE OF USABILITY TEST

A key decision before beginning a UX assessment is determining the type of study to conduct in a specific case. This section expands on work by Rubin and Chisnell and uses the system's life cycle to organize the types of tests available.[24]

Determining User Needs and Requirements

At the beginning of the systems life cycle, during initial design or redesign process, informaticians determine user needs and requirements from the following:
- Users' characteristics
- Tasks (including cognitive tasks)
- Work design
- Interactions among workers and tasks and products
- Requirements about the specific environments and particular needs related to the context of interactions

Studies can be conducted with limited resources if the scope of the investigation is focused. As the complexity increases, resource consumption increases concomitantly. Assessments early in the systems life cycle seek to answer the following questions:
- Who are the users and what are their characteristics?
- What are basic activities and tasks in this context?
- How do users cognitively process information?
- What information processing can be supported by products?
- What special considerations should be made for users in this environment?
- What attributes need to be in place for an initial design?

Observations using think-aloud protocol and task analysis can be used to determine users' needs and requirements and answer the questions listed previously.

Example of a Requirements Determination Usability Study

Researchers completed a series of studies focused on nurses' acute care handoffs or change of shift reports to determine the

TABLE 21.3   Sample Usability Measures

Usability Focus	Usability Measures
User behaviors (performance)	Task times (speed, reaction times) Percentage of tasks completed Number, kinds of errors Percentage of tasks completed accurately Time, frequency spent on any one option Number of hits and/or amount of time spent on a website Training time Eye tracking Facial expressions Breadth and depth of application usage in actual settings Quality of completed tasks (e.g., quality of decisions) Users' comments (think-aloud) as they interact with technology System setup or installation time, complexity of setup Model of tasks and user behaviors Description of problems when interacting with an application
User behaviors (cognitive)	Description of or systems fit with cognitive information processing Retention of application knowledge over time Comprehension of system Fit with workflow
User behaviors (perceptions)	Usability ratings of products Perceptions about any aspect of technology (speed, effectiveness) Comments during interviews Questionnaires and rating responses (workload, satisfaction)
User behaviors (physiologic)	Heart rate EEG Galvanic skin response Brain-evoked potentials
User behaviors (perceptions about physiologic reactions)	Perceptions about anxiety, stress
User behaviors (motivation)	Willingness to use system Enthusiasm
Expert evaluations (performance)	Model predictions for task performance times, learning, ease of understanding Observations of users as they use applications in a setting to determine fit with work
Expert evaluations (conformance to guidelines)	Level of adherence to guidelines, design criteria, usability principles (heuristic evaluation)
Expert evaluations (perception)	Ratings of technology, informal or formal comments
Context (organization)	Economic costs (increased FTEs for the help desk for a new application) Number of support staff, time needed to support product Number of training staff, time needed to support product Costs (for support, training, loss of productivity) Observations about the fit with work design and workflow in departments, organizations, networks of institutions
Combined	Videotaping and audiotaping users as they interact with an application and capturing keystrokes. Can capture any combination of the above.

EEG, Electroencephalography; *FTE*, full-time equivalent.
Adapted from Staggers N. Human-computer interaction. In: Englebardt S, Nelson R, eds. *Information Technology in Health Care: An Interdisciplinary Approach*. Philadelphia, PA: Harcourt Health Science Company; 2001:321-345; Staggers N. Improving the usability of health informatics applications. In: Hebda T, Czar P, eds. *Handbook of Informatics for Nurses and Health Professionals*. Upper Saddle River, NJ: Pearson Education; 2012:170-193.

current state of the activity and to develop requirements to support handoff tasks.[5,88,89] Handoffs are highly complex and cognitively intensive periods where nurses going off shift synthesize information about patients and communicate it to nurses coming on shift. Methods that would generate rich details about the process, such as observation, field notes,

and interviews, were selected. The HHCI framework guided the thinking about requirements analysis for different aspects of the handoff process. For example, researchers considered nurses (expertise levels, regular vs. travel nurses), types of units (critical care, emergency department, medical, and surgical), and types of product support in place (EHRs, CPOE, eMAR). Handoff tasks can be completed in a variety of ways, including audio recordings, face-to-face interactions, and bedside reports. The researchers completed a focused ethnography across available medical and surgical units in different facilities. They observed change of shift reports, audiotaped nurses, photographed nurses' tools, and took field notes about nurses' interactions with the existing EHRs in the facilities. From the findings, the researchers were able to derive detailed information about requirements for computerized support for change of shift activities.[89]

Formative Tests

Formative tests are conducted earlier in the systems life cycle after requirements are determined. These tests are conducted on preliminary designs/redesigns when fewer resources have been committed to programming the product. Methods are often more informal and involve extensive interactions between the evaluator and user. Results often produce rich data (e.g., from think-alouds). The objective of a very early formative test is to assess the effectiveness of emerging design concepts by asking the following:

- Is the basic functionality of value to users?
- Is basic navigation and information flow intuitive?
- Is fundamental content missing?
- How much computer experience does a user need to use this module?[24]

The usability focus is on the effectiveness goal. Users are asked to perform common tasks with the prototype or step through paper mockups of the application using the think-aloud method. At this assessment, researchers strive to understand *why* users are behaving as they do with the application rather than how quickly they perform.[5] To assess effectiveness, the researcher is interested in finding cognitive disconnects with basic functions, missing information or steps, and assessing how easily users understand the task at hand.

Nielsen recommends having at least five users perform think-aloud protocols as an observer watches them and records any issues. This number of users can detect as much as 60% to 80% of design errors.[64,90] Later research confirmed that as few as five to eight users are sufficient for most early usability tests.[91,92]

Examples of Formative Tests

A public health researcher wanted to develop an application to display reportable patient conditions across jurisdictions. After researching available applications and completing requirements, she developed a prototype using PowerPoint to meet initial requirements and to assess usability for the following sample tasks: (1) find out whether chlamydia is a reportable condition in Utah, Colorado, or Washington; (2) determine the time frame for reporting the condition; and (3) ascertain whether a specimen must be submitted and the location for the submission. She selected key public health, clinical, and laboratory users as participants in the test. These users were asked to think aloud as they completed common tasks. The researcher took notes to record the data related to their responses. Using these data, several iterations of the prototype were designed to improve the UX in completing the tasks.[93]

A second example of a formative test is one conducted midway through the development of a product application.[24] After the organization and general design were determined, this type of test assessed lower-level operations of the application, stressing the efficiency goals of the product (vs. effectiveness in the above example) and how well the task is presented to users. The researcher assessed a subsequent version of the public health application described previously. She asked the same key users to use the same tasks, but now participants commented on operations, icons, and the arrangement of the radio buttons.

Questions during this test might include the following:

- How quickly and accurately can users perform selected tasks?
- Are the terms in the system consistent across modules?
- Are operations displayed in a manner that allows quick detection of critical information?

Users performed common tasks with a product that was partially developed. Usability measures (see Table 21.3) such as performance time and errors are often selected. Users can perform tasks silently or researchers can use think-aloud methods to elicit issues. Again, designers use the results to craft a redesigned prototype to correct issues.

Validation Test

A validation test is completed later in the systems life cycle using a more mature product. This type of test assesses how this particular product compares to a predetermined standard, benchmark, or performance measure. A second purpose might be to assess how all modules in a technology application work as an integrated whole. For instance, a validation test can be useful in a system selection process to decide how a new vendor supports critical tasks such as medication barcoding or medication reconciliation. Questions for a validation test might include the following:

- Can 80% of users retrieve the correct complete blood count (CBC) test results within 10 seconds of interacting with the system?
- How many heuristic violations are identified for this product?
- Can users complete admission orders for a trauma patient with no errors?

This type of test is more structured, so it precludes interactions between testers and users. Performance measures mentioned earlier are employed as users interact to complete the benchmark testing. The methods are carefully structured.

Example of a Validation Test

A nurse researcher wanted to ensure that a new mobile device for rural care in Tanzania mirrored the established algorithms on paper. The goal was to assess whether the algorithms used with the mobile device were 100% accurate. She enlisted key users and informaticians to interact with each pathway in the device. Deviations from the established algorithms were documented and corrected.[94]

Comparison Test

Readers can conduct comparison tests at any point in the systems life cycle, but they are more commonly done to compare an existing design with a redesign or to compare two different design solutions for the same application. The major objective of this usability test is to determine which application, design, or product is more effective, efficient, and satisfying.[24] The study design can range from an informal side-by-side comparison with structured tasks or use of a classic experimental study design. Results are more dramatic if the designs are substantially different.

Examples of a Comparison Study

The purpose of this study was to determine whether a new user interface for orders management was different than an older interface in terms of performance times, errors, and user satisfaction.[74] The tasks and interactions were planned to minimize the amount of time that nurses would be away from patient care. The informaticians used an HCI framework to guide elements in the study. Users interacted on identical computers to test both interfaces. Tasks were "real-world" orders and identical for the two designs. The environment was a computer training room away from patient care units and distractions. The developmental trajectory was considered in this study to ensure that results were not affected by practice time. Therefore 40 tasks for each interface allowed nurses to become practiced at each user interface. (The threshold of task numbers was determined in pilot work.) Tasks, keystrokes, and errors were captured automatically by the computer. The QUIS was administered after each interface to assess user satisfaction. Each nurse interacted with both interfaces, but the order in which they were presented was randomized. The results showed the new interface was significantly faster, had fewer errors, and produced high user satisfaction.

In a second study, a nurse researcher wanted to compare the traditional design of physiologic monitors and other products to a new design that integrated data across physiologic parameters, medication management, and communication.[95,96] His target population was intensive care unit (ICU) nurses. The tasks were designed so that the study could be completed in about 20 to 30 minutes in each of two sessions. Paper prototypes were used to assess effectiveness, efficiency, and satisfaction before resources were expended to code bidirectional interfaces to the devices. Tasks were defined, and nurses interacted with the prototypes. Findings were that the new, integrated monitor view resulted in faster task times, higher detection of potential medication interactions, lower perceived mental workload, and higher satisfaction.

Identifying Usability Issues With Fielded Health IT Products

As organizations begin to understand the importance of the UX, leaders may be unsure where to begin identifying usability issues in their current environments. The following list includes symptoms of potential strategic usability issues and provides a framework for determining where initial energy and resources could be focused[19]:

- Products or applications requiring long training times
- Support calls categorized by product or application
- Adverse events related to product interactions
- Lists of requested system change requests typically tracked in a database of system change requests across users and products
- User group requests for updates or changes
- Users' descriptions of their most vexing applications and interactions
- Users' identified delays or errors when they interact with complex applications, especially any requiring information synthesis such as eMARs, clinical summaries, and handoffs

Once a usability problem is suspected, researchers or students begin assessing the issue more systematically using the techniques described previously.

Steps for Conducting User Experience Tests

At some point in their careers, readers will likely want to conduct a usability project. Step-by-step guides are available.[1,24,97] The texts by Crandell, Klein, and Hoffman;[72] Rubin and Chisnell;[24] and Tullis and Albert[98] can act as specific guides. HIMSS[1] and the National Institute of Standards and Technology (NIST)[97] have published guides for conducting usability tests on EHRs. For instance, the NIST suggests using both HE and summative testing to evaluate products, especially EHRs.

The basic steps for conducting usability tests can be summarized as follows:

1. *Define a clear purpose.* The specific purpose guides testers to determine the type of study, methods, and users required. For example, if the purpose relates to assessment of a redesign of a CPOE module for an intraoperative surgical team, an exploratory test may be indicated.

2. *Assess constraints.* Testers are always mindful of study constraints: time; resources; availability of the software to be evaluated; and availability of other equipment such as video cameras, testing labs, or users, especially if the users are specialists. These constraints may drive the type of usability test. For example, if the tester's goal is to evaluate an application to support anesthesiologists, these time-constrained physicians may not be willing to spend more than 15 to 20 minutes participating in a usability test. Tasks, methods, and products are defined to work within this constraint.

3. *Use an HCI framework to define pertinent components.* Use a framework to assess each component against the planned study. Who are the key users? What are typical tasks? What information needs to be exchanged? What product characteristics and which actions are needed? What is the setting or context? Will it be a naturalistic setting to determine exactly how an application will be used or a laboratory setting to control interruptions? What is a representative time in the developmental trajectory? How much practice time needs to be considered, especially if the design is new? Be sure to examine the latter component carefully to ensure a valid comparison between users'

interactions with a new product and a current one by including practice time in the study.

4. *Match methods to the purpose, constraints, and framework assessment.* Methods that produce rich results such as a think-aloud protocol will match a purpose of understanding key user requirements, while a more structured method will allow a comparison of new and old designs. Long training and practice times for complex devices may constrain the number of tasks testers can offer. Other basic methodological steps are as follows:

- Select representative end users.
- Select a usability test appropriate to the purpose and point in the systems life cycle.
- Define and validate tasks.
- Measure key elements and control for others (e.g., measure performance time but control interruptions unless the effect of interruptions is the focus).
- Define the context to be used.
- Consider training and practice for new products.
- Pilot test methods before running the main study to smooth out procedures and bugs.

Once the methods are defined, all of these pieces can be put into action and the evaluation can be conducted.

CONCLUSION AND FUTURE DIRECTIONS

UX issues have clear impacts on health IT users. In the United States, agencies are engaging in activities to improve the UX for health IT products (e.g., NIST, the Office of the National Coordinator for Health Information Technology, and AMIA). The Food and Drug Administration has required usability testing on medical devices for over 20 years, but other health IT vendors and health organizations are only beginning to employ the principles and processes for improving UX. The most immediate future direction concerns UX education and understanding action steps to be taken. Organizations need to increase their knowledge and skills related to improving the UX. One way is to use the material outlined by the HIMSS Usability Task Force in 2011 on a Health Usability Maturity Model.[19] The material can guide organizations in assessing their current level of UX, employing methods to market usability to the organization, and increasing the UX to reach a strategic level.

Future UX directions are both strategic and tactical. Strategic directions might include the development of a national clearinghouse or organization to track UX issues and solutions. In particular, tracking for issues related to patient safety and health IT use is needed. AMIA usability recommendations should be implemented to include an expanded research agenda for health IT and UX. UX issues should also have a "home" within respective professional organizations (e.g., nurses might collaborate with HIMSS or the American Nurses Association on a repository for UX solutions). Tactically, the future might include the use of automated methods to ensure that designs conform to known standards, especially basic screen designs. Best practices in UX and implementations should be employed. The future must include a focus on health IT products that support the way users think and work in health settings.

This chapter described current issues with technology, definitions, or terms and the potential benefits of improving the UX in health organizations. Axioms of usability were defined: an early and central focus on users in the design and development of systems, iterative design of applications, and systematic usability measures. Across HCI frameworks, these major elements exist: users, products, contexts, tasks, information, interactions, and a developmental trajectory. Common usability methods and tests were discussed, and examples were provided. Readers are now prepared to conduct discount usability tests and several types of formative, summative, validation, and comparison usability tests. Readers have examples of performance and benchmark measures and four steps outlining the planning and conducting of usability tests.

REFERENCES

1. Health Information Management and Systems Society (HIMSS) User Experience Committee. *Defining and Testing EMR Usability: Principles and Proposed Methods of EMR Usability Evaluation and Rating*; 2009. http://www.himss.org/ResourceLibrary/ContentTabsDetail.aspx?ItemNumber=41050/.
2. Beuscart-Zephir MC, Borycki E, Carayon P, Jaspers MW, Pelayo S. Evolution of human factors research and studies of health information technologies: the role of patient safety. *Yearb Med Inform.* 2013; 8(1):67–77.
3. Carayon P, Xie A, Kianfar S. Human factors and ergonomics as a patient safety practice. *BMJ Qual Saf.* 2014; 23(3):196–205.
4. TJC. The Joint Commission. *Safe Use of Health Information Technology*; 2015. www.jointcommission.org/.
5. Staggers N, Clark L, Blaz JW, Kapsandoy S. Why patient summaries in electronic health records do not provide the cognitive support necessary for nurses' handoffs on medical and surgical units: insights from interviews and observations. *Health Inform J.* 2011; 17(3):209–223.
6. Pew Charitable Trust. *Conference on Issues and Solutions to Electronic Health Record Usability*, Washington DC: Pew Charitable Trust; 2015.
7. Stead W, Lin H. *Computational Technology for Effective Healthcare: Immediate Steps and Strategic Directions.* Washington, DC: National Academies Press; 2009.
8. Committee HUE. *Issues and Solutions to Nurses' User Experiences with Health IT*; 2016. http://www.himss.org/library/user-experience-healthcare-it/.
9. Staggers N, Jennings BM, Lasome CE. A usability assessment of AHLTA in ambulatory clinics at a military medical center. *Mil Med.* 2010; 175(7):518–524.
10. Staggers N, Iribarren S, Guo JW, Weir C. Evaluation of a BCMA's Electronic Medication Administration Record. *West J Nurs Res.* 2015; 37(7):899–921.
11. Guo J, Iribarren S, Kapsandoy S, Perri S, Staggers N. eMAR user interfaces: a call for ubiquitous usability evaluations and product redesign. *Appl Clin Inform.* 2011; 2(2):202–224.
12. ACP. American College of Physicians and American EHR Partners. *Survey of Clinicians: User Satisfaction with Electronic Health Records has Decreased Since 2010*; 2013. http://www.acponline.org/pressroom/ehrs_survey.htm/.

13. AMA. American Medical Association. *AMA Calls for Design Overhaul of Electronic Health Records to Improve Usability*; 2014. http://www.ama-assn.org/ama/pub/news/news/2014/2014-09-16-solutions-to-ehr-systems.page/.

14. Staggers N, Elias BL, Hunt JR, Makar E, Alexander GL. Nursing-centric technology and usability a call to action. *Comput Inform Nurs*. 2015; 33(8):325–332.

15. Kuniavsky M. *Observing the User Experience: A Practitioner's Guide to User Research*. San Francisco, CA: Morgan Kaufmann Publishers (Elsevier); 2003.

16. ISO. *International Organization of Standards 9241-11*; 1998. http://www.usabilitynet.org/tools/r_international.htm#9241-11/.

17. HFES. *Definitions of Human Factors and Ergonomics*; 2012. http://www.hfes.org/Web/EducationalResources/HFEdefinitionsmain.html#govagencies/.

18. Schaffer E. Is usability different than the user experience? *HFI Connect: User Experience for a Better World*; 2010. http://connect.humanfactors.com/profiles/blogs/is-user-experience-different/.

19. HIMSS. *Promoting Usability in Health Organizations: Initial Steps and Progress Toward a Healthcare Usability Maturity Model*. Health Information Management Systems Society: Chicago, IL; 2011.

20. NN Group. User experience—our definition. *Strategies to Enhance the User Experience*; 2007. http://www.nngroup.com/about/userexperience.html/.

21. Gurses AP, Carayon P. Performance obstacles of intensive care nurses. *Nurs Res*. 2007; 56(3):185–194.

22. Norman D. *The Psychology of Everyday Things*. New York: Basic Books; 1988.

23. Dix A, Finlay JE, Abowd GD, Beale R. *Human-Computer Interaction*. 3rd ed. Prentice-Hall: Essex, England; 2004.

24. Rubin J, Chisnell D. *Handbook of Usability Testing: How to Plan, Design and Conduct Effective Tests*. New York: John Wiley & Sons; 2008.

25. Stanford University. *Design Thinking*; 2015. http://designprogram.stanford.edu/design-thinking.php/.

26. Bias RG, Mayhew DJ. *Cost-Justifying Usability: An Update for the Internet Age*. San Francisco, CA: Morgan Kaufman; 2005.

27. Nielsen J, Gilutz S. *Usability Return on Investment*. Nielsen Norman Group: Fremont, CA; 2003.

28. Dey Consulting. *Return on Investment Discussion Articles*; 2009. http://www.deyalexander.com.au/resources/uxd/roi.html/.

29. Philpott T. Doctors See Bigger Role in Electronic Health Record Reform. *Stars and Stripes*; 2009. http://www.stripes.com/.

30. Saitwal H, Feng X, Walji M, Patel V, Zhang J. Assessing performance of an electronic health record (EHR) using cognitive task analysis. *Int J Med Inform*. 2010; 79(7): 501–506.

31. Souza R, Sonderegger P, Roshan S, Dorsey M. *Get ROI from Design*. Cambridge, MA: Forrester Research; 2001.

32. IOM. Institute of Medicine. *Health IT and Patient Safety: Building Safer Systems for Better Care*. Washington, DC: The National Academies Press; 2011.

33. Ash JS, Sittig DF, Poon EG, Guappone K, Campbell E, Dykstra RH. The extent and importance of unintended consequences related to computerized provider order entry. *J Am Med Inform Assoc*. 2007; 14(4):415–423.

34. Ash JS, Sittig DF, Dykstra R, Campbell E, Guappone K. The unintended consequences of computerized provider order entry: findings from a mixed methods exploration. *Int J Med Inform*. 2009; 78(Suppl 1):S69–S76.

35. Kushniruk A, Triola M, Stein B, Borycki E, Kannry J. The relationship of usability to medical error: an evaluation of errors associated with usability problems in the use of a handheld application for prescribing medications. *Stud Health Technol Inform*. 2004; 107(Pt 2):1073–1076.

36. Nielsen J, Levy J. Measuring usability-preference vs performance. *Commun ACM*. 1994; 37(4):66–75.

37. Dray SM, Karat C. Human factors cost justification for an internal development project. In: Bias RG, Mayhew DJ, eds. *Cost-Justifying Usability*. San Francisco: Morgan Kauffman Publishers; 1994:111–122.

38. Drews FA, Westenskow DR. The right picture is worth a thousand numbers: data displays in anesthesia. *Hum Factors*. 2006; 48(1):59–71.

39. Syroid ND, Agutter J, Drews FA, et al. Development and evaluation of a graphical anesthesia drug display. *Anesthesiology*. 2002; 96(3):565–575.

40. Wachter SB, Johnson K, Albert R, Syroid N, Drews F, Westenskow D. The evaluation of a pulmonary display to detect adverse respiratory events using high resolution human simulator. *J Am Med Inform Assoc*. 2006; 13(6):635–642.

41. Koch SH, Weir C, Haar M, et al. Intensive care unit nurses' information needs and recommendations for integrated displays to improve nurses' situation awareness. *J Am Med Inform Assoc*. 2012; 19(4):583–590.

42. Pressman RS. *Software Engineering: A Practitioner's Approach*. New York: McGraw-Hill; 1992.

43. Bias RG, Mayhew DJ. *Cost-Justifying Usability*. San Francisco, CA: Morgan Kaufmann Publishers; 1994.

44. IBM. *Cost Justifying Ease of Use: Complex Solutions Are Problems*; 2001. http://www.usabilitynet.org/management/c_cost.htm.

45. Marcus A. *Return on Investment for Usable User-Interface Design: Examples and Statistics*. Aaron Marcus and Associates, Inc; Berkeley, CA; 2004.

46. Bosert JL. *Quality Function Deployment: A Practitioner's Approach*. New York: ASQC Quality Press; 1991.

47. Karat C. *Iterative testing of a security applications*. Paper presented at Proceedings of the Human Factors Society; 1989. Denver, CO.

48. Landauer TK. *The Trouble with Computers: Usefulness, Usability and Productivity*. Cambridge. MA: MIT Press; 1995.

49. Ammenwerth E, Iller C, Mahler C. IT-adoption and the interaction of task, technology and individuals: a fit framework and a case study. *BioMed Cent*. 2006; 6(3):1–13.

50. Kushniruk AW, Triola MM, Borycki EM, Stein B, Kannry JL. Technology induced error and usability: the relationship between usability problems and prescription errors when using a handheld application. *Int J Med Inform*. 2005; 74(7-8):519–526.

51. Borycki EM, Kushniruk AW, Bellwood P, Brender J. Technology-induced errors. The current use of frameworks and models from the biomedical and life sciences literatures. *Methods Inf Med*. 2012; 51(2):95–103.

52. Despont-Gros C, Mueller H, Lovis C. Evaluating user interactions with clinical information systems: a model based on human-computer interaction models. *J Biomed Inform*. 2005; 38(3):244–255;

53. Hollnagel E, Woods D. *Joint Cognitive Systems: Foundations of Cognitive Systems Engineering*. Boca Raton, FL: Taylor & Francis Group; 2005.

54. Johnson CM, Johnson TR, Zhang J. A user-centered framework for redesigning health care interfaces. *J Biomed Inform*. 2005; 38(1):75–87.

55. Staggers N. Human-computer interaction. In: Englebardt S, Nelson R, eds. *Information Technology in Health Care: An Interdisciplinary Approach*. Orlando, FL: Harcourt Health Science Company; 2001:321–345.

56. Yusof MM, Kuljis J, Papazafeiropoulou A, Stergioulas LK. An evaluation framework for health information systems: human, organization and technology-fit factors (HOT-fit). *Int J Med Inform*. 2008; 77(6):386–398.

57. Yusof MM, Stergioulas L, Zugic J. Health information systems adoption: findings from a systematic review. *Stud Health Technol Inform*. 2007; 129(Pt 1):262–266.

58. Zhang J, Butler KA. *UFuRT: A Work-Centered Framework and Process for Design and Evaluation of Information Systems. Paper presented at Proceedings of HCI International*; 2007: July 22–27. Beijing, China.

59. Zhang J, Walji MF. TURF: toward a unified framework of EHR usability. *J Biomed Inform*. 2011; 44(6):1056–1067.

60. Holden RJ, Carayon P, Gurses AP, et al. SEIPS 2.0: a human factors framework for studying and improving the work of healthcare professionals and patients. *Ergonomics*. 2013; 56 (11):1669–1686.

61. Staggers N, Parks PL. Collaboration between unlikely disciplines in the creation of a conceptual framework for nurse-computer interactions. *Proc Annu Symp Comput Appl Med Care*. 1992; 661–665.

62. Middleton B, Bloomrosen M, Dente MA, et al. Enhancing patient safety and quality of care by improving the usability of electronic health record systems: recommendations from AMIA. *J Am Med Inform Assoc*. 2013; 20(e1):e2–e8.

63. Thompson CB, Snyder-Halpern R, Staggers N. Analysis, processes, and techniques. Case study. *Comput Nurs*. 1999; 17(5):203–206.

64. Nielsen J. *Usability Engineering*. Cambridge, MA: AP Professional; 1993.

65. Nielsen J. Heuristic evaluation. In: Nielsen J, Mack RL, eds. *Usability Inspection Methods*. New York: John Wiley & Sons Inc; 1994:25–62.

66. Nielsen J. Finding usability problems through heuristic evaluation. In: *Paper presented at Proceedings of the SIGCHI Conference on Human factors in Computing Systems*; 1992. Monterey, CA.

67. Nielsen J. *10 usability heuristics for interface design*; 1995. http://www.nngroup.com/articles/ten-usability-heuristics/.

68. Zhang J, Johnson TR, Patel VL, Paige DL, Kubose T. Using usability heuristics to evaluate patient safety of medical devices. *J Biomed Inform*. 2003; 36(1-2):23–30.

69. Shneiderman B, Plaisant K. *Designing the User Interface: Strategies for Effective Human-Computer Interaction*. 4th ed. Pearson/Addison-Wesley: Boston, MA; 2005.

70. Hackos JT, Redish JC. *User and Task Analysis for Interface Design*. New York: John Wiley & Sons; 1998.

71. Courage C, Redish J, Wixon D. Task analysis. In: Sears A, Jacko J, eds. *The Human-Computer Interaction Handbook*. New York: Lawrence Erlbaum Associates; 2008:928–937.

72. Crandall B, Klein G, Hoffman R. Incident-based CTA: helping practitioners "Tell Stories." In: Crandall B, Klein G, Hoffman RR, eds *Working Minds: a Practitioner's Guide to Cognitive Task Analysis*. Cambridge, MA: The MIT Press; 2006:69–90.

73. Wei J, Salvendy G. The cognitive task analysis methods for job and task design: review and reappraisal. *Behav Inform Technol*. 2004; 23(4):273–299.

74. Staggers N, Kobus D, Brown C. Nurses' evaluations of a novel design for an electronic medication administration record. *Comput Inform Nurs*. 2007; 25(2):67–75.

75. Hammersley M, Atkinson P. *Ethnography: principles in practice*. 3rd ed. London: Routledge; 2007.

76. Viitanen J. Contextual inquiry method for user-centred clinical IT system design. *Stud Health Technol Inform*. 2011; 169: 965–969.

77. Ash JS, Sittig DF, Dykstra R, Campbell E, Guappone K. Exploring the unintended consequences of computerized physician order entry. *Stud Health Technol Inform*. 2007; 129(Pt 1):198–202.

78. Ash JS, Berg M, Coiera E. Some unintended consequences of information technology in health care: the nature of patient care information system-related errors. *J Am Med Inform Assoc*. 2004; 11(2):104–112.

79. Staggers N. The April 2011 hearing on EHR usability. Column on crucial conversations about optimal design column. *Online J Nurs Inform*. 2011; 15(2).

80. Staggers N. Improving the usability of health informatics applications. In: Hebda T, Czar P, eds. *Handbook of informatics for nurses and health professionals*. Upper Saddle River, NJ: Pearson; 2013:170–193.

81. Sweeney M, Maguire M, Shackel B. Evaluating user-computer interaction: a framework. *Int J Man-Machine Stud*. 1993; 38:689–711.

82. Virzi RA. Refining the test phase of usability evaluation: how many subjects is enough? *Hum Factors*. 1992; 34(4):457–468.

83. Bangor A, Kortum P, Miller JT. An empirical evaluation of the system usability scale. *Int J Hum-Comput Interact*. 2008; 24 (6):574–594.

84. Sauro J. *Measuring Usability With the System Usability Scale (SUS)*; 2011. http://www.measuringusability.com/sus.php/.

85. Norman K, Shneiderman B, Harper B, Slaughter L. *Questionnaire for User Interaction Satisfaction, version 7.0.1*; 1998. http://lap.umd.edu/quis/.

86. Lin H, Choong Y, Salvendy G. A proposed index of usability: A method for comparing the relative usability of different software systems. *Behav Inf Technol*. 1997; 16(4-5):267–278.

87. Kirakowski J, Corbett M. SUMI: the software measurement inventory. *Br J Educ Technol*. 1993; 24:210–212.

88. Staggers N, Jennings BM. The content and context of change of shift report on medical and surgical units. *J Nurs Adm*. 2009; 39 (9):393–398.

89. Staggers N, Clark L, Blaz JW, Kapsandoy S. Nurses' information management and use of electronic tools during acute care handoffs. *West J Nurs Res*. 2012; 34(2):153–173.

90. Nielsen J. *Why You Only Need to Test with Five Users*; 2000. http://www.nngroup.com/articles/why-you-only-need-to-test-with-5-users/.

91. Shneiderman B, Plaisant C. *Designing the User Interface: Strategies for Effective Human-Computer Interaction*. 5th ed. Boston: Addison-Wesley; 2010.

92. Dumas JS, Fox JE. Usability testing: current practice and future directions. In: Sears A, Jacko J, eds. *The Human-Computer Interaction Handbook: Fundamentals, Evolving Technologies and Emerging Applications*. 2nd ed. New York: Lawrence Erlbaum; 2008.

93. Rajeev D. *Development and Evaluation of New Strategies to Enhance Public Health Reporting*. Salt Lake City, UT: University of Utah; 2012.

94. Perri S. *Using Electronic Decision Support to Enhance Provider-Caretaker Communication for Treatment of Children Under Five in Tanzania*. Salt Lake City, UT: University of Utah; 2012.

95. Koch S, Westenskow D, Weir C, et al. *ICU nurses' evaluations of integrated information integration in displays for ICU nurses on user satisfaction and perceived mental workload;* 2012. Paper presented at the Medical Informatics Europe. Pisa, Italy.

96. Koch SH, Weir C, Westenskow D, et al. Evaluation of the effect of information integration in displays for ICU nurses on situation awareness and task completion time: a prospective randomized controlled study. *Int J Med Inform.* 2013; 82 (8):665–675.

97. Lowry SZ, Quinn MT, Ramaiah M, et al. *Technical Evaluation, Testing and Validation of the Usability of Electronic Health Records.* Rockville, MD: National Institute of Standards and Technology; 2012.

98. Tullis T, Albert B. *Measuring the User Experience: Collecting, Analyzing and Presenting Usability Metrics.* New York: Elsevier; 2008.

DISCUSSION QUESTIONS

1. Discuss critical user experience issues in your own organization. Describe one example in more detail.
2. Outline how to apply the heuristic evaluation technique to analyze where the major violations exist for a selected health IT product.
3. Search the internet for current policies on the user experience in health IT by searching the Centers for Medicare and Medicaid (CMS), the Office of the National Coordinator for Health Information Technology, and the National Institute of Standards and Technology websites. Analyze how one of these current policies will affect your organization.
4. Outline a usability test for one module of your current EHR. Include the elements discussed in the chapter in your proposed usability test. Describe why you chose the methods you did.
5. Your organization is planning to purchase new physiologic monitors for the adult ICUs. You are the clinical/informatics person assigned to this project. Describe how you would include usability in the purchase process. Outline participants, methods, and tasks to be tested.

CASE STUDY

A tertiary care center in the western United States has an installed base of EHRs supported by Cerner Corporation for inpatient areas and by Epic for outpatient areas. Other technology includes a suite of about 300 different applications supported by the IT department. The current environment, while including robust capabilities such as computerized provider order entry, is "siloed" with information. Healthcare providers complain that they have difficulty obtaining the "big picture" of the patient across systems and they have to remember information located in disparate systems. They are burdened with integrating information themselves. Not only is this time consuming; it is potentially prone to error. Providers have developed numerous workarounds to the different systems in ambulatory and inpatient areas, including "shadow" files for patients they see frequently. Nurses complain that they have to "jump around" the inpatient system to find information they need for activities such as patient handoffs.

The organization responds by developing a vision for the future that centered on the concept of knowledge management (KM). This concept is defined as the systematic process of identifying, capturing, and transferring information and knowledge that people can use to create, compete (with other organizations), and improve. A crucial aspect of KM is improving the user experience. As the leaders in the organization begin to address KM and improve the user experience, they are employing the same tactics described in this chapter.

Discussion Questions

1. Assume that you are the leader for UX for your discipline in your organization. Where would you start to improve the user experience?
2. Pharmacists supporting the ICUs are asking for your help to improve their situation (their user experience) because they are forced to use nonintegrated systems. What methods would you use to examine this issue?
3. The institution is in the process of purchasing new physiologic monitors for their step-down unit. Describe how usability should be incorporated as part of the purchasing process. Design a brief usability test to support the purchasing process.

22

Informatics-Related Standards and Standards-Setting Organizations

Tae Youn Kim and Susan A. Matney

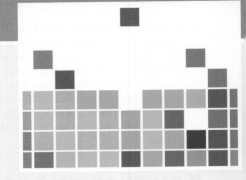

The use of standardized clinical terminology can allow patient data to be available across the full spectrum of healthcare settings.

OBJECTIVES

At the completion of this chapter, the reader will be prepared to:

1. Use basic terms and resources available to health professionals regarding data standardization, health information exchange, and interoperability.
2. Examine selected standard-setting organizations and their foci.
3. Explain the difference between a standardized reference terminology and an interface terminology.
4. Apply adopted evaluation criteria in assessing the quality of different standard terminologies.
5. Compare and contrast the similarities and differences among standardized healthcare terminologies relevant to patient care.
6. Examine how the adoption of standardized terminologies can assist in the implementation of Meaningful Use criteria of electronic health records (EHRs).
7. Describe the importance of data exchange across settings and the role of standardized terminologies in the development process of data exchange.
8. Discuss the areas of future research and development in relation to data standardization and exchange from a nursing perspective.

KEY TERMS

ABSTRACT ❖

The current health information technology (health IT) environment is rapidly changing worldwide. There is increasing evidence that the adoption of health IT will ensure the use of best practices and improve quality of care in a cost-efficient manner. However, shaping a cost-effective, quality healthcare system based on best practices is only possible if interoperability within and between all aspects of the healthcare delivery system has been achieved. Achieving interoperability requires a system-wide consensus concerning the standards for the operating of that system. This chapter begins with an explanation of standards and the standard development process in health informatics, including the relationship between standards and interoperability as these concepts relate to health informatics. The chapter then focuses on standardized terminologies, which are one of the fundamental components of standards and in turn interoperability. These terminologies facilitate coherent communication as well as the collection and aggregation of healthcare data across settings. The advantages of adopting standard terminologies in practice include (1) an enhanced user interface in electronic health records (EHRs), (2) effective data retrieval and exchange, (3) improved monitoring of quality of care, and (4) discovered knowledge through clinical research. The role of standardized terminologies in the process of exchanging healthcare data across systems is also discussed. The chapter concludes with a discussion of topics for future research and development, including data summarization and mining, knowledge management and decision support, linkage of professional vocabulary and consumer vocabulary, and clinical translational and comparative effectiveness research.

INTRODUCTION

The Institute of Medicine (IOM) identified health IT as critical to closing the quality chasm and shaping a better healthcare delivery system in the 21st century.[1] Achieving this goal of closing the quality chasm and shaping a better healthcare delivery system, however, is only possible if interoperability within and between all aspects of the healthcare delivery system has been achieved. Interoperability is defined as the extent to which healthcare systems and devices can exchange data and users can interpret that shared data.[2] Standards are imperative for the achievement of interoperability. A standard is defined as an established specification, guideline, or characteristic that describes the measurement, material, product, processes, and/or services required for a specific purpose.[3] Standards can be as basic as the distance between the prongs on a plug for a household appliance or as complex as the standards of practice for the treatment of a major health problem.

The simple household plug provides an excellent example of the relationship between standards and interoperability. There are very few rooms within any home in North America that do not have a wall outlet. Plugged into those outlets are an unbelievable variety of electrical devices produced by companies across the world. Yet all of these devices have the same size plug, thereby meeting the specific standards required to connect to the electrical grid for all of North America. Achieving this level of standardization involves both a process for establishing and maintaining the standards and an organizational infrastructure for implementing that process. For example, in the case of the electrical grid for North America, the North American Electric Reliability Corporation (NERC) develops and enforces reliability standards.[4]

In health informatics, a number of such organizations exist, referred to as either standards development organizations (SDO) or standards-setting organizations (SSO).[a] In turn, there are a significant number of standards developed by these organizations. The SSOs and the standards themselves evolve from three primary sources: (1) standards related to the technology used in health informatics, (2) standards related to healthcare in general, and (3) standards specific to health informatics. In most cases, these standards have evolved when the need for a specific standard has been identified and refined. For example, the Digital Imaging and Communications in Medicine (DICOM) standard was developed in 1985 when the National Electrical Manufacturers Association identified the need for a nonproprietary data interchange protocol, digital image format, and file structure for biomedical images and image-related information. As this example demonstrates, groups identifying the need for standards are usually focused on a specific need. As a result of the diverse needs and fragmentation of the standard development process, a number of SDOs have focused on consensus building and coordination in healthcare standards. For example, the American National Standards Institute (ANSI) has emerged as "the 'accreditor and coordinator of the U.S. private sector voluntary standardization system ensuring that its guiding

principles—consensus, due process, and openness—are followed by the entities accredited by this organization."[5]

Not all standards are established by an accredited SSO. Standards are established primarily through one of two different processes:

1. *Dominant vendors.* With this process, the standard becomes the de facto established standard due to market dominance of the vendor. Examples of this process for establishing standards are demonstrated by both the Microsoft and Apple operating systems. Today several companies unrelated to either Microsoft or Apple have designed their applications to run on top of one or both of these operating systems. While there are other computer operating systems, the vast majority of applications for personal computing use one or both of these operating systems.

2. *Official SSO.* These organizations are founded with the mission of developing or coordinating specific standards. They use a formal process that stresses the building of consensus through open communication. Standards established by an official SSO are referred to as *de jure* standards. Table 22.1 includes several examples of SSOs of importance in health informatics.

A great deal of work needs to be done on standards, as there are many existing standards to choose from in healthcare. Given this reality, learning about and understanding standards related to health informatics cannot be done by studying lists of standards. Such an approach would be the equivalent of reading a textbook on diagnostic tests, such as a lab manual, with no background or understanding of the disorders being diagnosed. Likewise, developing an understanding of standards in health informatics is best done by learning individual standards in the context of their specific purpose. In the rest of this chapter, the focus is on standard languages and their purpose in communicating health related data, especially across EHRs.

STANDARDIZED HEALTHCARE TERMINOLOGIES RELEVANT TO PATIENT CARE

The use of health IT, including EHRs, has become a component of a funded national agenda in the United States, as it is considered a tool to support patient-centered care and improve quality and safety of treatments during the last decade.[6] Of the various health IT products, EHRs are lauded as a means to collect longitudinal data, provide best evidence for practice, support efficient care delivery, and promote electronic access by authorized users for quality care, research, and policy development.[7] To make EHRs optimally beneficial, however, data standardization and data exchange are needed as fundamental components, in that they facilitate clear, concise communication as well as the collection and aggregation of healthcare data across settings.

The Centers for Medicare and Medicaid Services (CMS) established an incentive program for the use of a certified

---

[a]The terms *standards development organizations (SDO)* or *standards-setting organizations (SSO)* are used interchangeably in the literature and this chapter.

TABLE 22.1 Select Standards-Setting Organizations Impacting Health Information Technology

Name	Description	Health IT Standards	Website
Accredited Standards Committee (ASC) X12N Insurance subcommittee	Develops electronic data interchange (EDI) standards that facilitate electronic interchange relating to business transactions.	X12N Insurance Subcommittee: Develops components of the ASC X12 Standards related to the insurance industry's business activities, including those related healthcare insurance.	http://www.x12.org/x12org/subcommittees/sc_home.cfm?strSC=N
American National Standards Institute (ANSI) NOTE: ANSI is the U.S. representative to International Organisation for Standardization (ISO).	Promotes the use of U.S. standards internationally; advocates for U.S. policy and technical positions in international and regional standards organizations; encourages the adoption of international standards as national standards where these meet the needs of the user community; and provides a process for the accreditation of standards development organizations.	Primarily focused in health IT is on establishing communications among standards development organizations concerned with Health IT.	http://www.ansi.org/default.aspx
American Society for Testing and Materials (ASTM) International	Provides a forum for the development of international standards for materials, products, systems, and services.	E31 Healthcare Informatics develops standards related to the architecture, content, storage, security, confidentiality, functionality, and communication of information used within healthcare.	http://www.astm.org/COMMIT/SCOPES/E31.htm
Clinical Data Interchange Standards Consortium (CDISC)	Establishes standards to support the acquisition, exchange, submission, and archive of clinical research data and metadata.	—	http://www.cdisc.org
Digital Imaging and Communications in Medicine (DICOM)	Provides the international standard for the electronic exchange of medical images and related information.	—	http://dicom.nema.org
Health Level Seven (HL7) International	Provides a framework and related standards for the exchange, integration, sharing, and retrieval of electronic health information that supports clinical practice, and management, delivery, and evaluation of health services.	Clinical Document Architecture Release 2 (CDA) Fast Health Interoperability Resources (FHIR)	http://www.hl7.org/index.cfm
Institute of Electrical and Electronics Engineers (IEEE) Standards Association	Develops industry standards in a broad range of technologies.	IEEE Engineering in Medicine and Biology Society Technical Committee on Biomedical and Health Informatics focuses on standards for medical devices (http://tc-bhi.embs.org).	http://standards.ieee.org
Integrating the Healthcare Enterprise (IHE) International	Promotes the coordinated use of established standards in Health IT.	—	http://www.ihe.net
International Organization for Standardization (ISO)	Develops international standards by working with their 162 national standards bodies.	ISO Technical Committee (TC) 215 on Health Informatics has published over 154 standards (http://www.iso.org/iso/iso_technical_committee?commid=54960)	http://www.iso.org/iso/home.htm
MedBiquitous Consortium	Develops information technology standards for healthcare education and quality improvement.	—	http://www.medbiq.org
National Council for Prescription Drug Programs (NCPDP)	Develops standards supporting the information exchange of prescribing, dispensing, monitoring, managing, and paying for medications and pharmacy services.	—	https://www.ncpdp.org
Working Group for Electronic Data Interchange (WEDI)	Supports the development of transaction standards with the goal of enhancing the quality of care, improving efficiency, and reducing costs of the American healthcare system.	—	http://www.wedi.org/home

EHR system to meet the standards and criteria of Meaningful Use.[8,9] EHRs should, for example, support e-prescribing, maintaining patient problems and medication lists, and care management, and demonstrate interoperability according to the Health Information Technology for Economic and Clinical Health (HITECH) Act.[9] Standards that facilitate data capture and data sharing play a key role in achieving Meaningful Use of healthcare data. This chapter first examines current healthcare data standardization and exchange efforts. Applications of standardized health terminologies are further discussed, along with future directions. Additional information concerning Meaningful Use and HITECH Act regulations is available in Chapter 27.

HEALTHCARE DATA STANDARDIZATION

Definitions

Patient records contain words, terms, and concepts that are used in a variety of ways. A *word* is a unit of language, while a *term* is a linguistic label used to represent a particular concept.[10] A *concept* is defined as a construct representing the unique meaning for one or multiple terms. For example, *sudden pain in lower back* is composed of five words, and the term *sudden pain* is identical to the term *acute onset pain*, consisting of three words. In this case, both terms can be denoted with the concept *acute pain*. Also, the concept *pressure ulcer* can be represented with diverse terms such as *bedsore, decubitus, pressure sore, decubitus ulcer,* and *pressure ulcer*. These examples indicate that various expressions (including abbreviations) used with identical meanings can be characterized using a representative concept in patient records.

When a list of words or phrases is organized alphabetically, such a collection is called a *vocabulary*. In contrast, a collection of representative concepts in a specified domain of interest is defined as a *terminology*, which is often organized in a hierarchical or tree structure according to semantic relationships among concepts. Continuing our example, the concept *acute pain* is a type of *pain* and presents a narrower meaning than the parent concept *pain* in a terminology.

Identifying a representative concept for terms with the same meaning is particularly important when communicating healthcare data. Natural language, with its diverse expressions of terms with equivalent meanings, cannot be used to share information within or across systems in a consistent way. Incongruent descriptions of patient care contribute to poor quality care and hinder the Meaningful Use of EHRs. Accordingly, a number of healthcare terminologies have been developed by different disciplines and specialties. When a terminology meets specific requirements established by an SDO, it is referred to as a standardized terminology. A reference terminology serves as a resource to represent domain knowledge of interest and thus facilitate data collection, processing, and aggregation. Such a terminology, however, may not be sufficient to design and structure documentation forms used by healthcare providers in daily practice.[11] Task-oriented terms with abundant synonyms can assist documentation by enhancing expressivity and usability of standard concepts.

An interface terminology is a collection of task-oriented terms considered to support data entry and display in EHRs.[11]

A terminology is often called a classification when concepts or expressions are organized according to their conceptual similarities rather than semantic (meaning) resemblances. For example, a set of concepts related to the human body could be arranged by physiologic function or body structure. For instance, *chest pain* and *growing pain* are semantically close in that both are considered a type of *pain*. Therefore both terms can be categorized as a finding of the sensory nervous system. However, they could also be classified by the location of pain (i.e., body structure); *chest pain* can be categorized as a finding of trunk structure and *growing pain* can be categorized as a finding of limb structure.

A concept refers to a class in ontology, where the meaning of a concept is formally specified using properties and its relationships with other concepts through inheritance.[12] While a terminology often presents only a broad–narrow relationship between two adjacent concepts, an ontology contains multiple subsumptions or subclass relationships of a concept based on its formal definition. A reasoner or classification software can be used to assist in this process by automatically determining logical placements of asserted concepts and creating an inferred hierarchy.[13] An example of how ontology is structured is demonstrated by the BioPortal sponsored by the National Center for Biomedical Ontology, including more than 500 terminologies, classifications, and ontologies maintained by various organizations and individuals.[14] Fig. 22.1 presents a hierarchical organization of sample concepts (or classes) related to human organ systems and a graphic view of the hierarchy in BioPortal.[14]

Evaluation of the Quality of Terminology

Healthcare terminologies have a long history of research and development. Currently, the Unified Medical Language System (UMLS®) Metathesaurus® contains more than 190 source terminologies, classifications, and ontologies used in the healthcare domain.[15] Regardless of the structure of a source terminology, the UMLS consolidates all source concepts in a unified framework so that it is possible to examine lexical and semantic relations within and across source terminologies.[16] The UMLS Metathesaurus is distributed by the National Library of Medicine (NLM) every 6 months and includes more than 3.2 million concepts and 13 million unique concept names, available for browsing through UMLS Terminology Services.[15] Any source concepts with semantically equivalent meanings are assigned to the same concept unique identifier in the UMLS Metathesaurus.[16] Fig. 22.2 displays a search result for the keyword "comfort alteration" in the UMLS browser. An online resource, "NLM Resource for Standards and Interoperability," developed by the NLM provides introductions to the terminologies used by nursing and a tutorial on how to find a map between two different terminologies.[17]

Given the complexity of the healthcare delivery system in the 21st century, the health IT industry demands a comprehensive solution to promote data standardization and exchange. One terminology is unlikely to meet the needs of the wide range

Foundational Model of Anatomy

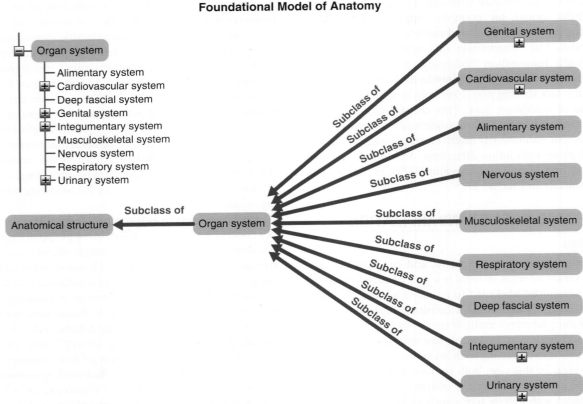

FIG 22.1 An example ontology. (From the Foundational Model of Anatomy in BioPortal. http://bio portal.bioontology.org/ontologies/FMA.)

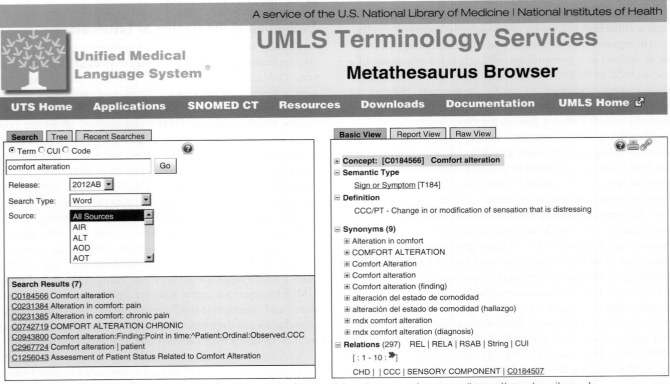

FIG 22.2 The Unified Medical Language System Metathesaurus browser. (https://uts.nlm.nih.gov/home.html.)

of disciplines within healthcare, yet adopting quality terminologies is crucial for Meaningful Use of EHRs. Assessing the quality of a terminology is not a simple task, as each terminology evolves according to its *terminology life cycle* linked to structural and development processes.[18-21]

A terminology life cycle contains three major phases: change requests, terminology editing, and terminology publication.[21] A *terminology change request* is a formal mechanism for users to submit requests for any changes or additions with respect to a given terminology.[20,22,23] *Terminology editing* begins with the activation of a new concept, revision of an existing concept, or inactivation of a concept, and follows formal concept change and version management guidelines. When terminology editing is completed with subsequent documentation, a series of tasks is performed throughout the *terminology publication* phase to release a new version of terminology for public use. Any products (such as terminologies, cross-maps, translations, subsets, and educational materials) generated through the terminology life cycle should be easily accessible, usable, and interoperable in EHRs.[21]

Requirements for maintaining healthcare terminology quality address the terminology structure, content, mapping, and process management in alignment with the terminology life cycle.[21,24-30] The International Organization for Standardization (ISO) has developed international terminology standards. Specifically, ISO/TS 17117:2002, Health Informatics—Controlled Health Terminology—Structure and High-Level Indicators, describes technical specifications for high level evaluation of a controlled health terminology. According to the specifications, the purpose, scope, and content coverage of a terminology should be explicitly stated for a specified domain of use. Each concept should be clearly defined with a unique identifier; hence there should be no redundancy, ambiguity, or vagueness.[31]

Further, ISO/TS 18104:2014, Categorical Structures for Representation of Nursing Diagnoses and Nursing Actions in Terminological Systems, provides a framework to promote terminology development and mapping, data analytics, and interoperability of nursing diagnoses and actions across healthcare settings.[32] This standard defines categories of healthcare entities for nursing diagnoses, including clinical course, clinical findings, degree, focus, judgment, potential, site, anatomical structure, subject of information, and timing.[32,33] For example, the nursing diagnosis *severe pain* meets this standard, as it consists of the finding concept *pain* and the degree concept *severe*. The ISO standard also requires that a nursing intervention be composed of at least two categories of healthcare entities, including action, means, route, subject of record, and target.[32] For example, the nursing intervention *patient education about pain management* comprises a nurse's *education* (action) on *pain management* (target).

Building on these standards, the American Nurses Association (ANA) recognizes 10 healthcare terminologies appropriate for use in nursing.[34,35] Of these, seven are designed specifically for nursing and the other three are considered multidisciplinary terminologies (Table 22.2). The ANA also recognized two minimum datasets: (1) the Nursing Minimum Data Set (NMDS) as a framework for collecting nursing care data, and (2) the Nursing Management Minimum Data Set (NMMDS) as a framework for collecting nursing service data elements. That is, the NMDS requires patient demographics, nursing process data (i.e., assessments, diagnoses, interventions, and outcomes), and service elements (e.g., agency and admission and discharge dates) to assess the quality of care.[36] The NMMDS focuses on collecting variables associated with nursing environment, nurse resources, and financial resources to support administrative analysis and decision making of nurse executives.[37-39]

TABLE 22.2	An Overview of Standardized Terminologies Relevant to Nursing Practice					
Terminology or Classification[a]	Developer	Discipline or Specialty	Release Time (Current Version)	ANA Recognized	Cross-maps Available	Web-Based Terminology Browser[b] (Language)
Clinical Care Classification (CCC)	SabaCare	Nursing	As needed (Version 2.5)	Yes	ICNP SNOMED CT LOINC	http://sabacare. com/ (English)
International Classification for Nursing Practice (ICNP)	International Council of Nurses (ICN)	Nursing	Every 2 years in ICN conference (2015)	Yes	CCC ICF SNOMED CT	http://www.icn.ch/ ICNP-Browser-NEW.html (multilingual)
NANDA International (NANDA-I)	NANDA-I	Nursing	Every 2 years (2015–2017)	Yes	—	Not publicly available (member only)
Nursing Interventions Classification (NIC)	University of Iowa	Nursing	Every 4 years (2013; 6th ed.)	Yes	—	Not publicly available (member only)

Continued

TABLE 22.2   An Overview of Standardized Terminologies Relevant to Nursing Practice—cont'd

Terminology or Classification	Developer	Discipline or Specialty	Release Time (Current Version)	ANA Recognized	Cross-maps Available	Web-Based Terminology Browser (Language)
Nursing Outcomes Classification (NOC)	University of Iowa	Nursing	Every 4 years (2013; 5th ed.)	Yes	—	Not publicly available (member only)
Omaha System	Martin, KS	Nursing	As needed (2005; 2nd ed.)	Yes	SNOMED CT LOINC	http://www.omahasystem.org (English)
Perioperative Nursing Data Set (PNDS)	Association of Perioperative Registered Nurses (AORN)	Perioperative nursing	As needed (2011; 3rd ed.)	Yes	SNOMED CT	Not publicly available (member only)
Logical Observation Identifiers Names and Codes (LOINC)	Regenstrief Institute, Inc.	Multidiscipline	Biannual (Version 2.56)	Yes	CCC Omaha System	http://loinc.org/downloads/relma (multilingual; note that it can be browsed after installing RELMA)
Systematized Nomenclature of Medicine—Clinical Terms (SNOMED CT)	International Health Terminology Standards Development Organisation (IHTSDO)	Multidiscipline	Biannual (July 2016)	Yes	ICD-10 ICD-9-CM ICNP	http://browser.ihtsdotools.org (multilingual)
ABC Codes	ABC Coding Solutions	Multidiscipline	Annual (2016)	Yes	—	Not publicly available (member only)
Current Procedural Terminology (CPT)	American Medical Association (AMA)	Medicine	Annual (2016)	—	LOINC	Not publicly available (member only)
International Classification of Diseases (ICD)	World Health Organization (WHO)	Medicine	As needed (10th ed.) (2016)	—	SNOMED CT	http://apps.who.int/classifications/icd10/browse/2016/en (English)
International Classification of Functioning, Disability and Health (ICF)	WHO	Multidiscipline	As needed (2008)	—	—	http://apps.who.int/classifications/icfbrowser/ (multilingual)
RxNorm	National Library of Medicine (NLM)	Multidiscipline (drug)	Monthly (July 2016)	—	—	http://rxnav.nlm.nih.gov/ (English)

HL7, Health Level Seven; *RELMA*, Regenstrief LOINC Mapping Assistant.
[a]All terminologies and classifications are accessible through the Unified Medical Language System (UMLS) released every 6 months by the National Library of Medicine (NLM). Available at https://uts.nlm.nih.gov/home.html.
[b]All of the web browsers listed are publicly available at no cost. Also, personal digital assistant (PDA) versions of terminology browsers may be available as knowledge resources.

Multidisciplinary Terminologies

Terminologies are essential to communicate and document patient care data in alignment with the care process. Various types of data are critical to clinical care, such as lab results, medications, medical diagnoses and procedures, and billing information. Accordingly, multidisciplinary terminologies as described in this section are essential.

Logical Observation Identifiers Names and Codes

Logical Observation Identifiers Names and Codes (LOINC), established in 1994 by the Regenstrief Institute, is a standardized coding system for laboratory and clinical measurements (observations).[40] Each LOINC observation is created using six axes: (1) the name of the observation (or analyte); (2) property (e.g., substance concentration, mass, volume); (3) timing of

TABLE 22.3   Coding Structure and Application of LOINC

Code	Description	
	Length: 3 to 7 characters	
	The last digit (ranging from 0 to 9) of the LOINC code preceded by a hyphen is required to avoid errors in transcription of the code.	
Fully specified name	<component/analyte>:<kind of property>:<time aspect>:<system/sample type>:<scale>:<method>	
Example coding of laboratory tests	2339-0:Glucose:MCnc:Pt:Bld:Qn This example includes a LOINC code and four attributes: 1. Code = 2339-0 2. Name of component = Glucose 3. Property = Mass concentration (MCnc[a]) 4. Type of system/sample = Patient's blood (Pt:Bld[a]) 5. Measurement scale = Quantitative (Qn[a])	2341-6:Glucose:MCnc:Pt:Bld:Qn:Test strip manual This example includes a LOINC code and five attributes: 1. Code = 2341-6 2. Name of component = Glucose 3. Property = Mass concentration (MCnc[a]) 4. Type of system/sample = Patient's blood (Pt:Bld[a]) 5. Measurement scale = Quantitative (Qn[a]) 6. Method = Test strip manual

LOINC, Logical Observation Identifiers Names and Codes.

[a]Details on the abbreviations can be found in McDonald C, Huff S, Mercer K, Hernandez J, Vreeman DJ, eds. *Logical Observation Identifiers Names and Codes (LOINC) Users' Guide.* Indianapolis, IN: Regenstrief Institute, Inc.; 2016. http://loinc.org/downloads/files/LOINCManual.pdf.

the measurement; (4) the type of system or sample (e.g., serum, urine, patient, family); (5) scale (e.g., qualitative, quantitative); and (6) the method used to make the observation (optional).[41]

All LOINC names are case sensitive. Table 22.3 presents an example of blood glucose tests coded using the LOINC system. Actual values of observations need to be documented using numeric values or other standardized terms. LOINC contains more than 80,000 terms (as of 2016) and is widely adopted for ordering and exchanging laboratory and clinical observations in the communication protocol called Health Level Seven International (HL7).[41] The laboratory portion of the LOINC database contains the usual laboratory categories, such as chemistry, hematology, and microbiology. The domain and scope of clinical LOINC are extremely broad. Some of the sections include terms for vital signs, obstetric measurements, clinical assessment scales, outcomes from standardized nursing terminologies, and research instruments.[42] LOINC is also used for document and section names.[43] Nursing content is one of the scientific domains with a special focus on clinical LOINC.[44] Nursing assessments can be structured in LOINC as a "Panel." For example, the Skin Assessment Panel (LOINC ID 72284-3) contains "Skin Color," "Skin Temperature," "Skin Turgor," and "Skin Moisture." Nursing assessment development is an ongoing project for the Nursing Clinical LOINC Subcommittee.

Systematized Nomenclature of Medicine—Clinical Terms

Systematized Nomenclature of Medicine—Clinical Terms (SNOMED CT) is the most comprehensive clinical terminology and has become an international standard for coding healthcare data.[45,46] The International Health Terminology Standards Development Organisation (IHTSDO) has developed a set of principles to guide SNOMED CT development

and quality improvement. SNOMED CT is continually updated to meet users' needs. The governments of member countries fund IHTSDO; therefore healthcare institutions in IHTSDO member countries are able to use SNOMED CT without additional costs. For example, there are no fees for use in the United States, whose national release center is responsible for managing concept requests and distributing and supporting IHTSDO products. The NLM, which also maintains and distributes the UMLS, is the U.S. member of the IHTSDO.

SNOMED CT contains preferred terms and the related synonyms (including Spanish translations of preferred terms) organized in a hierarchical tree structure with top-level concepts, such as body structure, clinical finding (e.g., diseases, disorders, drug actions), event, observable entity, procedure (e.g., treatment or therapy, surgical procedure, laboratory procedure), specimen, and substance.[47] Concepts lower in the hierarchy are more specific in meaning than those higher in the hierarchy, creating multiple levels of granularity. Defining attribute relationships using description logics further details the meaning of a concept by relating all necessary and sufficient conditions.

In general, clinical questions for assessment and measureable outcomes (e.g., pain level) can be coded using concepts placed under *observable entity*. Most nursing diagnoses and outcomes can be found under *clinical finding* and *event*, while nursing interventions and actions are found under *procedure*. An example of SNOMED CT coding of the clinical question "*ability to manage medication?*" with the answer "*unable to manage medication*" is presented in Fig 22.3. This set of questions and answers coded using standardized terminologies is ready for data exchange using messaging standards such as HL7.

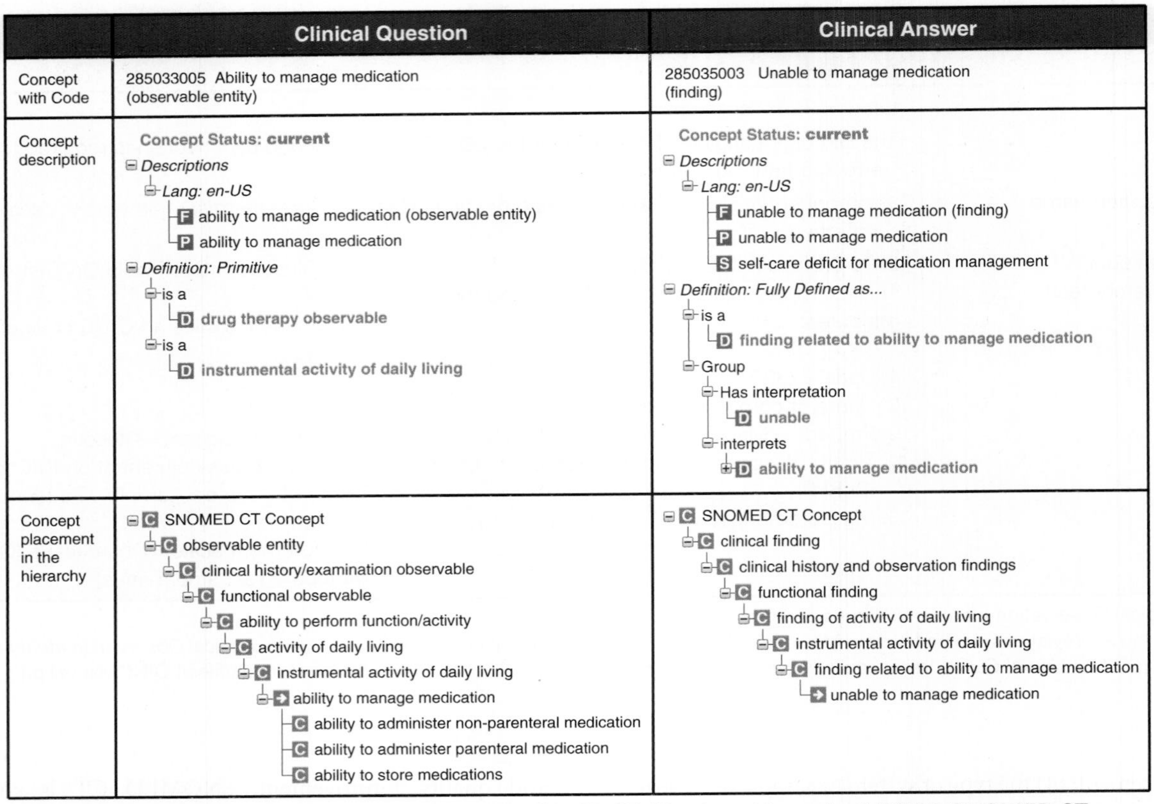

	Clinical Question	**Clinical Answer**
Concept with Code	285033005 Ability to manage medication (observable entity)	285035003 Unable to manage medication (finding)
Concept description	Concept Status: **current** ⊟ *Descriptions* 　⊟ *Lang: en-US* 　　F ability to manage medication (observable entity) 　　P ability to manage medication ⊟ *Definition: Primitive* 　⊟ is a 　　D drug therapy observable 　⊟ is a 　　D instrumental activity of daily living	Concept Status: **current** ⊟ *Descriptions* 　⊟ *Lang: en-US* 　　F unable to manage medication (finding) 　　P unable to manage medication 　　S self-care deficit for medication management ⊟ *Definition: Fully Defined as...* 　⊟ is a 　　D finding related to ability to manage medication 　⊟ Group 　　⊟ Has interpretation 　　　D unable 　　⊟ interprets 　　　D ability to manage medication
Concept placement in the hierarchy	⊟ C SNOMED CT Concept 　⊟ C observable entity 　　⊟ C clinical history/examination observable 　　　⊟ C functional observable 　　　　⊟ C ability to perform function/activity 　　　　　⊟ C activity of daily living 　　　　　　⊟ C instrumental activity of daily living 　　　　　　　⊟ ▶ ability to manage medication 　　　　　　　　C ability to administer non-parenteral medication 　　　　　　　　C ability to administer parenteral medication 　　　　　　　　C ability to store medications	⊟ C SNOMED CT Concept 　⊟ C clinical finding 　　⊟ C clinical history and observation findings 　　　⊟ C functional finding 　　　　⊟ C finding of activity of daily living 　　　　　⊟ C instrumental activity of daily living 　　　　　　⊟ C finding related to ability to manage medication 　　　　　　　▶ unable to manage medication

FIG 22.3 The structure and application of SNOMED CT. (Retrieved from the IHTSDO SNOMED CT browser. http://browser.ihtsdotools.org.)

Classifications Used for Reimbursement

The International Classification of Diseases (ICD), copyrighted by the World Health Organization (WHO), is used to report mortality and morbidity data worldwide and to compare statistics across settings, regions, or countries over time.[48] Further, ICD is used for billing, reimbursement, and allocation of health service resources for approximately 70% of the world's health expenditures.[48] The current version of ICD-10 (10th edition) was endorsed by the WHO in 1990 and implemented in the United States as of October 1, 2015.[49] Additional information concerning the structure and function of ICD-10 is included in Chapter 19. With the advancement of information technology and EHRs, ICD-11 has been developed and is currently in a revision process, with an anticipated release in 2018. ICD-11 provides more detailed information (such as definitions, signs, and symptoms) on disease in a structured way.

Depending on the focus of specialty areas, additional classifications can be used for ordering, billing, and reimbursement of medical procedures and diagnostic services. ICD Clinical Modification (ICD-CM) is a coding system developed to encode medical diagnoses and procedures (such as surgical, diagnostic, and therapeutic procedures) performed in U.S. hospital settings.[50] ICD-10-CM, a modified version of ICD-10, is updated annually by the National Center for Health Statistics (NCHS) and CMS. The Current Procedural Terminology (CPT) classification system is used extensively in the United States, as CMS mandates its use for reporting outpatient hospital surgical procedures as part of the

Omnibus Budget Reconciliation Act.[51] Diagnosis Related Groups (DRG) is a patient classification scheme designed to cluster similar cases using ICD and CPT codes as well as patient characteristics for reimbursement purposes according to the inpatient prospective payment system (IPPS).[52]

Other healthcare providers may use a different coding system for ordering, billing, and reimbursement for care delivered. For example, the *Diagnostic and Statistical Manual of Mental Disorders*, Fourth Edition (DSM-IV), developed by the American Psychiatric Association, has been widely used by clinicians to code mental and behavioral health–related conditions. All DSM-IV diagnostic codes have been integrated into ICD-9-CM.[53] Due to differences between the two coding systems, however, cross-map between DSM-IV and ICD-10-CM is under development. Another example is the ABC Coding Solutions, which provides more than 4500 codes for integrative healthcare services and products.[54] In other words, the ABC coding system covers clinical services related to nursing, behavioral health, alternative medicine, ethnic and minority care, midwifery, and spiritual care. An ABC code consists of five characters representing types of services, remedies, supplies, and practitioners.[54]

RxNorm

RxNorm is a normalized drug-naming system derived from 14 drug terminologies containing drug names, ingredient, strength, and dose form.[55] Example source terminologies within RxNorm include Micromedex RED BOOK, Food

TABLE 22.4 Structure and Application of CCC In Relation to the Nursing Process for Pressure Ulcer

Nursing Process	CCC Structure	Example Concepts
Assessment	Healthcare pattern	Physiologic
	Care component	R. Skin Integrity
Diagnosis	Nursing diagnosis	
	• Major category	R.46.0 Skin Integrity Alteration
	• Subcategory	R.46.2 Skin Integrity Impairment
Outcome	Expected outcome	R.46.2.1 Skin Integrity Impairment Improved
Planning	Nursing intervention	
	• Major category	R.51.0 Pressure Ulcer Care
	• Subcategory	R.51.1 Pressure Ulcer Stage 1 Care
Implementation	Nursing action type	R.51.1.2 Perform/Direct Care/Provide/Assist Pressure Ulcer Stage 1 Care
Evaluation	Actual outcome	R.46.2.1 Skin Integrity Impairment Improved

CCC, Clinical Care Classification.

and Drug Administration (FDA) National Drug Code Directory, SNOMED CT, and the Veterans Health Administration National Drug File. Due to different naming systems used in each terminology, the NLM produces normalized generic and brand names of prescription drugs and over-the-counter drugs available in the United States.[55] The NLM uses the UMLS framework to maintain and distribute RxNorm, allowing consistent communication among various hospital and pharmacy systems. RxNorm preserves original drug names as synonyms and semantic relationships among drugs. It also serves as a knowledge resource to advance e-prescribing systems with decision support functionality, as RxNorm contains pharmacologic knowledge such as drug interactions.[56]

World Health Organization Family of International Classifications

The WHO formed a Family of International Classifications (WHO-FIC), containing a suite of WHO-endorsed classifications, including three reference classifications, five derived classifications, and five related classifications.[57] ICD and International Classification of Functioning, Disability and Health (ICF) are core reference classification systems in WHO-FIC.[57] While the ICD system provides a set of diagnosis codes to encode causes of death and health conditions, ICF (formerly known as the International Classification of Impairments, Disabilities, and Handicaps) is a classification system that focuses on functional status as a consequence of disease or health conditions.[58] Although ICF has been used mainly in physical therapy and rehabilitation professions, previous studies demonstrated the usefulness of ICF in documenting nursing practice in acute care hospitals and early postacute rehabilitation settings.[59-62] Knowing that these core classifications lack in covering other specialty areas, the WHO recognizes an additional 10 classifications or terminologies in WHO-FIC.[63] For example, ICD-10 Classification of Mental and Behavioral Disorders and ICF Version for Children and Youth are derived from the core classification systems (i.e., ICD and ICF). International Classification of Primary

Care and International Classification for Nursing Practice (ICNP®) are considered related classifications in WHO-FIC.

Nursing Terminologies

As shown in Table 22.2, the ANA recognized seven nursing terminologies or classifications supporting nursing practice as they conform to the terminology development standards.[64] All of the ANA-approved nursing terminologies have been integrated into the UMLS Metathesaurus and widely adopted nationally and internationally. This section briefly introduces the nursing terminologies and describes their purpose, scope, content coverage, and structure.

Clinical Care Classification

The Clinical Care Classification (CCC) has been used for more than 20 years in nursing across the care continuum since its development as the Home Health Care Classification System in 1991.[65] CCC is a classification system of nursing diagnoses and interventions organized under 21 care components to support documentation of the nursing process.[66] In this classification, a nursing care component is a navigation or high-level abstract concept, clustering the nursing practice with similar patterns. These care components are further aggregated into four healthcare patterns of patient care: functional, health behavioral, physiologic, and psychological.

CCC Version 2.5 includes 176 nursing diagnoses (60 major categories and 116 subcategories), from which 528 nursing outcomes can be derived using three modifiers: (1) improved, (2) stabilized, and (3) deteriorated.[67] As such, 201 nursing interventions (77 major categories and 124 subcategories) can be expanded to as many as 804 nursing actions by combining four action types: (1) monitor/assess/evaluate/observe, (2) perform/direct care/provide/assist, (3) teach/educate/instruct/supervise, and (4) manage/refer/contact/notify. This compositional ability of CCC allows users to express nursing care in any care setting while maintaining a simple classification structure (Table 22.4). Each nursing diagnosis, intervention, and outcome is assigned to a code with alphanumeric characters.

BOX 22.1   Structure and Application of ICNP

ICNP Structure: Asserted Hierarchy		Example Concepts
Article I.	Process	The concept *Acute pain* is a precoordinated nursing diagnosis composed of the
Article II.	Body process	primitive concepts *pain, acute,* and *actual.*10000454 Acute pain
Article III.	Nervous system process	= has focus "10013950 pain" +
Article IV.	Perception	has onset "10001739 acute" +
Article V.	Impaired perception	has potentiality "10000420 actual"
Article VI.	Pain	The concept *Acute abdominal pain* can be postcoordinated if needed by selecting
Article VII.	Acute pain[a]	the nursing diagnosis *Acute pain* and the body location *Abdomen.* Acute
Article VIII.	Chronic pain	abdominal pain
Article IX.	Labor pain	=10000454 Acute pain +
Article X.	Musculoskeletal pain	10000023 Abdomen

ICNP, International Classification for Nursing Practice.
[a]This example shows the placement of the nursing diagnosis Acute pain in the ICNP asserted hierarchy.

International Classification for Nursing Practice

The ICNP is a nursing terminology designed to represent nursing diagnoses, outcomes, and interventions capturing the delivery of nursing care across settings.[68] The ICNP is an entity of the International Council of Nurses (ICN) eHealth Programme that was launched to transform nursing through the use of health information and communication technology.[69] The ICN is a federation of more than 130 national nurses associations that represent millions of nurses worldwide. Since 1989, the ICNP has evolved from a collection of nursing-related concepts to a logic-based nursing terminology system maintained in an ontology development environment.[68] The ICNP has been developed using a sophisticated language (i.e., Web Ontology Language, or OWL) to ensure the sustainability of the ever-expanding terminology and maintain the quality of the terminology.[70]

In conformance with ISO standards (ISO/TS 18104:2014), nursing diagnosis, outcome, and intervention statements are precoordinated with primitive concepts such as focus, judgment, and action concepts. Each precoordinated concept is assigned a unique identifier, and it is possible for practitioners to postcoordinate primitive concepts to meet their needs.[70] For example, as shown in Box 22.1, the nursing diagnosis *acute pain* is a precoordinated concept with an assigned code (10000454), but *acute abdomen pain* does not exist in ICNP, meaning that the concept could be postcoordinated with two concepts: *acute pain* (10000454) in *abdomen* (10000023). All ICNP primitive and precoordinated concepts are organized in a hierarchical tree structure. The 2015 release included 805 nursing diagnoses/outcomes and 1019 intervention statements. A new version of ICNP is released every 2 years in conjunction with the ICN conference. Due to the size and complexity of ICNP, subsets are created to promote the utility of ICNP in practice.[71] That is, ICNP catalogs or subsets with select nursing diagnoses and interventions have been developed and distributed in collaboration with national nurses associations, health ministries and governments, and expert nurses worldwide.[72–75]

NANDA International Nursing Diagnoses

The North American Nursing Diagnosis Association (NANDA) dates back to 1970, and its terminology was the first to be recognized by the ANA.[76] The membership organization was renamed NANDA International (NANDA-I) to reflect worldwide use of the terminology and established network teams in Latin America, Europe, Asia, and Africa.[77] In NANDA-I, a nursing diagnosis is defined as "a clinical judgment about actual or potential individual, family, or community experiences/responses to health problems/life processes."[77, p. 134] The purpose of NANDA-I is to ensure consistent, accurate documentation of nurses by clinical reasoning judgments and drive nursing interventions and outcome evaluations. As shown in Table 22.5, a three-level structure was adopted to place diagnoses according to conceptual similarities.[77] That is, a nursing diagnosis (Level 3) is located in a class (Level 2) according to its definition, defining characteristics and related factors, or risk factors. A class is further clustered into a domain (Level 1). The NANDA-I 2015–2017 release includes 235 nursing diagnoses organized in 47 classes and 13 domains, along with the evidence to support knowledge-based diagnostic decisions.

Nursing Interventions Classification

The Nursing Interventions Classification (NIC) is a funded research-based standardized classification of interventions describing nursing activities performed directly or indirectly. An intervention is defined as "any treatment, based upon clinical judgment and knowledge that a nurse performs to enhance patient/client outcomes."[78, p. 2] This means that choosing a nursing intervention is based on the characteristics of nursing diagnosis and expected patient outcomes. The NIC is designed to support the communication and documentation of nurses

TABLE 22.5   Structure and Application of NANDA-I With Knowledge Content to Reference

NANDA-I Structure	Example Nursing Diagnosis
Domain (Level 1)	11. Safety/Protection
Class (Level 2)	2. Physical Injury
Nursing Diagnosis Label (Level 3):	00045. Impaired Oral Mucous Membrane
Axis 1: Diagnostic concept (i.e., root of the diagnostic statement)	Axis 1: Mucous membrane
Axis 2: Subject of the diagnosis	Axis 2: Individual
Axis 3: Judgment (i.e., modifier specifying the meaning)	Axis 3: Impaired
Axis 4: Location (i.e., body parts or their functions)	Axis 4: Oral
Axis 5: Age	Axis 5: Adult
Axis 6: Time (i.e., duration)	Axis 6: Acute
Axis 7: Status of the diagnosis (i.e., potentiality, wellness/health promotion)	Axis 7: Actual
Definition	Disruption of the lips and/or soft tissue of the oral cavity
Defining characteristics	Bleeding, coated tongue, fissures, gingival pallor, halitosis, oral lesions, white patches, etc.

NANDA-I, North American Nursing Diagnosis Association International.

TABLE 22.6   Structure and Linkage of NANDA-I, NIC, AND NOC

Structure	Example Nursing Diagnosis	Example Nursing Intervention	Example Nursing Outcome
Domain (Level 1)	11. Safety/Protection	1. Physiological: Basic care that supports physical functioning	II. Physiologic Health
Class (Level 2)	2. Physical Injury	F. Self-Care Facilitation	L. Tissue Integrity
Label (Level 3)	00045. Impaired Oral Mucous Membrane	1710. Oral Health Maintenance	1100. Oral Hygiene
NANDA-I description,	Defining characteristics: bleeding, coated tongue, fissures, gingival	• Establish a mouth care routine.	110011. Color of mucous membranes
NIC activity, or NOC indicator	pallor, halitosis, oral lesions, white patches	• Apply lubricant to moisten lips and oral mucosa as needed.	110012. Oral mucosa integrity

NANDA-I, North American Nursing Diagnosis Association International; *NIC*, Nursing Interventions Classification; *NOC*, Nursing Outcomes Classification.

and other healthcare providers with the exception of physicians.[78] The current release (2013) includes more than 550 interventions clustered into 30 classes and 7 domains. Each intervention concept includes a definition, a code, and a list of detailed activities ranging from 10 to 30 statements. An intervention concept may appear in more than one class, resulting in approximately 13,000 narrative activity statements.[78]

Nursing Outcomes Classification

The Nursing Outcomes Classification (NOC) is also a funded research-based standardized classification of patient and caregiver outcomes that can be used in the course of care delivery for any specialty and setting.[78,79] An outcome is "a measurable individual, family, or community state, behavior or perception that is measured along a continuum and is responsive to nursing interventions."[79, p. 35] The current release (2013) includes 490 outcomes clustered into 32 classes and 7 domains. Each outcome concept consists of a definition,

a list of indicators, and five-point Likert-type scales. The scales, ranging from 1 to 5, are used to measure the existing level, patients' preferred level, and subsequent evaluation longitudinally to determine change scores in patients. The Center for Nursing Classification and Clinical Effectiveness (CNC) at the University of Iowa College of Nursing has an ongoing collaboration and alliance with NANDA-I to establish linkages among the three nursing classification systems—NANDA-I, NIC, and NOC—for use in EHRs.[79] An example linkage of the three classifications is presented in Table 22.6.

Omaha System

The Omaha System is a standardized classification designed to document nursing practice across the continuum of care. (Details about home health and the Omaha System are provided in Chapter 9.) Work on the Omaha System began in the 1970s and was further expanded with the release of the 2005 version. The Omaha System is structured with three schemes—Problem Classification, Intervention, and the

TABLE 22.7   Structure and Application of Omaha System

| | **EXAMPLE LINKAGE** | | |
Structure	Problem	Intervention	Outcome
Level 1	Domain: 02 Physiological		Knowledge (1 ~ 5): • did not recognize worsening condition
Level 2	Problem: 29 Circulation	07 Cardiac care	
Level 3	Modifiers: • Actual • Individual	Category: 01 Teaching, guidance, and counseling	Behavior (1 ~ 5): • Not taking daily weights and elevating legs
Level 4	Signs and symptoms: • Edema • Abnormal cardiac laboratory results	Specific actions: • Relief of edema • Elevate legs • Schedule fluid intake	Status (1 ~ 5): • Significant fatigue, edema in lower extremities, and dyspnea

TABLE 22.8   Structure and Application of PNDS in Relation to the Nursing Process

Nursing Process	Example Statements	
Assessment	Domain: A.350	Safety Assesses susceptibility for infection
Diagnosis	00004	Risk for Infection (from NANDA-I)
Implementation	Im.300 Im.300.1 Im.360	Implements aseptic technique Protects from cross-contamination Monitors for signs and symptoms of infection
Evaluation	E.330	Evaluates for signs and symptoms of infection through 30 days following the perioperative procedure
Outcome	O.280	Patient is free from signs and symptoms of infection

NANDA-I, North American Nursing Diagnosis Association International; *PNDS*, Perioperative Nursing Data Set.

Problem Rating Scale for Outcomes.[80] The Problem Classification Scheme (i.e., assessment) consists of four components: domains, problem statements, modifiers, and signs and symptoms (Table 22.7). Forty-two problem statements are neutral until two modifiers are attached to the problems. One set of modifiers is related to potentiality (i.e., actual and potential) and health promotion; the other set of modifiers is related to health problems (i.e., individual, family, and community). A problem is considered actual if signs and symptoms associated with the problem are selected from a predefined list. All problems are grouped into one of four domains: environmental, psychosocial, physiological, or health-related behaviors. The Intervention Scheme (i.e., care plans and services) consists of 75 target interventions and 4 action categories: (1) teaching/guidance/counseling, (2) treatments/procedures, (3) case management, and (4) surveillance. Patient problems are evaluated throughout the course of care using a Likert-style measurement scale ranging from 1 to 5 in the areas of client knowledge, behavior, and status.

Perioperative Nursing Data Set

The Perioperative Nursing Data Set (PNDS) is a standardized classification system designed specifically to support the perioperative nursing process in documenting patient experience from preadmission to discharge.[81] The PNDS (2011) is composed of 74 nursing diagnoses adopted from NANDA-I, 153 nursing interventions, and 38 nurse-sensitive patient outcomes. All nursing interventions consist of three different types of actions: assessment, implementation, and evaluation. These statements are clustered into one of four domains: safety, physiologic responses, behavioral responses (of family and individual), and health system (which is not directly related to nursing process).[81,82] Using the Perioperative Patient Focused Model, the PNDS provides a systematic approach for identifying the contributions of perioperative nursing care by reporting and benchmarking. Table 22.8 shows example statements selected from the PNDS in relation to the nursing process.

DATA EXCHANGE EFFORTS

Health terminologies keep evolving to incorporate changes in clinical practice, health policy, and advances in science. It is unlikely that in the future any one standard language will be able to support all clinical practices within the different disciplines functioning within the healthcare system. A key concern is how to communicate and exchange data collected through the various clinical practices across settings while preserving terminology-related standards. HL7 standards have been established to regulate data exchange and integration using standardized terminologies and other terminology harmonization efforts.

HL7 Standards

Since 1987, HL7 has served as a standards-developing organization to promote data retrieval, exchange, and integration across different health information systems.[83] HL7 provides a comprehensive framework and the standards necessary to foster interoperability (or exchange) of healthcare data. This chapter focuses on the two standards most commonly used in clinical practice: Clinical Document Architecture (CDA) and Fast Health Interoperability Resources (FHIR).

CDA is used to represent clinical documents using eXtensible Mark-up Language (XML) and standard terminologies in defined reusable patterns called templates.[84] CDA markup standards specify the structure of clinical documents and semantic relations among the subcomponents of clinical documents.[84] CDA is used to exchange documents such as patient assessments, discharge summaries, imaging reports, and quality reports between healthcare providers.[85] The Consolidated Clinical Document Architecture (C-CDA) Release 1.1 is an implementation guide required by Meaningful Use stage 2 for the exchange of patient information within the following measures: transitions of care, data portability, patient engagement, view, download and transmit to a third party, and clinical summary.[86-88]

FHIR is designed to enable the exchange of clinical, healthcare-related administrative, public health, and research data.[89] FHIR is intended to be useable worldwide in various contexts, including in-patient, skilled nursing, and long-term care. *Resources* are the most important parts of the FHIR specification to understand because they simulate paper "forms" by replicating different types of clinical and administrative information that can be captured and shared. The FHIR specification defines a generic "form template" for type of clinical information such as demographics, health conditions, and procedures.[89] The FHIR data repositories contain completed "forms" (resource instances) that describe patient-related information as well as administrative information such as practitioners, organizations, and locations. Each resource defines a small amount of specific data. A single resource does not provide much information, but a compilation of resources taken together constructs a useful clinical record. Information systems map actions that a user takes (e.g., record vital signs, add a nursing diagnosis) to operations on the relevant resources.

While the C-CDA and FHIR specify structural components, HL7 messaging standards address rules to communicate detailed information about patient care. Regardless of coding rules employed in individual departments or organizations, messaging specifications prevent any misclassification of data communicated between senders and receivers of clinical data.[83] The messaging standards thus ensure consistent descriptions of patient care among disparate systems. Standardized terminologies reviewed earlier in this chapter are the basic elements of the messaging standards.

Terminology Harmonization

Interoperability is defined as "the ability of health information systems to work together within and across organizational boundaries in order to advance the effective delivery of healthcare for individuals and communities."[90, p. 75] The U.S. Department of Health and Human Services (HHS) recommends the implementation of a health IT infrastructure to enhance interoperability of healthcare data.[91] The Healthcare Information Technology Standards Panel (HITSP), founded in 2005 through a contract with the HHS, has contributed to enabling interoperability among EHRs through the development of technical specifications.[92]

Standards harmonization is an effort to consolidate and enhance the coverage of domain knowledge of interest. Terminology harmonization is regarded as one way to support interoperability, considering variations in terminology adoption in practice. Cross-mapping healthcare terminologies is essential to preserve the meaning of exchanged information and facilitate integration of clinical data in a disparate information system so that the comprehensive picture of healthcare delivery can be understood.

As described previously, numerous health and nursing terminologies exist, resulting in various harmonization activities within and across disciplines. The scope of these harmonization activities ranges from a simple survey designed to understand the characteristics of terminologies adopted in clinical practice to harmonization agreements between two standards organizations. Harmonization of the multidisciplinary terminologies includes maps between SNOMED CT and ICD-10, SNOMED CT and ICD-10-CM, and LOINC and HL7 vocabulary. These cross-maps are publicly available through the NLM. A draft cross-map of LOINC Version 2.15 and CPT Version 2005 is available in the UMLS.[93]

Since LOINC and SNOMED CT are widely adopted and considered data standards nationally and internationally, nursing has participated actively in harmonization efforts through terminology cross-mapping and integration of nursing terminologies into SNOMED CT and LOINC. The ANA further recommends using SNOMED CT and LOINC for a C-CDA exchange with another setting for problems and care plans.[94] The recommendation promotes standard terminologies and also suggests that all care settings create a plan for mapping ANA-recognized nursing terminology to national standards such as SNOMED CT or LOINC.

Both the CCC and Omaha System outcomes are mapped into LOINC.[17] All ANA-recognized nursing terminologies are mapped to SNOMED CT to some extent.[77,95–97] This means that nursing diagnoses, interventions, and outcomes have been modeled in SNOMED CT and assigned to a unique identifier according to the SNOMED CT development guidelines. Equivalency tables between ICNP and SNOMED CT are distributed through ICN and IHTSDO. Table 22.9 presents examples of nursing concepts mapped to SNOMED

TABLE 22.9   Mapping Nursing Concepts to SNOMED CT

Source Terminology	Example Concepts in Source Terminology	Target Terminology: SNOMED CT (Type)
CCC	K25.5 Infection risk K30.0.1 Teach infection control	78648007 At risk for infection (finding) 385820004 Teach infection control (procedure)
ICNP	10021941 Lack Of Knowledge Of Medication Regime	129866007 Deficient knowledge of medication regimen (finding)
NANDA-I	00004 Risk for infection	78648007 At risk for infection (finding)
NIC	6540 Infection control	77248004 Infection control procedure (procedure)
NOC	1807 Knowledge: Infection control	405111006 Knowledge: Infection control (observable entity)
Omaha System	71 Infection precautions (Qualifier: Treatment/procedure)	77248004 Infection control procedure (procedure)
PNDS	A.350 Assesses susceptibility for infection O.280 Patient is free from signs and symptoms of infection	370782005 Assessment of susceptibility for infection (procedure) 397680002 Absence of signs and symptoms of infection (situation)

CCC, Clinical Care Classification; *ICNP*, International Classification for Nursing Practice; *NANDA-I*, North American Nursing Diagnosis Association International; *NIC*, Nursing Interventions Classification; *NOC*, Nursing Outcomes Classification; *PNDS*, Perioperative Nursing Data Set; *SNOMED CT*, Systematized Nomenclature of Medicine—Clinical Terms.

TABLE 22.10   Mapping CCC Concepts to ICNP

Source Terminology	Example Concepts in source Terminology	Target Terminology: ICNP
CCC Nursing Diagnoses	Q45.0 Comfort alteration K25.5 Infection risk	10023066 Discomfort 10015133 Risk for infection
CCC Nursing Interventions	U.75.4.4 Manage postpartum care R54.0.1 Assess skin care	10031931 Managing postpartum care 10030747 Assessing self-care of skin

CCC, Clinical Care Classification; *ICNP*, International Classification for Nursing Practice.

CT and shows a potential opportunity for collaboration in harmonizing all of the nursing terminologies and SNOMED CT. In addition, ICNP has been mapped to CCC, ICF, and other local terminologies to enhance data capture and sharing and to develop national nursing datasets.[98-102] Harmonization agreement between ICN and SabaCare resulted in cross-maps between CCC and ICNP, presenting different yet complementary solutions to advance standardization of nursing process data across specialties and settings (Table 22.10).

APPLICATION OF STANDARDIZED TERMINOLOGIES

There are multiple ways of communicating and recording patient care data in EHRs. Many clinical records (e.g., physical assessments) are documented using prestructured clinical templates with discrete data elements and predefined value sets. Yet massive volumes of narrative text data (e.g., clinical notes from various disciplines, progress notes, discharge notes) are also documented in free-text forms in EHRs. Developing quality terminologies and classifications to cover domain-specific content is of critical importance for system design, data retrieval and exchange, quality improvement, and clinical research.[103-111]

Choosing one among the various terminologies is not immediately straightforward. Although informatics and professional organizations endorse various terminologies, they do not recommend single taxonomies for use. Informaticians will need to evaluate their organizational, professional, and contextual needs to determine the most appropriate terminologies to deploy. In many cases with EHRs, vendors have embedded local terminologies and used particular communication standards (e.g., HL7), so any decisions about terminologies will need to be evaluated at the system selection stage or just be accepted as part of the purchasing package. For other applications, informaticians will want to consider the context (e.g., home health) and evaluate existing terminologies for that setting. At this point in the time, the onus is still on the purchaser to evaluate terminologies for the extent of use, completeness, and appropriateness to the module at hand.

Designing User Interfaces Using Terminologies

The comprehensiveness and completeness of a standardized health terminology vary depending on the domain of interest and the facility. When designing prestructured clinical templates for clinical documentation, interface terminologies can be used to facilitate data entry and storage of clinical data at the point of care. An interface terminology is considered a solution to enhance the user interface in EHRs because of its ability to cover clinicians' preferred terms with rich synonyms and conceptual relations among the terms.[11] An interface terminology either can be derived from standardized reference terminologies and classifications reviewed in this chapter or can be developed locally to support the documentation practice. However, if not careful, local systems might result in numerous duplicate and ambiguous concepts without development guidelines.[11] Accordingly, a systematic approach should be undertaken to map any local interface terminology to standardized reference terminologies. Otherwise, clinical data cannot be communicated as intended.

Supporting Data Retrieval and Exchange

Storing clinical data using standardized terminologies means that data are encoded using concept unique identifiers or alphanumeric codes to prevent any inconsistencies created by typing errors. Prestructured clinical templates can be a vehicle to help users pick and choose from a predefined value set and encode accurately selected values. Retrieving these coded data is much easier than free-text data that are documented using natural language that contains numerous variations in expressions for the same concept or meaning.

While coded data can be easily retrieved and transferred to other facilities using messaging standards (such as HL7), exchanging free-text data requires multiple steps for processing.[112] For instance, assume that no structured form exists to document a skin and wound assessment but only narrative text. To identify a patient who developed a pressure ulcer during hospitalization in the narrative statements, natural language processing of clinical notes would be required. This requires computing resources and human verification of the machine-aided findings (i.e., patients with a pressure ulcer). Many natural language processing tools used in the healthcare domain adopt standardized terminologies to map terms extracted from clinical notes or scientific articles. For example, MetaMap, developed and distributed by the NLM, uses UMLS Metathesaurus to extract certain expressions in a standardized way.[113]

Monitoring the Quality of Care

Clinical databases hold massive amounts of structured and unstructured data along with date and time stamps. Once clinical data are coded in a standardized way, it is possible to monitor the quality of care by joining multiple data sources, including administrative databases. Clinicians and administrators can examine gaps between current practice and best practice, trends in patient outcomes associated with changes in the organization's policy, practice patterns, and nurse staffing ratios. This type of investigation can be summarized and shared for ongoing quality monitoring and benchmarking.[114] Example quality-monitoring activities include identification of the following:

- Medication errors associated with reconciliation, prescription, and administration
- Degree of clinicians' adherence to best evidence and guidelines supported through reminders and alerts

- Healthcare resource use (e.g., length of stay, 30-day readmission rate of select population)

Using a standardized terminology facilitates the aggregation of patient care data based on predefined conceptual and semantic relationships of the coded data. An administrator may want an overview of staffing to support various types of patient populations. The highest-level construct of each terminology (e.g., functional, physiologic, or psychosocial) could be used to aggregate diagnoses and interventions implemented by unit.[45] Next, the administrator could examine the types of patient problems most prevalent in each unit by sorting according to the next level of hierarchical structure of the given terminology. Practitioners can also benefit from data summarization and presentation produced at both high and granular levels to understand their level of individualized care for accreditation processes or to guide local clinical education to address the major problems, risks, and needs for health promotion for the patient population.

To ensure patient safety and reduce healthcare costs, CMS developed various initiatives to collect quality measures such as smoking cessation and hospital-acquired pressure ulcer development.[9] CMS is collaborating with public agencies and private organizations to support the use of such quality measures, including, for example, the National Quality Forum, The Joint Commission on Accreditation of Healthcare Organizations, the National Committee for Quality Assurance, the Agency for Healthcare Research and Quality, and the American Medical Association.[115] Reporting these quality measures requires the adoption of standardized terminology.

Discovering Knowledge Through Research

Clinical researchers can benefit from EHRs with the functionality and capacity to access complete coded data across the care continuum. Current barriers, including that data are coded with multiple terminologies, could be removed as more standardized terminologies are harmonized to support data exchange and reuse. Ideally healthcare terminologies can complement each other to enhance the coverage of domain knowledge and thus promote Meaningful Use of clinical data. Coded data enable comparative effectiveness research and healthcare transformation using standardized data retrieved from multiple EHRs.[116]

Huge volumes of clinical and administrative data reside in large repositories, providing additional opportunities for clinical research, as discussed in Chapter 23. When paper-based records are used for clinical research, the number of reviewed charts is restricted because of the major resource requirements and the time-intensive chart abstraction process. In contrast, clinical research using current EHRs can involve thousands or even millions of patient records, offering the potential to identify new relationships among the data. Standardized terminologies in EHRs facilitate this kind of research. Even so, using current EHRs for research creates additional challenges and costs for data queries, processing, and analysis to handle the many inconsistent descriptions of patient care and large volumes of missing data.

CONCLUSION AND FUTURE DIRECTIONS

Since the release of the IOM report on the U.S. quality chasm in 2001, health IT has been seen as a promising solution for improving patient safety, delivering patient-centered care, and reducing healthcare costs.[1] However, a fundamental requirement for health IT is information exchange across systems. The use of standardized terminologies facilitates information exchange and is one of the requirements for Meaningful Use and healthcare interoperability.

Health practitioners recognize the benefits of using standardized terminologies and are actively participating in the development of both discipline-specific terminologies and multidisciplinary terminologies. As patient engagement with electronic records increases, the health practitioner needs to be involved in the development of consumer health vocabulary as well. With standardized clinical terminology, patient data will be available across the full spectrum of healthcare settings. Also, these data are and will be shared with individual patients, requiring additional efforts to translate professional vocabulary to consumer vocabulary. Patient-centered records maintained jointly by consumer and health professionals will provide opportunities to enhance public health surveillance by enabling a clinician's ability to track a patient's health maintenance, follow-up activity, engagement, and progress. The health professions should continue to participate in current and future endeavors to ensure that the domain concepts are represented in the approved manner within health IT.

Data standardization and exchange efforts were reviewed at various levels. Historically, coding requirements were associated with billing and reimbursement. Clinically focused coding efforts have advanced with the expansion of electronic health information. With the advancement of health IT and health sciences, data standardization and exchange are key elements for improving the nation's healthcare. Many benefits of using data standards have yet to be realized, but progress is evident. While terminology developers will continue to put their efforts into further enhancements, terminology users also need to evaluate the quality of terminologies and provide feedback to terminology developers.

REFERENCES

1. Institute of Medicine. *Crossing the Quality Chasm: A New Health System for the 21st Century.* Washington, DC: National Academies Press; 2001.
2. Healthcare Information and Management Systems Society (HIMSS). *Interoperability & Standards: What Is Interoperability?* (n.d.) <http://www.himss.org/library/interoperability-standards>.
3. International Organization for Standardization (ISO). *Standards: What Is a Standard?* (n.d.) http://www.iso.org/iso/home/standards.htm.
4. North American Electric Reliability Corporation (NERC). *About NESC.* (n.d.) http://www.nerc.com/AboutNERC/Pages/default.aspx.
5. HIMSS. *Evolution of Healthcare Informatics Standards.* (n.d.) http://www.himss.org/library/interoperability-standards/Evolution-of-Healthcare-Informatics-Standards.
6. Agency for Healthcare Research and Quality (AHRQ). *Health IT at AHRQ.* AHRQ; 2014. http://healthit.ahrq.gov/program-overview.
7. Institute of Medicine. *Health IT and Patient Safety: Building Safer Systems for Better Care.* Washington, DC: National Academies Press; 2012.
8. Blumenthal D, Tavenner M. The "Meaningful Use" regulation for electronic health records. *N Engl J Med.* 2010;363 (6):501–504.
9. Centers for Medicare & Medicaid Services (CMS). *EHR Incentive Programs.* CMS; 2015. http://www.cms.gov/Regulations-and-Guidance/Legislation/EHRIncentivePrograms.
10. de Keizer NF, Abu-Hanna A, Zwetslook-Schonk JHM. Understanding terminological systems I: terminology and typology. *Methods Inf Med.* 2000;39:16–21.
11. Rosenbloom ST, Miller RA, Johnson KB, Elkin PL, Brown SH. Interface terminologies: facilitating direct entry of clinical data into electronic health record systems. *J Am Med Inform Assoc.* 2006;13(3):277–288.
12. Gruber T. Toward principles for the design of ontologies used for knowledge sharing. *Int J Hum Comput Syst.* 1995;43 (5–6):907–928.
13. Tsarkov D, Horrocks I. FaCT++ description logic reasoner: system description. *Lecture Notes Comput Sci.* 2006;4130:292–297.
14. The National Center for Biomedical Ontology. *BioPortal*; 2016. http://bioportal.bioontology.org/.
15. Wilder V. UMLS 2016 AA release available. *NLM Technical Bulletin.* 2016;410:e2. https://www.nlm.nih.gov/pubs/techbull/mj16/mj16_umls_2016aa_release.html.
16. McCray AT, Nelson SJ. The representation of meaning in the UMLS. *Methods Inf Med.* 1995;34(1–2):193–201.
17. U.S. National Library of Medicine. *Nursing Resources for Standards and Interoperability*; 2015. https://www.nlm.nih.gov/research/umls/Snomed/nursing_terminology_resources.html.
18. Rogers JE. Quality assurance of medical ontologies. *Methods Inf Med.* 2006;45(3):267–274.
19. Bakhshi-Raiez F, Cornet R, de Keizer NF. Development and application of a framework for maintenance of medical terminological systems. *J Am Med Inform Assoc.* 2008;15 (5):687–700.
20. de Coronado S, Wright LW, Fragoso G, et al. The NCI thesaurus quality assurance life cycle. *J Biomed Inform.* 2009;42 (3):530–539.
21. Kim TY, Coenen A, Hardiker N. A quality improvement model for healthcare terminologies. *J Biomed Inform.* 2010;43 (6):1036–1043.
22. International Health Terminology Standards Development Organisation (IHTSDO). *Customer Guidance for Requesting Changes to SNOMED CT®.* IHTSDO; 2015. http://www.ihtsdo.org/resource/resource/174.
23. NANDA International. *Defining the Knowledge of Nursing.* NANDA International; 2015. http://www.nanda.org/DiagnosisDevelopment.aspx.
24. Cimino JJ, Clayton PD, Hripcsak G, Johnson SB. Knowledge-based approaches to the maintenance of a large controlled medical terminology. *J Am Med Inform Assoc.* 1994;1(1):35–50.
25. Tuttle MS, Olson NE, Campbell KE, Sherertz DD, Nelson SJ, Cole WG. Formal properties of the Metathesaurus. *Proc Annu Symp Comput Appl Med Care.* 1994;145–149.

26. Campbell JR, Carpenter P, Sneiderman C, Cohn S, Chute CG, Warren J. Phase II evaluation of clinical coding schemes: completeness, taxonomy, mapping, definitions, and clarity. CPRI Work Group on Codes and Structures. *J Am Med Inform Assoc.* 1997;4(3):238–251.

27. Chute CG, Cohn SP, Campbell JR. A framework for comprehensive health terminology systems in the United States: development guidelines, criteria for selection, and public policy implications. ANSI Healthcare Informatics Standards Board Vocabulary Working Group and the Computer-Based Patient Records Institute Working Group on Codes and Structures. *J Am Med Inform Assoc.* 1998;5(6):503–510.

28. Cimino JJ. Desiderata for controlled medical vocabularies in the twenty-first century. *Methods Inf Med.* 1998;37(4-5):394–403.

29. Oliver DE, Shahar Y. Change management of shared and local versions of health-care terminologies. *Methods Inf Med.* 2000;39(4–5):278–290.

30. Elkin PL, Brown SH, Carter J, et al. Guideline and quality indicators for development, purchase and use of controlled health vocabularies. *Int J Med Inform.* 2002;68(1–3):175–186.

31. International Organization for Standardization. *Health Informatics—Controlled Health Terminology—Structure and High-Level Indicators (ISO/TX17117:2002).* Geneva, Switzerland: ISO; 2002.

32. International Organization for Standardization. *Health Informatics— Categorical Structures for Representation of Nursing Diagnoses and Nursing Actions in Terminological Systems (ISO/TX 18104:2014).* Geneva, Switzerland: ISO; 2014.

33. Goossen W. Cross-mapping between three terminologies with the international standard nursing reference terminology model. *Int J Nurs Terminol Classif.* 2006;17(4):153–164.

34. Warren JJ, Bakken S. Update on standardized nursing data sets and terminologies. *J AHIMA.* 2002;73(7):78–83. quiz 85–86.

35. American Nurses Association. *ANA Recognized Terminologies that Support Nursing Practice.* Nursing World; 2012. http://www.nursingworld.org/npii/terminologies.htm.

36. Ryan P, Delaney C. Nursing minimum data set. In: Fitzpatrick JJ, Stevenson JS, eds. *Annual Review of Nursing Research.* Vol. 13; New York: Springer Publishing Company; 1995:169–194.

37. Huber D, Schumacher L, Delaney C. Nursing Management Minimum Data Set (NMMDS). *J Nurs Adm.* 1997;27(4):42–48.

38. Westra BL, Subramanian A, Hart CM, et al. Achieving "Meaningful Use" of electronic health records through the integration of the Nursing Management Minimum Data Set. *J Nurs Adm.* 2010;40(7–8):336–343.

39. Kunkel DE, Westra BL, Hart CM, Subramanian A, Kenny S, Delaney CW. Updating and normalization of the Nursing Management Minimum Data Set element 6: patient/client accessibility. *Comput Inform Nurs.* 2010;30(3):134–141.

40. Vreeman DJ. *Logical Observation Identifiers Names and Codes.* Regenstrief Institute, Inc; 2016. http://loinc.org/.

41. McDonald C, Huff S, Mercer K, Hernandez J, Vreeman DJ, eds. Logical Observation Identifiers Names and Codes (LOINC®) users' guide. In: *Regenstrief Institute, Inc*; 2016. http://loinc.org/downloads/files/LOINCManual.pdf.

42. Scichilone RA. The benefits of using SNOMED CT and LOINC in assessment instruments. *J AHIMA.* 2008;79(7):56–57.

43. Hyun S, Shapiro JS, Melton G, et al. Iterative evaluation of the Health Level 7—Logical Observation Identifiers Names and Codes clinical document ontology for representing clinical document names: a case report. *J Am Med Inform Assoc.* 2009;16(3):395–399.

44. Matney S, Bakken S, Huff SM. Representing nursing assessments in clinical information systems using the logical observation identifiers, names, and codes database. *J Biomed Inform.* 2003;36(4–5):287–293.

45. Cornet R, de Keizer N. Forty years of SNOMED: a literature review. *BMC Med Inform Decis Mak.* 2008;8(suppl 1):S2.

46. International Health Terminology Standard Development Organisation (IHTSDO). *History of SNOMED CT.* IHTSDO; 2016. http://www.ihtsdo.org/snomed-ct/what-is-snomed-ct/history-of-snomed-ct.

47. International Health Terminology Standard Development Organisation (IHTSDO). *SNOMED CT Starter Guide.* IHTSDO; 2014. http://www.ihtsdo.org/resource/resource/41.

48. World Health Organization (WHO). *International Classification of Diseases (ICD).* WHO; 2016. http://www.who.int/classifications/icd/en/.

49. Centers for Medicare & Medicaid Services (CMS). *ICD-10.* CMS; 2016. http://www.cms.gov/Medicare/Coding/ICD10/index.html?redirect=/ICD10/.

50. Centers for Disease Control and Prevention (CDC). *International Classification of Diseases, Tenth Revision, Clinical Modification (ICD-10-CM).* CDC; 2016. http://www.cdc.gov/nchs/icd/icd10cm.htm.

51. American Medical Association (AMA). *CPT—Current Procedural Terminology.* AMA; 2015. http://www.ama-assn.org/ama/pub/physician-resources/solutions-managing-your-practice/coding-billing-insurance/cpt.page.

52. Centers for Medicare & Medicaid Services (CMS). *Acute Inpatient PPS.* CMS; 2016. http://www.cms.gov/Medicare/Medicare-Fee-for-Service-Payment/AcuteInpatientPPS/index.html.

53. American Psychiatric Association (APA). *Covered Diagnoses & Crosswalk of DSM-IV Codes to ICD-9-CM Codes.* APA; 2003. http://www.apapracticecentral.org/reimbursement/billing/icd-9-cm.aspx.

54. ABC Coding Solutions. *ABC Code Structure.* ABC Coding Solutions; 2016. http://www.abccodes.com.

55. National Library of Medicine (NLM). *RxNorm Overview.* NLM; 2005. http://www.nlm.nih.gov/research/umls/rxnorm/overview.html.

56. Nelson SJ, Zeng K, Kilbourne J, Powell T, Moore R. Normalized names for clinical drugs: RxNorm at 6 years. *J Am Med Inform Assoc.* 2011;18(4):441–448.

57. Madden R, Skyes C, Ustrun TB. *World Health Organization Family of International Classifications: Definition, Scope, and Purpose.* World Health Organization; 2007. http://www.who.int/classifications/en/FamilyDocument2007.pdf.

58. World Health Organization (WHO). *International Classification of Functioning, Disability and Health.* Geneva, Switzerland: WHO; 2001.

59. Heerkens Y, van der Brug Y, Napel HT, van Ravensberg D. Past and future use of the ICF (former ICIDH) by nursing and allied health professionals. *Disabil Rehabil.* 2003;25(11–12):620–627.

60. Heinen MM, van Achterberg T, Roodbol G, Frederiks CM. Applying ICF in nursing practice: classifying elements of nursing diagnoses. *Int Nurs Rev.* 2005;52(4):304–312.

61. Van Achterberg T, Holleman G, Heijnen-Kaales Y, et al. Using a multidisciplinary classification in nursing: the International

Classification of Functioning Disability and Health. *J Adv Nurs.* 2005;49(4):432–441.

62. Mueller M, Boldt C, Grill E, Strobl R, Stucki G. Identification of ICF categories relevant for nursing in the situation of acute and early post-acute rehabilitation. *BMC Nurs.* 2008;7:3.

63. World Health Organization (WHO). *Derived and Related Classifications in the WHO-FIC.* WHO; 2012. http://www.who.int/classifications/related/en/index.html.

64. Coenen A, McNeil B, Bakken S, Bickford C, Warren JJ. Toward comparable nursing data: American Nurses Association criteria for data sets, classification systems, and nomenclatures. *Comput Nurs.* 2001;19(6):240–246. quiz 246–248.

65. Saba V. Nursing classifications: home health care classification system (HHCC): an overview. *OJIN.* 2002;7(3). http://www.nursingworld.org/MainMenuCategories/ANAMarketplace/ANAPeriodicals/OJIN/TableofContents/Volume72002/No3Sept2002/ArticlesPreviousTopic/HHCCAnOverview.aspx.

66. Saba V. *Clinical Care Classification (CCC) System Manual: A Guide to Nursing Documentation.* New York, Springer Publishing Company; 2007.

67. Saba V. *Clinical Care Classification (CCC) System Version 2.5 User's Guide.* 2nd ed. New York, Springer Publishing Company; 2012.

68. International Council of Nurses. *ICNP® Version 2.* Geneva, Switzerland: ICN; 2009.

69. International Council of Nurses (ICN). *ICN eHealth Programme.* ICN; 2015. http://www.icn.ch/what-we-do/ehealth/.

70. Hardiker NR, Coenen A. Interpretation of an international terminology standard in the development of a logic-based compositional terminology. *Int J Med Inform.* 2007;76(suppl 2):S274–S280.

71. Coenen A, Kim TY. Development of terminology subsets using ICNP. *Int J Med Inform.* 2010;79(7):530–538.

72. International Council of Nurses (ICN). *Partnering with Patients and Families to Promote Adherence to Treatment.* Geneva, Switzerland: ICN; 2008.

73. International Council of Nurses (ICN). *Palliative Care for Dignified Dying.* Geneva, Switzerland: ICN; 2009.

74. International Council of Nurses (ICN). *Nursing Outcome Indicators.* Geneva, Switzerland: ICN; 2011.

75. International Council of Nurses (ICN). *Scottish Government, National Health Service Scotland, Community Nursing.* Geneva, Switzerland: ICN; 2012.

76. Gordon M. *Nursing Diagnosis: Process and Application.* 3rd ed. St. Louis, MO: Mosby; 1994.

77. Herdman TH, ed. *North American Nursing Diagnosis Association International (NANDA-I) Nursing Diagnoses 2012–2014: Definitions and Classification.* Oxford, England: Wiley-Blackwell; 2012.

78. Bulechek GM, Butcher HK, Dochterman JM, Wagner CM, eds. *Nursing Interventions Classification.* 6th ed. St. Louis: Mosby; 2013.

79. Moorhead S, Johnson MM, Maas M, Swanson E, eds. *Nursing Outcomes Classification.* 5th ed. St. Louis: Mosby; 2013.

80. Martin KS. *The Omaha System: A Key to Practice, Documentation, and Information Management.* 2nd ed. Omaha, NE: Health Connections Press; 2005.

81. Association of Operating Room Nurses. *Perioperative Nursing Data Set.* 3rd ed. Denver, CO: AORN Inc; 2011.

82. Petersen C, Kleiner C. Evolution and revision of the Perioperative Nursing Data Set. *AORN J.* 2011;93(1):127–132.

83. Health Level Seven International (HL7). *Introduction to HL7 Standards.* HL7; 2015. http://www.hl7.org/implement/standards/index.cfm?ref=nav.

84. Dolin RH, Alschuler L, Boyer S, et al. HL7 clinical document architecture, release 2. *J Am Med Inform Assoc.* 2006;13(1):30–39.

85. D'Amore JD, Sittig DF, Wright A, Iyengar MS, Ness RB. The promise of the CCD: challenges and opportunity for quality improvement and population health. *AMIA Annu Symp Proc.* 2011;285–294.

86. Centers for Medicare & Medicaid Services. *Electronic Health Record Incentive Program—Stage 2. Federal Registe,* Vol 77. CMS; 2012: 53967–54132.

87. Centers for Medicare & Medicaid Services. *Stage 2 Eligible Professional Meaningful Use Core Measures. Measure 15 of 17;* 2015. http://www.cms.gov/Regulations-and-Guidance/Legislation/EHRIncentivePrograms/downloads/Stage2_EPCore_15_SummaryCare.pdf.

88. Centers for Medicare & Medicaid Services. Medicare and Medicaid programs; modifications to the Medicare and Medicaid Electronic Health Record (EHR) Incentive Program for 2014 and other changes to EHR Incentive Program; and health information technology: revision to the certified EHR technology definition and EHR certification changes related to standards. Final rule. *Fed Regist.* 2014;79(171):52909–52933.

89. HL7. *Welcome to FHIR®;* 2016. http://hl7.org/fhir/index.html.

90. Healthcare Information and Management Systems Society (HIMSS). *HIMSS Dictionary of Healthcare Information Technology Terms, Acronyms and Organizations.* 3rd ed. Chicago, IL: HIMSS; 2013. p. 75.

91. U.S. Department of Health & Human Services. *A Shared Nationwide Interoperability Roadmap. HealthIT.gov;* 2015. http://www.healthit.gov/policy-researchers-implementers/interoperability.

92. *Healthcare Information Technology Standards Panel;* 2009. http://www.hitsp.org/default.aspx.

93. National Library of Medicine (NLM). *LOINC to CPT Mapping.* NLM; 2015. http://www.nlm.nih.gov/research/umls/mapping_projects/loinc_to_cpt_map.html.

94. American Nurses Association. *Inclusion of Recognized Terminologies Within EHRs and Other Health Information Technology Solutions.* American Nurses Publishing; 2015.

95. Lu DF, Park HT, Ucharattana P, Konicek D, Delaney C. Nursing outcomes classification in the systematized nomenclature of medicine clinical terms: a cross-mapping validation. *Comput Inform Nurs.* 2007;25(3):159–170.

96. College of American Pathologists (CAP). *SNOMED CT® Mappings to NANDA, NIC, and NOC Now Licensed for Free Access through National Library of Medicine.* CAP; 2005. http://www.cap.org.

97. Kim TY, Hardiker N, Coenen A. Inter-terminology mapping of nursing problems. *J Biomed Inform.* 2014;49:213–220.

98. Canadian Nurses Association (CNA). *Mapping Canadian Clinical Outcomes in ICNP.* CNA; 2008. http://c-hobic.cna-aiic.ca/documents/pdf/ICNP_Mapping_2008_e.pdf.

99. Matney SA, DaDamio R, Couderc C, et al. Translation and integration of CCC nursing diagnoses into ICNP. *J Am Med Inform Assoc.* 2008;15(6):791–793. 96.

100. Dykes PC, Kim HE, Goldsmith DM, Choi J, Esumi K, Goldberg HS. The adequacy of ICNP version 1.0 as a

representational model for electronic nursing assessment documentation. *J Am Med Inform Assoc.* 2009;16(2):238–246.

101. Hannah KJ, White PA, Nagle LM, Pringle DM. Standardizing nursing information in Canada for inclusion in electronic health records: C-HOBIC. *J Am Med Inform Assoc.* 2009;16(4):524–530.

102. Kim TY, Coenen A. Toward harmonising WHO International Classifications: a nursing perspective. *Inform Health Soc Care.* 2011;36(1):35–49.

103. Andison M, Moss J. What nurses do: use of the ISO Reference Terminology Model for Nursing Action as a framework for analyzing MICU nursing practice patterns. *AMIA Annu Symp Proc.* 2007;2007:21–25.

104. Badalucco S, Reed KK. Supporting quality and patient safety in cancer clinical trials. *Clin J Oncol Nurs.* 2011;15(3):263–265.

105. Bernhart-Just A, Lassen B, Schwendimann R. Representing the nursing process with nursing terminologies in electronic medical record systems: a Swiss approach. *Comput Inform Nurs.* 2010;28(6):345–352.

106. Bouhaddou O, Warnekar P, Parrish F, et al. Exchange of computable patient data between the Department of Veterans Affairs (VA) and the Department of Defense (DOD): terminology mediation strategy. *J Am Med Inform Assoc.* 2008;15(2):174–183.

107. Cho I, Park HA, Chung E. Exploring practice variation in preventive pressure-ulcer care using data from a clinical data repository. *Int J Med Inform.* 2011;80(1):47–55.

108. Leung GY, Zhang J, Lin WC, Clark RE. Behavioral health disorders and adherence to measures of diabetes care quality. *Am J Manag Care.* 2011;17(2):144–150.

109. Monsen KA, Newsom ET. Feasibility of using the Omaha System to represent public health nurse manager interventions. *Public Health Nurs.* 2011;28(5):421–428.

110. Watkins TJ, Haskell RE, Lundberg CB, Brokel JM, Wilson ML, Hardiker N. Terminology use in electronic health records: basic principles. *Urol Nurs.* 2009;29(5):321–326. quiz 327.

111. Kim TY, Marek KD, Coenen A. Identifying care coordination interventions provided to community-dwelling older adults using electronic health records. *Comput Inform Nurs.* 2016;34(7):304–312.

112. Friedman C, Shagina L, Lussier Y, Hripcsak G. Automated encoding of clinical documents based on natural language processing. *J Am Med Inform Assoc.* 2004;11(5):392–402.

113. Aronson AR, Lang FM. An overview of MetaMap: historical perspective and recent advances. *J Am Med Inform Assoc.* 2010;17(3):229–236.

114. Dunton N, Montalvo I, eds. *Transforming Nursing Data into Quality Care: Profiles of Quality Improvement in U.S. Healthcare Facilities.* Silver Spring, MD: American Nurses Association Inc; 2007.

115. Centers for Medicare & Medicaid Services (CMS). *Quality Measures.* CMS; 2016. http://www.cms.gov/Medicare/Quality-Initiatives-Patient-Assessment-Instruments/QualityMeasures/index.html?redirect=/QualityMeasures/.

116. Westra BL, Latimer GE, Matney SA, et al. A national action plan for sharable and comparable nursing data to support practice and translational research for transforming health care. *J Am Med Inform Assoc.* 2015;22(3):600–607.

DISCUSSION QUESTIONS

1. A cost-effective, quality healthcare system requires interoperability, which in turn requires standards. However, "healthcare standards developed by specific vendors often do not rise to dominance because there are no truly dominant vendors in the industry, nor are there industry action groups powerful enough to achieve voluntary convergence."[5] Given this reality, how can healthcare providers and health informatics specialist support the development of standards?

2. You are the only informatician at your small community hospital and have been asked to choose terminologies within your EHR for interdisciplinary care planning. What terminologies would you use and why?

3. Discuss the benefits of using standardized terminologies within your EHR.

4. Discuss the major local, national, and international obstacles to implementing standardized terminologies within EHRs.

5. As a researcher, you have been assigned to obtain data from two different facilities. Both facilities have mapped their data to standardized terminologies within their data warehouses. Discuss how this will benefit your research. Alternatively, what if the data in both facilities were not coded using standards? What obstacles would need to be overcome?

CASE STUDY

A small community hospital in the Midwest has used a homegrown information system for years. The system began in the early 1970s with a financial module. Over time, additional modules were added. A limited number of departments selected a commercial system, and interfaces were used to integrate these into the overall functionality of the hospital information system. Except for physicians, most in-house clinical or care-related documentation is online. However, about 15% to 20% of this documentation is done by free text

and is not effectively searchable. In addition, the screens, including the drop-down and default values, were built using terms selected by the in-house development team in consultation with clinical staff; thus there is no data dictionary or specific standard language. In the last few years the hospital has purchased two outpatient clinics (obstetrics and mental health) and a number of local doctor practices. The clinics and doctors' offices are now being converted to the hospital administrative systems as described in Chapter 7. A few of the clinical applications that are tied directly to the administrative systems such as order entry and results reporting are also being installed.

A major change is being planned. A new chief information officer (CIO) was hired last year, and she has appointed a chief medical information officer (CMIO) and a chief nursing information officer (CNIO). No other significant staff changes were made. With her team in place, one of the CIO's first activities was to complete an inventory of all applications. As part of this process, each application and the system as a whole were assessed for the ability to meet Meaningful Use criteria. Based on this analysis, the CMS modified Stage 2 criteria are currently met; however, meeting Stage 3 criteria will require a significant investment in hardware, software, and additional staff. Rather than continue to build, a decision has been made to switch to a commercial vendor. The hospital is now in the process of selecting a commercial system. Because of your background as a member of the clinical staff with informatics education, you have been appointed to the selection committee. It is also anticipated that you will serve on the implementation committee.

Discussion Questions

1. What role, if any, should standard language play in the selection process?
2. What key standard languages and coding systems should be incorporated in the new system?
3. Can the work done in building the screens and developing the terms that are used for documentation of care in the old system be used in the new system, or will this delay customizing the new system applications?
4. It is expected that clinical staff will participate in site visits and vendor displays. What, if any, preparation related to standard languages should be given before these activities?
5. How should clinical staff who will be using the new system be prepared for the introduction of new or different terms in the clinical documentation system?

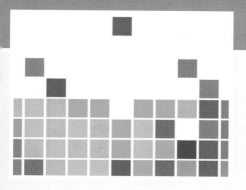

23

Data Science and Analytics in Healthcare

Mollie R. Cummins, Louis Luangkesorn, and Nancy Staggers

OBJECTIVES

At the completion of this chapter, the reader will be prepared to:

1. Analyze the meanings of various terms and concepts related to big data.
2. Define the goals, objectives, and uses of big data, healthcare analytics, including knowledge discovery and data mining (KDDM).
3. Describe three categories of analytics.
4. Interpret characteristics of big data.
5. Discuss the key elements of model development.
6. Outline the steps in Knowledge, Discovery and Data Mining (KDDM) as well as current challenges to the process.
7. Describe three categories of analytics platforms.
8. Identify the roles and activities of the informatics specialist related to data management and use in healthcare environments.

KEY TERMS

big data, 392
classification matrix, 399
data analytics, 392
data governance, 404
data mining, 398
data science, 392

exploratory data analysis, 394
knowledge discovery and data mining (KDDM), 394
machine learning, 395
natural language processing (NLP), 397
predictive analytics, 394
prescriptive analytics, 394

ABSTRACT ❖

Availability of extremely large repositories of healthcare data and new analytic tools have revolutionized efficient access to comprehensive data across large numbers of patients. Advances in tools and methods for analyzing large stores of data enable detection of subtle patterns in these data, even with missing or less than optimal data quality. This chapter introduces approaches to data science, analytics, and knowledge building from health data, including details on a process known as knowledge discovery and data mining (KDDM). Data science or "big data" concepts are introduced, and the fundamentals of data analytics are discussed. The chapter explores the application of data analytic processes in healthcare and describes organizational needs for data science such as personnel and data governance. The chapter concludes with recent advances and challenges in the field and a discussion of future directions in data science, data analytics, and KDDM.

INTRODUCTION

Leaders must foster a shared learning culture for improving healthcare. This includes extending improvement efforts beyond individual units or healthcare organizations to create more generalizable knowledge development. Sound, rigorous methods are needed by leaders, analysts, researchers, informaticians, and health professionals to (1) create knowledge for learning organizations and (2) address practical questions about risks, benefits, and costs of interventions as they occur in actual clinical practice. A powerful tool for accomplishing this is the use of data science to answer questions such as:

- Are treatments used in daily practice associated with intended outcomes?
- Can adverse events be predicted in time to prevent or ameliorate them?
- Which data elements are key to predicting patient behaviors for population health management?

- How can evidence-based practice be used in providing individualized patient care?
- What planning for individualized patient care and which potential interventions are most likely provide the greatest value?
- What groups of individuals are at risk for certain conditions?
- How can available resources be best used to deliver care to patient population?
- Which available tools and methods best meet the needs of an organization or individual who is analyzing large datasets?

DATA SCIENCE IN HEALTHCARE

U.S. healthcare expenditures exceed one-sixth of the U.S. gross domestic product.[1] Health information technology (IT) can help leverage those monies by reducing costs and improving outcomes. However, routine use of IT, in and of itself, does not automatically lead to these benefits. Rather, these benefits are tied to specific uses of health IT within and across healthcare organizations, including the use of data science to improve care.

Data science, also called data analytics or "big data," offers a systematic approach to answering interesting questions across large datasets. Simply put, big data is a colloquial term for extremely large datasets that are analyzed using computerized techniques to reveal patterns, trends, and associations.[2] New and specific analysis techniques allow managing and processing across a combination of data types. These are analyses that are not possible with conventional research and database analysis methods.

The volume and size of big datasets are often in the range of terabytes and typically above one petabyte. One petabyte can be explained using the following analogy: If an average MP3 song on a mobile device lasts 4 minutes, then a petabyte of songs would play continuously for 2000 years. Likewise, a petabyte has enough space to store the DNA of the entire population of the United States, including one clone of each person.[3]

The amount of data being generated today is enormous. Over 2.5 quintillion terabytes of data were generated each day in 2012. The data generated in two days is now estimated to be as much as was created from the dawn of civilization through 2003.[4] Kaiser Permanente estimated it had already generated 26.5-44 petabytes from its electronic health records (EHRs) alone by 2013.[5] As organizations continue to install EHRs, integrate patient-generated data, and move toward precision medicine (with its inherent requirement of integrating genomic, environmental, health, and other data), datasets will continue to grow exponentially.

Data science involves the analysis within and across types and categories of data. Examples of these categories are listed in Table 23.1.[6]

Big data in healthcare are a mixture of structured (e.g., laboratory values) and unstructured information (e.g., clinical notes). Using analytical techniques, data science has the potential to provide powerful insights across and within patients,

TABLE 23.1   Data Categories and Examples of Big Data[6]

Data Category	Examples of Collected Data
Web and social media	Facebook, LinkedIn, Twitter, health enterprise websites, mHealth apps
Machine to machine	Uploads and readings from sensors and other devices
Big transaction	Claims data and billing records
Biometric	Vital signs, medical imaging, fingerprints, genetics, retinal scans, handwriting
Human generated	Electronic health records, e-mail, paper documents

Data from Institute for Health Technology Transformation. *Transforming Health Care Through Big Data: Strategies for Leveraging Big Data in the Health Care Industry.* Institute for Health Technology Transformation. http://c4fd63cb482ce6861463-bc6183f1c18e748a49b87a25911a0555.r93.cf2.rackcdn.com/iHT2_BigData_2013.pdf; 2013.

institutions, regions, and nations. For example, clinical records can be linked to repositories of genetic or familial data.[7-9] These data constitute an incredible resource that is currently underused for scientific research in healthcare.

Analyses can be conducted to support the decision-making process at the population or individual patient level. For example, the United States Veterans Health Administration (VHA) has a repository storing nationwide EHR data. Analyses using this repository enabled the VHA to recognize the dangers (such as cardiovascular events) of Vioxx, a nonsteroidal antiinflammatory drug, among its patients. The VHA then initiated a policy to restrict Vioxx use well before the drug was finally removed from the market.[10] Other questions useful to analyze the population health management across millions of patients might include:

- Which treatments are associated with better outcomes for patients with kidney disease or specific carcinomas?
- How does obesity affect the need for joint replacement surgery at younger ages and at what costs?
- How do patients' physiologic parameters compare for newer and previous cardiac medications?

Unlike traditional reports, these analyses require information across multiple sources such as patients' problem lists, histories, medications, and lab and imaging results, as well as claims data.[11]

Data science analyses for individual patients can allow for more personalized care (precision medicine). For instance, a patient with diabetes might have metabolic rates, biochemical reactions, and responses to insulin that could be analyzed against norms to pinpoint specific, individualized medication delivery doses and times, along with tailored nutritional guidance.[11] In another example, Tamoxifen is 70% to 80% effective for the population of patients with breast cancer. However, at the individual level, Tamoxifen is 100% effective in 70% to 80% of patients but 100% ineffective for 20% to 30%. Thus individualized data are required to determine what treatment is effective for a particular patient. A final example is the IBM

BOX 23.1   Sample Data Science Projects

- **Neonatal infections**. Real-time analyses of neonates' physiologic data predicted nosocomial infections 24 hours before clinical symptoms were evident. These kinds of early detection may be applied to any ICU setting and lead to improved patient outcomes.[14]
- **National influenza rates**. Google Flu Trends in late 2013 showed the rate of influenza across the United States as "intense." Two weeks later, in early 2014, the Centers for Disease Control (CDC) confirmed the rating. The reason Google data surfaced earlier is because Google mined its data for terms that would likely be related to influenza, while the CDC relied on reports from physician visits.[15]
- **Big Data to Knowledge Program**. The **Big Data to Knowledge** (BD2K) Center for Causal Discovery, part of the BD2K program, is developing and making available a set of open-source tools for modeling and discovering knowledge from large health and biomedical datasets. Initial work is integrating real data from lung disease, cancer driver mutations, and functions and connections of the human brain.[16] Information about the BD2K program is available at http://datascience.nih.gov/bd2k.
- **Alzheimer's Disease Neuroimaging Initiative**. This multicenter, collaborative effort is gathering clinical and imaging data for a large cohort of patients.[17] Researchers have already developed dementia risk stratification based on these data.[18]

BOX 23.2   The Five Vs of Big Data

- Volume
- Velocity
- Variety
- Veracity
- Value

Watson project that combines information from the entire corpus of published medical journals along with individuals' health records from healthcare organizations to suggest treatment pathways tailored to the individual, a method of personalized medicine.[12] Similar individualized questions could be completed for genetic test results.[13] The same data used for personalized medicine can also then be analyzed to identify population health trends, enabling a healthcare organization to monitor emerging health trends and issues among its patient population.

Other obvious data science applications are quality improvement initiatives and learning systems projects. In fact, the potential for knowledge development is seemingly unlimited. Sample data science projects are listed in Box 23.1.

CHARACTERISTICS OF BIG DATA

Five data characteristics are important in understanding big data in healthcare, as seen in Box 23.2.

The first three characteristics are important to data in any field.[19] *Volume* refers to the sheer quantity of data generated and analyzed. In practical terms, data are often stored in distributed locations, so techniques for working with distributed data storage, such as cloud computing or clusters, need to be employed. *Velocity* refers to the speed at which data are generated and change over time. The important implication here is that the environment generating the data changes rapidly, and any analysis must be completed quickly enough to support decisions relevant to that data. Otherwise, decisions may not be useful or timely.

Variety means that the data come from many different sources simultaneously and in many different formats, as seen in Table 23.1. These include varied forms of storing or sharing data, different types of media (e.g., such as visual, audio, text, molecular), different rules surrounding data (e.g., security for data protected under HIPAA), and different sources (e.g., census data, billing, public health, EHRs, and social media). For example, payment data provided by the Centers for Medicare and Medicaid Services, hospital patient data, and hospital billing data are all from different sources and have different rules for use, as well as different levels of data validity and reliability.

Veracity and *value* are two issues that need to be addressed to make data useful to a healthcare organization. Veracity refers to the accuracy and completeness (the "truth") of the data or its opposite, the messiness of the data. The quality of individual data elements can vary greatly, especially when they are from various sources. Data processing must then include normalizing data so varied elements related to a single subject are identified and matched. That allows the processing of data to proceed so unstructured data such as voice or freely chosen text can be analyzed in ways similar to structured data.

Value recognizes that the purposes of collecting, processing, and analyzing data are to fill a need. For example, an acute care staffing mix that emphasizes more highly educated nurses can result in fewer patient complications; however, there is a point beyond which increased labor costs do not produce fewer complications (or produce value). Considering value, a key component of any data project is the question the data are expected to answer and how a healthcare organization will respond to the results of the analysis.

A data scientist or analyst needs to be able to manage data with mindful consideration of the five Vs of big data (see Box 23.2). An analyst or analytic team member should have computer programming skills to manage the data and have expertise to recognize how to test for the veracity of the data, perform correct analyses, and present the results in a meaningful format to provide value to the organization.

DATA SCIENCE FOR CLINICAL AND TRANSLATIONAL RESEARCH

Big data can be used for decision making and/or research. The gold standard research design for answering questions about the efficacy of treatments is an experimental design, often referred to as a randomized controlled trial (RCT). An RCT requires random assignment of patients to treatment conditions as well as other design features, such as tightly controlled inclusion criteria to ensure, as much as possible, that the only difference between the experimental and control groups is the treatment (or placebo) that each group receives. The strength of the RCT is the degree of confidence in causal inferences. In other words, how confident can one be that the therapeutic intervention caused the clinical effects (or lack of effects), as opposed to some other variable? Drawbacks of the RCT include the time and expense required to conduct a comparison of a small number of treatment options and the limited generalizability of the results to patients, settings, intervention procedures, and measures that differ from the specific conditions in the study condition. Further, RCTs have little value in generating unique hypotheses and possibilities.

BENEFITS OF DATA SCIENCE

Data science benefits come from using data across a wide range of resources that are beyond the ability of an individual person to aggregate and synthesize. Data analytics is a powerful tool with the ability to inform healthcare delivery decisions based on complex information. Various forms of data analytics and tools are used to systematically analyze healthcare operations across healthcare areas, including financial, operational, and clinical data. They can be used to coordinate care and/or business decisions over time and venues. For instance, analysts can examine the process of care and generate insights on how to improve those processes.

General benefits of data science include the advancement of science and improvements in healthcare, treatments, and the economics of healthcare.[20] Clearly, the projects described earlier show how advances in science, healthcare, and treatments can be made. Other benefits cross typical healthcare areas (e.g., healthcare costs and treatments). Newer cost models like value-based payment are based on the effectiveness of medical treatments for individuals or groups of patients in contrast to the traditional model of fee for service (i.e., volume of treatment). Fee for service can result in the administration of treatments that may not be effective for a particular individual.[21] Through data science and analytics, particularly methods of knowledge discovery and data mining (KDDM), knowledge models can be developed to identify optimal treatments for individuals and groups of patients according to their characteristics, such as diabetic diet and exercise regimens for inner-city, underserved patients. Components of computerized clinical decision support (CDS) systems with these knowledge models become routinely available as part of the clinicians' toolset and can allow care to be delivered at a lower cost.[5] Thus adding data science to the healthcare provider's toolset can offer a more cost-effective and less time-consuming approach to building knowledge.

However, insights from data are not realized automatically through installation of an analytics IT infrastructure and/or an EHR system. To derive the benefits of analytics, a healthcare organization needs to (1) identify the required analytic capabilities at all levels of the organization, (2) ensure that the system has the required capabilities, and (3) commission appropriately educated personnel to plan and implement the analytic process from data to deployment, thereby ensuring ultimate translation.[10]

No matter whether data analytics are used for research or decision making, the approaches to analyses are similar. In the next section, these sample approaches are outlined.

APPROACHES TO ANALYSES

Data analytics can be approached in three general ways: exploratory, predictive, and prescriptive.[21]

Exploratory Data Analysis

Exploratory data analysis (EDA) prepares and analyzes retrospective data to identify patterns or trends. The process of EDA includes the use of descriptive statistics (including summaries and data visualizations) and statistical analysis. The goal of EDA is to understand the state of a system, such as the distribution of inpatient stays among current patients in a hospital or the outcome of all patients' diagnoses or treatments over the past year. Information and knowledge gained by revealing patterns and trends through EDA can be used to support more effective administrative or clinical decision making. EDA can also be used to generate hypotheses that can be answered by analyzing available system data (e.g., the frequency of lab tests and their costs over the past year). The information discovered through the use of EDA produces data reports or information dashboards using spreadsheets or web-based applications to view and interpret specific information to aid decision makers.

Predictive Analytics

Predictive analytics is the development of analytic models that predict future trends based on retrospective or real-time data. KDDM methods including machine and statistical learning methods are commonly used in predictive analytics. Other methods can include:

- *Regression.* Predicting an outcome or a new observation (e.g., predicting which patients can be expected to experience a fall).
- *Classification.* Predicting the category for a new outcome (e.g., predicting which patients will respond to a specific medication or treatment protocol).
- *Clustering.* Grouping observations into similar groups (e.g., seeing that women who smoke have a higher rate of premature infants).
- *Association rules.* Determining a new characteristic based on known characteristics of an observation (e.g., noting that people in a lower socioeconomic group have a higher rate of health literacy problems).[9]

Prescriptive Analytics

Prescriptive analytics refers to the use of models to evaluate and determine new ways of operating in a health system. These work through modeling the system and potential alternatives, both assessing the value of the business objective and tracking constraints. Methods used in prescriptive analytics include queuing models, mathematical programming methods for optimization, and simulation. These methods have the advantage of being able to predict system output under a range of system configurations, allowing decision makers to choose the best of potential alternatives.

KNOWLEDGE DISCOVERY AND DATA MINING

KDDM is a process of data analytics where machine learning (ML) and statistical methods are applied to identify patterns in large sets of data. It entails the use of specialized software tools that facilitate the (1) extraction, (2) sampling, (3) large-scale cleaning, and (4) preprocessing of data. Frequently, KDDM is used to infer missing information based on available data and to develop models that predict future events. Methods of KDDM are preferred because these methods are effective for analyzing very large repositories of clinical data and for analyzing complex, nonlinear relationships. The level of analysis far exceeds the types of descriptive summaries typically presented by dashboard applications, such as a clinical summary for a patient. Instead, KDDM is used to build tools that support clinical decision making, generate hypotheses for scientific evaluation, and identify links between genotype and phenotype. KDDM can also be used to "patch" weaknesses in clinical data that pose a barrier to research. For example, if poor data quality is a barrier to automatic identification of patients with type II diabetes from diagnostic codes, an ML approach could be used to more completely and accurately identify the patients on the basis of text documents and laboratory and medication data.

Models developed for use with routinely collected clinical data have several advantages:

1. KDDM models access and leverage the valuable information contained in large repositories of clinical data.
2. Models can be developed from very large sample sizes or entire populations.
3. Models based on routinely collected data can be implemented in computerized systems to support decision making for individual patients.
4. Models induced directly from data using ML methods often perform better than models manually developed by human experts.

For example, Walton et al. developed a model that forecasts an impending respiratory syncytial virus (RSV) outbreak.[22] RSV is a virus that causes bronchiolitis in children, and severe cases warrant hospitalization. RSV outbreaks cause dramatic increases in the census at pediatric hospitals, so advance warning of an impending RSV outbreak would allow pediatric hospitals to plan staffing and supplies. Some evidence indicates that weather is related to outbreaks of RSV, and RSV outbreaks are known to follow a biennial pattern, information that may be useful for predicting outbreaks in advance. Given these circumstances, the authors built a model using historical data that predicts RSV outbreaks up to 3 weeks in advance. In addition to planning for events such as RSV, these types of models can be especially effective in designing CDS systems.

The design of individual CDS systems based on KDDM methods varies and can be as simple as an alert that warns about potential drug-drug interaction.[23] Every CDS system is based on some underlying algorithm or set of rules that are applied to existing or entered patient data. These rules must be specified in machine-readable code that is compatible with patient data stored in an EHR or other applications.

Historically, clinical practice guidelines have not been expressed as a set of adequately explicit rules and could not be executed by a machine. See, for example, Lyng and Pederson and Isern and Moreno for a detailed discussion of this issue.[24,25] While a human being can reason on the basis of conditions such as "moderate improvement" or "diminished level of consciousness," a machine has difficulty working with "fuzzy data." The term *fuzzy data* refers to data that are vague and lack a precise meaning. The interpretation or meaning of fuzzy data can vary greatly in different settings. CDS models must consist of rules, conditions, and dependencies described in terms of machine-interpretable relationships and specific data values. Moreover, the algorithms and rules must be executable over the data as they are coded in the information system. For example, gender may be included in a set of rules. If the rule is based on a gender variable coded with the values male, female, or unknown, it will not work in a system where gender is coded as 0, 1, 2, 3, or null, where $0 = $ male, $1 = $ female, $2 = $ transgender, $3 = $ unknown, and null $ = $ missing. While relatively simple changes could adapt the rule set for use in a system with different coding of gender, other variables pose a greater challenge. Some necessary variables may not exist as coded data in an information system or may be represented in a variety of ways that cannot be resolved as easily as gender can be.

A substantial effort is underway to develop computer-interpretable guidelines—guidelines that are expressed as an adequately explicit set of rules—with some success.[26] KDDM is also advantageous in this situation because it develops *only* machine-executable algorithms or rules, based on native data. Native data are data that have been coded for a specific system. Therefore using KDDM to develop a set of rules will result in rules that can be applied to the data within that system. Moreover, in situations where there is insufficient evidence to fully specify rules, the rules can be induced from a large sample of real-life examples using KDDM.

Retrieving a Dataset for Analysis

The process of KDDM depicted in Fig. 23.1 encompasses multiple steps and actions. Although KDDM projects increasingly use streams or feeds of data, data are more commonly extracted from a data warehouse. Data warehouses are complex, retrospective collections of data that originate from a variety of different sources. KDDM projects almost never use all of the data. Instead, analysts use queries to select a subset of relevant data. To accomplish this, analysts must collaborate closely with data warehouse personnel to develop effective queries, queries that select the clinical data relevant to the specific KDDM project with a sufficient but not overwhelming sample size.

To request the appropriate data, investigators and clinicians first need to understand how the concepts of interest are represented (coded) in the data. Clinical concepts are typically represented in EHRs in a way that supports healthcare delivery but not necessarily research or broader analytics. For example, pain might be qualitatively described in a patient's

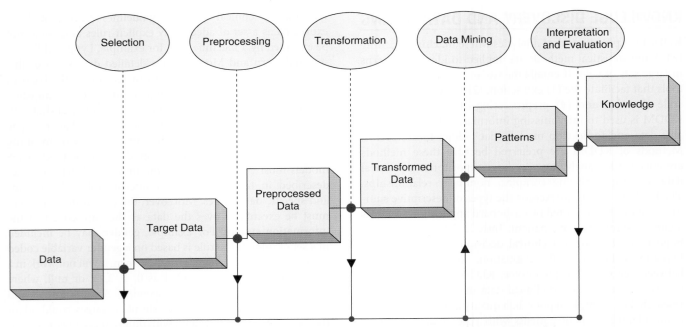

FIG 23.1 Steps of the KDDM process. *KDDM*, Knowledge discovery and data mining.

note and EHR as "mild" or "better." This may meet the immediate need for documentation and care, but it does not allow the analyst or researcher to measure differences in pain over time and across patients, as does measurement using a pain scale. Another example is one where coded data is available. In many healthcare organizations, laboratory tests and many other types of data relevant to healthcare are coded according to the standard Logical Observation Identifier Names and Codes (LOINC) terminology.[27] To ensure that the extracted dataset contains urinalysis data, for instance, it would be necessary to first determine how and where a urinalysis is coded. In the case of VHA data, this may entail identification of the LOINC codes used to represent urinalysis results. For concepts with greater coding variability, such as mental health diagnoses, multiple codes may be relevant and applicable. Some data may not be structured and may be captured only in text documents such as discharge summaries. Information extraction from these documents can be accomplished and represents an active area of research and development with increasingly available commercial solutions.[28]

Queries written in a specialized programming language such as structured query language (SQL) are used to retrieve data from a data warehouse according to a researcher's specifications. Currently, investigators and healthcare organization IT personnel collaborate to develop effective queries. The code used to execute the query is saved as a file and can be reused in the future or repeatedly reused on a scheduled basis. In some cases, healthcare organizations opt to support ongoing investigator data needs by creating separate repositories of aggregated, processed clinical data that relate to a particular clinical domain. In the VHA, investigators in infectious disease have developed procedures to aggregate a specialized set of nationwide patient data related to methicillin-resistant *Staphylococcus aureus* (MRSA).[29] These specialized repositories of data can be more readily analyzed

on an ongoing basis to support quality improvement, health services research, and clinical research.

The amount of data retrieved from clinical data warehouses can be enormous, especially when data originate from multiple sites. Investigators will want to define a sampling plan that limits the number of selected records, according to the needs of the study or project. For KDDM, it may not be possible to import the data fully into analytic software as a single flat file. Fortunately, many statistical and ML software packages can be used to analyze data contained within an SQL database. For example, SAS Enterprise Miner can be used to analyze data within an SQL database using open database connectivity (ODBC).[30] Clinicians or investigators who are new to KDDM should collaborate with statistical and informatics personnel to plan an optimal approach.

Preprocessing Clinical Data

To illustrate preprocessing, this section uses EHR data as an example. The process can be extrapolated to other datasets. EHRs include both coded (structured) data and unstructured text data that must be cleaned and processed prior to analysis. EHRs collect and store data according to a coding system consisting of one or more terminologies. While standard terminologies exist, many systems make use of a local terminology, a distinct set of variables, and a distinct coding system for those variables that are not necessarily shared across systems. Different sites, clinics, or hospitals within a healthcare organization could use different terminologies, coding data in different ways. Within a single site, changes in information systems and terminologies over time can also result in variations in data coding. When data are aggregated across time and across sites, the variations in terminology result in a dataset that represents similar concepts in multiple ways. For example, one large healthcare organization recognized that within its clinical data, the relatively simple concepts of "yes" and "no" were represented using

30 unique coding schemes.[31] Unlike data collected using a prospective approach, clinical data often require extensive cleaning and preprocessing. Thus preprocessing constitutes the majority of effort in the clinical KDDM process shown in Fig. 23.1. See Box 23.3 for information concerning tools that can be used in this process.

Preprocessing Text Data

In clinical records, the richest and most descriptive data are often unstructured, captured only in the text notes entered by clinicians. Text data can be analyzed in a large number of clinical records using a specialized approach known as **natural language processing (NLP)** or, more specifically, information extraction.[32] Methods of information extraction identify pieces of meaningful information in sequences of text, pieces of information that represent concepts and can be coded as such for further analysis. Machine interpretation of text written in the form of natural language is not straightforward because natural language is rife with spelling errors, acronyms, and abbreviations, among other issues.[33] Consequently, information extraction is usually a computationally expensive, multistep process in which text data are passed through a pipeline of sequential NLP procedures. These procedures deal with common NLP challenges such as word disambiguation and negation and may involve the use of ML methods. However, each pipeline may differ according to the NLP task at hand.[33] Unstructured Information Management Architecture (UIMA) (http://uima.apache.org) is one example of an NLP pipeline framework. Information extraction for clinical text is an active area of research and development. Information extraction tools are maturing and increasingly available. However, more advanced applications of semantic NLP typically require custom software and/or collaboration with NLP specialists.

Preprocessing Coded (Structured) Data

In a set of consistently coded clinical data, the data should be analyzed using descriptive statistics and visualization with respect to the following:

- *Distribution.* Normally distributed data are most amenable to modeling. If the data distribution is not normally distributed, the data can be transformed using a function of the original data or analyzed using nonparametric statistical methods.
- *Frequency.* The frequency of specific values for categorical variables may reveal a need for additional preprocessing. It is not uncommon for identical concepts to be represented using multiple outcome values. Also, some values are so rare that their exclusion from analysis should be considered as outliers.
- *Missing data.* Missing data can be meaningful. For example, a missing hemoglobin A1c (HgA1c) laboratory test may indicate that a patient does not have diabetes. In that case, a binary variable indicating whether or not HgA1c values are truly missing can be added to the dataset. In other circumstances, the values are simply missing at random. If values are missing at random, they can be replaced using a number of statistical imputation approaches.
- *Sparsity.* Sparse data are data for which binary values are mostly zero. Categorical variables with a large number of possible values contribute to sparsity. For example, a field called "primary diagnosis" has a set of possible values equal to the number of diagnoses found in the International Classification of Diseases (ICD)-10 coding system. Upon 1 of n encoding, the number of possible values becomes the number of new columns added to the dataset. Some diagnoses will be more common than others. For uncommon diagnoses, the value of "primary diagnosis" will almost always equal zero. The value of "1" will be found in only a small percentage of records.
- *Outliers.* Outliers, data points that fall far outside the distribution of data, should be considered for elimination or further analysis prior to modeling.
- *Identifiers.* Codes or other values that uniquely identify patients should be excluded from the modeling process.
- *Erroneous data.* Absurd, impossible data values are routinely found in clinical data. These can be treated as randomly missing values and replaced.

Descriptive analysis is facilitated by many software packages. Weka, a freely available data mining software package, is an example.[34] In this software, when a variable from the dataset is selected, basic descriptive statistics and a graph of the frequency distribution are displayed. A variety of filters can then be applied to address issues with the data.

The considerations in preprocessing the data at this stage are numerous and beyond the scope of this chapter. Preprocessing is always best accomplished through a joint effort by the analyst and one or more domain experts, such as clinicians who are familiar with the concepts the data represent. The domain experts can lend valuable insight to the analyst, who must develop an optimal representation of each variable. Review of the data at this point may reveal conceptual gaps, the absence of data, or the lack of quality data that represent important concepts. For example, age and functional status (e.g., activities of daily living) might be important data to include in a project related to predicting patient falls in the hospital. By mapping concepts to variables, or vice versa, teams can communicate about gaps and weaknesses in the data as well as potential solutions.

Sampling and Partitioning

Once the data have been fully cleaned and preprocessed, they must be sampled and partitioned. Sampling is the step in which a smaller subset of the data is chosen for analysis. Sampling is important because excessive amounts of data slow computer processing time during analysis. Sampling for classification tasks is typically random or stratified on class membership.

Partitioning refers to the assignment of individual records or rows in a dataset for a specific purpose: model development (training, incremental testing of models during development) or model validation (data held out from the development process for the purpose of unbiased performance estimation). There are multiple approaches to sampling and partitioning, and the suitability of the approach depends on the nature of the project and the quantity of available data. If very large amounts of data are available, large sets can be sampled for model development and validation. If more limited amounts of data are available, it will be necessary to optimize the use of that data through resampling approaches. Two common resampling approaches are termed *bootstrapping* and *cross-validation*.[35] Bootstrapping involves repeatedly calculating the mean from multiple samples to increase the data available for training.

Within the model development dataset, cross-validation can be used to maximize the amount of data used for both training and testing. In cross-validation, the data are partitioned into n folds. Then, in a series of n experiments, $n-1$ folds are used to train models, and the remaining fold, which is unique in each experiment, is used for testing. In that way, each record is available for both training and testing, but there is no duplication of records in the testing dataset. Cross-validation is commonly performed with either 10 or 100 folds. In very small datasets, leave-one-out cross-validation can be implemented, wherein the number of folds equals the number of records. This maximizes the amount of data available for training within each of the n experiments.

Data Mining

Data mining is the step in the knowledge discovery process where patterns are enumerated over a set of data.[36] The methods used to accomplish this are varied and include both ML and statistical approaches. Examples of these approaches are outlined in the following sections.

Statistical Approaches

Statistical approaches fit a model to the data. Bayesian networks, a class of models based on Bayes theorem, constitute one popular approach. Bayesian models are robust, tolerate missing data, and can be computed quickly over a set of data. The simplest implementation, Naive Bayes, has been shown to perform well despite its assumption of independence between input variables. Another important approach is logistic or linear regression, which represents the observed relationship between input variables and a classification or a dependent variable.

Machine Learning

ML methods are computer algorithms that learn to perform a task on the basis of examples. In data mining, the task is typically prediction or regression (predict a real number) or classification (predict class membership). ML algorithms vary in the way they learn to perform tasks. Many algorithms begin with an initial working theory of how a set of input data predict an output (a.k.a. target), a future event, or an unknown value. The algorithm then makes incremental adjustments to the working theory, based on examples of both the input and the target. The examples are contained in a set of training data. A complete discussion of ML and specific ML algorithms is beyond the scope of this chapter. However, key methods and characteristics are summarized in Table 23.2.

TABLE 23.2	Examples of Data Mining Methods
Method	**Description**
Decision trees	Recursive partitioning of data based on an information criterion (entropy, information gain, etc.) Common algorithms: C4.5, CART Easily interpreted Require pruning based on coverage to avoid overfit More difficult to calibrate to new populations and settings
Decision rules	Classification rules in the form of if-then-else rule sets Easily interpreted Require pruning based on coverage to avoid overfit Closely related to decision trees; decision trees can be easily converted to decision rules
Artificial neural networks	Networks of processing units Output a probability of class membership Computationally expensive Effective for modeling complex, nonlinear solutions Not easily interpreted
Support vector machines	Linear functions implemented in a transformed feature space Computationally efficient Effective for modeling complex, nonlinear solutions Not easily interpreted
Random forests	"Ensemble" method that combines the output of multiple decision trees Scalable (computationally feasible even with very large amounts of data) Not easily interpreted
Bayesian networks	Probabilistic models based on Bayes theorem Models are easily calibrated for use with new settings and populations Models may assume conditional independence among variables Not as scalable as other methods; may not work well with very large amounts of data due to the way in which Bayesian networks are computed

CART, classification and regression trees.

All of the methods listed in this table are commonly implemented in general-purpose data mining software.

Multiple variant algorithms can be used to implement each approach, and specialized method-specific software is available to support more flexible configurations. ML algorithms also can be implemented in a variety of programming languages. Data mining software allows users to implement versions of these algorithms via point-and-click graphic user interfaces. However, these algorithms can also be written and executed using analytical environments such as R, MATLAB, or Python. It is important that users understand how to apply each unique method properly in order to produce optimal models and avoid spurious results.

Evaluating Data Mining Models

The most critical step in evaluation, the partitioning of data, occurs early in KDDM (Fig. 23.2). Performance estimates are calculated by comparing a model's predictions to actual values on a set of data for which the actual values are known. If this comparison is made using the training data—that is, the same data used to parameterize the model—the performance estimates will be optimistically biased. It is critical that a sizable sample of the original data is set aside and not used in any way to train or calibrate models. This held-out sample of data is often termed the validation set or testing set. Used solely for performance estimation, the held-out data will yield unbiased estimates.

Performance measures are based on a comparison of the predicted and actual values in a set of held-out testing data. In classification, this comparison yields a **classification matrix** that can be used to derive performance measures, similar to the performance measures used in evaluating clinical diagnostic tests, such as true-positive rate, false-positive rate, true-negative rate, false-negative rate, sensitivity, specificity, and likelihood ratios (Fig. 23.3). The specific performance measures should be selected with respect to the goals of the KDDM project. For example, if a model is developed as a screening tool, sensitivity may be of particular interest. If a model is developed for a CDS tool, alert fatigue is an important consideration, and so the false-positive rate may be of particular interest.

To evaluate and compare overall model performance, the receiver operating characteristic (ROC) curve and the area under the ROC curve are important measures of performance. The ROC curve, depicted in Fig. 23.4, is obtained by plotting the false-positive fraction and true-positive fraction, based on cumulative comparison of predicted and actual values at increasing values of probability. The resulting curve shows the trade-off between sensitivity and specificity exhibited by a classifier at any given threshold. The area under the ROC curve is the probability that a randomly chosen positive case will be selected as more likely to be positive than a randomly selected negative case.[37] As such, it serves as an overall measure of model performance. An area under the ROC curve ($A_z = 0.5$) is equivalent to random chance. Better performance is indicated by higher values of A_z. Interpretation of the area under the ROC curve, especially in relation to other models or classifiers, requires the calculation of confidence intervals.

For models that predict a real number (e.g., glucose level), performance measures are simply based on the difference between the predicted value and the true value in a set of held-out testing data for which the true values are known. From these differences various measurements of error can be calculated, such as mean squared error and root mean squared error. Measurement of correlation is also important (e.g., r^2), as is visualization of predicted and actual values.

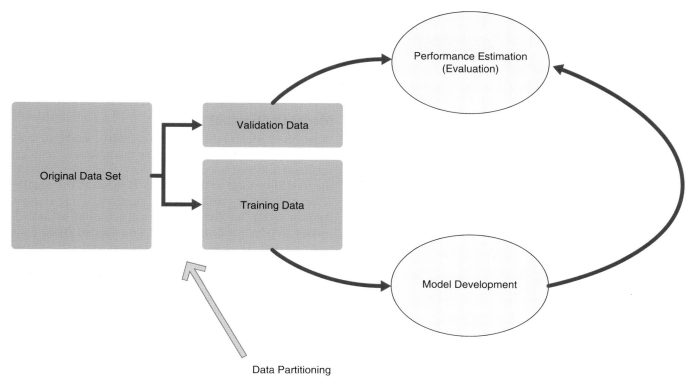

FIG 23.2 The relationship of data partitioning to both model development and evaluation.

A model has been developed to predict whether or not a patient is colonized with MRSA upon admission to a tertiary health care facility. The model outputs a probability of MRSA colonization, from which a prediction of MRSA status can be generated . . . The model's predictions are compared to actual patient MRSA status in order to estimate the model's performance.

Case ID	Known MRSA Status	Probability of MRSA	Predicted MRSA Status
5478	0	0.23	0
2222	1	0.85	1
6123	1	0.85	1
0805	1	0.46	0

False negative

The comparison of predicted and actual values yields a confusion matrix, from which most performance metrics for classifiers (models that predict class membership) are calculated.

	Actual value = 0 (no MRSA)	Actual value = 1 (MRSA)
Model predicts value = 0 (no MRSA)	True-negative count	False-negative count
Model predicts value = 1 (MRSA)	False-positive count	True-positive count

Measures of performance for classification models:

False-positive fraction
True-negative fraction
Positive-predictive value
Negative-predictive value
Sensitivity or true-positive fraction
False-positive fraction
Specificity
Positive and negative diagnostic likelihood ratios
Receiver operating characteristic (ROC) curve

FIG 23.3 The process of calculating performance estimates from a comparison of predicted and actual values for a classification model of MRSA status on admission. *MRSA,* Methicillin-resistant *Staphylococcus aureus*; *ROC,* receiver operating characteristic.

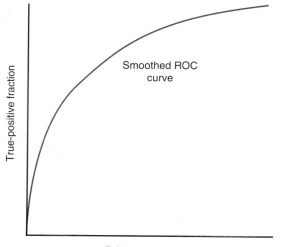

Smoothed ROC curve

True-positive fraction

False-positive fraction

FIG 23.4 Smoothed ROC curve. *ROC,* receiver operating characteristic.

Model Deployment

Deployment refers to the actual use of analytic models or tools. In this step, analysts determine how the models or tools are optimally delivered to a decision maker—that is, they translate the models or tools to the problem at hand. In the simplest sense, deployment could consist of merely reporting analyses. Another model involves routine prospective use of analytic models to offer predictions or decision support based upon real-time data. The latter entails either configuring the system such as an EHR or adding a module that functions to provide analyses within the live information system. Examples of analytic models functioning with live data outside healthcare are the live recommendations offered by Netflix or Amazon.com as well as credit card fraud detection alerts.

A key aspect of deployment is the ability of an analyst to adapt models to changes in the nature of the data and to calibrate models for different settings and patient populations. Sometimes, the analyst and the developer are the same. In other cases, the developer works in response to analyst needs and feedback. Often, analysts will request changes to the model to address a specific need or issue. These types of changes are best developed and tested in conjunction with a source code version of the model. Once the changes are well tested in the source code environment, these changes can be examined for potential inclusion into the main model functioning in a live system. The concept of "make one to throw it away" is well known in software development,[20,38] but in analytics it is common to have many iterations to allow institutional knowledge to grow as initial, rough results are shared with decision makers.

Another method of deployment is the direct delivery of results to a decision maker without explicit analyst intervention. One way to accomplish this is through delivery of spreadsheets such as Microsoft Excel, with graphical user interfaces (GUIs) that can be operated by the decision maker to select the data and generate predeveloped summaries and charts. For example, a display may show registered nurse (RN) staffing patterns and projected infection rates occurring within the next few days. The user may drill down into the data looking at education level of the staff or into the type or location of specific infections.

A third deployment method is the intranet delivery of reports, where decision makers access a site that allows them to tailor a report request or details. Their requested details are run on a remote server and delivered through an internet browser, including generated tables, charts, and explanations on how they should be interpreted.

A fourth method is automated report generation. Programming can be embedded into statistical software such as Sweave[39] or knitr,[40] platforms such as IPython[41] and Jupyter,[42] notebooks, or other reproducible research tools.[43] These can be used to specify the subject of the analysis, directed to run the analysis in the hosted data analysis software and produce a report in Adobe PDF or word processor formats with tables, charts, and other results embedded. A descriptive narrative can be included so that the analysis can be reproduced with the same or new datasets as needed. For instance, one neurological practice uses a combination of R and Sweave to analyze the data and deliver a customized, comprehensive report immediately after the completion of a series of neuropsychological tests.[44] Sweave is a tool that uses the R code for data analyses within a document, thereby creating dynamic reports that can be updated automatically if data or analyses change. Another example is shown in Fig. 23.5, which displays intensive care unit (ICU) and step-down unit usage over time.[45] The explanatory text indicates that the step-down unit is often at capacity, while the ICU is rarely so.

Modern software development methodologies such as the spiral development model incorporate multiple rounds of feedback. Once deployed, this model is in continual use in a live environment with constant feedback within its cycle. That is, as decision makers' stated requirements change and as the organization builds experience using this approach, new information is incorporated into the analysis used in making decisions. This process can improve business and data understanding, which changes the way that analysis

products are used, as well as decision makers' future requirements.

The spiral model approach is demonstrated in a project undertaken by one of the authors (llk).[46] The analysis was conducted using data from a health screening clinic. The author wanted to determine optimal clinic design to increase the efficiency of patient processing in the clinic. The first step was to understand the structure of the clinic, the activities of the workers, and the procedures used as clients arrived and were processed through their clinic visit. While developing this understanding, we found that the data about clinic times were rounded to the nearest whole minute, so in the data preparation and analysis phase, we used methods to deal with this kind of altered time data. Several forms of models were applied to determine parameters for a simulation to model the current system. This model was shared with employees in charge of the clinic, which both confirmed our understanding of the clinic workflow process and generated questions that improved our understanding of the clinic and pertinent data. The resulting simulation was then used to explore different clinic configurations, run analyses, and ultimately identify the best clinic design and management of resources for optimal patient processing in the clinic.

Organizational Considerations for Data Science

Organizations can mature over time in their use of data science and analytics. A model showing this progression is in Fig. 23.6. Organizations begin with retrospective analysis (exploratory data analyses discussed earlier in the chapter) and gradually move up the scale of difficulty and value toward prescriptive analytics. As organizations gain maturity, several elements are important in this growth: data science personnel, tools and platforms, data standardization, and data governance.

Data Science Personnel

An analytics group needs to be established and grown over time. Analytics has a superficial overlap with traditional data analysis and/or software engineering, but requirements for modern analytics cannot be satisfied by a traditional data analyst or a pure programmer. Traditional data analysts are normally asked to perform descriptive analysis or to run standard summary or review procedures on standard datasets (e.g., to produce a chart for a report or to produce summary statistics using statistical software). An analytics group, on the other hand, is generally asked to be creative in developing analytics procedures across a range of datasets to meet the specific needs of decision makers and to present the results in ways that enhance decision makers' understanding of problems as they make decisions.

An example of this kind of project would be predicting the impact of adding another operating room to the current suite of rooms. Analytics could show decision makers data such as number of projected new cases to be added, the downtime in all rooms, the number and kinds of new staff required, the case mix, and projected revenue or loss. Similarly, software engineers and programmers may be asked to develop software

```
In [13]:  pyl.figure(figsize=(5.5,4))
          pyl.plot(hospNonstatEmp.icu.actMon.tseries(),hospNonstatEmp.icu.actMon.yseries())
          pyl.plot(hospNonstatEmp.icu.actMon.tseries(),
                  [G.icubeds for xi in hospNonstatEmp.icu.actMon.tseries()])
          pyl.title("ICU Utilization over time",
                  fontsize=12,fontweight="bold")
          pyl.xlabel("time",fontsize=9,fontweight="bold")
          pyl.ylabel("Beds",fontsize=9,fontweight="bold")
          pyl.grid(True)
          pyl.savefig(r".\icuutilization.png")
          pyl.show()
          pyl.clf()
```

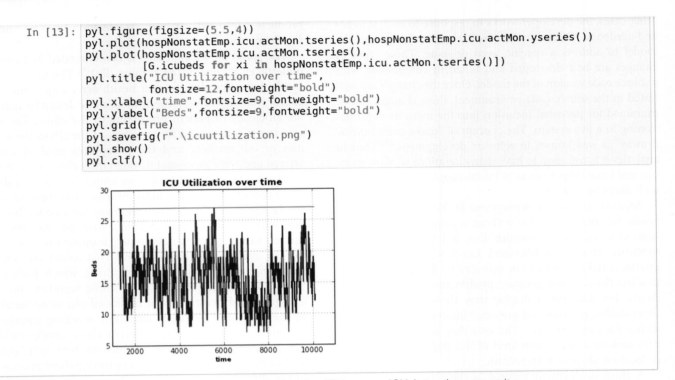

FIG. 23.5 A sample report showing ICU usage. *ICU,* Intensive care unit.

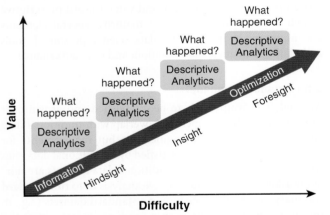

FIG. 23.6 Gartner Analytics Maturity Model. (Reprinted with permission of Gartner, Inc.)

products, and their workflow bears a resemblance to an analytics workflow, but software engineers do not require the same level of business domain understanding as an analytics professional.

Recommended Skills for a Data Science/Health Analytics Professional. To be of the most benefit to a healthcare system, a health analytics professional, a newer specialty in healthcare, is required to be bilingual in the skills of computer information systems and in healthcare operations.[47] Drew Conway describes the requirements of analytics professionals as a three-part Venn diagram (Fig. 23.7).[48] The three areas of knowledge required by analytics professionals are mathematics and statistics, computer hacking (programming), and subject matter expertise.

Computer hacking skills are required because of the way the data used in analytics is electronically stored and because of potential errors in the collection and recording of data. Without the ability to manipulate electronic data, including various types of numerical and text data, and to think algorithmically, this data is essentially closed off. This means that the analytics professional needs a fair proficiency in programming data, although a formal degree in programming may not be necessary. In addition, the analytics professional needs enough understanding of IT infrastructure to discuss issues with computer and IT engineers who manage the IT infrastructure and databases.

To develop true insight from data, the analytics professional requires mathematical and statistical understanding. Although the computational work of mathematical and statistical methods may be done through computer packages, an understanding of mathematical and statistical concepts is necessary to identify what is valid for a given situation, how to interpret

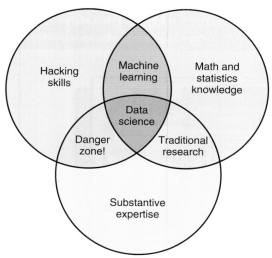

FIG. 23.7 Data scientist skills. (Copyright © 2015 Drew Conway Data Consulting, LLC.)

TABLE 23.3	Examples of Analytics Tools
Class	**Examples**
Spreadsheets and business intelligence tools	MS Excel, LibreOffice, Actuate BIRT, Pentaho
Statistical analysis programs	SAS, SPSS, Stata, Weka, KNIME, Rapidminer
Programming language	R, Python, Matlab, Scala, Julia

the results, and how to determine if the results are of practical significance.

The need for subject matter expertise is the biggest divergence from most quantitative professionals. This expertise is required for examining the healthcare business process to identify important values, translate the business requirements to mathematical and statistical models, and interpret the results in terms that make sense in the business setting. Drew Conway indicated this separates data science from academic fields such as ML, which are typically developed separately from the subject matter of potential applications.[49]

One issue is the difficulty in finding someone with the combination of all these skills. Each of the three knowledge areas could be a career in its own right, so finding a person who embodies strength in all three of these knowledge areas is often compared to looking for a mythical unicorn.[50] But what is often truly needed is a team of people who each have a minimum level of skills and understanding in all aspects and as a team collectively have strength and depth in every aspect of the analytics role.

Tools and Platforms

A second decision the organization needs to make in conjunction with the analytics group is the choice of computer platform. While many of the platforms are made to interact well with others, forming synergy across different types of capabilities, a basic understanding of choices is helpful.

A common platform for analytics is spreadsheet software such as MS Excel and business intelligence platforms such as Actuate BIRT and Pentaho. These are known for being able to connect or import data from databases and perform basic summaries and charting. As they are ubiquitous as part of software office suites or through

intranet interfaces, these are often used for descriptive analytics or as a delivery platform for more sophisticated methods, which can create databases as output then can use spreadsheets or business intelligence platforms as means to deliver the results. Table 23.3 illustrates categories of analytics tools and provides examples.

Another class of analytics platforms is stand-alone analytical programs. These can be driven through GUI menus or custom batch programming languages. These include many traditional statistical platforms such as SAS, SPSS, and Minitab, as well as graphical ML platforms such as Rapidminer,[51] KNIME,[52] or Weka.[53] These packages are specialized for statistics and data analysis and include ways of connecting to common databases. Often they include graphical model building capabilities to specify the data processing and analytical workflow. These graphical and menu-based workflows can significantly ease the initial development of models for use in analysis.

A third platform class is based on programming languages with special facilities for data analysis. Two characteristics are common to these languages:

1. Data frame data structure that stores information about entities and features that are based on a functional programming paradigm (as opposed to the more common object-oriented programming paradigm). These languages include R,[54] Python,[55] and Scala.[56] One advantage of the programming language–based platforms is that they are often extensible, meaning that capabilities not originally considered by the initial developer can be created and added to the platform.
2. Applications written using these languages can be connected to other applications. For example, the big data platforms of Apache Hadoop can embed the ML capabilities of Apache Spark,[57] which can be scripted (programmed) using Java, R, Python, or Scala. Similarly, the cloud data platform MS Azure[58] can include the Azure ML extension, which can be scripted using Python or R. Obviously, applicable computer programming knowledge and skills in addition to a mathematical and statistical background are needed to master these.

In the end, the choice of platform is dependent on the type of expected deployment for analytical products and the people available to the analytics group.

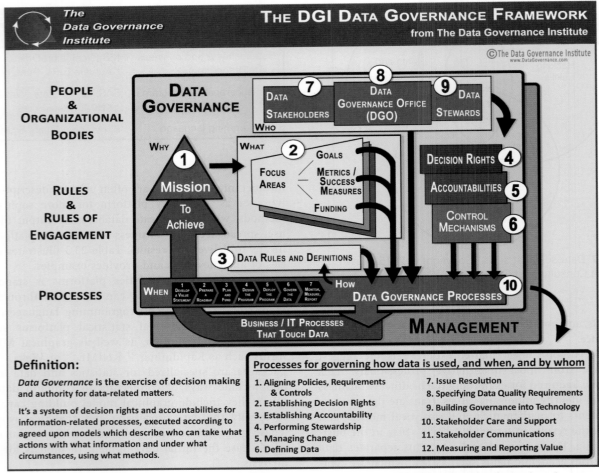

FIG. 23.8 Data governance framework. (Reprinted with permission of The Data Governance Institute.)

Data Standardization

Data quality affects the feasibility of secondary analysis and is critical to data science and analytics. Data quality can be enhanced through standardized data and the use of terminologies, as discussed in Chapter 22. The lack of data standardization and interoperability challenges are an ongoing issue in healthcare locally and nationally. Healthcare organizations need to make decisions about the extent of data standardization they will employ and enforce locally. This directly affects their data repository/data warehouse construction and usage. Nationally, recent initiatives such as PCORnet and federal policy changes such as the Medicare and Medicaid Meaningful Use incentive programs are improving the standardization and interoperability of clinical data.[59,60]

Data Governance

Organizations need to make myriad decisions around managing and obtaining value from data, such as minimizing cost and complexity, managing risk, and ensuring adherence to regulations and legal requirements. As organizations mature in their data science analyses, they need formal mechanisms, called data governance, to oversee these analytic processes. Data governance means decision making and authority over data-related matters. The concept can have many nuances

such as organizational structures for managing data, rules and policies, data decision rights, methods for accountability, and methods enforcement for data-related processes.[61]

Thus organizations need a structure for enterprise-wide data management.[62] This is a first step in transforming an organization's adoption of data science.

Data governance typically addresses these types of vendor-agnostic topics:

- Tools
- Techniques
- Models
- Best practices

Readers are referred to an excellent resource, the Data Governance Institute (DGI), at: http://www.datagovernance.com to learn more about this topic. The DGI provides a data governance framework seen in Fig. 23.8 that includes 10 components every data governance program should employ.[61]

CONCLUSIONS AND FUTURE DIRECTIONS

Data science, data analytics, and methods of KDDM are processes that can be used to glean important insights and develop useful, data-driven output and models from collected healthcare data. With each patient and each healthcare event, data describing numerous aspects of care accumulate. Large warehouses of clinical data are now commonplace, and as time passes, the data will become increasingly longitudinal in nature. This future direction presents an enormous opportunity, as large repositories of clinical data can be used to gain insight into the relationship between the characteristics of patient, diagnoses, interventions, outcomes, and other elements such as costs and operational processes. Data can also be used to identify prospective patient cohorts for scientific research. They can be used to assist healthcare providers with clinical decisions and avoid medical error. However, the sheer size and complexity of the data necessitate specialized approaches to data management and analysis. The methods of KDDM enable us to analyze the data efficiently and effectively and develop clinical knowledge models for decision support.

Accountable care organizations and shared risk reimbursement models require that organizations fundamentally understand the cost and outcomes of providing care, and this capability depends on data science. As more healthcare systems install EHRs and other health IT, data acquisition will become easier and less costly; data elements needed for analyses can be hard-coded in health IT in structured, exportable formats while also being used for clinical documentation of care. This concept has been implemented already in health systems in Israel and in various studies in the United States.[63] However, health IT transitions present challenges. While health IT can facilitate data acquisition, systems are not always data analytic or research-friendly. Many important clinical concepts are stored only in narrative text format, such as clinical notes, and cannot be easily analyzed. Textual data must be abstracted manually or via NLP, both labor-intensive and costly approaches. Systems for rapidly fulfilling data requests for aggregated retrospective data are not commonly well developed, and so data requests can be costly and consume an enormous amount of time. Subsequently, the extracted data requires validation and extensive cleaning.

Using data science and data analytics, informaticians and health professionals can leverage the vast amounts of data generated in the course of providing healthcare in order to improve healthcare. Leaders are now focusing on building and leveraging predictive analytics. Data science and KDDM can yield systematic cost, process, and outcomes information that complement the largely anecdotal and informal knowledge base underlying clinical practice. These tools are essential in contemporary healthcare organizations and necessary to optimize patient and organizational outcomes.

REFERENCES

1. Hyattsville M. *Health, United States, 2014: With Special Feature on Adults Aged 55–64*. National Center for Health Statistics: Atlanta, Georgia; 2015.
2. Oxford Dictionaries. *Definition of Big Data*; 2016. http://www.oxforddictionaries.com/us/definition/american_english/big-data?q=big+data.
3. McKenna B. What does a petabyte look like? 2015. *Computer Weekly*. http://www.computerweekly.com/feature/What-does-a-petabyte-look-like.
4. Shah ND, Pthak J. Why healthcare may finally be ready for big data. *Harv Bus Rev*. December 3, 2014. https://hbr.org/2014/12/why-health-care-may-finally-be-ready-for-big-data.
5. Hartzband DD. Using ultra-large data sets in healthcare: New questions, new answers. In: *Presentation at the Congressional Luncheon Seminar Series: unlocking the value of health data: transforming care using information securely to improve efficiency and quality, advance biomedical and health systems research, and promote population-health*, Institute of e-health policy; 2011. http://www.e-healthpolicy.org/seminarsSessions_20111005.asp.
6. Institute for Health Technology Transformation. *Transforming Health Care Through Big Data: Strategies for Leveraging Big Data in the Health Care Industry*. Institute for Health Technology Transformation. http://c4fd63cb482ce6861463-bc6183f1c18e748a49b87a25911a0555.r93.cf2.rackcdn.com/iHT2_BigData_2013.pdf; 2013.
7. Duvall SL, Fraser AM, Rowe K, Thomas A, Mineau GP. Evaluation of record linkage between a large healthcare provider and the Utah Population Database. *J Am Med Inform Assoc*. 2012;19(e1):e54–e59.
8. Slattery ML, Kerber RA. A comprehensive evaluation of family history and breast cancer risk: the Utah Population Database. *J Am Med Assoc*. 1993;270(13):1563–1568.
9. Hu H, Correll M, Kvecher L, et al. DW4TR: a data warehouse for translational research. *J Biomed Inform*. 2011;44(6):1004–1019.
10. Trotter F, Uhlman D. *Hacking Healthcare*. Sebastopol, CA: O'Reilly Media; 2013.
11. Peters SG, Buntrock JD. Big data and the electronic health record. *J Ambul Care Manag*. 2014;37:206–210.
12. IBM. *IBM Watson Health*. https://www.ibm.com/smarterplanet/us/en/ibmwatson/health/. Accessed April 13, 2016.
13. O'Reilly T, Steele J, Loukides M, Hill C. *How Data Science is Transforming Health Care: Solving the Wanamaker Dilemma*. Sebastopol, CA: O'Reilly Media; 2012.
14. Blount M, Ebling MR, Eklund JM, et al. Real-time analysis for intensive care: development and deployment of the artemis analytic system. *IEEE Eng Med Biol Mag*. 2010;29:110–118.
15. Poeter D. Google called the current flu outbreak two weeks ago. *PC Mag*. January 10, 2013. http://www.pcmag.com/article2/0,2817,2414156,00.asp.
16. Cooper GF, Bahar I, Becich MJ, et al. The center for causal discovery of biomedical knowledge from big data. *J Am Med Inform Assoc*. 2015;22:1132–1136.
17. Kansagra AP, Yu JP, Chatterjee AR, et al. Big data and the future of radiology informatics. *Acad Radiol*. 2016;23:30–42.
18. McEvoy LK, Holland D, Hagler Jr DJ, et al. Mild cognitive impairment: baseline and longitudinal structural MR imaging measures improve predictive prognosis. *Radiology*. 2011;259:834–843.
19. Eaton C, Deroos D, Deutsch T, Lapis G, Zikopoulos P. Understanding big data: analytics for enterprise class Hadoop and streaming data. NY: McGraw-Hill; 2012.

20. Culbertson R. The ethics of big data. There's a fine line between patient privacy and identifying better forms of treatment. *Healthc Exec.* 2015;30(44):6–7.

21. INFORMS. *Analytics Section of INFORMS.* https://www. informs.org/Community/Analytics; 2014.

22. Walton NA, Poynton MR, Gesteland PH, Maloney C, Staes C, Facelli JC. Predicting the start week of respiratory syncytial virus outbreaks using real time weather variables. *BMC Med Inform Decis Mak.* 2010;10:68.

23. Smithburger PL, Buckley MS, Bejian S, Burenheide K, Kane-Gill SL. A critical evaluation of clinical decision support for the detection of drug-drug interactions. *Expert Opin Drug Saf.* 2011;10(6):871–882.

24. Lyng KM, Pedersen BS. Participatory design for computerization of clinical practice guidelines. *J Biomed Inform.* 2011;44(5):909–918.

25. Isern D, Moreno A. Computer-based execution of clinical guidelines: a review. *Int J Med Inform.* 2008;77(12):787–808.

26. Sonnenberg FA, Hagerty CG. Computer-interpretable clinical practice guidelines: where are we and where are we going? *Yearb Med Inform.* 2006;145–158.

27. McDonald CJ, Huff SM, Suico JG, et al. LOINC, a universal standard for identifying laboratory observations: a 5-year update. *Clin Chem.* 2003;49(4):624–633.

28. Meystre S, Haug PJ. Natural language processing to extract medical problems from electronic clinical documents: performance evaluation. *J Biomed Inform.* 2006;39(6): 589–599.

29. Jones MM, DuVall SL, Spuhl J, Samore MH, Nielson C, Rubin M. Identification of methicillin-resistant Staphylococcus aureus within the nation's Veterans Affairs Medical Centers using natural language processing. *BMC Med Inform Decis Mak.* 2012;12(1):34.

30. SAS Institute. *SAS/ACCESS Interface to Teradata (white paper);* 2002. 1-42.

31. Lincoln MJ. *VA Enterprise Terminology Project (presentation).* Salt Lake City, UT: University of Utah Department of Biomedical Informatics Seminar Series; 2006.

32. Meystre SM, Savova GK, Kipper-Schuler KC, Hurdle JF. Extracting information from textual documents in the electronic health record: a review of recent research. *Yearb Med Inform.* 2008;128–144.

33. Nadkarni PM, Ohno-Machado L, Chapman WW. Natural language processing: an introduction. *J Am Med Inform Assoc.* 2011;18(5):544–551.

34. Hall M, Frank E, Holmes G, Pfahringer B, Reutemann P, Witten IH. The WEKA Data Mining Software: An Update. *SIGKDD Explorations.* 2009;11(1):10–18.

35. Sahiner B, Chan HP, Hadjiiski L. Classifier performance estimation under the constraint of a finite sample size: resampling schemes applied to neural network classifiers. *Neural Netw.* 2008;21(2-3):476–483.

36. Fayyad UMP-SG, Smyth P. From data mining to knowledge discovery: an overview. In: Fayyad UMP-SG, Smyth P, Uthurasamy R, eds. *Advances in Knowledge Discovery and Data Mining.* Menlo Park, CA: AAAI Press/The MIT Press; 1996:1–34.

37. Hanley JA, McNeil BJ. The meaning and use of the area under a receiver operating characteristic (ROC) curve. *Radiology.* 1982;143(1):29–36.

38. Brooks FP. *The Mythical Man Month: Essays on Software Engineering.* Boston: Addison-Wesley Pub. Co; 1995.

39. Leisch F. Sweave: dynamic generation of statistical reports using literate data analysis. In: *Compstat.* Heidelberg: Physica-Verlag HD; 2002:575–580. http://dx.doi.org/10.1007/978-3-642-57489-4_89.

40. Xie Y. *Dynamic Documents with R and knitr.* 2nd ed. USA: Chapman and Hall/CRC; 2015.

41. Perez F, Granger BE. IPython: A System for Interactive Scientific Computing. *Comput Sci Eng.* 2007;9(3):21–29. http://dx.doi.org/10.1109/MCSE.2007.53.

42. Perez F, Granger BE. *Project Jupyter: Computational Narratives as the Engine of Collaborative Data Science. Grant Proposal to Helmsley Charitable Trust, the Alfred P Sloan Foundation, and the Gordon and Betty Moore Foundation;* 2015. http://blog.jupyter.org/2015/07/07/project-jupyter-computational-narratives-as-the-engine-of-collaborative-data-science/.

43. Stodden V, Leisch F, Peng RD. *Implementing Reproducible Research.* New York: Chapman and Hall/CRC; 2014.

44. Garbade S, Burgard P. Using R/Sweave in Everyday Clinical Practice. *R News.* 2006;6(2). https://cran.r-project.org/doc/Rnews/Rnews_2006-2.pdf.

45. Luangkesorn KL, Bountourelis L, Schaefer A, Nabors S, Clermont G. The case against utilization: deceptive performance measures in in-patient care capacity models. In: Laroque C, Pasupathy R, Rose O, Uhramcher AM, eds. *Proceedings of the 2012 Winter Simulation Conference (WSC)* Berlin, DE: IEEE; 2012:847–858. http://dx.doi.org/10.1109/WSC.2012.6465104.

46. Luangkesorn KL, Norman BA, Zhuang Y, Falbo M, Sysko J. Practice summaries: designing disease prevention and screening centers in Abu Dhabi. *Interfaces.* 2012;42(4):406–409. http://dx.doi.org/10.1287/inte.1110.0617.

47. Meer D. Educating the Next Analytics "Bilinguals." *Strategy +Business;* 2016. http://www.strategy-business.com/blog/Educating-the-Next-Analytics-Bilinguals.

48. Conway C. *The Data Science Venn diagram;* 2013. http://drewconway.com/zia/2013/3/26/the-data-science-venn-diagram.

49. Conway D. *The Data Science Venn Diagram. drewconway.com;* 2010. http://www.dataists.com/2010/09/the-data-science-venn-diagram/.

50. Bertolucci J. Are you recruiting a data scientist, or unicorn? *Inf Week.* Nov 21, 2013.

51. RapidMiner. *RapidMiner;* 2015. https://rapidminer.com/.

52. KNIME.COM AG. *KNIME.* https://www.knime.org. Accessed February 3, 2016.

53. Frank E, Hall M, Reutemann P, et al. *Weka 3: Data Mining Software in Java;* 2015. http://www.cs.waikato.ac.nz/~ml/weka/.

54. R Core Team. *R: A Language and Environment for Statistical Computing.* Vienna, Austria: R Foundation for Statistical Computing; 2015.

55. Oliphant TE. Python for scientific computing. *Comput Sci Eng.* 2007;9(3):10–20. http://dx.doi.org/10.1109/MCSE.2007.58.

56. École Polytechnique Fédérale de Lausanne. *Scala;* 2016. http://www.scala-lang.org/.

57. Meng X, Bradley J, Yavuz B, et al. *MLlib: Machine Learning in Apache Spark.* 2015

58. Microsoft Corp. *Microsoft Azure Machine Learning;* 2016. https://azure.microsoft.com/en-us/services/machine-learning/.

59. Warren JJ, Matney SA, Foster ED, Auld VA, Roy SL. Toward interoperability: a new resource to support nursing terminology standards. *Comput Inform Nurs.* 2015;33(12):515–519. http://dx.doi.org/10.1097/CIN.0000000000000210.

60. Fleurence RL, Curtis LH, Califf RM, Platt R, Selby JV, Brown JS. Launching PCORnet, a national patient-centered clinical research network. *J Am Med Inform Assoc.* 2014;21(4):578–582. http://dx.doi.org/10.1136/amiajnl-2014-002747.

61. The DGI. *The Data Governance Institute.* http://www.datagovernance.com/. Accessed April 26, 2016.

62. IHTT. *Transforming Health Care Through Big Data.* The Institute for Health Technology Transformation; 2014. http://ihealthtran.com/big-data-in-healthcare.

63. Deutscher D, Hart DL, Dickstein R, Horn SD, Gutvirtz M. Implementing an integrated electronic outcomes and electronic health record process to create a foundation for clinical practice improvement. *Phys Ther.* 2008;88(2):270–285.

DISCUSSION QUESTIONS

1. Write a statement outlining the three top big data or data analytics questions you would want to consider in your work setting.

2. Compare and contrast the types and methods that are available for EDA, predictive, and prescriptive analytics. Give examples of each.

3. Why is it necessary to process coded and text data before using data mining methods?

4. When discussing KDDM, what is the meaning of the following adage: "Garbage in, garbage out"?

5. Fig. 23.7 includes 10 components every data governance program should employ. For each component, provide one implication of that component within a healthcare setting.

CASE STUDY

You are a new hire in a regional office that oversees 35 long-term care facilities. One of your goals is to build a regional knowledge development program. You have support from your supervisor in developing this new program. Your supervisor went to a recent conference and now understands the potential of using data across facilities for improved decision making. But your supervisor does not understand how to even begin such a program and is looking to you to provide some guidance. Using the information in this chapter, answer the following questions:

1. Thinking about the Gartner model that outlines how analytics mature in organizations, what would be your initial goals for a knowledge development program? Discuss initial characteristics of output for a beginning program.

2. One of your first steps would be to assess the health IT capabilities in each of your facilities and at the regional level. Think about what you would want to know about each of these. Consider available local functions, interoperability (information transfer) of systems, repositories at the local or regional level, and support personnel.

3. Thinking about the skills needed for data science analysts, outline an initial team of people you would need to begin the program.

4. Discuss marketing efforts for this program targeted to the executive staff of the long-term care facilities. Create a list of the kinds of questions that might be answered by using data science.

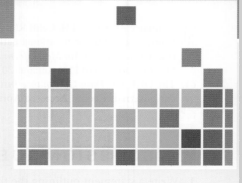

24

Patient Safety and Quality Initiatives in Health Informatics

Patricia C. Dykes and Kumiko O. Schnock

Due to the complexity of the errors in healthcare, multifaceted strategies including health information technology tools are needed to realize improvement in clinical processes and patient outcomes when striving to improve quality and safety.

OBJECTIVES

At the completion of this chapter, the reader will be prepared to:

1. Define patient safety and quality of care from a health informatics prospective.
2. Describe the role of health information technology (IT) in advancing the quality and safety of healthcare in the United States.
3. Analyze three national initiatives driving adoption and use of health IT to improve safety and quality of care in the United States.
4. Explore two national initiatives related to promoting quality data standards in the United States.
5. Discuss the three components of the Framework for Patient Safety and Quality Research.
6. Describe how the Framework for Patient Safety and Quality Research can be used to evaluate quality and patient safety interventions.

KEY TERMS

adverse event, 411
American Recovery and Reinvestment Act, 409
Bar Code Medication Administration, (BCMA), 414
Electronic Medication Administration Record (eMAR), 414

health information technology (health IT), 409
patient safety, 409
pay for performance, 416
quality of care, 409
workarounds, 414

ABSTRACT ❖

The focus of this chapter is patient safety and quality of care in health informatics. The chapter begins by defining these concepts and by discussing key regulatory initiatives for improving the quality and safety of healthcare in the United States. The Framework for Patient Safety and Quality Research Design (PSQRD) is then introduced as a means to classify and evaluate adverse patient safety and quality events. The application of the PSQRD Framework is demonstrated with a focus on medication safety, chronic illness screening and management, and nursing sensitive quality outcomes. The chapter ends with a discussion of success factors, lessons learned, and future directions that will assist with using the PSQRD Framework as a guide for both practice and research.

INTRODUCTION

In this chapter, the use of health IT to improve quality of care and patient safety is examined. The concepts *quality of care* and *patient safety* are defined, and selected key regulatory initiatives that are driving a focus on quality of care and patient safety in the United States are discussed. The Framework for Patient Safety and Quality Research Design[1] is then introduced and used to classify adverse patient safety and quality events, discuss key success factors and lessons learned, and then make recommendations for implementation and future research.

For more than a decade, a series of Institute of Medicine (IOM)[a] reports on the quality of healthcare have led to widespread recognition that errors occur far too often and that the

---

[a]Effective July 1, 2015, the National Academy of Science, Engineering, and Medicine voted to change the name of the Institute of Medicine to the National Academy of Medicine. In March 2016, the National Academy of Sciences announced that the division of the National Academies of Sciences, Engineering, and Medicine (the Academies) that focuses on health and medicine was renamed the Health and Medicine Division (HMD) in place of the name Institute of Medicine (IOM). In this textbook, you may see any of these three names used, depending on the date of the publication or report.

BOX 24.1   **Examples of Specific ARRA Requirements for Improving the Quality of Care**

Meaningful Use Requirement	Rationale
Use of a certified EHR	Ensures that EHRs in practice have the capability of achieving the goals of Meaningful Use (e.g., they are not simply used as "word processors")
Facilitation of care coordination and quality by participating in the exchange of electronic health information	Ensures that the correct data is available to support evidenced-based care at each encounter across the healthcare continuum
Submission of data for quality reporting	To improve the quality of care in the United States, consistent data are needed to support measurement and quality improvement

quality of patient care is variable across the U.S. healthcare system.[2–7] Evidence generated from several different studies[8–10] now demonstrate that health information technology (health IT) can be used to improve communication and reduce errors.[8,9] Widespread adoption of health IT is a recommended strategy to facilitate effective, high-quality, and safe patient care.[10]

The passage of the American Recovery and Reinvestment Act (ARRA) of 2009 was expected to improve the quality of care by promoting the adoption of electronic health records (EHRs) and by supporting Meaningful Use of EHRs[11] to achieve widespread improvement in the ability to detect and reduce clinical errors.[12] Examples of specific ARRA requirements directed at improving the quality of care are included in Box 24.1.

Early data indicate that Meaningful Use was effective in promoting use of certified EHRs. As of 2014, 83% of ambulatory providers have adopted an EHR, and as of 2015, 95% of hospitals demonstrated Meaningful Use of certified health EHRs.[13] However, improved care coordination, routine exchange of electronic health information, and automated submission of quality data have not been universally achieved and will likely be the focus of future health IT related legislation.[14,15] For example, the Medicare Access and CHIP Reauthorization Act of 2015 (MACRA), which is discussed in additional detail in Chapter 27, includes several provisions related to patient safety.[16,17]

DEFINITIONS

Inconsistent use of language and variations in definitions are barriers to understanding the concepts of quality care and patient safety, as well as to benchmarking beyond the organizational level.[18] The definitions of *quality of care* and *patient safety* put forth by the IOM and the World Health

Organization (WHO) World Alliance for Patient Safety provide a solid foundation for the consistent use of these terms.

Quality of Care

In its 1990 report titled *Medicare: A Strategy for Quality Assurance*, the IOM defined quality of care as "the degree to which health services for individuals and populations increase the likelihood of desired health outcomes and are consistent with current professional knowledge."[4, p. 21] In 2001, in its report titled *Crossing the Quality Chasm*, the IOM proposed six aims as a means to narrow the quality chasm that exists in the U.S. healthcare system.[2] It proposed that healthcare should be:

- *Safe.* Prevents injury or other adverse outcomes
- *Effective.* Ensures that evidence-based interventions are used, with patients always receiving the treatments most likely to be beneficial
- *Patient-centered.* Ensures that patient preferences, needs, and values are front and center in the process of clinical decision making
- *Timely.* Delivered when needed and without harmful delays
- *Efficient.* Prevents the waste of valuable human and material resources
- *Equitable.* Provided to all individuals without regard for ethnic, racial, socioeconomic, or other personal characteristics

The WHO World Alliance for Patient Safety adopted the IOM definition of quality of care in its International Classification for Patient Safety (ICPS) released in 2009.[18]

Patient Safety

The IOM defines patient safety as "freedom from accidental injury due to medical care, or medical errors," where error is defined as "the failure of a planned action to be completed as intended or the use of a wrong plan to achieve an aim."[3, p. 4]

The ICPS defines safety as "the reduction of risk and unnecessary harm to an acceptable minimum" and patient safety as "the reduction of risk of unnecessary harm associated with healthcare to an acceptable minimum."[18, p. 21] The ICPS defines error as "failure to carry out a planned action as intended or application of an incorrect plan" and healthcare-associated harm as "harm arising from or associated with plans or actions taken during the provision of healthcare, rather than an underlying disease or injury."[18, pp. 19, 21]

These definitions highlight the multifaceted nature of quality and safety and the notion that failures of both omission (e.g., failure to provide evidence-based care) and commission (e.g., providing care incorrectly) can compromise the quality and safety of healthcare.

NATIONAL INITIATIVES DRIVING ADOPTION AND USE OF HEALTH IT

A key lesson learned from the IOM's *Quality Chasm Series* is that achievement of higher quality and safer care in the United States requires systemic redesign of established clinical processes and that health IT is needed to support and maintain the transition to best practices.[1-3,5,19,20] Several initiatives on the national level have maintained a steady focus on quality and patient safety. Recent U.S. policy is aligning incentives with the goal of adoption and widespread use of health IT to ensure a healthcare system characterized by uniform high quality and safe patient care.[21]

In 2011, the Office of the National Coordinator for Health Information Technology (ONC) published a report titled *Federal Health Information Technology Strategic Plan: 2011–2015*.[22] This report defined the ONC's plan for working with the private and public sectors to achieve the nation's health IT agenda. Specific examples of accreditation and policy efforts designed to achieve the six quality aims defined by the IOM through a focus on redesign of clinical processes and adoption and Meaningful Use of health IT are included in Table 24.1.

As of 2015, the majority of providers and hospitals adopted EHRs;[12] however, not all Meaningful Use aims were achieved, largely due to lack of interoperability.[13,14] Without interoperability, the larger vision of achieving a learning healthcare system is in peril. In response, the ONC has released its first version of its shared nationwide interoperability roadmap, *Connecting Health and Care for the Nation*, which lays out a plan to achieve interoperable of health IT and to support a functional learning health system by 2024.[23]

The ONC also released an updated *Federal Health Information Technology Strategic Plan: 2015–2020*,[14] highlighting both the achievements of Meaningful Use (e.g., widespread adoption of health IT) and those areas where the U.S. IT infrastructure is lacking (e.g., interoperability, patient-centeredness). In this report, the ONC calls on public, private,

TABLE 24.1   Accreditation and Policy Initiatives Focusing on Improving Quality of Care and Patient Safety Through Health Information Technology (Health IT)

Initiative	Description
The Joint Commission National Patient Safety Goals (NSPG)[17]	Program established in 2002 by The Joint Commission to assist accredited organizations in addressing patient safety concerns.[20] Examples of 2012 NPSG facilitated by health IT include the following: • Reduce the likelihood of patient harm associated with the use of anticoagulant therapy (NPSG.03.05.01). (1) EMR-based clinical decision support to alert and manage potential food and drug interactions, (2) use of "smart pumps" to provide consistent and accurate dosing, and (3) use of MedlinePlus to educate patients about the importance of follow-up monitoring, compliance, drug–food interactions, and the potential for adverse drug reactions and interactions. • Maintain and communicate accurate patient medication information (NPSG.03.06.01). (1) Use of an electronic medication reconciliation system to obtain information on the medications the patient is currently taking at all care transitions and (2) use of MedlinePlus to provide the patient (or family) with written information about the medications prescribed.
The Leapfrog Group[75]	Initiative led by healthcare purchasers designed to improve the quality, safety, and affordability of healthcare by reducing preventable medical mistakes.[74] Examples of 2015 Leapfrog goals facilitated by health IT include the following: • Prevent medication errors: Use of CPOE. • Avoid harm: Use of clinical decision support in EMR decision support to prevent medical mistakes. • Reduce pressure ulcers: Electronic assessment and plan of care application to link areas of risk with tailored interventions to prevent pressure ulcers from occurring. • Reduce in-hospital injuries: Electronic assessment and plan of care application to link areas of risk with tailored interventions to prevent falls and related injuries.
CMS Hospital-Acquired Conditions[9]	In response to the Deficit Reduction Act of 2006, CMS identified a list of preventable hospital-acquired conditions for which hospitals would no longer receive additional payment.[10] Examples of hospital-acquired conditions that could be prevented through use of health IT include the following: • Pressure ulcers: Electronic assessment and plan of care application to link areas of risk with tailored interventions to prevent pressure ulcers from occurring • Patient falls with injury: Electronic assessment and plan of care application to link areas of risk with tailored interventions to prevent falls and related injury • Manifestations of poor glycemic control: Use of clinical decision support in EMR for postoperative insulin dosing

TABLE 24.1 Accreditation and Policy Initiatives Focusing on Improving Quality of Care and Patient Safety Through Health Information Technology (Health IT)—cont'd

Initiative	Description
Pay for Performance (P4P)[19]	Medicare initiative designed to improve quality of care in all healthcare settings through collaboration with providers and other stakeholders to ensure that valid reliable measures of quality and determine levels of reimbursement for care provided.[22] Examples of P4P measures facilitated by health IT include the following: • Cholesterol management–LDL control <100: Patient use of self-management tools through patient portal • HbA1c control <7.0%: Patient use of self-management tools through patient portal • Implement drug–drug and drug–allergy interaction checks: Use of clinical decision support in EMR for automated interaction checking
Meaningful Use[20]	American Recovery and Reinvestment Act (ARRA) of 2009 initiative designed to provide incentives for providers and healthcare organizations to improve quality of care through meaningful use of EHRs. Examples of meaningful use of health IT performance measures include the following: • Use CPOE. • Use Emar. • Provide online access to health information to patients.[28]
National Committee for Quality Assurance (NCQA)	A nonprofit organization established in 1990 by the Robert Wood Johnson Foundation to improve the consumer's ability to evaluate health plans through voluntary public reporting.[26] The Healthcare Effectiveness Data and Information Set (HEDIS) was developed and is maintained by NCQA.
Utilization Review Accreditation Commission (URAC)	An independent, nonprofit organization that aims to promote continuous improvement in the quality and efficiency of healthcare management through processes of accreditation and education.[27]

CMS, Centers for Medicare and Medicaid Services; *CPOE*, computerized provider order entry; *EHR*, electronic health record; *eMAR*, Electronic Medication Administration Record; *EMR*, electronic medical record; *LDL*, low-density lipoprotein.

consumer, and industry stakeholders to align to achieve the federal health IT vision of high-quality care, lower costs, a healthy population, and engaged people.[14]

In discussing safety-related initiatives, the *Federal Health Information Technology Strategic Plan: 2015–2020* links to the *Health Information Technology Patient Safety Action and Surveillance Plan: June 2013.*[24] This plan addresses health IT through two objectives: (1) to use health IT to make care safer and (2) to improve the safety of health IT. In September 2014, ONC issued an update on the progress achieved by implementing the plan. "The report explains that we now have a better understanding of the types of safety events related to health IT and, more importantly, the interventions available to prevent unintended consequences of the use of health IT tools."[25] Information about this plan and continuing progress can be found at http://www.healthit.gov/policy-researchers-implementers/health-it-and-patient-safety.

Key areas of focus for ongoing accreditation and policy efforts include improving the quality of care and preventing adverse events. An adverse event is any undesirable experience associated with the use of a medical product in a patient. Evidence suggests that the United States may be making progress in the quest for higher quality and safer care, but there is much room for improvement. Cohen et al. (2015)[26] examined national trends in surgical outcomes from 2006 to 2013. They reported long-term improvement in surgical outcomes

for hospitals participating in the American College of Surgery National Surgical Quality Improvement Program. Improved outcomes included mortality, morbidity, and surgical site infections.[27] Downey et al. evaluated national trends in patient safety indicators (PSI) such as postoperative pulmonary embolism, deep vein thrombosis, and pressure ulcers. They found significant PSI trends for the decade 1998 to 2007. PSIs with the greatest levels of improvement during that period included birth trauma injury to neonates, postoperative physiologic and metabolic derangements, and iatrogenic pneumothorax. The PSIs with the greatest increase in incidence included pressure ulcers, postoperative sepsis, and infections due to improper medical care. Downey et al. noted that health IT holds potential for decreasing PSIs through standard reporting requirements and by supporting evidence-based practices through decision support and the use of order sets.[27]

NATIONAL EFFORTS RELATED TO QUALITY DATA STANDARDS

As mentioned in the previous section, the Meaningful Use initiative aimed to improve the quality of care in the United States through routine exchange of electronic health information for care delivery and quality reporting purposes. However, much work is needed to build the informatics infrastructure required to support the interoperability of systems and routine data exchange.[13,14,23] An important component of the informatics infrastructure is establishing and adopting standards at multiple levels to support semantic interoperability. Semantic interoperability means that data are exchanged without a loss of context or meaning and therefore can be reused without special effort on part of the user.[23] Semantic interoperability is only possible when all organizations adopt the same standards for quality measurement and reporting and use those standards in their electronic systems. The ultimate goal is to capture data for quality reporting in the context of existing documentation workflows. This requires that standard clinical content is adopted and used in electronic systems, standard taxonomies or vocabularies are used to encode that content, and messaging standards are used to transfer information from one healthcare organization to another.

To automatically track the quality of care, standard quality measures are needed to ensure that all organizations are using consistent metrics for benchmarking and that organizations are using the same types of data to populate the quality metrics. For data to be collected as a by-product of documentation, the standard quality metrics must define standard value sets (allowed values), taxonomies (standard terminologies), concept codes (codes assigned by the terminology developer), attributes (characteristics that provide context), and data structures, and these same standards must also be used to encode the content in the electronic record.

The ongoing work that maps (links) specific quality concepts to recommended terminologies for Center for Medicare and Medicaid Services (CMS) quality measures is published on the electronic Clinical Quality Improvement (eCQI) website. The eCQI website is coordinated by the CMS and ONC to provide the most up-to-date measures, tools, and resources for applying existing standards to specify measures electronically.[28]

Defined standards to support Meaningful Use are included in Table 24.2. As mentioned previously, representation of the complete data element set (e.g., the entire question-answer pair) by standardized terminologies and codes within an EHR system is required for full automation of quality reporting. Adoption and use of the same standards by all organizations are required for quality reporting and benchmarking beyond the organizational level. Many of these standards were included in the Stage 2 Meaningful Use initiative that aimed to provide incentives for their use in EHR systems and subsequently to provide the informatics infrastructure needed

TABLE 24.2 A Sample of Categories and Types of Data Elements Common to High-Priority Measures and Adopted Terminologies*

Data Categories	Data Types		2016 Interoperability Standards Vocabulary Standards to Support Meaningful Use
Adverse drug event	Allergy	Intolerance	National Drug File - Reference Terminology (NDF-RT)
Communication	Provider-provider	Provider-patient	
Diagnostic study	Order	Result	CPT 4/ICD-10 CM, CPT 4
Diagnosis	Outpatient (billing) Outpatient (problem list)	Inpatient	SNOMED CT/ICD-10 CM, SNOMED CT
History	Behavioral (smoking) Birth Care classification Death Enrollment trial Ethnicity/race	Language Payment source Primary care provider Sex Symptoms	SNOMED CT
Laboratory	Order	Result	LOINC
Location	Source/current/target	Transfer type	HL7 2.x ADT message
Medication	Discontinue order Inpatient administered Inpatient ordered	Outpatient duration Outpatient order Outpatient filled	RxNorm
Opt out	Other reason		
Physical exam	Vitals		LOINC
Procedure	Inpatient end Inpatient start Order	Outpatient Past history Consult results	ICD-10 CM, CPT 4

Adapted with permission from American Medical Informatics Association and based on Dykes PC, Caligtan C, Novack A, et al. Development of automated quality reporting: aligning local efforts with national standards. *AMIA Annu Symp Proc.* 2010; 2010:187-191.
*For a complete list of data elements and codes, see the 2016 Interoperability Standards Advisor at https://www.healthit.gov/standards-advisory/2016.
CPT, Current Procedural Terminology; *ICD,* International Classification of Diseases; *LOINC,* Logical Observation Identifier Names and Codes; *SNOMED,* Systematized Nomenclature of Medicine.

across the United States to collect and report quality data as a by-product of documentation. Stage 3 Meaningful Use proposes to focus on outcomes and is scheduled to begin in 2017.[29] However, recent policy changes to MACRA may affect the start date.

EVALUATING QUALITY AND PATIENT SAFETY

The foundation for the approach used to evaluate quality and patient safety in healthcare organizations in the United States is based on the work of Avedis Donabedian. Donabedian developed a framework for measuring quality based on organizational structure, processes, and their linkages to patient outcomes.[30] Donabedian's model provides the underpinnings for the framework used to assess patient safety and quality research design (PSQRD). Box 24.2 provides definitions of the primary concepts of the Donabedian model in terms of healthcare. Fig. 24.1 demonstrated the links and interactions between the concepts.[17]

Conceptual Framework for Patient Safety and Quality

The framework for PSQRD builds on Donabedian's structure-process-outcome model to support evaluation of an intervention from the preimplementation testing phase through implementation and evaluation.[17] In the case of a health IT intervention, the expanded framework supports

---

BOX 24.2 Definitions of the Primary Concepts for the Donabedian Model in Terms of Healthcare

Structure — The healthcare setting and its attributes including buildings, staffing ratios, available equipment, and the care provision budget. Includes exogenous factors not completely under the local control of a hospital or healthcare organization. Examples include:
- The Joint Commission (TJC) accreditation standards
- Meaningful Use requirements
- Accreditation, licensing, and payment directives

Process — The managerial and clinical processes in place to support the provision of care. Includes both managerial and clinical processes. Managerial process interventions have a latent effect on outcomes, as they influence communication and care practices that aim to affect patient care delivery. Clinical process interventions may have an immediate effect on patient outcomes.

Outcomes — The end result of the structures and processes in place. May include both clinical outcomes and throughput. The outcomes are often the aim of health IT and other interventions implemented to improve patient status.

---

understanding where the health IT intervention is most likely to have an effect, within the organizational causal chain of quality and safety events (see Fig. 24.1). The PSQRD framework provides a means to categorize interventions according to areas of the causal chain targeted (e.g., the structure, the management or clinical processes, and the patient outcomes or throughput targeted by the intervention or that drive adoption and use of the intervention in clinical practice).

The PSQRD framework is pertinent for evaluating the effect of health IT interventions on quality and patient safety, as it provides a means to better explain why a health IT intervention was successful (or not). There are many reasons why health IT interventions are not adopted in practice.[31,32] Health IT tools not widely adopted and used will have a limited effect on patient outcomes. In the sections that follow, we use the PSQRD framework to first evaluate health IT interventions designed to improve quality and patient safety. We then use it to make recommendations for improving the implementation and evaluation of health IT interventions aimed at enhancing quality and patient safety.

Within the PSQRD framework, quality and safety issues are not mutually exclusive entities but exist on a "vector of egregiousness" (Fig. 24.2). Quality is at one end of the vector, representing frequent events with lower levels of immediacy. Causality and patient safety are at the opposite end of the vector, encompassing more immediate events with high levels of causality. Errors or events that do not fall on or close to the vector are included within the quality–safety continuum and classified as having components of both. The PSQRD framework defines causality as "the confidence with which a bad outcome, if it occurs, can be attributed to an error" and defines immediacy as "immediate or rapid."[17, pp. 158-159] For example, there is good evidence on the population level that screening mammography decreases breast cancer mortality in women.[33,34] When an unscreened woman develops end-stage breast cancer, the adverse outcome was preventable. However, the causal link is low, and the time over which breast cancer occurs is typically not immediate or rapid.

Using this model as a framework, a hospital-acquired infection from poor hand-washing practices has a high degree of causality and a low to moderate degree of immediacy. For example, there is a lot of evidence that poor hand-washing causes infections, though there is typically a time delay between exposure and onset of the infection. Patient falls and pressure ulcers are located midway up the vector of egregiousness, with lack of tailored interventions to mitigate risk, placing patients at risk for injury with moderate degrees of causality and immediacy. Serious medication errors are higher on the vector, as they may occur due to inadequate adherence to the "five rights" for medication safety (right patient, right time, right drug, right dose, and right route). Medication errors are the most common adverse event (an unintended and unfavorable effect of medical care or treatment) in hospital settings and are largely preventable through use of health IT systems with decision support at the bedside (i.e., closed loop barcoding, medication administration, and

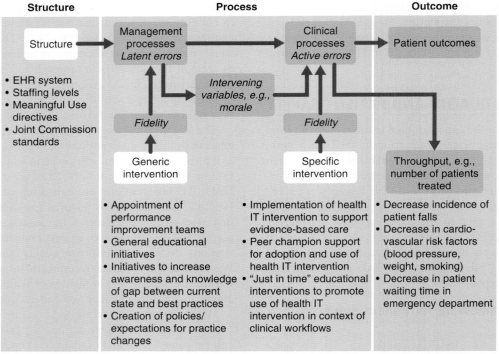

FIG. 24.1 A framework for patient safety and quality research design. *EHR*, Electronic health record. (Modified from Brown C, Hofer T, Johal A, et al. An epistemology of patient safety research: a framework for study design and interpretation. Part 1. Conceptualising and developing interventions. *Qual Saf Health Care.* 2008;17[3]:160.)

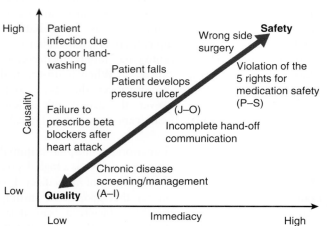

FIG. 24.2 The quality–safety continuum. (Modified from Brown C, Hofer T, Johal A, et al. An epistemology of patient safety research: a framework for study design and interpretation. Part 1. Conceptualising and developing interventions. *Qual Saf Health Care.* 2008;17[3]:159.)

smart pumps).[35] Medication errors are high on the vector of egregiousness toward safety because these types of errors are preventable through adherence to the "five rights" and, when they occur, have the potential to cause immediate and significant patient harm.

Medication Safety

Health IT systems hold promise for improving the quality and safety of care, particularly in the area of medication safety. To date, computerized provider order entry (CPOE) and clinical decision support (CDS) systems have been used successfully in clinical practice to reduce errors during the process of ordering medications.[7,8] In addition, **Bar Code Medication Administration (BCMA)** and **Electronic Medication Administration Record (eMAR)** systems have been adopted in a number of hospitals to improve patient safety and streamline clinical workflow, focusing in particular on improving administration processes at the point of care.[36-38] These systems leverage barcoding applications, with barcode labels placed on patient wristbands and on medications. The systems can ensure adherence to the "five rights" to reduce medication errors and to document administration of drugs in real time. BCMA and eMAR systems are effective when implemented and used properly.[39–41] For example, after BCMA system implementation, the scanning compliance rate is often suboptimal for scanning both drugs and patient IDs.[42,43] One study found that compliance with scanning medications was only 55.3%.[42] Another study revealed that nurses may bypass scanning processes and create workarounds to reduce workloads or prevent delay of medication administration.[41] **Workarounds** are defined as any use of an operating system outside its designed protocol.[41] This problem occurs most often in the system implementation stage

TABLE 24.3 The Joint Commission Standards and National Patient Safety Goals

	Requirements	Elements of Performance
National Patient Safety Goals (NPSG): NPSG.01.01.01	Use at least two patient identifiers when providing care, treatment, and services	Use at least two patient identifiers when administering medications, blood, or blood components; when collecting blood samples and other specimens for clinical testing; and when providing treatments or procedures. The patient's room number or physical location is not used as an identifier.
NPSG.03.04.01	Label all medications, medication containers, and other solutions on and off the sterile field in perioperative and other procedural settings*	In perioperative and other procedural settings both on and off the sterile field, label medications and solutions that are not immediately administered. This applies even if there is only one medication being used.
Medication Management: MM.06.01.01	The hospital safely administers medications	Before administration, the individual administering the medication does the following: • Verifies that the medication selected matches the medication order and product label • Verifies that the medication has not expired • Verifies that no contraindications exist • Verifies that the medication is being administered at the proper time, in the prescribed dose, and by the correct route

*Medication containers include syringes, medicine cups, and basins.
Data from The Joint Commission. National Patient Safety Goals. Effective January 1, 2015. <http://www.jointcommission.org/assets/1/6/2015_NPSG_HAP.pdf>.

and may create potential new paths to medical errors or other negative effects, such as inefficiency.[40,44]

Another important medication safety system that functions at the point of care is a smart infusion pump. Smart infusion pumps (also known as "smart pumps" or computerized patient infusion devices) include features designed to reduce administration errors and represent transformational clinical tools with the potential to greatly decrease the rate of IV medication errors in hospitals.[45] This technology provides medication error reduction capabilities via a preprogrammed drug library with dose limit alerts and audio/visual feedback to users regarding entries programmed beyond predetermined dose, concentration, and duration thresholds. Smart pumps have been widely used in the United States and other regions, and the adoption rate in the United States has doubled from 2005 to 2012.[45] The growing adoption rate corresponds with the implementation of other technologies for quality and safety improvement, such as EHRs, CPOE, and BCMA.[39] One review paper found that smart pumps could reduce programming error rates, but other types of errors may persist after implementing smart pumps (e.g., wrong drug errors, administration timing errors, and wrong patient errors).[46] A combination of smart pumps along with other clinical systems can prevent these errors, and interoperability between currently implemented clinical systems and smart pumps is key to making meaningful improvements in IV medication safety. A lack of smart pump integration with other clinical systems in practice may limit the benefit of smart pumps.

The IOM reports, The Joint Commission Standards, and the National Patient Safety Goals (NPSG) represent structural incentives for use of health IT to improve medication safety.[9,20] The Joint Commission is an international nonprofit organization that provides motivation through accreditation for healthcare organizations to excel in providing safe and effective care of the highest quality and value. The NPSG and The Joint Commission Standards relevant to medication administrations (Table 24.3) are requirements for institutions in the United States and other countries that seek The Joint Commission accreditation.

Published studies suggest that successful implementation of BCMA and eMAR systems that improve patient safety depends on several factors, including the following:[36–38]

1. A positive workplace culture (leadership, teamwork, and clinician ownership)
2. Training and support
3. Acceptance of the major impact of work practices by all team staff
4. A usable system with adequate decision support

Systems implemented using these principles can meet TJC Standards and NPSG and are likely to improve patient safety.

Chronic Illness Screening and Management

Health IT has demonstrated potential in improving the quality of care with regard to chronic illness screening and management.[47–54] As noted in Fig. 24.2, health IT interventions that target chronic illness screening and management fall on the quality end of the vector of egregiousness, with lower levels of causality and immediacy.

Examples of structural incentives for use of health IT to improve clinical processes include clinical decision support based on practice guidelines such as the U.S. Preventive Services Task Force (USPSTF) recommendations on screening for breast cancer[55] and depression,[56] pay-for-performance measures,[57] and CMS core measures.[58] Analysis of these types of external programs on process improvement and patients' outcomes suggests that the long-term effect is limited and that tailoring quality improvement programs (e.g., the management and clinical processes) based on organization-specific situations is recommended.[57]

One strategy that is successful in improving quality outcomes is the use of health IT interventions that target patients to improve access to treatment,[49] adherence with medication, diet and exercise regimens,[59,60] adherence to recommended screening guidelines,[47] and engagement in symptom management.[52] Engagement of patients using health IT is a successful strategy for improving adherence with screening and best practices management of chronic illness and improved quality outcomes.[61,62]

Nursing Sensitive Quality Outcomes: Patient Falls and Pressure Ulcers

Health IT interventions are also effective for improving quality of care and patient safety related to fall and pressure ulcer prevention.[59,63–67] The patient characteristics and factors related to risks for falls and pressure ulcers are multifaceted. For example, the patient's risks increase when skin surveillance is inadequate or when fall prevention interventions are not ordered and taught to the patient and family. As noted previously and in Fig. 24.2, patient falls and pressure ulcers are located midway on the vector of egregiousness between quality and safety, with moderate levels of causality (failure to consistently implement tailored interventions) and immediacy (time to patient fall or development of pressure ulcer). An important structural component present for hospitals in the United States was the Deficit Reduction Act of 2006, through which CMS identified a list of preventable, hospital-acquired conditions for which hospitals would no longer receive additional payment.[10] The regulations regarding nonpayment for hospital-acquired conditions included both patient falls and pressure ulcers.[10] The regulations provided an external directive (e.g., structure) that created a sense of urgency within organizations to eliminate preventable patient falls and pressure ulcers.

Management processes, including an administrative focus on fall and pressure ulcer prevention, are key factors in improving quality of care. At the organizational level, interventions such as training, the use of health IT systems for decision support, and involvement of peer champions in identifying and implementing interventions that are both feasible and effective provide an environment conducive to fall and pressure ulcer prevention.[64,67] The use of clinical experts to improve the knowledge base of nurses and other healthcare providers[59] and the use of a peer champion model[59,64,67–69]

support fidelity of both management processes (e.g., communication, importance of behavior change, advocacy for fall and pressure ulcer prevention initiatives) and clinical processes (e.g., end user training, support, modeling the intervention set on patient care units).

When implementing complex practice changes, as required for fall and pressure ulcer prevention, health IT is often a single component of a multifaceted performance improvement intervention, and leadership support for the practice change is essential. Health IT interventions are most effective when both clinical and management processes are addressed and where organizational leadership demonstrates strong support for improvement strategies.[59,64,67]

SUCCESS FACTORS AND LESSONS LEARNED

The effects of health IT interventions aimed at improving quality and patient safety using the PSQRD framework have been evaluated to identify key success factors and to provide a foundation for making recommendations for health IT implementation and future research. The PSQRD framework is useful for exploring the relationships between the organization's structural forces (e.g., setting attributes, exogenous factors) that support organizational change, including adoption and use of health IT as a tool to improve clinical processes and patient outcomes. External accreditation or regulatory requirements provide structural incentives for the changes in clinical processes that are supported by health IT interventions. The PSQRD framework expands the process component of the Donabedian model to include both management and clinical processes. The expanded process components underscore the relationship between managerial interventions, improved clinical processes, and patient outcomes. Management interventions are effective in maximizing stakeholder support for a project. An example of a management intervention is the appointment of a task force to address poor adherence with best practice guidelines. The task force is charged by management with identifying and overcoming barriers to best practice. These types of interventions improve overall adherence to practice changes and improve fidelity with health IT interventions. In addition, the PSQRD framework includes a focus on intervening variables that improve staff commitment to process changes such as incentive payments and morale.[68] Additional examples of management strategies to improve fidelity with the intervention include the use of peer champion support networks[59,70,71] and end user education.[67,68,71]

The PSQRD framework provides a means to plan for and evaluate health IT interventions designed to improve quality and patient safety. Characteristics of successful health IT implementation projects are provided in Box 24.3. The PSQRD framework is a useful guide for development of a comprehensive implementation and evaluation plan that addresses these success factors and provides an effective strategy for evaluating the effect of health IT on quality of care and patient safety outcomes.

The PSQRD framework is recommended as a guide for implementation and evaluation of health IT interventions.

BOX 24.3 Characteristics of Successful Health IT Implementation Projects Supporting Quality and Safety

Factor	Description
Leadership support	Leaders support adoption and use of health IT to improve patient care and facilitate practice changes.
Comprehensive health IT implementation and adoption strategy	Attention to both management and clinical processes to promote fidelity with the intervention.
Health IT as a "tool"	Health IT applications considered a tool or a single component of a multifaceted intervention to improve the underlying clinical processes and, ultimately, patient outcomes.
Patient engagement	Patients engaged in clinical process changes to deliver evidenced-based care, to improve safe practices, and to improve patient outcomes. Health IT is one tool to support process changes.
End user involvement	End users involved in iterative development and implementation of health IT interventions to improve quality and safety.
Peer champion support	The use of peer support to facilitate adoption and proper use of health IT applications within clinical workflows.

The PSQRD framework provides a means to introduce health IT interventions in a systematic way, and it serves as a reminder to incorporate measures of success across the causal chain. This approach supports implementation, performance improvement, and research projects with an appreciation for the effects and the limitations of health IT and other intervention components.

Adoption of the PSQRD framework for both research and organizational implementations will provide a means to plan for successful implementation and to collect data on the structural and process factors that may affect adoption and use of health IT interventions and ultimately patient outcomes. This type of measurement is appropriate for both research-based and operational implementations of health IT.

Even well-designed health IT interventions require a comprehensive plan that includes a focus on structure, management and clinical processes, and intervening variables to address fidelity with the intervention. Failure to address these factors may prevent adoption and use of health IT tools and serve as a barrier to patient safety and quality in clinical

practice. For example, Schnipper et al. describe a Smartforms application, a clinical documentation tool designed to facilitate real-time, documentation-based decision support to capture structured, coded data in the context of documentation.[72] A randomized controlled trial demonstrated a limited impact of the Smartforms on patient outcomes, because only 5.6% of eligible healthcare providers used the application.[69] Investigators summarized their lessons learned, stating that in addition to well-designed health IT tools, improvements in chronic disease management require a comprehensive approach that includes the following:

- Financial incentives (structure)
- Multifaceted quality improvement efforts (management processes including interventions to promote fidelity with the intervention)
- Reorganization of patient care activities (clinical processes) across care team members[69]

This is one example where the PSQRD framework used during project planning could have highlighted strategies to promote adoption and use of the health IT intervention and potentially led to a more significant outcome. While many frameworks exist, this chapter introduced one framework that has been successfully used; however, others are available and deserve consideration. A process of thoughtful consideration of each setting and its characteristics is needed to identify what frameworks, models, and techniques should be considered to improve the quality and safety of patient care.

CONCLUSION AND FUTURE DIRECTIONS

Medical errors and poor quality care continue to occur far too often in healthcare organizations. The evidence presented in this chapter demonstrates that the United States is making progress toward addressing suboptimal care through recognition of the problem (i.e., IOM reports), an emphasis on quality reporting, and Meaningful Use of EHRs. Health IT innovations continue to be associated with improved patient safety and quality related to chronic illness care and the prevention of patient falls, pressure ulcers, and medication errors.

Further improvements require that healthcare organizations use a comprehensive and thoughtful approach to health IT evaluation. The PSQRD framework takes into consideration the supporting structures and processes (management and clinical) that drive healthcare outcomes. This approach can facilitate adoption and Meaningful Use of health IT tools that will systematically drive patient safety and quality in clinical practice and inform effective research.

Because of the complexity of the errors in healthcare, multifaceted strategies, including evaluation frameworks and innovative health IT tools, are needed to realize additional improvement in clinical processes and patient outcomes by improving the quality and safety of healthcare.[36-38,53,54,59,63,64,69,70] Prerequisites for health IT systems that will improve quality and patient safety include strong clinical leadership and a solid informatics infrastructure. Clinical leadership characterized by technical skill, experience with managing IT projects, and a vision for the value of technology for improving patient care are associated with successful IT adoption.[73] Such attributes are needed to lead the clinical team from planning to implementation, where the optimal benefits of health IT can be realized. A solid informatics infrastructure across healthcare organizations, where standards are adopted and used by all, is vital to the improvement of safety and quality. In addition to standardized measures and benchmarks, standard clinical content used in electronic systems, standard taxonomies or vocabularies to encode that content, and messaging standards to transfer information from one healthcare organization to another are the foundational requirements for improved quality and safety of care.

The Meaningful Use initiative as well as newer legislation continues to develop standards that will create an informatics infrastructure to support quality and patient safety across the United States.[74] However, standards are often the minimum required, and much more than the minimum is necessary to advance best practices in each setting. Standards are a place to ensure quality and safety at a very basic level, but patients often define (and expect) quality at a much higher level. Moving forward, all healthcare organizations and institutions must strive to meet and exceed patient expectations of quality and safety through the adoption and use of health IT.

REFERENCES

1. Brown C, Hofer T, Johal A, et al. An epistemology of patient safety research: a framework for study design and interpretation. Part 4. One size does not fit all. *Qual Saf Health Care.* 2008;17(3):178–181.
2. Adams K, Corrigan J. *Priority Areas for National Action: Transforming Health Care Quality.* Washington, DC: Institute of Medicine; 2003.
3. Institute of Medicine. *Crossing the Quality Chasm: A New Health System for the 21st Century.* Washington, DC: Institute of Medicine; 2001.
4. Kohn L, Corrigan J, Donaldson M. *To Err Is Human: Building a Safer Health System.* Washington, DC: IOM; 1999.
5. Lohr K. *Medicare: A Strategy for Quality Assurance, Volume I.* Washington, DC: Institute of Medicine; 1990.
6. Page A. *Keeping Patients Safe: Transforming the Work Environment of Nurses.* Washington, DC: Institute of Medicine; 2004.
7. National Academies of Sciences, Engineering, and Medicine. *Improving Diagnosis in Health care.* Washington, DC: The National Academies Press; 2015.
8. Bates DW, Gawande AA. Improving safety with information technology. *N Engl J Med.* 2003;348(25):2526–2534.
9. Kaushal R, Shojania KG, Bates DW. Effects of computerized physician order entry and clinical decision support systems on medication safety: a systematic review. *Arch Intern Med.* 2003;163(12):1409–1416.
10. The Joint Commission. *National Patient Safety Goals;* 2016. http://www.jointcommission.org/standards_information/npsgs.aspx.
11. Centers for Medicare and Medicaid Services. *Hospital-Acquired Conditions (Present on Admission Indicator);* 2009. http://www.cms.hhs.gov/HospitalAcqCond/01_Overview.asp#TopOfPage.
12. Bradley R, Pratt R, Thrasher E, Byrd T, Thomas C. An Examination of the Relationships Among IT Capability Intentions, IT Infrastructure Integration and Quality of Care: A Study in U.S. Hospitals. In: *Paper presented at: 45th Hawaii International Conference on System Sciences;* 2012. Hawaii.
13. Healthit.gov. *Health IT Quick Stats;* 2015. http://dashboard.healthit.gov/quickstats/quickstats.php.
14. Agency for Healthcare Research and Quality. *A Robust Health Data Infrastructure.* Rockville, MD; 2014. AHRQ Publication No. 14-0041-EF 14-0041-EF. https://www.healthit.gov/sites/default/files/ptp13-700hhs_white.pdf.
15. Office of the National Coordinator for Health Information Technology. *Federal Health IT Strategic Plan 2015–2020;* 2015. https://www.healthit.gov/sites/default/files/federal-healthIT-strategic-plan-2014.pdf.
16. *Better, Smarter, Healthier: In Historic Announcement, HHS Sets Clear Goals and Timeline for Shifting Medicare Reimbursements from Volume to Value.* http://www.hhs.gov/news/press/2015pres/01/20150126a.html. Accessed January 26, 2015.
17. *Medicare Access and CHIP Reauthorization Act of 2015.* H.R.2. EN. http://thomas.loc.gov/cgi-bin/query/D?c114:4:/temp/~c1144daAw2::&gt.
18. Runciman W, Hibbert P, Thomson R, Van Der Schaaf T, Sherman H, Lewalle P. Towards an International Classification for Patient Safety: key concepts and terms. *Int J Qual Health Care.* 2009;21(1):18–26.
19. Aspden P, Wolcott J, Bootman J, Cronenwett L. *Preventing Medication Errors: Quality Chasm Series.* Washington, DC: National Academies Press; 2007. 463.
20. The Joint Commission. *The Joint Commission E-dition;* 2015. https://e-dition.jcrinc.com/MainContent.aspx.
21. Centers for Medicare and Medicaid Programs; electronic health record incentive program; Final Rule. *Fed Regist.* 2010;75(144).
22. Office of the National Coordinator for Health Information Technology. *Federal Health Information Technology Strategic Plan 2011 – 2015.* Washington, DC: Office of the National Coordinator for Health Information Technology; 2011.
23. Office of the National Coordinator for Health Information Technology. *Connecting Health and Care for the Nation:A 10-Year Vision to Achieve an Interoperable Health IT Infrastructure.* Washington, DC: Office of the National Coordinator for Health Information Technology; 2014. https://www.healthit.gov/sites/default/files/ONC10yearInteroperabilityConceptPaper.pdf.
24. Office of the National Coordinator for Health Information Technology. *Health Information Technology Patient Safety Action & Surveillance Plan: June 2013.* Washington, DC: Office of the National Coordinator for Health Information Technology; 2013. https://www.healthit.gov/sites/default/files/safety_plan_master.pdf.
25. Office of the National Coordinator for Health Information Technology. *ONC Health IT Safety Program – Progress on Health IT Patient Safety Action and Surveillance Plan.* Washington, DC: Office of the National Coordinator for Health Information Technology; 2014. https://www.healthit.gov/sites/default/files/ONC_HIT_SafetyProgramReport_9-9-14_.pdf.
26. Cohen ME, Liu Y, Ko CY, Hall BL. Improved Surgical Outcomes for ACS NSQIP Hospitals Over Time: Evaluation of Hospital Cohorts With up to 8 Years of Participation. *Ann Surg.* Feb 26 2015.

27. Downey JR, Hernandez-Boussard T, Banka G, Morton JM. Is patient safety improving? National trends in patient safety indicators: 1998-2007. *Health Serv Res.* Feb 2012;47(1 Pt 2):414–430.

28. Office of the National Coordinator for Health Information Technology. *The One-Stop Shop for the Most Current Resources to Support Electronic Clinical Quality Improvement;* 2015. https://ecqi.healthit.gov/.

29. Centers for Medicare and Medicaid. Medicare and Medicaid Programs; Electronic Health Record Incentive Program—Stage 3; 2015 Edition Health Information Technology (Health IT) Certification Criteria, 2015 Edition Base Electronic Health Record (EHR) Definition, and ONC Health IT Certification Program Modifications; Proposed Rules. *Fed Regist.* 2015;80 (60). 2015.

30. Donabedian A. The quality of care. How can it be assessed? *J Am Med Assoc.* 1988;260(12):1743–1748.

31. Jha AK, Bates DW, Jenter C, et al. Electronic health records: use, barriers and satisfaction among physicians who care for black and Hispanic patients. *J Eval Clin Pract.* 2009;15(1):158–163.

32. Jha AK, DesRoches CM, Campbell EG, et al. Use of electronic health records in U.S. hospitals. *N Engl J Med.* 2009;360 (16):1628–1638.

33. Moss SM, Cuckle H, Evans A, Johns L, Waller M, Bobrow L. Effect of mammographic screening from age 40 years on breast cancer mortality at 10 years' follow-up: a randomised controlled trial. *Lancet.* 2006;368(9552):2053–2060.

34. Moss SM, Wale C, Smith R, Evans A, Cuckle H, Duffy SW. Effect of mammographic screening from age 40 years on breast cancer mortality in the UK Age trial at 17 years' follow-up: a randomised controlled trial. *Lancet Oncol.* 2015;16 (9):1123–1132.

35. Garrouste-Orgeas M, Philippart F, Bruel C, Max A, Lau N, Misset B. Overview of medical errors and adverse events. *Ann Intensive Care.* 2012;2(1):2.

36. Paoletti RD, Suess TM, Lesko MG, et al. Using bar-code technology and medication observation methodology for safer medication administration. *Am J Health Syst Pharm.* 2007;64 (5):536–543.

37. Sakowski J, Leonard T, Colburn S, et al. Using a bar-coded medication administration system to prevent medication errors in a community hospital network. *Am J Health Syst Pharm.* 2005;62(24):2619–2625.

38. Yates C. Implementing a bar-coded bedside medication administration system. *Crit Care Nurs Q.* 2007;30(2):189–195.

39. Mills PD, Neily J, Mims E, Burkhardt ME, Bagian J. Improving the bar-coded medication administration system at the Department of Veterans Affairs. *Am J Health Syst Pharm.* 2006;63(15):1442–1447.

40. Patterson ES, Cook RI, Render ML. Improving patient safety by identifying side effects from introducing bar coding in medication administration. *J Am Med Inform Assoc: JAMIA.* 2002;9(5):540–553.

41. van Onzenoort HA, van de Plas A, Kessels AG, Veldhorst-Janssen NM, van der Kuy PH, Neef C. Factors influencing bar-code verification by nurses during medication administration in a Dutch hospital. *Am J Health Syst Pharm.* 2008;65(7):644–648.

42. Franklin B, O'Grady K, Donyai P, Jacklin A, Barber N. The impact of a closed-loop electronic prescribing and administration system on prescribing errors, administration errors and staff time: a before-and-after study. *Qual Saf Health Care.* 2007;16(4):279–284.

43. Koppel R, Wetterneck T, Telles JL, Karsh BT. Workarounds to barcode medication administration systems: their occurrences, causes, and threats to patient safety. *J Am Med Inform Assoc: JAMIA.* 2008;15(4):408–423.

44. Patterson E, Rogers M, Chapman R, Render M. Compliance with intended use of Bar Code Medication Administration in acute and long-term care: an observational study. *Hum Factors.* 2006;48(1):15–22.

45. Pedersen CA, Schneider PJ, Scheckelhoff DJ. ASHP national survey of pharmacy practice in hospital settings: dispensing and administration—2011. *Am J Health Syst Pharm.* 2012;69 (9):768–785.

46. Ohashi K, Dalleur O, Dykes PC, Bates DW. Benefits and risks of using smart pumps to reduce medication error rates: a systematic review. *Drug Saf.* 2014;37(12):1011–1020.

47. Atlas SJ, Grant RW, Lester WT, et al. A cluster-randomized trial of a primary care informatics-based system for breast cancer screening. *J Gen Intern Med.* 2011;26(2):154–161.

48. Cebul RD, Love TE, Jain AK, Hebert CJ. Electronic health records and quality of diabetes care. *N Engl J Med.* 2011;365 (9):825–833.

49. Knaevelsrud C, Maercker A. Long-term effects of an internet-based treatment for posttraumatic stress. *Cogn Behav Ther.* 2010;39(1):72–77.

50. Kwok R, Dinh M, Dinh D, Chu M. Improving adherence to asthma clinical guidelines and discharge documentation from emergency departments: implementation of a dynamic and integrated electronic decision support system. *Emerg Med Australas.* 2009;21(1):31–37.

51. Park MJ, Kim HS. Evaluation of mobile phone and Internet intervention on waist circumference and blood pressure in post-menopausal women with abdominal obesity. *Int J Med Inform.* 2012;81(6):388–394.

52. Ruland CM, Andersen T, Jeneson A, et al. Effects of an internet support system to assist cancer patients in reducing symptom distress: a randomized controlled trial. *Cancer Nurs.* 2013;36 (1):6–17.

53. Simon GE, Ralston JD, Savarino J, Pabiniak C, Wentzel C, Operskalski BH. Randomized trial of depression follow-up care by online messaging. *J Gen Intern Med.* 2011;26(7):698–704.

54. Saposnik G, Teasell R, Mamdani M, et al. Effectiveness of virtual reality using Wii gaming technology in stroke rehabilitation: a pilot randomized clinical trial and proof of principle. *Stroke.* 2010;41(7):1477–1484.

55. U.S. Preventative Services Task Force. *Breast Cancer Screening Draft Recommendations;* 2015. http://screeningforbreastcancer.org/.

56. U.S. Preventative Services Task Force. *Depression in Adults: Screening;* 2009. http://www.uspreventiveservicestaskforce.org/Page/Document/RecommendationStatementFinal/depression-in-adults-screening.

57. Werner RM, Kolstad JT, Stuart EA, Polsky D. The effect of pay-for-performance in hospitals: lessons for quality improvement. *Health Aff.* 2011;30(4):690–698.

58. Chassin M, Loeb J, Schmaltz S, Wachter R. Accountability measures: using measurement to promote quality improvement. *N Engl J Med.* 2010;363(7):683–688.

59. Carson D, Emmons K, Falone W, Preston AM. Development of pressure ulcer program across a university health system. *J Nurs Care Qual.* 2012;27(1):20–27.

60. Park MJ, Kim HS. Evaluation of mobile phone and Internet intervention on waist circumference and blood pressure in

post-menopausal women with abdominal obesity. *Int J Med Inform.* Jan 20 2012.

61. Shade SB, Steward WT, Koester KA, Chakravarty D, Myers JJ. Health information technology interventions enhance care completion, engagement in HIV care and treatment, and viral suppression among HIV-infected patients in publicly funded settings. *J Am Med Inform Assoc: JAMIA.* 2015;22(e1):e104–e111.

62. Bowles KH, Dykes P, Demiris G. The use of health information technology to improve care and outcomes for older adults. *Res Gerontol Nurs.* 2015;8(1):5–10.

63. Dowding DW, Turley M, Garrido T. The impact of an electronic health record on nurse sensitive patient outcomes: an interrupted time series analysis. *J Am Med Inform Assoc: JAMIA.* Jul-Aug 2012;19(4):615–620.

64. Dykes PC, Carroll DL, Hurley A, et al. Fall prevention in acute care hospitals: a randomized trial. *JAMA.* 2010;304(17):1912–1918.

65. Fossum M, Alexander GL, Ehnfors M, Ehrenberg A. Effects of a computerized decision support system on pressure ulcers and malnutrition in nursing homes for the elderly. *Int J Med Inform.* 2011;80(9):607–617.

66. Fossum M, Ehnfors M, Svensson E, Hansen LM, Ehrenberg A. Effects of a computerized decision support system on care planning for pressure ulcers and malnutrition in nursing homes: an intervention study. *Int J Med Inform.* 2013;82(10):911–921.

67. Garrett J, Wheeler H, Goetz K, Majewski M, Langlois P, Payson C. Implementing an "always practice" to redefine skin care management. *J Nurs Adm.* 2009;39(9):382–387.

68. Riggio J, Sorokin R, Moxey E, Mather P, Gould S, Kane G. Effectiveness of a clinical-decision-support system in improving compliance with cardiac-care quality measures and supporting resident training. *Acad Med.* 2009;84(12):1719–1726.

69. Schnipper JL, Linder JA, Palchuk MB, et al. Effects of documentation-based decision support on chronic disease management. *Am J Manag Care.* 2010;16(12 Suppl HIT): SP72–SP81.

70. Day R, Roffe D, Richardson K. Implementing electronic medication management at an Australian teaching hospital. *Med J Aust.* 2011;195(9):498–502.

71. Dykes P, Carroll DAH. Fall TIPS: strategies to promote adoption and use of a fall prevention toolkit. Paper presented at *AMIA Annual Symposium.* 2009.

72. Schnipper JL, McColgan KE, Linder JA, et al. Improving management of chronic diseases with documentation-based clinical decision support: results of a pilot study. *AMIA Annu Symp Proc.* 2008;1050.

73. Ingebrigtsen T, Georgiou A, Clay-Williams R, et al. The impact of clinical leadership on health information technology adoption: systematic review. *Int J Med Inform.* 2014;83 (6):393–405.

74. Office of the National Coordinator for Health Information Technology. *Interoperability Standards Advisory, Draft for Comment*; 2015. https://www.healthit.gov/standards-advisory/ 2016.

75. *The Leapfrog Group*; 2015. http://www.leapfroggroup.org/home.

DISCUSSION QUESTIONS

1. The U.S. Department of Health and Human Services Agency for Healthcare Research and Quality has identified seven Portfolios of Research. The full list can be viewed at http://www.ahrq.gov/cpi/portfolios/index.html. Two of the Portfolios of Research that are of key importance to this chapter are (1) Health Information Technology and (2) Patient Safety. Describe how these two Portfolios of Research relate to the ONC's *Health Information Technology Patient Safety Action and Surveillance Plan: June 2013* (Washington, DC: Office of the National Coordinator for Health Information Technology, 2013).

2. What is the utility of Donabedian's structure-process-outcome model as the basis for evaluating quality of care and patient safety associated with a health IT application? Describe two limitations. Discuss how the framework for patient safety and research design can be used to overcome these limitations.

3. Use the framework for patient safety and quality research design to create a comprehensive plan to support successful implementation of Bar Code Medication Administration.

4. The Office of the National Coordinator (ONC) is taking actions on health IT and patient safety as described in their *Health IT Patient Safety Action and Surveillance Plan* by *improving* the safe use of health IT, *learning* more about the impact of health IT on patient safety, and *leading* to create a culture of shared responsibility among all users of health IT. A description of this initiative is located at https://www.healthit.gov/policy-researchers-implementers/health-it-and-safety. Describe the implications of this initiative from an interprofessional prospective for either your current work setting or that of the case study presented later.

CASE STUDY

Western Heights Hospital (WHH) is a 1125-bed, 5-hospital academic healthcare system servicing central and western Massachusetts. WHH is the only designated Level I Trauma Center for adults and children in the area and is home to New England's first hospital-based air ambulance and the region's only Level III Neonatal Intensive Care Center. WHH launched a 5-year strategic plan with a fundamental goal of a system-wide move from a predominately paper environment to an electronic one. Phase I included implementation of an EHR system consisting of order entry for all laboratory, radiology, and patient care orders. Additionally, clinical documentation was implemented, including admission assessments and all nursing flow sheets. The nursing informatics counsel, a 25-member group of nurses representing all disciplines, developed the clinical content. The clinical content was custom built using both free text and structured data entry fields within the application.

Three months after go-live, hospital leadership is reporting that it is unable to report on various state and federally mandated quality measures. These measures track healthcare quality based on national standards, are compared to nationally accepted benchmarks, and are used to plan ways to improve quality. Leadership has communicated that the reports generated by the system are incomplete and are putting the hospital at financial risk due to lower reimbursement rates.

Clinicians are eager and excited to continue to develop content in the application. However, the project's program manager is proposing a stabilization and optimization approach and does not want to go forward with content development until the issue of reporting has been assessed and addressed.

Discussion Questions

1. Assuming that you are the clinical content manager and lead all reporting efforts, what approach would you take to address the reporting problem?
2. Preadmission testing data are currently collected on paper. The chief of surgery has identified an opportunity to have these data collected in the new EHR system by the preadmission testing area in the outpatient setting. Many of the collected data elements are shared with the current admission assessment. Describe how this effort can be approached. What methods can be used to implement the process?
3. Using the PSQRD methodology, identify an area of quality improvement in the hospital setting, develop a process plan, and identify the expected outcomes.

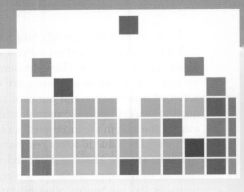

25

Legal Issues, Federal Regulations, and Accreditation

Jonathan M. Ishee, Shannon Majoras, and Robin L. Canowitz

OBJECTIVES

At the completion of this chapter, the reader will be prepared to:

1. Describe the U.S. governmental processes and structure for regulating health information technology (health IT).
2. Explain the difference between laws, regulations, and subregulatory guidance.
3. Discuss the intersection of federal fraud and abuse regulations as they relate to electronic health records (EHRs) and health IT.
4. Discuss the impact of informatics-related regulations on payment reform.
5. Outline accreditation measures and agencies in the United States.

KEY TERMS

accreditation, 422
Anti-Kickback statute, 426
donation safe harbor, 427
False Claims Act, 427
liability, 425

mHealth, 431
privacy, 423
Stark law, 426
wearable devices, 432

ABSTRACT ❖

This chapter provides (1) a brief synopsis of the legal system of the U.S. government as a basis for understanding how healthcare and specifically informatics is regulated; (2) an overview of selected laws and regulations impacting health informatics; (3) an overview of the accreditation process for healthcare entities, focusing specifically on health information systems management; and (4) insight on emerging uses of technology in the healthcare arena, with the potential for new or increased regulations.

INTRODUCTION

The U.S. healthcare system functions within the context of the legal system of the U.S. government. Healthcare, and in turn health informatics, is heavily regulated by federal and state governments. Therefore understanding health informatics-related legal issues, federal regulations, and accreditation begins with an understanding of the basic structure of the legal system in the United States.

The federal government consists of the three branches of government: legislative, executive, and judicial. Each plays a role in health IT laws and regulations. Bills (proposed laws) are passed by the U.S. legislature and become law. Administrative agencies within the executive branch implement these laws by establishing regulations or rules. Disagreements about how those laws and regulations should be interpreted are settled by the courts, the judicial branch. These judicial interpretations become precedent and are binding on future actions. Through these processes each of the three branches of the U.S. government has significant impact on the day-to-day operations within the American healthcare system and health IT. In addition to laws and regulations, many healthcare systems must also meet accreditation requirements to be eligible for participation in healthcare programs administered by the government. While there are a variety of accrediting agencies in healthcare, the two primary agencies that accredit hospitals and other healthcare-related institutions are The Joint Commission (TJC) and Det Norske Veritas (DNV) Healthcare.

LEGAL SYSTEM

Federalism and the Constitution

The government of the United States functions as a federal system. There is a distribution of power between the federal government and the state and municipal governments. The U.S. Constitution, the supreme law of the land, defines the basic composition of the three branches of government and sets forth the powers of each branch. It also provides the state governments with governing authority. State governments have their own rule-making authority and do not need to have federal approval before passing a state law. However, any laws or regulations that states pass must comply with the Constitution and be within the scope of power granted to them by the Constitution. Ultimately, the states and municipal governments are subject to both the federal government and the Constitution, despite having some autonomy.

Within the Constitution, there are two types of grants of powers, express or implied. *Express*, or enumerated powers, are powers explicitly granted to Congress. Examples of express powers include the powers to regulate interstate commerce, to create requirements for states or individuals who receive federal funding, or to levy taxes. *Implied powers* do not define the exact scope of the authority granted. An example of an implied power is the necessary and proper clause, which gives Congress the power to enact any laws "necessary and proper" to execute its responsibilities under the Constitution. Both express and implied powers have been used by Congress to implement laws that ultimately impact informatics and health IT, including Health Information Portability and Accountability Act (HIPAA), Meaningful Use requirements for EHRs, and the Patient Protection and Affordable Care Act (PPACA).

Powers expressly delegated to the federal government may not be exercised by the state governments.[1] Any law a state passes that encroaches upon the federal government's scope of authority would be preempted by the federal law, and the state law would be invalid. For example, a state could not pass a law to establish its own system to patent new health IT. The federal government alone has the power to issue patents and trademarks, so the state law would be overturned.

There are also powers that are given both to the federal government and to the state governments. These are called *concurrent powers*. For instance, both the federal government and the state government have the ability to regulate the **privacy** of personal health information in EHRs. When both the federal and the state governments have the authority to regulate a particular industry, the question of which law controls in the event that state and federal laws conflict becomes more complex. Typically, a federal law will control and preempt a conflicting state law absent special circumstances. An example of when federal law would not preempt state law occurs when a state enacts a health privacy law that provides more privacy protections than HIPAA, such as California's Confidentiality of Medical Information Act.[2]

The state and federal governments also occasionally collaborate so that laws passed in various states do not create a hostile environment for health IT nationwide where different states have conflicting regulations that make the use of health IT across states impractical. Two current examples of collaboration are the Health Information Exchange (HIE) Consensus Project and the Health Information Security and Privacy Collaboration.[3] Both of these projects seek to minimize the differences in laws and regulations between the states that govern HIE and health IT privacy and security. Regulations with different requirements in every state for the same subject matter can be burdensome to comply with for an entity that operates nationwide. It should be noted that while collaborations may produce model laws (a proposed series of laws pertaining to a specific subject), it is still up to individual state legislatures to pass legislation implementing the model law.

State governments have significant regulatory power related to healthcare and health informatics. Sometimes this power has been expressly granted to the states by the federal government through legislation, as is the case with Medicaid.[4] In other cases, the state derives their power to regulate the healthcare industry through the Tenth Amendment (that of reserved powers) and the state police power to establish laws to protect the health and safety of the public. For example, state governments may pass stricter regulations for health IT security and privacy than what the federal government mandates through HIPAA.

Federal Healthcare Regulatory Framework

The healthcare regulatory system, on a federal level, is shaped like a pyramid (Fig. 25.1). At the base, on the broadest level, are laws passed by Congress. On the next level are regulations, or rules, which are promulgated by administrative agencies.[5] Finally, at the top of the pyramid are advisory opinions and subregulatory guidance documents issued by administrative agencies.

Laws

Laws passed through Congress are often written in broad terms and establish only general objectives that must be met. For an overview of the process of passing a law through Congress, see Table 25.1. Congress does not typically provide the specific means to implement the law. As part of the legislative process, Congress may choose to delegate authority to implement those laws to the executive branch. This delegation may carry with it the power to pass separate, legally binding regulations, or rules, to facilitate compliance with the laws.

For example, Congress may pass a law that states that healthcare entities need to establish a quality control system. The law that Congress passes may not provide the specifications that such a system must meet or determine a specific timeline to implement such a system, but the law does mandate participation in the quality control program. Congress, in order to fully execute the law, turns to administrative agencies. For the executive branch of the government to assist with what would ordinarily be a legislative duty, Congress must first grant the administrative agency a specific authority to

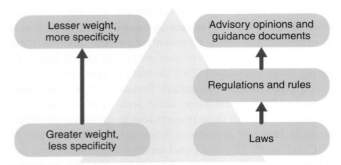

FIG 25.1 The healthcare regulatory system at the federal level.

TABLE 25.1 The Legislative Process

Bill is introduced in the Senate.	Bill is introduced in the House.
Bill is sent to committee or subcommittee for hearing, debate, and amendment. Health IT bills would typically be sent to the Senate Committee on Health, Education, Labor, and Pensions.	Bill is sent to committee or subcommittee for hearing, debate, and amendment. Health IT bills would typically be sent to the House Committee on Commerce and Energy, which has a Health Subcommittee.
Bill is sent to the floor of the Senate for a vote.	Bill is sent to the floor of the House for a vote.
Bill goes to a conference committee to reconcile the Senate and House versions of the bill to form one compromise bill.	
Compromise bill goes back to both the House and Senate floors for a vote.	
Compromise bill is sent to the president for a signature.	
If the president vetoes the bill, it may still become a law if two-thirds of Congress vote in favor of the bill.	

TABLE 25.2 Administrative Agencies

Agency	Purpose
Food and Drug Administration (FDA)	Regulates and approves new drugs and medical devices. Issues regulations about drug interactions, safe storage and handling of drugs, and counterfeiting of drugs or devices. Responsible for producing a new report proposing a new risk-based regulatory framework for health IT.
Centers for Medicaid and Medicare Services	Issues regulations for Medicaid and Medicare, including information about appropriate billing and coding. Issues the Conditions of Participation, which govern the accreditation standards. Responsible for some enforcement of Stark and Anti-Kickback laws.
Office of the National Coordinator for Health Information	Responsible for establishing programs and regulations to improve safety, quality of care, and efficiency through health IT. Establishes standards and certification criteria for EHRs.
Office of Civil Rights	Enforces HIPAA and HITECH compliance.
Department of Justice	Enforces False Claims Act and Anti-Kickback statutes.
Federal Trade Commission	Regulates development of new health IT devices. Responsible for enforcement of competition in the healthcare market.
National Labor Relations Board	Issues regulations that can govern the interaction of healthcare and social media.

EHRs, electronic health records; *FDA,* Food and Drug Administration; *HITECH,* Health Information Technology for Economic and Clinical Health.

create regulations. Once an agency has been granted authority to pass regulations under a particular law, it can begin the rule-making process.[6]

Regulations and Rule Making

The burden of creating regulations to carry out legislation often falls to the executive branch and the administrative agencies because they are more experienced than Congress in working within a particular industry or regulatory system. There are several agencies that play significant roles in regulating health IT. Table 25.2 provides several examples.

The rule-making process starts with the drafting of a proposed rule. The agency is required to submit that proposed rule for publication and a comment period. This comment period is open to anyone who might have an interest in the proposed rule. A key responsibility of health informaticians either working through their professional organizations and/or as individuals is to take advantage of this opportunity to participate in the rule-making process. Comments are generally made through a government website. The agency reads the comments and either publishes a final rule or issues another proposed rule if significant changes will be made to the initial rule. A final rule is typically published with responses to comments submitted during the proposed rule's comment period. Through its response to the comments, the agency provides some insight into how it will be enforcing the rule or what result is expected from a particular regulation. This commentary is not binding authority, but it does provide valuable information for entities looking to fulfill their obligations under newly promulgated rules. Once a final rule is passed and published, it becomes a regulation, which is legally binding.

Guidance and Advisory Opinions

In addition to rule making, agencies also provide *advisory opinions* and *guidance documents* on regulations they enforce. Advisory opinions are responses to a written request by a regulated party for an interpretation of whether its action is in compliance with a particular regulation. These advisory opinions are only legally binding on the particular entity that has asked for the opinion and involve a very narrow issue. Agencies publish advisory opinions to provide assistance and information on the application of a regulation to particular facts. These advisory opinions are another way to understand the agency's rationale behind enforcement.

Guidance documents are official agency publications designed to help subjects understand and comply with specific regulations. Guidance documents are often significant and can appear similar to rule making in their scope. Typically, guidance is issued to clarify potentially ambiguous sections of a rule or to explain how an agency intends to enforce a rule. Guidance documents are much narrower in scope than rules, and there may be several guidance documents that relate to different subsections, or even words, of a single rule.

Guidance documents may be issued by the administrative agency without a specific authorization from Congress because they are not legally binding. This means that guidance documents may be issued at any time by the administrative agency without having to comply with the formal requirements of the rule-making process. Despite their seemingly informal nature, guidance documents can sometimes have just as much impact on an industry as a rule because, in practice, agencies tend to treat the two similarly.

Enforcement

The final step of the healthcare regulatory process is enforcement. There are two possible mechanisms for regulatory enforcement. The first is through the administrative agencies that promulgate the regulations. The second mechanism is through the court system.

Administrative Enforcement

Administrative enforcement can be initiated in several ways. Oftentimes enforcement mechanisms will be built into the law or regulation. The Health Information Technology for Economic and Clinical Health (HITECH) Act, passed in 2009, called for the Office for Civil Rights to implement an audit program to evaluate compliance with HIPAA standards. Compliance issues that are identified during the audit program may then trigger an initiation of a formal investigation. Similarly, the Physician Self-Referral (Stark) law now

contains a mechanism for healthcare entities to self-disclose possible violations of the law once the entity discovers a potential compliance issue. Another way an enforcement action may be initiated is through a complaint from an individual.

Once an enforcement action has been initiated, an administrative agency investigates the allegations of noncompliance. The administrative agency investigating the complaint may be the same agency that issued the regulation, or it may be a separate agency that is generally tasked with enforcement, like the Department of Justice, the Office of the Inspector General, or the Office for Civil Rights. The agencies have the authority to enact a wide range of penalties, from monetary penalties to exclusion from participating in federal programs to a demand for corrective action. Several examples of penalties for HIPAA-related violations can be seen in Chapter 26.

Typically, an agency will negotiate and try to reach a settlement with a potentially noncompliant entity before initiating a formal proceeding. If the entity reaches a settlement agreement with the agency, there will be no finding of **liability** against the entity. However, settlement agreements may still result in monetary penalties or expulsion from federal programs.

If a settlement agreement cannot be reached, then a formal proceeding will be initiated. Once a formal proceeding is initiated, the entity has a right to have a hearing in front of an administrative law judge if monetary penalties are involved. An administrative law judge is a decision maker who is independent from the agency and has authority under the agency's procedural rules to issue a binding decision. An administrative proceeding in front of an administrative law judge is typically less formal and less strict procedurally than a comparable proceeding in front of a federally appointed judge. The exact nature of the proceedings will be governed by the agency's rules. Once a final decision is issued, a formal appeal of the decision is permitted. Generally, before the appeal may go before a federal court, it must be appealed through the agency, usually in front of a review board.

Court System

An enforcement proceeding may also be initiated in the federal court system, either at the beginning of the process or as an appeal of an administrative decision. If the allegations involve a criminal indictment, then the proceedings must be started in the federal court system. The federal court system is composed of three levels of courts. A case is initially brought in a district court. If a case is appealed, it is appealed to the circuit court that oversees the district court. It is possible to petition for an appeal from the circuit court to the Supreme Court through a writ of certiorari, but the Supreme Court hears very few appeals during a year because it has the sole discretion whether to grant any particular appeal.

A court proceeding is more formal than an administrative proceeding. In addition, a court proceeding and an administrative proceeding may follow different procedural rules. Another important difference between a court and an administrative hearing is the length of time it takes to reach a decision. Bringing an action in a federal court generally takes much longer to resolve than would be the case in an administrative proceeding.

A court and an administrative proceeding are functionally equivalent. The federal court judge and the administrative law judge have the same remedies available in the event that the entity is found guilty of noncompliance. The administrative law judge and the federal court judge issue binding decisions, although there is an additional route to appeal if the decision is issued in an administrative proceeding as opposed to a federal court proceeding.

FRAUD AND ABUSE AND BILLING ISSUES RELATED TO ELECTRONIC HEALTH RECORD USE

Although the federal government has incentivized the use of EHRs, there are pitfalls for the unwary user. EHRs can make some clinical documentation easier for users, but use of an EHR can lead to fraud and abuse claims by the federal government that may include hefty fines and jail time if violations are proven. Chief among the potential pitfalls are EHR purchase transactions. EHR systems are expensive. Hospitals and health systems are usually able to cover these expenses within their budget, but it is often financially difficult for independent practitioners including medical group practices to purchase these systems. The systems purchased by these practitioners need to be interoperable with other healthcare entities such as hospitals, long-term care, laboratories, and other healthcare institutions. It may seem logical for these practitioners to approach hospitals, laboratories, and other large corporations to ask them to help fund these purchases. However, legal and regulatory hurdles must be understood and purchasers need to be wary before moving forward with these types of transactions.

In the area of fraud and abuse, there are three laws that should be considered before providers purchase EHR systems—the Stark law, the federal Anti-Kickback statute, and the federal False Claims Act (FCA). It is important to have a general understanding of what these laws prohibit, and to examine transactions related to and within the EHR while keeping these laws in mind.

Stark Law

The Stark law, passed in 1992, is named after its sponsor, U.S. Congressman Peter Stark. It is a combination of statutes and regulations that were promulgated in three phases.[7] The Stark law governs physician self-referral for Medicare and Medicaid patients.[8] This law generally prohibits a physician from referring patients for certain designated health services (DHS) to entities with whom the physician has a financial relationship. DHS includes following services (other than those provided as emergency physician services furnished outside of the United States):

- Clinical laboratory services
- Physical therapy services
- Occupational therapy services
- Outpatient speech-language pathology services
- Radiology and certain other imaging services
- Radiation therapy services and supplies
- Durable medical equipment and supplies
- Parenteral and enteral nutrients, equipment, and supplies
- Prosthetics, orthotics, and prosthetic devices and supplies
- Home health services
- Outpatient prescription drugs
- Inpatient and outpatient hospital services.[9]

The Stark law's central tenet is that there is a conflict of interest created when referring physicians or their families can benefit from the referral. It is believed that allowing self-referrals encourages over-utilization of services, increasing healthcare costs. Therefore healthcare providers must be careful when they enter into business relationships with family members, or with companies where the physician has a financial interest.

There are two types of financial relationships that trigger the Stark law. The first is when there is physician or family "ownership or investment interest" in the entity furnishing the DHS.[10] The second type of arrangement is a compensation arrangement with the physician or the physician's immediate family.[11] This relationship can be either direct or indirect. The only way to avoid the requirements of Stark is to fall under an exception or a "safe harbor." The penalties for not complying with the Stark law are discussed in more detail later, but may include civil monetary penalties, denial of payment, or exclusion from the federal healthcare program.

Federal Anti-Kickback Statute

The federal Anti-Kickback statute is a criminal statute that prohibits the exchange or offer to exchange anything of value in an effort to induce referral of a federal healthcare program beneficiary.[12] Because this is a criminal statute, the government must prove its case beyond a reasonable doubt. A typical situation where a violation of the Anti-Kickback statute might occur is when physicians lease space within their office to another provider who is in a position to refer business to the landlord physician. Another situation often arising in the Anti-Kickback context is when physicians receive remuneration from a drug company when they are in a position to prescribe a drug manufactured by that company. In the EHR context, the Anti-Kickback statute could be triggered when a hospital or other healthcare provider offers to purchase or to help fund an EHR for a provider who refers patients to the hospital or other healthcare provider for testing, surgery, lab work, or other clinical services.

The statute requires a knowing and willful offer of payment, solicitation, or receipt of any remuneration to induce someone to refer patients or to purchase, order, or recommend any item of service that may be paid for under a federal healthcare program.[13] The PPACA added a provision clarifying the intent requirement of the Anti-Kickback statute. Under the PPACA, actual knowledge of an Anti-Kickback statute violation or the specific intent to commit a violation of the Anti-Kickback statute is *not* necessary for conviction under the statute.[14]

Remuneration and inducement generally involve exchanges that are direct or indirect, overt or covert, or cash or in kind. The threshold for triggering the Anti-Kickback statute is low. "If one purpose of the payment was to induce future referrals, the Medicare statute has been violated."[15]

The penalties for violating the Anti-Kickback statute apply to those on both sides of the transaction. A single violation can result in a fine of up to $25,000 and up to 5 years imprisonment. Additionally, a violation can result in mandatory exclusion from the federal healthcare program. The government may also assess civil monetary penalties, which could result in treble damages plus an additional $50,000 for each violation.[16]

Safe Harbors

The Office of Inspector General and the U.S. Department of Health and Human Services (HHS) have been given the authority to adopt safe harbors that protect against criminal and civil prosecution for Stark and Anti-Kickback violations in certain situations. To qualify for safe harbor protection, the arrangement must cover all parameters of the safe harbor as written. There are common criteria that must be met to meet safe harbor requirements under the Anti-Kickback statute. These generally include the following:

- Written and signed agreements are in effect for more than 1 year.
- Agreement specifies all services, products, and space to be provided.
- Agreement specifies part-time intervals and/or charges.
- Payment is set in advance, is fair market value, and does not take into account the volume or value of referrals.
- Agreement terms do not exceed commercially reasonable terms.
- Agreement does not involve counseling or promotion of illegal activity.

Health and Human Services Donation Safe Harbor

In 2006, a donation safe harbor exception was created, allowing certain referral recipients to donate an EHR system to referral sources. This safe harbor was originally scheduled to end in 2014 but was revised and extended until 2021.[16] It was designed to facilitate physician adoption of EHR technology, as many physician practices were unable to purchase and support the technology due to its high cost.

Under this exception, a donor may donate EHR technology and services to persons in a position to refer to the donor. The donor may only pay up to 85% of the cost to purchase and implement the technology. This allows hospitals and other large healthcare entities to transfer or assist with the purchase of EHRs for physicians and other practices that refer patients to them at a large discount without violating Stark or the Anti-Kickback statute. Under the latest iteration of the safe harbor, laboratory providers are not allowed to donate EHR technology. In order to qualify for the safe harbor, the

TABLE 25.3 Electronic Health Record Donation Safe Harbor

Type of Expense	Hospital or MA Donor	Physician Recipient
Software (includes training costs and internet connectivity)	85%	15%
Hardware	0%	100%

Additional Requirements:
Donor cannot finance any portion of the costs required to be paid by the physician.
Donor cannot impose any additional requirements that would hinder the software being interoperable with other community providers.

EHR, electronic health record; *MA,* Medicare Advantage.

EHR must meet current EHR certification criteria as of the date of the donation. This means the EHR must be certified by a certifying body authorized by the National Coordinator for Health IT. This certification process is further explained in Chapter 19. Table 25.3 includes the basic safe harbor requirements.

False Claims Act

The False Claims Act (FCA) imposes civil liability on any person who submits a claim to the federal government that he or she knows or should know to be false, and imposes certain monetary penalties for violations of the act. The FCA essentially prohibits fraudulent or false claims submitted to the government for payment and also fraudulent or false claims that would decrease an amount owed to the government. Monetary penalties are imposed by the FCA, including a penalty of three times the amount of the claim submitted to the government for payment plus $11,000 per claim.[17] In the healthcare arena, the FCA creates an issue with EHRs because each clinical encounter generates a bill. If that bill is not accurate and is sent to a governmental payor (such as Medicare, Medicaid, or the military's health insurance program [Tricare]) for payment, it is considered a false claim. This can present an added challenge with coding systems being changed, such as the recent move from International Classification of Diseases (ICD)-9 to ICD-10. Each individual bill would be a separate violation of the FCA, and the fines and penalties can add up very quickly. No intent to defraud the government is required to violate the law. Although the statute uses the word "knowingly," it does not require that a person submitting a claim have actual knowledge that the claim he is submitting is false. Acting in reckless disregard, or in deliberate ignorance of the truth or falsity of the information, can also lead to liability under the statute.[18]

The PPACA expanded the scope of the FCA. Medicare and Medicaid providers may discover that they have received payment on a mistaken claim that they submitted to Medicare or Medicaid. The claim may have been improperly coded, or there was a clerical error, resulting in an overpayment to the provider. Under the PPACA, a provider receiving a Medicare overpayment has 60 days to report and return the money before facing civil charges once the overpayment has been identified, or reasonably should have been identified.[19] If providers retain overpayments past the 60-day deadline, this creates an "obligation" under the FCA, and the provider faces liability under the FCA as well. Each individual overpayment is a separate false claim and triggers the penalties and fines discussed previously. When an overpayment situation occurs, it is very important to act quickly to return the money to the government to avoid the FCA fines and penalties.

Private citizens may also bring suits to enforce the FCA. These suits are called *Qui Tam* suits, and the person who brings them is referred to as the *Qui Tam* relator. These *Qui Tam* relators can potentially recover a portion of any judgment or settlement. The U.S. Department of Justice reviews all cases brought by *Qui Tam* relators and determines whether the government should join in the lawsuit. When the government joins, the amount that is recoverable by the *Qui Tam* relator is diminished but is still significant.

In addition to civil penalties,[20] the federal government can also prosecute and fine those engaging in healthcare fraud from a criminal perspective. An example of this is the general Healthcare Fraud statute. This statute provides that any person who knowingly and willfully executes, or attempts to execute, a scheme or artifice to (1) defraud any healthcare benefit program, or (2) obtain, by means of false or fraudulent pretenses, representations, or promises, any of the money or property owned by, or under the custody or control of, any healthcare benefit program in connection with the delivery of or payment for healthcare benefits, items, or services shall be fined under this title or imprisoned not more than 10 years, or both.[21] It is important to note that this criminal statute applies to any healthcare payor, public or private, and is not just limited to federal healthcare programs. Additionally, there is a criminal FCA statue that can be used against healthcare providers, but unlike the general healthcare fraud discussed previously, the criminal FCA only applies to a claim for payment from the federal government.[22]

Wire/Mail Fraud

Mail fraud and wire fraud are additional issues that need to be considered during claims submission by providers. Mail fraud includes healthcare fraud that occurs through use of the U.S. mail system or common delivery services such as FedEx or UPS. Mail fraud can occur when paper claims with improper coding are sent to patients or their insurers. If these paper-based claims for payment contain fraudulent information, charges of criminal mail fraud can be brought against the provider.[23]

Improper computerized claims submission can lead to charges of wire fraud. The statute addressing wire fraud provides criminal penalties for devising a scheme to defraud or "for obtaining money or property by means of fraudulent or false pretenses."[24] Wire fraud involves interstate use of wire, radio, or TV communication to commit fraud, and would clearly encompass computerized claim submission.

Each claim submitted would create a separate count of wire fraud. Both mail and wire fraud are punishable by fines of up to $1000 and up to 5 years imprisonment per violation. For example, assume a physician upcoded 50 claims and submitted those claims electronically to Medicare via the EHR billing module. In addition to the civil penalties any physicians would face through the FCA, they may face criminal charges for 50 counts of wire fraud and one or more counts of Medicare fraud.

Fraud and Abuse and the Electronic Health Record

Each entry in an EHR helps determine what a healthcare provider will bill to an insurer or to Medicare or Medicaid. When these entries are inaccurate, fraudulent billing may occur. Each time a fraudulent claim is submitted to a government payor, there is a separate claim of fraud the government can make. Therefore it is very important that those who use EHRs are educated regarding steps they can take to ensure that fraud does not occur.

Healthcare fraud can include such things as billing for services not rendered, billing for services that were unnecessary, or unbundling services that are generally billed as one Current Procedural Terminology (CPT) code in order to increase revenue. Over-documentation is the practice of inserting false or irrelevant documentation to create the appearance of support for billing at a higher level of service. Some EHRs autopopulate fields when using templates that may be inaccurate if not appropriately edited. For example, if a provider pulls up an order set for a particular diagnosis and several of the orders are pre-checked, including some procedures that have already been performed, this may lead to additional testing that is not necessary.

Most EHRs allow providers to create macros and templates for documentation. These macros and templates should be edited each time they are used to accurately reflect what occurred at each visit. Providers often do not take the time to edits these templates. For example, pediatricians may have a template they use for an adolescent well-child visit. The template may say that a mental health screening was done when it was not done at a particular visit. The physician then bills for the mental health screening, resulting in fraudulent billing. Features in the EHR resulting in over-documentation to meet reimbursement requirements can cause problems for providers when the services were not medically necessary or were not delivered.

One of the biggest fraud and abuse issues the government is targeting within the EHRs is the use of copy and paste functionality. When used appropriately, copy and paste can be a valuable tool. However, it can also result in creating a flawed medical record that could result in poor patient care. Consider a situation where the phrase "family history of breast cancer" is copied and pasted into a medical record as "history of breast cancer." This history is then reviewed by providers on each additional visit, which could lead to unnecessary care and testing that would not otherwise be needed by this patient.

The Centers for Medicare and Medicaid Services (CMS) published a toolkit that advises providers about ways they can ensure EHR fraud and abuse detection. Some of their key recommendations are as follows:[25]

- Providers should purchase systems that incorporate anti-fraud features.
- Software should have operational audit logs that always remain operational.
- Systems should have the ability to show who modified a record and when.
- Providers utilizing EHRs should have robust compliance programs that include standards of conduct that ensure that employees act in an appropriate and lawful manner.
- Employees should be trained regarding risks associated with EHRs. The training should emphasize the importance of accurate record-keeping and the potential criminal and disciplinary issues that can arise if there are issues with the integrity of the health record.
- Providers should audit their EMRs or EHRs to ensure that audit logs are functioning appropriately and users are appropriately utilizing the system. Fraud detection software is available to perform pattern matching that would identify text that is cloned or copied from other sections. Unusually high usage of these features should be addressed with employees. If issues are identified, an appropriate investigation should occur.

A 2013 report issued by the Department of HHS Office of Inspector General found that most hospitals with EHR technology had audit functions in place, but not all were using them to the full extent.[26] This report noted that although most hospitals were analyzing audit log data, their efforts were aimed at HIPAA privacy issues, and not on the prevention of fraud and abuse.

It is important for those who are utilizing EHRs to recognize and understand the risks they face related to fraudulent billing. Audit controls should be in place to help providers ensure that the records they are creating are accurate.

State Law

In addition to federal law, each state has its own laws regarding fraud and abuse in the healthcare system. When providers are billing their states through Medicaid, they must also be cognizant of their local laws related to fraud and abuse, and how those laws might impose civil or criminal penalties on unwary healthcare providers.

ACCREDITATION

CMS has designated TJC and DNV as third-party agencies able to accredit hospitals for participation in Medicare and Medicaid programs.[27,28] TJC and DNV each have separate accreditation programs, but both accreditation programs use the Medicare Conditions of Participation as baseline requirements in order for hospitals to achieve accreditation.[29] TJC uses a survey and audit program called TJC Standards that it developed specifically for the healthcare industry. It provides more detailed, care-based requirements that a hospital must satisfy.[30] Additionally, TJC provides guidance

documents on the implementation of its care requirements and publishes alerts and recommendations for coping with new issues that may impact the quality of patient care in the future.[31]

DNV uses the National Integrated Accreditation for Healthcare Association Organization program, which evaluates hospitals based on compliance with the Medicare Conditions of Participation and the International Organization of Standard's (ISO) 9001 Quality Management Program, an internationally recognized quality control program that is used across many industries.[32] DNV does not set specific care-based requirements, instead requiring only the satisfaction of the Medicare Conditions of Participation. It then uses the ISO 9001 program to evaluate other quality metrics.

While both TJC and DNV offer accreditation programs, only TJC provides a specific health information management chapter.[33] DNV addresses health IT only through the broader Medicare Conditions of Participation. The remainder of this section will take a closer look at TJC standards and its specific recommendations for health information management.

The Joint Commission Health Information Management Standards

TJC has developed a specific chapter of its accreditation standards dealing with information management. The goal of TJC's information management standards is to ensure that healthcare providers have a well-planned information management system that assists practitioners with the provision of safe and high quality care. There are four primary categories of responsibilities a hospital will have to address in order to ensure full performance of the TJC Standards for information management:

1. Planning for management of information,
2. Using health information,
3. Using knowledge-based information, and
4. Monitoring the data and health information process.

Included within those broader categories are provisions for protecting the privacy of health information and managing the capture, storage, and retrieval of health data.

Each larger category is divided into separate elements of performance that TJC uses to evaluate hospitals' compliance when it performs accreditation surveys. The elements of performance are specific actions that a hospital must take to satisfy the overall standard. For example, within the planning for management of information category, elements of performance include the organization identifying the information needed to provide quality, safe care; the organization identifying how data and information will flow through the organization; the organization using that identified information to develop a process to manage information; and staff and practitioners participating in the assessment, integration, and use of information management systems in the delivery of care. In other examples, elements of performance related to patient privacy and security of patient information track the HIPAA standards, requiring specific privacy and security policies and procedures to be in place. For a summary of TJC's standards relating to information management, see Table 25.4.

TABLE 25.4 The Joint Commission Information Management Accreditation Standards

Category	Examples of Standard
Planning for Management of Information	Organization plans for managing information. Organization plans for continuity of its information management processes.
Using Health Information	Organization protects the privacy of health information. Organization protects the security and integrity of health information. Organization effectively manages the collection of health information. Organization retrieves, disseminates, and transmits health information in useful formats.
Using Knowledge-Based Information	Knowledge-based information resources are available, current, and authoritative.
Monitoring Data and Health Information Processes	Organization maintains accurate health information.

From The Joint Commission. Information Management. *2016 Comprehensive Accreditation Manual for Ambulatory Care (CAMAC).* Accessed August 1, 2016.

During an accreditation survey, TJC surveyors evaluate the hospitals on each element of performance to determine whether the overall standard is met. Every element of performance is given a scoring category, and the elements of performance are ranked based on the threat to patient safety and quality of care.[34] Whether or not a hospital fails to meet the standard for accreditation, based on its failure to meet an element of performance, depends on the particular nature of an incomplete element of performance.

Sentinel Event Alerts

The TJC also issues Sentinel Event Alerts, describing potential hazards to the quality of care and patient safety. TJC will identify actions that may serve to minimize the risk associated with those hazards. Since 2008 TJC has issued two major Sentinel Event Alerts related to health IT.

The earlier of the two, Sentinel Event Alert 42, was issued in December 2008.[35] In Alert 42, TJC identified the two primary factors that led to preventable adverse events related to, or caused by, health IT. The first factor was the human–machine interface and the second was the overall organization and design of the health IT system. Contributing to these factors was a general failure to perform adequate due diligence before investing in and implementing health IT—including failing to involve practitioners in the discussion on the best

uses of and the care-related needs for health IT, an overreliance on vendor advice regarding health IT, and an inability to integrate feedback from providers into the end user experience. TJC advised hospitals to take more time to receive input from providers before investing into any health IT, to continuously monitor the use of the health IT, and to implement adequate training programs prior to initiating the use of any new IT programs.

Sentinel Event Alert 54 was issued in March 2015.[36] This alert built upon the conclusions of Alert 42. Again TJC found that the use of health IT had inherent risks for preventable adverse events after they analyzed over 3375 adverse events reports. TJC identified eight areas of weakness that contribute to adverse events within health IT. The three largest areas of weakness came from (1) the human-computer interface (a full one-third of health IT–related events), (2) workflow and communication issues relating to health IT support, and (3) design issues related to clinical content and decision support. To understand more about health IT design, usability, and interaction outcomes, readers are referred to Chapter 21. To help resolve these issues, TJC recommended action through three pathways.

The first pathway is an increased culture of safety. A safety-minded culture includes active internal reporting and identification of possible health IT hazards. In addition to internal reporting, hospitals should not hesitate to make reports to external organizations, such as patient safety organizations, to reduce the aggregate risk throughout the healthcare system. The focus in reporting should be identifying risks rather than apportioning blame to individuals involved in any adverse events. Hospitals should also conduct an analysis of any adverse event to determine if health IT had been involved in the adverse event. Any analysis or identification of an adverse event or risk of an adverse event should be communicated globally, including with vendors, so that the overall hazard related to health IT is decreased.

The second pathway is process improvement. This involves implementing strategies to make the health IT programs themselves safer and free from malfunction, as well as using the health IT programs to monitor patient safety. TJC recommends using the SAFER (Safety Assurance Factors for EHR Resilience) guides, an EHR checklist produced by the ONC to address the safety of the installed IT programs. The SAFER checklist includes items such as backing up hardware systems, conducting extensive testing of systems before implementation, and using standardized codes across all platforms. TJC also recommends ensuring that providers and other health IT users have adequate training on the use of IT programs and that IT programs are structured to be user-friendly and to minimize the effect of human error.

The third and final pathway is through hospital and facility leadership. The leadership of the hospital should encourage the culture of safety and responsibility related to potential adverse events caused or contributed to by health IT. The identification and reporting of adverse events should be done in a manner to encourage reporting and not assign blame. Additionally, leadership should be proactive in engaging health IT users to provide feedback and recommendations for improvements to IT interfaces and hazard identification. Furthermore, leadership should be proactive about evaluating IT programs for safety risks and inefficiencies. If leadership believes a change to IT programs is in the best interest of patient safety and quality of care, any modifications or improvements to the system should be implemented only after appropriate due diligence and training of all end users.

THE INTERSECTION OF NEW TECHNOLOGY AND REGULATION

The explosion of mobile health (mHealth) technology and consumer-driven health applications has taxed an outdated regulatory framework that was never designed for these new types of technologies. This section presents a discussion of the current regulatory framework and recent efforts to update this framework, given the impact of exploding innovate technology in healthcare. Currently, no one agency is tasked with regulating health IT or applications. Regulatory authority is spread over agencies such as the Food and Drug Administration (FDA), Federal Trade Commission (FTC), state medical boards, Federal Communications Commission (FCC), CMS, and the Office of the National Coordinator (ONC) for health IT.

Medical Devices

The FDA has authority over the Food Drug and Cosmetic Act (FDCA). As the title of the FDCA suggests, the FDA generally has regulatory authority over foods, drugs, cosmetics, herbal supplements, and medical devices (including certain health IT and embedded medical device software). The FDA is also tasked with assuring the safety and effectiveness of medical devices. Specifically, Section 201(h) of the Act defines a "Device" as

> ... an instrument, apparatus, implement, machine, contrivance, implant, in vitro reagent, or other similar or related article, including a component part, or accessory which is: recognized in the official National Formulary, or the United States Pharmacopoeia, or any supplement to them, intended for use in the diagnosis of disease or other conditions, or in the cure, mitigation, treatment, or prevention of disease, in man or other animals, or intended to affect the structure or any function of the body of man or other animals, and which does not achieve its primary intended purposes through chemical action within or on the body of man or other animals and which is not dependent upon being metabolized for the achievement of any of its primary intended purposes.[37]

Table 25.5 illustrates the various classes of medical devices and FDA oversight.

Initially it appears the FDCA regulates any type of health IT since the majority, if not all, of health IT is intended to be used "in the diagnosis of disease or other conditions, or in the cure, mitigation, treatment, or prevention of disease, in man."[38] However, FDA has taken a risk-based approach

TABLE 25.5 Food and Drug Administration Classes of Medical Devices

	Class I	Class II	Class III
Patient safety risk	Low	Medium	High
FDA requirements	General controls	General controls and special controls	General controls and premarket approval
Percentage of medical devices that fall into this category	47%	43%	10%
Examples	Dental floss	Power wheelchair	Replacement heart valve

FDA, Food and Drug Administration.

and not exercised its authority over certain health information technologies such as EHRs, even if such EHRs have computer decision support (CDS) or computerized physician order entry (CPOE) functionality.

Congress passed the Food and Drug Administration Safety and Innovation Act (FDASIA) in 2012 in recognition of the need for federal agencies to work together to come up with a new regulatory framework related to emerging health IT.[39] Specifically, Section 618 of the FDASIA required that the FDA in consultation with ONC and FCC create "a report that contains a proposed strategy and recommendations on an appropriate, risk-based regulatory framework pertaining to health IT, including mobile medical applications, that promotes innovation, protects patient safety, and avoids regulatory duplication."[38] In issuing its final report, the agencies divided health IT into three categories: (1) administrative health IT functions, (2) health management health IT functions, and (3) medical device health IT functions, with corresponding recommendations on each.[40]

The report suggests no additional FDA oversight on technology primarily engaged in administrative health IT functions, and no increased oversight activities for technology classified as a medical device serving a health management health IT function outside of the FDA's current focus "on medical device health IT functionality, such as computer aided detection software, remote display or notification of real-time alarms from bedside monitors, and robotic surgical planning and control."[40] The report recommended setting up a Health IT Safety Center in which federal agencies could convene stakeholders to discuss patient safety issues and the other topics described in Fig. 25.2. Since the report does not recommend that the FDA regulate any new technologies that are not currently the focus of FDA regulation, the practical results of the recommendation is that new consumer-focused mHealth technologies discussed later are in effect unregulated from a patient safety standpoint.

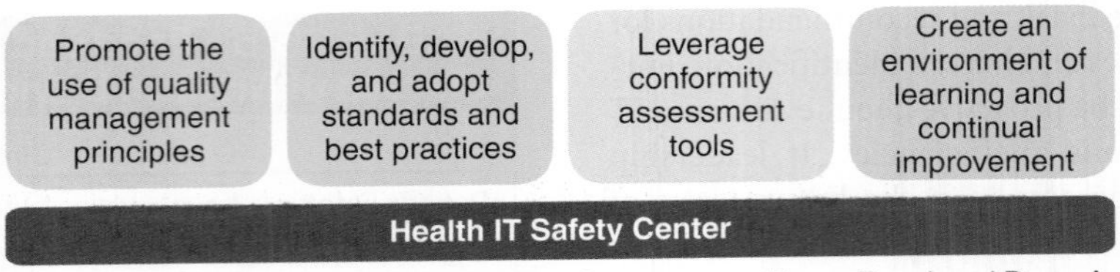

Promote the use of quality management principles	Identify, develop, and adopt standards and best practices	Leverage conformity assessment tools	Create an environment of learning and continual improvement

Health IT Safety Center

FIG 25.2 FDASIA recommendation for health IT safety center. (From Food and Drug Administration Safety and Innovation Act, Pub. Law 112-144.)

mHealth Wearable Devices and Telehealth

The development and use of mHealth applications and wearable devices has exploded with the advent of smartphones and broadband cellular technology. Patients can now open an application on their phone and be immediately connected to a physician for treatment, or ask the mHealth app a question about a health issue and be immediately given an answer, including a course of treatment. Some insurers now provide premium discounts to individuals who use wearable devices and agree to share the information collected with the insurer. While these applications provide convenience to patients, they also raise potential regulatory and liability issues.

As discussed previously, regulators seem to have taken a hands-off approach when it comes to mHealth applications and wearable devices. This perception was reinforced in January 2015 when the FDA issued draft guidance titled "General Wellness: Policy for Low Risk Devices."[41] This guidance reaffirmed the idea that the FDA generally will not regulate wearable devices used for general wellness under the FDCA. The FDA uses a two-part test in determining whether a wearable device is a low-risk general wellness product and not subject to regulation: (1) the project makes only general wellness claims, and (2) the product does not present inherent risks to a user's safety. Under the first part of the test, the FDA examines whether the device is designed and intended to maintain healthy lifestyles or promote healthy activities and does not make any reference to diseases or conditions unless it is well understood that healthy lifestyle choices may help reduce the risk of or help living with a certain disease or condition (such as making a claim that a wearable device will cure or mitigate diabetes). If a device uses an intervention or technology that requires device controls such as implants or raises novel questions of biocompatibility, the second part of the two-part test may trigger FDA scrutiny. Many mHealth applications have the functionality of connecting a patient in real time to a physician who may be physically located in a different state and may not be licensed in the same state of the patient. Some states like California require all physicians who provide telehealth services to California residents hold an active, unrestricted California Medical License or face the potential charge of the unauthorized practice of medicine.[42] Other jurisdictions such as the District of Columbia have more flexibility for physicians licensed out-of-state to provide telehealth services to District of Columbia residents.[43] Finally, some jurisdictions such as Texas allow for a limited scope telehealth license for specialist consults[44] but require some type of preexisting relationship between the physician and patient before a remote telehealth visit can occur.[45] For more traditional telehealth applications, interstate licensure issues continue to be a challenge to the broader use of this form of health IT. For a more detailed discussion of telehealth challenges, see Chapter 8.

Privacy and Ownership of Data Collected by mHealth and Wearable Devices

The privacy of health data that is collected by mHealth applications and wearable devices is also an issue of intense debate. Since these applications are not covered entities under HIPAA, there is no healthcare specific federal prohibition on the collection, use, and disclosure of personal health information that is collected by the app. Recently, the FTC has recognized the need for more transparency regarding how information collected by mobile applications is used by application developers and has published some subregulatory guidance on this issue, but such guidance does not have the force of law.[46] This does not mean that there are no regulations related to the privacy of data collected by these types of applications and devices. Some state privacy laws expand the prohibition of the collection and use of personally identifiable information related to health information, but most states do not have these types of protections.[47]

Another unresolved issue involves the ownership of data collected by mHealth applications and wearable devices in the era of big data and the data analytics. The data collected by these devices are valuable to both the developer of the device or application and to third parties such as researchers or pharmaceutical companies.[48] This has led many developers to monetize the sale of aggregated data to third party researchers as part of the developer's business plan. Patients should read the terms and conditions that accompany a particular device before use to determine whether the device manufacturer will share users' personal information with third parties.

Liability Issues

Finally, only mHealth applications that are regulated by the FDA are those considered medical devices, such as electrocardiograms or physiologic monitoring. The majority of the more than 165,000 available health apps are generally not considered medical devices, and they are not regulated by the FDA (or any other federal agency) from a patient safety perspective. This can be problematic when there is incorrect or grossly false data in the application and a patient relies on this information in lieu of seeking professional medical advice and suffers an injury. Adding to this problem is that many of the developers of mHealth applications are located in foreign countries, with varying legal systems making it difficult for an injured patient to recover damages from a developer.

Furthermore, the data collected by mHealth applications and wearable devices are becoming more and more combined with patient data stored in EHRs, which can lead to reliance on the accuracy of this data by providers when creating a treatment plan or treating a chronic disease.[49] If a provider relies on this information and such reliance results in harm to the patient, should the developer be held accountable, in addition to the provider? Also, if a developer is held liable, should the developer now be able to argue that it should have the benefit of the monetary caps many states have enacted related to medical malpractice tort reform?

Alternatively, if this type of information is available to a provider but is not reviewed, is the provider liable? These issues all play into whether or not the standard of care owed a patient should take technology into account. For a more detailed discussion about these issues and current research, see Chapter 15 on mHealth.

Social Media and Informatics

Another hot button issue in healthcare and informatics is the role of social media in balancing the rights of employees and free speech against the privacy rights of patients. More recently the National Labor Relations Board (NLRB) made this balancing act more difficult by publishing model social media polices for employers that might, if enforced, effectively prohibit employers from implementing social media policies that protect patient privacy.

Historically, one way employers would protect patient privacy on social media was to create and enforce employment policies that prohibited employees from posting patient information on social media. These types of policies were enacted after a spate of high-profile incidents in which employees posted patient information to social media. Here are some examples:

- A 2012 Chicago Daily Herald article detailed incidents such as a physician who on his blog called a patient "lazy" and "ignorant" because the patient had made several visits to the emergency room after failing to monitor her sugar levels.[50]
- In yet another case, a medical student filmed a doctor inserting a chest tube into a patient, whose face was clearly visible, and posted the footage on YouTube.[50]
- An incident in which a temporary employee assigned to the Providence Holy Cross Medical Center in Los Angeles posted a photo of a patient's medical record (clearly showing the patient's name), accompanied by the comment, "funny but this patient came in to cure her VD and get birth control."[51]

Section 7 of the National Labor Relations Act (NLRA) protects the right of employees to "engage in … concerted activities for the purpose of … mutual aid or protection" and gives the NLRB authority to investigate such behavior even if the employee filing a claim is not a union member or the employer is located in a right-to-work state.[52] On May 30, 2012, NLRB's Acting General Counsel published a memo that disapproved of a social media policy that prohibited employees "from posting information … that could be deemed material non-public information or any information that is considered confidential or proprietary."[53] Similarly, the NLRB found unlawful a social media policy that prohibited an employee from sharing "confidential information with another team member unless they have a need to know the information to do their job." These memos (if they were to be enforced) would effectively prohibit healthcare employers from implementing prudent social media policies that prohibit employees from engaging in activities that might expose the employer to violations of HIPAA or state privacy laws. After widespread condemnation by healthcare providers, the NLRB may revise these memos and guidance documents, but this has not been finalized.

CONCLUSION AND FUTURE DIRECTIONS

The healthcare system in the United States is highly regulated, and these regulations have a significant impact on the practice of health informatics. As a result, for their own safety, health professionals, health informaticians, the providers they serve, and the patients who depend on the healthcare system must understand and utilize the regulatory framework associated with health IT and informatics. This is especially important as the use of the technology becomes more widespread in the delivery of healthcare and the implementation of new consumer-focused technologies. Additionally, health informaticians must become proactive as the law and regulators struggle to catch up with health technology–related innovations as well as providers' and patients' reliance on these new technologies.

REFERENCES

1. McCulloch v. Maryland, 17 U.S. 316 (1819). *JUSTIA: U.S. Supreme Court*; 2016. https://supreme.justia.com/cases/federal/us/17/316/.
2. California Civil Code §§ 56 *et seq.*
3. Office of the National Coordinator for Health Information Technology. *Policymaking, regulation, & strategy. Federal-State Health Care Coordination.* https://www.healthit.gov/policy-researchers-implementers/federal-state-health-care-coordination/. Accessed December 7, 2015.
4. 42 U.S.C. §§ 1396 *et seq.* http://www.gpo.gov/fdsys/pkg/USCODE-2010-title42/pdf/USCODE-2010-title42-chap7-subchapXIX-sec1396d.pdf. Accessed July 5, 2016.
5. Administrative Procedure Act, Pub. L. 79-404, 60 Stat. 237; 1946. http://legisworks.org/sal/60/stats/STATUTE-60-Pg237.pdf.
6. 5 U.S.C. §§ 551 *et seq.* http://www.archives.gov/federal-register/laws/administrative-procedure/. Accessed July 5, 2016.
7. National Mining Association v. Jackson, 816 F.Supp. 2d 37 (D.D.C. 2011). JUSTIA: U.S. Law; 2016. http://law.justia.com/cases/federal/district-courts/district-of-columbia/dcdce/1:2010cv01220/143120/167/.

8. Section 1877 of the Social Security Act. https://www.ssa.gov/OP_Home/ssact/title18/1877.htm. Accessed July 5, 2016.

9. 42 U.S.C. § 1395nn. A list of CPT codes associated with Designated Health Services can be found at https://www.cms.gov/medicare/fraud-and-abuse/physicianselfreferral/list_of_codes.html.

10. 42 U.S.C. § 1395nn(a)(2)(A).

11. 42 U.S.C. § 1395nn(a)(2)(B).

12. 42 U.S.C. § 1320a-7b.

13. 42 U.S.C. § 1320a-7b(a).

14. *Section 6402(f)(2) of the Patient Protection and Affordable Care Act*, Pub. L. No. 111-148, 124 Stat 119 (2010).

15. U.S. v. Greber, 760 F.2d 68, 69 (3rd Cir. 1985), cert. denied, 474 U.S. 988 (1985).

16. 78 Fed. Reg. 79202 (December 27, 2013).

17. 31 U.S.C. § 3729(a)(1).

18. 31 U.S.C. § 3729(b)(1).

19. 42 U.S.C. § 1320a-7 k(d)(1).

20. 42 U.S.C. § 1320a-7a.

21. 18 U.S.C. § 1347.

22. 18 U.S.C. § 287.

23. 18 U.S.C. § 1341.

24. 18 U.S.C. § 1343.

25. Centers for Medicare and. *Detecting and responding to fraud, waste and abuse associated with the use of electronic health records (July 2015)*; 2015. https://www.cms.gov/Medicare-Medicaid-Coordination/Fraud-Prevention/Medicaid-Integrity-Education/Downloads/ehr-detect-fwabooklet.pdf.

26. U.S. Department of Health and Human Services. Office of Inspector General (December, 2013). *Not all recommended fraud safeguards have been implemented in hospital EHR technology*; 2013. http://www.oig.hhs.gov/oei/reports/oei-01-11-00570.pdf.

27. Centers for Medicare & Medicaid Services. Continued approval of the Joint Commission's (TJC) hospital accreditation program. *79 Federal Register 36524*. June 26, 2014.

28. Centers for Medicare & Medicaid Services. Continued approval of Det Norske Veritas Healthcare's (DNVHC) Hospital Accreditation Program. *77 Federal Register 51537*. September 26, 2012.

29. Kenney L. American Society for Healthcare Engineering. *Hospital accrediting organizations offer different approaches to the survey process*. http://www.ashe.org/resources/ashenews/2013/hosp_ao_article_131011.html#.Vjd2-t_lupo. Accessed November 2, 2015.

30. The Joint Commission. *Facts About Joint Commission Standards*. http://www.jointcommission.org/facts_about_joint_commission_accreditation_standards/; 2016.

31. The Joint Commission. *Benefits of Joint Commission Accreditation*; 2015. http://www.jointcommission.org/about_us/accreditation_fact_sheets.aspx.

32. DNV GL Healthcare. *DNV GL's pioneering NIAHO program integrates ISO 9001 with the Medicare conditions of participation*. http://dnvglhealthcare.com/accreditations/hospital-accreditation. Accessed November 2, 2015.

33. The Joint Commission. *The Joint Commission standards edition: information management*; 2014. http://foh.hhs.gov/tjc/im/standards.pdf.

34. The Joint Commission. *Facts about scoring and certification decision*. http://www.jointcommission.org/facts_about_scoring_and_certification_decision/; 2015.

35. The Joint Commission. *Sentinel Event Alert 42: Safely Implementing Health Information and Converging Technologies*. http://www.jointcommission.org/sentinel_event_alert_issue_42_safely_implementing_health_information_and_converging_technologies/; 2008.

36. The Joint Commission. *Sentinel Event Alert 54: Safe Use of Health Information Technology*. http://www.jointcommission.org/assets/1/18/SEA_54.pdf; 2015.

37. 21 U.S.C. § 201(h).

38. *Food and Drug Administration Safety and Innovation Act*, Pub. Law 112-144.

39. *Section 618 of the Food and Drug Administration Safety and Innovation Act*, Pub. Law 112-144.

40. FDASIA Health IT Report. *Proposed strategy and recommendations for a risk-based framework*. http://www.fda.gov/AboutFDA/CentersOffices/OfficeofMedicalProductsandTobacco/CDRH/CDRHReports/ucm390588.htm; 2014.

41. Food and Drug Administration. *General Wellness: Policy for Low Risk Devices. Draft Guidance for Industry*. http://www.fda.gov/MedicalDevices/DeviceRegulationandGuidance/GuidanceDocuments/ucm418408.htm.

42. Sections 2220-2319 of the California Business and Professions Code. http://www.leginfo.ca.gov/cgi-bin/displaycode?section=bpc&group=02001-03000&file=2220-2319. Accessed July 5, 2016.

43. *District of Columbia Statute § 3-1205.02*. http://doh.dc.gov/sites/default/files/dc/sites/doh/publication/attachments/Medicine_Health_Occupations_Revision_Act_%28HORA%29.pdf. July 5, 2016.

44. 22 TAC § 172.12.

45. 22 TAC §§ 174.1-174.12.

46. Federal Trade Commission. *Location, location, location*. https://www.ftc.gov/news-events/blogs/business-blog/2015/02/location-location-location?utm_source=govdelivery; 2015.

47. Tex. Health and Safety Code § 181.100 *et seq.*

48. Business Insider. *Senator warns Fitbit is a 'Privacy Nightmare' and could be 'Tracking' your movements*; 2014. http://www.businessinsider.com/senator-warns-fitbit-is-a-privacy-nightmare-2014-8#ixzz3A5M2nn17.

49. *Mobile & Device Integration*. http://www.cerner.com/Solutions/Workplace_Health/Wellness_Solutions_and_Services/Mobile_and_Device_Integration/.

50. Being Facebook Friends and Doctors May Cross Line. Chicago Daily Herald. Published at 2012 WLNR 14380254; July 9, 2012.

51. Patient Info on Facebook Traced to Temp Staff. Same-Day Surgery. Published at 2012 WLNR 7485830; May 1, 2012.

52. 29 U.S.C. §§ 151-169.

53. The National Labor Relations Board. *The NLRB and social media fact sheet*. https://www.nlrb.gov/news-outreach/fact-sheets/nlrb-and-social-media; July 5, 2016.

DISCUSSION QUESTIONS

1. How does the U.S. regulatory framework work to ensure patient safety?
2. Describe two express powers and one implied power given to the federal government in the Constitution that has implications for health-related technology.
3. Name two federal agencies and describe their role in the regulatory oversight of health IT.
4. What are the different types of healthcare fraud and abuse statutes?
5. What are three major issues with mHealth applications and wearable devices?
6. How are patient privacy rights impacted by labor and employment regulations?

CASE STUDY

A 50-member multispecialty medical practice has decided to implement a new EHR system. The practice chooses the new EHR system based on both clinical functionality and the practice management and billing functionality that is demonstrated specifically because the EHR sales representative repeatedly states that the new EHR can reduce patient visit times (thus increasing the number of patients a provider can see in a day) and increase reimbursement to the practice by helping the practice "correctly code" to the highest E/M (evaluation and management) code available. While the healthcare providers and practice administrator are impressed with the new EHR, the new system will cost $2,000,000 for the EHR software and $250,000 for the associated hardware, plus yearly maintenance fees of $125,000. These costs exceed the practice's budget. One day, while meeting with the vice president of a community hospital, the practice administrator mentions this issue and how the practice will have to delay purchasing an EHR due to the budget constraints. The VP states that the hospital will be happy to cover 85% costs for the new EHR system if the practice agrees to (1) consider their hospital first before sending a patient to any other potential competitors including not just ER or inpatient admission but outpatient diagnostic services and hospital-owned specialty practices, (2) include the hospital's logo on patient education materials printed from the system, (3) use the hospital's template for designing data entry pages for practitioners, and (4) use the hospital's template for the patient portal in the design of their patient portal.

Discussion Questions

1. Explain the basic requirements for a hospital to help finance the purchase of an EHR system by a provider.
2. Discuss whether the proposed course of action would be permissible under current fraud and abuse regulations.
3. If the structure of the proposed donation is not permitted under current fraud and abuse regulations, explain what steps the parties would need to take to make the transaction compliant.
4. Explain common issues related to use of EHR and healthcare fraud.
5. Discuss how the proposed new EHR could potentially facilitate healthcare fraud.

26

Privacy and Security

David L. Gibbs, Nancy Staggers, Ramona Nelson, and Angel Hoffman

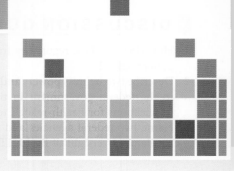

Neither patients nor healthcare providers will fully accept electronic healthcare systems unless they trust that private patient data are accurate and held in confidence through effective policies and procedures and secure information systems.

OBJECTIVES

At the completion of this chapter, the reader will be prepared to:

1. Describe and explain the following informatics concepts: privacy, security, confidentiality, integrity, availability, covered entity, and business associate.
2. Analyze current federal and state laws and regulations and their implications for privacy and security practices and procedures.
3. Use appropriate resources in establishing and implementing both privacy- and security-related policies and procedures.
4. Apply common procedures for securing sensitive health information.

KEY TERMS

ABSTRACT ❖

This chapter begins by explaining how the concepts of privacy and security apply to electronic health information. International, national, and state security and privacy-related practices, guidelines, and principles are then outlined. Current regulatory processes are discussed. The chapter concludes with an examination of security concepts and procedures necessary to ensure the safety and integrity of electronic health data.

INTRODUCTION

A primary responsibility of healthcare providers and their business associates is to ensure that the health data for which they are responsible is held in the strictest confidence. However, the reality is that the risks to confidentiality are significant for electronic health data. The importance of protecting and safeguarding protected health information (PHI) has grown exponentially as health-related device use has expanded for mobile devices, electronic health records (EHRs), sensors, biomedical devices, telehealth, personal health records, personal health devices, and health information exchanges (HIEs). Increased usage brings increased risk for data breaches. The increase in the number of users, types of use, and volumes of health IT-based data is directly proportional to the increased opportunities for privacy and confidentiality breaches. Patients as well as healthcare providers typically support concepts related to the use of data for research purposes, electronic health data storage, and communication. However, concerns regarding data security persist.[1]

As the volume of privacy breaches increased in recent years, health information privacy and information security became a top priority for contemporary healthcare organizations. Over 720 health information breaches occurred in 2015, with the top 7 affecting 193 million records. At this writing, the largest was Anthem (health insurance), with a breach of 78.8 million patient records.[2] To put this number in perspective it may be helpful to realize that the population of California, the largest in the United States, was 38.8 million in

2014.[3] The Office for Civil Rights (OCR) lists over 130 breaches (at greater than 500 people per breach) for electronic health data during 2015.[4] In two of these events, hacking incidences at a medical center in California and a health plan in New York resulted in a breach of 4.5 million and 10 million individuals' records, respectively. Readers can access the list of the most recent breach reports at https://ocrportal.hhs.gov/ocr/breach/breach_report.jsf.[4]

DEFINITIONS AND CONCEPTS

Privacy is the right of individuals to control access to their person (body privacy) or information about themselves (information privacy).[5] In informatics, the concern is focused primarily on privacy of information. Designing systems to ensure the security of information privacy is one of the most difficult challenges for institutions and individuals living in our digital age.[6] Health records can contain information on any or all aspects of an individual's life and as a result may contain highly sensitive information (e.g., sexually transmitted diseases, behavioral health information, or financial information). Health data and information must be kept private if such data are to be considered trusted information and a primary resource for building new knowledge. Also, the information must be protected from access and misuse by unauthorized persons. Moreover, specific policies and procedures must be implemented to prevent disclosures or breaches that encroach on the privacy of the data's primary owner—the patient.[7]

The difference between privacy, confidentiality, and security can be confusing. Terms central to these concepts are defined in Table 26.1. Privacy concerns who has access to information, a patient's right to keep information private, and what constitutes inappropriate or unauthorized access. Confidentiality relates to protecting and safeguarding health information from inappropriate access, use, and disclosure. In short, privacy is about the *person*, while confidentiality is about the *information*. Privacy speaks to the rights of patients, as they have a right to their privacy. Confidentiality speaks to the responsibility of healthcare providers because they are responsible for keeping patients' information private. Security relates to the administrative, technical, and physical safeguards implemented to prevent privacy and confidentiality breaches and also to ensure integrity and availability of information.

LEGAL AND HISTORICAL CONTEXT

Today's focus on health information security is built on a long history of concern with the privacy of information obtained during a caregiver–patient encounter. Even in the fourth century, the Hippocratic oath addressed the privacy of communications between patients and their healthcare providers.[5,8] In 1860, Florence Nightingale's *Notes on Nursing* addressed various uses of health information, including the importance of its proper acquisition for the benefit of the patient first and foremost, a concern that exists today.[9] Privacy and confidentiality continue today as global concerns. After all, the

TABLE 26.1 Distinctions Among Terms

Terms	Definitions
Accountability	The requirement for actions of an entity to be traced uniquely to that entity.[64]
Authenticity	Able to be verified and trusted; confidence in the validity of a transmission, a message, or message originator.[64]
Availability	Data or information is accessible and useable on demand by an authorized person.[39]
Confidentiality	Data or information is not made available or disclosed to unauthorized persons or processes.[39]
Integrity	Data or information have not been altered or destroyed in an unauthorized manner.[39]
Privacy	Restricting access to subscriber or relying party information in accordance with federal law and agency policy.[64]
Safeguard	Protective measures prescribed to meet the security requirements (i.e., confidentiality, integrity, and availability) specified for an information system. Safeguards may include security features, management constraints, personnel security, and security of physical structures, areas, and devices. Synonymous with security controls and countermeasures.[40]
Security	Protecting information and information systems from unauthorized access, use, disclosure, disruption, modification, or destruction in order to provide confidentiality, integrity, and availability.[39]

information that individuals share with their caregivers as part of that trusted relationship may not have been shared with their families or even close friends.[10]

Fair Information Practice Principles

Fair information practices (FIPs), also referred to as fair information practice principles (FIPPs), are a set of internationally recognized practices for addressing privacy of information. The principles are the result of joint work by U.S., Canadian, and European government agencies over time and are available in reports, guidelines, and legal codes that ensure that information practices are fair and provide adequate privacy protection to individuals.[11,12] Although these statements can vary according to the source, typical FIPs are included in Table 26.2.

Since the 1970s, many government agencies addressed the impact of computerization of health records. Some industrialized countries codified FIPs into a privacy law at the federal level, although this has not yet occurred in the United States. Instead, in the United States, FIPs are the basis of many

TABLE 26.2	Fair Information Practice Principles
Principle	**Description**
Transparency	Organizations should be transparent and notify individuals regarding collection, use, dissemination, and maintenance of personally identifiable information (PII).
Individual participation	Organizations should involve the individual in the process of using PII and, to the extent practicable, seek individual consent for the collection, use, dissemination, and maintenance of PII. Organizations should also provide mechanisms for appropriate access, correction, and redress regarding use of PII.
Purpose specification	Organizations should specifically articulate the authority that permits the collection of PII and specifically articulate the purposes for which PII is intended to be used.
Data minimization	Organizations should only collect PII that is directly relevant and necessary to accomplish the specified purpose(s) and only retain PII for as long as is necessary to fulfill the specified purpose(s).
Use limitation	Organizations should use PII solely for the purposes specific in the notice. Sharing PII should be for a purpose compatible with the purpose for which the PII was collected.
Data quality and integrity	Organizations should, to the extent practicable, ensure that PII is accurate, relevant, timely, and complete.
Security	Organizations should protect PII in all media through appropriate security safeguards against risks such as loss, unauthorized access or use, destruction, modification, or unintended or inappropriate disclosure.
Accountability and auditing	Organizations should be accountable for complying with these principles, providing training to all employees and contractors who use PII and auditing the actual use of PII to demonstrate compliance with these principles and all applicable privacy protection requirements.

Source: *Fair Information Practice Principles*. National strategy for trusted identities in cyberspace. Appendix A. National Institute for Standards and Technology. <http://www.nist.gov/nstic/NSTIC-FIPPs.pdf>.

individual laws at federal and state levels. The value of the FIPs is that they provide a framework for privacy laws and also can form the foundation for an organization's or an industry's privacy policy. For example, although the Health Insurance Portability and Accountability Act of 1996 (HIPAA) does not formally codify FIPs in the legislation, it implements all FIPs in some way.[13]

Code of Ethics for Health Informatics Professionals

When we discuss ethics in healthcare, biomedical ethics come to mind; however, a discussion on ethics in healthcare should involve business ethics as well. Business ethics are how we conduct ourselves, our organizational culture, and leadership. In informatics, sample business ethics are codified by the International Medical Informatics Association (IMIA).

International Medical Informatics Association

The IMIA published a Code of Ethics for Health Informatics Professionals that is closely related to the FIPs.[14] This code has two major sections. The first addresses fundamental ethical principles: autonomy, equality and justice, beneficence, nonmalfeasance, impossibility, and integrity as applied to informatics (Table 26.3). The second section concerns the rules of ethical conduct for health informatics professionals. As this code demonstrates, FIPs are now an integral aspect of ethical practices in health informatics.

PRINCIPLES, LAWS, AND REGULATIONS GUIDING PRACTICE

Over the centuries, health professionals used a combination of ethical codes, including a set of guidelines or guiding principles,

and applicable laws and regulations to maintain patient confidentiality. The introduction of computers into healthcare offered new challenges and opportunities for securing health-related data and maintaining patient confidentiality.

The U.S. federal government recognized the need for legislation to protect privacy in an electronic environment with the passage of the Privacy Act in 1974. This act protects certain personal information held by federal agencies in computerized databases.[15] It includes three important factors. First, privacy of health data is considered within the larger context of privacy in general. The Privacy Act is not specific to the protection of health data but provides for protection of health-related data in federal agencies with health-related databases such as the Veterans Health Administration (VHA), Military Health System (MHS), and Medicare.

Second, this legislation reflected the code of FIPs described previously. Third, the Privacy Act included specific legislation about cross-referencing data in multiple federal and state databases because combining databases could create information that clearly identifies individuals. Later in this chapter, we will review how this has changed in more recent years, as HIEs were created within and among states and regions in the U.S. Health and informatics professionals play a key role in understanding these complexities and developing policies and procedures to protect patient privacy within and across health-related databases.

The use of federal legislation to protect health data began in narrowly defined areas. For example, in 1975, the Department of Health, Education, and Welfare published rules and regulations governing the confidentiality of patient records containing information related to alcohol and drug use.[16] HIPAA was the first federal U.S. legislation to broadly address

TABLE 26.3 General Principles of Informatics Ethics Included in the IMIA Code of Ethics for Health Informatics Professionals

Principle	Description
1. Information—privacy and disposition	All persons have a fundamental right to privacy and hence control over the collection, storage, access, use, communication, manipulation, and disposition of data about themselves.
2. Openness	The collection, storage, access, use, communication, manipulation, and disposition of personal data must be disclosed in an appropriate and timely fashion to the subject of those data.
3. Security	Data that have been legitimately collected about a person should be protected by all reasonable and appropriate measures against loss, degradation, unauthorized destruction, access, use, manipulation, modification, or communication.
4. Access	The subject of an electronic record has the right of access to that record and the right to correct the record with respect to its accurateness, completeness, and relevance.
5. Legitimate infringement	The fundamental right of control over the collection, storage, access, use, manipulation, communication, and disposition of personal data is conditioned only by the legitimate, appropriate, and relevant data needs of a free, responsible, and democratic society, and by the equal and competing rights of other persons.
6. Least intrusive alternative	Any infringement of the privacy rights of the individual person, and of the individual's right to control over person-relative data as mandated under Principle 1, may only occur in the least intrusive fashion and with a minimum of interference with the rights of the affected person.
7. Accountability	Any infringement of the privacy rights of the individual person, and of the right to control over person-relative data, must be justified to the affected person in good time and in an appropriate fashion.

IMIA, International Medical Informatics Association.
From *International Medical Informatics Association (IMIA).* IMIA Code of Ethics for health information professionals. *IMIA.* <http://www.imia-medinfo.org/new2/node/39>.

the privacy and security of health data.[17] This act set a standard in the United States for protecting an individual's health information, although other countries already had such laws. HIPAA began in 1996 with subsequent revisions and effective dates: HIPAA Privacy Rule in 2003, Electronic Data Interchange in 2003, and the Security Rule in 2005. Additional privacy-related legislation was included in the HITECH Act in 2009 and in the HIPAA Omnibus Rule, which went into effect in early 2013. Critical aspects of PHI and HIPAA are discussed next.

National Privacy and Security Framework for Health Information Laws and Regulations

When consumers think of HIPAA, they often think that it covers all of their privacy rights. However, HIPAA only addresses those rights as they relate to PHI. PHI is individually identifiable health information transferred in any medium (e.g., demographics, health and mental conditions, and their treatments as well as payment information).[18] The following section outlines international efforts and then focuses on U.S. laws and regulations related only to PHI under HIPAA.

International Laws

On an international level, many countries instituted privacy laws prior to HIPAA. While there are differences between countries in how privacy is conceived and in the value placed on privacy of health data, privacy of health data is increasingly being recognized as an international value.[19] Becoming familiar with these laws is critical for conducting international business to avoid violations. Whether conducting domestic

business in the United States or conducting international business, readers need to know what is addressed in each law and then conduct business accordingly to mitigate risks of privacy breaches.

The European Union (EU) has historically been more protective of personal information than the United States. One of the earliest and most recognized agreements and legislation supporting the transfer of health data across their borders was created by the EU in 1995. It passed a comprehensive data privacy law titled the "EU Directive on the Protection of Individuals with Regard to the Processing of Personal Data and on the Free Movement of such Data."[20] The EU selected a "directive" approach that required each EU member state to enact its own law based on the fair principles outlined in the directive. As each EU member state developed and implemented its legislation, it implemented the 1995 rules differently, resulting in divergences in enforcement and a number of related problems.

1. In late 2015, the EU's General Data Protection Regulation (GDPR) was enacted to provide consumers with more input about how their digital information is collected and managed, strengthening the privacy rights of Europeans. The changes take effect in early 2017 across the 28 members of the EU. One of the unique concepts in the GDPR is the "right to be forgotten," which provides individuals in a region the right to ask companies to remove data about them. The law also requires companies to inform national regulators within three days of any reported data breach. This goes beyond what is required by U.S. authorities currently. Another

GDPR issue is in regard to children under 16 years old. The rule requires young children to obtain parental consent before using popular internet services such as social media applications.[21]

2. In a similar vein, the EU and the United States agreed to a framework for data sharing in early 2016. This new framework will protect the more stringent rights of EU citizens when their data are sent to the United States. It includes safeguards and opportunities for redress should personal data be compromised.[22] These regulations are important for readers to know, especially if they are employed by companies with international sites.

A number of other countries, in addition to those in the EU, have developed international agreements and legislation related to privacy of personal data. What does not exist at this point is a single set of standards, rules, or legislation that could be used in designing information systems storing health-related data, although both EU and Canada show evidence of being progressive in that direction. Other countries have adopted privacy standards (e.g., Philippines in 2011, Vietnam in 2008, and South Africa in 2002).[23] Readers may find a list of these countries at http://www.bakerlaw.com/files/Uploads/Documents/Data%20Breach%20documents/International-Compendium-of-Data-Privacy-Laws.pdf.

Informaticians should approach each international situation on an individual basis. Both the Electronic Frontier Foundation (EFF) (https://www.eff.org/issues/international-privacy-standards) and the Electronic Privacy Information Center (https://epic.org/privacy/intl/) maintain websites listing privacy-related international accords and agreements. Neither list is comprehensive but can be used as a starting point in exploring international privacy agreements pertinent to the privacy of health-related data.

U.S. Federal Law

U.S. federal efforts to protect and safeguard PHI are based on various federal and state laws and regulations. A list of related laws and regulations is provided in Box 26.1. The primary U.S. federal legislation dealing with privacy is HIPAA.[18]

HIPAA has multiple sections and subparts related to maintaining the confidentiality of health information, whether in paper or electronic format, and addressing privacy, security, and electronic data interchange standards. Here the discussion of HIPAA is limited to its importance in designing and implementing health information systems.

The History of HIPAA

In 1996, HIPAA was enacted by Congress.[17] Subsequently, several associated rules emerged: the Privacy Rule, Security Rule, Transactions and Code Sets, National Provider Identifier (NPI), Enforcement Rule, and Breach Notification Rule to increase safeguards. Of note, HIPAA applies to "covered entities" (healthcare providers, health plans, and healthcare clearinghouses) and their "business associates." Much debate and legal definitions exists about the term "business associate" as it relates to HIPAA, and a complete definition is lengthy. An example of the subtle implications with the use of this term can be seen in Box 26.2. For this chapter, we will use the term in its generic sense to mean an organization supporting the work of a covered entity having access to its PHI. For example, an external billing service (the business associate) may process specialized insurance requests for an emergency department in a medical center (the covered entity). Through this association, the billing company is considered a covered entity because the firm has access to PHI. All entities are responsible for protecting and safeguarding PHI. This section discusses pertinent and more recent HIPAA-related rules or laws.

HITECH Act

The 2009 HITECH Act included requirements for privacy breaches by covered entities and/or business associates.[24] Breaches are defined as an impermissible use or disclosure of PHI.[25] Specific new requirements were outlined in 2009 for notifying individuals, the media, and the HHS.[24] Any individuals affected by a breach must be notified about the details of the breach within a specific time frame. When a breach affects more than 500 residents of a state or jurisdiction, the covered entity or business associate is required to provide notice to prominent media in addition to notifying the affected individuals. For breaches affecting 500 or more individuals, the secretary of the HHS also must be notified. A summary of provisions expanded by the HITECH Act are in Box 26.3.

HIPAA Omnibus Final Rule of 2013

In January 2013, the Department of Health and Human Services (HHS) announced the HIPAA Omnibus Final Rule, based on statutory changes under the HITECH Act and the Genetic Information Nondiscrimination Act of 2008 (GINA).[26] Major provisions are summarized in Box 26.4. Modifications include a number of provisions to expand and strengthen the privacy and security protections for health information first established under HIPAA.[26] Specifically, this final rule adds patients' privacy protections, provides individuals new rights to their health information, and strengthens the government's ability to enforce the law. Current provisions are outlined in Box 26.5.

Under the rule, business associates who receive PHI (e.g., contractors, subcontractors, and other third parties) are also liable for noncompliance based on the level of negligence up to a maximum penalty of $1.5 million. The rule clarifies when breaches of unsecured health information must be reported to

the Department of Health and Human Services. Individual rights were also expanded. Importantly, patients can ask for a copy of their electronic medical record in an electronic form, and if they choose to pay cash for services provided, the patient can instruct the healthcare provider *not* to share information about their treatment with their health plan. The challenge lies in the processes healthcare providers have in place to honor this request.

This rule describes new limits on how information is used and disclosed for marketing and fundraising purposes.[26] It prohibits the sale of an individual's health information without their permission. A covered entity must request and obtain written authorization from an individual to use or disclose his or her PHI for marketing purposes. Specific exceptions exist when the provider receives no compensation for the communication, when the communication is face to face, or if the communication involves a drug or biologic the patient is currently being prescribed and the payment is

---

BOX 26.5   HIPAA Regulations: Individuals' Rights to Access Their Personal Health Information

With limited exceptions, HIPAA provides individuals with a legal, enforceable right to see and receive copies of the information in their medical and other health records maintained by their healthcare providers and health plans, as well as to direct the covered entity to transmit a copy to a designated person or entity of the individual's choice.

Key Terms

- **Covered Entity.** Includes (1) healthcare providers such as hospitals, physicians, clinics, psychologists, dentists, nursing homes, and pharmacies if they transmit any information in an electronic format; (2) insurance companies, HMOs, and government plans that pay for healthcare; and (3) healthcare clearinghouses that process nonstandard health information they receive from another entity into a standard format or vice versa.
- **Designated Record Sets.** The group of records maintained by the covered entity and/or business associate used to make decisions about the diagnosis, management, and treatment of the patient. This includes medical records, billing records, enrollment, payment, claims adjudication, and any other records used to make decisions about the patient.
- **Personal Representative.** A person with authority under state law to make healthcare decisions for the individual.

What Patient Rights Are Included?

- The right to receive copies of all information in the medical records, including clinical laboratory test results, medical images such as X-rays, wellness and disease management program files and clinical case notes, all billing and payment records, and insurance information.
- The right to request a change to any information the individual believes is wrong as well as to add information the individual believes is missing or incomplete. If the covered entity believes the information is correct or complete, the individual has the right to have the disagreement noted in their file within 60 days.

- The right to receive test results directly from clinical laboratory that is a covered entity. The designated record set includes not only the laboratory test reports but also the underlying information generated as part of the test, as well as other information concerning tests a laboratory runs on an individual. Patients may still obtain their results from their physician's office, but are not required to use that option.
- A personal representative also has the right to access PHI in a designated record set as well as the right to direct the covered entity to transmit a copy of the PHI to a designated person or entity of the individual's choice.

Exceptions

- PHI that is not part of a designated record set because the information is not used to make decisions about individuals. This includes records that are used for business decisions more generally rather than to make decisions about individuals such as quality assessment data.
- Psychotherapy notes, which are the personal notes of a mental healthcare provider documenting or analyzing the contents of a counseling session that are maintained separate from the rest of the patient's medical record.
- PHI is in a designated record set that is part of a research study that includes treatment that is still in progress, provided the individual agreed to the temporary suspension of access when consenting to participate in the research.

Source

U.S. Department of Health and Human Services: Office of Civil Rights. (2016). *Individuals' Right under HIPAA to Access their Health Information 45 CFR § 164.524*. Retrieved 11.01.16, from HIPAA for Professionals: Privacy: Guidance: http://www.hhs.gov/hipaa/for-professionals/privacy/guidance/access/index.html

U.S. Department of Health and Human Services: Office of Civil Rights. (n.d.). *Your Health Information privacy Rights*. Retrieved 08.01.16, from U.S. DHHS Office of Civil Rights: http://www.hhs.gov/sites/default/files/ocr/privacy/hipaa/understanding/consumers/consumer_rights.pdf

---

limited to reasonable reimbursement of the costs of the communication (at no profit).

ONC Tool for Integrating Privacy and Security into Health Practices

Individuals and healthcare providers are not willing to share complete and accurate health-related data unless they can trust that the data have been secured in a protected environment. As noted in Chapters 6 and 25, HIEs combine information from multiple databases, introducing new information from other practitioners or organizations and integrated elements such as medications, treatments, and therapies into a more comprehensive patient plan of care. This may, of course, include PHI. This is another area where informatics professionals play a key role in understanding these types of issues and complexities to develop policies and procedures to safeguard and protect PHI both internally and externally to an organization.

In April 2015, the Office of the National Coordinator for Health Information Technology (ONC) released a document titled, "Guide to Privacy and Security of Electronic Health Information," version 2.0.[27] The purpose of this tool is to assist providers and organizations, especially smaller organizations and practices, in understanding how to integrate federal health information privacy, security, and breach notification requirements into their practices. The tool answers practical questions such as, "Do I have to inform patients how I disclose their health information?" It summarizes patients' rights to their information and provides sample questions to ask of vendors, such as, "Does software installation include ePHI encryption, auditing and unique, individual identifications with strong passwords?"[27] Readers may view the full guide at https://www.healthit.gov/sites/default/files/pdf/privacy/privacy-and-security-guide.pdf.

While HIPAA protects PHI from misuse, the law also enables disclosing or sharing information when needed for patient care. To help clarify when PHI may be disclosed without obtaining an individual's authorization, ONC and the OCR developed easy-to-read fact sheets, released in February 2016:

- *Permitted Uses and Disclosures: Exchange for Health Care Operations* is available from https://www.healthit.gov/sites/default/files/exchange_health_care_ops.pdf.
- *Permitted Uses and Disclosures: Exchange for Treatment* is available from https://www.healthit.gov/sites/default/files/exchange_treatment.pdf.

In addition to federal laws, health plans, healthcare clearinghouses, and healthcare providers must follow state laws and regulations. State laws are further complicated when health services and institutions cross state lines, such as with telehealth services.

Federal-State Collaboration

The Health Information Security and Privacy Collaboration (HISPC) was established in 2006. In 2008, HISPC moved into its third and final phase, with 42 states and territories addressing the privacy and security challenges presented by electronic HIE through multistate collaboration.[28] Phase 3 projects included the following:

- Studying intrastate and interstate consent policies
- Developing tools to help harmonize state privacy laws
- Developing tools and strategies to educate and engage consumers
- Developing a toolkit to educate healthcare providers
- Recommending basic security policy requirements
- Developing interorganizational agreements[26]

Each project was designed to develop common, replicable multistate solutions for reducing variation in and harmonizing privacy and security practices, policies, and laws. A number of products and reports have been produced as a result of these efforts and can be accessed at http://www.healthit.gov/policy-researchers-implementers/health-information-security-privacy-collaboration-hispc. Each covered entity is required to interpret and apply these rules, as applicable to their organization and the state in which they reside.

HIPAA and Secondary Uses of Electronic Health Data

In addition to being used in the provision of healthcare, PHI can be used for a number of other activities. This is referred to as the secondary use of health data, and it presents its own special set of privacy and security issues. The three most common secondary uses of personal health information are public health monitoring or surveillance, research, and marketing.

Public Health Monitoring or Surveillance and HIEs

Public health agencies, which frequently must work within states and across state lines, are required to follow applicable federal and specific state laws and regulations. In addition to HISPC, discussed previously, the Public Health Data Standards Consortium (PHDSC) provides information, education, and tools for protecting the privacy of personal health data.[29] PHDSC is a national, nonprofit, membership-based organization of federal, state, and local health agencies; professional associations; academia; public and private sector organizations; international members; and individuals. Its mission focuses on promoting health IT standards to empower health communities to improve individual and community health. The PHDSC Privacy, Security, and Data Exchange Committee addresses individual and organizational privacy and security standards related to maintaining and sharing health information in electronic form for public sector health programs and health services research purposes. The goals include the following:

- To represent and educate broad public sector health and health services research interests on privacy and security issues
- To focus on priorities related to privacy, security, and data standardization
- To balance the need for individual privacy, confidentiality, and security with the need for use of data for public health and research activities

For additional information regarding PHDSC, go to www.phdsc.org.

PHDSC conducted a survey on privacy-related variations, solutions, and implementation plans directly involving or affecting public health practice. Two reports were issued. The first report summarizes the variations in privacy and security policies, practices, and state laws affecting the interoperability of public HIEs. The second report focuses on the analysis of solutions and implementation plans proposed by states and aimed at addressing barriers to public HIEs. Both reports are available from PHDSC at www.phdsc.org.

With the information in these reports, PHDSC developed a Privacy Toolkit for Public Health Professionals (PRISM). PRISM consists of a series of tables that outline different types and purposes of information use and disclosure and the general legal requirements relevant to each type of use or disclosure. The tables describe the baseline privacy requirements for disclosure of health information using HIPAA, other federal laws affecting health privacy, and common state privacy laws and related requirements. The PRISM tables can be accessed at http://phdsc.org/privacy_security/prismtool.asp.

De-identification of Data

The 2013 HIPAA Omnibus Rule provided clarification regarding the use of patient information for marketing purposes. Health data used for marketing (and some research) are almost always de-identified; that is, PHI is removed so that remaining information neither identifies nor provides a reasonable basis to identify an individual. HIPAA includes no restrictions on the use or disclosure of de-identified health information.[29] However, there are regulations concerning the specific procedures that can be used to de-identify protected data.[30] These two procedures, the safe harbor method and the expert determination method, are outlined in Fig. 26.1.

The next section discusses why information security is critical to today's organizations and individuals and provides an overview of critical security procedures.

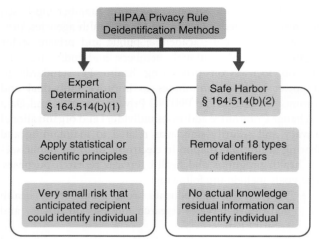

FIG 26.1 Two methods to achieve de-identification in accordance with the Health Insurance Portability and Accountability Act's (HIPAA's) Privacy Rule. (Copyright *U.S. Department of Health and Human Services [HHS] Office for Civil Rights.* Guidance regarding methods for de-identification of protected health information in accordance with the Health Insurance Portability and Accountability Act [HIPAA] Privacy Rule. HHS. <http://www.hhs.gov/hipaa/for-professionals/privacy/special-topics/de-identification/> Accessed January 13, 2016.)

THE IMPORTANCE OF INFORMATION SECURITY

While privacy and confidentiality are important, they are not the only issues that arise when dealing with health data. The HIPAA Security Rule requires safeguards be in place to ensure the *confidentiality, integrity,* and *availability* of PHI.[31] This triad is frequently mentioned together and often labeled *CIA* by cybersecurity professionals. Definitions for these and related terms may be found in Table 26.1.

As health data increasingly move from paper to electronic storage and transmission, they can become more vulnerable to unauthorized disclosure and modification, either accidentally or intentionally. Health professionals should be familiar with various safeguards, also known as controls or countermeasures, to protect the CIA of data. Likewise, ensuring health information confidentiality and security is facing new challenges as technology is introduced. One of the promises of EHRs is improved accessibility, especially through simultaneous access by multiple authorized persons and distributed across geographic locations. While electronic information systems do deliver this benefit, they also introduce new obstacles to availability such as system downtime, network outages, authentication, and access control. Just as modern healthcare is dependent on electrical cabling to bring power to medical devices, it also is dependent on networks (wired or wireless) to carry data. Safeguards are required to address availability of patient data. (See Chapter 20 for detailed information on downtime and disaster recovery.)

The HITECH Act, Meaningful Use, and subsequent efforts by government agencies to accelerate electronic exchange of health information make it virtually impossible for eligible providers to avoid having an internet connection. HITECH requirements such as exchanging patient data, submitting claims electronically, generating electronic records for patients' requests, and e-prescribing make an internet connection an absolute necessity. The existence of such a connection requires that these providers devise methods to safeguard data being shared via the internet. Effective cybersecurity practices are needed to protect the confidentiality, integrity, and availability of EHR systems, regardless of how they are delivered, whether installed in a small provider office or accessed over the internet by large organizations.[27]

Three areas emphasize the importance of health information security today: (1) the public trust, (2) legal requirements and fines, and (3) increasing security threats to healthcare data.

The Public Trust

A balance is needed for patients' requirements for privacy and society's need for improved efficiency and reduced costs.[32] With increased connectivity comes the sharing of highly sensitive data as well as social and political pressure to avoid inappropriate sharing. Healthcare institutions and providers earn patients' trust by guaranteeing the privacy and security of their health information. Patients entrust their most intimate information to healthcare providers, and they do not expect their health information or their identities to be exposed publicly.[33] Thus breaches of privacy and security undermine patients' confidence in their healthcare institutions and providers. On the other hand, adequate security measures can bolster the public trust and perhaps boost EHR adoption rates.[34] The following paragraphs identify efforts to establish and maintain public trust in EHR systems by applying formal risk management frameworks (RMFs).

To help healthcare organizations address the complex array of standards and regulations related to privacy and security, the Common Security Framework (CSF) was developed by the Health Information Trust Alliance (HITRUST). The framework provides a proven approach to risk management and regulatory compliance. Through the HITRUST CSF Assurance Program, healthcare organizations may perform internal assessments of their privacy and security practices or contract with a third-party assessor to achieve CSF certification.[35]

HITRUST was founded in 2007, and the CSF v.1 was released in 2009, with certification based on 35 security controls. The 2014 CSF v6 framework consisted of 135 control specifications organized into 13 categories. Box 26.6 lists the HITRUST CSF control categories. In 2015, version 7 was released with the framework expanded to incorporate cross-references related to privacy in addition to security. The additional privacy standards include the HIPAA Privacy Rule and NIST SP 800-53 R4 Security and Privacy Controls for Federal Information Systems and Organizations, among several others.[36]

Some health plans require their business associates to become HITRUST certified. HITRUST certification is also

BOX 26.6   HITRUST CSF Control Categories

- Information Security Management Program
- Access Control
- Human Resources Security
- Risk Management
- Security Policy
- Organization of Information Security
- Compliance
- Asset Management
- Physical and Environmental Security
- Communications and Operations Management
- Information Systems Acquisition, Development and Maintenance
- Information Security Incident Management
- Business Continuity Management

HITRUST Common Security Framework v6 brochure. https://hitrustalliance.net/content/uploads/2014/02/HITRUST-CSF-Brochure.pdf

BOX 26.7   NIST Cybersecurity Framework Functions and Categories

Function Unique Identifier	Function	Category Unique Identifier	Category
ID	Identify	ID.AM	Asset Management
		ID.BE	Business Environment
		ID.GV	Governance
		ID.RA	Risk Assessment
		ID.RM	Risk Management Strategy
PR	Protect	PR.AC	Access Control
		PR.AT	Awareness and Training
		PR.DS	Data Security
		PR.IP	Information Protection Processes and Procedures
		PR.MA	Maintenance
		PR.PT	Protective Technology
DE	Detect	DE.AE	Anomalies and Events
		DE.CM	Security Continuous Monitoring
		DE.DP	Detection Processes
RS	Respond	RS.RP	Response Planning
		RS.CO	Communications
		RS.AN	Analysis
		RS.MI	Mitigation
		RS.IM	Improvements
RC	Recover	RC.RP	Recovery Planning
		RC.IM	Improvements
		RC.CO	Communications

NIST Cybersecurity Framework v1.0, http://www.nist.gov/cyberframework/upload/cybersecurity-framework-021214.pdf. Accessed February 8, 2016.

occurring at the state government level. For example, the Texas Health Services Authority partnered with HITRUST to establish standards for sharing PHI and maintaining compliance with federal and state law.[37]

The U.S. federal government recognizes the importance of cybersecurity and has taken steps to help organizations across all industries, including healthcare, to understand and manage cybersecurity risks. The National Institute of Standards and Technology (NIST) is one agency heavily involved with cybersecurity. The NIST Computer Security Resource Center (CSRC) publishes a series of special publications (SPs) on computer security available at http://csrc.nist.gov/publications/PubsSPs.html. These are documents of interest to the security community and include current topics such as security measures for cloud computing and mobile devices. The collection is known as the SP 800 series because the documents, like SP 800-53 mentioned previously, are identified with a number beginning with the prefix 800. For example, NIST publishes SP 800-66, "An Introductory Resource Guide for Implementing HIPAA Security Rule." Other relevant NIST documents are outside the SP 800 series. One example is the Cybersecurity Framework created by the NIST in 2014.[38]

The Cybersecurity Framework consists of three parts that work together to manage cybersecurity risk. The first part, *Framework Core*, includes activities, desired outcomes, and references common across multiple industries. Best practices, industry standards, and guidelines are organized and presented. These are organized into five *functions*: Identify, Protect, Detect, Respond, and Recover. Each function is further organized into subcategories and aligned with *Informative References*. Box 26.7 shows the Cybersecurity Framework functions and categories.[38] Box 26.8 provides information about the HIPAA Security Rule Crosswalk to the NIST Cybersecurity Framework.

BOX 26.8   Security Rule Crosswalk to Cybersecurity Framework

In February 2016, the Office of Civil Rights (OCR) released a crosswalk developed with the National Institute of Standards and Technology (NIST) and the Office of the National Coordinator for Health IT (ONC), providing a helpful mapping of the HIPAA Security Rule and the Cybersecurity Framework, along with other commonly used security frameworks.

The crosswalk is available at http://www.hhs.gov/hipaa/for-professionals/security/nist-security-hipaa-crosswalk.

The second part is the *Framework Implementation Tiers* characterizing an organization's risk management practices as Partial (Tier 1), Risk Informed, Repeatable, or Adaptive (Tier 4). The framework recognizes varying target profiles and bases success on an organization achieving its cybersecurity goals versus progression to a higher tier.[38]

The third part is the *Framework Profile*, which represents the organization's business needs and priorities. The profile enables the organization to establish a roadmap to address cybersecurity risk in alignment with the organization's goals, regulatory requirements, and best practices. Comparing the current profile to the target profiles reveals gaps to be addressed.[38]

The previously provided frameworks are significantly influenced by the NIST RMF, as is the HIPAA Security Rule. The NIST RMF provides a structured, disciplined, extensible, and repeatable process built around continuous monitoring. NIST SP 800-66, "An Introductory Resource Guide for Implementing the HIPAA Security Rule," includes specific mapping of RMF phases to HIPAA Security Rule requirements.[39] The NIST RMF was initiated in 2005 and has been expanded to describe over 230 specific security controls organized into 17 families. Fig. 26.2 illustrates how the security controls are applied throughout the RMF Security Life Cycle.[40] Selected security controls will be highlighted later in this chapter.

More federal guidance is forthcoming. The Cybersecurity Act of 2015 included nine pages dedicated to healthcare-related security. Included in the language is the requirement for a task force to be formed with representatives from HHS, Homeland Security, and NIST. The task force is to examine the actions and safeguards used in other industries for application to healthcare cybersecurity. It is also tasked with analyzing EHR and interoperability issues.[41]

Another requirement of the Cybersecurity Act of 2015 is that agencies continue to improve preparedness by educating stakeholders and sharing cyber threat indicators and defensive measures between government and other entities. Also included is the Cybersecurity Information Sharing Act that establishes the personal data to be removed before data are shared and the notification rules for individuals whose information is shared.[41]

Legal Requirements and Fines

Legal requirements and potential fines make information security even more critical to organizations. In 2011, the largest fine was $4.3 million for an organization that refused to release health records to several patients and then did not cooperate with the government's investigation of the matter.[34] Today penalties and other costs related to security breaches have far exceeded the 2011 example. In fact, 2015 was considered to be a record year for privacy breaches. According to the Identity Theft Resource Center, the number of total breaches in 2015 was 781, about the same as in 2014, while the number of records compromised almost doubled from 85 million to 169 million. Of those numbers, 35.5% of the breaches and 66.7% of the records compromised were for healthcare organizations.[42] Financial penalties affected organizations in the form of fines; organizations are also faced with the costs of notifying affected customers as well as civil litigation.[43]

As can be seen in Table 26.4, security breaches are costly to organizations. The average cost of a health record breach in 2010 was $301 per compromised record.[44] In 2015, that figure grew to $363 per record.[45] Healthcare data breaches have become the most costly type of breach to remediate and are over twice the average cost across all industries. Considering that a single breach can include thousands or millions of records, even one breach is expensive. The average cost of a breach at a healthcare organization is estimated at over

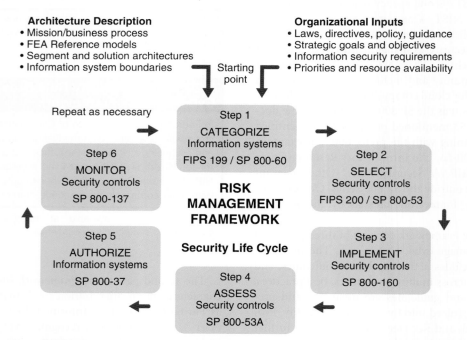

Architecture Description
- Mission/business process
- FEA Reference models
- Segment and solution architectures
- Information system boundaries

Organizational Inputs
- Laws, directives, policy, guidance
- Strategic goals and objectives
- Information security requirements
- Priorities and resource availability

Starting point

Repeat as necessary

Step 1
CATEGORIZE
Information systems
FIPS 199 / SP 800-60

Step 6
MONITOR
Security controls
SP 800-137

Step 2
SELECT
Security controls
FIPS 200 / SP 800-53

RISK MANAGEMENT FRAMEWORK

Security Life Cycle

Step 5
AUTHORIZE
Information systems
SP 800-37

Step 3
IMPLEMENT
Security controls
SP 800-160

Step 4
ASSESS
Security controls
SP 800-53A

Note: CNSS Instruction 1253 provides guidance for RMF Steps 1 and 2 for National Security Systems (NSS).

FIG 26.2 NIST Risk Management Framework. (From *NIST Special Publication 800-53 Revision 4 Security and Privacy Controls for Federal Information Systems and Organizations*. Joint task force transformation initiative; April 2013. Found at <http://nvlpubs.nist.gov/nistpubs/SpecialPublications/NIST.SP.800-53r4.pdf> [p. 8].)

TABLE 26.4 Examples of HIPAA Violations and Related Fines

News Release Date	Institution or Company	Violations	Settlement Agreement
November 30, 2015	Triple-S Management Corporation (an insurance holding company in Puerto Rico)	• Failure to implement appropriate administrative, physical, and technical safeguards to protect the privacy of its beneficiaries' PHI • Impermissible disclosure of its beneficiaries' PHI to an outside vendor with which it did not have an appropriate business associate agreement • Use or disclosure of more PHI than was necessary to carry out mailings • Failure to conduct an accurate and thorough risk analysis that incorporates all IT equipment, applications, and data systems utilizing ePHI • Failure to implement security measures sufficient to reduce the risks and vulnerabilities of its ePHI to a reasonable and appropriate level	$3.5 million fine and develop robust correction actions to comply with HIPAA and privacy and security rules.
May 7, 2014	New York Presbyterian and Columbia University	• Failure to secure electronic patient record PHI on their shared network, affecting 6800 individuals • Failure to conduct accurate and thorough security risk assessments	$4.8 M and create a substantive corrective action plan, which includes undertaking a risk analysis, developing a risk management plan, revising policies and procedures, training staff, and providing progress reports
April 22, 2014	Concentra Health Services, Springfield, MA	• Lack of encryption on laptops, desktop computers, medication equipment (an unencrypted laptop was stolen) • Insufficient security management processes	$1.98 M and adopt a corrective action plan including retraining employees

$2 million, while a breach at a business associate averages over $1 million.[46] The largest healthcare breach to date, Anthem, could exceed $1 billion in costs.[47] Therefore multiple organizations have either purchased or are exploring the purchase of cyber insurance.

Increasing Security Threats to Healthcare Data

The security threats to healthcare data are increasing for a variety of reasons, including the expanding volume of healthcare data being stored, proliferation of EHRs interconnected by HIEs, the internet of things (IoT), and increasing attractiveness of health data to hackers.

Recent health practices increase the risk of a security breach, including increased electronic health data access and transmission due to the use of mobile devices and expanded health data sharing within and across health organizations. Mobile devices are attractive to healthcare providers because they support increased health data access and increased individual productivity. However, these devices also increase opportunities for interception of health data and, in turn, data loss.

Health data are being increasingly shared. EHR information is no longer tied to one institution, and traditional stakeholders are transitioning to having patients inputting information in their own records.[48] HIE, by design, is meant to enable data sharing within a region and between regions. Population-based research is growing and, with it, the need for increased security for "big data."[1] Authors are now publishing material about how to share health data nationally and internationally.[49] Sharing and transmission of health data is also increasing on local networks. Each of these has security implications and opportunities for breaches.

The IoT is the term used to refer to the collective set of sensors and mobile devices connected to the internet and exchanging data. The IoT is improving the healthcare experience for patients and providers while also increasing the risks to privacy and security. For example, patients may be discharged to home sooner by using technology that permits remote monitoring by nurses and physicians.[50] Inside hospitals, IoT technology such as radio frequency identification (RFID) and real-time location services (RTLS) enables the location of movable items, including people, to be tracked.

While these wireless, remote technologies provide tremendous value, they also bring new security vulnerabilities.

In 2015, external criminal attacks became the leading cause of healthcare data breaches.[46] One reason is that stolen medical identity may now be worth 10 to 20 times the value of a stolen credit card number.[51] Criminals may use a stolen medical identity to obtain expensive health services or equipment that they can sell on the black market. It may take months or years for victims to learn that their medical identity has been compromised. Healthcare professionals must be aware that they are targets of attack from cybercriminals, simply due to their access to PHI.

CURRENT SECURITY VULNERABILITIES

Current security vulnerabilities can be classified into three types of events: natural events such as floods or hurricanes, external events such as malicious messages or hacking, and events internal to an organization.[52] Obviously, natural events such as lightning strikes can disable whole systems, networks, or security servers. In one example, a health organization abandoned a building but left clinical data in a locked closet. A power loss unlocked the door; nine servers containing clinical data were stolen.[34] Although natural events are dramatic, these events account for only a few of the reported security events.

External Events

Examples of external security events include outside attempts to access an organization's network (hacking), intrusions though a firewall, and installing malicious code or sending malicious messages via e-mail. Recent security conferences such as DefCon and BlackHat featured sessions about hacking into health systems.[34,53]

Large health systems have long protected their information systems and data using security controls described later in this chapter. Small organizations are more vulnerable[44] because they may lack the knowledge and resources necessary to implement security measures and information security may not be a high priority for them. For example, the network for a surgeons' group in California was hacked and data were stolen and encrypted to prevent access. Subsequently, the hackers sent a ransom note to the surgeons for return of their data; the surgeons refused to pay and lost all of their patients' data.[34] *Ransomware* has emerged as a new threat targeting the security of healthcare data.

Other targets for external hackers include systems readily accessible on the internet. Cloud-based services such as fitness trackers, personal health records, and even cloud-based EHRs may have many layers of protection from hackers but are extremely vulnerable to the simple compromise of a user's password.

Other methods of healthcare data access can be concerning. For example, a state-level agency may be a collector of healthcare data, but not a provider of services as a covered entity, and thus not required to comply with the HIPAA Privacy Rule. Some states offer collected healthcare data for sale to the public with less than effective de-identification of the data. Data collected by states may be subject to data mining and analysis that has been shown to reveal sensitive healthcare information.[54]

Internal Vulnerabilities

Prior to 2015, most security events in the healthcare industry were from internal sources, either unintentional or intentional.[44,52] This has changed so that today external threats are greater than internal ones. For internal events, security policies and procedures may be lacking in some organizations, or HIPAA compliance may not be a high priority,[32] especially in smaller organizations. Even if internal policies exist, current practices may not comply with either internal or external policies. Although security risk assessments or risk analyses are required under HIPAA, some organizations have never completed one and others do not complete them regularly.[44] In the latest available annual survey of professionals in health organizations, only 75% of respondents indicated that their organizations completed required risk analyses. This number was constant over the previous 4 years of surveys.[4] Since the 326 respondents do not represent all U.S. health organizations, the number of noncompliant organizations is likely much higher. Also, third-party organizations may not be using due diligence, even if main health organizations are compliant.

Many internal breaches are lapses in judgment. They may involve management decisions based on an understanding of relative priorities and constraints of limited resources. Other internal breaches are due to ineffective training.

Medical Devices

Medical devices present special security concerns because they interface directly with patients and therefore may cause immediate harm. This security concern was highlighted in 2011 when Jay Radcliffe, a security researcher with diabetes, described and demonstrated at a conference for security professionals how he was able to wirelessly hack into his insulin pump and remotely change the insulin dosage to potentially lethal levels.[55] Since that revelation, other researchers and investigators have been inspired to explore the cybersecurity vulnerabilities of medical devices and associated threats to patient health.[56]

Medical devices are proliferating and are being used for (1) monitoring (e.g., glucometers, oximetry, home blood pressure devices), (2) resuscitating (e.g., defibrillator, IV pumps), (3) surgical procedures (e.g., lasers, robotics such as da Vinci), (4) imaging (e.g., computed tomography, magnetic resonance imaging, echograms), and (5) diagnostic procedures (e.g., ultrasound, endoscopy). A growing number of life-sustaining devices, such as pacemakers and defibrillators, are implanted into patients and controlled externally via wireless communications.[56,57] Many of these devices have the capability to connect and share data through networks or even operate remotely through wireless or cellular networks.

Because these devices can connect to a network and share data, they also can be hacked. Multiple government agencies took notice of these potential cybersecurity and health impacts. The U.S. Department of Homeland Security Industrial Control Systems Cyber Emergency Response Team is investigating dozens of potential vulnerabilities in medical devices.[56] The U.S. Food and Drug Administration (FDA) is also engaged and in 2013 issued statements recommending manufacturers review cybersecurity aspects of medical devices to prevent unauthorized access or modification.[56] In 2015, the FDA issued a safety communication regarding vulnerabilities of specific infusion pump systems and confirmed the ability to access one specific infusion system remotely via a hospital network.[58] At this writing, the FDA has issued draft guidance for safe data exchange for medical devices. Readers are encouraged to access the FDA website for the latest material on medical device design and security recommendations.

In addition to the risks to patient health, medical devices also open a link to sensitive information about patients. The medical device itself can store sensitive data, including PHI that are often not encrypted.[59] Many medical devices are sold without common security controls such as antivirus software. In health organizations, medical devices are typically deployed and managed by biomedical or clinical engineering staff who may operate separately from the IT department. This can create issues about the number and kinds of devices deployed, as well as confusion about which are connected to the IT network.

Health professionals must also be aware of devices that may hold PHI in ways that are not obvious. For example, many modern photocopiers and multipurpose office machines include internal storage that may retain PHI related to jobs processed. If the device is returned at the end of a lease, or is removed for maintenance, the data on the internal storage must be properly erased. In 2013, HHS announced a settlement with Affinity Health Plan Inc. for a breach that occurred in 2010 when multiple photocopiers were returned to a leasing agent without hard drives being properly erased. One of the returned copiers was acquired by the CBS Evening News and found to contain PHI. After an investigation, the OCR found PHI for up to 344,579 individuals was impermissibly disclosed. Affinity Health Plan Inc. settled the potential violations with a payment of $1,215,780.[60]

CURRENT SECURITY CHALLENGES

Healthcare data have become the leading target for hackers due to the ease of availability. Until recently, not much attention was paid to the theft of medical information. Healthcare data contains much more than just financial information and can be used in multiple ways (e.g. identity theft, insurance fraud, ransom, exploiting details about VIPs, and even diverting information for uses such as gambling on sporting events).

Challenges to health data security can be grouped into the following three main areas:

- The competing goals of gaining access to patient data to support care and limiting access to patient data to support security

- Competing institutional priorities and competition for institutional resources
- Multiple and evolving regulations

Health information access and security constitutes a balancing act. The activities carried out by healthcare organizations involve communications in shared workspace, work under time constraints, and the need to transmit sensitive data quickly across settings. These kinds of needs can conflict with security goals. Even with privacy and security training, care goals or productivity losses may discourage clinicians from adhering to security-related procedures and policies. The Healthcare Information and Management Systems Society (HIMSS) conducted surveys indicating that the adoption of security technologies by healthcare organizations was slow until 2015.

MANAGING SECURITY RISKS WITH SECURITY CONTROLS

Healthcare shares the need for information security with many other industries. While no system can ever be completely secure, the ongoing effort to maintain a system in the most secure state possible is called *risk management*. Most solutions to security are relatively simple and not costly to implement once their need is understood.[34]

The ONC Guide to Privacy and Security of Electronic Health Information v2.0 published in 2015 compiles guidance from various authoritative sources applicable to healthcare organizations of all sizes. Chapter 4 of the guide summarizes the HIPAA Security Rule that organizes safeguards required to secure PHI into three categories: *administrative, technical*, and *physical*. NIST SP 800-53 provides a comprehensive list of over 230 security safeguards or controls spanning these areas.

Administrative

Administrative safeguards are policies, procedures, and administrative actions that prevent, detect, contain, and correct violations of security. These include selection, development, implementation, and maintenance of security measures and also management of the people involved. One core requirement is to conduct a risk assessment to identify security risks and to then implement safeguards to address the risks.[27]

Administrative controls include establishing and adhering to security policies and procedures as well as dedicating resources to security. Formal policies and procedures set internal rules about how an organization and its employees will protect PHI. These should be based on federal guidelines for HIPAA and the HITECH Act, as well as the NIST SP 800 series guidelines mentioned previously. Although the health community is not mandated to adhere to the NIST 800 series guidelines, they can be used for HIPAA compliance.[34]

Internal policies should include processes such as installing software service packs, installing antivirus software, and testing. While most organizations do install service packs, the issue may be timing and completeness. Installation of required software patches is sometimes delayed due to other priorities. Patches require continuous monitoring and updating to protect patient data.[44] Organizations should also have policies and procedures in place for intrusion protection to avoid malware and malicious attacks such as ransomware. Finally, policies need to be in place to encrypt mobile devices used for PHI.[34] Wireless handheld devices should be encrypted, as they are vulnerable to loss.[33] Given the increased attention to the vulnerabilities of medical devices, organizations should assess the security capabilities of these devices before purchase. Probably most important, health organizations need to educate their employees on their existing policies and procedures and conduct security risk assessments on an ongoing basis.

Conducting Risk Assessments or Risk Analysis

Risk assessment, also called risk analysis, is required by the HIPAA Security Rule and by Meaningful Use.[44] The purpose of these assessments is to identify gaps or weaknesses that could lead to security breaches. These also assist in prioritizing risk remediation efforts.[34] More formally, security risks are assessed by examining vulnerabilities and threats where

- Risk is the likelihood that something adverse will happen to cause harm to an informational asset (or its loss).
- Vulnerability is a weakness in the information system, device, or environment that could endanger or cause harm to an informational asset.
- Threat is a human act or an act of nature that has the potential to cause harm to an informational asset.[61]

Risk assessments should be conducted regularly, with at least one complete assessment done annually. A comprehensive risk assessment can cost between $10,000 and $100,000, depending on the complexity of the environment.[44] Risk assessments include an evaluation of how and where PHI is stored within the organization, who is managing these data, how these data are being used, and where data are transmitted. A risk assessment includes a review of the security measures and technical architecture.[34,44]

A number of toolkits are available for conducting risk assessments in a healthcare setting. A suite of toolkits is available from the HIMSS Privacy and Security Committee as well as the Agency for Healthcare Research and Quality (AHRQ) website (URLs are available at the end of the chapter). These toolkits include, for example, risk assessments for small practices, mobile devices, and cybersecurity.

Technical

Technical safeguards involve protecting the confidentiality, integrity, and availability of PHI. Common technical security controls for technology include authentication, access management and control, encryption, protection from malware and hacking attacks, disaster recovery planning, and privacy-enhancing technologies.

Authentication is defined as the technology and techniques for verifying the identity of human users of an information or computer system.[61] Authenticating a person means verifying that the person is who he or she claims to be. Reliable authentication is essential for access control and

auditing. Similar to the critical step of validating patient identity before administering medications, users must be authenticated before accessing PHI. Methods are evolving beyond traditional passwords that may be easily compromised. Biometrics such as fingerprint, iris, palm vein, and face recognition have been available for some time. Tokens such as access cards with accompanying PIN codes are widely used, similar to ATM cards. Such "two-factor authentication" requires users to both *know* something (the PIN code) and *have* something (the card) in order to authenticate. Two-factor authentication is much more secure than a password alone. Modern wireless technology permits the token for authentication to simply be nearby, or within proximity, rather than requiring insertion into a reader.

Encryption is the mathematical conversion of data into a form, called ciphertext, that cannot be easily understood by unauthorized people.[61] This technical method protects PHI against unauthorized access. To be able to access the data, an authorized person has to decrypt the data—that is, change the ciphertext back into the original, understandable data. This is accomplished through the use of a security key such as a password. This functions much like a padlock protects physical access: only someone with the key can unlock the padlock. Likewise, encryption keys must be carefully controlled to ensure data security. Encryption is a primary method of rendering PHI unusable, unreadable, or indecipherable to unauthorized individuals, either when the data are stored (at rest) or traversing a network (in transit).

Encryption is not required by HIPAA but often makes the difference in determining whether an incident constitutes a breach or not. The Final Breach Notification Rule indicates that if data are unusable, unreadable, or indecipherable to unauthorized individuals, then notification is not required following an impermissible use or disclosure. To qualify for this "safe harbor," the data must have been encrypted in compliance with NIST guidelines.

Encryption is available for use on many technology platforms (e.g., EHRs, desktop computers, laptops). Facilities can also encrypt PHI on mobile devices, e-mail, and files. This technology is not currently available for all platforms; for example, not all cellphone devices contain encryption capability. However, users can purchase encryption software separately and download it for use on devices. In some cases, the software is free for individual users but not for enterprise contracts. When cellphones are used to store PHI, use of encryption capability is critical.

Physical

The third category of security safeguards is physical. This involves physical methods to protect inappropriate access to PHI.[61] Examples are controlled access to buildings, workstation security, and securing portable devices such as medical devices or laptops with a cable and locking them to a desk.[59] Defined by administrative controls, actual physical devices or measures are put into place for improved security. Additional examples of physical security safeguards are: requiring two forms of identification for access, security guards and alarm systems, fire detection and suppression systems, redundancy for power and network connections, securing output from devices, and logging access to secured equipment.

RESOURCES

A number of resources are available to guide organizations in the administrative, technical, and physical aspects of information security. Examples include the following:

- AHRQ security toolkits available at http://healthit.ahrq. gov/portal/server.pt/community/health_it_tools_and_ resources/919/the_health_information_security_and_ privacy_collaboration_toolkit/27877
- HIMSS Privacy and Security Committee website at http:// www.himss.org/get-involved/committees/privacy-and-security.
- HIMSS Privacy and Security Toolkit—risk assessments, small provider privacy and security guides, and mobile devices cloud computing security—available at http:// www.himss.org/library/healthcare-privacy-security/toolkit
- HIPAA Security Rule Guidance from HHS available at http://www.hhs.gov/hipaa/for-professionals/security/guidance/index.html
- HIPAA Security Rule to NIST Cybersecurity Framework Crosswalk available at http://www.hhs.gov/hipaa/for-professionals/security/nist-security-hipaa-crosswalk
- NIST Computer Security Resource Center (CSRC) website at http://csrc.nist.gov
- NIST Guidelines for Media Sanitization available at http://nvlpubs.nist.gov/nistpubs/SpecialPublications/NIST.SP.800-88r1.pdf
- NIST security guidelines available at http://csrc.nist.gov/publications/PubsSPs.html, including the NIST Cybersecurity Practice Guides from 2015

CONCLUSIONS AND FUTURE DIRECTIONS

Confidentiality, integrity, and availability are critical to patient care and for improving outcomes. Practitioners and patients need to be confident that patient data are accurate and accessible when needed.

Given record privacy breaches in recent years, the need for information security will continue to be an urgent topic in the future. Currently the healthcare system is heavily dependent on legislation and regulations to ensure health information privacy, confidentiality, and security. However, this approach presents its own set of problems. Innovations in technology constantly offer the opportunity to improve healthcare delivery. But until these innovations are available and in use, it is impossible to develop legislation or regulation ensuring their adherence to ethical principles. Thus safeguards can lag behind innovations. In addition, "markets can incentivize irresponsible behaviors. Companies need to build their trustiness to gain our trust."[62, p. 24] Legislative attempts to prevent these irresponsible behaviors can act to limit the development of new and innovative approaches to improve healthcare delivery.

One approach to this challenge is for the industry to proactively consider the ethical, social, and legal implications in the design of innovative technologies. An example of this approach can be seen in the "Guidelines for Personalized Health Technology Final Report" developed under the direction of the Vitality Institute (http://thevitalityinstitute.org). These guidelines seek to build collaboration across the public and private sectors. They have the goal of creating a dialogue for personalized health technologies and promoting shared values for all stakeholders. The guidelines are built around five critical principles:

1. Build health technologies informed by science
2. Scale affordable health technologies
3. Guide interpretation of health data
4. Protect and secure health data
5. Govern the responsible use of health technology and data[62]

Another approach is the newer models for security being developed in lieu of current role-based models. For example, one model being developed places information control and release in the hands of patients.[63] These types of security frameworks allow patients to give informed consent for access to any data. Every data element is tagged with a unique identification code to prevent linking to unauthorized data. The framework provides a link to access control with a device such as a smart card and traceable information flow through the use of data on a central server should the mobile device be lost. This is more flexible than HIPAA security, where blanket consent is given.

In summary, privacy and security have been and will continue to be concerns for patients and healthcare providers. Health informaticians need a solid grounding in the concepts and solutions for these important principles.

REFERENCES

1. Stevenson F, Lloyd N, Harrington L, Wallace P. Use of electronic patient records for research: views of patients and staff in general practice. *Fam Pract.* 2012;30(2):227–232.
2. Davis J. 7 largest data breaches of 2015. *Healthcare IT News.* December 11, 2015. http://www.healthcareitnews.com/news/7-largest-data-breaches-2015?mkt_tok=3RkMMJWWfF9wsRonu6%2FBc%2B%2FhmjTEU5z16ewsXaayg4kz2EFye%2BLIHETpodcMTcNmPbjYDBceEJhqyQJxPr3MLtINwNlqRhPrCg%3D%3D. Accessed January 5, 2016.
3. *Census Data.* U.S. Census 2014. http://quickfacts.census.gov/qfd/states/06000.html. Accessed February 9, 2016.
4. Breach Portal. *Department of Health and Human Services, Office of Civil Rights. Notice to the Secretary of HHS Breach of Unsecured Protected Health Information Rights*; January 5, 2016. https://ocrportal.hhs.gov/ocr/breach/breach_report.jsf.
5. Soares NV, Dall'Agnol CM. Patient privacy: an ethical question for nursing care management. *Acta Paul Enferm.* 2011; 24(5):683–688. http://www.scielo.br/scielo.php?pid=S0103-21002011000500014&script=sci_arttext. Accessed July 5, 2016.
6. Hartzog W. Information privacy: chain-link confidentiality. *Ga L Rev.* 2012;46(3):657–704.

7. Neuhaus C, Polze A, Chowdhuryy M. *Survey on Health Care IT Systems: Standards, Regulation and Security.* Potsdam, NY: Potsdam University; 2011.

8. Rothstein MA. The Hippocratic bargain and health information technology. *J Law Med Ethics.* 2010;38(1):7–13.

9. Nightingale F. *Notes on Nursing*; 1860. http://quickfacts.census.gov/qfd/states/06000.html.

10. Olsen DP, Dixon JK, Grey M, Deshefy-Longhi T, Demarest JC. Privacy concerns of patients and nurse practitioners in primary care: an APRNet study. *J Am Acad Nurse Prac.* 2005;17 (12):527–534.

11. *Privacy Policy Guidance.* The fair information practice principles: framework for privacy policy at the Department of Homeland Security. http://www.dhs.gov/xlibrary/assets/privacy/privacy_policyguide_2008-01.pdf. Accessed January 13, 2016.

12. *Fair Information Practice Principles.* National strategy for trusted identities in cyberspace. Appendix A. National Institute for Standards and Technology. http://www.nist.gov/nstic/NSTIC-FIPPs.pdf. Accessed July 5, 2016.

13. Gellman R. *Fair information practices: a basic history. Version 2.15.* BobGellman.com; 2015. http://bobgellman.com/rg-docs/rg-FIPShistory.pdf.

14. International Medical Informatics Association (IMIA). *IMIA code of ethics for health information professionals.* IMIA; 2002. 2002. *http://www.imia-medinfo.org/new2/pubdocs/Ethics_Eng. pdf.* Accessed January 5, 2016.

15. *The Privacy Act of 1974 5 U.S.C. § 552a.* U.S. Department of Justice; 1974. http://www.justice.gov/opcl/privstat.htm.

16. Department of Health, Education and Welfare. Confidentiality of alcohol and drug abuse patient records. *Fed Regist.* 1975;40–127. http://archive.hhs.gov/ohrp/documents/19750701.pdf.

17. Office of the National Coordinator for Health Information Technology. *Nationwide privacy and security framework for electronic exchange of individually identifiable health information.* U.S. Department of Health & Human Services; 2008. https://www.healthit.gov/sites/default/files/nationwide-ps-framework-5.pdf.

18. *Health Information Privacy.* Health and human services. http://www.hhs.gov/hipaa/index.html. Accessed January 12, 2016.

19. Kay M, Santos J, Takane M. *Global Observatory for eHealth Series: Legal Frameworks for eHealth*, vol. 5. Geneva, Switzerland: World Health Organization; 2012.

20. *European Parliament and the Council of 24 October.* Directive 95/46/EC of the European Parliament and of the Council of 24 October 1995 on the protection of individuals with regard to the processing of personal data and on the free movement of such data. EUR-LEX Access to European Union Law. http://eur-lex.europa.eu/LexUriServ/LexUriServ.do?uri=CELEX:31995L0046:en:NOT.

21. Scott M. Europe approves tough new data protection rules. *New York Times.* 2015. http://www.nytimes.com/2015/12/16/technology/eu-data-privacy.html?_r=0.

22. European Commission. *EU Commission and United States agree on new framework for transatlantic data flows;* 2016. http://europa.eu/rapid/press-release_IP-16-216_en.htm.

23. *International Privacy Laws.* Information shield, Inc. http://www.informationshield.com/intprivacylaws.html. Accessed January 13, 2016.

24. HITECH Act Enforcement Interim Final Rule. *Health information privacy.* U.S. Department of Health & Human Services; 2009. http://www.hhs.gov/hipaa/for-professionals/special-topics/HITECH-act-enforcement-interim-final-rule/index.html.

25. *HIAA Definition of Breach.* HIPAA regulation. http://www.hipaasurvivalguide.com/hipaa-regulations/164-402.php. Accessed January 13, 2016.

26. *Omnibus HIPAA Rulemaking.* Health Information Privacy. U.S. Department of Health & Human Services. http://www.hhs.gov/hipaa/for-professionals/privacy/laws-regulations/combined-regulation-text/omnibus-hipaa-rulemaking/index.html. Accessed January 13, 2016.

27. Office of the National Coordinator for Health Information Technology. *Guide to privacy and security of electronic health information, version 2.0;* 2015. https://www.healthit.gov/sites/default/files/pdf/privacy/privacy-and-security-guide.pdf.

28. *HealthIT.gov.* Federal-state security & privacy coordination (HISPC). HealthIT.gov. http://www.healthit.gov/policy-researchers-implementers/federal-state-privacy-security-collaboration-hispc. Accessed January 13, 2016.

29. *U.S. Department of Health & Human Services (HHS) Office for Civil Rights.* Summary of the HIPAA privacy rule. *Health Information Privacy.* http://www.hhs.gov/hipaa/for-professionals/privacy/laws-regulations/. Accessed January 13, 2016.

30. *U.S. Department of Health & Human Services (HHS) Office for Civil Rights.* Guidance regarding methods for de-identification of protected health information in accordance with the Health Insurance Portability and Accountability Act (HIPAA) privacy rule. HHS. http://www.hhs.gov/hipaa/for-professionals/privacy/special-topics/de-identification/. Accessed January 13, 2016.

31. *U.S. Department of Health & Human Services (HHS) Office for Civil Rights.* Summary of the security rule. http://www.hhs.gov/hipaa/for-professionals/security/laws-regulations/index.html. Accessed January 23, 2016.

32. Neubauer T, Heurix J. A methodology for the pseudonymization of medical data; *Int J Med Inform.* 2011;80(3):190–204.

33. Huang C, Lee H, Lee DH. A privacy-strengthened scheme for E-health care monitoring system. *J Med Syst.* 2012;36(5):2959–2971.

34. McMillan M. A national perspective on helping IT play a meaningful role in health care reform. Paper presented at: Summer Insight Educational Session, Salt Lake City, UT; August 16, 2012.

35. *Health Information Trust Alliance (HITRUST).* HITRUST CSF. https://hitrustalliance.net/hitrust-csf Accessed January 25, 2016.

36. *HITRUST.* What's new in CSF v7. https://hitrustalliance.net/whats-new-csf-v7/. Accessed January 31, 2016.

37. *Texas Health Services Authority.* SECURETexas background. http://securetexas.org/about/background. Accessed January 25, 2016.

38. NIST. *Framework for improving critical infrastructure cybersecurity, version 1.0;* 2014. http://www.nist.gov/cyberframework/upload/cybersecurity-framework-021214-final.pdf.

39. Scholl MA, Stine KM, Hash J, et al. *SP 800-66 Rev. 1. An introductory resource guide for implementing the Health Insurance Portability and Accountability Act (HIPAA) security rule.* NIST; 2008. http://csrc.nist.gov/publications/nistpubs/800-66-Rev1/SP-800-66-Revision1.pdf.

40. Ross R. *NIST SP 800-53, Revision 4. Security and Privacy Controls for Federal Information Systems and Organizations.* NIST; 2013.

41. Davis J. 5 key takeaways from Cybersecurity Act of 2015. *Healthcare IT News;* December 28, 2015. http://www.healthcareitnews.com/news/5-key-takeaways-cybersecurity-act-2015.

42. Identity Theft Resource Center. 2015 data breach category summary; 2016. http://www.idtheftcenter.org/images/breach/ITRCBreachStatsReportSummary2015.pdf.
43. McMillan M. The cost of IT security. *Healthc Financ Manage*. 2015;69(4):44–48.
44. McMillan M. HITECH security mandates for health care organizations. *Healthc Financ Manage*. 2011;65(11):118–122. 124.
45. Conn J. Healthcare data breaches are costliest: study. *Mod Healthc*. 2015. http://www.modernhealthcare.com/article/20150528/NEWS/150529899.
46. Ponemon Institute. *Fifth annual benchmark study on privacy & security of healthcare data*; May 2015. http://media.scmagazine.com/documents/121/healthcare_privacy_security_be_30019.pdf.
47. Redspin. *Breach Report 2014: Protected Health Information (PHI)*. Carpinteria, CA: Redspin, Inc; February 2015.
48. Haas S, Wohlgemuth S, Echizen I, Sonehara N, Muller G. Aspects of privacy for electronic health records. *Int J Med Inform*. 2011;80(2):e26–e31.
49. Li JS, Zhou TS, Chu J, Araki K, Yoshihara H. Design and development of an international clinical data exchange system: the international layer function of the Dolphin Project. *J Am Med Inform Assoc*. 2011;18(5):683–689.
50. Harpham B. How the internet of things is changing healthcare and transportation. *CIO*; 2015. http://www.cio.com/article/2981481/healthcare/how-the-internet-of-things-is-changing-healthcare-and-transportation.html.
51. Humer C, Finkle J. *Your medical record is worth more to hackers than your credit card*. Reuters.com; 2014. http://www.reuters.com/article/us-cybersecurity-hospitals-idUSKCN0HJ21I20140924.
52. Liu CH, Chung YF, Chen TS, Wang SD. The enhancement of security in health care information systems. *J Med Syst*. 2012;36(3):1673–1688.
53. Blake A. Medical devices too prone to hackers, researchers warn. *Wash Post*; 2015. http://www.washingtontimes.com/news/2015/aug/6/medical-devices-too-prone-hackers-researchers-warn.
54. Sweeney L. Only you, your doctor, and many others may know. *Technology Science*; 2015. http://techscience.org/a/2015092903.
55. Radcliffe J. *Hacking medical devices for fun and insulin: breaking the human SCADA system. Black Hat Conference*; January 23, 2016. https://media.blackhat.com/bh-us-11/Radcliffe/BH_US_11_Radcliffe_Hacking_Medical_Devices_WP.pdf.
56. Klonoff D. Cybersecurity for connected diabetes devices. *J Diabetes Sci Technol*. 2015;9(5):1143–1147.
57. Sametinger J, Rozenblit J, Lysecky R, Ott P. Security challenges for medical devices. *Commun ACM*. 2015;58(4):74–82.
58. *U.S. Food and Drug Administration*. Medical devices: cybersecurity. http://www.fda.gov/MedicalDevices/DigitalHealth/ucm373213.htm. Accessed February 13, 2016.
59. Swim R. Keeping data secure: protected health information and medical equipment. *Biomed Instrum Technol*. 2012;46(4):278–280.
60. *Department of Health and Human Services*. HHS settles with health plan in photocopier breach case. http://www.hhs.gov/hipaa/for-professionals/compliance-enforcement/examples/health-plan-photocopier-breach-case/index.html. Accessed January 31, 2016.
61. Brown GD, Patrick TB, Pasupathy K. *Health Informatics: A Systems Perspective*. Chicago, IL: Health Administration Press; 2012.
62. Christie GP, Patrick K, Yach D. *Guidelines for Personalized Health Technology: Final Report*. The Vitality Group & the Vitality Institute; 2016. http://thevitalityinstitute.org/projects/personalized-health-technology/.
63. Health care Information and Management Systems Society (HIMSS). *HIMSS Security Survey*. Chicago, IL: HIMSS; 2011.
64. Kissel R, ed. *Glossary of Key Information Security Terms (NIST IR 7298, revision 1)*. Washington, DC: U.S. Department of Commerce & National Institute of Standards and Technology; 2011.

DISCUSSION QUESTIONS

1. Hospitals usually have a policy and related procedure for responding when patients request a copy of their records. Select a procedure from your current place of employment or a local hospital. Compare and contrast the selected procedure with the principles of fair information practice (FIPs).
2. The European Union created privacy agreements across their 28 members. What are the challenges and resources for creating an agreement to share health data across the borders of countries near you (e.g., Canada and the United States or Mexico and the United States)?
3. The following websites include toolkits for completing a risk assessment:
   a. www.himss.org/ASP/topics_pstoolkitsDirectory.asp?faid=569&tid=4
   b. https://healthit.ahrq.gov/health-it-tools-and-resources/health-information-security-and-privacy-collaboration-toolkit

   Review the risk assessment guides available at these sites and then answer the following question: Since HIPAA requires that a covered entity appoint a security officer, what is the role of the health professional or informatics specialist in working with the security officer to complete a risk assessment? In your discussion, consider who has access to the information required to complete the assessment and how the information should be collected.
4. Providing access to healthcare providers and securing a system from inappropriate access can be a difficult balancing act. In many cases, the more secure a system is, the more restricted access to that system becomes. Discuss situations where this balancing act has created conflict or might create conflict within the clinical area and how that conflict was (or could be) managed.
5. Increasingly patients are creating and maintaining personal health records (PHRs) with data from a variety of healthcare providers, as well as data they have generated about their health. What provisions should be included in a model privacy and security policy that patients might use in making decisions related to their privacy and the security of their PHRs?

CASE STUDY

Last month you were hired with the title Health Informatics Specialist at an independent community care hospital with 350 beds. The hospital includes a comprehensive outpatient clinic, a rehabilitation center with both inpatient and outpatient services, a cardiac care center, and an emergency room. In addition, four family health centers are located throughout the community. More than 930 primary care and specialty physicians are associated with the hospital, which has a staff of just over 2000 employees. The hospital has an EHR in place.

The hospital has a working relationship with a major academic medical center located 23 miles away. Acute care patients who need more extensive treatment are usually transferred to the medical center. These are often emergency situations, and data are freely shared among the institutions with the best interests of the patient in mind.

Located directly beside the hospital is a 194-bed skilled nursing home. While the nursing home has its own medical staff consisting of a physician and two nurse practitioners, patients needing consults or additional care are usually seen at the hospital with follow-up at physicians' offices. While the nursing home, most of the physicians' offices, and the hospital are independent institutions, there is a long history of sharing health-related data when treating patients who live at the nursing home and are seen at the hospital or in the physicians' offices. This coordination is seen as a general benefit for a number of patients. It appears that most patients have signed a form giving the hospital permission to send information to the nursing home. However, these forms have been stored in individual offices, so it is difficult to determine who has signed what forms and what permission has or has not been given to share information among the nursing home, hospital, and independent medical practices.

Discussion Questions

1. What additional information is needed to clarify what problems may exist and what changes may be needed in terms of data that are shared among the institutions?
2. Can the EHR system and/or e-mail be used to share data among these different institutions more effectively and securely? If yes, how would this be done? For example, what agreements, policies, and procedures might need to be developed?
3. In your position as Health Informatics Specialist, how would you go about determining whether there are other potential security issues that now need to be managed by the hospital?

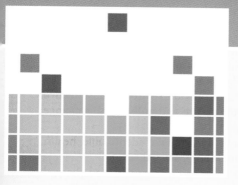

27

The Health Information Technology for Education and Clinical Health Act, Meaningful Use, and Medicare Access and CHIP Reauthorization Act of 2015

Michele P. Madison

As federal legislation continues to drive changes in how healthcare is provided and how payment is received, using information technology will facilitate enhanced and creative models for new healthcare delivery designs.

Michele P. Madison

OBJECTIVES

At the completion of this chapter, the reader will be prepared to:

1. Discuss key federal legislative initiatives related to the adoption of health information technology.
2. Describe the Centers for Medicare and Medicaid Services (CMS) financial incentive program to encourage the adoption of electronic health records (EHRs).
3. Describe the objectives for each stage of the Meaningful Use (MU) program.
4. Analyze the progression and impact of the MU program.
5. Describe the Medicare Access and CHIP Reauthorization Act of 2015 (MACRA) and its potential impact on value-based payment models.

KEY TERMS

Children's Health Insurance Program (CHIP), 472
eligible professional (EP), 460
meaningful objectives, 461

Meaningful Use (MU), 455
modified Stage 2, 466

ABSTRACT ❖

Healthcare reform and economic stimulus legislation are rapidly advancing regulations that incentivize the adoption and Meaningful Use (MU) of electronic health records (EHRs) with the goal of improving the health of Americans. However, in order to obtain financial incentives, healthcare providers must perform specific tasks that demonstrate the provider is meaningfully using a certified EHR. The MU standards also merge into the changes driven by the healthcare reform legislation. Throughout the stimulus funding and healthcare reformation laws, the federal government's policies for improving care coordination by reducing costs and engaging patients and families remain constant elements, and the initiatives are the basis for changing healthcare providers' behavior. This chapter explores these key legislative initiatives and describes their impact on the healthcare delivery processes.

INTRODUCTION

A new era of government support for health information technology (IT) began on April 27, 2004, when President George W. Bush addressed the topic in his State of the Union address: "an electronic health record (EHR) for every American by the year 2014…by computerizing health records, we can avoid dangerous medical mistakes, reduce costs and improve care."[1] Commencing with the American Recovery and Reinvestment Act of 2009, commonly referred to as the "Stimulus Act," the federal government began using legislation supporting financial incentives to change how healthcare services would be delivered. The Health Information Technology for Education and Clinical Health (HITECH) Act portion of the Stimulus Act dedicated billions of dollars to change how healthcare providers documented the services rendered and communicated with both patients and payers. The MU program has now grown from capturing and entering specific forms of data into a certified EHR to communicating and transferring that data with other providers and patients with the longer-range goal of building a Nationwide Health Information Network (NwHIN). Building on these achievements, the federal government is moving forward with the development of programs and regulations to implement the Medicare Access and CHIP Reauthorization Act of 2015 (MACRA) that will change how providers are reimbursed by Medicare.

FEDERAL INITIATIVES TO DRIVE HEALTH INFORMATION TECHNOLOGY

The challenge for the healthcare system in the United States is to improve the quality of care for patients while reducing the costs of delivering such care, with the ultimate goal of achieving improved health and healthcare outcomes. Implementing health IT has been lauded as a critical element to address this challenge. Promoting the adoption and implementation of health IT is a bipartisan initiative that has been endorsed by both Republican and Democratic presidents, beginning with President George W. Bush's State of the Union address in 2004. Bipartisan support continues today with the approval of MACRA, which includes advanced practitioners and requires physicians to expand their use of health IT to maximize Medicare reimbursement.

Executive Order 13335

President Bush followed up on his 2004 State of the Union address by signing Executive Order 13335. This Executive Order outlined the federal initiative granting federal dollars to incentivize healthcare providers to implement and use health IT. The Executive Order created the position of Office of the National Coordinator for Health Information Technology (ONC) with the goal of facilitating the widespread adoption and implementation of EHRs across the United States. Ultimately the goals were to develop a NwHIN and to ensure that all residents of the United States had access to a clinical health record by 2014.

The federal initiative was built on six key components that have continued to serve as the foundation of the revolutionary changes to the healthcare delivery system. In 2004, the fundamental policies set forth by President Bush were as follows:

1. Ensure that appropriate information to guide medical decisions is available at the time and place of care.
2. Improve healthcare quality, reduce medical errors, and advance the delivery of appropriate, evidence-based medical care.
3. Reduce healthcare costs resulting from inefficiency, medical errors, inappropriate care, and incomplete information.
4. Promote a more effective marketplace, greater competition, and increased choice through the wider

availability of accurate information on healthcare costs, quality, and outcomes.
5. Improve the coordination of care and information among hospitals, laboratories, physician offices, and other ambulatory care providers through an effective infrastructure for the secure and authorized exchange of health information.
6. Ensure that patients' individually identifiable health information is secure and protected.[2]

While Executive Order 13335 created the ONC and charged this office with implementing an interoperable health IT system in both the public and the private healthcare sectors in order to reduce medical errors, improve quality, and produce greater value for healthcare expenditures, it was not until 2009, when the federal government passed the American Recovery and Reinvestment Act of 2009 (Stimulus Act), that the initiative was actually funded.[3]

The American Recovery and Reinvestment Act of 2009

The HITECH portion of the Stimulus Act was designed to (1) encourage health providers to adopt EHRs, (2) achieve MU of these EHRs, and (3) support the exchange of health information. These goals and the specific approaches for achieving them are illustrated in Fig. 27.1 and are explained later in this section.

To achieve these goals, the HITECH Act dedicated billions of dollars to change how healthcare providers documented the services rendered and communicated with both patients and payers. For example, taking a concept as simple as paying providers for implementing a certified EHR and requiring specific actions (called Meaningful Use) when using the certified HER began the process of changing healthcare providers' behavior. In order to obtain financial incentives, healthcare providers were required to perform specific tasks, thereby demonstrating that the provider was using a certified EHR in a meaningful way. The MU standards merge into the changes being driven by the healthcare reform legislation. Throughout the funding and reformation laws, the federal government's policies of improving care coordination by reducing costs and engaging patients and families remain constant elements. The sections of this legislation are outlined in Box 27.1.

Sections 3001, 3002, and 3003 of the HITECH Act establish the administrative structure for achieving the goals of the act by defining the responsibilities of (1) the ONC, (2) the Health IT Policy Committee, and (3) the Health IT Standards Committee.

Office of the National Coordinator for Health Information Technology

The HITECH Act established the ONC as a funded position with powers and authority granted by statutory support. Establishing the ONC through federal statutes instead of an executive order emphasized the fact that this position and its operations were approved and endorsed by both parties in Congress and represented a critical component of the

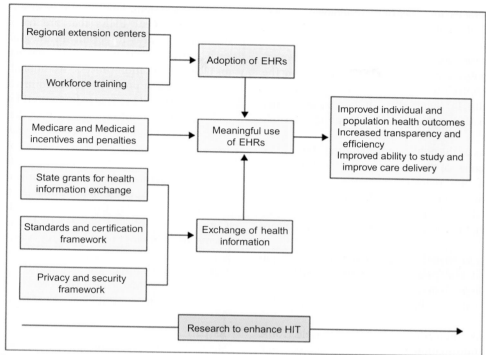

FIG 27.1 The HITECH Act's Framework for Meaningful Use of Electronic Health Records. (From Blumenthal, D. Launching HITECH. *N Engl J Med.* 2010;362(5):382–385. Used with permission of the *New England Journal of Medicine*.)

BOX 27.1 Sections of the Health Information Technology for Education and Clinical Health Act

Title XXX—Health Information Technology and Quality
Sec. 3000. Definitions.

Subtitle A—Promotion of Health Information Technology
Sec. 3001. Office of the National Coordinator for Health Information Technology.
Sec. 3002. HIT Policy Committee.
Sec. 3003. HIT Standards Committee.
Sec. 3004. Process for Adoption of Endorsed Recommendations; Adoption of Initial Set of Standards, Implementation Specifications, and Certification Criteria.

Sec. 3005. Application and Use of Adopted Standards and Implementation Specifications by Federal Agencies.
Sec. 3006. Voluntary Application and Use of Adopted Standards and Implementation Specifications by Private Entities.
Sec. 3007. Federal Health Information Technology.
Sec. 3008. Transitions.
Sec. 3009. Miscellaneous Provisions.

From the American Recovery and Reinvestment Act of 2009. 111th United States Congress. Page 123 STAT. 115 (February 17, 2009). *HIT*, health information technology; *HITECH*, health information technology for economic and clinical health.

BOX 27.2 Duties of the National Coordinator

- Standards
- HIT policy coordination
- Strategic plan
- Website

- Certification
- Reports and publications
- Assistance
- Governance for NwHIN

Data from the Health Information Technology for Economic and Clinical Health Act. 42 U.S.C. § 300jj-11. 2009. *HIT*, health information technology; *NwHIN*, nationwide health information network.

---

federally mandated strategic plan. Section 3001 lists the duties of the ONC and groups these duties into eight areas (Box 27.2). As shown in Box 27.2, Section 3001 of the HITECH Act directed the ONC to create a strategic plan to address the following federal initiatives:

1. The electronic exchange and use of health information and the integration of such information

2. The use of an EHR for each person in the United States by 2014
3. The incorporation of privacy and security protections for the electronic exchange of individually identifiable health information
4. Security methods (a) to ensure appropriate authorization and electronic authentication of health information and

(b) for specifying technologies or methodologies rendering health information unusable, unreadable, or indecipherable

5. A framework for coordination and flow of recommendations and policies under the HITECH Act among the secretary, the ONC, the Health IT Policy Committee, and the Health IT Standards Committee, and other health information exchanges (HIEs) among other relevant entities

6. Methods to foster the public understanding of health IT

7. Strategies to enhance the use of health IT in improving the quality of care, reducing medical errors, reducing health disparities, improving public health, increasing prevention and coordination with community resources, and improving the continuity of care among healthcare settings

8. Specific plans to ensure that populations with unique needs, such as children, are appropriately addressed in the technology design, which may include technology that automates enrollment and retention for eligible individuals[3]

To establish national uniform standards for the electronic exchange of health information and to facilitate the strategic plan, the HITECH Act included in the duties of the ONC responsibility for creating two committees that report to the ONC. These are the Health IT Policy Committee and the Health IT Standards Committee.

Health Information Technology Policy Committee

The Health IT Policy Committee was charged with making policy recommendations to the ONC relating to the implementation of a nationwide health IT infrastructure, including implementation of the eight components of the strategic plan listed previously. This committee is composed of individual stakeholders representing the full spectrum of the healthcare delivery system. These stakeholders include individual healthcare providers, patients, healthcare payer plans, legislative representatives, technology vendors, privacy and security experts, and other interested parties. Each stakeholder brings unique expertise and ultimately creates the policies defining MU of certified EHR systems. Additional opportunities to participate in the work of the Health IT Policy Committee are offered via workgroups. As of 2016, the workgroups include

• Advanced Health Models and MU
• Consumer
• Interoperability and HIE
• Privacy and Security

Health IT Standards Committee

The Health IT Standards Committee was charged with recommending standards, implementation specifications, and certification criteria for EHRs, electronic exchange, and use of health information. Specific standards for the electronic exchange of health information enable each healthcare provider, regardless of location, to transmit healthcare information and allow the receiving party to receive the data directly

in its EHR system. However, to ensure that healthcare providers implement EHRs that are based on the uniform national standards to permit meaningful exchange of data, each provider must use an EHR that has been certified by an ONC certification process. Additional information about this certification process is included in Chapter 19.

The Health IT Standards Committee is also a multistakeholder committee that includes healthcare providers, insurance companies, health IT companies that translate billing claims in nonstandard forms to a format that complies with specific electronic transaction standards (clearinghouses), academic institutions, and individuals who have specific health IT expertise and knowledge. In coordination with the Health IT Policy Committee, the Health IT Standards Committee established the standards and uniform requirements for technology to exchange data and to be deemed "certified" by the federal government. The Health IT Standards Committee task forces are

• Precision Medicine Task Force
• 2017 Interoperability Standards Advisory (ISA) Task Force

As part of their responsibility related to the standards, the Health IT Standards Committee, along with the ONC, is also responsible for recommending standards, including the necessary infrastructure to the state-funded HIEs and the privately run exchanges. Rather than using rule making through a top-down process for vetting and selecting the data transport, content exchange, and vocabulary standards, they chose a consensus-based bottom-up approach through the Standards and Interoperability (S&I) Framework Initiatives, working in collaboration with standards development organizations.

Office of the National Coordinator for Health Information Technology Standards and Interoperability Framework

Interoperability is the ability of health information systems to work together within and across organizational boundaries to improve the health and healthcare for individuals and communities by sharing data between all types of health IT. To achieve interoperability, standards for data transport, content exchange, and vocabulary management are needed. This is why standards development is so important; it enables the interoperability needed for regional and nationwide health data exchange and is essential to the development of patient-centric records. Additional information about specific standards is included in Chapter 22.

Launched in January 2011, the ONC-sponsored Standards and Interoperability ("S&I") Framework is a set of harmonized interoperability specifications to support national health outcomes and healthcare priorities, including MU and the ongoing mission to drive better care, better population health, increased patient engagement, and cost reduction through delivery improvements. The S&I Framework creates a forum for healthcare stakeholders to focus on solving real-world interoperability challenges. Each S&I Initiative focuses on a single interoperability challenge with a set of value-creating goals and outcomes that will enhance efficiency, quality, and effectiveness of the delivery of healthcare through the development or modification of standards for data transport, content exchange, and vocabulary management.

The S&I Framework started with three initiatives but now has 11 active and completed initiatives. Active initiatives include work on data access, data provenance, electronic submission of medical documentation, clinical quality, electronic long-term services and supports, and lab order interfaces. Each S&I Initiative has a rigorous process that includes the following:

- Development of clinically oriented user stories and robust use cases
- Harmonization of interoperability specifications and implementation guidance, including synchronization among the initiatives
- Provision of real-world experience and implementer support through new initiatives, workgroups, and pilot projects
- Mechanisms for feedback and testing of implementations, often in conjunction with ONC partners such as the National Institute of Standards and Technology (NIST)[4]

The work is done online through a moderated wiki with more than 2300 volunteer participants.[5] The focus of the S&I Framework is on delivering guidance to the health IT community through the development of standards content and technical specifications, the development of reusable tools and services, and the effort to unite stakeholders on common healthcare challenges. This work is necessary to move forward on data exchange between venues of care and to take healthcare delivery to the next level in creating a patient-centric rather than facility-centric healthcare record.

With the recognition that local and regional electronic exchange of health information is essential to the successful implementation of a nationwide exchange and to the success of national healthcare reform in general, the HITECH Act authorized and funded a State HIE Cooperative Agreement Program. This state-based grant program offered local and regional assistance and technical support to healthcare providers while enabling coordination and alignment within and among states. The State HIE program funding began winding down in 2014, with the HIEs creating sustainability models with mixed success. Concurrently, private exchanges with varying business models and value propositions are being established. Ultimately this will allow information to follow patients anywhere they go within the U.S. healthcare system.

In addition to the activities described here, both the Health IT Policy Committee and the Health IT Standards Committee engaged in research and workgroups that facilitated the development of specific policies and standards required for the foundational components of the NwHIN. To ensure coordination between the two committees, the Health IT Policy and Standards Committees meet jointly and collaborate in making recommendations to the National Coordinator for Health IT.

As pointed out previously in this chapter, the HITECH Act was designed to improve healthcare by encouraging healthcare providers to adopt and use EHRs in a meaningful

manner. While sections 3001, 3002, and 3003 established the ONC and related committees, additional sections of the HITECH Act define how both technical assistance provided by Regional Extension Centers (RECs) and financial incentives are designed to support the achievement of this goal.

Regional Extension Centers

In addition to financial incentives, HITECH supported the use of EHRs by establishing RECs and a national Health Information Technology Research Center (HITRC). This program funded 60 local organizations to create 62 RECs located in virtually every geographic region of the United States. RECs provided technical assistance to providers concerning EHR implementation and project management, training, vendor selection and financial consultation, workflow redesign, and privacy and security.[6] The HITRC promoted communication and learning among the RECs and collaborated with them by offering technical assistance, guidance, and information on best practices to support and accelerate healthcare providers' efforts to become meaningful users of EHRs.

The REC program funding began winding down in 2014. Currently, many of the RECs are working to become sustainable through fee-for-service models. As of August 2015, over 157,000 providers are enrolled with a REC; of these, more than 146,000 are live on an EHR, with more than 116,000 having demonstrated MU.[7]

In 2016, a report documenting the positive impact of RECs was published with the following key findings:

- REC participation was positively associated with EHR adoption among primary care physicians working in small practices or practices with a large underserved patient base.
- REC participation was positively associated with achieving MU at the level required to receive financial incentives.
- RECs provided needed technical assistance for physicians who were unable or ineligible to receive assistance from payers or health systems in their local area.
- The REC program likely helped many physicians who were more skeptical about EHRs and added these physicians to the pool of physicians with EHRs.[6]

Financial Incentives

The purpose of the health IT incentives outlined in the HITECH Act is to promote reform in the delivery, cost, and quality of healthcare in the United States. Dr. David Blumenthal, former national coordinator for health IT, emphasized this point when he said that health IT is the means but not the end. Getting health IT up and running in doctors' offices is not the main objective behind the incentives provided by the federal government under the American Recovery and Reinvestment Act—improving health is.[8]

The ultimate goal of the NwHIN is to support significant and measurable improvements in population health by an improved healthcare system. The vision includes engaging patients in their healthcare and ensuring that providers have immediate access to health information and tools to improve the quality and safety of care delivery. NwHIN also includes provisions for improved access and decreased healthcare disparities. To achieve this vision, healthcare providers must adopt and implement certified EHRs. Due to the cost of an EHR, many healthcare providers were reluctant to purchase a system. The HITECH Act amended the Social Security Act (42 U.S.C. 1395w-4) to provide financial incentives directly to healthcare providers that adopt, implement, and engage in MU of certified EHR technology. In the first year of the MU program, if an eligible professional (EP) or entity achieved and demonstrated to the satisfaction of the Secretary of the Department of Health and Human Services (HHS) that they had adopted, implemented, upgraded, and used a certified EHR technology in a meaningful manner, the EP or entity was entitled to receive financial incentives.

Eligible Entities and Eligible Professionals

Some healthcare providers are eligible to participate in both the Medicare and the Medicaid programs, while others are limited to only one potential program. Eligible entities for the Medicare program include the following:

1. All licensed hospitals that are reimbursed based on the prospective payment system
2. Critical access hospitals (CAHs)

An EP in the Medicare program is a doctor of medicine or osteopathy legally authorized to practice medicine and surgery, a doctor of dental surgery, a doctor of podiatric medicine, a doctor of optometry, or a chiropractor (see HITECH Act, Section 4101). All physicians participating in the Medicare program are eligible to participate in the financial incentive program regardless of the total percentage of Medicare patients treated by each physician.

To be eligible to participate in the Medicaid program, an individual physician must have a 30% Medicaid patient population. Pediatricians with a 20% Medicaid patient population are also eligible; however, these pediatricians will be eligible only for two-thirds of the financial incentives (see HITECH Act, Section 4201). The Medicaid program's eligible provider category also extends to certified nurse midwives and nurse practitioners. Physician assistants practicing in rural health clinics and federally qualified health centers are also eligible to participate.

Children's hospitals are eligible to participate in the Medicaid program and do not require a specific volume of Medicaid patients; other hospitals must have at least a 10% Medicaid patient volume to be eligible to participate in the Medicaid incentive program. Hospitals that satisfy the eligibility requirements may participate in both the Medicare and the Medicaid programs. However, individual physicians may participate in only one financial incentive program. Physicians are allowed to change from one program to the other, but this change is permitted only one time during the program.

Medicare and Medicaid Payments

Medicare payments are based on 75% of an individual physician's allowable Medicare charges for the payment year to a maximum cap per year. To encourage healthcare providers to adopt and implement EHRs early, physicians are eligible for Medicare incentives up to $18,000 in the first two payment years, and then the amounts decline each year thereafter, with a total capped amount of $44,000 during the entire program. If a physician is providing services in a Health Professional Shortage Area (HPSA), the physician is eligible for a 10% increase in payments.

Medicaid payments for EPs are based on 85% of the costs attributed to the purchase of a certified EHR. In the first year, the total payment to a physician by the state Medicaid program is capped at $25,000 and then is $10,000 for each subsequent year, with a total capped amount of $63,750.

For hospitals that participate in the Medicare program, the payment amount is based on a calculation that will result in a different amount for each hospital. Each hospital must calculate its payment based on the mathematical formula created by the Centers for Medicare and Medicaid Services (CMS), as described in Table 27.1. For the Medicaid program, the calculation for hospitals is based on a different formula than the one described in Table 27.1 and depends on how many Medicaid patients receive care at the hospital.

The financial incentives provided through the Stimulus Act are carrots to encourage healthcare providers to adopt and implement EHRs in an expedited manner. As of October 2015, the CMS had paid over $21,041,137,966 to EPs and

TABLE 27.1 Hospital Medicare Payment Calculation		
	Hospitals With 1149 or Fewer Discharges During the Payment Year	Hospitals With at Least 1150 But No More Than 23,000 Discharges During the Payment Year	Hospitals With 23,001 or More Discharges During the Payment Year
Base amount	$2,000,000	$2,000,000	$2,000,000
Discharge-related amount	$0	$200 × (n – 1149) (n is the number of discharges during the payment year)	$200 × (23,001 – 1149)
Total initial amount	$2,000,000	Between $2 M and $6,370,400, depending on the number of discharges	Limited by law to $6,370,400

Source: Centers for Medicare and Medicaid Services (CMS). EHR incentive program for Medicare hospitals. CMS. <https://www.cms.gov/Regulations-and-Guidance/Legislation/EHRIncentivePrograms/Downloads/MLN_TipSheet_MedicareHospitals.pdf/>. Accessed December 15, 2015.

hospitals for achieving the MU measures through the Medicare program and over $10,184,919,115 for the Medicaid program. By 2016, these amounts increased to $23.5 billion for the Medicare program and $10.9 billion for the Medicaid program.[9]

The downside following the financial incentives period is that if healthcare providers have failed to adopt and implement certified EHR systems by 2015, their Medicare reimbursement decreases. Specifically, if a physician or chiropractor has failed to adopt and implement a certified EHR by 2015, his or her Medicare reimbursement is decreased by 1% for each year thereafter, to a maximum of 5% decrease (42 USC 1395w-4). If an EP failed to achieve Stage 1 MU measures by 2015, that EP could apply for a hardship exception to avoid the payment decrease. However, the EP must file for a hardship exception annually.

The applicable reasons to receive a hardship exception are limited to the following scenarios:

1. The EP does not have adequate infrastructure, including sufficient internet access to report on the MU measures.
2. The EP is a new practitioner who does not have adequate time to become a meaningful user.
3. The EP suffered unforeseen circumstances such as a hurricane or other natural disaster.
4. The EP switched vendors during the reporting period.
5. The EP is adversely impacted because the rule was published late in 2015 and the EP did not have adequate time to achieve the measures.

Other providers may also be exempt because their specialty does not provide sufficient follow-up face to face with patients or if the provider practices in multiple locations and the provider does not control the certified EHR at the practice location. For example, anesthesiologists, pathologists, and radiologists do not have to apply for a hardship exception, and they will likely receive a waiver of the penalty.

Meaningful Use

Notwithstanding the monetary incentive plans to ensure that healthcare providers would electronically enter and exchange patient information to improve patient outcomes, the federal government determined that healthcare providers' behavior must change. Therefore to obtain Medicare payments, the EP or entity must use certified EHRs "meaningfully." Section 4101 of the HITECH Act defines MU as ePrescribing (eRx), engaging in HIE, and submitting information on clinical quality measures and other measures specified by the Secretary of HHS. Therefore by requiring healthcare providers to adopt certified EHRs and perform and report on specific measures, the end goal is to change provider behavior and increase the electronic exchange of patient information.

As described previously, the Health IT Policy Committee and the Health IT Standards Committee focused on establishing the underlying policies and standards to establish the NwHIN. The ultimate goal identified by the Health IT Policy Committee was to enable significant and measurable improvements in population health through a transformed healthcare delivery system. The goal of the financial incentive program is to encourage eligible healthcare providers to

change their behavior to achieve the strategic goals of electronically exchanging health information to improve patient care while supporting the NwHIN. However, adoption of certified EHRs without using the EHRs in a meaningful manner was insufficient to facilitate the NwHIN. Therefore the financial incentives were only remitted to healthcare providers that became meaningful EHR users. The criteria for meeting MU are divided into the following five initiatives, adapted from the work of the National Priorities Partnership (NPP)[10]:

1. Improve quality, safety, and efficiencies, and reduce health disparities.
2. Engage patients and families.
3. Improve care coordination.
4. Improve population and public health.
5. Ensure adequate privacy and security protections for personal health information.[10,11]

In general, each policy conforms to the initiatives from both the 2004 and the 2009 legislation designed to reduce medical errors, improve communication, and facilitate secure electronic transmission of patient information. The Health IT Policy Committee and the Health IT Standards Committee developed specific measures for each healthcare provider to perform and report on to successfully be deemed a meaningful EHR user. Each measure is directly related to driving the use of IT in the clinical care setting. Because individual healthcare providers have different types of practices, the Health IT Policy Committee and the Health IT Standards Committee divided the MU metrics into "core" required elements and "menu" elements. Permitting healthcare providers an opportunity to report on required core elements and then choose to report on a select few "menu" elements addressed the unique aspects of each provider's practice or facility and added flexibility to the financial incentives program. Table 27.2 provides a detailed description of the Stage 1 core and menu elements. As the stages of MU progressed, the menu elements were removed and standard meaningful objectives controlled the MU requirements. The Health IT Policy Committee is instrumental in developing and commenting on the MU requirements. Specifically, the Health IT Policy Committee in May 2012 provided comments on the Stage 2 MU requirements and in March 2014 recommended Stage 3 MU measures.[12] The Health IT Policy Committee has consistently modified the MU measures to conform to the underlying policy initiatives of the committee established in 2009.

Although each year the Medicare program requires attesting to the MU metrics, the Medicaid program is much more flexible. In the first year, healthcare providers under the Medicaid program do not have to satisfy the MU metrics. Instead, if a provider adopts, implements, or upgrades an EHR system during the first payment year, the individual physician will be eligible to receive payments to a maximum of approximately $21,000 to $25,000 during that first year. Because Medicaid is a state program, each state may require different forms of verification that the healthcare provider adopted, implemented, or upgraded an EHR system. For each subsequent year, providers must attest to achieving the MU metrics to obtain Medicaid incentives. The Medicaid program also extends

TABLE 27.2 Meaningful Use

Health Outcomes Policy Priority	CORE SET		
	STAGE 1 OBJECTIVES		
	Eligible Professionals	Eligible Hospitals and CAHS	Stage 1 Measures
Improve quality, safety, and efficiency, and reduce health disparities	Use CPOE for medication orders directly entered by any licensed healthcare professional who can enter orders into the medical record per state, local, and professional guidelines	Use CPOE for medication orders directly entered by any licensed healthcare professional who can enter orders into the medical record per state, local, and professional guidelines	More than 30% of unique patients with at least one medication in their medication list seen by the EP or admitted to the eligible hospital's or CAH's inpatient or emergency department (POS 21 or 23) have at least one medication order entered using CPOE
	Implement drug-drug and drug-allergy interaction checks	Implement drug-drug and drug-allergy interaction checks	The EP/eligible hospital/CAH has enabled this functionality for the entire EHR reporting period
	Generate and transmit permissible prescriptions electronically (eRx)	More than 40% of all permissible prescriptions written by the EP are transmitted electronically using certified EHR technology	—
	Record demographics • Preferred language • Gender • Race • Ethnicity • Date of birth	Record demographics • Preferred language • Gender • Race • Ethnicity • Date of birth • Date and preliminary cause of death in the event of mortality in the eligible hospital or CAH	More than 50% of all unique patients seen by the EP or admitted to the eligible hospital's or CAH's inpatient or emergency department (POS 21 or 23) have demographics recorded as structured data
	Maintain an up-to-date problem list of current and active diagnoses	Maintain an up-to-date problem list of current and active diagnoses	More than 80% of all unique patients seen by the EP or admitted to the eligible hospital's or CAH's inpatient or emergency department (POS 21 or 23) have demographics recorded as structured data
	Maintain active medication list	Maintain active medication list	More than 80% of all unique patients seen by the EP or admitted to the eligible hospital's or CAH's inpatient or emergency department (POS 21 or 23) have at least one entry (or an indication that the patient is not currently prescribed any medication) recorded as structured data
	Maintain active medication allergy list	Maintain active medication allergy list	More than 80% of all unique patients seen by the EP or admitted to the eligible hospital's or CAH's inpatient or emergency department (POS 21 or 23) have at least one entry (or an indication that the patient is not currently prescribed any medication) recorded as structured data
	Record and chart changes in vital signs: • Measure height • Record weight • Measure blood pressure • Calculate and display BMI	Record and chart changes in vital signs: • Measure height • Record weight • Measure blood pressure • Calculate and display BMI	For more than 50% of all unique patients aged 2 years and over seen by the EP or admitted to eligible hospital's or CAH's inpatient or emergency department (POS 21 or 23), height, weight, and blood pressure are recorded as structured data

TABLE 27.2	Meaningful Use—cont'd		

	CORE SET		
Health Outcomes Policy Priority	**STAGE 1 OBJECTIVES**		
	Eligible Professionals	**Eligible Hospitals and CAHS**	**Stage 1 Measures**
	• Plot and display growth charts for children 2–20 years, including BMI	• Plot and display growth charts for children 2–20 years, including BMI	
	Record smoking status for patients aged 13 years or older	Record smoking status for patients aged 13 years or older	More than 50% of all unique patients aged 13 years or older seen by the EP or admitted to the eligible hospital's or CAH's inpatient or emergency department (POS 21 or 23) have smoking status recorded as structured data
	Implement one clinical decision support rule relevant to specialty or high clinical priority, along with the ability to track compliance with that rule	Implement one clinical decision support rule relevant to specialty or high clinical priority along with the ability to track compliance with that rule	Implement one clinical decision support rule
	Report ambulatory clinical quality measures to CMS or the state	Report hospital clinical quality measures to CMS or the state	For 2011, provide aggregate numerator, denominator, and exclusions through attestation, as discussed in section II(A)(3) of this final rule. For 2012, electronically submit the clinical quality measures as discussed in section II(A)(3) of this final rule
Engage patients and families in their healthcare	Provide patients with an electronic copy of their health information (including diagnostic test results, problem list, medication lists, medication allergies) upon request	Provide patients with an electronic copy of their health information (including diagnostic test results, problem list, medication lists, medication allergies, discharge summary, procedures) upon request	More than 50% of all patients of the EP or the inpatient or emergency departments of the eligible hospital or CAH (POS 21 or 23) who request an electronic copy of their health information are provided it within 3 business days
	—	Provide patients with an electronic copy of their discharge instructions at time of discharge upon request	More than 50% of all patients who are discharged from an eligible hospital's or CAH's inpatient department or emergency department (POS 21 or 23) and who request an electronic copy of their discharge instructions are provided it
	Provide clinical summaries for patients for each office visit	—	Clinical summaries provided to patients for more than 50% of all office visits within 3 business days
Improve care coordination	Capability to exchange key clinical information (e.g., problem list, medication lists, medication allergies, diagnostic test results) among providers of care and patient authorized entities electronically	Capability to exchange key clinical information (e.g., discharge summary, procedures, problem list, medication lists, medication allergies, diagnostic test results) among providers of care and patient authorized entities electronically	Performed at least one test of certified EHR technology's capacity to electronically exchange key information

Continued

TABLE 27.2   Meaningful Use—cont'd

	CORE SET		
Health Outcomes Policy Priority	STAGE 1 OBJECTIVES		
	Eligible Professionals	Eligible Hospitals and CAHS	Stage 1 Measures
Ensure adequate privacy and security protections for personal health information	Protect electronic health information created or maintained by the certified EHR technology through the implementation of appropriate technical capabilities	Protect electronic health information created or maintained by the certified EHR technology through the implementation of appropriate technical capabilities	Conduct or review a security risk analysis per 45 CFR 164.308 (a)(1) and implement security updates as necessary and correct identified security deficiencies as part of its risk management process
Improve quality, safety, and efficiency, and reduce health disparities	Implement drug-formulary checks	Implement drug-formulary checks	The EP/eligible hospital/CAH has enabled this functionality and has access to at least one internal or external drug formulary for the entire EHR reporting period
	—	Record advance directives for patients aged 65 years or older	More than 50% of all unique patients aged 65 years or older admitted to the eligible hospital's or CAH's inpatient department (POS 21) have an indication of an advance directive status recorded
	Incorporate clinical lab test results into certified EHR technology as structured data	Incorporate clinical lab test results into certified EHR technology as structured data	More than 40% of all clinical lab test results ordered by the EP or by an authorized provider of the eligible hospital or CAH for patients admitted to its inpatient or emergency department (POS 21 or 23) during the EHR reporting period whose results are either in a positive/negative or numerical format are incorporated in certified EHR technology as structured data
	Generate lists of patients by specific conditions to use for quality improvement, reduction of disparities, research, or outreach	Generate lists of patients by specific conditions to use for quality improvement, reduction of disparities, research, or outreach	Generate at least one report listing patients of the EP, eligible hospital, or CAH with a specific condition
	Send reminders to patients per patient preference for preventative/follow-up care	—	More than 20% of all unique patients aged 65 years or older or 5 years or younger were sent an appropriate reminder during the EHR reporting period
Engage patients and families in their healthcare	Provide patients with timely electronic access to their health information (including lab results, problem list, medication lists, medication allergies) within 4 business days of the information being available to the EP	—	More than 10% of all unique patients seen by the EP are provided timely (available to the patient within 4 business days of being updated in the certified EHR technology) electronic access to their health information subject to the EP's discretion to withhold certain information
	Use certified EHR technology to identify patient-specific education resources and provide those resources to the patient if appropriate	Use certified EHR technology to identify patient-specific education resources and provide those resources to the patient if appropriate	More than 10% of all unique patients seen by the EP or admitted to the eligible hospital's or CAH's inpatient or emergency department (POS 21 or 23) are provided patient-specific education resources

TABLE 27.2 Meaningful Use—cont'd

	CORE SET		
Health Outcomes Policy Priority	STAGE 1 OBJECTIVES		
	Eligible Professionals	Eligible Hospitals and CAHS	Stage 1 Measures
Improve care coordination	The EP, eligible hospital, or CAH who receives a patient from another setting of care or provider of care or believes an encounter is relevant should perform medication reconciliation	The EP, eligible hospital, or CAH who receives a patient from another setting of care or provider of care or believes an encounter is relevant should perform medication reconciliation	The EP, eligible hospital, or CAH performs medication reconciliation for more than 50% of transitions of care in which the patient is transitioned into the care of the EP or admitted to the eligible hospital's or CAH's inpatient or emergency department (POS 21 or 23)
	The EP, eligible hospital, or CAH who transitions their patient to another setting of care or provider of care or refers their patient to another provider of care should provide a summary of care record for each transition of care or referral	The EP, eligible hospital, or CAH who transitions their patient to another setting of care or provider of care or refers their patient to another provider of care should provide a summary of care record for each transition of care or referral	The EP, eligible hospital, or CAH who transitions or refers their patient to another setting of care or provider of care provides a summary of care record for more than 50% of transitions of care and referrals
Improve population and public health[a]	Capability to submit electronic data to immunization registries or immunization information systems and actual submission in accordance with applicable law and practice	Capability to submit electronic data to immunization registries or immunization information systems and actual submission in accordance with applicable law and practice	Performed at least one test of certified EHR technology's capacity to submit electronic data to immunization registries and followed up submission to determine if the test was successful (unless none of the immunization registries to which the EP, eligible hospital, or CAH submits such information have the capacity to receive the information electronically)
	—	Capability to submit electronic data on reportable (as required by state or local law) lab results to public health agencies and actual submission in accordance with applicable law and practice	Performed at least one test of certified EHR technology's capacity to provide electronic submission of reportable lab results to public health agencies and followed up submission to determine if the test was successful (unless none of the public health agencies to which eligible hospital or CAH submits such information have the capacity to receive the information electronically)
	Capability to submit electronic syndromic surveillance data to public health agencies and actual submission in accordance with applicable law and practice	Capability to submit electronic syndromic surveillance data to public health agencies and actual submission in accordance with applicable law and practice	Performed at least one test of certified EHR technology's capacity to provide electronic syndromic surveillance data to public health agencies and followed up submission to determine if the test was successful (unless none of the public health agencies to which eligible hospital or CAH submits such information have the capacity to receive the information electronically)

BMI, Body mass index; CAH, critical access hospital; CMS, Centers for Medicare and Medicaid Services; CPOE, computerized provider order entry; EHR, electronic health record; EP, eligible professional; eRx, ePrescribing; POS, place of service.
Source: Centers for Medicare & Medicaid Services. Department of Health and Human Services: Medicare and Medicaid programs; Electronic Health Record Incentive Program; Final rule. *Federal Register.* 2010;75(144).
aUnless an EP, eligible hospital, or CAH has an exception for all of these objectives and measures, they must complete at least one part of their demonstration of the menu set in order to be a meaningful EHR user.

payments for 5 years as long as the healthcare provider begins by 2016. Thus Medicaid funding may continue until 2021.

Further, to effectively change healthcare provider behavior, the reporting obligations have been divided into three stages. The first stage, which commenced in 2011 with an end date of 2014, required reporting on specific measurements to achieve MU. The intention of Stage 1 was to enable the collection of meaningful data in a coded format to permit tracking of key clinical conditions and communication of that information for care coordination purposes. Stage 1 metrics also required the implementation of clinical decision support tools to facilitate disease and medication management, reporting clinical quality measures and public health information. Stage 1 established a foundation of adopting technology with uniform functions that enable healthcare providers to change their behavior. Stage 2 measures were delayed until 2014 and were designed to encourage continuous quality improvement and the exchange of information. Stage 2 focused on the structured formats created to electronically transmit patient data between healthcare providers.[13] Stage 2 took the Stage 1 objectives that were optional and incorporated these measures into the required core elements. The final rules for Stage 2 were announced in August 2012 and make it clear that no healthcare providers will be required to follow the Stage 2 requirements before 2014.

In late 2015, CMS published a new "modified Stage 2" that was applied in 2015 for any EP or hospital seeking to start the MU program in 2015. The modified Stage 2 removed measures from Stage 1 that were considered "redundant, duplicative or topped out." Table 27.3 provides a listing of the measures that were removed for the modified Stage 2. Table 27.4 provides an overview of the modified Stage 2 objectives and measures for EPs, and Table 27.5 provides an overview of the modified Stage 2 hospital objectives and measures. In order to achieve the MU criteria, the EP must report on nine core objectives and one public health objective. Hospitals, including CAHs, must report on eight core objectives and one public health objective. In 2015 only, the reporting requirements for all providers was any continuous 90-day period. For EPs the reporting period was January 1, 2015, through December 31, 2015, and for eligible hospitals, the reporting period was October 1, 2014, to December 31, 2015. After 2015, the eligible providers are required to report for the full calendar year. All of the objectives are designed to build upon the initial data captured in a certified EHR to advance the clinical processes by using the data to make informed decisions when establishing treatment plans.

In light of the changes in late 2015, CMS provided more flexibility to EPs and hospitals attempting to achieve MU measures. CMS focused on the fact that healthcare information technology is the tool to achieve improved patient outcomes and population health. CMS also pushed the Stage 3 measures to be voluntary in 2017 and mandatory in 2018. Stage 3 measures will focus on the interoperability of sharing patient information among providers and patients. Therefore the delay in implementing Stage 3 will provide technology developers and providers more time to implement the

TABLE 27.3	Objectives Are Redundant, Duplicative, or Topped Out
Provider Type	**Objectives and Measures**
EP	Record demographics
	Record vital signs
	Record smoking status
	Clinical summaries
	Structured lab results
	Patient list
	Patient reminders
	Summary of care: Measure 1—any method; Measure 3—Test
	Electronic notes
	Imaging results
	Family health history
Eligible hospital/CAH	Record demographics
	Record vital signs
	Record smoking status
	Structured lab results
	Patient list
	Summary of care: Measure 1—any method; Measure 3—test
	Electronic medication administration record
	Advanced directives
	Electronic notes
	Imaging results
	Family health history
	Structure labs to ambulatory providers

CAH, critical access hospital; *EP*, eligible professional.
Source: *Federal Registry*. Medicare and Medicaid Programs; Electronic Health Record Incentive Program-modifications to Meaningful Use in 2015 through 2017. Table 3—Objectives and Measures Identified by Provider Type Which Are Redundant, Duplicative or Topped Out. Located <https://www.federalregister.gov/articles/2015/04/15/2015-08514/medicare-and-medicaid-programs-electronic-health-record-incentive-program-modifications-to#table_of_tables>. Accessed December 21, 2015.

technology necessary to facilitate the electronic exchange of information to improve patient information.

Stage 3 will require higher standards for healthcare providers to be deemed meaningful users of certified EHRs. The optional standards under Stage 2 will be mandatory measures in Stage 3. If a provider elects to achieve Stage 3 in 2017, the reporting period will be 90 days during the year, but 2018 will require reporting for the entire year. In addition, Stage 3 promotes improvements in quality, safety, and efficiency. Stage 3 goes beyond merely exchanging data electronically and focuses on improving the general population health. Instead of healthcare providers changing their behavior in the practice setting, Stage 3 intends to use technology to engage in decision support analysis for studying chronic disease and best practices. The eight objectives of the Stage 3 MU measures focus on the following:

1. Protecting patient health information
2. Electronic prescribing

TABLE 27.4   Eligible Professional Objectives and Measures for 2015 Through 2017

Objectives for 2015, 2016, and 2017	Measures for Providers in 2015, 2016, and 2017	Alternate Exclusions and/or Specifications for Certain Providers
Objective 1: Protect patient health information	*Measure:* Conduct or review a security risk analysis in accordance with the requirements in 45 CFR 164.308 (a)(1), including addressing the security (to include encryption) of ePHI created or maintained by Certified EHR Technology in accordance with requirements in 45 CFR 164.312(a)(2)(iv) and 45 CFR 164.306(d)(3), and implement security updates as necessary and correct identified security deficiencies as part of the EP's risk management process.	None
Objective 2: Clinical decision support	*Measure 1:* Implement five clinical decision support interventions related to four or more clinical quality measures at a relevant point in patient care for the entire EHR reporting period. Absent four clinical quality measures related to an EP's scope of practice or patient population, the clinical decision support interventions must be related to high-priority health conditions. *Measure 2:* The EP has enabled and implemented the functionality for drug–drug and drug–allergy interaction checks for the entire EHR reporting period.	If for an EHR reporting period in 2015, the provider is scheduled to demonstrate *Stage 1: Alternate Objective* and *Measure 1: Objective*, implement one clinical decision support rule relevant to specialty or high clinical priority, along with the ability to track compliance with that rule. *Measure:* Implement one clinical decision support rule.
Objective 3: CPOE	*Measure 1:* More than 60% of medication orders created by the EP during the EHR reporting period are recorded using computerized provider order entry. *Measure 2:* More than 30% of laboratory orders created by the EP during the EHR reporting period are recorded using computerized provider order entry. *Measure 3:* More than 30% of radiology orders created by the EP during the EHR reporting period are recorded using computerized provider order entry.	*Alternate Measure 1:* For Stage 1 providers in 2015 only, more than 30% of all unique patients with at least one medication in their medication list seen by the EP during the EHR reporting period have at least one medication order entered using CPOE, or more than 30% of medication orders created by the EP during the EHR reporting period during the EHR reporting period are recorded using computerized provider order entry. *Alternate Exclusion for Measure 2:* Providers scheduled to be in Stage 1 in 2015 may claim an exclusion for Measure 2 (laboratory orders) of the Stage 2 CPOE objective for an EHR reporting period in 2015, and providers scheduled to be in Stage 1 in 2016 may claim an exclusion for Measure 2 (laboratory orders) of the Stage 2 CPOE objective for an EHR reporting period in 2016. *Alternate Exclusion for Measure 3:* Providers scheduled to be in Stage 1 in 2015 may claim an exclusion for Measure 3 (radiology orders) of the Stage 2 CPOE objective for an EHR reporting period in 2015, and providers scheduled to be in Stage 1 in 2016 may claim an exclusion for Measure 3 (radiology orders) of the Stage 2 CPOE objective for an EHR reporting period in 2016.
Objective 4: Electronic prescribing	*EP Measure:* More than 50% of all permissible prescriptions written by the EP are queried for a drug formulary and transmitted electronically using CEHRT.	*Alternate EP Measure:* For Stage 1 providers in 2015 only, more than 40% of all permissible prescriptions written by the EP are transmitted electronically using CEHRT.
Objective 5: HIE	*Measure:* The EP that transitions or refers their patient to another setting of care or provider of care (1) uses CEHRT to create a summary of care record and (2) electronically transmits such summary to a receiving provider for more than 10% of transitions of care and referrals.	*Alternate Exclusion:* Provider may claim an exclusion for the measure of the Stage 2 Summary of Care objective, which requires the electronic transmission of a summary of care document if for an EHR reporting period in 2015 they were scheduled to demonstrate Stage 1, which does not have an equivalent measure.

Continued

TABLE 27.4 Eligible Professional Objectives and Measures for 2015 Through 2017—cont'd

Objectives for 2015, 2016, and 2017	Measures for Providers in 2015, 2016, and 2017	Alternate Exclusions and/or Specifications for Certain Providers
Objective 6: Patient-specific education	*EP Measure:* Patient-specific education resources identified by CEHRT are provided to patients for more than 10% of all unique patients with office visits seen by the EP during the EHR reporting period.	*Alternate Exclusion:* Provider may claim an exclusion for the measure of the Stage 2 Patient-Specific Education objective if for an EHR reporting period in 2015 they were scheduled to demonstrate Stage 1 but did not intend to select the Stage 1 Patient-Specific Education menu objective.
Objective 7: Medication Reconciliation	*Measure:* The EP performs medication reconciliation for more than 50% of transitions of care in which the patient is transitioned into the care of the EP.	*Alternate Exclusion:* Provider may claim an exclusion for the measure of the Stage 2 Medication Reconciliation objective if for an EHR reporting period in 2015, they were scheduled to demonstrate Stage 1 but did not intend to select the Stage 1 Medication Reconciliation menu objective.
Objective 8: Patient Electronic Access (VDT)	*EP Measure 1:* More than 50% of all unique patients seen by the EP during the EHR reporting period are provided timely access to view online, download, and transmit to a third party their health information subject to the EP's discretion to withhold certain information. *EP Measure 2:* For 2015 and 2016: At least one patient seen by the EP during the EHR reporting period (or patient-authorized representative) views, downloads, or transmits his or her health information to a third party during the EHR reporting period. For 2017: More than 5% of unique patients seen by the EP during the EHR reporting period (or patient-authorized representative) view, download, or transmit their health information to a third party during the EHR reporting period.	*Alternate Exclusion Measure 2:* Providers may claim an exclusion for the second measure if for an EHR reporting period in 2015 they were scheduled to demonstrate Stage 1, which does not have an equivalent measure.
Objective 9: Secure messaging	*Measure:* For 2015: For an EHR reporting period in 2015, the capability for patients to send and receive a secure electronic message with the EP was fully enabled. For 2016: For at least one patient seen by the EP during the EHR reporting period, a secure message was sent using the electronic messaging function of CEHRT to the patient (or patient-authorized representative), or in response to a secure message sent by the patient (or patient-authorized representative) during the EHR reporting period. For 2017: For more than 5% of unique patients seen by the EP during the EHR reporting period, a secure message was sent using the electronic messaging function of CEHRT to the patient (or the patient-authorized representative), or in response to a secure message sent by the patient (or the patient-authorized representative) during the EHR reporting period.	*Alternate Exclusion:* An EP may claim an exclusion for the measure if for an EHR reporting period in 2015 they were scheduled to demonstrate Stage 1, which does not have an equivalent measure.
Objective 10: Public health	*Measure 1—Immunization Registry Reporting:* The EP is in active engagement with a public health agency to submit immunization data. *Measure 2—Syndromic Surveillance Reporting:* The EP is in active engagement with a public health agency to submit syndromic surveillance data. *Measure 3—Specialized Registry Reporting:* The EP is in active engagement to submit data to a specialized registry.	Stage 1 EPs in 2015 must meet at least 1 measure in 2015; Stage 2 EPs must meet at least 2 measures in 2015, and all EPs must meet at least 2 measures in 2016 and 2017.

CPOE, computerized provider order entry; *EHR,* electronic health record; *HIE,* health information exchange.
Source: *Federal Registry.* Meaningful Use Final Report, Electronic Health Record Incentive Program: Stage 3. Table 7—Eligible Professional (EP) Objectives and Measures for 2015 through 2017. <https://www.federalregister.gov/articles/2015/10/16/2015-25595/medicare-and-medicaid-programs-electronic-health-record-incentive-program-stage-3-and-modifications>. Accessed December 21, 2015.

TABLE 27.5   Eligible Hospital and Critical Access Hospitals Objectives and Measures for 2015 Through 2017

Objectives for 2015, 2016, and 2017	Measures for Providers in 2015, 2016, and 2017	Alternate Exclusions and/or Specifications for Certain Providers
Objective 1: Protect patient health information	*Measure:* Conduct or review a security risk analysis in accordance with the requirements in 45 CFR 164.308(a)(1), including addressing the security (to include encryption) of ePHI created or maintained in CEHRT in accordance with requirements in 45 CFR 164.312(a)(2)(iv) and 45 CFR 164.306(d)(3), and implement security updates as necessary and correct identified security deficiencies as part of the eligible hospital or CAHs risk management process.	None
Objective 2: Clinical decision support	*Measure 1:* Implement five clinical decision support interventions related to four or more clinical quality measures at a relevant point in patient care for the entire EHR reporting period. Absent four clinical quality measures related to an eligible hospital or CAH's scope of practice or patient population, the clinical decision support interventions must be related to high-priority health conditions. *Measure 2:* The eligible hospital or CAH has enabled and implemented the functionality for drug-drug and drug-allergy interaction checks for the entire EHR reporting period.	If for an EHR reporting period in 2015 the provider is scheduled to demonstrate *Stage 1: Alternate Objective* and *Measure 1: Objective,* implement one clinical decision support rule relevant to specialty or high clinical priority, along with the ability to track compliance with that rule. *Measure:* Implement one clinical decision support rule.
Objective 3: CPOE	*Measure 1:* More than 60% of medication orders created by authorized providers of the eligible hospital's or CAH's inpatient or emergency department (POS 21 or 23) during the EHR reporting period are recorded using computerized provider order entry. *Measure 2:* More than 30% of laboratory orders created by authorized providers of the eligible hospital's or CAH's inpatient or emergency department (POS 21 or 23) during the EHR reporting period are recorded using computerized provider order entry. *Measure 3:* More than 30% of radiology orders created by authorized providers of the eligible hospital's or CAH's inpatient or emergency department (POS 21 or 23) during the EHR reporting period are recorded using computerized provider order entry.	*Alternate Measure 1:* For Stage 1 providers in 2015 only, more than 30% of all unique patients with at least one medication in their medication list seen by the EP during the EHR reporting period have at least one medication order entered using CPOE; or more than 30% of medication orders created by the EP during the EHR reporting period during the EHR reporting period are recorded using computerized provider order entry. *Alternate Exclusion for Measure 2:* Providers scheduled to be in Stage 1 in 2015 may claim an exclusion for Measure 2 (laboratory orders) of the Stage 2 CPOE objective for an EHR reporting period in 2015, and providers scheduled to be in Stage 1 in 2016 may claim an exclusion for Measure 2 (laboratory orders) of the Stage 2 CPOE objective for an EHR reporting period in 2016. *Alternate Exclusion for Measure 3:* Providers scheduled to be in Stage 1 in 2015 may claim an exclusion for Measure 3 (radiology orders) of the Stage 2 CPOE objective for an EHR reporting period in 2015, and providers scheduled to be in Stage 1 in 2016 may claim an exclusion for Measure 3 (radiology orders) of the Stage 2 CPOE objective for an EHR reporting period in 2016.
Objective 4: Electronic prescribing	*Eligible Hospital/CAH Measure:* More than 10% of hospital discharge medication orders for permissible prescriptions (for new and changed prescriptions) are queried for a drug formulary and transmitted electronically using CEHRT.	*Alternate EH Exclusion:* The eligible hospital or CAH may claim an exclusion for the eRx objective and measure if for an EHR reporting period in 2015 if they were either scheduled to demonstrate Stage 1, which does not have an equivalent measure, or if they are scheduled to demonstrate Stage 2 but did not intend to select the Stage 2 eRx objective for an EHR reporting period in 2015, and the eligible hospital or CAH may claim an exclusion for the eRx objective and measure if for an

Continued

TABLE 27.5   Eligible Hospital and Critical Access Hospitals Objectives and Measures for 2015 Through 2017—cont'd

Objectives for 2015, 2016, and 2017	Measures for Providers in 2015, 2016, and 2017	Alternate Exclusions and/or Specifications for Certain Providers
		EHR reporting period in 2016 if they were either scheduled to demonstrate Stage 1 in 2015 or 2016, or if they are scheduled to demonstrate Stage 2 but did not intend to select the Stage 2 eRx objective for an EHR reporting period in 2015.
Objective 5: HIE	*Measure:* The eligible hospital or CAH that transitions or refers their patient to another setting of care or provider of care (1) uses CEHRT to create a summary of care record and (2) electronically transmits such summary to a receiving provider for more than 10% of transitions of care and referrals.	*Alternate Exclusion:* Provider may claim an exclusion for the measure of the Stage 2 Summary of Care objective, which requires the electronic transmission of a summary of care document if for an EHR reporting period in 2015 they were scheduled to demonstrate Stage 1, which does not have an equivalent measure.
Objective 6: Patient-specific education	*Eligible Hospital/CAH Measure:* More than 10% of all unique patients admitted to the eligible hospital's or CAH's inpatient or emergency department (POS 21 or 23) are provided patient-specific education resources identified by CEHRT.	*Alternate Exclusion:* Provider may claim an exclusion for the measure of the Stage 2 Patient-Specific Education objective if for an EHR reporting period in 2015 they were scheduled to demonstrate Stage 1 but did not intend to select the Stage 1 Patient-Specific Education menu objective.
Objective 7: Medication reconciliation	*Measure:* The eligible hospital or CAH performs medication reconciliation for more than 50% of transitions of care, in which the patient is admitted to the eligible hospital's or CAH's inpatient or emergency department (POS 21 or 23).	*Alternate Exclusion:* Provider may claim an exclusion for the measure of the Stage 2 Medication Reconciliation objective if for an EHR reporting period in 2015 they were scheduled to demonstrate Stage 1 but did not intend to select the Stage 1 Medication Reconciliation menu objective.
Objective 8: Patient electronic access (VDT)	*Eligible Hospital/CAH Measure 1:* More than 50% of all unique patients who are discharged from the inpatient or emergency department (POS 21 or 23) of an eligible hospital or CAH are provided timely access to view online, download, and transmit their health information to a third party their health information. *Eligible Hospital/CAH Measure 2:* For 2015 and 2016: At least 1 patient who is discharged from the inpatient or emergency department (POS 21 or 23) of an eligible hospital or CAH (or patient-authorized representative) views, downloads, or transmits to a third party his or her health information during the EHR reporting period For 2017: More than 5% of unique patients discharged from the inpatient or emergency department (POS 21 or 23) of an eligible hospital or CAH (or patient-authorized representative) view, download, or transmit to a third party their health information during the EHR reporting period.	*Alternate Exclusion Measure 2:* Provider may claim an exclusion for the second measure if for an EHR reporting period in 2015 they were scheduled to demonstrate Stage 1, which does not have an equivalent measure.
Objective 9: Secure messaging	Not applicable for eligible hospitals and CAHs	Not applicable for eligible hospitals and CAHs.
Objective 10: Public health	*Measure 1—Immunization Registry Reporting:* The eligible hospital or CAH is in active engagement with a public health agency to submit immunization data. *Measure 2—Syndromic Surveillance Reporting:* The eligible hospital or CAH is in active engagement with a public health agency to submit syndromic surveillance data.	Stage 1 eligible hospitals and CAHs must meet at least 2 measures in 2015, Stage 2 eligible hospitals and CAHs must meet at least 3 measures in 2015, all eligible hospitals and CAHs must meet at least 3 measures in 2016 and 2017.

TABLE 27.5   Eligible Hospital and Critical Access Hospitals Objectives and Measures for 2015 Through 2017—cont'd

Objectives for 2015, 2016, and 2017	Measures for Providers in 2015, 2016, and 2017	Alternate Exclusions and/or Specifications for Certain Providers
	Measure 3—Specialized Registry Reporting: The eligible hospital, or CAH, is in active engagement to submit data to a specialized registry. *Measure 4—Electronic Reportable Laboratory Result Reporting:* The eligible hospital or CAH is in active engagement with a public health agency to submit ELR results.	

CAH, critical access hospitals; *eRx*, ePrescribing; *EHR*, electronic health record; *HIE*, health information exchange; *POS*, place of service.
Source: *CMS*. EHR Incentive Programs for Eligible Hospitals and CAHs: What You Need to Know for 2015 Tipsheet <https://www.cms.gov/Regulations-and-Guidance/Legislation/EHRIncentivePrograms/Downloads/Stage3_EH.pdf>. Accessed December 21, 2015.

3. Clinical decision support
4. Computerized provider order entry (CPOE)
5. Patient electronic access to health information
6. Coordination of care through patient engagement
7. HIE
8. Public health and clinical data registry reporting

Stage 3 is the final phase for the MU incentive program and is intended to transition providers to the new payment methodology. The payment adjustments to providers that fail to achieve MU will be superseded by MACRA. The incentives for the providers will transform to merit-based reimbursement under MACRA. In order to successfully achieve reimbursement for services on a merit-based payment schedule, providers will need to improve patient outcomes and reduce health disparities through the use of health IT.

Medicare Access and Children's Health Insurance Program Reauthorization Act of 2015

MACRA was passed with strong bipartisan support in both the U.S. House of Representatives and the Senate and was signed into law on April 16, 2015, by President Obama.[14.] The legislation established significant changes in how Medicare pays physicians and demonstrates meaningful support for and progress toward paying physicians for value or the quality of the care provided and not the volume of care provided.[15,16.] MACRA replaces the sustainable growth rate (SGR) formula based on fee for service, sunsets the Physician Quality Reporting System (PQRS) and the value modifier, and transitions from MU with two value-based payment options. These are the Merit-Based Incentive Payment System (MIPS) and the Alternative Payment Models (APM).

With the MIPS approach, MACRA calculates a composite performance score for providers, using four categories of measurements that are weighted to determine an overall MIPS score. The four categories include:

- Quality (50% of total adjustment in 2019, shrinking to 30% of total adjustment in 2021)
- Resource use (10% of total adjustment in 2019, growing to 30% of total adjustment by 2021)
- Clinical Practice Improvement Activities (15% of total adjustment)

- Advancing Care Information (formerly MU) (25% of total adjustment)

The score is then used to positively or negatively impact the physician payment. By 2022, the impact will range from −9% up to +27%.[17]

Providers that are subject to the MIPS payment may receive an increase in the fee-for-service Medicare reimbursement if the provider participates in an APM that does not have a financial risk share element. For example, by participating in an Accountable Care Organization in the one-sided track that does not have any financial risk, the provider's reimbursement will be scored under the MIPS program, and the provider may be eligible for a slight increase in the fee-for-service model.

Advanced APMs are those in which clinicians accept the risk for providing coordinated, high-quality care. The proposed rule includes examples of models that could qualify as Advanced APMs: (1) Comprehensive End Stage Renal Disease Care Model (Large Dialysis Organization arrangement), (2) Comprehensive Primary Care Plus, (3) Medicare Shared Savings Program—Track 2 or Track 3, (4) Next Generation ACO Model, and (5) Oncology Care Model Two-Sided Risk Arrangement (available in 2018). Providers who have a sufficient patient volume participating in the Advanced APM will be considered a "Qualifying Provider." However, in order to be a Qualifying Provider, the provider must utilize a certified EHR. Qualifying Providers are exempt from the MIPS adjustment and will receive a 5% quality bonus through the Advanced APM model.[17a]

The Advanced APM tract provides an alternative to MIPS by offering incentives and a pathway for physicians to develop and participate in new models of healthcare delivery and payment. MACRA calls for the creation of an advisory panel to consider physicians' proposals for new models. However, the proposed list of Advanced APMs was initially very limited. By November 1, 2016, the secretary must establish criteria focused for the advisory panel to use in making recommendations on APMs.[18] These criteria will be used in determining if (1) the proposed model is a qualified APM, and (2) quality measures are clearly described and the physician assumes a reasonable financial risk. However, while there are major incentives for providers to engage in APMs, currently there are no clear definitions in the statute other than a few criteria listed.[15] The need for healthcare providers, health informatics specialists, and healthcare consumers to become actively involved in developing the specific regulations and criteria is obvious.

While HITECH offered incentives to both physicians and hospitals, MACRA is for the most part focused on physician payments. However, there are implications for hospitals and other health systems. Hospitals that employ physicians directly could bear some implementation costs related to physician performance reporting requirements, as well as be at risk for any payment adjustments. Moreover, physicians may call upon hospitals to participate in APMs so that the physicians with whom they partner can qualify for the APM track.[18] However, until the regulations have been implemented, these implications will be somewhat unclear.

In addition to changes in how Medicare will pay physicians, MACRA also extended funding for the Children's Health Insurance Program (CHIP) and community health centers for two years. CHIP provides low-cost health coverage to children in families that earn too much money to qualify for Medicaid. Each state offers CHIP coverage and works closely with its state Medicaid program, resulting in coverage variations between states.

CONCLUSION AND FUTURE DIRECTIONS

The three foundational stages of the MU program are designed to modify provider behavior and transform how healthcare information is shared to improve patient outcomes, supporting reimbursement in the future. The incentivized adoption of EHRs continues to be at the core of reform initiatives to improve care quality and better manage care costs, meeting clinical and business needs by capturing, storing, and displaying clinical information when and where it is needed to improve individual patient care and provide aggregated, cross-population data analysis. EHRs manage healthcare data and information in ways that are patient centered and information rich. Improved information access and availability enable both the healthcare provider and the patient to better manage the patient's health by using capabilities provided by enhanced clinical decision support and customized education materials. The Stimulus Act took the federal policy EHRs leading to NwHIN to a new and elevated level that, among other initiatives, dedicated $27 billion to incentivize healthcare providers to adopt and use EHRs by providing the needed funding

At the time of this writing, MACRA is fairly new legislation. Many of the related regulations and criteria that will be used in implementing this legislation are currently in development. However, it is clear at this point that the incentives leading to the adoption and MU of EHRs are just the beginning of a process whereby the federal government is encouraging the use of health IT to improve access, decrease cost, and improve quality of healthcare and in turn the health of all Americans.

REFERENCES

1. Bush GW. *The 2004 State of the Union Address*; 2004. http://www.washingtonpost.com/wp-srv/politics/transcripts/bushtext_012004.html.
2. Executive Order 13335. *Incentives for the Use of Health Information Technology & Establishing the Position of the NHI IT Coordinator*; April 27, 2004.
3. 111th Congress. *The American Recovery and Reinvestment Act of 2009*; 2009.
4. *Standards & Interoperability Framework*. What is the S&I Framework? http://www.siframework.org/whatis.html. Accessed January 3, 2016.
5. Standards & Interoperability Framework. *Wiki*; 2015. http://wiki.siframework.org/.
6. Farrar B, Wang G, Bos H, et al. *Evaluation of the Regional Extension Center Program: Final Report* [Prepared By The American Institutes For Research Under Contract No. Hhsps23320095626wc.].Washington, D.C: Office of the National Coordinator for Health Information Technology; 2016. https://www.healthit.gov/sites/default/files/Evaluation_of_the_Regional_Extension_Center_Program_Final_Report_4_4_16.pdf.
7. *Health.gov*. Regional Extension Centers (RECs); 2015. https://www.healthit.gov/providers-professionals/regional-extension-centers-recs.
8. Blumenthal D. *National HIPAA Summit in Washington, DC*; 2009. http://www.healthcareitnews.com/news/healthcare-it-means-not-end-says-blumenthal.
9. CMS.gov Centers for Medicare & Medicaid Services. *Data and Program Reports*; 2016. https://www.cms.gov/Regulations-and-Guidance/Legislation/EHRIncentivePrograms/DataAndReports.html.
10. National Priorities Partnership. *National Priorities and Goals: Aligning Our Efforts to Transform America's Healthcare*. Washington, DC: National Quality Forum; 2008.
11. Office of the National Coordinator for Health Information Technology. *HIT Policy Committee Meaningful Use Matrix (August 10, 2009)*; 2009. https://www.healthit.gov/sites/faca/files/final_mu_recommendations_table_7_2009.pdf.
12. Office of the National Coordinator for Health Information Technology. HIT Policy Committee Meaningful Use Stage 3 final recommendations. https://www.healthit.gov/sites/faca/files/HITPC_MUWG_Stage3_Recs_2014-04-01.pdf. Accessed December 15, 2015.
13. U.S. Department of Health & Human Services. Medicare and Medicaid programs; Electronic Health Record Incentive Program—Stage 2; Final rule. *Fed Regist*. 2012;77(171).
14. Conway PH, Gronniger T, Pham, et al. *MACRA: New Opportunities for Medicare Providers through Innovative Payment Systems (Updated)*. HealthAffairs Blog; 2015. http://healthaffairs.org/blog/2015/09/28/macra-new-opportunities-for-medicare-providers-through-innovative-payment-systems-3/.
15. Glover S. *Overview of the Medicare Access and CHIP Reauthorization Act (MACRA)*. The National Partnership for Women & Families; 2015. http://www.nationalpartnership.org/research-library/health-care/CBC/npwf-macra-webinar.pdf.
16. *CMS.Gov*. The Merit-Based Incentive Payment System (MIPS) & Alternative Payment Models (APMs). https://www.cms.gov/Medicare/Quality-Initiatives-Patient-Assessment-Instruments/

Value-Based-Programs/MACRA-MIPS-and-APMs/MACRA-MIPS-and-APMs.html. Accessed April 16, 2016.

17. Cragun E. *The Most Important Details in the SGR Repeal Law.* The Advisory Board Company; 2015. https://www.advisory.com/research/health-care-advisory-board/blogs/at-the-helm/2015/04/sgr-repeal.

17a. *Medicare Access and CHIP Reauthorization Act of 2015.*[Public Law No: 114-10]. https://www.congress.gov/114/plaws/publ10/PLAW-114publ10.pdf. Accessed August 3, 2016.

18. American Hospital Association. *Physician Payment Reform: What is MACRA.* http://www.aha.org/advocacy-issues/physician/index.shtml. Accessed April 16, 2016.

DISCUSSION QUESTIONS

1. Describe how the NwHIN is facilitated by the MU program.
2. List and describe the federal agencies and committees that are responsible for facilitating electronic exchange of health information in the United States.
3. What are the current time periods for the MU program under Medicare and Medicaid, respectively?
4. How do providers avoid payment penalties for failing to satisfy MU requirements?

CASE STUDY

A health system owns and operates a hospital and employs primary care physicians, general surgeons, and oncologists. The hospital purchased a surgical practice in 2012. Part of the purchase of the practice included the purchase of the electronic medical record system that was a certified EHR. In January 2014, the hospital transitioned the primary care physicians, surgeons, and the radiologists in the hospital to a new certified electronic health record, the implementation of which was completed 10 months later in October 2014. The physicians did not satisfy the MU criteria from January 1, 2014, to December 31, 2104, because of the transition to a new certified EHR system. In addition, in 2015 the hospital's electronic medical record vendor informed the hospital that it would not be able to satisfy the Stage 3 interoperability and technology standards by January 2018.

Discussion Questions

1. Determine which (if any) of the following physicians will be subject to a payment penalty in 2015: (a) primary care physicians, (b) surgeons, or (c) radiologists.
2. Describe the timeline of the program and its potential financial impact on the individual healthcare providers who are involved in MU.
3. Describe the process the physicians must complete to avoid the payment penalties.
4. Describe the time frame for the provider to achieve modified Stage 2 and Stage 3 measures.
5. Discuss what the hospital must do to achieve the MU objectives for interoperability.

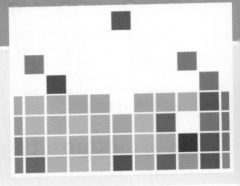

28

Health Policy and Health Informatics

Joyce Sensmeier and Judy Murphy

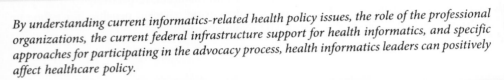

By understanding current informatics-related health policy issues, the role of the professional organizations, the current federal infrastructure support for health informatics, and specific approaches for participating in the advocacy process, health informatics leaders can positively affect healthcare policy.

OBJECTIVES

At the completion of this chapter, the reader will be prepared to:

1. Identify key health policy issues of importance to the practice of health for informatics.
2. Explain the process for developing and utilizing informatics principles and concepts in developing health policy.
3. Differentiate the Institute of Medicine (IOM) recommendations in the *HIT and Patient Safety* and *The Future of Nursing* reports.

KEY TERMS

ABSTRACT ❖

To improve health delivery and health outcomes, all health practitioners require an understanding of current health policy initiatives as well as knowledge about the process for influencing the development of health policy. Informatics and heath professional leaders must be knowledgeable about current technology-related public policy initiatives in order to positively impact healthcare practice and care delivery by leveraging informatics principles and technology within that policy.[1] This chapter begins by identifying informatics-related health issues driving policy initiatives of the U.S. government. Understanding the driving forces and the resulting initiatives provides a foundation for understanding the leadership role of health practitioners in influencing health policy to improve health and healthcare delivery.

Health practitioners and information specialists understand that the effective and efficient use of health information technology (health IT), when combined with best practice and evidence-based care, can improve health and healthcare for all. As leaders, health professionals and informaticians can maximize the use of health IT for bringing practice standards and decision-making evidence to the point of care, thereby empowering patients and healthcare consumers as partners.

INTRODUCTION

Informatics focuses on technology as a tool with the goal of an efficient, cost-effective healthcare system that ensures health and healthy communities for individuals, families, groups, and communities. Therefore policy goals and issues in health informatics are grounded in broader field of health policy. Health policy refers to the decisions, plans, and actions that are undertaken to manage healthcare delivery and to achieve specific healthcare goals.[2]

Healthcare leaders in the Unites States are being challenged on multiple fronts by an ever-changing healthcare landscape. The many challenges to cost-effective, efficient healthcare delivery are the driving forces in creating current health policy. Current health policy has developed in response to the challenges faced by the multiple stakeholders and healthcare leaders within the American healthcare system and by their vision of what is possible.

In this chapter, current health policy initiatives of major importance in health informatics are explored. The chapter begins by describing first the structure and then an example of the process by which a driving force leads to health IT policy. The concepts of safety and quality in the healthcare setting are used as examples of the process by which a driving

- Preventing Medication Errors: Quality Chasm Series—July 20, 2006
- Improving the Quality of Health Care for Mental and Substance-Use Conditions: Quality Chasm Series—November 1, 2005
- First Annual Crossing the Quality Chasm Summit: A Focus on Communities—September 14, 2004
- Crossing the Quality Chasm: A New Health System for the 21st Century—March 1, 2001
- To Err is Human: Building A Safer Health System—November 29, 1999

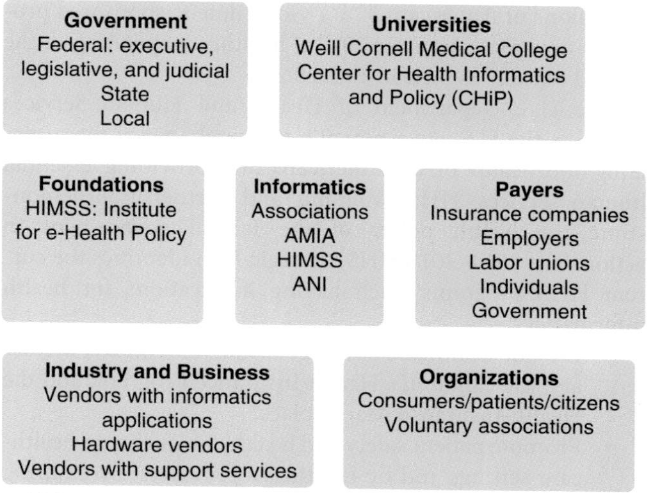

FIG 28.1 Examples of Health Informatics Stakeholders.

force leads to health policy. In many of the reports and studies dealing with the American healthcare system, the use of health IT is recommended as an effective tool to manage challenges facing healthcare delivery. The Quality Chasm Series from the IOM is an excellent example. Box 28.1 provides examples from this series. The complete list of reports in the series can be seen at https://www.nap.edu/catalog/21895/quality-chasm-series-health-care-quality-reports. The chapter concludes by describing the leadership role of healthcare providers and health informatics specialists in influencing the development and implementation of health policy. Included are specific actions that are effective in moving health policy forward. These actions are built on foundational competencies that all practitioners and students should possess to meet the goals of providing safe, quality, and competent care.

DEVELOPING AND IMPLEMENTING HEALTH INFORMATION TECHNOLOGY POLICY

A clearly stated health policy can achieve several things. It defines a vision for the future, which in turn helps establish targets and points of reference for both short- and medium-term planning. Health policy outlines priorities and expected roles of different groups. It both builds consensus and informs people.[2]

While several research studies and reports over the previous decades have identified health problems and healthcare delivery issues in the United States, no unified clear statement or consensus identifies the primary health problems or the primary healthcare delivery issues impacting the health status of individuals, families, communities, or the country as a whole. In addition, strong differences of opinion exist on the responsibilities and rights of the individuals, families, groups, and societal institutions around questions of health and healthcare delivery. As a result, health policy in the United States is an ever-changing reflection of the interactions and negotiations between the many health IT–related stakeholders. Fig. 28.1 provides several examples of stakeholders who impact and are affected by health IT policy, including the government, which plays a primary role in establishing the health IT policy of the United States.

BOX 28.2 Federal and State Healthcare Expenditures

- **Medicare** covers seniors (65+) and some individuals with disabilities.
- **Medicaid** covers low-income families, children, and individuals with physical and developmental disabilities.
- **CHIP** (Children's Health Insurance Program) covers kids who would not otherwise qualify for Medicaid.
- **VA** (Veterans Health Administration) provides services to veterans.
- **TRICARE** covers members of the military, families, and military retirees across the Department of Defense.
- **FEHBP** (Federal Employees Health Benefits Program) covers government employees and retirees.
- **Indian Health Service (IHS)** provides healthcare to American Indians and Alaskan Natives.
- **Federal Refugee Health Promotion Program** helps refugees resettling in the United States.
- **Inmates** are cared for in state and federal prisons.
- **SAMHSA** (Substance Abuse and Mental Health Services Administration) provides programs and funding for people with behavioral health needs.
- **Tax exemption** is provided for businesses and individuals with private insurance from their employer.
- **Subsidies** provide premium and cost sharing for individuals who are under 400% of the federal poverty level.
- Public health, research, and infrastructure, which includes activities to detect and prevent disease outbreaks, biomedical research, and the construction and improvement of structures to improve the delivery of healthcare.

Source: James E, Hughes M. Government-sponsored programs make up 52% of what we spend on healthcare. *Forbes;* Jul 29, 2015. <http://www.forbes.com/sites/realspin/2015/07/29/for-the-first-time-government-programs-make-up-the-majority-of-u-s-health-spending/#4b3f205d8e1c> Accessed April 23, 2016.

Role of the Federal Government

"Federal agencies are purchasers, regulators, developers, and users of health IT. In their various roles, they set policy and insure, pay for care, or provide direct patient care for tens of millions of Americans."[3, p. 5] Government-sponsored programs now make up over 50% of healthcare spending in the United States,[4] as seen in Box 28.2.

The U.S. Department of Health and Human Services (HHS) is the U.S. government's principal agency for protecting the health of all Americans and providing essential human services. HHS programs and partnerships demonstrate the health policy of the federal government in action. The 2014–2018 HHS Strategic Plan identifies the current HHS programs, each having implications for health informatics.[5]

- Provide healthcare coverage through Medicare, Medicaid, the Children's Health Insurance Program, and the Health Insurance Marketplace.
- Promote patient safety and healthcare quality in healthcare settings and by healthcare providers, by assuring the safety, effectiveness, quality, and security of foods, drugs, vaccines, and medical devices.
- Eliminate disparities in health, as well as healthcare access and quality.
- Conduct health, public health, and social science research.
- Leverage health IT to improve the quality of care, and use HHS data to drive innovative solutions to health, public health, and human services challenges.
- Improve maternal and infant health as well as promote the safety, well-being, and healthy development of children and youth.
- Promote economic and social well-being for individuals, families, and communities.
- Support wellness efforts across the life span.
- Prevent and manage the impacts of infectious diseases and chronic diseases and conditions, including the top causes of disease, disability, and death.
- Protect Americans from and provide comprehensive responses to health, safety, and security threats.
- Serve as responsible stewards of the public's investments.

The work of HHS is carried out by 11 divisions and 14 offices, including the Office of the National Coordinator (ONC) for Health IT Fig. 28.2. The ONC serves as the Secretary's principal advisor, charged with coordinating nationwide efforts to implement and use the most advanced health IT and the electronic exchange of health information.[6] The "ONC is at the forefront of the administration's health IT efforts and is a resource to the entire health system to support the adoption of health IT and the promotion of nationwide health information exchange (HIE) to improve healthcare."[6] But this does not mean that every federal health informatics project is under the direction of the ONC. Several federal health informatics projects are based in other government divisions, especially in the HHS. For example, the Center for Surveillance, Epidemiology and Laboratory Services (CSELS) is under the direction of the CDC (http://www.cdc.gov/ophss/).

The Health Information Technology for Economic and Clinical Health (HITECH) Act, which became law in 2009,

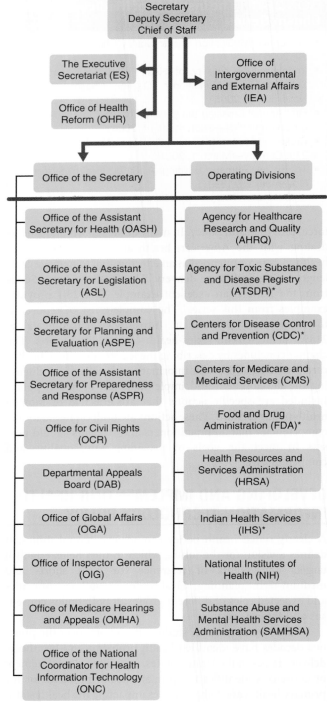

FIG 28.2 Department of Health and Human Services organizational chart.

played a key role in informing the HHS Strategic Plan covering the years 2010–2015 and in turn is the basis for many of the current programs and activities of the ONC.[7] The 2014–2018 HHS Strategic Plan continues to build on these programs and is now beginning to incorporate MACRA (Medicare Access and CHIP Reauthorization Act), which became law in 2015 (see Chapter 27 for details). In both strategic plans, *strength healthcare* is the first strategic goal. Each plan lists the following specific objectives for achieving this goal:

2010–2015: Promote the adoption and Meaningful Use of health information technology.

2014–2018: Improve healthcare and population health through Meaningful Use of health information technology.

Each plan then lists the strategic actions for achieving the objectives. The strategic actions for both plans are listed in Table 28.1, including several examples of current health informatics initiatives under the direction of the ONC as well as other initiatives supporting the various HHS programs. Table 28.1 demonstrates that while the ONC is the lead agency for health informatics–related projects and programs, these types of initiatives can be found throughout the federal government (and in several other chapters of this book). As a result, coordination and cooperation is imperative to the development and implementation of effective health policy. Or, as stated in the ONC Strategic Plan, "Federal plans now benefit from engagement and coordination by a wider spectrum of government agencies and private sector stakeholders."[3, p. 1]

Office of the National Coordinator for Health Information Technology

The ONC has submitted a budget appropriation request of $82 million for fiscal year 2017. As pointed out in this document, the "ONC leads the U.S. Government's work to ensure that actionable electronic health information is available when and where it matters most so that we move expeditiously to an open, connected community of health."[8, p. 1] The document goes on to describe a list of key activities, including health policy. The health policy activities are described as follows: "ONC develops and coordinates federal health IT policy to achieve national health priorities set forth by the White House and Secretary of HHS, and to implement statutory requirements such as those identified in the HITECH Act and the Medicare Access and CHIP Reauthorization Act (MACRA)."[8, p. 24]

The ONC Federal Health IT Strategic Plan for 2015–2020 provides an overview of the current and future health IT policy directions. Its vision is focused on four areas and four overarching goals, as shown in Figs. 28.3 and 28.4. These set the priorities for the plan. In viewing Fig. 28.3, note that the vision is focused on health and not technology. Health

TABLE 28.1 Examples of Government Initiatives With Policy Implications for Health Informatics

2014–2018 DHHS Strategic Plan ONC Strategies	2010–2015 DHHS Strategic Plan ONC Strategies	Example of Federal Initiatives	Chapter	URL
Inform, engage, empower, and partner with patients	Endorse the active participation of consumers	Blue Button	14	https://www.healthit.gov/patients-families/your-health-data
		—	Unit 3 chapters	https://www.healthit.gov/policy-researchers-implementers/consumer-ehealth-program
	—	FDA Office of Health Informatics	25	http://www.fda.gov/AboutFDA/CentersOffices/OC/OfficeofScientificandMedicalPrograms/ucm480020.htm
Encourage the health IT vendor community to build security into their products (i.e., privacy by design) Work to ensure privacy and security	Inspire confidence and trust by ensuring the privacy and security of electronic health information	HIPAA	26	http://www.hhs.gov/hipaa/
	—	HITECH Act	27	https://www.healthit.gov/sites/default/files/hitech_act_excerpt_from_arra_with_index.pdf
	—	Office of the National Coordinator for Health Information Technology	27	https://www.healthit.gov/policy-researchers-implementers/select-portions-hitech-act-and-relationship-onc-work

Continued

TABLE 28.1   Examples of Government Initiatives With Policy Implications for Health Informatics—cont'd

2014–2018 DHHS Strategic Plan ONC Strategies	2010–2015 DHHS Strategic Plan ONC Strategies	Example of Federal Initiatives	Chapter	URL
Engage stakeholders to accelerate development, and support effective use of standards Improve accessibility and integration of healthcare databases	Encourage innovation; support pilots and develop policies, standards, and services that enable the appropriate reuse of information	HIE	5	https://www.healthit.gov/HIE
Increase interoperable health information Support electronic information exchange among public health and clinical entities Promote the use of health IT to help ensure continuity of appropriate care during disasters	—	A Shared Nationwide Interoperability Roadmap version 1.0	28	https://www.healthit.gov/policy-researchers-implementers/interoperability
Encourage widespread meaningful use of health IT by providers Assess provider adoption and use of health IT Promote the use of electronic data, measurement, and clinical decision support tools Provide the tools and infrastructure for providers to see local trends in quality and safety using their certified electronic health record technology Provide tools to improve quality at the patient level	Use incentives, grants, and technical assistance to encourage widespread adoption and meaningful use	The Center for Medicare and Medicaid Services EHR Incentive Programs	27	https://www.cms.gov/Regulations-and-Guidance/Legislation/EHRIncentivePrograms/index.html
Use health IT to support the business requirements of alternative and innovative health delivery and payment models (e.g., accountable care organizations and patient-centered medical homes)	—	MACRA of 2015	27	https://www.cms.gov/Medicare/Quality-Initiatives-Patient-Assessment-Instruments/Value-Based-Programs/MACRA-MIPS-and-APMs/MACRA-MIPS-and-APMs.html
	—	ICD-10	22	http://www.cdc.gov/nchs/icd/icd10cm_pcs_background.htm
Enhance capacity for electronic surveillance of healthcare-associated infections	—	PHSIPO	11	http://www.cdc.gov/surveillancepractice/
	—	National Patient-Centered Clinical Research Network (PCORnet)	4	http://www.pcornet.org

Continued

TABLE 28.1 Examples of Government Initiatives With Policy Implications for Health Informatics—cont'd

2014–2018 DHHS Strategic Plan ONC Strategies	2010–2015 DHHS Strategic Plan ONC Strategies	Example of Federal Initiatives	Chapter	URL
Expand the adoption of telemedicine Increase the use of telemedicine to make specialized and emergency care more available to American Indians and Alaska Natives and to other vulnerable and underserved populations	Support and promote use of telehealth	The HHS: Health Resources and Services Administration Telehealth Program	8	http://www.hrsa.gov/healthit/toolbox/RuralHealthITtoolbox/Telehealth/
Enhance public awareness about the value and use of health IT	Enhance communication and support a public awareness campaign	—	—	—
	Explore the use of mobile technology	Mobile Devices Roundtable	15	https://www.healthit.gov/policy-researchers-implementers/overview-federal-role-mobile-health

DHHS, Department of Health and Human Services; *EHR,* electronic health record; *HHS,* Health and Human Services; *health IT,* health information technology; *HIE,* health information exchange; *HIPAA,* Health Insurance Portability and Accountability Act; *HITECH,* Health Information Technology for Economic and Clinical Health; *ICD-10,* International Classification of Diseases-10; *MACRA,* Medicare Access and CHIP Reauthorization Act; *ONC,* Office of the National Coordinator; *PHSIPO,* Public Health Surveillance and Informatics Program Office.

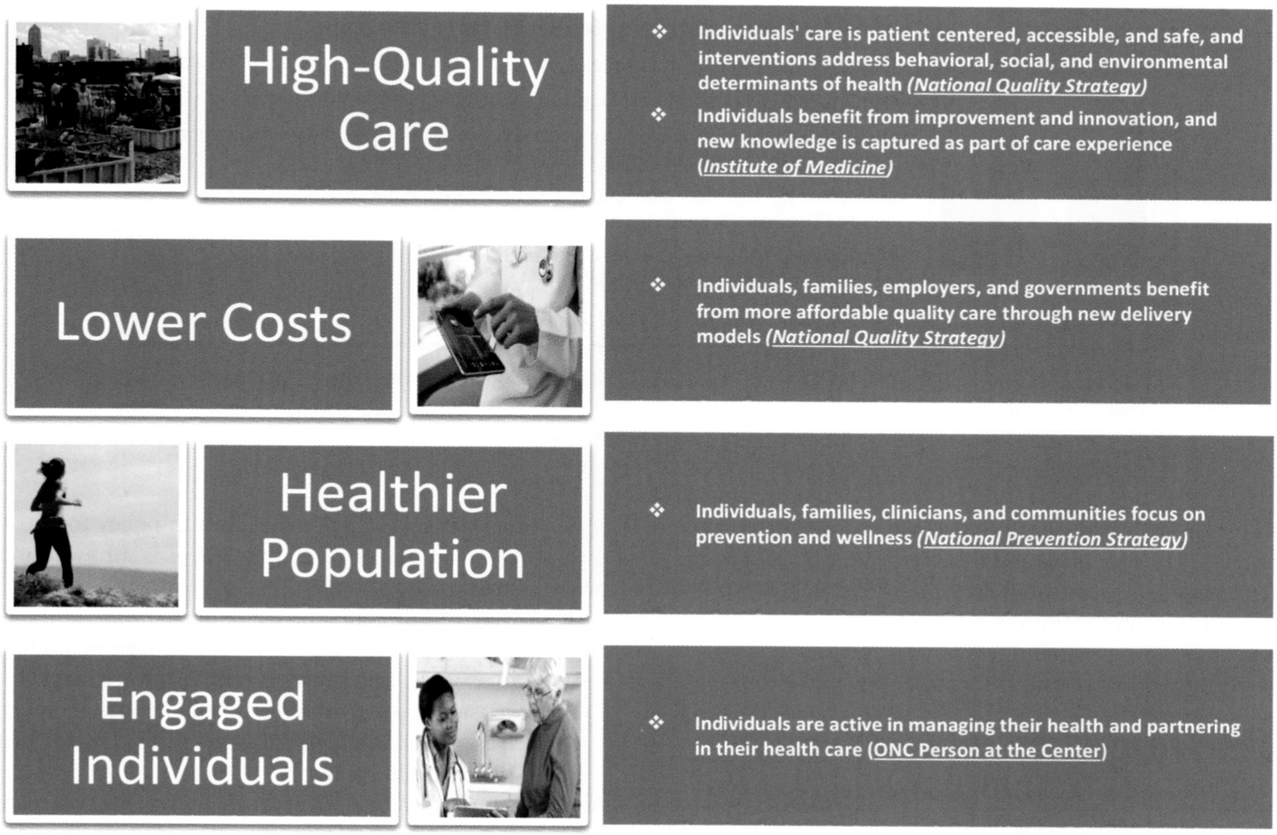

High-Quality Care

❖ Individuals' care is patient centered, accessible, and safe, and interventions address behavioral, social, and environmental determinants of health (*National Quality Strategy*)

❖ Individuals benefit from improvement and innovation, and new knowledge is captured as part of care experience (*Institute of Medicine*)

Lower Costs

❖ Individuals, families, employers, and governments benefit from more affordable quality care through new delivery models (*National Quality Strategy*)

Healthier Population

❖ Individuals, families, clinicians, and communities focus on prevention and wellness (*National Prevention Strategy*)

Engaged Individuals

❖ Individuals are active in managing their health and partnering in their health care (*ONC Person at the Center*)

FIG 28.3 The vision and expected results guiding the Federal Health IT Strategic Plan 2015–2020. (From *The Office of the National Coordinator for Health Information Technology (ONC). Federal health IT strategic plan; 2015–2020,* p 13. <https://www.healthit.gov/sites/default/files/9-5-federalhealthitstratplanfinal_0.pdf>. Accessed April 24, 2016.)

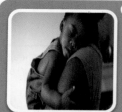

Goal 1: Advance Person-Centered and Self-Managed Health
- **Objective A:** Empower individual, family, and caregiver health management and engagement
- **Objective B:** Foster individual, provider, and community partnerships

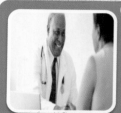

Goal 2: Transform Health Care Delivery and Community Health
- **Objective A:** Improve health care quality, access, and experience through safe, timely, effective, efficient, equitable, and person-centered care
- **Objective B:** Support the delivery of high-value health care
- **Objective C:** Protect and promote public health and healthy, resilient communities

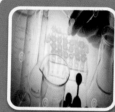

Goal 3: Foster Research, Scientific Knowledge, and Innovation
- **Objective A:** Increase access to and usability of high-quality electronic health information and services
- **Objective B:** Accelerate the development and commercialization of innovative technologies and solutions
- **Objective C:** Invest, disseminate, and translate research on how health IT can improve health and care delivery

Goal 4: Enhance Nation's Health IT Infrastructure
- **Objective A:** Finalize and implement the Nationwide Interoperability Roadmap
- **Objective B:** Protect the privacy and security of health information
- **Objective C:** Identify, prioritize, and advance technical standards to support secure and interoperable health information and health IT
- **Objective D:** Increase user and market confidence in the safety and safe use of health IT products, systems, and services
- **Objective E:** Advance a national communications infrastructure that supports health, safety, and care delivery

FIG 28.4 Federal Health IT Goals from the Federal Health IT Strategic Plan 2015–2020. (Source: *The Office of the National Coordinator for Health Information Technology [ONC]. Federal health IT strategic plan; 2015–2020.* <https://www.healthit.gov/sites/default/files/9-5-federalhealthit stratplanfinal_0.pdf>. Accessed April 24, 2016.)

IT is a tool to achieve the goals of the plan and not the purpose of this plan. The four goals and their respective objectives and strategies are not sequential but interdependent with the vision and purpose of improving the health and well-being of individuals and communities.

DRIVING FORCES FOR CREATING HEALTH INFORMATION TECHNOLOGY POLICY

As pointed out in the introduction to this chapter, there are a number of challenges to cost-effective, efficient healthcare delivery. When a problem or challenge is first recognized,

society does not magically create a health policy to deal with that problem or challenge. Rather, there is an evolutionary progress that includes:

1. Analysis leading to a better understanding of the issue
2. Increased public awareness and education leading to both a public and professional push for change
3. Proposed approaches from multiple stakeholders, as well as political and legislative action leading to changes in public health policy

As new approaches to deal with the issue are implemented, improvements typically exist but also new challenges are introduced by the technology. Issues related to patient safety and quality of care are used here to illustrate this process.

Patient Safety

An increased focus on patient safety began with the 1999 IOM report *To Err Is Human*. The report estimated that 44,000 to 98,000 lives were lost every year due to medical errors in hospitals, which in turn led to the widespread recognition that healthcare is not safe enough and catalyzed a revolution to improve the quality of care.[9] Despite considerable effort, patient safety has not yet improved to the degree hoped for in the follow-up IOM report, *Crossing the Quality Chasm*.[10] In 2012, the IOM proposed new strategies to advance quality and safety in yet another report, *Best Care at Lower Cost: The Path to Continuously Learning Health Care in America*.[11] However the challenge of creating a safe healthcare system continues. In 2013, John T. James published one of the latest studies to date. "The number of premature deaths associated with preventable harm to patients was estimated at more than 400,000 per year. Serious harm seems to be 10- to 20-fold more common than lethal harm."[12, p. 122] Each of the IOM reports identifies health IT as an effective strategy for safer, more effective care in all settings.

When designed and implemented appropriately, health IT can improve healthcare providers' performance, support better communication between patients and healthcare providers, and enhance patient safety, all of which ultimately leads to better care.[13] For example, the number of patients who receive the correct medication in hospitals increases significantly when hospitals implement computerized prescribing and use barcoded medication administration.[14] However, poorly designed and implemented health IT can actually create new hazards in the already complex delivery of healthcare. To protect patients, health IT must be designed and used in ways that maximize patient safety while minimizing harm. Information technology can better help patients if it becomes more usable, more interoperable, and easier to implement and maintain.

Institute of Medicine Report on Health Information Technology and Patient Safety

In the wake of more widespread use of health IT and to mitigate the risks posed by these safety concerns, the U.S. Department of HHS asked the IOM to evaluate health IT safety concerns and to recommend ways in which both the government and the private sector can make patient care safer using health IT. The resulting 2011 IOM report, *HIT and Patient Safety*, states that safe use of health IT relies on several factors, including clinicians and patients.[15] Safety analyses should not look for a single cause of problems but should consider the system as a whole and consider the interplay of people, process, and technology when looking for ways to make it safer. Vendors, users, government, and the private sector all have roles to play. The IOM's recommendations include improving transparency in the reporting of health IT safety incidents and enhancing monitoring of health IT products. A summary of these recommendations follows:

- HHS should ensure that vendors support users in freely exchanging information about health IT experiences and issues, including safety.
- ONC should work with the private sector to make comparative user experiences publicly available.
- HHS should fund a new Health IT Safety Council within an existing standards organization to evaluate criteria for judging the safety of health IT.
- HHS should establish a mechanism for vendors and users to report health IT–related deaths, serious injuries, or unsafe conditions.
- HHS should recommend that Congress establish an independent federal entity, similar to the National Transportation Safety Board, to perform investigations in a transparent, nonpunitive manner.

According to the report, these would be the first stages for action, to advance current understanding of the threats to patient safety. The IOM report also examined a broad range of health information technologies, including electronic health records (EHRs), secure patient portals, and HIEs. While some organizations had very good tracking databases to prioritize technical issues and human factors issues related to technology, others were doing little to track health IT problems and resolutions. The report also asked that the Secretary of HHS publish a plan within 12 months to minimize patient safety risks associated with health IT and report annually on the progress being made. As a result, the Health IT Patient Safety Action and Surveillance Plan was finalized in 2013.[16] As part of the Safety Plan, a new Health IT Safety Center Roadmap was published by ONC in 2015, laying out a 5-year plan for creating a federal center, as a public–private partnership, to focus on aggregating data from health IT–related adverse events. The road map grew out of a series of meetings with selected stakeholders, including federal agencies, patient safety organizations (PSOs), researchers, and clinicians. The center's three major tasks will be (1) convening groups of stakeholders to learn more about health IT–related risks; (2) researching hazards and disseminating information gleaned from these activities, which could include real-world pilot testing and implementation; and (3) evaluation of health IT safety solutions.[17]

Unintended Consequences of Health Information Technology Implementation

The unprecedented funding provided by the HITECH Act spawned a flurry of EHR implementations. While expectations were high for achieving all of the quality, safety, and cost benefits anticipated from these implementations, experience and research shows that unplanned and unexpected consequences have resulted from major policy and technological changes.[18,19] Unintended consequences are defined as positive, negative, or neutral unanticipated outcomes occurring as a result of a planned activity or event. Thus it is important to consider the potential unintended consequences that may be produced by adoption of health IT, particularly when implementations are accelerated.[20]

Government-sponsored research in this area of health IT began in 2004 with the Agency for Healthcare Research and Quality (AHRQ) grants for planning, implementing, and testing the value of both EHRs and HIEs. Yet there is still a great deal that has not yet been explored or understood. However, health IT implementation science continues to expand (see Chapters 17 and 19 on project management and system implementation). Monitoring for and tracking of the unplanned or unexpected consequence, especially when it has an undesirable outcome, is important. Enhanced communication among multiple stakeholders in different venues and disciplines will strengthen the collective ability to identify and address unintended consequences of health IT. Federal and organizational leadership can facilitate the sharing of information about technical and organizational safeguards that address unintended consequences. Further, mechanisms are needed to share findings of health IT system implementers so that data captured by individual organizations can have a broader impact.

One Meaningful Use criterion for both hospitals and healthcare providers at all three stages is to report Clinical Quality Measures (CQMs) to the Centers for Medicare and Medicaid Services (CMS) (for Medicare) or to the state (for Medicaid). As with the other Meaningful Use criteria, the CQMs mature during each stage of Meaningful Use, with increasing numbers of measures required and increasing numbers of National Quality Strategy domains covered. In addition, the CQMs moved from legacy quality measures to electronically specified measures. These eMeasures seek to standardize performance and include specific reporting requirements. Going forward, the CQMs are incorporated into MARCA.

Quality Initiatives

Quality initiatives provide a second example of the process by which health IT policy continues to evolve. The Stage 1 Meaningful Use objectives were organized around five quality initiatives adapted from the work of the National Priorities Partnership (NPP) and are fundamental to each stage of Meaningful Use. The NPP is a collaborative effort of 51 major national organizations that brings together public- and private-sector stakeholder groups as partners in a forum that balances the interests of consumers, purchasers, health plans, clinicians, providers, communities, states, and suppliers in achieving the aims of better care, affordable care, and healthy people and communities.

Under contract to provide input to the Secretary of HHS on the 2012 National Quality Strategy, NPP published its report on national priorities in 2011.[21] To provide more input on each priority, the structure for this work allowed the full NPP to serve as an overarching committee, while its partners divided into three subcommittees responsible for advising on goals, measures, and strategic opportunities specific to three domains of the National Quality Strategy: healthy people and healthy communities, better care, and affordable care. This important work evolved from

NPP's previous input to HHS on national priorities and goals, including a report submitted in 2010 as well as its 2008 report, *Aligning Our Efforts to Transform America's Healthcare.*

National Quality Strategy

In March 2011, HHS released the National Quality Strategy for health improvement, the first effort to create a national framework to help guide local, state, and national efforts to improve the quality of care in the United States.[22] The National Quality Strategy recognizes health IT as critical to improving the quality of care, improving health outcomes, and ultimately reducing costs. Each year, an annual Progress Report to Congress[23] on achievement of the quality goals is published.

Putting the National Quality Strategy into action, HHS subsequently launched the following two key initiatives that set specific national targets:

- Partnership for Patients, which is working with a wide variety of private and public stakeholders to make hospital care safer by reducing hospital-acquired conditions by 40% and improving care transitions upon release from the hospital so that readmissions are reduced by 20%
- Million Hearts campaign, which is a public-private initiative to prevent 1 million heart attacks and strokes between 2012 and 2016 by improving access to care and increasing adherence to basic preventive medicine

The evidence shows that health IT, along with delivery system improvements, should be a key ingredient in the success of these campaigns and other efforts around the country to improve health outcomes. One study published in *The New England Journal of Medicine* looked at diabetes care in Cleveland and found the following:

- 51% of patients being treated by physician practices using an EHR received care that met all endorsed standards of diabetes care, compared to 7% of patients treated by practices not using an EHR.
- 44% of patients treated by practices using an EHR met at least four of five outcome standards for diabetes, compared to 16% of patients treated by paper-based practices with similar outcomes.[24]

This study speaks volumes about the positive impact that well-implemented health IT that supports clinical decisions can have on the quality of clinical practice. With clinical decision support applications, health IT can facilitate the consistent execution of evidence-based best practices by healthcare providers, including both nursing and medicine.

LEADERSHIP COMPETENCIES FOR DEVELOPING AND IMPLEMENTING HEALTH INFORMATION TECHNOLOGY POLICIES

Healthcare professionals and informaticians have a professional responsibility to participate in the development and implementation of effective health policies that maximize the use of health IT and empower clinicians and patients as partners for health. The following section of the chapter makes frequent use of nursing as one example of leadership activities for developing effective health IT policy and for illustrating the impact such activities can have on healthcare. However, as pointed on in the IOM report, *Assessing Progress on the Institute of Medicine Report "The Future of Nursing"*: "The nursing profession is making a wide-reaching impact by providing quality, patient-centered, accessible, and affordable care."[25, p. 1] However, "No single profession, working alone, can meet the complex needs of patients and communities."[25, p. 3] To truly create a cost-effective quality healthcare for all, each of the healthcare disciplines must "continue to develop skills and competencies in leadership and innovation and collaborate with other professionals in health care delivery and health system redesign."[25, p. 3]

Ensuring That Health Practitioners Are Positioned on Key Committees and Boards

Over the past few decades, health professionals and health informaticians have become increasingly engaged with health policy efforts. This is especially true within the nursing and nursing informatics community, where nursing leaders are claiming a seat at the policy table and are being sought after for key national appointments as well as being hired for executive positions. In 2014 The American Nurses Association (ANA), the American Academy of Nursing, and the American Nurses Foundation launched a national coalition to place 10,000 nurses on governing boards by 2020.[26] The Nurses on Boards Coalition is a group of national nursing organizations working together to increase nurses' presence on corporate and non-profit health-related boards of directors throughout the country. The goal of this effort is to bring nurses' valuable perspectives to governing boards as well as state-level and national commissions with an interest in health. Through this effort, an awakening occurred about the importance of recognizing opportunities to communicate and collaborate with others to produce favorable outcomes.[27]

Another notable change is that nurses today proactively reach out to other colleagues and leaders in positions of influence, including government agencies, national organizations, professional societies, and committees, to share knowledge and offer expertise, and they have learned a great deal from these discussions. One key takeaway is that national leaders and groups respond positively to nursing's large population. For example, the Alliance for Nursing Informatics (ANI) and the American Nurses Association (ANA) are working closely to articulate a unified voice that more broadly represents the profession, consisting of more than 3 million nurses. ANA works in collaboration with ANI and AAN to identify and endorse qualified individuals in response to calls for participation in national activities and testimony opportunities that advance policies focused on improving quality, patient safety, and outcomes.[28]

An example of the ANI and ANA efforts was demonstrated when ONC launched a consumer campaign to empower and educate patients, caregivers, and individuals in managing their day-to-day health and acting as partners in their health through the use of health IT.[29] This campaign includes "Innovation Challenges," which consist of public contests for technology developers to create tools related to a particular problem or need. ONC periodically issues these innovation challenges to spur innovation related to consumer health information. In support of this effort, ANI and ANA jointly pledged to coordinate a campaign with other national nursing organizations to promote use of personal health records (PHRs) and patient portals. The ultimate goal of the ANI Pledge to Support the Consumer eHealth Program[30] is to help clinicians offer a wider range of considerations and options for patients, while also providing patients with resources that encourage proactive behavior, thus empowering them to be active partners in their health plan.

An additional example is that the ANA, which continually tracks calls for nominations for agencies and organizations, reported that as of 2015, 11 nurses were appointed to 13 positions at the U.S. ONC for Health IT.[31]

Responding to Requests for Comments

With the increasing numbers of policies and regulations for healthcare and health IT, a growing number of opportunities exist for organizations and individuals to submit comments on the ensuing regulations and other related federal guidance documents. Laws passed by Congress rarely contain enough specific language to fully guide their implementation.[32] Regulations and the rule-making process are used to clarify definitions, authority, eligibility, benefits, and standards. Their development is shaped by the monitoring, involvement, and input of professional societies, healthcare providers, third-party payers, consumers, and other special interest groups. (The process for developing regulations from legislation is explained in Chapter 25.)

Each organization's internal policies may offer direction as to whether or when a formal written response to federal policy-makers is warranted. As one example, ANI has developed a policy that describes its process for member organizations to achieve consensus on policy issues affecting nursing informatics.[30] This policy states:

> ANI, as a collaboration that represents multiple nursing informatics organizations, responds as one voice to federal health policy initiatives by sharing nursing informatics perspectives for shaping health policy. Due to limited timing to respond, it is not always possible to have a full review by all members within each of the ANI member organizations. ANI will make every effort to provide notification about its intent to respond to a call for comments for healthcare reform initiatives, requirements and rulings from ONC or other government agencies and organizations, as soon as ANI decides to pursue a specific call. The length of time available to respond will determine the steps in the procedure for obtaining comments.[32]

The ANA has offered the following guidance on how individual nurses can affect federal rules and regulations:

- Learn about the federal rule-making process and how to make your voice heard.
- Become informed about the public policy and health policy issues currently under consideration at the federal level of government.
- Check out the *Federal Register*. It is the very best source of information about proposed rules and changes to existing rules for federal programs. It is posted every day and contains complete directions on where to send comments and deadlines for the public comment period.
- Work with your state nurses association by offering your expertise to assist in developing new regulations, modifying existing regulation, or preparing comments on proposed regulations.[33]

Other tips are offered to individuals. To enhance the credibility of submitted comments, address any questions in the notice and take the time to offer positive feedback on points of agreement with the proposed regulation. If a template is provided, use it for the response submissions. Finally, be sure to publicize the response via various media channels, including social media, and use it as an opportunity to increase awareness and provide education about the public policy effort and related publications or activities.

Developing Position Statements

Another mechanism for advancing health policy is through the development and publication of position statements (sometimes called policy briefs). A position statement is an explanation or a recommendation for a course of action that reflects an organization's stance on an issue of concern. Position statements are typically developed after an internal discussion with content experts, then advanced to the broader membership for review and input, and finally submitted to the oversight governance group or board for approval. This development, review, and approval process allows interested parties to voice their concerns and opinions on the issue at hand and enables the group to reach consensus.

One example is the Healthcare Information and Management Systems Society (HIMSS) Nursing Informatics Position Statement titled *Transforming Nursing Practice through Technology and Informatics*. This HIMSS Position Statement was developed by the HIMSS Nursing Informatics Community and subsequently reviewed and approved by the HIMSS board of directors. Position statements may also be created in collaboration with other groups and issued as joint statements. An example of this type of effort is the ANA Position Statement on the Inclusion of Recognized Terminologies within EHRs and other Health IT Solutions.[34] The purpose of this position statement is to reaffirm the ANA's support for the use of recognized terminologies supporting nursing practice as valuable representations of nursing practice and to promote the integration of those terminologies into information

technology solutions. The ANA worked in collaboration with attendees of the Nursing Knowledge Big Data Science Conference sponsored by the University of Minnesota to develop and review this position statement, which was subsequently approved by the ANA board of directors on March 19, 2015.

LEADING POLICY ACTIVITIES THROUGH ORGANIZATIONAL WORK AND LEADERSHIP

Health informatics–related organizations actively influencing health informatics policy through organizational work and leadership include the ANI, AAN, American Health Information Management Association (AHIMA), American Medical Informatics Association (AMIA), HIMSS, and others. A brief summary of the public policy focus of selected informatics-related organizations is provided in Table 28.2.

Strategies

Health informaticians working together within professional associations bring to the health policy table a deep understanding of clinical processes, technology, and health IT systems in addition to experience as advocates for patients, groups, communities, and overall populations. Using the contacts and structure provided with a professional association, these leaders have a unique opportunity and a professional responsibility to share this knowledge with the goals of advancing an improved health system that is increasingly focused on value-based care. Changes in health policy are one part of necessary reform,[35] but how do healthcare providers and health informaticians prepare to engage in public policy efforts? The beginner must acquire a basic knowledge of health policy and funding.

An understanding of health policy principles can be gained through formal coursework, continuing education, reviewing the literature, or even self-study of the myriad resources available on the internet.[36] Getting involved with the policy efforts within one's own organization is a simple way to get started. Professional colleagues with the organization are often willing to act as coaches to offer advice, criticism, information, encouragement, and support. For example, HIMSS believes that nurses must lead and be visible, vocal, and present at the table for all significant healthcare reform initiatives.[37] In addition, volunteering to participate in state-level advocacy activities can provide experience in meeting with legislators. Applying for a committee appointment at the local and state levels offers other opportunities to learn how to influence policy.

Beyond acquiring knowledge of basic policy principles, demonstrating leadership skills and leveraging a professional network are necessary to achieve success. Health practitioners require certain skills to be able to communicate effectively with policy-makers and take advantage of relevant advocacy opportunities. According to Alexander and Halley, to advocate, health professionals and informaticians must be strategists, leaders, and great communicators, and they must engage stakeholders across multiple spectrums to ensure that

TABLE 28.2 Professional Association in Informatics Influencing Health Policy

Name	Mission Statement or Focus	Examples of Current Activities	Website
AMIA Public Policy Committee	To improve health in the United States and globally, we are engaging with policy-makers and other thought leaders to holistically improve health and healthcare with use of informatics' science, research and practice….AMIA Public Policy exists to improve the legislative and regulatory environment for health informatics research, practice, and education through AMIA member expertise. Priorities include: 1. Health IT patient safety 2. Workforce and education 3. Data sharing in research 4. Health IT standards and interoperability 5. Patient data access 6. Electronic clinical quality measurement	• Letter of support to the chairman and members of the HELP Committee in crafting the Improving Health Information Technology Act of 2015, with specific mention of regulatory and administrative burden related to clinical documentation and data capture; publicity demonstrating certification process for health IT; clearly defining interoperability; providing patients access to their health information maintained in an EHR and ensuring accurate patient information for the correct patient (February 9, 2016) • Submitted comments to the CMS with recommendations for improving quality measurement in an electronic environment (February 2, 2016) • Submitted comments to CMS asking that regulators change stage 3 Meaningful Use requirements to better align with programs required by MACRA (December 14, 2015)	https://www.amia.org/public-policy
HIMSS Policy Center	HIMSS believes that the appropriate use of IT and management systems can transform healthcare to save lives, improve outcomes of care, and reduce costs. Key issues include: 1. Health Information Exchange (Interoperability and Standards) 2. Meaningful Use 3. Privacy and Security 4. User Experience	• Weekly update via health IT policy newsletter • Annual HIMSS Policy Summit • 2014–2016 Policy Principles • HIMSS IT Value Suite • Policy Committee • Legislative Action Center • 2015–2016 Congressional Asks include expand access to telehealth services for Medicare beneficiaries, support for robust interoperability and health information exchange, and support for healthcare's efforts to combat cyber threats • Sent a letter to Senate HELP Committee outlining policy recommendations related to achieving interoperability, public process for certification of EHRs, and patient access to their personal health information along with a number of other topics	http://www.himss.org/library/health-it-policy
AHIMA The Advocacy and Public Policy Center	AHIMA's advocacy and public policy team actively monitors, responds to, and participates in national policy and industry initiatives to shape and guide issues that are important to the health information management profession.	• Provided comments to the National Quality Forum (NQF) concerning their report, *Identification and Prioritization of Health IT Patient Safety Measures* • Provided comments to the ONC on the ONC 2016 Interoperability Standards Advisory • Provided comments to CMS on proposed Procedure Code Modifications Presented at the ICD-10 Coordination and Maintenance Committee Meeting Held March 2016	http://www.ahima.org/about/advocacy
American Academy of Nursing Expert Panel on Informatics and Technology	The expert panel gathers health policy data and information, then disseminates information, advises, and represents the AAN on issues related to health information management, implementation of informatics and technology through EHRs and PHRs, HIPAA, patient safety initiatives, consumer and personal health,	• Released a policy brief that endorsed the capturing of social and behavioral determinants of health in the EHR • Published in *Nursing Outlook*: "Putting 'health' in the electronic health record: A call for collective action" (volume 63, page 614–616, September 2015)	https://aan.memberclicks.net/ep-informatics–technology

Continued

TABLE 28.2	Professional Association in Informatics Influencing Health Policy—cont'd		
Name	**Mission Statement or Focus**	**Examples of Current Activities**	**Website**
	workforce issues and training, bioterrorism and bio surveillance, evidence-based practice, clinical decision support, and other areas of concern related to the use of informatics and technology in nursing education, practice, and research.		
ANI	To advance nursing informatics leadership, practice, education, policy, research, and leadership through a unified voice of nursing informatics organizations	• Provided NINR with comments concerning the NINR Strategic Plan • Provided comments to ONC 2016 Interoperability Standards Advisory • Provided comments to Senate HELP bill • Provided comments to NQF HIT & Patient Safety Project concerning identification and prioritization of Health IT Patient Safety Measures	http://www.allianceni.org/statements.asp
JPHIT	A coalition of nine national public health associations that help U.S. governmental public health agencies build modern information systems across a spectrum of public health programs.	• Develops policy positions that articulate IT priorities shared across the U.S. public health system • Maintains an action agenda to help alert public health professionals of national activities that impact their informatics work	http://www.jphit.org/about/

AAN, American Academy of Nursing; *AHIMA,* American Health Information Management Association; *AMIA,* American Medical Informatics Association; *ANI,* Alliance for Nursing Informatics; *CMS,* Centers for Medicare and Medicaid Services; *EHR,* electronic health record; *Health IT,* health information technology; *HELP,* health, education, labor and pensions; *HIPAA,* Health Insurance Portability and Accountability Act; *HIMSS,* Healthcare Information and Management Systems Society; *ICD-10,* International Classification Of Diseases-10; *IT,* information technology; *MACRA,* Medicare Access and CHIP Reauthorization Act; *NINR,* National Institute of Nursing Research; *NQF,* National Quality Forum's; *ONC,* Office of the National Coordinator; *PHRs,* personal health records.

the needs of patients and professionals are met.[27] Communication skills are essential to be able to craft and articulate key points that will "make the case" as well as to capture and engage the target audience. Exemplary leadership activity will move the cause forward in an actionable way toward policy improvement.[30] Demonstrating such leadership requires more than showing passion for an issue. It also involves being able to connect evidence to the policy agenda and frame it in a logical context. Collaboration and unified messaging among all stakeholders are keys to success.

DISCIPLINE-SPECIFIC POLICIES: NURSING

This section provides an example of current influences within the specific discipline of nursing. All health disciplines are encouraged to research current policies specific to their areas. Readers in other health disciplines are encouraged to note the outline and content provided here as a model.

Use of Health Information Technology to Advance the Future of Nursing

In 2008, The Robert Wood Johnson Foundation (RWJF) and the IOM launched a 2-year initiative to assess and offer recommendations for transforming the nursing profession. In 2010, the Committee appointed by the IOM to complete this task released their report entitled *The Future of Nursing: Leading Change, Advancing Health.*[38] The published report offered bold recommendations for transforming the nursing profession, leading to advanced roles and leadership positions for nurses in the redesign of the healthcare system.

The Future of Nursing Report Recommendations

Many leading nursing organizations, including ANI, provided testimony to the Committee. These contributions from ANI, along with others from national nursing leaders, were used by the Committee in the development of the report, which has been described by some as the "tipping point in nursing care," calling for the nursing profession to be reengineered with a more educated workforce capacity.[39] *The Future of Nursing* report outlined several opportunities to transform nursing practice through informatics and technology.

Implications for Time and Place of Care. Care supported by interoperable digital networks will shift in the importance of time and place. It is likely that a significant subset of care delivery will be independent of physical location when health IT is fully implemented. Nurses provide care in every setting, particularly in the community; therefore nurses should be involved in shaping the effective use of health IT and related policies wherever they practice. Nurses have identified that lack of an integrated EHR is a barrier to success.[37] National initiatives to address EHR adoption and integration challenges are being advanced. Nurses should become increasingly more engaged in national, regional, and local policy efforts in order to drive this agenda of person-centric, location-independent healthcare information.

Expand Opportunities for Nurses to Lead and Diffuse Collaborative Efforts. Interoperable EHRs linked with patient portals influence how collaborative care teams are able to work and share clinical information. Care teams are no longer bound by physical space but rather can engage in virtual learning environments to support the care delivery of the future. The increasing use of communication tools, the proliferation of mobile devices, and the increasing availability of online health tools are offering multiple opportunities for healthcare providers to collaborate with each other and to engage with patients.[40] Personal health information is a valuable resource for individuals, their families, and healthcare professionals who provide treatment and deliver care in institutional and community settings. Examples of personal health information management systems and tools that can be leveraged include personal health devices, PHRs, and web-based portals linked to EHRs or clinical information systems. Well-defined policies are necessary to ensure that the security and confidentiality of protected health information is safeguarded in this rapidly evolving virtual healthcare environment. Nurses should seek opportunities to participate in efforts to define policies that affect patient care, including volunteering for policy development committees within their own organizations.

While health IT will have an increasing influence on how nurses plan and document their care, all facets of care are becoming increasingly digital. From the expanded use of tracking devices and smart beds, data capture is being automated, and nurses are more able to focus on complex cognitive decisions using knowledge management and decision support. Policy-makers should and do work with nurse leaders to leverage these opportunities to transform nursing practice through the use of new and existing technologies intended to support decision making and care delivery. For example, nurses can provide input as to how the proposed use of health IT may affect their workflow or offer guidance on the optimal use of these technologies to improve care delivery.

A recent effort to engage consumers in compiling their own health information is the GetMyHealthData effort. This is a collaborative activity among leading consumer organizations, healthcare experts, clinicians, policy-makers, and technology organizations that believe passionately that consumer access to digital health information is an essential cornerstone of better health and better care. The ANI joined these efforts. ANI organizations have joined forces to ask their members, nurses, and clinical colleagues to broadly share and give feedback to GetMyHealthData. The goal of this effort is to liberate healthcare data for the benefit of consumers and the health

system as a whole so they can use it to improve their health and care.[41]

Prepare and Enable Nurses to Lead Change to Advance Health. Other key recommendations in *The Future of Nursing* report emphasize the importance of preparing and enabling nurses to lead change to advance health. Public, private, and governmental healthcare decision makers should include nurses at every level. Nurses consistently rank at the top of the Annual Gallup Poll on Honesty/Ethics in Professions, doing so each year since they were first included in the poll in 1999, except in 2001 when firefighters were included on a one-time basis to recognize their heroic actions on September 11.[42] But frequently they do not recognize that power or work as a group to leverage opportunities to influence policy or strategic direction.

The TIGER (Technology Informatics Guiding Education Reform) Initiative's goal of engaging more nurses in leading both the development of a national health IT infrastructure and healthcare reform is referenced in *The Future of Nursing*, as is its goal to accelerate adoption of smart, standards-based, interoperable technology that will make healthcare delivery safer, more efficient, timely, accessible, and patient centered, while also reducing the burden on nurses.[43] Through efforts such as TIGER, nurses are mastering informatics competencies to better influence policy efforts in today's rapid EHR adoption. The TIGER initiative report on the Leadership Imperative emphasizes that now, more than ever, innovative nurse leaders are positioned to work closely with local and national policy leaders and lawmakers through public policy engagement. Effective engagement requires a comprehensive understanding of policy processes and the knowledge and skill to effectively evaluate the interconnections between policy, nursing, and health outcomes, as well as the critical role of health IT. Using this knowledge to develop programs of action grounded in the principles of professional nursing, the innovative nurse leader plays a major role in effecting positive change as our system of healthcare continues to evolve.

The Future of Nursing report emphasizes that the United States has the opportunity to transform its healthcare system, and nurses must play a fundamental role in this transformation. However, this transformation will require that nurses embrace technology as a necessary tool to innovate the delivery of nursing care.

Center to Champion Nursing in America

The Future of Nursing: Campaign for Action is an initiative to advance comprehensive healthcare change. It envisions a healthcare system in which all Americans have access to high-quality care, with nurses contributing to the full extent of their capabilities.[44] The campaign is coordinated through the Center to Champion Nursing in America (CCNA), an initiative of American Association of Retired People (AARP), the AARP Foundation, and the RWJF. The Center includes 50 state action coalitions, a wide range of healthcare providers, consumer advocates, policy-makers, and business, academic, and philanthropic leaders. The Campaign for

Action is moving forward simultaneously on national, state, and local levels through efforts to accomplish the following:

- Strengthen nurse education and training
- Enable nurses to practice to the full extent of their education and training
- Advance interprofessional collaboration among healthcare professionals to ensure coordinated and improved patient care
- Expand leadership ranks to ensure that nurses have a voice on management teams, in boardrooms, and during policy debates
- Improve healthcare workforce data collection to better assess and project workforce requirements[45]

State-level action coalitions are also working to advance the campaign's efforts at the local, regional, and state levels. These action coalitions will capture best practices, determine research needs, track lessons learned, and identify replicable models that can be embedded in national policy efforts. Yearly, the campaign is analyzing established datasets to evaluate where we are gaining ground and areas that require additional emphasis. Examples of campaign progress are discussed in the following sections.[45]

Advancing Education Transformation.

- From the fall of 2010 to 2014, the number of students enrolled in RN-to-BSN programs increased from 77,259 to 130,345, a 69% increase.
- For the first time in its history, Medicare is paying to support the training of nurses with the Graduate Nurse Education Demonstration, a $200 million demonstration project in five hospital systems. This historic legislation is designed to prepare more advanced practice registered nurses to care for people across all healthcare settings.

Fostering Interprofessional Collaboration. Three major foundations—the RWJF, the Gordon and Betty Moore Foundation, and the Josiah Macy Jr. Foundation—collaborated to support the Health Resources and Services Administration's National Center for Interprofessional Practice and Education at the University of Minnesota. The center is working to provide leadership, scholarship, evidence, coordination, and national visibility to advance interprofessional education and practice as a viable and efficient healthcare delivery mode.

Healthcare Information and Management Systems Society Nursing Informatics Position Statement

To further advance recommendations in *The Future of Nursing* report, HIMSS published a position statement in 2011 titled *Transforming Nursing Practice Through Technology and Informatics.* This statement asserts that:

Nurses are key leaders in developing the infrastructure for effective and efficient HIT [health IT] that transforms the delivery of care. Nurse informaticians play a crucial role in advocating both for patients and fellow nurses who are often the key stakeholders and recipients of these evolving solutions. Nursing informatics professionals are the liaisons to successful interactions with technology in healthcare. As clinicians who focus on transforming

information into knowledge, nurse informaticians cultivate a new time and place of care through their facilitation efforts to integrate technology with patient care. Technology will continue to be a fundamental enabler of future care delivery models and nursing informatics leaders will be essential to transforming nursing practice through technology.[1]

To achieve the goals of this position statement, nurse leaders should be engaged at all levels in health IT policy and strategy-setting committees and initiatives. In addition, they must be knowledgeable and well versed in current public policy initiatives and seek opportunities to participate in advocacy and educational efforts directed toward policy-makers. Through the efforts of the Nursing Knowledge: Big Data Conference, a workgroup has been formed to engage and equip all nurses in health IT policy.[46] This effort will make strides in providing nurses with the education, tools, and resources to equip them as knowledgeable advocates for policy efforts that are important to nursing.

Assessing Progress on the Institute of Medicine Report *The Future of Nursing*

Five years after the IOM's Future of Nursing report, the RWJF asked the IOM to convene a committee to examine the progress made in implementing the report's recommendations. The resulting report, *Assessing Progress on the Institute of Medicine Report The Future of Nursing,*[31] summarizes progress and offers recommendations for the future campaign to accelerate implementation of recommendations. The report includes information about the following:

- **Removing barriers to practice and care**. Significant barriers still exist to allowing the full practice of Advanced Practice Registered Nurses. Nurses should work with other professions to remove scope of practice scope-of-practice restrictions.
- **Transforming education.** Recommendations are to provide pathways to the BSN degree; create and fund residency programs; promote doctoral degrees, emphasizing the PhD; and promote interdisciplinary and life-long learning.
- **Collaborating and leading.** Nurses are encouraged to serve in executive and leadership positions. Continued efforts are needed for interdisciplinary collaborations and leadership development.
- **Promoting diversity.** While many organizations have increased diversity, continued emphasis is needed.
- **Improving data.** Data collection is needed about numbers and types of health professionals, their roles and places of employment. More robust and organized datasets are needed.

As described earlier, many of these strategies have implications for health informatics specifically about improving data and leadership efforts. In addition, *Recommendation 2: Expand Opportunities for Nurses to Lead and Diffuse Collaborative Improvement Efforts* speaks specifically to health informatics by continuing the following recommendation from the initial report:

Health care organizations should engage nurses and other front-line staff to work with developers and manufacturers in the design, development, purchase, implementation, and evaluation of medical and health devices and health information technology products.[31, p. 191]

CONCLUSION AND FUTURE DIRECTIONS

This chapter describes current health policy initiatives with a focus on health IT and the health policy leadership responsibilities of the health professionals and informaticians. By understanding current informatics-related health policies issues, the role of the professional organizations, the current federal infrastructure support for health informatics, and specific approaches for participating in the advocacy process, health professionals and informatics leaders can positively affect health policy. As demonstrated by a variety of nursing initiatives, leadership makes a difference. Health practitioners can and must take on leadership roles and influence policy to improve safety and efficiency, thereby bringing evidence for decision making to the point of care and empowering patients and consumers as partners. Collectively, health practitioners must respond to the policy challenges outlined in this chapter to advance the health of individuals, families, groups, and communities. Whatever their role, healthcare providers and informatics specialists must be confident that they can influence health policy at the local and organizational, regional, state, and national level.

Where are we now, several decades after starting the implementation of health IT in healthcare? Winston Churchill put it best when he said, "Now this is not the end. It is not even the beginning of the end. But it is, perhaps, the end of the beginning."[47, p. 264] We have much more to do. Through strong leadership and active participation we will be able to organize and complete the hard work necessary to create the policy changes that will transform healthcare.

REFERENCES

1. Healthcare Information and Management Systems Society (HIMSS). *Position Statement on Transforming Nursing Practice Through Technology and Informatics.* Chicago, IL: HIMSS; 2011.
2. *World Health Organization (WHO) Health Policy.* http://www.who.int/nationalpolicies/about/en/. Accessed July 17, 2016.
3. The Office of the National Coordinator (ONC) for Health Information Technology. *Federal health IT strategic plan 2015–2020.* https://www.healthit.gov/sites/default/files/9-5-federalhealthitstratplanfinal_0.pdf.
4. James E, Hughes M. Government-sponsored programs make up 52% of what we spend on healthcare. *Forbes.* 2015;29.http://www.forbes.com/sites/realspin/2015/07/29/for-the-first-time-government-programs-make-up-the-majority-of-u-s-health-spending/#4b3f205d8e1c.
5. U.S. Department of Health & Human Services. *HHS strategic plan FY 2014–2018: Introduction;* 2014. http://www.hhs.gov/about/strategic-plan/introduction/index.html.
6. Health.gov. *Newsroom: About ONC*; 2014. https://www.healthit.gov/newsroom/about-onc.
7. U.S. Department of Health & Human Services. *HHS Strategic Plan FY 2010–2015.* http://www.hhs.gov/sites/default/files/secretary/about/priorities/strategicplan2010-2015.pdf. Accessed April 25, 2016.
8. The Office of the National Coordinator (ONC) for Health Information Technology. *Fiscal year 2017: justification of estimates for appropriations committee.* https://www.healthit.gov/sites/default/files/final_onc_cj_fy_2017_clean.pdf.
9. Institute of Medicine. *To Err Is Human: Building a Safer Health System.* Washington, DC: National Academy Press; 1999.
10. Institute of Medicine. *Crossing the Quality Chasm: A New Health System for the 21st Century.* Washington, DC: National Academy Press; 2001.
11. Institute of Medicine. *Best Care at Lower Cost: The Path to Continuously Learning Health Care in America.* Washington, DC: National Academy Press; 2012.
12. John TJ. A new, evidence-based estimate of patient harms associated with hospital care. *J Patient Saf.* 2013;9(3):122–128. 2013. http://journals.lww.com/journalpatientsafety/Fulltext/2013/09000/A_New,_Evidence_based_Estimate_of_Patient_Harms.2.aspx.
13. Sensmeier J. Patient safety and IT trends. *Nurs Manag.* 2015;46 (11):24–26.
14. Wulff K, Cummings GG, Marck P, Yurtseven O. Medication administration technologies and patient safety: a mixed-method systematic review. *J Adv Nurs.* 2011;67(10):2080–2095.
15. Institute of Medicine. *HIT and Patient Safety: Building Safer Systems for Better Care.* Washington, DC: The National Academies Press; 2011.
16. Office of the National Coordinator for Health IT. *Health IT Patient Safety Action and Surveillance Plan*; 2013. https://www.healthit.gov/sites/default/files/safety_plan_master.pdf.
17. Prepared by RTI International for Office of the National Coordinator for Health IT. *Health IT safety center roadmap.* http://www.healthitsafety.org/uploads/4/3/6/4/43647387/roadmap.pdf.
18. Ash JS, Berg M, Coiera E. Some unintended consequences of information technology in health care: the nature of patient care information system-related errors. *J Am Med Inform Assoc.* 2004;11(2):104–112.
19. Koppel R, Metlay JP, Cohen A, et al. Role of computerized physician order entry systems in facilitating medication errors. *J Am Med Assoc.* 2005;293(10):1197–1203.
20. Bloomrosen M, Starren J, Lorenzi NM, Ash JS, Patel VL, Shortliffe EH. Anticipating and addressing the unintended consequences of health IT and policy: a report from the AMIA 2009 Health Policy Meeting. *J Am Med Inform Assoc.* 2011;18 (1):82–90.
21. National Priorities Partnership. *Input to the Secretary of Health and Human Services on the Priorities for the National Quality Strategy.* Washington, DC: National Quality Forum; 2011.
22. National Quality Strategy. *Report to Congress: National Strategy for Quality Improvement in Health Care*; 2011. http://www.ahrq.gov/workingforquality/nqs/nqs2011annlrpt.htm.
23. National Quality Strategy. *Working for quality: NQS Reports and Annual Updates.* http://www.ahrq.gov/workingforquality/reports.htm.
24. Cebul R, Love TE, Jain AK, Hebert CJ. Electronic health records and quality of diabetes care. *N Engl J Med.* 2011;365 (9):825–833.

25. Institute of Medicine. *Assessing Progress on the Institute of Medicine Report—the Future of Nursing: Report in Brief*; 2015. http://www.nationalacademies.org/hmd/~/media/Files/Report%20Files/2015/AssessingFON_releaseslides/Nursing-Report-in-brief.pdf.

26. American Academy of Nursing. *Nurses on Boards Coalition*; 2014. http://www.aannet.org/index.php?option=com_content&view=article&id=742:nurses-on-boards-coalition&catid=23:news&Itemid=133.

27. Alexander D, Halley EC. Establishing nursing informatics in public policy. In: Saba V, McCormick KA, eds. *Essentials of Nursing Informatics*. 6th ed. New York, NY: McGraw-Hill; 2015:281–291.

28. Alliance for Nursing Informatics. *Nursing Informatics Leaders Impacting Health IT Policy*; 2014. http://allianceni.org/documents/NursingInformaticsLeadersImpactingHealthITPolicy.pdf/.

29. Office of the National Coordinator for Health Information Technology. *Individuals' Access to their Own Information: ONC Policy Brief*; 2012. https://www.healthit.gov/sites/default/files/pdf/individual-access-06-03-2012.pdf.

30. Alliance for Nursing Informatics (ANI). *Alliance for Nursing Informatics Pledge to Support the Consumer eHealth Program*. ANI; 2011. http://www.allianceni.org/documents/ANIPledgetoSupportONCConsumereHealthProgram_000.pdf.

31. National Academies of Sciences, Engineering, and Medicine. *Assessing Progress on the Institute of Medicine Report The Future of Nursing*. Washington, DC: The National Academies Press; 2016. http://www.nap.edu/catalog/21838/assessing-progress-on-the-institute-of-medicine-report-the-future-of-nursing. Accessed April 26, 2016.

32. *Alliance for Nursing Informatics (ANI) Prioritization and Procedures for Obtaining and Integrating Health Policy Comments*. http://allianceni.org/docs/ANI_Policy_ProcedureCommentsHealthPolicy.pdf; 2015.

33. American Nurses Association. *Agencies & Regulations; Nursing World*; 2015. http://www.nursingworld.org/MainMenuCategories/Policy-Advocacy/Federal/Agencies.

34. American Nurses Association. *Inclusion of Recognized Terminologies within EHRs and Other Health Information Technology Solutions*; 2015. http://www.nursingworld.org/MainMenuCategories/Policy-Advocacy/Positions-and-Resolutions/ANAPositionStatements/Position-Statements-Alphabetically/Inclusion-of-Recognized-Terminologies-within-EHRs.html.

35. Gillis CL. Developing policy leadership in nursing: three wishes. *Nurs Outlook*. 2011;59(4):179–181.

36. Milstead JA. *Health Policy and Politics: A Nurse's Guide*. 5th ed. Jones & Bartlett Learning: USA; 2016.

37. Healthcare Information and Management Systems Society (HIMSS). *2011 HIMSS Nursing Informatics Workforce Survey*; 2011. http://s3.amazonaws.com/rdcms-himss/files/production/public/HIMSSorg/Content/files/2011HIMSSNursingInformaticsWorkforceSurvey.pdf.

38. Institute of Medicine. *The Future of Nursing: Leading Change, Advancing Health*. Washington, DC: The National Academies Press; 2011.

39. Sensmeier J, Murphy J. Health Policy and Informatics. In: Nelson R, Staggers N, eds. *Health Informatics: An Interprofessional Approach*. Mosby, St Louis: Elsevier; 2014.

40. California HealthCare Foundation (CHCF). *What's Ahead for EHRs: Experts Weigh in*. CHCF; 2012. http://www.chcf.org/publications/2012/02/whats-ahead-ehrs.

41. The National Partnership for Women & Families. *Get My Health Data*; 2015. http://getmyhealthdata.org/2015.

42. *Gallup Poll*; 2014. http://www.gallup.com/poll/180260/americans-rate-nurses-highest-honesty-ethical-standards.aspx.

43. TIGER Initiative. *The Leadership Imperative: TIGER's Recommendations for Integrating Technology to Transform Practice and Education*; 2014. http://www.thetigerinitiative. http://www.thetigerinitiative.org/docs/TIGERReportTheLeadershipImperative.pdf.

44. *Center to Champion Nursing in America*; 2015. http://campaignforaction.org/about-us/campaign-history.

45. *Future of Nursing Campaign for Action*. Campaign overview; 2016. http://campaignforaction.org/resource/campaign-action-overview/.

46. Nursing Knowledge: Big Data Conference. *Engage and Equip all Nurses in Health IT Policy Workgroup*; 2016. https://www.nursing.umn.edu/centers/center-nursing-informatics/events/2016-nursing-knowledge-big-data-science-conference.

47. Churchill WS. *The End of the Beginning*; London, England: Cassel; 1943. http://www.winstonchurchill.org/resources/speeches/1941-1945-war-leader/987-the-end-of-the-beginning.

DISCUSSION QUESTIONS

1. Outline the basic health policy competencies for health informatics leaders.
2. Discuss how the Federal Health IT Strategic Plan could impact future health IT policy and, in turn, future projects and programs supporting the use of health IT in the United States.
3. Describe the policy concerns regarding the use of health IT to improve healthcare quality and control costs as the American healthcare system moves from HITECH to MACRA.
4. Discuss the interprofessional health IT policy implications of *The Future of Nursing* report.
5. Outline the process for developing and implementing informatics policy.
6. Describe four strategies for leading policy activities through organizational work and leadership.

CASE STUDY

Mr. Smith Goes to Washington is a 1939 American film starring James Stewart and Jean Arthur about one man's effect on American politics. Today, health practitioners make their own trips to our nation's capital, and while the focus may be somewhat different, the experience is no less exciting. Here is a case study outlining one possible scenario.

It all started with a phone call requesting that a nurse testify at a congressional hearing on Standards for Health IT: Meaningful Use and Beyond, hosted by the House Subcommittee on Technology and Innovation. The testimony would include both written and oral comments. The call launched a flurry of activity aimed at ensuring that the testimony would be successful, and Johnson was selected to testify. Multiple documents were prepared in advance, including a draft of the testimony and Johnson's curriculum vitae, biography, and financial disclosure form. The team worked to create testimony that addressed the House Subcommittee's two questions:

1. What progress has ONC made since the HITECH Act was passed in meeting the need for interoperability and information security standards for EHRs and health IT systems?

2. What are the strengths and weaknesses of the current health IT standards identification and development process, and what should the top standards-related priorities be for future health IT activities?

During preparation of the written comments, previous testimony, position statements, and background materials were leveraged. Several board members, leaders in privacy and security efforts, leaders in standards and standards harmonization efforts, and volunteer leaders from the HIMSS EHR Association were interviewed. Multiple rounds of editorial and content review took place prior to calling the testimony "final" and ready for submission.

Next, oral comments were prepared, keeping them to a maximum of 5 min. The testimony was boiled down to the key points that could be delivered in that brief time frame yet still make sense. Repeated practice sessions drove home the realization that 5 min is very little time!

Then came the "murder squad," a dry run facing a team of experts who drilled Johnson with questions that she might be asked by House Subcommittee members. She said later that it may have been more nerve-racking to face peers than to face the House Subcommittee itself! In this practice session, the key lessons learned were to get to the point quickly and use the responses to panel members' questions as an opportunity to reemphasize key points from the testimony. Other homework included reviewing the list of House Subcommittee members to recognize their faces and learn their districts, political parties, recent activities, and any relevant legislation they had recently introduced or supported.

On the day of the testimony, a meeting was held with the team in the House of Commons cafeteria to share last-minute updates and further refine the strategy. Johnson then proceeded to the office of the House Subcommittee chairman, where the panelists were introduced to each other. The chairman joined the panelists at the prehearing session, facilitating the dialog in a casual setting to put the panelists more at ease. During this session, the panelists learned that the hearing had been at risk of cancellation since the House had adjourned the night before and many of the House Subcommittee members had left Washington for their home states. However, the chairman's staff commented that the chairman is very committed to the advancement of health IT as well as to the House Subcommittee's HITECH Act oversight role, and therefore he did not cancel the hearing.

At the scheduled time, the panelists entered the hearing room and took their seats at a row of tables on the main floor. The House Subcommittee chairman, members, and staff were seated at the front of the room, one level above the main floor, and the public audience was seated at the back of the room. In front of each panelist was a microphone, timer, and stop light that tracked each speaker's time limit. During the testimony, the stop light changed from green to yellow and then to red when each speaker's 5-min time limit was reached.

Throughout the hearing, the chairman was very gracious, noting his appreciation of the panelists' contributions. In part because of her thorough preparation, Johnson gave her prepared oral testimony flawlessly. Although not asked any direct questions, she chimed in to help answer several other questions that were asked of other panelists in order to offer key points germane to the discussion. The hearing was broadcast live on the internet; a transcript of the testimony is available in the public record of the hearing, and a video clip of the testimony can be found on YouTube.

While *Mr. Smith Goes to Washington* made James Stewart a major movie star, Johnson's aspirations were quite simple: that the recommendations on how to improve patient care and reduce costs would be heard and that steps toward implementation would be taken.

Discussion Questions

1. How can healthcare providers best leverage their clinical background when providing testimony as expert witnesses?

2. When preparing testimony, should a healthcare expert witness focus primarily on healthcare delivery, or should his or her clinical background be used more as a context for the discussion? What are the advantages and disadvantages of each approach?

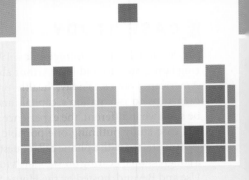

Health Information Technology Governance

Jim Turnbull and Kensaku Kawamoto

Given the rapidly changing healthcare environment, it is critical that healthcare organizations develop a health information technology (health IT) governance structure that allows priorities and direction to be promptly adapted to these changes.

OBJECTIVES

At the completion of this chapter, the reader will be prepared to:

1. Describe why health information technology (health IT) governance is needed.
2. Assess a health IT governance structure.
3. Discuss challenges to establishing effective health IT governance.
4. Describe key considerations for the establishment of health IT governance.
5. Evaluate the effectiveness of health IT governance approaches.

KEY TERMS

ABSTRACT ❖

Health information technology (health IT)—the leveraging of information systems to improve health and healthcare—represents a critical enabler for healthcare organizations to achieve strategic objectives and operational excellence. To optimize the value of health IT resources, a healthcare organization must have in place effective governance to ensure IT's alignment with institutional strategic objectives and the effective prioritization of limited resources. This chapter provides direction and insight into various issues that must be considered in establishing that governance structure. In addition, recommendations are provided for establishing an effective health informatics governance structure that is aligned with institutional strategic objectives, effectively prioritizes competing health IT needs, and is tailored to the unique culture and characteristics of the organization. In particular, effective health IT governance will be critical for healthcare organizations to survive and thrive as healthcare payments shift from a pay-for-volume to a pay-for-value paradigm.

INTRODUCTION

As an emerging element of our healthcare delivery system, the concept of **health IT governance** is far from mature in all but the most advanced healthcare facilities. There are some relevant resources on health IT governance available in the literature, such as a book by Kropf and Scalzi published by the Healthcare Information and Management Systems Society.[1] However, a search of MEDLINE and the general web reveals relatively little literature on this topic, and much of the existing literature focuses on the tactical implementation of transactional (operational) IT systems rather than on the growing need to optimize information management broadly within and across organizations by leveraging health IT. Consequently, the authors of this chapter offer a perspective based primarily on their extensive experience in providing administrative leadership in organizations ranging from large multi-hospital systems to academic medical centers (AMCs). These organizations demonstrate varying degrees of sophistication with regard to electronic health record (EHR) systems and associated health IT capabilities. Because establishing operational processes (e.g., for proposing and reviewing project proposals) is much more straightforward compared to establishing an effective governance structure that appropriately owns and uses these processes, this chapter focuses on health IT governance structure rather than on the processes used to operationalize the governance. This chapter focuses on health IT governance of larger healthcare organizations such as AMCs because of the expertise of the authors. However, we believe the general principles and recommendations provided in this chapter should be equally applicable to other healthcare settings, such as small and medium-sized healthcare organizations and postacute facilities.

HEALTH INFORMATION TECHNOLOGY GOVERNANCE: NEED AND CORE COMPONENTS

Given that healthcare is an information-intensive endeavor, health IT represents a core pillar that enables and supports a modern healthcare organization's ability to achieve its strategic and operational objectives. Indeed, health IT encompasses virtually all aspects of a healthcare organization's clinical and business activities, including clinical care delivery, billing, human resource management, staffing, financial management, population health management, research, education, and the tracking and improvement of care value. In larger organizations, the numbers of systems and applications can be in the hundreds. Given the broad and deep involvement of health IT in all aspects of an organization's mission and operations, healthcare organizations must ensure that their health IT efforts are aligned with their key objectives. Moreover, a healthcare organization's strategic and operational initiatives often require health IT resources to be optimally effective. Whether it is care pathway implementation, population health management, or medication safety, it is rare for a key healthcare initiative to *not* require health IT support. Thus the need for health IT resources (e.g., analysts and software developers) will often significantly exceed the available capacity of such resources. The critical nature of effective health IT governance then arises from the following fundamental interrelated needs:

1. The need to ensure alignment of health IT resources with institutional priorities
2. The need to effectively prioritize the use of health IT resources in the face of numerous competing demands for these limited resources

Healthcare enterprises are often recognized as being one of the most complex of all organizational structures. Consequently, when one speaks of "institutional priorities," the list is often long and generated from multiple sources. Historically, beyond priorities established by senior leadership, requests for health IT resources are received from researchers, the finance and quality departments, specialists who are refining clinical processes or investigating clinical variances, and so forth. More recently, increasing requests from institutional stakeholders are being submitted as they work on emerging areas of priority in healthcare, such as payment reform,

personalized medicine, and more sophisticated costing methodologies. In summary, the demand for health IT resources and expertise is growing rapidly, the requests are coming from a broader group of constituencies, and the institutional priorities are becoming much less clear. Without effective governance, key stakeholders—including healthcare providers—will be frustrated by delayed or inadequate IT support and a resource allocation rationale they do not understand. Moreover, the overall resource allocation is likely to be suboptimal for addressing institutional strategic priorities, and organizations may even be supporting conflicting and overlapping projects.

The role of health IT governance is to help clarify priorities, allocate resources and, if necessary, approve the funding to support the expansion of available health IT resources. Health IT governance should also be accountable to track and monitor the benefits of these investments.

To meet these needs, effective health IT governance must include the following components:

- Organizational structures responsible for clearly defining institutional priorities. Typically, this function is primarily the responsibility of the board of directors and senior leadership of a healthcare organization.
- Organizational structures responsible for ensuring that health IT efforts are aligned with institutional priorities and used optimally.
- Accompanying processes to operationalize the governance. For example, health IT governance typically incorporates the processes in Box 29.1.

Establishing such operational processes is much more straightforward compared to establishing a governance structure that appropriately owns and uses these processes; therefore the remainder of the chapter will focus on health IT governance structure rather than on the processes used to operationalize the governance.

A sample health IT governance structure, adapted from recommendations by Hoehn, is as follows:

- Board of directors and executive management, responsible for setting the overall health IT strategy and clear expectations within the context of institutional priorities
- Clinical IT governance committee, including chief medical officer, chief nursing officer, chief medical informatics officer, chief nursing informatics officer, chief information officer, other relevant operational executives (e.g., chief operating officer, chief financial officer), and appropriate clinical and administrative department chairs, responsible for establishing and overseeing the implementation of the health IT strategic plan

BOX 29.1 Health Information Technology Governance Activities and Processes

- Formal processes for proposing new projects requiring health IT resources (e.g., formal submission templates outlining major aspects of a project such as purpose, scope, estimated timelines, and resources; see Chapter 17 for details about project management)
- Planning future directions and investments

- Evaluating and prioritizing potential projects; evaluating, approving, and prioritizing changes to the EHR system (e.g., the introduction of new clinical decision support alerts and reminders)
- Approving funding
- Monitoring return on investment for projects

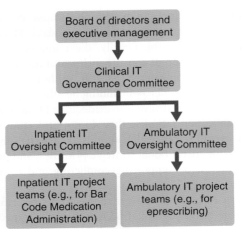

FIG 29.1 Sample health IT governance structure. *IT*, information technology.

- Various committees reporting to clinical IT governance committee, responsible for overseeing operational execution of clinical IT initiatives consistent with institutional priorities and the health IT strategic plan[2]

Fig. 29.1 shows an example of an organizational chart demonstrating this kind of health IT governance structure. The figure shows one of many potential approaches an institution may take to create IT governance. Each institution may need to adapt this governance structure to incorporate other committees with overlapping responsibilities. The next section discusses this and other relevant issues that should be considered in establishing any health IT governance.

KEY INSIGHTS

Respect Current Decision-Making Structures

In establishing a health IT governance, strong consideration and respect should be given to the governance structures and decision-making processes that are already in place within the organization. For example, if the culture is for clinical department chairs to have a strong voice in institutional decisions, then the health IT governance should ensure adequate representation of such chairpersons. Furthermore, it is important that strong alignment be demonstrated between the initiatives of the broader organization and the focus of the health IT program. For example, if understanding and improving care value is a key focus of the institution, then supporting the measurement and improvement of value (versus only profit) should be a key priority of the health IT program. If a health IT governance model does not demonstrate this alignment between organizational priorities and the priorities of the health IT program, barriers to effective communication could be erected needlessly.

Time invested in determining who "owns" health IT governance is time well spent. In some fortunate cases, an existing committee can be modified to embrace the requirements for health IT governance. A much more likely scenario is that the topic has not been addressed. In those situations, the health IT team typically responds to "he who yells the loudest is best heard." Clearly the governance structure needs to be tightly aligned with the position within the organization that is perceived to be "highest in the food chain" when it comes to health IT priorities and resource allocation.

Shift in Organizational Mindset

For several decades, healthcare organizations focused on developing IT infrastructure and implementing a plethora of applications. The latter have consisted primarily of transaction-based applications that support the revenue cycle, back-office functions such as payroll, and the delivery of clinical care (e.g., EHRs). More recently data warehouses with an array of decision support and reporting tools developed by both vendors and in-house resources have emerged. These allow analysis across specialty systems—for example, robust queries can be made across clinical, financial, and staffing systems to more accurately understand the value of care delivered (i.e., outcomes achieved in relation to costs incurred). The increasing sophistication of the IT environment has enabled both clinical and administrative leaders to leverage data in support of their programs and services, while also increasing the expectations that such leaders have on their colleagues in IT. For example, an institution could conduct analyses about a new warfarin clinic and its impact on patient outcomes as well as its associated operational costs to the institution for staffing, supplies, and management. Litigation avoidance costs could be also considered in these analyses.

Almost in lockstep, the emergence of the internet in the early 1990s led to customer expectations that information about all topics should be at the fingertips of both clinicians and customers (often with little consideration being given as to whether the information is accurate or can be trusted). As a result, patients and families have new expectations in terms of both access to and transparency of data from their caregivers, with the expectations of patients, families, and other healthcare consumers often exceeding that of healthcare providers and institutions.

More recently, the era of Meaningful Use and health reform has brought regulatory mandates and incentives, as well as new market pressures, to the forefront. For example, healthcare is increasingly being reimbursed for the value provided to patients, rather than simply on the volume of services rendered. To effectively respond to these changes, organizations have had to commit significant capital to health IT while requiring ever more sophisticated data analyses to refine clinical care delivery processes and improve outcomes.

These internal and external forces are causing organizations to rethink their priorities and how both capital and operational and human resources are focused. This requires a change in health IT governance for which many organizational leaders are not prepared. Information has become a strategic asset that is essential to survival within the current healthcare context, and the demands on those with health IT expertise are expanding quickly. As the demands rapidly outstrip the internal capacity to meet the need, prioritization of projects becomes imperative. This is the role of governance.

The Continual Increase in Demand for Health Information Technology

Due in large part to the successful implementation of core enabling technologies such as EHR systems and computerized provider order entry (CPOE) systems, a continual increase is evident in the demand for health IT resources by providers and administrators who increasingly see health IT as a key tool for achieving their goals. Indeed, the implementation of core clinical information systems is just the beginning of an institution's health IT road map, as the availability of these core infrastructure components opens up the possibility of ever more advanced uses of health IT, whether it be data mining, point-of-care decision support, or population health management. Moreover, especially within AMCs, a growing demand exists for health IT resources to support research missions such as health services research, outcomes research, and personalized healthcare research. Readers are referred to Chapters 8 (telehealth), 12 (ePatients), 15 (mHealth), 23 (data science and analytics), and 24 (patient safety initiatives) as examples of this growing demand for IT support. Again, the need to prioritize and manage the continuously growing demand for health IT resources is a core role of health IT governance.

Governance Does Not Depend on Specific Technology Choices

The selection of specific health IT solutions, such as an EHR system, is certainly a critical health IT decision for an institution. However, health IT governance should be independent of any particular technology choices made. Instead, health IT governance should guide those types of technologies and technology choices. For example, the selection of an EHR system, population health management tool, or business intelligence platform should be within the scope of the expected responsibility of a health IT governance structure. In particular, it is imperative that the governance structure has mechanisms in place to obtain the perspectives of all relevant stakeholders and make decisions in a manner that fosters stakeholder buy-in and sustained support for these oftentimes long-term health IT investment decisions. For instance, providers and pharmacists are obvious key stakeholders for EHR governance structures, while financial analysts are clearly needed for business intelligence initiatives.

Coordination and Collaboration with Diverse Stakeholders

Because of their very nature, health IT initiatives require the close coordination and collaboration of various institutional stakeholders. For example, an EHR system implementation will affect virtually every area of a healthcare organization. This need for multi-stakeholder engagement is discussed in detail in Chapters 16 (selecting a system) and 19 (implementing systems). Thus a traditional governance structure that is informatics centered by nature may present a barrier to the kind of integrated, cross-stakeholder coordination and collaboration required. A medication safety initiative, for example, may need the close engagement of the pharmacy and therapeutics committee and other relevant stakeholders from groups such as pharmacy and nursing, perhaps more so than a health IT governance committee. As discussed earlier, substantial consideration must be given to how the health IT governance takes into account and coordinates with existing governance structures outside health IT. For instance, Chapters 16 (strategic planning and selecting systems) and 17 (project management) discuss the need for interdisciplinary project management to ensure projects fulfill the needs of diverse stakeholder groups.

RECOMMENDATIONS

One of the biggest challenges for organizations addressing health IT governance is deciding where to begin. As mentioned, there is very little literature to provide guidance on the effective governance of health IT. The following recommendations are provided with the understanding that this is an evolving area of focus in the industry. Organizations may well need to make course corrections or experiment with different approaches until a more permanent solution emerges.

Conduct a Health Information Technology Capability Maturity Assessment

A good starting point in developing a health IT governance model is obtaining an understanding of the current health IT structure and culture. A well-defined resource that can be used for conducting such an assessment is the Informatics Capability Maturity Model developed by the United Kingdom's National Health Service.[3] This qualitative model (Table 29.1) assesses an organization's capabilities with respect to five dimensions, measured on a scale of 1 (basic) to 5 (innovative).

Of note, the effectiveness of health IT governance is measured both directly and indirectly across each of these dimensions. For example, the following are governance-related characteristics across the five dimensions that scored 5 in each category for an organization with an innovative health IT capability (level 5):

- *Managing information.* Senior management sees information as being core to business success and exploits it to improve service quality, efficiency, and productivity.
- *Using business intelligence.* Executives and managers embrace business intelligence and use it to set and manage business strategy.
- *Using information technology.* IT is a key focus of the business strategy encompassing all aspects and elements of its business provision.
- *Aligning business and informatics.* Governance processes support and sustain the integration of strategic business planning and health IT planning.
- *Managing change.* Governance arrangements are a core aspect of organizational control, with demonstrable reporting lines to the executive board level and with clear ownership and control responsibilities embedded within the organization.

The Informatics Capability Maturity Model includes a self-assessment tool[4] that can be completed in approximately 2 hours in a forum that allows sufficient time for discussion and debate. To understand an organization's baseline state with regard to its health IT capabilities generally and its health

IT governance specifically, an organization looking to enhance its health IT governance should first complete this self-assessment in a process led by its senior leadership. As part of this self-assessment, an organization should explicitly identify the current health IT governance structure and processes, including in particular the various channels through which committees and institutional stakeholders currently request informatics resources and how those institutional needs are prioritized.

Upon completing this baseline assessment, an organization should be able to identify the current maturity of its health IT

TABLE 29.1	Informatics Capability Maturity Model Dimensions
Dimension	Definition
Managing information	The degree to which users have access to the right information at the right time
Using business intelligence	The degree to which business data are effectively analyzed and presented to inform business and clinical decision making
Using information technology	The degree to which IT is innovatively leveraged to enable leaner processes and seamless information flows
Aligning business and informatics	The degree to which an organization values health IT as a strategic asset and has the capability to ensure that it can be exploited to deliver against its business objectives
Managing change	The degree to which an organization has a structured and effective approach to realizing the full benefits of health IT to enable business change

IT, Information technology.

governance and how improvements in that governance could advance the organization's ability to achieve its strategic objectives. If, for instance, the assessment reveals a low score across all five dimensions, the establishment of a health IT governance structure is probably urgently needed, albeit with a somewhat less mature model than one might find at a more advanced institution. The next step would be to identify potential health IT governance models that could be appropriate for the organization, given its current health IT maturity level.

Investigate Peer Informatics Governance Models

There is unfortunately no single model for health IT governance, just as there is no single model for other areas of organizational governance. Rather than offering a prescriptive solution, the organization needs to investigate health IT governance models that are already in place at organizations of similar size and complexity. Key questions to consider when investigating other organizations' health IT governance include the following:

- How mature is the health IT capability at the organization? What are the potential implications to governance if an organization has a significantly different health IT capability?
- What is the official governance structure and process?
- Are there ad hoc governance processes in place, for example, in terms of individual institutional leaders requesting health IT governance support and prioritizing informatics activities?
- What works well with the governance? What could be improved?
- Are there aspects of the governance that are dependent on unique characteristics of the organization, such as its culture or specific individuals?

Fig. 29.2 provides a sample health IT governance structure that may be appropriate for a large academic health system. Note that this structure is significantly more complicated than the one in Fig. 29.1, which may be more feasible and appropriate for a smaller healthcare system or a healthcare system

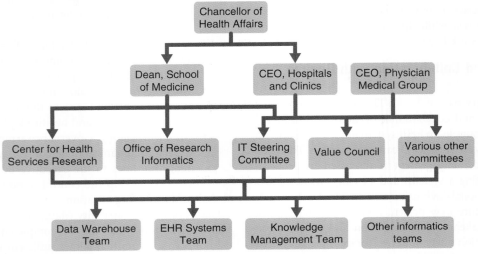

FIG 29.2 Sample informatics governance structure for an academic health system.

with fewer competing needs related to research and education. In this sample governance structure there are three main sources of authority: the dean of the school of medicine, the chief executive officer (CEO) of the hospitals and clinics, and the CEO of the physician medical group, which in this case is independent of the university. In this organizational structure, the primary health IT governance is intended to be the IT steering committee, which oversees the creation and implementation of the health IT governance strategic plan. However, other committees and organizational subunits also make significant demands on health IT resources, including a center for health services research, an office of research informatics, a value council with oversight of initiatives to improve care value, and various other committees such as for finance and population health management. The key to enabling effective prioritization in this environment is global prioritization of the various competing initiatives by the senior leadership and, perhaps more importantly, determination of what will need to wait until the priority initiatives are completed. Also critical to enabling this sample health IT governance structure to work effectively is empowering the IT steering committee to adjudicate competing demands in terms of large-scale initiatives that require significant capital funding and operational resources.

Design, Implement, and Iteratively Enhance Informatics Governance

Following the baseline assessment of current health IT governance and the evaluation of the benefits and limitations of the governance models in place at peer institutions, the findings should be synthesized, and a small number of candidate governance approaches should be generated for consideration by senior leaders and other key informatics stakeholders. In developing these candidate approaches, the following principles should be considered:

- Balance the sophistication of the health IT governance model with the organization's health IT capability maturity assessment.
- Develop a health IT governance structure that is reflective of the high level of organizational collaboration required for an effective health IT governance program.
- Propose a health IT governance structure that reports to the highest strategic body within the organization, whether that is an executive-level committee or a senior-level executive position.
- Consider and align with the unique characteristics and culture of the institution. For example, take into account the viewpoints and preferences of key senior leaders and whether the organization has a centralized culture with top-down decision making or a decentralized culture with consensus-driven decision making.

Following an open discussion of the candidate health IT governance model by senior leaders and other key stakeholders, the candidate approach deemed to be most suitable for the organization should be refined with operational details. Moreover, to the extent possible, consensus regarding the candidate approach should be developed across all stakeholder groups, in particular with groups and individuals that have traditionally had a central role in the use and prioritization of health IT governance resources.

When sufficient institutional consensus has been attained, the new health IT governance model should be implemented. The impact of the new model, including unintended consequences, should be actively evaluated. The health IT governance should then be iteratively assessed and refined as needed, with the ultimate goal of ensuring that health IT is fully aligned with the strategic direction of the institution and that limited health IT resources are used optimally.

CONCLUSION AND FUTURE DIRECTIONS

Looking forward, healthcare organizations are likely to face ever more opportunities and challenges that require the effective leveraging of health IT. Given the rapidly changing healthcare environment, it will be critical for healthcare organizations to develop a health IT governance structure that allows priorities and direction to be rapidly adapted to these changes. Moreover, given the increasingly vital role of health IT in almost all aspects of a healthcare organization, it is important for health IT governance to incorporate the viewpoints of relevant stakeholders, such as providers, from across the enterprise. The governance approach needs to be balanced and collaborative yet still capable of focusing on strategic priorities without being pulled in a thousand directions by various competing demands. In looking toward the numerous opportunities and challenges ahead for healthcare organizations, a key factor in an organization's ability to survive and thrive will be its ability to implement effective health IT governance.

REFERENCES

1. Kropf R, Scalzi G. *IT Governance in Hospitals and Health Systems.* Chicago, IL: Healthcare Information and Management Systems Society; 2012.
2. Hoehn BJ. Clinical information technology governance. *J Healthc Inf Manag.* 2010;24(2):13–14.
3. United Kingdom Health and Social Care Information Centre. *Informatics Capability Maturity Model.* http://www.hscic.gov.uk/article/4931/Informatics-Capability-Maturity-Model-ICMM. Accessed August 4, 2016.
4. United Kingdom Health and Social Care Information Centre. *Informatics Capability Maturity Model tool.* http://www.hscic.gov.uk/article/4933/ICMM-tool. Accessed August 4, 2016.

DISCUSSION QUESTIONS

1. What unique characteristics within the organizational culture at your institution are relevant in terms of their impact on health IT governance?
2. Using the Informatics Capability Maturity Model as a guide, describe the current state of health IT governance at your organization.
3. In what ways has health IT governance at your organization been affected by the Health Information Technology for Economic and Clinical Health (HITECH) Act?
4. How does the current health IT structure at your institution support or hinder the effectiveness of informatics specialists in nursing, medicine, and other disciplines?
5. What opportunities do you see for health IT governance to facilitate the achievement of strategic priorities at your institution?

CASE STUDY

Imagine that you have been hired as the chief information officer (CIO) of an academic healthcare system. The healthcare system consists of several large hospitals and several dozen outpatient clinics, all using the same EHR system. There is an affiliated but independent physician practice group as well as a School of Medicine with a strong research focus. The current health IT governance structure is as described in Fig. 29.2, except that the current committees function independently of one another, and as a result, health IT resources are being overwhelmed by requests coming from a variety of sources, each with its own priority list. As one of your first tasks on the job, you have been asked to lead the formulation and implementation of a new health IT governance structure. The effectiveness of the new governance structure will be critical to your success and the success of your team and the institution as a whole.

Discussion Questions

1. How would you go about assessing the current state of health IT governance and your organization's health IT governance capabilities?
2. What issues would you need to consider in recommending improved health IT governance at your institution?
3. How could the informatics governance at your institution be more centralized to allow an enterprise-wide approach to prioritizing informatics efforts?

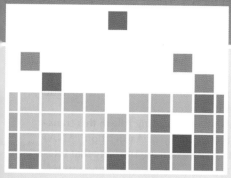

30

Informatics in the Curriculum for Healthcare Professionals

E. LaVerne Manos, Helen B. Connors, Judith J. Warren, and Teresa Stenner

OBJECTIVES

At the completion of this chapter, the reader will be prepared to:
1. Summarize the forces driving the integration of informatics into the curriculum for health professionals.
2. Recommend appropriate pedagogic approaches for the incorporation of informatics competencies for generalist and specialist.
3. Articulate the importance of continued professional development.
4. Analyze the challenges of informatics education.
5. Operationalize the interprofessional team approach to informatics education and practice.

KEY TERMS

health information exchange (HIE), 500
interprofessional education (IPE), 507

Learning Health System (LHS), 500

ABSTRACT ❖

Health and healthcare in this country and around the world are being transformed by advances in information and communication technology (ICT). Increasingly these industries are turning to digital information and the use of electronic communication to fundamentally change the services they provide. The Health Information Technology for Economic and Clinical Health (HITECH) Act of 2009 laid the foundation to operationalize the infrastructure for a digital healthcare system. This unprecedented change has major implications for the workforce and workforce development. The widespread adoption of electronic health records (EHRs), digital communications between patients and healthcare providers, accessible web-based health information, remote diagnosis and treatment, and the availability of large health data repositories necessitate widespread training and upgrading of skills for health practitioners and support for workers who will interface with patients and these technological advances. Health professional education is a vital component of the Learning Health System (LHS).[1] This chapter focuses on the interface between the LHS and a health professional curriculum that will help drive that system.

INTRODUCTION AND BACKGROUND

Overview of Informatics and Health Information Technology

To understand the discipline of informatics and the various roles within informatics, it is important to understand the national, regional, and local contexts of the use of health information and the political agenda for the use of health information technology (health IT). Health information and health IT have received significant federal strategic attention for more than a decade. Since 1999, the various Institute of Medicine (IOM) reports have linked health IT to the improvement of healthcare. In the first IOM report, *To Err Is Human*, one of the main conclusions is that the majority of medical errors are caused by faulty systems, processes, and conditions that lead people to make mistakes or fail to prevent mistakes.[2] The report emphasized the importance of IT in implementing safe systems to ensure safe practices at the point of care. The next IOM report, *Crossing the Quality Chasm*, not only addressed the importance of health IT but also noted how crucial it is to all aspects of clinical decision making, the delivery of population-based care, consumer education, professional development, and research.[3] In 2003, the

IOM issued a third report, *Health Professional Education: A Bridge to Quality*.[4] This report called for including informatics as a core competency in the educational programs of all health professionals.

After slow but steady progress over a decade in converting paper-based health records to electronic delivery, President Obama signed into law the American Recovery and Reinvestment Act (ARRA) on February 17, 2009.[5] Among other initiatives, the HITECH Act, enacted as part of ARRA, put resources behind the Office of the National Coordinator for Health IT (ONC). The widespread meaningful use of EHRs and health information exchanges (HIEs) encouraged by this act has expanded greatly in the past few years.

In 2010, to better understand the impact of health IT on patient safety, the ONC commissioned the IOM to summarize the existing knowledge of the effects of health IT on patient safety and to make recommendations for both federal and private sector organizations to maximize health IT and patient safety. The resulting report, *Health IT and Patient Safety: Building Safer Systems for Better Care* ("IOM Report"), was released in 2012.[6] Building upon the 2011 IOM Report, in July 2013, the ONC published the Health IT Patient Safety Action and Surveillance Plan and established ONC's Health IT Safety Program to coordinate activities related to the plan.[7] Although much progress has been made in adoption and meaningful use of health IT across the nation, much work needs to be done to see that every person and their care provider can get appropriate health information when and how they need it. To this end, in June 2014, the ONC released *Connecting Health and Care for the Nation: A 10-Year Vision to Achieve an Interoperable Health IT Infrastructure*.[8] This paper described ONC's broad vision and framework and was the springboard for the Shared Interoperability Roadmap and the ONC Strategic Plan, both released in 2015.

The HITECH Act and its funding positioned informatics and health IT at the forefront of all healthcare sectors, including health professional education. The major foundational trends to watch are Meaningful Use (MU), quality measures, interoperability, patient engagement, data analytics, and the Learning Health System (LHS), all of which can be expected to have a major impact on the informatics-related education of all health professionals. A Learning Health System (also referred to as a Learning Healthcare System) is defined as one with "goal-oriented feedforward and feedback loops that create actionable information with the potential to effect marked improvements in population health and decreases in the cost of evidence-based care if implemented correctly."[1, p 20.]

Education Reform Initiatives

For the past decade, the previously mentioned driving forces have spurred health professional organizations and special interest groups to call for transformation in education. This transformation includes the addition of health informatics and health IT competencies in the curriculum for all health professionals. As the United States continues to transform its healthcare system to be safe, efficient, patient centered, timely, equitable, and effective, it must invest in the education

of individuals to ensure that the workforce is poised to meet the challenge of this newly integrated health system. The demand for an increasingly technological and integrated health system requires educators to use an interprofessional approach to education while continuing to meet the specific needs of the different health workers.

Nursing in particular has played a leading role in this transformation. In 1992, the American Nurses Association (ANA) recognized nursing informatics as a nursing specialty that integrates nursing science, computer science, and information science to manage and communicate data, information, and knowledge in nursing practice. The definition was further articulated and roles and responsibilities were defined in the first editions of *The Scope of Practice for Nursing Informatics*[9] and *The Standards of Practice for Nursing Informatics*.[10] As technology and informatics developed over time, these documents were combined into the ANA's *Scope and Standards of Nursing Informatics Practice*[11] and expanded in 2008 and again in 2015 as *Nursing Informatics: Scope and Standards of Practice*[12,13] to reflect the growing changes in nursing informatics roles and responsibilities brought about by the dramatic bolstering of the nation's health IT agenda.

The Technology and Informatics Guiding Education (TIGER) and the Quality and Safety Education in Nursing (QSEN) initiatives, launched in 2005, spearheaded the development of informatics competencies across the nursing curriculum. Later, with the emphasis on interprofessional competencies (IPE),[14] the TIGER and QSEN quality and safety competency model was adapted by other health professional organizations. Additionally, accrediting agencies for health professional education programs added core informatics knowledge and skills as a curriculum requirement. This is congruent with the IOM's specification that education for healthcare professionals includes the use of informatics in the clinical area.[15] Currently, the American Medical Informatics Association (AMIA) Academic Forum and the Health Informatics Accreditation Committee are working to delineate these competencies for graduate health professional education. More recently, other health professional organizations and credentialing agencies have established initiatives to emphasize the inclusion of core informatics, as well as interprofessional practice, knowledge, and skill in all undergraduate, graduate, and continuing education programs for health professionals.

Accreditation, Certification, and Credentialing

Accreditation, certification, and credentialing are quality indicators for ensuring accountability in a specific field of study. As the field of informatics expands, it is imperative to ensure a standard of education, training, and continuing endorsement of informatics professionals. This standard of excellence is accomplished through three activities: educational program accreditation, individual certification, and organization/individual credentialing. These three activities, while working independently, work synergistically to achieve the goal of quality. Table 30.1 lists these activities and examples of various professional associations involved in these activities in health informatics.

TABLE 30.1   Quality Indicators

Quality Indicator	Definition	Organizations	Scope
Accreditation	Accreditation in the United States is a means to ensure and improve higher education quality, assisting institutions and programs using a set of standards developed by peers. An institution or program that has successfully completed an accreditation review has in place the needed instructional, student support, and other services to assist students to achieve their educational goals.[15]	Commission on Accreditation for Health Informatics and Information Management Education (CAHIIM), www.cahiim.org	Health informatics
		Liaison Committee on Medical Education (LCME), www.lcme.org	Medicine
		Commission on Collegiate Nursing Education (CCNE), www.aacn.nche.edu/ccne-accreditation	Nursing
		Accreditation Commission for Education in Nursing (ACEN), www.acenursing.org	Nursing
		Commission on Accreditation in Physical Therapy Education (CAPTE), www.capteonline.org	Physical therapy
		American Occupational Therapy Association (AOTA), www.aota.org/education-careers/accreditation.aspx	Occupational therapy
		Accreditation Council for Education in Nutrition and Dietetics, www.eatrightacend.org/ACEND/content.aspx?id=73	Nutrition
		Council on Social Work Education (CSWE) Commission on Accreditation, www.cswe.org/accreditation.aspx	Social work
		Council on Academic Accreditation in Audiology and Speech-Language Pathology (CAA), www.asha.org/academic/accreditation	Speech pathology and audiology
		Commission on Dental Accreditation, www.ada.org/en/coda	Dentistry and oral hygiene
		Accreditation Council for Pharmacy Education, www.acpe-accredit.org	Pharmacy
Certification	A person is certified as being able to competently complete a job or task, usually by the passing of an examination and/or the completion of a program of study.[54]	American Nurses Credentialing Center, www.nursecredentialing.org/InformaticsNursing	Nursing informatics
		American Board of Medical Specialties, www.abms.org/board-certification	Medical informatics
		Certified Professional in Health Information and Management Systems (CPHIMS), www.himss.org/health-it-certification/cphims	Chief information officers and other health professionals
		College of Healthcare Information Management Executives (CHIME) Certified Healthcare CIO (CHCIO), www.chimecentral.org/chcio	Chief information officers and information technology executives only
Credentialing	Credentialing is the process of establishing the qualifications of licensed professionals, organizational members or organizations, and assessing their background and legitimacy.[16] Many healthcare institutions and provider networks conduct their own credentialing, granting and reviewing specific clinical privileges and allied health staff membership.[55]	No official organization for this effort; conducted by the organization concerning their employees	—

Accreditation of educational programs and institutions in the United States is a means to ensure and improve the quality of higher education through the use of a set of standards developed by peers. An institution or program that has successfully completed an accreditation review has in place the needed curriculum, qualified faculty, student support and other services to assist students in achieving their educational goals.[16] The primary accreditation organization for accrediting health informatics programs is the Commission on Accreditation for Health Informatics and Information Management Education (CAHIIM). As accreditation moves to a student outcomes focus, the development of health informatics competencies is critical. Competencies are developed by professional organizations, such as the AMIA, and then used by the accrediting organization. The CAHIIM standard concerning curriculum states that the curriculum must build on health informatics competencies. However, at this point in time, many informatics-related programs exist within university programs that are accredited as part of the specialty accreditation for that program. For example, a nursing informatics tract offered as part of a school of nursing graduate program could be accredited by either Accreditation Commission for Education in Nursing Inc. (ACEN), the Commission on Collegiate Nursing Education (CCNE), or the NLN Commission for Nursing Education Accreditation (CNEA).

Certification is a process that indicates that an individual or institution has met predetermined standards. Many specialty areas, such as informatics, have professional organizations that provide certification to individual practitioners to ensure that the individuals are qualified in terms of knowledge and skills. A person is certified as being able to competently complete a job or task, usually by the passing of an examination. Certification examinations are developed from job analyses and professional competencies. Additional information about the history of the certification process in health informatics is included in Chapter 35.

Credentialing is the process of establishing the qualifications of licensed professionals, organizational members or organizations, and assessing the professional's and/or organization's background and legitimacy.[17] In this process, the individual or the organization presents evidence that they are prepared to practice in a competent and safe manner. The evidence may be graduation from an accredited program, individual certification, demonstration of continuing education, and other forms of scholarship.

These three quality indicators of health informatics practice depend on the professional association to develop practice competencies. The professional organization describes the discipline through these competencies. Accreditation defines standards and peer review to determine standard achievement. Certification is accomplished through examination of the individual's ability to demonstrate competency and job mastery. Credentialing requires evidence that includes accreditation and certification. These activities form a three-legged stool that defines and promotes the knowledge and skills for the discipline of health informatics.

One of the primary professional organizations engaged in activities to support accreditation and certification in health informatics is the AMIA. AMIA became a member of CAHIIM in 2015 and, in cooperation with CAHIIM, established the Health Informatics Accreditation Committee to coordinate the development of health informatics competencies to be used in the accreditation of health informatics programs.

In addition, AMIA established the Advanced Interprofessional Informatics Certification (AIIC) task force to develop a certification process for professionals who practice clinical/health informatics at an advanced level.[18] AMIA also collaborated with the American Board of Medical Specialties (ABMS) and American Board of Pathology (ABP) to develop a certification examination for board certified physicians in the subspecialty of clinical informatics.

Challenges of Technology-Enhanced Education

Several challenges must be overcome to teach informatics and assist students at all levels to develop appropriate competencies. The paucity of faculty prepared to teach informatics competencies is well documented.[19] Although advanced informatics education programs are accelerating, finding qualified faculty to teach in these programs is extremely difficult. At the same time, health IT tools and applications in the curriculum are no longer a luxury but a necessity. Teaching informatics requires knowledge of the content, experience in the use of informatics skills in clinical practice, and access to health IT tools for the curriculum.

Faculty Expertise

Any strategy to include informatics in health professionals' education must involve attention to faculty informatics expertise. The ability for faculty to teach informatics competencies at the appropriate level depends on (1) faculty understanding of the informatics competencies needed by their students; (2) faculty ability to understand the parallels of health, healthcare, and health IT as well as quality and safety; (3) faculty ownership of the need for informatics; and (4) support from their schools and department leadership, including infrastructure and help with technology needs as they arise.

"AMIA considers informatics when used for healthcare delivery to be essentially the same regardless of the health professional group involved (whether dentist, pharmacist, physician, nurse, or other health professional)."[20] The focus is not the profession but improving the use of information with the assistance of technology. Health informatics is a relatively new subject in healthcare and recently has received more recognition as a specialty area. A growing number of health profession certifying bodies understand the importance of and the need for students to learn the concepts and competencies of health informatics and have started including this information in their national exams. As is not unusual for a newer specialty, the only alternative is often to recruit willing but untrained personnel from the existing faculty or healthcare team and appoint them to cover informatics. These practitioners or faculty are then expected to teach students and/or colleagues clinical informatics concepts and methodologies or to begin building or optimizing an EHR.

All programs educating direct and indirect care providers at the various competency levels need to prepare professionals to "be able to synthesize knowledge; integrate evidence into practice; work collaboratively and in interdisciplinary teams; use clinical information and decision support systems, and provide safe and ethical care"[25, p. IX.] Faculty in all healthcare education programs need formal informatics education or faculty development that matches the level of learner they teach. The Competencies Matrix of Health Information Technology and Informatics Skills is displayed in Box 30.1.

Despite these efforts to bring informatics to the forefront and increase informatics knowledge and competencies in the curriculum, a number of studies demonstrated slow progress on integrating these competencies in the curriculum.[21-24] Faculty have been cited as the largest barrier to greater IT integration in education because they lack the knowledge and skills regarding new technologies and their potential.[25] However, recent federal initiatives to coordinate efforts for the implementation and use of advanced health IT have included support for faculty development in the use and integration

---

BOX 30.1 Competencies Matrix of Health Information Technology and Informatics Skills

Direct Patient Care

Generalist (All students and health professionals need this information.)

- Demonstrate skills in using patient care technologies, information systems, and communication devices that support safe practices.
- Use telecommunication technologies to assist in effective communication in a variety of healthcare settings.
- Apply safeguards and decision-making support tools embedded in patient care technologies and information systems to support a safe practice environment for both patients and healthcare workers.
- Understand the use of CIS to document interventions related to achieving positive outcomes.
- Use standardized terminology in a care environment (e.g., functional independence measures, nursing diagnosis terminology).
- Evaluate data from all relevant sources, including technology, to inform the delivery of care.
- Recognize the role of IT in improving patient care outcomes and creating a safe care environment.
- Uphold ethical standards related to data security, regulatory requirements, confidentiality, and clients' rights to privacy.
- Apply patient care technologies to address the needs of a diverse patient population.
- Advocate for the use of new patient care technologies for safe, quality care.
- Recognize that redesign of workflow and care processes should precede implementation of care technology to facilitate practice.
- Participate in evaluation of information systems in practice settings through policy and procedure development.

Direct and Indirect Patient Care

Graduate Level

Master's

- Analyze current and emerging technologies to support safe practice environments and optimize patient safety, cost effectiveness, and health outcomes.
- Evaluate outcome data using current communication technologies, information systems, and statistical principles to develop strategies to reduce risks and improve health outcomes.
- Promote policies that incorporate ethical principles and standards for the use of health and information technologies.

- Provide oversight, guidance, and leadership in the integration of technologies to document patient care and improve patient outcomes.
- Use information and communication technologies, resources, and principles of learning to teach patients and others.
- Use current and emerging technologies in the care environment to support lifelong learning for self and others.

Practice Doctorate (DPT, DDS, DNP, MD, DOT, PharmD, etc.)

- Design, select, use, and evaluate health IT programs, including consumer use of healthcare information systems.
- Analyze and communicate critical elements necessary to the selection, use, and evaluation of healthcare information systems and patient care technology.
- Demonstrate the conceptual ability and technical skills to develop and execute an evaluation plan involving data extraction from practice information systems and databases.
- Provide leadership in the evaluation and resolution of ethical and legal issues within healthcare systems relating to the use of information, IT, communication networks, and patient care technology.
- Evaluate consumer health information sources for accuracy, timeliness, and appropriateness.

Indirect Patient Care

Health IT Support

Workflow and Information Management (IM) Specialist

- Document workflow and IM models of practice.
- Conduct user requirements analysis.
- Develop revised workflow and IM models based on Meaningful Use of a certified EHR product.
- Develop a set of plans to keep the practice running if the EHR system fails.
- Work directly with practice personnel to implement the revised workflow and IM model.
- Evaluate the new processes, identify problems and solutions, and implement changes.
- Design processes and information flows that accommodate quality improvement and reporting.

Implementation Support Specialist

- Install hardware and software to meet practice needs.
- Incorporate usability principles in software configuration and implementation.
- Test the software against performance specifications.

Continued

BOX 30.1 **Competencies Matrix of Health Information Technology and Informatics Skills—cont'd**

- Interact with the vendors to rectify technical problems that occur during the deployment process.
- Proactively identify software or hardware incompatibilities.
- Assist the practice in identifying a data backup and recovery solution.
- Ensure that the mechanism for hardware and software recovery and related capabilities is appropriately implemented to minimize system downtime.
- Ensure that privacy and security functions are appropriately configured and activated.
- Document IT problems and evaluate the effectiveness of problem resolution.
- Assist end users with audits.

Technical and Software Support Staff
- Interact with end users to diagnose IT problems and implement solutions.
- Document IT problems and evaluate the effectiveness of solutions.
- Support systems security and standards.
- Assist end users with the execution of audits and related privacy and security functions.
- Incorporate usability principles into ongoing software configuration and implementation.
- Ensure that the hardware and software "fail-over" and related capabilities are appropriately implemented to minimize system downtime.
- Ensure that privacy and security functions are appropriately configured and activated in hardware and software.
- Interact with the vendors as needed to rectify technical problems that occur during the deployment process.
- Work with the vendor and other sources of information to find the solution to a user's questions or problems as needed.

Informatics Specialists
Consultant
- Analyze and recommend solutions for health IT implementation problems in clinical and public health settings.
- Advise and assist clinicians in taking full advantage of technology, enabling them to make best use of data to drive improvement in quality, safety, and efficiency.
- Assist in selection of vendors and software by helping practice personnel ask the right questions and evaluate answers.
- Advocate for users' needs, acting as a liaison between users, IT staff, and vendors.
- Ensure that the patient and consumer perspective is incorporated into the EHR, including privacy and security issues.
- Train practitioners in best use of the EHR system, conforming to the redesigned workflow.
- Provide leadership, ensuring that implementation teams function cohesively.

Implementation Project Manager
- Apply project management and change management principles to create implementation project plans to achieve the project goals.

- Interact with diverse personnel to ensure open communication across end users and with the support team.
- Lead implementation teams consisting of workers in the roles described previously.
- Manage vendor relations, providing schedule, deliverable, and business information to health IT vendors for product improvement.
- Coordinate implementation-related efforts across the implementation site and with the health information exchange partners, troubleshooting problems as they arise.
- Apply an understanding of health IT, Meaningful Use, and the challenges practice settings will encounter in achieving Meaningful Use.

Trainer
- Be able to use a range of health IT applications, preferably at an expert level.
- Communicate clearly both health and IT concepts as appropriate, in language the learner or user can understand.
- Apply a user-oriented approach to training, reflecting the need to empathize with the learner or user.
- Assess training needs and competencies of learners.
- Accurately assess employees' understanding of training, particularly through observation of use both in and out of the classroom.
- Design lesson plans, structuring active learning experiences for users and creating use cases that effectively train employees through an approach that closely mirrors actual use of the health IT in the patient care setting.
- Maintain accurate training records of the users and develop learning plans for further instruction.

Data Scientist
- Prepare the dataset using advanced analytics.
- Select appropriate analytics.
- Describe the dataset.
- Create and provide a visualization of the data.

Researcher and Innovator
- Conduct research on design, development, implementation, and impact of informatics solutions.
- Conduct research on mobile health and telehealth technologies and the impact on informatics.
- Conduct research on emerging patterns of care and outcomes.
- Analyze outcomes leading to new evidence-based guidelines.
- Develop new methods of organizing data to enhance research capacities.
- Design and develop informatics solutions.
- Develop new ways to interact with computer systems and access data.
- Assist in setting the future agenda for health informatics.
- Disseminate process and outcomes of research and product development.

Note: Competencies apply to both students and their faculty in each category.

of information and other technologies. In addition, private funders and professional organizations have developed initiatives to enhance informatics in the curriculum.

Health IT Tools

In addition to experienced faculty, many academic institutions do not have the infrastructure to support the integration of health IT tools, such as an academic electronic health record (AEHR), essential for informatics competencies in the curriculum. An AEHR is an adapted version of a clinical information system used in acute and ambulatory care facilities, with modifications that customize the product for the learning environment. To be competent, students need to use the tools that they will use in clinical practice. One such tool is an AEHR that incorporates point-of-care evidence-based practice information. In many instances, the cost of these tools is prohibitive in academic arenas or, if the tools are available, faculty members often lack the knowledge and expertise needed to strategically incorporate the tools in their teaching. Successful implementation requires integration in the curriculum and a change in workflow. Teaching students to be competent with health IT tools and practices cannot be an add-on to an already overcrowded curriculum. Faculty need to adjust their teaching practices to integrate the technology into teaching and learning across the curriculum. To achieve this goal, faculty need to critically examine what content is taught and how it contributes to a workforce that supports the evolving LHS. For example, if one of the goals of the LHS is to achieve the best outcome for every patient, we need better evidence at point of care on which to base healthcare decisions. However, with the current pace of change, the problem is the health professional's ability to acquire the needed evidence in a timely manner.[26] While knowledge of the importance of evidence-based practice is apparent in faculty publications, it has not yet found its way extensively into the curriculum framework of many health professional programs. As evidence-based healthcare practice evolves, educators need to be ready to transform curriculum to ensure that graduates have a new skill set that is recognized and used in the healthcare setting.[26] However, for the most part curriculum is not readily adaptable to change, thus creating a gap between education and practice that needs to be resolved in this rapidly changing healthcare environment. Curriculum that is agile, flexible, and up to date with employers' needs in a shifting healthcare environment will serve graduates well.

TEACHING AND LEARNING IN AN EVOLVING HEALTHCARE AND TECHNOLOGY ENVIRONMENT

Several reports and white papers published in the past decade suggest paradigm shifts in health professional education. As the technology-driven healthcare system continues to evolve, it is only right that we overhaul the educational platforms to prepare graduates who are the core of the healthcare

environment.[27] Health professionals, in all domains of practice and at all levels, must be "technology competent" to be able to participate in decision making and evaluation of health IT systems and their MU. These systems are patient centered and support healthcare providers in information management, knowledge development, and evaluation of evidence-based innovative practice strategies that support value-based care. Currently, the United States is facing transformative changes in healthcare and living through one of the most dynamic ages in the history of healthcare. Through technology advancements, drug discoveries, and new medical device innovations, along with the ability to communicate worldwide and deliver healthcare in different settings, graduates will witness more change in healthcare within the next few years than ever before. Awareness of the continued transformation in the healthcare environment is essential for practice.

The Role of Informatics in the Curriculum

The term *informatics* as it relates to healthcare is ubiquitous and ambiguous, largely because of the various health professionals and related disciplines that use health IT and health data.[28] AMIA and its classification of informatics domains—translational bioinformatics, clinical informatics, clinical research informatics, consumer health informatics, and public health informatics—provide one structure to the overall categories of health informatics.

As new health IT evolves to meet the demands of the healthcare system, informatics competencies need to be addressed at all levels of health professional curricula. Informatics competencies should be considered along a continuum from basic to advanced competencies. All health professionals will need some level of basic informatics knowledge and skills introduced in their curriculum, while certain clinicians and informaticians will need advanced specialty education.

The History of Informatics Competency Development

Several disciplines have completed foundational work on needed competencies: nursing, public health, and medicine. In the case of nursing in the United States, the Delphi work in 2002 by Staggers et al. spurred additional work on informatics competencies (e.g., for advanced practice nurses and BSN students).[24] The initial list of competencies was updated in 2011, and a review of informatics competencies was completed in 2012.[29,30] This work continued through QSEN[31] and the TIGER Informatics Competency Collaborative.[32] In 2007, the American Health Information Management Association (AHIMA) and AMIA convened a joint task force to identify basic core competencies expected of a healthcare workforce that uses EHRs in their daily work. The results of this work is a matrix tool that addresses cross-cutting core competencies required of all health professionals regardless of discipline.[33]

Likewise, public health experts completed a consensus list of informatics competencies in the mid-2000s, and their most current work from 2009 is available online at www.cdc.gov/informaticscompetencies.[34] More recently, in 2012 AMIA released a list of informatics competencies for physicians to be certified in clinical informatics. Information is available on the AMIA's general website and at https://www.amia.org/biomedical-informatics-core-competencies. Unfortunately, no consensus exists as of yet about informatics competencies despite the large amount of work in the area. Clearly more work is needed to harmonize informatics competencies across disciplines and reach consensus about required core competencies.

The Science of Informatics and Curriculum Design

The science of informatics is inherently interprofessional, drawing on (and contributing to) a large number of other component fields, including computer science, decision science, information science, management science, cognitive science, data science, and organizational theory. Discipline-specific sciences and practices, such as nursing, medicine, dentistry, and pharmacology, are what differentiate how informatics is applied. Knowledge of the interprofessional approach to informatics; the science that underpins informatics; the relationship among the elements of data, information, knowledge, and wisdom; and the corresponding automated support systems drive the framework for curriculum development.[12] Working in teams across disciplines provides a better understanding of the various roles of the informatics team and assists in placing the right competencies with the right role and educational level. In addition, providing informatics education in an interprofessional environment will assist in ensuring that health professionals in different disciplines understand and appreciate the different levels and types of competencies across disciplines.

FRAMEWORK FOR INFORMATICS CURRICULUM

The Learning Health System

The term *LHS* refers to the cycle by which the global health system learns from itself. In broad terms, the health system starts by absorbing information about patient treatment, then evaluates and applies the results to similar patients and researches this data to create clinical guidelines and policy. Finally, the health system incorporates the resulting recommendations into the electronic system to support clinical decisions in real time. The cycle continuously repeats and improves itself. In more specific terms, the LHS encompasses much more than the healthcare experience, and more than individual or patient-specific information. It incorporates the macro system where all stakeholders (patients, healthcare professionals, private payers, employers, public payers, researchers, population health analysts, quality measure stewards, technology developers, HIE, standards development organizations, hospitals and hospital systems, government—federal, state, tribal, and local, etc.) contribute, share, and/or analyze data to create information and new knowledge to benefit patient care. This knowledge is then consumed by stakeholders and becomes a continuous learning cycle in many dimensions. The end product of a successful LHS is the emergence of healthcare data that informs clinical decisions, reports on conditions or events, and measures the quality of care while providing evidence for the care of individuals and populations. A graphic of the LHS as visualized by the ONC is shown in Fig. 30.1.

As the LHS unfolds, this is an opportunity for health professional education to be guided by this national model. Since the release of the IOM's LHS series, the ONC has become one of the

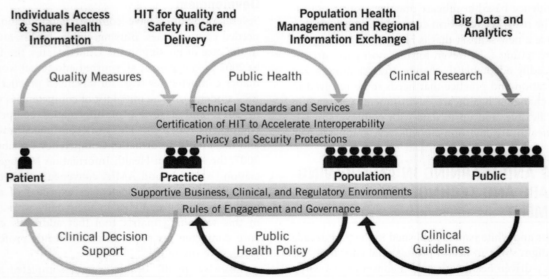

FIG 30.1 The Learning Health System. (Source: *ONC*. connecting health and care for the nation: a 10-year vision to achieve an interoperable health it infrastructure. https://www.healthit.gov/sites/default/files/ONC10yearInteroperabilityConceptPaper.pdf.)

prime promoters of the LHS. The ONC released two important documents for public in 2015: the interoperability roadmap and the strategic plan for 2015–20.[35] The roadmap contains the ONC's interoperability goal and is ONC's "vision for a future Health IT eco system where electronic health information is appropriately and readily available to empower consumers, support clinical decision-making, inform population and public health and value based payment, and advance science."[35] In this document, the ONC focuses on achieving interoperability for health IT. The purpose of the interoperability goal is to "support a broad scale learning health system by 2024." The LHS is a critical element in meeting the goals and outcomes in the proposed ONC strategic plan. In a system that increasingly learns from data collected at the point of care and applies the lessons learned to improve patient care, health professionals will be the cornerstone for assessing needs, directing approaches, ensuring integrity of the tracking and quality of the outcomes, and leading innovation.[36] However, practitioners and health professional educators need to know that how and what they learn will dramatically change as technology, evidence-based practices, and innovations evolve over time. Orienting the education system to meet the needs of an evolving LHS requires new ways of thinking about how we can create and sustain a healthcare workforce that recognizes the by-products of an LHS and uses these by-products to adjust curriculum and address lifelong learning needs. Therefore it is essential to have a nimble curriculum that can readily adapt to change.

Pedagogy

Pedagogy is a broad term that includes multiple theories of behavior based on the learning process. Modern pedagogy has been strongly influenced by three major categories of theory: behaviorist, cognitive, and constructivism. Behaviorists believe that learning is a change in behavior caused by external stimuli—the "know what." Early computer programs were based on behaviorist theory. This theory is useful in learning basic content and concepts. Cognitive psychology claims that learning involves memory, motivation, thinking, reflection, and abstraction. It is concerned with how to apply content, access and synthesize information, think critically, and make decisions—the "know how." Constructivism asserts that learners interpret information and the world according to their personal reality and that they learn by observing, processing, and interpreting information and then customizing the information into personal knowledge for immediate application. Learners use previous knowledge to create new knowledge and act on it—the "know why." The LHS model is built on the theory of constructivism.

Teaching Tools and Learning Strategies

Today's information age students are calling for learner-driven education environments that provide access to powerful learning tools, knowledge bases, and scholarly exchange networks for the delivery of learning. New tools and new approaches must be incorporated to teach fundamental concepts and methods that can be applied in different situations. For example, there is no doubt that health professional

students will encounter EHRs in clinical practice; however, in many instances, students in clinical practice settings are denied access to documenting in this record. This is a common but unsafe practice, since it forces the faculty, students, and staff to develop workarounds for documenting care that was provided by students. Integrating an AEHR in the curriculum as a teaching tool provides students a nonthreatening approach to interacting with health IT while learning discipline-specific content and processes. The interactive learning approach with this technology includes viewing and entering clinical documentation, viewing diagnostic results (lab, diagnostic imaging, reports, etc.), performing chart reviews, order management, medication administration and reconciliation, and developing plans of care. It is through these and other learning activities that the student begins to use evidence-based clinical practices, critical-thinking skills, and data-driven decision making.

The AEHR also can be used to promote learning about decision support tools, safety alerts, clinical workflow, population management, quality improvement, and interprofessional learning. Education programs can emphasize the importance of the EHR in healthcare, but unless there is an opportunity for students to use the EHR in the clinical setting, they will not develop the competencies required for practice in a progressive, technology-enriched healthcare environment.[37] Yet using an EHR alone is not sufficient for health professional students to learn the capabilities of the clinical information system. Health professional students need a theoretical base often provided via lectures, reading, and discussion to completely understand the full potential of an EHR and HIE and how both technologies can empower providers to be meaningful users of these systems. The AEHR provides a technology teaching platform that supports higher-order evidence-based teaching strategies such as active learning, time on task, rapid feedback, collaboration,[38,39] and interprofessional education (IPE) when it is integrated across the health professional's curriculum. Interprofessional education is education that provides students within the health disciplines "with opportunities to learn and practice skills that improve their ability to communicate and collaborate. Through the experience of learning with and from those in other professions, students also develop leadership qualities and respect for each other, which prepares them for work on teams and in settings where collaboration is a key to success."[39A, P 7] Other examples of teaching and learning strategies that should be incorporated in the curriculum are collaborative practice, knowledge management, simulation, and web tools. An example of a *collaborative practice tool* is TeamSTEPPS®,[40] an evidence-based teamwork system that improves communication and teamwork skills among health professionals. TeamSTEPPS is an established system for improving patient safety as well as the efficiency and effectiveness of the healthcare team. Because graduates are expected to work in interprofessional teams, this skill needs to be part of all health professional curricula. Additional information on TeamSTEPPS is located at http://www.ahrq.gov/professionals/education/curriculum-tools/teamstepps/index.html.

Similarly, *knowledge management tools* build individual and organizational intelligence by enabling people to improve the way in which they capture, share, and use knowledge. Knowledge management involves not only building your own knowledge repository (personal knowledge management) but also using the knowledge, ideas, and experience of others to improve the organization's performance. An LHS incorporates knowledge-based decision support tools to build on what works well and discover which evidence leads to better practice, strategy, and policy.

Simulation is a tool used to assist in resolving the patient safety issue while enhancing student learning. During the past decade, simulation in health professional programs has increased exponentially. Simulation is an educational process that replicates the clinical work environment, including informatics, and requires students to demonstrate an identified skill set. Simulation-based IPE is a new phenomenon with increasing evidence to support outcomes. Qualitative feedback regarding IPE indicates that participants report feeling comfortable learning with students from other professions and find value in the interprofessional simulation sessions. Additional information on how to understand and effectively use simulation can be found in Chapter 29.

Web tools (see Chapters 31 and 32) are on the rise in all aspects of our lives, including healthcare and education. The emergence of new classes of web-based applications has introduced new possibilities for healthcare delivery as well as new environments for teaching and learning. A variety of web tools is available, and the menu continues to grow. Some of these tools are blogs, podcasts, social media networks (e.g., Facebook, Twitter, YouTube), and virtual worlds (e.g., Second Life). For example, Second Life can be used to set up a virtual conference room so that remote informatics students can practice interviewing a hospital executive for a mock EHR installation.

Mobile and connected health technologies are changing the way in which consumers and healthcare providers access information and learn. The LHS is a multi-stakeholder collaboration across the public and private sector, including patients, consumers, caregivers, and families. Fundamental to the LHS is the full engagement of patients and the public. New mobile technologies and emerging health apps allow more patient access to healthcare than ever before and allow for on-demand treatment and health management. As the momentum for patient engagement builds, it will be imperative that we prepare health professionals in this world of connected health.[41] Seamlessly integrating mobile and digital technologies (smartphones, iPads, robots, patient portals, secure messaging, personal health records, mobile apps, social media, and patient-generated health data tools) in the curriculum is an efficient and effective mechanism for bringing health professional education into the digital age and assisting students to gain the competencies they need in practice. Table 30.2 shows some examples of suggested learning strategies to integrate the teaching tools in the curriculum.

IT TAKES A VILLAGE: ROLES AND COMPETENCIES

A standard list of informatics competencies does not exist. What is clear is that all undergraduate, graduate, and practicing health professionals need to have a certain level of knowledge about and competency in informatics and its impact on an LHS that supports evidence-based practice, quality care, and safety. In addition, informatics specialists are needed to work in interprofessional teams to provide vision, leadership, and management and to advance the science of health informatics through wisdom, research, and innovation. Informatics specialists, educated in informatics specialty programs at the master's or doctoral level (both the research doctorate [PhD] and the practice doctorate) will continue to be in high demand. Currently there are not enough health professionals in this specialty area of practice. In addition, subspecialties within health informatics with their own additional education needs are beginning to evolve. For example, a more recent key player on the informatics team is the "data scientist." These individuals bring structure to large quantities of "big data" generated by the LHS. Data scientists analyze large volumes of health data, often from various sources, in order to identify trends, extract knowledge, make discoveries, and visually communicate the data in a clear, competent, and meaningful manner. The goal is to leverage the power of analytics to improve care and lower cost. These subspecialists within informatics needed to be well prepared in the discipline of health informatics but must also receive additional education for their role as a data scientist.

Health IT Workforce Roles

Over the past few years, the HITECH Act programs have had a significant impact on health IT roles and competencies. In 2010, the U.S. Department of Health & Human Services (HHS) estimated a shortfall of approximately 51,000 qualified health IT workers over the next 5 years based on data from the Bureau of Labor Statistics, the Department of Education, and independent studies. In an attempt to address this shortfall, the ONC awarded grants totaling $84 million to 16 universities and junior colleges to help support the training and development of more than 50,000 new health IT professionals. A total of 12 key health IT workforce roles were identified. Each role has specific required educational preparation and outcomes. Six roles require 1-year university-based training and the remaining six roles require 6 months of intense training in a community college or distance-learning organization. As of October 2013, 20,777 graduates were reported to have completed the university-based (1704) and community college programs (19,773). This is not even close to the 51,000 shortfall projected in 2010. Recently, ONC issued $6.4 million in new funding to continue to train the health IT workforce. Specifically, awardees will update training materials from the original Workforce Curriculum Development Program and train 6000 incumbent healthcare workers to use new health information technologies in a variety of settings: team-based care environment, long-term care

TABLE 30.2 Examples of Teaching Tools and Strategies

Tools	Strategies
Academic Electronic Health Record (AEHR)	Integrate throughout the curriculum to teach informatics competencies from basic to complex, including documentation, navigation, best practice guidelines, quality measures, clinical decision support at point of care, order management, medication administration and reconciliation, data collection, data mining, privacy and security issues, population management, quality improvement, and so on. • http://www.kumc.edu/health-informatics/seeds.html Build case studies within the AEHR to use across disciplines to foster interprofessional education (IPE) and collaborative practice. • Warren, J. J., Manos, E. L., Meyer, M., & Roche, A. (2012). Integrating an academic electronic health record into simulations. In Campbell, S., & Daley, K. (Eds.), In Simulation scenarios for nursing educators. New York, NY: Springer.
Collaborative practice	Make TeamSTEPPS a part of your curriculum. Can be incorporated at all levels, basic to advanced. • http://www.ahrq.gov/professionals/education/curriculum-tools/teamstepps/index.html • http://www.qsen.org/docs/2012_conference/QSEN_2012_Warren.pdf Work with others to develop IPE case studies for education and practice. • The National Center for Interprofessional Practice and Education: https://nexusipe.org
Knowledge management	Engage students in communities of practice (CoP) to share clinical evidence and new knowledge among the various healthcare team members. Teach students to evaluate and/or develop clinical practice guidelines and clinical decision support tools.
Web tools	Web tools provide a rich set of technologies for engaging students and remove the logistical barrier for IPE. • Sabus, C., Sabata, D., & Antonacci, D. M. (2011). Use of a virtual environment to facilitate instruction of an interprofessional home assessment. *J Allied Health* 40(4). 199-205. Envisioning the possibilities of user created virtual worlds (e.g., Second Life) • Antonacci, D. M., & Modaress, N. (2008). Envisioning the educational possibilities of user-created virtual worlds. *AACE Journal*, 16(2), 115-126. Integrate the use of secure texting into your course. • https://text4baby.org
Simulation	Strategically plan and integrate simulation across the curriculum from basic to complex: • Simulation in healthcare education: a best evidence practice guide: http://wp.vcu.edu/adlt674/wp-content/uploads/sites/4095/2014/01/Simulation-best-practice-AMEE-guideline.pdf • Center for Interprofessional Education and Simulation: http://www.kumc.edu/center-for-interprofessional-education-and-simulation.html • Simulation Innovation Resource Center: http://sirc.nln.org
Mobile/connected health	Use standardized patient for Virtual home or clinic Visits. • http://www.nlnjournal.org/doi/pdf/10.5480/1536-5026-36.3.198 Conduct follow-up virtual visits with patients after discharge • http://www.sciencedirect.com/science/article/pii/S0738399115001007 Integrate mobile technologies including mobile apps in your learning activities. For example, you can have students work together to develop new or evaluate existing mobile technologies: • http://www.fda.gov/medicaldevices/digitalhealth/mobilemedicalapplications/default.htm

facilities, patient-centered medical homes, accountable care organizations, hospitals, and clinics. The workforce efforts will focus on four key topic areas: population health, care coordination, new care delivery and payment models, and value-based care.[42]

Box 30.1 organizes the competencies derived from the ANA's *Nursing Informatics: Scope and Standards of Practice*, QSEN, TIGER, and the ONC work role descriptions and categorizes the competencies across curriculum levels. It also includes health IT support professionals, recognizing that these individuals work closely with informatics specialists,

researchers, and innovators. In some organizations, these support roles may be subsumed by informatics specialists.

Community College Training Overview

The educational training materials developed for the community college training program were supported by the ONC Curriculum Development Centers Program's grants. The entire set of teaching materials for the curriculum components is available on the ONC website.[43] This is a great resource and foundation for a strong, short-term training program, but it should not replace the integration of the content and competencies across health professional curriculum or the need for advanced education in health informatics. Since the ONC workforce development plan is designed to rapidly increase the number of healthcare IT professionals who will be able to assist healthcare providers in reaching MU, these competencies need to be cross-mapped in higher education programs to reach the goal of an LHS. As academic institutions, healthcare organizations, and accrediting agencies establish competencies for health IT and health professionals, they need to look to these nationally defined workforce roles and competencies for guidance. For a health informatics curriculum to be relevant, it must encompass both current and future roles of health IT professionals in all types of health organizations. As the LHS continues to evolve, these roles and competencies will adjust to better align with the market demands of students, communities, and employers. The problem is that healthcare organizations are looking for seasoned health IT professionals, and those individuals are rare at this time. Specific roles designed for community college training include the following:

- *Implementation and support specialist.* Individuals in this role provide support before and during implementation of health IT systems in clinical and public health settings. They execute implementation plans by installing hardware and software, incorporating usability principles, testing software against performance specifications, and interacting with vendors to resolve issues during deployment. Backgrounds for these individuals include IT and information management.
- *Implementation managers.* Individuals in this role provide on-site management of adoption support teams before and during implementation of health IT systems. Backgrounds for this role include experience in health and/or IT environments as well as administrative and management experience. These individuals apply project management and change management skills to create implementation plans to achieve project goals, lead implementation support teams, and manage vendor relations.
- *Technical and software support staff.* Individuals in this role maintain health IT systems in clinical and public health settings. Previous backgrounds include IT and information management. Workers interact with end users to diagnose and document IT problems as well as implement solutions and evaluate their effectiveness.
- *Trainer.* Individuals in this role design and deliver training to employees in clinical and public health settings. Backgrounds for these workers include experience as a health professional or health information specialist. Experience as an educator or trainer is also valued.

University-Based Education Overview

Specific health IT roles requiring university-based education and training include the following:

- *Clinician and public health leader.* Individuals in this role are expected to lead the successful deployment and use of health IT to achieve transformational improvement in the quality, safety, outcomes, and value of health services. Training appropriate to this role will require at least 1 year of study, leading to a university-issued master's level certificate or master's degree in health informatics or health IT as a complement to the individual's prior clinical or public health academic training. The individual entering this program may already hold a master's or doctoral degree, or the program may be part of his or her existing program of study, leading to an advanced clinical practice or public health professional degree. Career opportunities include chief information officer and chief informatics officer.
- *Health information management and exchange specialist.* Individuals in this role support the collection, management, retrieval, exchange, and analysis of electronic information in healthcare and public health organizations. These individuals would require a bachelor's degree in health information management (HIM) but would not enter into leadership or management roles unless they had graduate-level or master's education in HIM or health informatics.
- *Health information privacy and security specialist.* Individuals in this role are charged with maintaining trust by ensuring the privacy and security of health information as an essential component of any successful health IT deployment in healthcare and public health organizations. Education for this role requires a computer science specialization within baccalaureate-level programs or a certificate of advanced studies or post-baccalaureate training in HIM or health informatics. Individuals in this role would be qualified to serve as institutional and organizational information privacy or security officers.
- *Research and development specialist.* Individuals in this role support efforts to create innovative models and solutions that advance the capabilities of health IT. They conduct studies on the effectiveness of health IT and its impact on healthcare quality. Education required for this role is a doctoral degree. Career opportunities include faculty roles as well as data science, enterprise-wide analytics, and research and development positions.
- *Program and software engineer.* Individuals in this role will be the architects and developers of advanced health IT solutions. They need to have knowledge and understanding of health domains to complement their computer and information science expertise. This knowledge will enable them to work with the healthcare team (including the patient) to develop solutions that address their specific concerns. Training appropriate to this role is specialization within a baccalaureate program or a certificate of advanced studies or a post-baccalaureate education in health informatics. A certificate of advanced study or a master's in health informatics may be very appropriate for individuals with IT backgrounds.
- *Health IT subspecialist.* A small subset of specialized individuals with a general knowledge of healthcare or public health and in-depth knowledge of disciplines that inform

health IT policy or technology is critical to the success of the health IT initiative. Such disciplines might include ethics, economics, business, policy and planning, cognitive psychology, and industrial and systems engineering. These individuals might expect to find employment in research and development organizations or teaching. These positions would require at least a master's degree but more likely a doctoral degree.

- *Practice workflow and information management redesign specialist.* Individuals in this role assist in reorganizing the work of a healthcare provider to take full advantage of meeting the MU criteria. These individuals may have backgrounds in healthcare or IT, but they are not licensed clinical professionals.
- *Clinician or practitioner consultant.* This role is similar to the redesign specialist discussed previously; however, these individuals have backgrounds and experience as licensed clinical or public health professionals. In addition to the responsibilities discussed previously, they address workflow and data collection issues, including quality outcomes and improvement, from a clinical perspective. They serve as a liaison between users, IT staff, and vendors.

Educating the Generalist

All health professionals at the generalist level need knowledge, skills, and attitudes related to informatics. According to QSEN, nurses at the prelicensure level, as well as other health professionals at the entry level, should be able to use information and technology to communicate, manage knowledge, mitigate error, and support decision making in a caring and secure environment.[44] These QSEN competencies, as well as some of the ONC health IT role competencies, are further delineated in the AACN's *The Essentials of Baccalaureate Education for Professional Nursing Practice* and the NLN position statement titled *Preparing the Next Generation of Nurses to Practice in a Technology-Rich Environment: An Informatics Agenda.*[45,46] Upon examination of these basic competencies, it is obvious that integrating an EHR into the academic environment is essential to fully prepare healthcare workers to use EHRs in clinical practice. Several schools use academic versions of EHRs in the classroom and simulated case scenarios to create powerful high-fidelity learning environments that promote informatics competencies.[27,37,47-50] Just as pilots are trained in simulators to fly airplanes, simulation, including the use of an EHR, can be used to teach health professionals IPE and informatics skills.

Educating Healthcare Specialists at the Graduate Level

While there is variation across the healthcare disciplines, the overall pattern is that increased levels of education correlate with increased specialization as well as advanced management and leadership. As the use of technology expands, all master's- or doctorate-prepared health practitioners, regardless of specialty, must have the knowledge and skills to meaningfully use current technologies to deliver and coordinate care across multiple settings and analyze point-of-care outcomes. In addition, they must have the expertise required to communicate with the media, the public, policy makers, and health professionals regarding health IT and the secure and trusted use of HIEs. Integral to these skills is an attitude of openness to innovation and continual learning, since information systems and care technologies are constantly changing.[51] For example, all nurses educated at the master's level should be prepared to use information and technology to communicate, manage knowledge, mitigate error, and support decision making.[52] The IOM and QSEN advanced practice competencies build on the prelicensure competencies and are embedded in the AACN's revised *The Essentials of Master's Education for Professional Nursing*[50] and *The Essentials of Doctoral Education for Advanced Nursing Practice.*[53] The need for an informatics skill set across all levels of the curriculum further points out the importance of integrating informatics tools in the curriculum and a shift in teaching approaches to include collaboration and teamwork. At this level, students use EHR data to monitor open-loop processes, generate research questions, look for links to evidence-based decision making, detect unanticipated events, and support clinical workflow and population management. Clinicians at this level use a variety of digital technologies to advance their skills as integrators, aggregating information from patients and their health records, recognizing patterns, making decisions, and translating those decisions into action.

Educating the Health Informatics Specialist

Informatics specialists are formally prepared at the graduate level (master's or doctorate) in health informatics programs. Informatics specialists design, manage, and apply discipline-specific data and information to improve decision making by consumers, patients, nurses, and other healthcare providers.[12] Informatics specialists must have strong communication and analytical skills as well as clinical knowledge and technical proficiency. Most health informatics specialists work in a hospital or healthcare setting in management or administrative positions; however, a significant percentage hold positions with health-related vendors, suppliers, insurance companies, and consulting firms. As EHRs and other information and communication technologies become increasingly important, informatics specialists will become even more vital in bridging the gap between clinical care skills and technology. These specialists are expected to practice in interprofessional team environments, interact with health IT support professionals, and lead change. They need to be knowledgeable about clinical information systems and how they support the work of clinicians.

The healthcare industry is looking for informatics specialists to correctly design, build, test, implement, and maintain health IT systems to meet MU criteria. The specific job description and activities of an informatics specialist in any setting will, of course, be determined by the employing organization, but these activities can be expected to include responsibilities such as analysis, project management, software tailoring and development, designing and implementing educational programs, administration, management and leadership, consulting, and program evaluation and research.

Educating the Health Informatics Researcher and Innovator

The role of the informatics researcher is prominent in the emergence of an LHS that focuses on best care practices and the generation and application of new knowledge. Constant innovation is needed to keep pace with evolving technologies and ever-changing regulatory mandates. As new health technologies emerge, innovations will grow, and research and development will be essential to support commercialization. Preparation for the researcher and innovator role is at the doctoral level. Education for the researcher focuses on discovering knowledge and analyzing evidence; at the practice level, the focus is on evaluating, applying, and implementing evidence.

The role of an informatics researcher includes knowledge of research designs and applications to develop better and more efficient ways of entering, retrieving, and using health informatics to improve health outcomes and engage consumers. An informatics researcher has a key role in developing new data collection methods and assisting with finding the appropriate data to collect for various projects and research grants. This research ranges from experimental research to process improvement and from informal evaluation to evidence-based practice.[12] Informatics researchers must be effective written and oral communicators, as dissemination of their work through consultation, publication, and presentation is an important part of their role. They should have a clear understanding of research design and how to develop accurate and correct questions for surveys and research projects. The ability to work in a team environment with those both familiar and not as familiar with research is essential. Excellent computer skills and knowledge of databases and software programs available for research are important. A healthcare background and experience working with patients and consumers in some capacity are helpful. Knowledge of healthcare organizations, state and federal regulations and policies regarding healthcare practices, data collection, data stewardship, and confidentiality is critical. In addition, a spirit of entrepreneurship along with knowledge of commercialization and technology transfer are important to the innovator role.

Continuing Professional Development

Lifelong learning is a key component of an LHS. The acceleration of national efforts to increase adoption of health IT across all healthcare arenas (including consumer engagement, public health surveillance, and research) affects all health professionals. As practice changes and new technology evolves, continuous learning is necessary to have competent, up-to-date, skilled professionals who are able to respond quickly to the needs of the system. Health professionals who are interested in expanding their education to include informatics have many opportunities for learning through formal academic education as well as continuing education programs. The HITECH Act, federal and private initiatives, professional organizations, the health IT industry, and universities have increased opportunities for health IT and informatics in continuing education. A web search for health IT or health informatics seminars and webinars or conferences will provide a variety of opportunities to help meet the learner's specific needs.

CONCLUSION AND FUTURE DIRECTIONS

Health, healthcare, and education in this country are going digital, setting the stage for an LHS dependent on continuous learning and facilitated by information and communication technologies. This developing potential presents opportunities and challenges for health professional education. It is forcing educators to redefine and rethink how they educate health professionals.

Health informatics specialty programs will continue to expand, and core informatics competencies will be taught across all levels of the curriculum for health professionals. In the future, health informatics education will see a move to baccalaureate as entry level. The practice doctorate (DNP, MD, DOT, DPT, etc.) will dominate practice and leadership in health informatics. The LHS will require a new skill set that will necessitate a major redesign of educational programs for health professionals, including a focus on interprofessional collaborative education and practice. Informatics competencies and new workforce roles will continue to evolve as the continuous learning loop and new technologies change the way in which healthcare and education are delivered. Continuous learning through formal academic programs, short-term courses, conferences, workshops, and seminars is core to ensuring that clinical practice reflects the current best evidence. In the future, one can expect to see continued learning and just-in-time learning incorporated directly into the information systems used to provide care. For example, as standards of care change, healthcare providers may not need to attend a workshop to learn about these new standards but rather will be brought up to date on these new standards through the decision support systems incorporated in the EHR.

REFERENCES

1. Grossman C, Powers B, McGinnis M, eds. Digital Infrastructure for the Learning Health System. In: *The Foundation for Continuous Improvement in Health and Health Care: Workshop Series Summary*. Washington, DC: The National Academies Press; 2011.
2. Kohn LT, Corrigan JM, Donaldson MS, eds. *To Err Is Human: Building a Safer Health System*. Washington, DC: The National Academies Press; 2000.
3. Committee on Quality of Health Care in America, Institute of Medicine. *Crossing the Quality Chasm: A New Health System for the 21st Century*. Washington DC: The National Academies Press; 2001.
4. Greiner AC, Knebel E, eds. *Health Professions Education: A Bridge to Quality*. Washington DC: The National Academies Press; 2003.

5. *American Recovery and Reinvestment Act (ARRA)*; 2009. http://www.gpo.gov/fdsys/pkg/PLAW-111publ5/html/PLAW-111publ5.htm.

6. IOM Report (Institute of Medicine). *Health IT and patient safety: building safer systems for better care*; 2012. http://www.nap.edu/catalog/13269/health-it-and-patient-safety-building-safer-systems-for-better.

7. IOM Report (Institute of Medicine). *Health information technology patient safety action surveillance plan*; 2013. https://www.healthit.gov/sites/default/files/safety_plan_master.pdf.

8. ONC. *Connecting health and care for the nation: A 10-year vision to achieve an interoperable health IT infrastructure.* <https://www.healthit.gov/sites/default/files/ONC10yearInteroperabilityConceptPaper.pdf> Accessed July 6, 2016.

9. American Nurses Association. *The Scope of Practice for Nursing Informatics.* Washington, DC: American Nurses Publishing; 1994.

10. American Nurses Association. *The Standards of Practice for Nursing Informatics.* Washington, DC: American Nurses Publishing; 1995.

11. American Nurses Association. *Scope and Standards of Nursing Informatics Practice.* Washington, DC: American Nurses Publishing; 2001.

12. American Nurses Association. *Nursing Informatics: Scope and Standards of Practice.* Washington, DC: American Nurses Publishing; 2008.

13. American Nurses Association. *Nursing Informatics: Scope and Standards of Practice.* 2nd ed. Washington, DC: American Nurses Publishing; 2015.

14. IPEC. *Core competencies for interprofessional collaborative practice, 2011*; 2012. https://ipecollaborative.org/uploads/IPEC-Core-Competencies.pdf. Accessed July 6, 2016.

15. IOM Report (Institute of Medicine). *Health professions education: a bridge to quality*; 2003. http://www.nap.edu/catalog/10681/health-professions-education-a-bridge-to-quality.

16. Eaton, J.S. *An Overview of U.S. Accreditation.* Council for Higher Education Accreditation (CHEA). http://www.chea.org/pdf/Overview%20of%20US%20Accreditation%202015.pdf; Accessed July 18, 2016.

17. National Academies of Sciences, Engineering, Medicine. *Future directions of credentialing research in nursing: a workshop*; 2014. www.nationalacademies.org/HMD.

18. AMIA. *Advanced Interprofessional Informatics Certification (AIIC).* https://www.amia.org/advanced-interprofessional-informatics-certification. Accessed July 6, 2016.

19. Committee on the Robert Wood Johnson Foundation Initiative on the Future of Nursing, Institute of Medicine. *The Future of Nursing: Leading Change, Advancing Health.* Washington, DC: The National Academies Press; 2010.

20. AMIA. *Informatics areas. Clinical informatics.* https://www.amia.org/applications-informatics/clinical-informatics. Accessed July 6, 2016.

21. Booth RG. Educating the future ehealth professional nurse. *Int J Nurs Educ Scholarsh.* 2006;3:13.

22. Healthcare Information and Management Systems Society (HIMSS). *Impact of the Informatics Nurse Survey.* HIMSS; 2015. http://s3.amazonaws.com/rdcms-himss/files/production/public/FileDownloads/2015%20Impact%20of%20the%20Informatics%20Nurse%20Survey%20Full%20Report.pdf.

23. Skiba D, Rizzolo MA. Education and faculty development. In: Hannah KJ, Ball MJ, eds. *Nursing Informatics: Where Technology and Caring Meet.* 4th ed. New York: Springer; 2011:65–80.

24. Staggers N, Gassert CA, Curran C. A Delphi study to determine informatics competencies for nurses at four levels of practice. *Nurs Res.* 2002;51(6):383–390.

25. Billings D. Forward. In Jefferies P, ed. *Simulation in nursing education.* New York: National League for Nursing; 2007.

26. Institute of Medicine. *Learning What Works: Infrastructure Required for Comparative Effectiveness Research.* Washington, DC: The National Academies Press; 2007.

27. Connors HR. Transforming the nursing curriculum: going paperless. In: Weaver CA, Delaney CW, Weber P, Carr RL, eds. *Nursing and Informatics for the 21st Century: An International Look at Practice, Trends and the Future.* Chicago, IL: HIMSS Press; 2006:183–194.

28. Connors H, Warren J, Popkess-Vawter S. Technology and informatics. In: Giddens JF, ed. *Concepts for Nursing Practice.* St. Louis, MO: Elsevier; 2012:443–452.

29. Chang J, Poynton MR, Gassert CA, Staggers N. Nursing informatics competencies required of nurses in Taiwan. *Int J Med Inform.* 2011;80(5):332–340. http://dx.doi.org/10.1016/j.ijmedinf.2011.01.011.

30. Goncalves L, Wolf LG, Staggers N. *Nursing informatics competencies: analysis of the latest research.* Paper presented at NI 2012: Advancing Global Health through Informatics. Montréal, Canada, June 2012.

31. Quality and Safety in Nursing Education (QSEN). *Competencies.* http://qsen.org/competencies/; July 6, 2016.

32. *Technology Informatics Guiding Education Reform (TIGER).* TIGER International Informatics Competency Synthesis Project. http://www.himss.org/professional-development/tiger-initiative/tiger-international-informatics-competency-synthesis-project. Accessed August 4, 2016.

33. American Medical Informatics Association (AMIA). *Joint work force task force: health information management and informatics core competencies for individuals working with electronic health records*; 2008. https://www.amia.org/sites/default/files/Joint-Work-Force-Task-Force-2008.pdf.

34. Centers for Disease Control and Prevention (CDC). *Competencies for public health informaticians*; 2009. http://www.cdc.gov/informaticscompetencies/pdfs/phi-competencies.pdf.

35. Office of the National Coordinator (ONC). *Federal health IT strategic plan. Final Published Version*; 2015. https://www.healthit.gov/sites/default/files/federal-healthIT-strategic-plan-2014.pdf.

36. Office of the National Coordinator (ONC). *Interoperability roadmap. Final Published Version 1.0*; 2015. https://www.healthit.gov/sites/default/files/hie-interoperability/nationwide-interoperability-roadmap-final-version-1.0.pdf.

37. Warren JJ, Meyer MJ, Thompson TL, Roche AJ. Transforming nursing education: integrating informatics and simulations. In: Weaver CA, Delaney CW, Weber P, Carr RL, eds. *Nursing and Informatics for the 21st Century: An International Look at Practice, Trends and the Future.* 2nd ed. Chicago, IL: HIMSS Press; 2010:145–161.

38. Chickering AE, Gamson ZF. Seven principles for good practice in undergraduate education. *AAHE Bull.* 1987;39(7):3–6.

39. Chickering AW, Ehrmann S. Implementing the seven principles: technology as lever. *AAHE Bull.* 1996;49:3–6.

39a. IOM (Institute of Medicine). Interprofessional education for collaboration: Learning how to improve health from interprofessional models across the continuum of education to practice. *Workshop summary.* Washington, DC: The National Academies Press; 2013.

40. *Agency for Healthcare Research and Quality (AHRQ).* TeamSTEPPS: strategies and tools to enhance performance and patient safety. http://teamstepps.ahrq.gov/. Accessed July 6, 2016.

41. Skiba DJ. Connected health: preparing practitioners. *Nurs Educ Perspect.* 2015;36(3):198.

42. HealthITBuzz. *New ONC grant funding opportunities help advance health IT in communities and workforce training.* https://www.healthit.gov/buzz-blog/from-the-onc-desk/grant-funding-healthit-communities-workforce-training/. Accessed February 3, 2015.

43. Workforce Development Programs. *Health IT curriculum resources for educators.* https://www.healthit.gov/providers-professionals/health-it-curriculum-resources-educators. Accessed July 6, 2016.

44. QSEN Institute. *Pre-licensure KSAS.* http://qsen.org/competencies/pre-licensure-ksas/; 2012.

45. American Association of Colleges of Nursing (AACN). The essentials of baccalaureate education for professional nursing practice. *AACN*; 2008. http://www.aacn.nche.edu/education/pdf/baccessentials08.pdf.

46. National League for Nursing (NLN) Board of Governors. *Preparing the next generation of nurses to practice in a technology-rich environment.* NLN; 2008. http://www.nln.org/docs/default-source/professional-development-programs/preparing-the-next-generation-of-nurses.pdf?sfvrsn=6.

47. Connors HR, Weaver C, Warren JJ, Miller KL. An academic-business partnership for advancing clinical informatics. *Nurs Educ Perspect.* 2002;23(5):228–233.

48. Fauchald SK. An academic-industry partnership for advancing technology in health science education. *Comput Inform Nurs.* 2008;26(10):4–8.

49. Jeffries PR, Hudson K, Taylor LA, Klapper SA. Bridging technology: academe and industry. In: Hannah KJ, Ball MJ, eds. *Nursing Informatics: Where Technology and Caring Meet.* 4th ed. New York: Springer; 2011:167–188.

50. Warren JJ, Connors HR. Health information technology can and will transform nursing education. *Nurs Outlook.* 2007;55(1):59–60.

51. American Association of Colleges of Nursing (AACN). *The essentials of master's education for professional nursing.* AACN; 2011. http://www.aacn.nche.edu/education-resources/MastersEssentials11.pdf.

52. Cronenwett L, Sherwood G, Pohl J, et al. Quality and safety education for advanced nursing practice. *Nurs Outlook.* 2009;37(6):338–348.

53. American Association of Colleges of Nursing (AACN). *The essentials of doctoral education for advanced practice nurses.* AACN; 2006. http://www.aacn.nche.edu/publications/position/DNPEssentials.pdf.

54. Certification. *In Wikipedia, the free encyclopedia*; September 27, 2015. https://en.wikipedia.org/w/index.php?title=Certification&oldid=683035080.

55. Credentialing. *In Wikipedia, the free encyclopedia*; December 27, 2014. https://en.wikipedia.org/w/index.php?title=Credentialing&oldid=639858662.

56. American Association of Health Centers (AAHC). *About AAHC.* <http://www.aahcdc.org/About.aspx>. Accessed August 29, 2016.

57. Institute of Medicine. *Health professions education: a bridge to quality.* Washington, DC: The National Academies Press; 2003.

DISCUSSION QUESTIONS

1. As with healthcare systems in many countries, the American healthcare system is moving from a fee-for-service model to a value-based model. What are the implications of this change in terms of informatics education and curriculum for healthcare professionals?

2. Compare and contrast informatics knowledge/competencies, information literacy, and computer literacy.

3. Compare and contrast the competencies in the Competencies Matrix of Health Information Technology and Informatics Skills (Table 30.1)—generalists, advanced practice, health IT support, informatics specialist, and researcher/innovator. Differentiate between direct and indirect patient care roles.

4. Describe a set of strategies that could be used to integrate informatics competences within an undergraduate curriculum as opposed to teaching this content as a separate course.

5. Describe how health informatics can be used to transform interprofessional education (IPE).

6. What resources would you need to integrate an academic electronic health record into healthcare simulations (with and without human patient simulators)? Include staff in the discussion.

7. Develop an action plan to improve informatics competencies for faculty; develop an action plan to improve informatics competencies for students.

8. Develop a plan of study for a researcher to be able to engage in Big Data analytics.

9. Discuss the Learning Health System in relation to developing a curriculum and assignments to assist students in gaining the competencies required for participating in this system.

10. The top health professional in your organization is challenged with implementing a healthcare information system for the organization and is putting together a committee for this purpose. The top health professional recognizes your talents and abilities to be a major contributor to this committee. What qualities, characteristics, intellectual strengths, and future ambitions would drive you to be influential in your role?

CASE STUDY

In affiliation with the University of Excellence Medical Center (UEMC), the University of Excellence (UE) is recognized as a major academic health center. As defined by Association of Academic Health Centers (AAHC), an academic health center "encompasses all the health-related components of universities, including their health professions schools, patient care operations, and research."[56] The UE includes schools of allied health, dentistry, medicine, nursing, pharmacy, and public health. The UEMC is a growing health system that consists of several patient care operations ranging from small rural hospitals to large multiple-specialty tertiary referral hospitals.

The health professional schools at UE have agreed to incorporate the five core competencies identified by the IOM in their report entitled *Health Professions Education: A Bridge to Quality.*[57] These core competencies include patient-centered care, interdisciplinary teams, evidence-based practice, quality improvement, and informatics. With this goal in mind, they are currently working together to integrate informatics throughout their revised curricula. The plan is to develop an interprofessional approach that incorporates informatics across the different educational programs within these schools. The schools have requested a meeting with clinical leaders from Best Memorial Hospital to gain a practice perspective on what information should be included in the curriculums. Best Memorial Hospital is part of the University of Excellence Medical Center (UEMC) system. Best Memorial Hospital has a long history of association with local universities, functioning mainly as a site for student clinical experiences:

- Undergraduate students enrolled at the UE College of Health Professions often complete a portion of their clinical work at the hospital.
- Each year the hospital hires a number of healthcare graduates from this university.
- Several clinicians in first-level management positions at the hospital are enrolled in graduate programs at the university.

The vice president for clinical practice at Best Memorial Hospital, where you work, has included you on the list of leaders to attend the meeting with UE. In preparation for this meeting, complete the tasks below.

Discussion Questions

1. Prepare a list of key references for using an interprofessional approach to integrating informatics into the curricula of healthcare professionals.

2. Prepare a list of competencies, concepts, and/or skills that should be included in the educational preparation of graduates of the healthcare educational programs at both the undergraduate and graduate levels. Give examples that include an interprofessional approach to the practice of informatics.

3. Describe how informatics competencies could be incorporated into the clinical experiences of students. Be specific. For example, how should student access to Best Memorial Hospital's clinical information systems be developed? Who should provide the needed instruction for orienting each group of students?

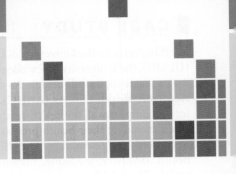

31

Distance Education: Applications, Techniques, and Issues

Irene Joos

Web 2.0 tools and the semantic web (Web 3.0) are enhancing educational opportunities for the diverse global community.

OBJECTIVES

At the completion of this chapter, the reader will be prepared to:

1. Discuss historical developments and their impact on today's distance education scene, including developments in nursing and other healthcare professional fields.

2. Evaluate course delivery systems using appropriate criteria.

3. Examine issues and trends related to development and implementation of distance education options in a college or university.

KEY TERMS

course delivery (management) system, 520
distance education, 518

distributed education, 518

ABSTRACT❖

The changes in our educational environment are reflective of shifts in our demographics, economic conditions, and technological developments. Technology (Web 2.0) tools and the semantic web (Web 3.0) are enhancing educational opportunities for lifelong learning within a diverse global community. This chapter presents a brief history of distance education, defines related terms, and discusses course delivery systems, including issues related to the selection of these systems. It concludes with a discussion of issues related to the development and implementation of distance education and lifelong learning.

INTRODUCTION

Technology developments and the internet are providing opportunities to examine how institutions of higher learning and healthcare corporations deliver instruction or training and how this delivery may be improved. Since the late 1990s and early 2000s, distance education has become an increasingly important part of education. It is one of the "most complex issues facing higher education institutions today."[1, p. v] While this statement was written years ago, it holds true today.[2] Most colleges and universities are now beyond asking whether they should offer distributive or distance learning options. They are instead addressing how to handle these offerings in an effective, efficient, and economic way. These discussions focus on questions such as how to increase enrollment, retain students, stay competitive, address the needs of a changing student population, and improve quality. In addition to the many educational institutions, many healthcare institutions and corporations provide continuing education and required training as well as patient education through distance education options.

Given the current work environment and the economic times, a growing number of health-related programs are offering part or all of their program content through distance education. Increasingly students come to school with work and family obligations or live in areas distant from educational opportunities. Distance education is a viable option for this demographic of health professions students.[3,4] It provides increased flexibility in meeting the educational needs of the changing student population, while influencing how publishers deliver textbooks and how instructors facilitate all learning styles through creative use of interactive activities, social media, videos, and podcasts, and other means.

Technological developments have an impact on institutions, student expectations, and how students learn. For example, most institutions provide wireless connections because students, patients, and family expect to be able to use their wireless devices in schools, hospitals, and outpatient facilities. Several recent books addressed how constant technology-facilitated connections may affect the brain; how constant connections can affect relationships between family members, friends, and colleagues; how we understand privacy, community, intimacy, and solitude; and how the digital revolution changes people.[5-8] Frand identified the following 10 attributes of the information age mindset that influences student expectations and learning. Think about how these influence your expectations and learning.

- Computers are not technology.
- The internet is better than TV.
- Reality is no longer real.
- Doing is more important than knowing.
- Trial and error and experimentation are preferable to logic.
- Multitasking is a way of life.
- Typing is preferable to handwriting.
- Staying connected is essential.
- There is zero tolerance for delays.
- There is a blurring of the lines between consumer and creator.[9]

Oblinger and Oblinger (2006) proposed that discussions about distance learning should not be about technology, but the activities that technology enables: working in teams or with peers, social networking, participatory learning, interaction, immediacy, and multimedia expression.[10] Think about the impact those mindsets and technology-enabled learning are having on the educational system and traditional methods of teaching.

This chapter presents a brief history of distance education, defines evolving terms, examines course management and learning management systems (LMSs) for delivering distance education, and presents issues related to development and implementation of distance education in colleges, universities, and organizations.

HISTORICAL DEVELOPMENT

Four phases divide the historical development of distance education and its changing nature. Correspondence education characterized the first phase, encompassing the mid- to late 1800s. Correspondence education involved receiving printed materials, reading those materials, and sending back any required assignments. The founding of the Society to Encourage Studies at Home in 1873 by Anna Ticknor[11] and the founding of the Chautauqua College of Liberal Arts in 1883[12] were two instrumental events that moved correspondence education forward, as both of these programs offered correspondence opportunities. They responded to the need for a more educated workforce and to the interest of women and the common man for an education. An inexpensive postal service facilitated this development. While the number of offered courses grew along with enrollment, so too did the concerns about quality education and the effectiveness of this means of delivery—a theme that continues today.

Phase 2, encompassing the 1960s through the early 1980s, enhanced the delivery method for distance education by involving the broadcast media: cable and satellite television.[13] The terms changed from *correspondence* to *telecourses* and from *correspondence education* to *distance education* during this time. While students were ready to embrace this method

of delivery because of family responsibilities, work responsibilities, geographic challenges in accessing academic institutions, and disability issues, the academic institutions continued to question the effectiveness of this new delivery method and the changes required in teaching methods.

Phase 3, which took place in the 1980s and 1990s, found many colleges and universities laying fiber optic cables on campus. This high-speed connection made possible live two-way video communication between local (main campus) distance education classrooms and remote (branch campus) classrooms. Students and faculty at both sites could see and hear each other, although with a slight transmission delay. This was education at a distance but in real time (synchronous). In addition, developing technology made it possible for more people to purchase home personal computers with dial-up internet access, enabling students to access course materials from a distance and to interact with faculty and other students through e-mail, telephone, or other communication systems.

Phase 4, which began in the late 1990s and continues to the present, saw advances in the internet and the development of Web 2.0 tools. This moved the focus from information retrieval to user-generated content, interactive learning, and virtual communities. This phase saw a surge in development of distance education courses and programs to meet the needs of a mobile society concerned about costs, currency, and life-long learning, as well as a need to stay competitive in the job market. In healthcare education, faculty have been providing distance education courses and programs for more than 35 years.[14,15] Early programs relied on mostly print materials and some audiotapes, with a few on-campus meetings during the semester. With changing technology developments, delivery system formats changed from mostly printed materials to broadcast courses (e.g., distance learning classrooms that broadcast live classes to remote sites). Computer-aided instructional programs and interactive videodiscs ran on free-standing computers.[16] The current generation of course delivery methods increasingly incorporates:

- Mobile devices
- Web 2.0 tools such as podcasts, wikis, blogs, and video conferencing
- Integrated campus LMSs, personal learning systems (PLS), and personal portals.

These systems integrate learner functions such as registration, billing, courses, library, tutoring, and other related learner services. Additional information about the growing interrelationships of these applications and systems can be seen in Chapter 32. What tools are in development that will facilitate delivery of courses and improved learner outcomes? The answers to these questions will become apparent as we move toward Web 3.0 tools and applications and ever-changing technological developments. What do you envision your learning environment to look like in 15 to 20 years?

TERMINOLOGY

Although the phrases *distributive (distributed) education*, *distance education*, *distributive (distributed) learning*, and *distance learning* are used interchangeably, the nuances that can exist between these terms have broad implications for higher education and related institutions.

Distance education is instruction and planned learning in which the teacher and the learner are separated by location, and possibly teaching and learning occurs asynchronously or at different times.[3] Others remove the time element, defining distance education as teaching and learning where the teacher and learner are geographically separated and rely on technology for instructional delivery.[17,18] Time is not a critical element in this definition of distance education, but rather distance and the use of communication technology are the critical elements. For example, Knebel's definition[17] fits with the distance learning *classrooms* that educational institutions use to provide instruction to remote locations through satellite connections and equipment that permits the teacher and learner to interact with and see one another in real time. The teacher and learner are separated by distance but not by time. Note that time here refers to when students attend to their learning, not the time frame surrounding start and end of semesters, due dates for completion of assignments, and so forth. The National Council of State Boards of Nursing (NCSBN) also provides an example of this definition. The Distance Learning Education Committee defines distance education as "instruction offered by any means where the student and faculty are in separate physical locations. Teaching methods may be synchronous or asynchronous and shall facilitate and evaluate learning in compliance with BON approval status/regulations."[19, p. 9] Note the focus on learning and expansion to include both views—at the same time (synchronous) or not at the same time (asynchronous). This definition aligns with that of Knebel's in that time is not the issue; distance is the issue. Given the variations in meaning, many accrediting bodies are defining distance education within their regulations.[20,21]

It is also critical to distinguish distance education from independent learning or programmed computer instruction in that distance education is planned, mediated instruction. This means that the teacher not only designs learning experiences to guide the student's learning but also provides direction, comments on coursework, and issues a grade on completion of the course.

Distributive (distributed) education is a change in pedagogy where one customizes the learning environment to the learning styles of the learners using technology; the learners may be taking distance, hybrid (combination of online and face to face), or on-site courses. This method includes interactive activities using available technologies. The pedagogy supports a hands-on learning-by-doing approach in which the learners interact and collaborate during the course of study using appropriate technology. For example, one might have the learners review a lesson and video on patient teaching, discuss critical elements of a good patient teaching guide on a discussion forum, and then work on a wiki to produce a project such as a patient teaching guide on some aspect of patient care where there is a written lesson, podcast, and demonstration video.

Dede's characteristics of distributive education:

- Supports different learning styles by using mixed media
- Builds on the learner's perspective though interactive experiences
- Builds learning and social skills through collaboration
- Integrates learning into daily lives.[22]

In 2004, Dede defined distributed education as "a term used to describe educational experiences that are distributed across a variety of geographical settings, across time and across various interactive media."[23, p. 16] Although the terms *distributed learning* and *distance education* are used interchangeably, distance education has a narrower definition. Since the primary characteristic of distance education is that learners and teachers are separated by time and distance, learners learn the material on their own time and in their own place. Distance education may or may not include the use of emerging technologies. The primary goal of distributed learning is the customization of the learning environment to better meet the learner's needs through the use of technologies and an interactive collaborative environment that can take place on or off campus—that is, through course enhancements embedded in traditional classroom settings, hybrid (combination of face-to-face and distance learning), or distance courses. Distributed learning is more inclusive in its delivery methods. Additional information concerning the next generation of learners, learning environments, personal learning assistant initiatives, and related research can be seen at the Office of the Undersecretary of Defense for Personnel and Readiness's Advanced Distributed Learning Network at https://www.adlnet.gov/adl-research/.

Three other useful terms one might encounter are *online education,* *eLearning,* and *mLearning.* Each will be defined here, but what is important is how these terms are used within the context of the content they are referencing.

- **Online education** requires the use of the internet or an intranet to deliver educational materials.
- **eLearning (eTraining)** is "an approach to teaching and learning that is based on the use of electronic media and devices."[24, p. 152] Some authors believe there are three major elements that make eLearning different from face-to-face learning: asynchronous learning, a different location, and use of electronic devices that provide for interaction and communications.[25] The consensus seems to be that eLearning requires a computer or other electronic device such as a smartphone or tablet. eLearning involves a greater variety of equipment than online resources or the internet in that any electronic device may be used: DVDs, CD-ROMs, and so forth.
- **mLearning** is the use of a mobile device (smartphone, tablet, iPad, etc.) as an educational tool for meaningful, just-in-time learning any place and time. Mobile devices refer to those devices that can be held in the hand. While some consider mLearning an extension of eLearning, there are differences between the two. These differences relate to time, information access, context, and assessment.[26,27] mLearning has short learning sessions, accessed when needed, driven by context, and applied immediately. As mobile devices

BOX 31.1   Outline for a Strategic Plan for Distributive Education

Executive Summary

This section sets the background for the plan and generally includes the following subsections:

- *Introduction.* This subsection sets the stage for why faculty and the school are doing this. It addresses what is happening in the broader world, then locally, and then within the institution. It should answer the following questions: Why is the institution and faculty doing this? What are the goals? How will faculty and the institution define related terms? Some include a strengths, weaknesses, opportunities, and threats (SWOT) analysis in the introduction. Others place it within the Details section as a separate subsection called *SWOT analysis.* Others place it in an appendix to the plan.
- *Mission statement.* What is the mission for this initiative? How does that fit with the mission of the college or university? The mission statement should include some of the language of the school's mission.
- *Goals.* What are the specific goals for this initiative in terms of students, faculty, programs, and so forth? This can include goals such as providing flexibility in helping students achieve their educational goals, targeting the adult and second-degree populations, and developing faculty. Areas to address in the goals are as follows:
  - *Students.* Who are the target students? What are the rules as to who can take these courses or enroll in the program? How will students be oriented to these means of learning?
  - *Faculty.* How will faculty be trained? What training will faculty need? How will ongoing support be provided? How will this count toward faculty teaching loads? Who will monitor quality?

- *Courses and programs.* What programs and courses will be offered in this delivery method? Who makes these decisions? How are decisions approved? How do faculty address issues such as the Technology, Education, and Copyright Harmonization (TEACH) Act and copyright? What is the target class size? How will that decision be made?
- *Support issues.* What course management systems (CMS) will be used? Can it interface with the school's other systems? When will faculty have access to a shell for course development? What library changes will be needed to support remote students? How will access to other support services such as registration, paying tuition, and accessing tutoring be handled? What support services will students need?
- *Policy and procedures.* Who will develop and approve them? When?

Details

This section provides the details for each of the goals identified.

- *Goals.* List and number each goal. For example, 1a, 1b, 2a, 2b, 2c, etc.
- *Recommendations.* After careful review, comparison, and research, what is the recommendation for each goal? For example, after careful review, Blackboard is the recommended CMS. Recommendations should also include who will be responsible for moving each goal forward.
- *Budget items.* Include projected costs for achieving each goal.
- *Time frame.* Include a target date for achievement of each goal.

---

continue to develop more capabilities, you will see more interactive, stimulating learning environments. What we need to focus on is the learning environment that mobile devices can facilitate.

With such variations and overlap in these definitions, schools that offer distance or distributive education must consistently define these terms and the related required technology to implement the program or course. This process should answer the question, "Will these terms be used interchangeably or not?" If not, what distinctions are faculty making, and why is that important? Students applying to educational programs need to know how these terms are being used and, in turn, what will be required from them.

Faculty should discuss and define these terms during their strategic planning process when developing distance or distributive education courses and programs. Box 31.1 provides a sample outline for a strategic plan, and Box 31.2 provides an outline for a progress report. These same questions and processes also apply when implementing training initiatives in the work world. Questions to ask and answer during strategic planning include:

- What terms are faculty and the school using to describe the distance learning initiative? You can turn this question around to say "Describe the distance training initiative." What terms do the accreditation agencies use? How are colleagues in other schools and accrediting

BOX 31.2   Content for a Progress or Status Report on a Strategic Plan

Plan name and date. For example, Distributive Education Plan 2016–2019.
Goal and objective. List each goal and objective.
Tasks, actions, or activities. What is needed to achieve the goal and objectives, coded to each goal and objective?
Persons responsible. Who is held responsible for this task?
Budget. Original or revised.
Due date. May include original and revised dates for completion of the task.
Progress note or description. Status of the task: what has been done and what needs to be done.

agencies defining the terms? How will these definitions be conveyed to the learner?

- What technology will the institution use to deliver these courses or training? How will the institution notify learners about the required technology—for example, a webcam and broadband connection or a tablet with broadband connection?
- Does enrollment in online and distance education courses mean that students will never be required to come to campus? Are faculty using some hybrid approach that may require some attendance on

campus? Will you use cohorts and, if so, how do you build them?

- What delivery system will the school use? Who will make that decision? What input do faculty have?
- What are the learning needs of the students? How will you maximize their learning with the use of technology and personalize learning environments?

Once the school decides to provide options for students regarding course delivery methods to complete their degrees, the selection of the course delivery system usually begins. This generally requires considering all available options.

COURSE DELIVERY SYSTEMS: COURSE MANAGEMENT SYSTEMS

Course delivery systems (CDS), also known by some as course management system (CMS) or learning management system (LMS), are software programs or applications that permit the development and delivery of a course or training program without requiring knowledge of programming code. These programs provide the tools necessary to plan, implement, and assess the learning process by giving the professor/trainer the ability to create and deliver content, monitor learner participation and progress, provide for interactive communications, and assess learning outcomes.[28] Many believe there are distinct differences between a CDS (CMS) and an LMS and that a CMS is a narrower term than an LMS. An LMS includes course management but also includes additional features that handle course registration, integration with HR systems, administrative features, and integration with other institutional information systems.[28,29] In other words, an LMS handles all aspects of eLearning or corporate training, while a CMS focuses on content delivery and learner interaction and communication. This distinction, however, is blurring as CMS vendors incorporate more of the management aspect into their products.

There are several CMS software programs available, and the market is constantly changing. See Table 31.1 for CMS usage rankings reported by Campus Computing in 2015.[30]

TABLE 31.1 Campus Computing Profile of the Course Management Systems Market, Fall 2014

CMS	Market Share (%)*
Blackboard	39.1
Moodle	21.6
Instructure (Canvas)	14.2
D2L	11.8
Sakai	3.1

Data from Green K. C. The Campus Computing Project. http://www.campuscomputing.net/sites/www.campuscomputing.net/files/CC2015%20-%20Exec%20Summary%20&%20Graphics.pdf; 2015 [p. 17].
CMS, Course management system, D2L, desire2learn.
*Rounded up.

However, it should be noted that three fifths (61.6%) of campuses responding to the survey report plans to review their current LMS strategy for budget or other reasons. Although Table 31.1 lists the most frequently used CMSs in the academic higher education world, the business world uses other CMSs for its training. Some of the more common examples include Cornerstone, SuccessFactors, Interactyx TOPYX, LearnUpon, SilkRoad, DigitalChalk, and Grovo, to name a few.[31] Other CMSs are popular with the K-12 institutions and still others with the international market.

The CMS selection decision often rests with administrators, information technology (IT) personnel, and faculty, although some institutions may have student representatives on the planning committee. The process for the selection of a CMS should be an integral part of the strategic plan for distance education or corporate training. CMS selection should never be delegated to the IT department with minor input from other stakeholders. Considerations for selection include the following:

- *Objectives or goals.* What are the goals/objectives for distance education or corporate training? How does a CMS fit with these goals/objectives? How does this fit with the school's philosophy and mission?
- *Features.* What features do faculty or trainers believe are essential to delivering the course or training? What are desirable features but not essential ones? What can the infrastructure support?
- *Integration with current institutional systems.* How important is this? Which information systems need to be addressed? Does the CMS support interoperability with third-party products (e.g., registrar's applications, billing, registration)? If interoperability is limited, an LMS may be a better choice.
- *Compatibility with different student systems* such as operating systems, mobile devices, and related security programs like firewalls and antivirus programs.
- *User base.* What is the installed user base (how many institutions and end users are using the product)? Is the installed user base important to your organization? Is there a local user group associated with the CMS?
- What type of support does it provide for the faculty, students, and IT department?
- How stable is the company offering the CMS? This question may require the financial department to investigate.
- *Customization/Maintenance.* Will the CMS require extensive custom programming or maintenance? Are sufficient resources in place for that work? Will this require a dedicated staff person?
- *Scalability.* How scalable is the CMS? Can it easily expand or contract based on varying needs?
- *Usability.* How user friendly is the CMS? Does it have the tool set that faculty or trainers need to deliver the courses? Are there data tracking and report features? Are those tools intuitive to use for both learners and faculty or trainers to complete typical tasks?

- *Outcome measures.* Does the CMS support outcome measures? Is this important to the organization?
- *Sharable Content Object Reference Model (SCORM) compliance.* Is the system SCORM compliant (encourages the standardization of LMSs)? Is that important? Are there other standards that are important like Aviation Industry CBT Committee (AICC)?
- *Cost.* What does it cost to buy the CMS; what does it cost to own the CMS? What is the cost of hosting versus housing the CMS? What are the mechanism for and frequency of upgrades? What are the costs of these upgrades?[31,32]

One way to start the selection process is to first decide on the type of system that will meet the needs of the institution and its students: campus-based portal, proprietary CMS, open-source system, Cloud-based, or partnership.[33] Many of these systems are moving toward the campus-based portal model and a better fit with most definitions of an LMS.

Portals

Portals are customized, personalized entries or gateways where users, including students and faculty, can access all of the content they typically need. A portal is a user-centric web page that includes access to a CMS. The portal integrates and provides a secure access point to the data, information, and applications that users need in their roles as a student or faculty. Portals generally include enterprise resource systems (finance, human relations, etc.), community building communications, admissions, retention, web-based academic counseling, CMSs, and metrics to measure success, to name a few features. Two examples of vendor-based portals are Ellucian and Jenzabar.

Ellucian

Ellucian's (www.ellucian.com) focus is assisting educational institutions to grow by offering applications that integrate and interface the systems that faculty and students need. Fig. 31.1 presents the homepage of their website with the software submenu showing. At Ellucian Live 2015, the CEO announced the acquisition of a competency-based education LMS called Helix and the movement of two of their products to the Cloud—Banner and Colleague by Ellucian.[34]

Jenzabar

Jenzabar (www.jenzabar.com) is another example of a portal system that supports a college or university across each department, including administrative offices and academic departments.[35] Jenzabar attempts to align the school's mission and goals with technology investments. Fig. 31.2 shows the Higher Education Solutions menu on the homepage and the range of offerings that Jenzabar provides. Notice the Cloud services on the left side of the screen. These products are similar for most portal systems. Their eLearning software includes the typical features of CMS: content management, course copy, a gradebook, exams, e-mail, calendars, chat, discussion forums, online meetings, test analytics, and usage statistics.

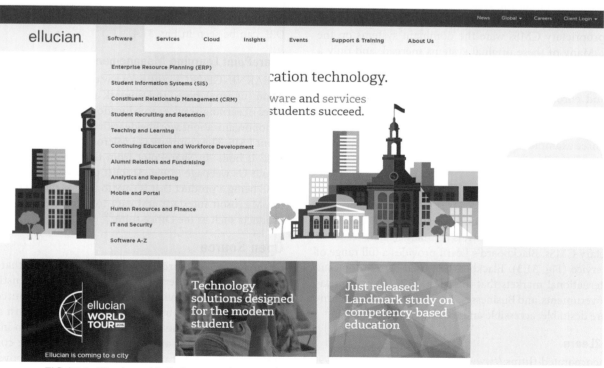

FIG 31.1 Ellucian with Software submenu displayed. (Used with permission.)

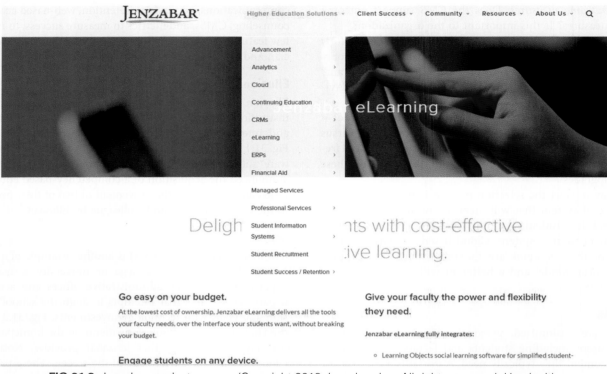

FIG 31.2 Jenzabar products menu. (Copyright 2013 Jenzabar, Inc. All rights reserved. Used with permission.)

Proprietary Course Management Systems and Learning Management Systems

Proprietary CMSs are "software products that are purchased or licensed by one vendor."[36, p. viii] These vendors provide a license either to install the system on the customer's servers or to host the customer's license on their servers. For many years, proprietary CMSs were the dominant systems on the market. Many of these original systems merged, and only a handful make up the current market of proprietary systems.

Most CMSs provide content management, user management and enrollment, assessment of learners, communications such as e-mail and discussion forums, and social learning tools such as wikis, blogs, journals, and mobile features. Three examples of proprietary CMSs and LMSs are presented in the following sections: Blackboard, Desire2Learn (D2L), and SharePoint LMS.

Blackboard

Blackboard (www.blackboard.com), founded in 1997 as a small educational technology company, is the market share leader in proprietary CMSs. Blackboard's Learn provides a full range of CMS service (Fig. 31.3). Blackboard is used across domestic and international markets that includes K-12, Higher Education, Governments, and Businesses. Their goal is "to make learning more desirable, accessible and meaningful for learners."[37]

Desire2Learn

D2L Incorporated (https://www.d2l.com/), founded in 1999, markets itself as providing innovative learning solutions to K-12, higher education, corporate, government, and healthcare organizations worldwide.[38] D2L's Brightspace includes a variety of modules for managing the creation, delivery, and management of courses. The functionality is robust, but the learning curve for novice users can be more challenging than Blackboard. An example of the products offered by D2L can be seen in Fig. 31.4.

SharePoint Learning Management System

ELEARNINGFORCE (http://www.elearningforce.com/Pages/About-us.aspx), based in Denmark and founded in 2003, provides eLearning services to educational, corporate, and public sector organizations worldwide with its primary product SharePoint LMS. The company is a Microsoft Gold Partner, and the LMS is built "in SharePoint from the ground up." (See their About Us webpage in Fig. 31.5.) It prides itself on SharePoint LMS being a product that is easy to use for those familiar with the Microsoft interface and easy to integrate with Microsoft products such as the Office suite.[39]

Open Source

Open-source software refers to software code that one is "free" to use and alter to match existing needs. Institutions interested in cost savings may select an open-source CMS. While the cost to buy may be very low, the cost to own can be very high. The development of the custom interface, the needed IT staff, and long-term maintenance costs of a custom-built CMS can push these costs well above initial expectation. Additionally, updates for new requirements

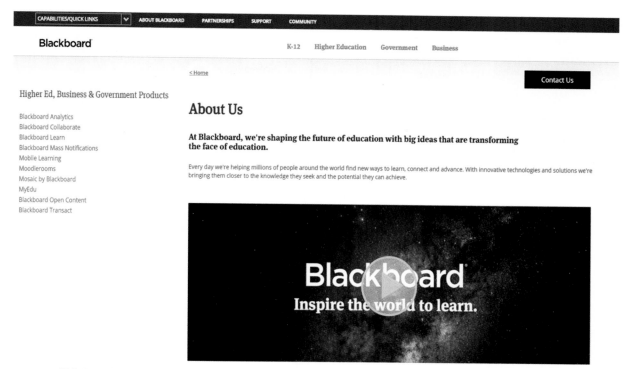

FIG 31.3 Blackboard home page with the platforms menu. (From www.blackboard.com. Property of Blackboard and used with permission.)

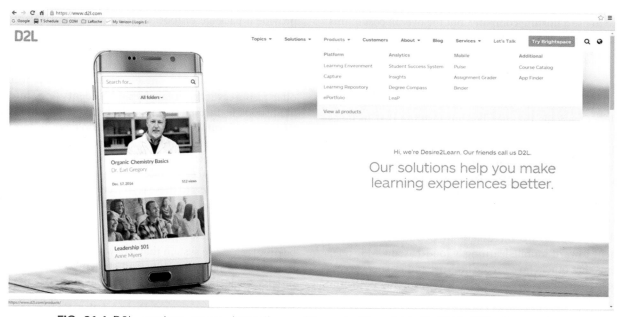

FIG 31.4 D2L product menu. https://www.d2l.com/. (Copyright © 2013 D2L Corporation. Used with permission.)

or security can take significant time and effort. Institutions must address the cost for IT department time, the skill set to manage server and network issues, and training time on open-source CMS. What is free is the code; there is no yearly license fee to pay. Two examples of open-source software are Moodle and Sakai.

Moodle

Moodle (https://moodle.com/) is popular among educators around the world as a tool for creating online websites for students. To work, Moodle must be on a web server, either on one of the school's servers or on a server at a web hosting company such as MoodleCloud (https://moodle.com/cloud/),

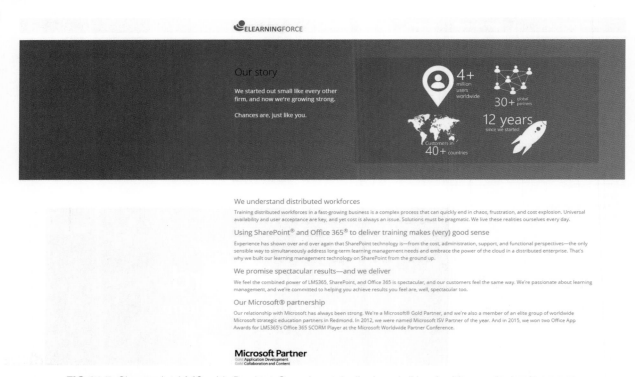

FIG 31.5 Sharepoint LMS with Product Overview tab displayed. (Used with permission.)

which services small schools and Moodle Partners like Class-roomRevolution LLC and eLerningExperts.[40] There is generally a fee to use a hosting company, but the overall cost of this approach may be less because of free access to the code.

Sakai

Sakai (https://www.sakaiproject.org/) is an international community that exists to enhance teaching, learning, and research.[41] One joins the membership institute that includes small colleges, universities, hospitals, government agencies, and political parties. The organization defines the needs of academic users, creates software tools, and shares best practices while pooling knowledge and resources in support of this goal.

Cloud Based

Cloud-based CMSs are increasing in popularity with the movement toward mobile learning. Cloud-based CMSs refer to systems that others host on the internet and learners access over the internet using their browser.[42] While many LMS now have Cloud services as one of their products, this group of CMSs focuses more on employee training. Some of the benefits of this approach are the same as for others, such as lower costs, security, and easy access from any device. One of the main advantages is that Cloud service vendors provide the needed technical support, thereby freeing up IT staff for other projects. The end user needs to provide only the internet access and developed courses. Some examples of Cloud-based CMSs include Litmos LMS (http://www.litmos.com/), Agylia (http://www.cm-group.co.uk/), TalentLMS (http://www.talentlms.com/), Docebo SaaS LMS (https://www.docebo.com/), and G-Cube (http://www.gc-solutions.net/).[43]

Partnerships

Book publishers often partner with software vendors to provide a package of tools to assist with the delivery of distance education. Elsevier's Evolve LMS and Pearson's learning environments (LearningStudio, MyLab, Mynursinglab) supply everything from customized, concept-to-completion LMSs to digital content. These online learning environments offer resources to both faculty and students (e.g., interactive grade book features, learning tools that simulate clinical experience and charting, Cloud-based technology). In most cases, the disadvantage to using this approach is that they may require you to use their textbook or may require students to purchase an access code. When you change textbooks, you may lose access to these resources. If students try to resell their textbooks on the used-textbook market, the access code is not valid.

With all of these options, how do faculty and the school begin to select the system that will work within their environment and with their faculty and students? The next section discusses selection criteria and the role of the faculty.

Selection Criteria and Role of the Selection Committee

From a faculty perspective, the criteria for the selection of a CMS or LMS fall into several categories: ease of use, stability, tool set, and support. Other school considerations relate to compatibility or integration and to cost issues that require financial and technical support.[32] While faculty can provide valuable insights about what they do best, developing and teaching courses in the area in which they are experts, to be an effective participant in system selection, they should review articles such as "The Top LMS Statistics and

Facts For 2015 You Need to Know" to gain a big picture perspective.[44]

- *Ease of use.* There is a learning curve to using CMS software. The interface should be intuitive to use. Does it use common educational terms to describe tools such as discussion forums or boards? Does its design support distance education or is it an adaptation of other products? Faculty should ask questions and complete typical educational tasks to assess ease of use for grading papers, projects, and tests; returning files; and setting up and using the grading center. Also important are tools such as wikis, blogs, conferencing, and chat that are available for collaboration activities for assignments such as group projects. How easy is it for students and faculty to learn to use these tools? This could include an analysis of the number of clicks it takes to upload content, what file formats are acceptable for upload, and what file size limits are enforced. Another area to analyze is the ease of content movement between courses and between semesters and the ease of archiving and exporting courses. Too many required clicks or difficulty in understanding the screen discourages faculty from using tools. Does the setup reduce time and effort or demand more time and effort in delivering the course? Additional information about usability is included in Chapter 21.
- *Stability.* How stable is the company offering the CMS? Will it be in business next year or will the school have to select another system next year if the company fails or another company acquires it? Stability also includes system reliability issues such as the frequency of system crashes and the turnaround time to restore the system after such a crash. Students and faculty require nearly 24/7 access.
- *Tool set (features).* What are the bundled tools in the CMS or LMS, and which ones require additional funds to access? For example, is Blackboard's Collaborate tool bundled with the basic version of Blackboard, or does access to that tool increase the price? Do faculty want collaborative tools such as video conferencing, podcasting, blogging, wiki abilities, chatting, and so forth? What "smart" features do faculty need? This may include alerts that the system automatically sends to students and tools that remember who the user is and where he or she left off in doing work. Do faculty want mobile computing as part of the tool set? Do they want textbook cartridge capabilities or online testing tools? Cartridges are files that a textbook publisher provides faculty who select its textbook. Once uploaded, the cartridge sets up the course in the CMS. These cartridges contain lessons, PowerPoint slides, discussion forums, tests, and so forth. It is the role of faculty to identify what tools they need to teach a course.[45]
- *Support.* Is implementation training provided? Is that part of the start-up costs? What training materials does the CMS offer? Does it have a 24/7 help system, either by phone or by chat? What support does it offer students?

After considering these factors, faculty are responsible for determining the essential criteria or features necessary to deliver a quality course using appropriate technology as well as any "nice to have" but not essential criteria or features. In many universities, CMS decisions are made for the academic environment as a whole. Thus knowing school- and profession-specific requirements is critical.

CMS and LMS products are improving with new technological developments and arrangements with partners that bring new tools to the product. For example, most products now provide access to Web 2.0 tools that facilitate collaboration efforts. These include tools such as wikis, blogs, conferencing, ePortfolio, and journaling. Most products now also offer mobile learning options.

The Future of Course Management Systems

What is the future of CMS software? Green and Spencer present the results of surveys regarding the top trends in eLearning for 2015 and beyond. These include:

- Mobile and wearable access to eLearning materials
- More sophisticated collaboration tools
- Growing Cloud-based LMS services
- Personalized learning using pull technologies putting the learner in control
- Augmented and gaming learning environments providing practical experiences[46,47]

What will this mean to faculty and students? What will this mean for the selection of CMSs?

Institutions are or have considered adding mobile ability in the criteria for selection of CMS or LMS software. Does this mean that colleges and universities that make this decision will require students to have a tablet or wearable device like glasses, watches, or bracelets of some sort? Think about how this might affect education of patients with articles like "Wearable Enhanced Learning for Healthy Ageing: Conceptual Framework and Architecture of the 'Fitness MOOC.'"[48] What will this mean for the design of learning materials and learning experiences? What will this mean for educating our learners in how to work with patient educational experiences?

Another area of growing technological development is collaborative tools that are smarter (i.e., remember who users are, what they like, and what they were doing [Web 3.0]) and provide relevant information to each user. Users should also see more lifelike virtual 3D worlds integrated into the LMS or CMS software. These virtual worlds will make use of the latest technological capabilities, such as Google's augmented reality 3D glasses and Corning's view of the future. The Corning vision integrates glass surfaces to access information and to interact in the virtual world. Imagine a time when bathroom mirrors remind students that work is due, when students can interact with their world on their TV screens, and when students can chat with classmates and the professor through their kitchen counter. (See YouTube video—"A Day Made of Glass.") What will this mean for the design and teaching of distance education and the new wave of distributive courses?

INSTRUCTIONAL DESIGN FOR DISTANCE EDUCATION AND LEARNING

While most of the principles of instructional design hold true for distance education, the principal teaching change in a learning environment is the use of technology to engage and empower the learner. This section is of this chapter is not a comprehensive treatise about instructional design concepts but rather a discussion of key factors that should be considered in the design of eLearning experiences.

Learners and How They Learn

The key is to know the learners and their skill sets. Are these undergraduate or graduate students? Are these older adults returning to the educational world? Are these working adults pursuing updated skills? What technology skills do they bring to the course? What comfort level do they have with new methods of course delivery and learning? Have they taken distance education or distributive courses before? Are they ready to take responsibility for their learning? Do they understand that they must be an active and not passive learner in this environment? What are their expectations of response time? For example, some learners expect the instant access and response that they experience when texting, while other learners wait much too long to ask for needed help.

As the introduction to this chapter pointed out, there can be a different mindset among digital natives (learners who grew up with technology) and students who were schooled using more historical methods. Table 31.2 gives a sense of how technology has evolved over the different generations. How do faculty design for those differences? Oblinger et al. identify the following implications for learning and the design of these courses:

- Using the web as an exploratory tool to access the wealth of information available
- Offering learners a comprehensive learning experience
- Engaging learners
- Empowering learners to take charge of their own learning[1]

Faculty will usually see a range of students with a range of abilities. Knowing this, faculty must provide a range of learning activities to meet the needs of current students. At the beginning of the course, faculty may assess students' learning styles and work with the students to develop strategies to deal with various learning styles. A faculty member may also develop interactive activities. For example, the faculty may provide a written lesson about some concept, a podcast with the same content, discussion questions to engage students in the content, and an exploratory WebQuest activity that requires students to explore the web for quality resources that cover this content. A WebQuest is an inquiry-oriented lesson format in which most or all the information that learners work with comes from the web. See Google's Teaching with Technology website (https://sites.google.com/site/learnteachtech/webquest-projects) for several examples. Fig. 31.6 provides examples of nursing-related WebQuests created using the website www.zunal.com. This example

TABLE 31.2	Who Were the Students, Who Are the Students, Who Will Be the Students?	
Age Range in 2016	Name of the Generation	Technology Development During Birth Years
51 to 73	Boomers	1943—ENIAC used plug boards and switches for programming, occupied more than 1000 square feet, used about 18,000 vacuum tubes and weighed 30 tons. 1964—Digital Equipment Corporation launch the 12-bit PDP-8, the first successful commercial minicomputer.
35 to 50	Gen X	1965—The Victor 3900 the first desktop calculator is available. 1981—The first IBM Personal Computer is released with a 4.77 MHz Intel 8088 microprocessor.
19 to 34	Millennials	1982—The personal computer was *Time*'s "Machine of the Year." The article was written on a typewriter, but *Time* was planning to upgrade the office to word processors within the year. 1990—The first web browser is invented. 42% of American adults have used a computer at some point. 1998—Apple releases the iMac with a 233-MHz G3 processor, 4GB hard drive, 32 MB of RAM, a CD-ROM drive, and a 15″ monitor.
0 to 18	Post-Millennial	1999—41% of adults are using the internet. 2008—75% of Americans are using the internet. 2016—88.5% of Americans use the internet 2015—Almost two thirds of American adults (64%) own a smartphone of some type.

Sources: <http://www.pewinternet.org/2014/03/11/world-wide-web-timeline/#2008>.; <http://www.computerhistory.org/timeline>; <http://www.pewresearch.org/fact-tank/2015/01/16/this-year-millennials-will-overtake-baby-boomers/>; <http://www.pewinternet.org/2015/04/01/chapter-one-a-portrait-of-smartphone-ownership/>; http://www.internetlivestats.com/internet-users/us/.

The Nurse Practitioner Mentor: The Basics

Mentoring has been used to support role development and clinical practice transitions in nursing. Mentoring advanced practice nurses will foster role transition, clinical competency, creativity, and innovative clinical practice. The NP mentor will pr

Subject: Professional Skills | **Grade:** College / Adult

Author(s): Patricia Bartley Daniele Phd(c), Fnp-Bc.

Views: 10,696 | **Favorited:** 2 | **Reviews:** ☆☆☆☆☆ (0)

End Of Life Care: Nursing Student Role

To assist graduate nursing students in providing compassionate and effective End of Life care to patients across care settings.

Subject: Health / PE | **Grade:** College / Adult

Author(s): Kimberly Augustine

Views: 6,751 | **Favorited:** 8 | **Reviews:** ☆☆☆☆☆ (0)

Functional Assessment In The Older Adult

This webquest will identify what functional decline in the older adult is along with exploring different functional status assessments using proven methodology. This will explore the different rationales for functional status assessment, provide pro

Subject: Professional Skills | **Grade:** College / Adult

Author(s): Kari Vastbinder

Views: 6,165 | **Favorited:** 5 | **Reviews:** ★★★★★ (1)

Medical Surgical Nursing: Hypertension

This webquest is designed to assist nursing students in developing an awareness of Hypertension, also known as High Blood Pressure, the causes, symptoms, and treatment.

Subject: Health / PE | **Grade:** College / Adult

Author(s): Yvonne Baird

Views: 5,241 | **Favorited:** 3 | **Reviews:** ☆☆☆☆☆ (0)

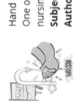

Hand Hygiene For Student Nurses

One of the most important, but too often ignored, practice health care workers can do for their patients is simply to treat them with just-washed hands. In this WebQuest, nursing students will learn the basics of hand hygiene & alcohol-based han

Subject: Professional Skills | **Grade:** College / Adult

Author(s): Rachel O'Connor, Rn, Bsn

Views: 4,163 | **Favorited:** 9 | **Reviews:** ☆☆☆☆☆ (0)

The Ins And Outs Of Mediports

Cancer is becoming a chronic illness and you may care for an oncology patient with a mediport. Nursing school may not have taught you about mediports or how to care for someone that has one. This webquest will teach you what a mediport is, how to acc

Subject: Professional Skills | **Grade:** College / Adult

Author(s): Lori Gofter

Views: 4,144 | **Favorited:** 3 | **Reviews:** ☆☆☆☆☆ (0)

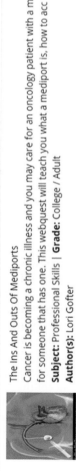

FIG 31.6 Nursing Webquest Examples. (Used with permission.)

was developed using the keyword "nursing" and limiting the search to "college/adult, all curriculum." As can be seen in Fig. 31.6, this search returned several different nursing-related WebQuests.

Goals and Objectives (Outcomes)

In distance education, writing clear, measurable goals and objectives or outcomes is critical to ensure that students know the course expectations and how faculty will assess their learning. Each lesson, module, or activity should identify the purpose, goals, and objectives; provide clear directions for what students are to do; and provide a scoring rubric or guide for evaluation of students' achievement of the objectives or outcomes. These should also include due dates and time periods.

Instructional and Learner Activities

Instructional and learner activities should provide learners with the skills, knowledge, and experience necessary to meet the course objectives. These activities or experiences should consider the learners' need for engagement, activity, and relevance to the content, objectives, and work world. This means that the professor will need to take advantage of the tool set available through the CMS software as well as tool sets available from outside sources. It may also mean that the professor must step outside his or her comfort zone in learning new ways to deliver the course and develop relevant learning experiences. Faculty should have access to a wide variety of collaborative tools that encourage interaction with the content and with others. These tools include wikis, blogs, discussion forums, journals, and WebQuests. Other learner activities could include developing podcasts, videos, and group projects. When designing course activities, keep in mind that active participation facilitates learning better than does passive participation. For training, the same applies, making it relevant to the work tasks. As an example, teaching how to use Excel and related features with activities that demonstrate common uses from the work setting is much more effective than a basic, intermediate, and advanced perspective for organizing the learning.

To help guide the selection of learning activities, one should consider the use of a model like the Community of Inquire Model, with its three main concepts of social presence, cognitive presence, and teaching presence.[49,50] Social presence refers to establishing a support learning community where students can engage in meaningful communication and develop social relationships. Cognitive presence is the development of learning materials where students construct knowledge through reflection and discussions. Teaching presence is the last concept that deals with designing the learning experiences, guiding the learning, and moving the students to the desired student learning outcomes.

Evaluation

Regular and timely feedback to learners on their progress is important to learner success and engagement with the content/concepts/skills. Learners benefit from frequent feedback as they master new content. But this can also be very time consuming for faculty or trainers.

Faculty members who design learning activities or projects where grading requires faculty judgment as opposed to "objective testing" should develop a grading rubric or guide for each activity and place it with the directions or guidelines file as well as attach it to the assignment in the CMS. These guidelines should also convey to learners when students will receive comments and grades on submitted work. When developing these guidelines, trainers should think carefully about how they will use these same guidelines during the grading process. How will they actually evaluate the learner's learning? Will there be feedback provided directly on the learners work, a review of a sample document from the work world, or follow-up once the learner is back in the work setting?

Once the grading is completed, faculty will also need to enter scores in the CMS so that these scores can be viewed in the online student grade sheet. Many online grade sheets now offer the students several ways they can sort and analyze their grades. Faculty should consider how students might interpret this information. For example, would a student learning new information be motivated or discouraged if they determine they have the lowest score in the class?

In addition to the evaluation of learner's learning, faculty should give consideration to evaluation of the course and related learning activities. Does the school have course evaluation or best practices guidelines? Are these guidelines appropriate for distance education courses? Many of these course evaluation forms link to faculty contracts and will not necessarily help improve the course. Does the faculty member use something like Quality Matters, which is a peer review process to certify the quality of online and blended courses?[51] It might be helpful to use a guide like Quality Matters as the course is developed. There is no one best practice guide for distance education, but all guides consider these points as being critical to quality:

- Institutional commitment and resources
- Curriculum and instructional rigor with interactivity and regular communication between faculty and learners
- Faculty support services
- Student support services
- Evaluation of the course and programs

In the corporate world, the trainer needs to give consideration to how a training session fits with the rest of the training provided by the corporation and the corporation's mission, goals, and values. For example, in a clinical setting, are the employees at the completion of the training able to safely use the electronic health record (EHR), or are there common data entry errors that are impacting patient care?

On a course-by-course basis, faculty may develop some activities that provide learner feedback to the professor. A student statement illuminating what the student learned from completion of the activity provides feedback as to what is working and what is not. For example, at the end of each blog entry, have the student identify up to three things that they have learned and why they found them to be important. As a final example, require the students to rate themselves on a scale of 1 to 5 on how well they achieved each course objective and to support that rating with some data (an activity or a resource that helped them learn, a product that they produced, etc.).

Equally important to a well-designed and well-delivered course are the support services available to learners.

STUDENT (LEARNER) SUPPORT SERVICES

Student support services are important to the achievement of learner outcomes, learner satisfaction, and learner retention. In planning for learner support services, the faculty may need to assess what support services online learners expect. Nelson states, "putting all student services online will not eliminate the need for support services specifically designed for distance education students."[52, p. 186] That statement is still relevant today. All learners, both on and off campus, must have access to the same resources, but they may be delivered in a different way.

Library

While most schools have online access to full text databases, interlibrary loans, and book borrowing, there is a wealth of other library resources of which the learner should be made aware. The following are two examples:

- Top Sites Blog contains a list of the top 10 free online libraries (http://topsitesblog.com/free-online-libraries). These online libraries contain mostly historical information but can assist students with their general education requirements as well as provide historical information about healthcare.
- Nursing on the Net: Health Care Resources You Can Use (https://nnlm.gov/training/nursing/sampler.html) includes a list of topics with links such as alternative medicine, drug information, evidence-based nursing, and mobile apps, to name a few. There is an extensive listing of links to resources under these categories. This site is maintained by the National Network of Libraries of Medicine and is updated regularly.

The Association of College and Research Libraries (ACRL) publishes a set of standards for libraries servicing the distance education population, initially approved on July 1, 2008, but referred to as a "living document."[53] Guidance in the use of these standards may be found at the DLS website (http://acrl.ala.org/DLS/). In addition, a bibliography of recent literature on distance learning library services can be accessed at https://distancelearningsection.wordpress.com/resources-publications/.

During the planning phase, the school should compare its services to those standards and develop a plan to acquire the services and materials that do not currently meet those standards. In addition, faculty must discuss what additional services online students may need that on-campus students do not. This can vary from institution to institution based on

how the course is delivered. For example, do learners need a different user ID and password to access the school's online full text databases, or do they have one user ID and password to access all resources whether on or off campus? Do they have access to an online librarian who can help them with their search strategy?

Tutoring Services

All learners studying at a distance should have the same access to tutoring services as on-campus learners. There are several online tutoring services that learners may use for a fee or that the school may provide. Some examples include Tutor.com (www.tutor.com), Smarthinking, Inc. (http://www.pearsoned.com/higher-education/products-and-services/services-and-solutions-for-higher-ed/services/smarthinking/), and Chegg Study (https://www.chegg.com/study). See also http://www.tutor.com/higher-education. The tutoring service must be similar to those that the school offers on campus and must have the same pricing structure. Faculty should ask questions about these services regarding the fees, live real-time help, hours of operation, and qualifications of the tutors. For example, does the service have tutors who can address the needs of healthcare students?

If there are peer tutoring services for on-campus learners, how will those same services be available to the distance education learner? What technology will be in place to provide for these services? For example, does the school provide a web-based video solution where the writing center peer tutor can interact with the student and the student's paper while talking about needed improvements? If a video conference system is not available, the learner could e-mail the paper to the tutor and arrange a phone conversation to discuss it.

Online Textbook Distributors

The cost and acquisition of required textbooks in a timely fashion merits attention. How is the campus bookstore responding to the growing student population that may not reside on campus or live nearby? Does it provide online ordering and shipping to the student's residence? What does that do to the costs? Does it provide eText options? Can learners rent their textbooks through the bookstore? Will open textbooks (licensed under an open copyright license) be used that are free to the students? Other options that learners may use are the growing number of online textbook distributors such as Chegg, Ecampus, and CourseSmart. Of course, the student has the option to order from websites like Amazon and Barnes & Noble College, as well as from traditional booksellers. The following are a few examples of distributors in the higher education market:

- *Follett* (www.follettbooks.com). Follett is a leading operator of college bookstores and a major distributor of textbooks. It operates a service called CafeScribe, which is a digital textbook platform; this is different from e-books, which are digital editions of traditional textbooks that students or faculty read on a computer, tablet, or smartphone. CafeScribe provides the ability for faculty and students to share notes and insights in line with the text, search the text for specific information, take notes directly in the text, bookmark places in the text, and highlight information.[54]

- *Chegg* (www.chegg.com). Chegg provides students with the ability to rent textbooks as well as buy new and used textbooks at a reduced cost. Students can also sell their books back to Chegg. It also offers homework help for many courses, scholarships, and course selection help. Chegg acquired several companies in 2010 and 2011: CourseRank, Cramster, Notehall, Student of Fortune, and Zinch.[55]
- *VitalSource* (https://www.vitalsource.com/). VitalSource provides eTextbook and digital learning tools. It provides both online and off-line access. It has a partnership arrangement with more than 50 publishers and offers more than 90% of the textbook market in higher education.[56]

What guidance should the school provide to learners in distance education courses with regard to acquisition of textbooks? For example, are these books that the student will need throughout their time in college? Depending on the answer, the students then must ensure that they are renting or using digital forms of the textbook that are available to them for the duration of their time in college. The Higher Education Opportunity Act (HEOA), discussed later in this chapter, mandates that students be provided with information about the required textbooks when they register for a course. What should they know about older editions? Are they acceptable or not? When will students actually need access to the textbooks? They may need certain textbooks immediately but may not need others until later in the course. Knowing this may help students balance the cost of textbooks. Will students need a code to access the textbook website? If so, does a used textbook come with the code or will the student need to buy that separately? Buying codes separately is generally more expensive and may not save students money when the used book costs and new code costs are combined. What is the return policy of these online distributors?

Help Desk

Given the nature of technology and that technical issues will arise during the course of the semester, the school will need to address technical assistance for off-campus learners. Should it provide for a university-based help desk, an outsourced help desk, or some combination? This is not an easy decision. It requires a cost analysis to assess staffing a help desk with staff and students versus outsourced staffing. Software will be necessary to run the help desk and a training budget allocated to train the staff. The school will need to make decisions about help desk staff's ability to reset passwords and access the CMS, with designated privileges for functions they can perform, such as configuring a student's browser and firewall and running virus checks. What is the range of help that a student working at the help desk can provide? Will more hours be allotted during the first few weeks of the semester when more help may be needed? Is there an orientation program for the students to the CMS?

Because distance learning occurs at any time (24/7) and any place, many schools are opting for outsourcing. Outsourcing can be offered by either the CMS vendor or be a freestanding service that is independent of the vendor. A key question to ask in the CMS selection process is whether a CMS provides a help desk service. Faculty may want to confirm that the school's CMS provider can effectively bundle a help desk product with its CMS product; many CMSs are moving in this direction (to a portal or bundled product). If so, what is the fee and what is the advantage of using that service for the distance education program?

Another approach is to use a general help desk provider. The following are a few examples of a portal and CMSs help desk services.

- *BlackBeltHelp* (www.blackbelthelp.com) is a freestanding help desk service that has been working with higher education institutions for the past 5 years. It offers 24/7, 365 days a year support to students, faculty, and staff. Support includes LMS and ERP issues, general IT help, and so forth.
- *Ellucian* (http://www.ellucian.com/Support-and-Train ing/Ellucian-Client-Support/). This portal solution also offers help desk services. It offers assistance 365 days per year to faculty, staff, and students. Since it knows the portal software, it may be in a better position to assist students than a freestanding help desk service.
- *Blackboard* (http://www.blackboard.com/higher-educa tion/student-services-and-technology-support/index. aspx). On July 8, 2014, Blackboard acquired Perceptis to enhance its help desk support service.

If outsourcing is the solution, then the college must ensure that it outsources the correct work and tasks. For example, will the help desk be able to reset passwords? Will it have remote access to see what the student is doing or to control the student's desktop? What should it know about the CMS or LMS? Will it have privileges to enter the CMS? What legal implications does CMS access have? In either case, the school will need to monitor the effectiveness of its contract in defining the services to be provided and the quality of the services provided. The efficiency and effectiveness of the help desk support must be subject to evaluation to validate that it is meeting the needs of this student population.

In summary, learners will need access to the help desk 24/7 or close to it, and this will necessitate a variety of communication channels: phone, chat, video conference, self-help website, and so forth.

Administrative Services, Academic Support, and Community Building

The retention rate for students who learn in their own space and time has been a problem. How should the school adjust certain traditional student services to provide for a feeling of connectedness and belonging for distance education students? Will this aid in retention and better student outcomes?

- *Administrative services.* These services include registration, financial aid, adds and drops, and admissions.

Since most schools provide these services online, the procedures for accessing them should be the same as those used by on-campus students. The key institutional issue here is whether this should be a portal solution with one interface or stand-alone systems.

- *Academic support.* This includes advising and career services. Many of these services are already extended to students through web portals or department websites and through social media tools such as Facebook and Twitter. The school may need to develop additional options for use of social media tools to extend the services in both time and space. For example, use of video conferencing or chat rooms for advising sessions with extended hours may be appropriate. It may also be important to put in place an alert and "job well done" system (such as Starfish, www. starfishsolutions.com) to keep students on track and motivate them to finish. Questions to ask are: Does the software integrate with the CMS? What are the issues if it does integrate? If it doesn't integrate? Some schools also have as a part of the student information system an online audit for ease of scheduling courses, reminders for requirements they met, and links to appropriate content.
- *Community building.* This is an area that schools may neglect more than other learner support services. How does the institution build a sense of belonging and identification with the program or school? Faculty and the school should consider services such as a cyber cafe either in or outside the CMS program (some CMSs have a community tab or feature separate from a course) or a blog that students can use to interact outside of the course. Faculty might also consider a regular newsletter or podcast that highlights an event, student, or opportunity. What about a webinar on an issue of concern to healthcare or nursing that is open to students in the program? What about an online student government community? There are other community-building options, but these must engage the students and help them identify with their online learning community.

ISSUES

This section addresses additional issues that relate to distance education—legal, disability, quality, and readiness.

Legal

Digital Millennium Copyright Act of 1998

The Digital Millennium Copyright Act (DMCA) addresses the demands of the digital and internet age and conformance to the requirements of the World Intellectual Property Organization.[57] This is a complex act that is generally outside the scope of this chapter. This chapter highlights those areas of the law that might affect a distance learning program. DMCA protects any copyrightable work. Copyrightable work includes written

text or literary works, visual works, graphic works, musical works, and codes that pass between computers.[58] Key sections that affect distance learning include the following:

- Prohibiting the circumvention of protection technologies, including encryption or password-breaking programs, and the manufacturing of devices that defeat such protection measures
- Limiting liability of online service providers because of the content that users transmit over their services
- Expanding existing exemptions for making copies of computer programs under certain conditions
- Updating rules and procedures for archival preservations
- Mandating studies to examine distance education in a networked world[59]

DMCA also established the Takedown Notice, through which copyright holders can demand removal of infringing content. This requires the copyright holder to follow the appropriate process and procedures.

Since this is a complex law, students and faculty should check with the school's legal counsel if they are in doubt about violating DMCA while preparing and posting educational materials for a distance course. Many schools also have a checklist that can be used as a guide to maintain compliance with this law. This checklist is often posted on the library website.

Technology, Education, and Copyright Harmonization Act

The Technology, Education, and Copyright Harmonization (TEACH) Act, passed in 2002 and signed into law by President George W. Bush, addresses some of the issues that require attention when planning and delivering distance education. The purpose of this act was to clarify acceptable use of copyrighted materials as it relates to distance education. Many of the responsibilities for compliance with this act are placed on the institution and its IT staff. The TEACH Act permits the performance and display of copyrighted materials for distance education under the following conditions:

- The institution is an accredited, nonprofit educational institution.
- Only students who have enrolled in the course can have access to these materials.
- The use must be for either "live" or asynchronous sessions (permits storage of the materials on a server).
- The institution must provide information to faculty and students stating that course materials may be copyrighted and provide access policies regarding copyright.
- The institution must limit access to the materials for the period of time necessary to complete the session or course.
- The institution must prevent further copying or redistribution of copyrighted materials.
- No part of the use may interfere with copy protection mechanisms.[59-61]

For the professor, the law includes the following:

- The materials must be part of mediated (systematic) instructional activities (i.e., relevant to the course).

- The use must not include the transmission of textbook materials or other materials generally purchased or works developed specifically for online uses.
- Faculty can use only reasonable and limited portions of such materials, as they would typically use in a live classroom.
- The materials must be available *only* to registered students and not to guests or observers.
- Faculty must post a notice or message in the CMS that identifies the copyrighted materials and therefore precludes the student from copying or distributing these materials to others, as that would be a breach of copyright law.
- Faculty must pay attention to "portion" limitations (how much one can use).[59-61]

The latest attempt at revisions to the TEACH Act is H.R. 3505, introduced on November 15, 2013, for the purpose of developing accessibility guidelines for electronic instructional materials and related information technologies in higher education institutions. Congress.gov's website (https://www.congress.gov/bill/113th-congress/house-bill/3505) provides a copy of the bill, a summary of the bill, as well as information on the progress of this bill, which is still in the Subcommittee on Higher Education and Workforce Training as of October 14, 2016.

Consult the school's policy and legal and library authorities when in doubt about materials necessary for the course. The American Library Association has an excellent website that further explains the roles of the institution (administrators or policy-makers and IT staff), faculty, and librarians.

Higher Education Opportunity Act

The Higher Education Opportunity Act (HEOA) of 2008 is a reauthorization of the Higher Education Act of 1965. It requires postsecondary institutions to be more transparent about costs and requires that the institution post a net price calculator as well as security and copyright policies on its website.[62] While many of the provisions in this act do not directly affect faculty (since they relate to administrative offices that deal with fees, growth, public relations, credits, etc.), the following do affect faculty: the textbook information provision, the definition of distance education, and the requirement to establish that students are indeed who they say they are.[63,64]

HEOA compliance entails the following:

- Faculty must select and submit textbook requirements to the campus bookstore *before* posting the next semester's schedule and registration. Each institution establishes the process for this. Under certain circumstances, the institution may post a "to be determined" notice if textbook selection was not practical before the school posts the next semester's schedule.
- Schools must pay attention to the change in terminology from distance learning to distance education. Education describes the process from the institution's perspective; it includes the use of one or more technologies to deliver instruction to students who are in a separate location and to support regular and substantive

interaction between faculty and students. Learning describes the process from the students' perspective; it focuses on how the student interacts with the course content, classmates, and instructor in mastering the course content.
- Institutions must have a process in place to verify that the enrolled student is actually the person completing the course. Faculty may assist in determining how this process will work and with the development of a policy to cover this provision.

There are periodic updates to HEOA and the related regulations. These changes can be found at sites such as https://www.naicu.edu/special_initiatives/hea101/publications/page/updates-on-regulations-and-regulatory-process. Most educational institutions keep abreast of these updates and notify faculty during faculty in-service days.

Intellectual Property

The issue of intellectual property is coming to the forefront as a major concern in the digital age. Faculty are increasingly concerned about the ownership of distributive course materials and the use of those materials. Many faculty assume that these course materials are their creative property, meaning that a requirement exists for others to obtain permission to use them. Since these materials exist in digital form on a school's accessible server, others may have access to these materials with or without faculty consent. In today's world, some of these materials may have commercial value, and institutions are increasingly taking ownership of these materials. A clear institutional policy will convey to all persons involved who owns what and what constitutes allowable use of the materials.

Some questions to consider in developing an intellectual property policy are:

- What works are included under the policy (e.g., artworks, writings, software, course learning objects, PowerPoint slides, podcasts)?
- To whom does the policy apply (e.g., all employees, professors, researchers, postdoctoral fellows, administrators, students)?
- Under what circumstances does the school own the materials? Under what circumstances does the faculty member own the materials? Can there be joint ownership? Is this a work for hire or within the scope of the faculty member's employment?
- What institutional resources did the faculty member use to create the materials?
- What key words should the policy clearly define?
- Is there a clear, definitive written agreement between the faculty member and the institution as to ownership and rights?
- Who is responsible for obtaining copyrights, trademarks, etc.?[65,66]

Family Educational Rights and Privacy Act

The Family Educational Rights and Privacy Act (FERPA) is a federal law that requires colleges and universities to give students access to their educational records. Colleges and universities must maintain the confidentiality of personally identifiable educational records. See www.ed.gov/policy/gen/guid/fpco/ferpa/index.html for the U.S. Department of Education's summary of FERPA. While distance education courses were not a direct concern to those who wrote the FERPA rules, any time a faculty member or a university generates student information electronically, you must take precautions.

Consider the following guidelines for distance education and student records:

- Only enrolled students and the faculty teaching the course should have access to the course. However, the CMS administrator also has access to the course to manage and troubleshoot problems in using the CMS. The school must make the administrator aware of FERPA policies.
- If a college uses a hosting client (someone off campus that maintains the CMS), this arrangement makes the hosting client a third-party vendor. While the client should not have access to information that links a student to a grade, the client's systems administrator does have access to the servers and ultimately to everything on them.
- Students should be able to view only their own grades in the online grade book. They should not be able to see other students' grades.
- Some issues may arise regarding discussion forums, depending on how the faculty use them. Faculty should *not* post evaluative comments or grades for students' comments in the discussion forum. Faculty should also state in the course requirements that students are required to post to the discussion forum, share their papers, and so on.
- If faculty use Excel to keep a record of student grades, they should remove the students' ID numbers from the spreadsheet, leave no storage devices where others may access them, password protect the spreadsheet (but faculty *must* remember the password), and use an encryption program that comes with some external drives. This will protect the confidentiality of student data.
- If faculty lose a portable device such as a thumb drive that contains student grade sheets where the student names and grades are identifiable, they must notify the proper college or university authorities to determine what additional action must be taken.
- If faculty require students to send or post information to sites outside the college (e.g., blogs; social networking sites such as LinkedIn, Facebook, and YouTube; etc.), a clear policy must be developed and followed. This type of assignment can be ripe for FERPA violations.

Disability Issues

Distance learning opportunities can open doors for millions of Americans with disabilities. When planning for the delivery of distance education courses, faculty must not create access barriers for the disabled. Laws such as the Americans with Disabilities Act (ADA) prohibit discrimination due to disability, and sections 504 and 508 of the Rehabilitation Act provide protections to learners with disabilities.[67]

What constitutes a reasonable accommodation for a particular learner will depend on the situation and the type of program. The accommodation, however, may not be unduly costly or disruptive for the school or be for the student's personal use only. In colleges and universities, the student has the primary responsibility to identify and document the disability and to request specific support, services, and other accommodations. Most schools have a person responsible for assessing students with disabilities and providing an accommodation letter to faculty. Each accommodation letter details modifications for each student with a disability. The modifications may include the following items:

- Providing extended time to turn in assigned work
- Providing extra time for timed exams
- Administering an exam in an alternative format, such as a paper exam when others will take the exam on a computer through the CMS
- Allowing spelling errors on papers or exams without deduction of points

Given the disability of the student and the nature of distance education, the student may need computer assistive devices. Students with disabilities may need adapted keyboards; magnification software; screen reader programs, such as Job Access With Speech (JAWS) (http://www.freedomscientific.com/products/fs/jaws-product-page.asp) or Dolphin's SUPERNOVA (http://www.yourdolphin.com/products.asp), that convert the text and images to speech; voice recognition; and alternative communication programs. Most operating systems support persons with disabilities by incorporating accessibility utilities into the system.

For faculty, this may mean providing alternative experiences for a student with a disability (e.g., use of a captioned video for the hearing-impaired student). Faculty that teach distance education courses should review the tutorial entitled Ten Simple Steps toward Universal Design of Online Courses (located at https://ualr.edu/pace/tenstepsud/) that addresses these issues. It lists 10 steps and provides examples and details for each one.

Quality

The traditional model of quality evaluation is site based, but distance and distributive education are not site based.[68] Distance education is changing the thinking about quality assessment methods. Pond suggests that this new paradigm creates opportunities and challenges for quality assurance and accreditation.[69] Pond further suggests that the traditional items of quality assurance, such as physical attendance, contact hours, proctored testing, and library holdings, are impractical or simply not rational in a distance education course. Pond makes the following three suggestions:

- Use a consumer-based means of judging quality much like Amazon or eBay.
- Accredit the learner by having the learner demonstrate competencies rather than earn credits or certify the teacher's competencies.

- Move quality assurance toward an outcomes- or product-based model.

This new model will look at quality indicators such as continuity between "advertising" and reality, personal and professional growth of the learner, relevance, and multidirectional interactions.

Eaton states that accreditation institutions or agencies need to do the following[70, p. 6]:

- Identify the distinctive features of distance learning delivery.
- Modify accreditation guidelines, policies, or standards to meet the needs of this distinctive environment.
- Pay attention to student achievement and learning outcomes.

In the Eaton article, Appendix A features guidelines for quality assurance in distance education, and Appendix B includes 12 important questions about external quality review that are worth examining.

Faculty must answer these questions: How will they evaluate quality in the distance education environment? How will the approach be the same as or different from that used for on-campus courses or programs? What are the current criteria that educational accrediting agencies will use to accredit or review the program? How do faculty address these criteria? What issues arise when states serve as the primary arbiters of policy and governance issues in U.S. education but the student population resides in one state and does not physically go to the campus in another state where the student is taking distance education courses?[71]

Readiness

This section examines both the institution's readiness and the learner's readiness for teaching and learning in a distance education model.

Institution

Some institutions may enter the distance education market to maintain competitiveness; others may do so because their recruitment staff identified a market need. Some see this movement as a means to increase revenues in these difficult financial times without the need for brick and mortar facilities. Regardless of the reason, the critical issues for readiness are as follows:

- Does the movement to distance education fit with the institution's missions and goals?
- Is the institution ready to invest in the technologies necessary to produce a quality program?
- Does the institution have the resources—people, money, and time—to develop and implement the program?
- Does the institution have faculty buy-in? Does it have administrative commitment? Does it have staff buy-in?
- Are faculty ready and prepared? Some institutions, such as Pennsylvania State University (PSU) and SUNY, have developed a faculty readiness assessment; the SUNY document is available at https://hybrid.commons.gc.cuny.edu/teaching/getting-started/faculty-self-assessment-preparing-for-online-teaching/. Does the institution have such an assessment or survey?

Without this readiness and commitment, distance education will not work or at best will result in a program of marginal quality. Just as the institution needs to be ready, it also needs to assess the students and potential student population for their readiness. That being said, the move to this method is moot for many institutions, because competition is forcing distance education solutions and most universities have already made this transition. In the corporate world (i.e., hospitals), it is also moot because of the need to provide mandatory training that takes into account employees working all shifts and all days. What is essential is the assessment of technologies necessary to deliver the training, resources necessary to make it happen, and trainer readiness to prepare the training materials.

Students (Learners)

Students who enter distance education courses need to consider their interest and ability to succeed in this learning environment. Inappropriate expectations about requirements for succeeding in these types of courses can lead to frustration and failure. Key questions include:

- What information does the institution provide to these learners to assess their readiness to learn in distance courses?
- Does the institution provide learners with a self-assessment tool such as Kizlik's readiness assessment (http://www.adprima.com/dears.htm) or Cypress College's readiness assessment (http://www.cypresscollege.edu/DistanceEdquiz/CCDERQ.aspx)?
- How will the institution make learners aware of the requirements for learning in this manner? For example, do learners know that distance courses require discipline and organization in setting aside time to complete the learning, as well as reading and comprehension skills to understand the concepts and develop the skills necessary for this program or course? Do students have the ability to follow directions and ask questions and the ability to work on their own under the guidance of a faculty member?
- How does the institution make eLearners aware of their responsibilities? For example, students will have to meet course deadlines, check in to the course regularly, interact with faculty and classmates, ask questions as necessary, and conduct themselves in a professional manner in all interactions.

The institution should list or outline learner requirements in a policy and procedures document and make this document available to students to ensure that they understand their responsibilities.

CONCLUSION AND FUTURE DIRECTIONS

The changes in our educational environment are reflective of shifts in our demographics, economic conditions, and technological developments. Web 2.0 tools are opening up educational opportunities for lifelong learning to a diverse global community. Emerging terms, course management and learning management systems, and issues related to the development and implementation of distance education and distributive learning are all elements resulting from these budding educational opportunities.

The next generation of CMSs and LMSs will be integrated portals that are smarter, track more information, and analyze learner data across functions such as e-mail, wikis, chats, forums, and so forth. They will include personal learning environments (PLEs), immersive, 3D learning worlds with better communication channels and collaboration for any time and any place learning with tablets and mobile devices.[72] This will result in just-in-time, customized learning environments where the focus is on outcomes rather than traditional credit hours. This emerging environment is about the learners, the learners' needs, and the integration and use of appropriate technologies.

REFERENCES

1. Oblinger D, Barone C, Hawkins B. *Distributed Education and Its Challenges: An Overview. American Council on Education, Center for Policy Analysis*; 2001. http://www.acenet.edu/newsroom/Documents/Distributed-Education-and-Its-Challenges-An-Overview.pdf.
2. Amirault R. Distance learning in the 21st century university: key issues for leaders and faculty. *Q Rev Distance Educ*. 2012;13(4):253–265.
3. Holly C. The case for distance education in nursing. *MERLOT J Online Learn Teach*. 2009;5(3):506–510. http://jolt.merlot.org/vol5no3/holly_0909.htm.
4. National Council of State Boards of Nursing. Distance Education; 2015. https://www.ncsbn.org/6662.htm.
5. Carr N. *The Shallows: What the Internet Is Doing to Our Brains*. New York: W.W. Norton & Company; 2011.
6. Turkle S. *Alone Together: Why We Expect More from Technology and Less from Each Other*. New York: Basic Books; 2011.
7. Lanier J. *You Are Not a Gadget: A Manifesto*. New York: Vintage Books; 2011.
8. Carr N. *The Glass Cage: How Our Computers Are Changing Us*. New York: W.W. Norton & Company; 2015.
9. Frand J. The information-age mindset: changes in students and implications for higher education. *EDUCAUSE Rev*. 2000;14–24. September/October, https://net.educause.edu/ir/library/pdf/ERM0051.pdf.
10. Oblinger D, Oblinger J. Is it age or IT: first steps toward understanding the net generation. *CSLA J*. 2006;29(2):8–16.
11. Eliot S, Agassiz E. *Society to Encourage Studies at Home*. Cambridge, MA: Riverside Press; 1897.
12. Moore M. *From Chautauqua to the Virtual University: A Century of Distance Education in the United States*. Columbus, OH: Center on Education and Training for Employment, Ohio State University; 2003. http://www.calpro-online.org/eric/docs/distance.pdf.
13. Jeffries M. Research in distance education. http://cmapspublic.ihmc.us/rid=1HZXXGY8W-1ZZ4DLF-137T/Research%20in%20Distance%20Education.docx. Accessed August 22, 2016.
14. Billings D. Optimizing distance education in nursing. *J Nurs Educ*. 2007;46(6):247–248.
15. American Association of Colleges of Nursing (AACN). *Distance Technology in Nursing Education White Paper. Provided by ERIC Document Reproduction Service ED448636*; 1999. http://files.eric.ed.gov/fulltext/ED448636.pdf.
16. Billings D. Distance education in nursing: 25 years and going strong. *Comput Inform Nurs*. 2007;25(3):121–123.
17. Knebel E. *The Use and Effect of Distance Education in Healthcare: What Do We Know?* Bethesda, MD: U.S. Agency for International Development, Quality Assurance Project; 2001. https://www.usaidassist.org/sites/assist/files/distance_education.pdf.
18. Moore M, Kearsley G. *Distance Education: A System View of Online Learning*. Belmotn, CA: Wadsworth Cengage; 2012.
19. Spector N, Lowery B. NCSBN's Distance Education Guidelines for Prelicensure Nursing Programs. In: *NCSBN's virtual conference on distance education in prelicensure programs*; 2015. https://www.ncsbn.org/2015_DLE_BLowery-NSpector.pdf.
20. SACS-COC. Distance and Correspondence Education Policy Statement; 2012. http://www.sacscoc.org/pdf/DistanceCorrespondenceEducation.pdf.
21. Lowery B, Spector N. Regulatory implications and recommendations for distance education in prelicensure nursing programs. *J Nurs Regul*. 2014;5(3):24–32.
22. Dede C. The evolution of distance education: emerging technologies and distributed learning. *Am J Distance Educ*. 1996;10(2):4–36. [ERIC Document Reproduction Services EJ534454].
23. Dede C. Enabling distributed learning communities via emerging technologies—Part one. *THEJ*. 2004;32(3):12–22.
24. Sangra A, Vlachopoulos D, Cabrera N. Building an inclusive definition of e-learning: an approach to the conceptual framework. *Int Rev Res Open Distance Learn*. 2012;13(2):145–159. [ERIC Document Reproduction Services EJ983277].
25. Koch L. The nursing educator's role in e-learning: a literature review. *Nurse Educ Today*. 2014;34(11):1382–1387.
26. Brown T, Mbati L. Mobile learning: moving past the myths and embracing the opportunities. *Int Rev Res Open Distrib Learn*. 2015;16(2):115–135.
27. Laouris Y, Eteokleous N. We need an educationally relevant definitions of mobile learning. In: *Proceedings of the 4th World Conference on Mobile Learning*; 2005. http://www.mlearn.org.za/CD/papers/Laouris%20&%20Eteokleous.pdf.
28. Watson W, Watson S. An argument for clarity: what are learning management systems, what are they not, and what should they become? *TechTrends*. 2007;51(2):28–34.
29. Ferriman J. *Course Management System vs Learning Management System*; July 12, 2012. http://www.learndash.com/course-management-system-vs-learning-management-system/.
30. Green K. *The campus computing survey. The Campus Computing Project*; October 2014. http://www.campuscomputing.net/sites/www.campuscomputing.net/files/CampusComputing2014-SummaryGraphics&Data.pdf.
31. *Business-Software.com*. 2016 Edition Top 10 learning management systems software report; 2016. http://landing.business-software.com/top-10-lms-vendors-v3.php.
32. Jafari A, McGee P, Carmean C. Managing courses, defining learning: what faculty, students, and administrators want. *EDUCAUSE Rev*. 2006;41(4):50–71. http://www.educause.edu/ero/article/managing-courses-defining-learning-what-faculty-students-and-administrators-want.

33. Wright C, Lopes V, Montgomerie T, Reju S, Schmoller S. Selecting a Learning Management System: Advice from an Academic Perspective. *EDUCAUSE*; 2014. http://er.educause.edu/articles/2014/4/selecting-a-learning-management-system-advice-from-an-academic-perspective.

34. Ellucian. *Ellucian Draws More Than 8,800 Attendees at Ellucian Live 2015 in New Orleans*; 2015. http://www.ellucian.com/News/Ellucian-Draws-More-Than-8-800-Attendees-at-Ellucian-Live-2015-in-New-Orleans/.

35. Jenzabar. Solutions for Higher Education; 2016. http://www.jenzabar.com/higher-ed-solutions/.

36. Simonson M. Course management systems. *Q Rev Distance Educ.* 2007;8(10):vii–ix. http://web2integration.pbworks.com/f/COURSE%2BMANAGEMENT%2BSYSTEMS.pdf.

37. Blackboard. *Who We Are*; 2016. http://www.blackboard.com/about-us/who-we-are.aspx.

38. D2L. *We're Transforming the Way the World Learns*; 2016. http://www.d2l.com/about/.

39. ELEARNINGFORCE. *Our Story*; 2016. http://www.elearningforce.com/Pages/About-us.aspx.

40. Moodle. Moodle Partners. https://moodle.com/partners/; 2016.

41. *Sakai.* About us; 2016. https://www.sakaiproject.org/about-sakai-project.

42. Kaplanis D. *8 Top Benefits of Using a Cloud Based LMS.* eLearning Industry; April 7, 2014. http://elearningindustry.com/8-top-benefits-of-using-a-cloud-based-lms.

43. Pappas C. *The Ultimate List of Cloud-Based Learning Management Systems.* eLearning industry; May 18, 2013. http://elearningindustry.com/the-ultimate-list-of-cloud-based-learning-management-systems.

44. Pappas C. *The Top LMS Statistics and Facts for 2015 You Need to know.* eLearning industry; 2015. http://elearningindustry.com/top-lms-statistics-and-facts-for-2015.

45. Dawson C. *LMS? SIS? SIF? LTI? Alphabet Soup and Blended Learning.* ZDNet; July 8, 2012. http://www.zdnet.com/lms-sis-sif-lti-alphabet-soup-and-blended-learning-7000000420/.

46. Green K. *The 2014 National Survey of Computing and Information Technology in US Higher Education. Campus Computing*; 2014. http://www.campuscomputing.net/item/campus-computing-2014.

47. Spencer R. *Top 10 eLearning trends for 2015.* eLearning industry; June 3, 2015. http://elearningindustry.com/top-10-elearning-trends-2015.

48. Buchem I, Merceron A, Kreutel J. Wearable enhanced learning for health ageing: conceptual framework and architecture of the "fitness MOOC". *Interact Des Archit J.* 2015;24:111–124.

49. Pecka S, Kotcherlakota S, Berger A. Community of inquiry model: advancing distance learning nurse anesthesia education. *AANA J.* 2014;82(30):212–218.

50. Garrison D. Online community of inquiry review: social, cognitive, and teaching presence issues. *J Asynchronous Learn Netw.* 2007;11(1):61–72.

51. Quality Matters Program. MarylandOnline; 2010. http://www.qmprogram.org.

52. Nelson R. Student support services for distance education students in nursing programs. In: Oermann M, Hernrich K, eds. *Annual Review of Nursing Education.* Vol 5. New York: Springer Publishing Company; 2007:183–206.

53. Association of College & Research Libraries (ACRL). Standards for distance learning library services. *ACRL*; 2008. http://www.ala.org/acrl/standards/guidelinesdistancelearning.

54. *Digital textbooks from CafeScribe.* follettbooks.com; 2015. http://www.follettbooks.com/fb3/ebooksMain.jsp.

55. Chegg. *Fact Sheet: About Chegg.* Chegg; 2015. http://www.chegg.com/factsheet.

56. Straumshein C. A New Course; 2014. https://www.insidehighered.com/news/2014/03/04/coursesmart-publishing-industrys-e-textbook-provider-acquired-vital-source.

57. American Library Association (ALA). DMCA: The Digital Millennium Copyright Act. *ALA*; 2015. http://www.ala.org/advocacy/copyright/dmca.

58. *The Digital Millennium Copyright Act of 1998: US Copyright Office Summary.* United States Copyright Office; 1998. http://www.copyright.gov/legislation/dmca.pdf.

59. Copyright Clearance Center. *The TEACH Act: new roles, rules and responsibilities for academic institutions.* Copyright Clearance Center; 2005. http://www.copyright.com/wp-content/uploads/2015/04/CR-Teach-Act.pdf.

60. American Library Association (ALA). TEACH Act best practices using Blackboard™. *ALA*; 2015. http://www.ala.org/advocacy/copyright/teachact/teachactbest.

61. Gassaway L. Balancing copyright concerns: the TEACH Act of 2001. *EDUCAUSE.* November/December 2001. http://er.educause.edu/~/media/files/article-downloads/erm01610.pdf.

62. EDUCAUSE. Implementing the Higher Education Opportunity Act: A checklist for business officers. *EDUCAUSE.* 2009. http://www.educause.edu/Resources/ImplementingtheHigherEducation/192839.

63. Middle States Commission on *Higher Education. Distance Education and the HEOA. Middle States Commission on Higher Education Newsletter*; January 2010. http://www.msche.org/news_newsletter.asp.

64. Middle States Commission on Higher Education. *New HEOA Regulations Impact Distance Education Programs, Substantive Change & Monitoring Growth, Transfer of Credit.* Middle States Commission on Higher Education Newsletter; 2009. Fall, http://www.msche.org/news_newsletter.asp.

65. Diaz V. *Distributed Learning Meets Intellectual Property Policy: Who Owns What? Campus Technology*; 2005. http://campustechnology.com/articles/2005/08/distributed-learning-meets-intellectual-property-policy-who-owns-what.aspx.

66. Ulius S. Intellectual property ownership in distributed learning. *EDUCAUSE*; 2003. http://net.educause.edu/ir/library/pdf/erm0346.pdf.

67. U.S. Department of Justice. *A Guide to Disability Rights Laws.* U.S. Department of Justice; July 2009. http://www.ada.gov/cguide.htm.

68. Baer MA. Forward. In: Eaton JS, ed. *Maintaining the Delicate Balance: Distance Learning, Higher Education Accreditation, and the Politics of Self-Regulation.* Louisville, CO: EDUCAUSE Publications; 2002. http://www.acenet.edu/news-room/Documents/Maintaining-the-Delicate-Balance-Distance-Learning-Higher-Education-Accreditation-and-the-Politics-of-Self-Regulation-2002.pdf.

69. Pond W. *Distributed Education in the 21st Century: Implications for Quality Assurance.* University of West Georgia; 2002. http://www.westga.edu/~distance/ojdla/summer52/pond52.html.

70. Eaton J. *Maintaining the Delicate Balance: Distance Learning, Higher Education Accreditation, and the Politics of Self-Regulation.* American Council on Education, Center for Policy Analysis; 2002. http://www.chea.org/pdf/Maintaining-the-Delicate-Balance-Distance-Learning-

Higher-Education-Accreditation-and-the-Politics-of-Self-Regulation-2002.pdf.

71. Levine A, Sun J. *Barriers to Distance Education.* American Council on Education, Center for Policy Analysis; 2002. http://

www.acenet.edu/news-room/Documents/Barriers-to-Distance-Education-2003.pdf.

72. Brown M, Dehoney J, Millichap N. What's next for the LMS. *EDUCAUSE Rev.* 2015;July/August;40–51.

DISCUSSION QUESTIONS

1. Research how constant connectivity affects you socially, cognitively, and physically. Refer to such books as Carr, N., *The Shallows*; Turkel, S., *Alone Together: Why We Expect More From Technology and Less From Each Other*; Lanier, J., *You Are Not A Gadget: A Manifesto*; and Carr, N., *The Glass Cage: How Our Computers Are Changing Us*. Ask yourself how technology is changing the way you think and focus, and how this affects your learning style. Provide two examples and resources that support how technology is changing how we socialize.
2. From a student or faculty perspective, develop criteria to use in comparing and evaluating two course management systems (CMS) or learning management systems (LMS) delivery systems. Select two systems and compare them using the developed criteria. Discuss what you learned in developing these criteria and in comparing two products against them. Include answers to the following questions: How useful were these criteria, what was missing, and how would you revise the criteria next time?
3. Think of a situation where distance education might be appropriate. Identify three technology tools that might be useful for the specific audience and how they would be used. What skills would the learner need to use them? What skills would the instructor/trainer need?
4. Research the future of higher education, distance learning, and the movement toward personal learning environments (PLEs). What will the day in the life of a nursing student be like in 2026? What impact will technologies have on license renewal?

CASE STUDY

You are a faculty member serving on the online learning committee. The university requires an assessment of which learning strategies are working and which are not and an examination of the current standards, emerging trends, and how the school should plan for the distance education and elearning movement. The committee is charged with setting the course for this initiative for the next 2 years. There are many subcommittees, each with a specific charge. You are serving on the subcommittee charged with developing the stakeholder matrix, a document identifying all "stakeholders"—those who have an interest in this initiative, how they fit in the organizational structure, what influence they exert, and so forth. These are the people from whom you will collect data and who you will involve in the process and many times in the decision making.

Create a five-column table with the following headings for the columns: Stakeholder Name and Organization; Organizational Role; Influence and Power; Unique Information About This Person/Organization; and Strategies for Communicating and Working With This Person. Each stakeholder will be entered as a new row in the matrix.

Once you design the stakeholder matrix, analyze its importance and how it will be used. Using what you learned in this chapter, create a strategy for each column. For example, determine how you would systematically identify each stakeholder. Develop up to three questions to guide your collection of the data for each column. Then complete this matrix for your college.

Discussion Questions

1. Discuss the pertinent laws that should be considered for this initiative.
2. Describe next steps in the process that would help assure the success of the initiative.
3. Using what you learned in this chapter and by searching the web for distance learning materials, list two likely future directions.

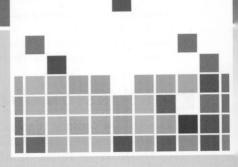

32

Informatics Tools for Educating Healthcare Professionals*

William Scott Erdley and Kay M. Sackett-Fitzgerald

In education, the final record of a student's learning is the limited information included on the transcript. In the manual world of education, for the most part, all other data collected by individual faculty and academic departments are maintained, if at all, in file cabinets or individual faculty files. This can be called the ultimate system for creating an island of lost data and information.

OBJECTIVES

At the completion of this chapter, the reader will be prepared to:

1. Discuss the effectiveness of computerized teaching tools that can be used to deliver education within the traditional classroom environment.
2. Explore computerized applications that can be used to manage educational information and support the work of health-related faculty.
3. Examine the increasing impact of automation, including comprehensive education information systems on the academic policies and procedures of the academy.
4. Outline the impact of computerization on the role and career development of healthcare faculty within the academy.
5. Analyze how technical tools and education information systems can be used to increase the effectiveness and efficiency of faculty.

KEY TERMS

academy, 539
avatar, 546
big data, 538
clicker, 543

comprehensive education information system (CEIS), 539
eBooks, 541
ePortfolio, 545
interactive whiteboard, 540

ABSTRACT ❖

While all levels of education are affected by computerization and the use of technology tools (e.g., course management systems, the internet, computer-based instructional games), it is at the collegiate level that the impact of technology is most keenly felt in health informatics. The educational preparation of healthcare providers is the foundation of a safe, effective, and efficient healthcare delivery system. This chapter addresses the use of education information systems and technical tools to support the work of healthcare faculty and educators charged with the preparation of competent healthcare providers. The impact of the computerization of higher education is described, computerized teaching tools are presented, the impact of computerization on the faculty role is discussed, and the implications for health-related faculty are explored. The increased computerization in institutions of higher education is now creating sets of big data (large datasets). In this chapter the implications of these data and the potential for predictive analytics are explored with a focus on future directions.

*Acknowledgments: We acknowledge the assistance of Dr. Veronica Outlaw, PhD, Director of Distance Learning at the University of South Carolina Aiken. We appreciate her thoughtful comments and suggestions from an instructional design and evidence-based perspective. We also acknowledge the assistance of Dr. Ernesto Perez, Dr. Mary Smith, Dr. Vincent Sperandeo, and Dr. Dara Warren from the DNP graduating class of 2011, Capstone College of Nursing, University of Alabama. We appreciate their thoughtful comments and suggestions for this chapter.

INTRODUCTION

Over the last several decades, the implementation of healthcare computer-based information systems has transformed the healthcare delivery system. That impact is now incorporated within the educational process of healthcare providers. A primary mission of higher education is the education of students to ultimately create an improved healthcare system. These may be students in current degree programs or continuing education. No matter the program, the educational process is supported by a complex administrative infrastructure. The computerization of the academy can be considered from academic and administrative perspectives. The academic perspective focuses on the delivery of learning and student assessment. The administrative perspective focuses on the development of systems and processes supporting the day-to-day operation of the institution. This includes student information systems, financial information systems, and human resources and payroll systems.[1] Both the education of students and the surrounding administrative infrastructure have benefited from the opportunities provided by technology integration. In addition, as new systems in both areas evolve, their functions increasingly overlap, moving toward a comprehensive education information system. Such a system creates the opportunity for increased effectiveness of the learning process and efficiency of the academy. For example, predictive analysis of big data can result in innovative curricula that may prevent academic problems for future students. In this chapter, the computerization of the academy is described, computerized teaching tools are presented, the impact of computerization on the faculty role is discussed, and the implications for health-related faculty are explored.

COMPREHENSIVE EDUCATION INFORMATION SYSTEM

Comprehensive education information systems (CEISs) include the hardware, applications, overlapping and integrated functionality, and data produced by all information systems within an academic setting. This is depicted in Fig. 32.1, which divides the CEIS into three overlapping areas. These are the administrative information systems, the learning management system (LMS), and the academic information tools used in teaching. Overlap of functionality and data flow occurs across the system. For example, a group of students preregisters for an online three-credit theory course and a five-credit related clinical course. As each student registers, the course shell roster for the online course is populated with the student's name. The faculty member then assigns the students to their clinical sections, and these data are sent back to the registration system for transcript and tuition purposes.

Increasingly a common database depicted on the model as big data allows data integration across the institution. The model demonstrates the concept of a CEIS as it applies to an academic institution; however, the concept can be applied to several educational institutions within a larger system. For example, in Ohio, the Higher Education Information (HEI) system (www.ohiohighered.org/hei) includes a comprehensive database with student enrollment, courses, financial aid, personnel, facilities, and finance data submitted by Ohio's colleges and universities. Data are used for a variety of purposes, including reporting on higher education outcomes, funding formula and financial aid, policy analysis, and strategic planning.

One module within the HEI system is the Course Inventory Expert System, which includes decision rules for classifying undergraduate courses with the goal of achieving consistent treatment of undergraduate courses across the system (https://transfercredit.ohio.gov/ap/1?12861140478913). This makes it possible to implement a comprehensive credit transfer system across Ohio's entire public higher education system of 14 universities, 24 regional campuses, and 23

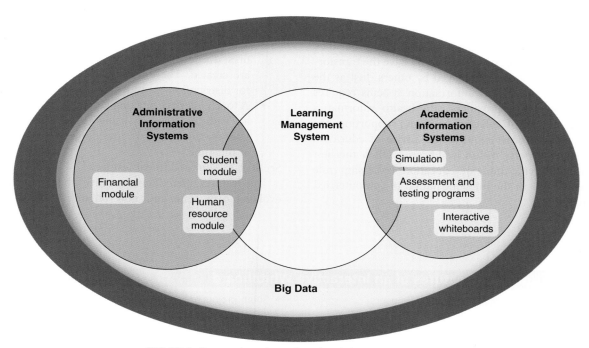

FIG 32.1 Comprehensive education information system.

community colleges. In contrast to traditional approaches, an individual faculty member does not need to review a syllabus and other course materials to decide whether a student can transfer a course.

A second example of how educational administrative systems are changing faculty responsibilities can be seen with the commercially available Typhon Group (http://www.typhongroup.com) products. This company offers a student tracking system targeted at health professional programs. Available packages include modules addressing a wide range of content, stretching from case logs to curriculum mapping to clinical site databases. These examples suggest the potential impact that academic systems will have on the roles and responsibilities of faculty within the academy.

To ensure information systems implemented in health-related education programs support the teaching-learning process and take full advantage of the potential for innovative opportunities offered by automation, health-related faculty must assume a proactive role. Nelson and others identified the following four key areas where faculty should become proactive:

- Identifying data elements and developing standard terminology needed to capture the essence of education with the healthcare professions
- Participating in the development of policies and procedures for securely collecting, accessing, and using faculty, staff, administrative, and student data
- Contributing to the process for selecting, implementing, and integrating education information systems
- Designing educational opportunities to ensure faculty clearly understand the potential of automated academic systems and the importance of participating in these activities[1]

Participating in these activities obviously requires time and effort; at the same time, these activities may not contribute to achieving tenure and promotions. Given this reality, faculty teaching in the health disciplines must decide whether they will play a leadership role or step back and have the transformation of higher education managed by others. Just as the design of effective healthcare information systems requires input from healthcare providers and health informatics experts, the design of effective systems supporting the teaching-learning process requires the advice of educators and informatics experts within healthcare.[1] Often the best way to begin moving into an education leadership role involves working with the implementation of computerized teaching tools.

COMPUTERIZED TEACHING TOOLS

Computerized teaching tools are hardware and software used in the design, implementation, and evaluation of student learning. These tools make it possible to develop creative and innovative learning experiences as well as assess and track student learning.

Hardware

Hardware refers to tangible physical items used in the educational process. These devices are used by students and faculty to engage with each other and educational content, with the goal of increased learning. Hardware includes computer-related tools used in all areas of society, such as laptop computers, tablets, cellphones, and tools specifically designed for education, such as interactive whiteboards and clickers.

Interactive Whiteboards

Historically conventional classrooms within a college or university setting included at minimum a chalkboard across the front of the room. Over time, the chalkboard was supplemented with the use of overheads. The computerization of these basic tools early in the 1990s resulted in the "smart whiteboard" or "interactive whiteboard," which offered innovative approaches to education and the related administrative functions.[2] The boards come in a wide variety of sizes to complement or meet general, and unique, user and environment requirements. These interactive whiteboards are sold with a variety of possible functions, allowing for real-time consultation between faculty and students, real-time editing of documents by geographically distinct persons, and the ability for videoconferencing. Typical features of these interactive tools include the following:

- The ability to project materials from a computer, a document camera, or the internet.
- The ability to write directly on the board, creating figures, documents, and notes that can be edited as they are created. These materials can be saved or printed for distribution to students.
- A touch interface, making it possible for a user to interact with the board by using a finger. A single digit is used for the most part; multifinger use is not common at this time.

See Box 32.1 for additional features.

The features offered on interactive whiteboards have been evolving over time and now often include collaborative

---

BOX 32.1 Common Features of an Interactive Whiteboard

- Wireless (Wi-Fi connectivity, interface with users)
- Touch, keyboard, and mouse capable
- Conferencing capable with multiple concurrent users
- Document editing with two or more concurrent users
- Short projection distance to eliminate walking in front of projection
- Multiple USB ports with easy access

functionality such as conferencing between users anywhere a connection is available. Faculty can use these boards for videoconferencing between classes held on different university campuses or with colleagues located in different areas of the world. However, not all universities provide an interactive whiteboard with a video camera available at both sites. As a result, videoconferencing may be one-sided. Other uses include note creation, thus allowing the instructor to insert notes into a document projected to both sites and create a collaborative distributed classroom. Because of the interactive capabilities, participants in the distance classroom are able to respond by entering their own viewable notes. On the downside, these tools can be expensive, ranging from $1500 for low-end models to $15,000 or more for models with all possible features.

Cheaper priced applications, with many of the same functions as interactive whiteboards, are also available. One example is Google Hangouts (https://plus.google.com), a part of Google+, which includes desktop sharing, Google docs, and other functionalities found on more costly hardware and/or software. However, the price is not without barriers. For instance, typically the number of concurrent videoconferencing attendees is capped. Additional technical issues are possible due to use of Java. Some browsers (for example Chrome) do not work well with Java due to inherent security policies that may conflict with Java. And perhaps not all have access or use of this application for whatever reason (company policy, security concerns, and so forth). Nonetheless, applications such as Hangouts may prove the most cost-effective approach for many users with proper IT support.

However, of special concern when using these types of apps is the issue of student privacy. In 2014, the U.S. Department of Education released guidance on protecting student privacy while using online educational services. Additional information about the Federal Education Records Privacy Act (FERPA) as it applies to institutions of higher education can be found at the U.S. Department of Education Privacy Technical Assistance Center (PTAC). PTAC functions as a resource for education stakeholders to learn about data privacy, confidentiality, and security practices related to student-level longitudinal data systems and other uses of student data. PTAC (http://ptac.ed.gov/) provides current information and updated guidance on privacy, confidentiality, and security practices. It offers a variety of resources, including training materials and opportunities to receive direct assistance with privacy, security, and confidentiality of student data systems.[3]

As educators and legislators become increasing aware of these issues, one can expect to see increasing state and federal legislation and regulations controlling the use of these types of apps. For example, in the fall of 2015, two Pennsylvania representatives, Dan Miller and Tedd Nesbit, introduced a two-bill package, whereby schools could use education technology products that amass, sell, or share student data, but only after notifying parents and allowing them to opt out. "The bills wouldn't ban apps like the poster-making program Glogster, which markets to teachers and indicates in its privacy policy that it may share 'personal information' with 'consumer products, telecom, financial, military, market research, entertainment, and educational services companies and their third party service providers.'"[4]

eReaders and Digital Books

eBooks are an emerging technology for educational users. Initially designed for reading books, eReaders are now branching out to challenge tablet computers. eBook readers have electronic "ink" or electronic paper to render a "page" similar to a printed page found in a book. Only a few technology companies have created digital ink, and many reading devices license the technology from these companies (e.g., Adobe and E Ink). Sony (Reader), Amazon (Kindle), and Barnes & Noble (Nook) are examples of suppliers of these digital reading devices. The advantages of using these media include portability, the ability to adjust font sizes for easier viewing, and large storage capabilities. Some disadvantages are limited backlighting of the page, a need to maintain adequate battery charge, and limited ability for text markup. In the past, these devices were single function, although this is changing. Newer versions of the Kindle (Fire) and Nook (Touch) are evidence of the shift toward multifunctional devices, as these now provide an ability to browse the internet, check e-mail, connect via cellular plan and Wi-Fi, and watch movies on the device, along with reading text-based content. Newer models also support text markup or highlighting.

Additional applications (or apps) are available, permitting eReader functions on non-eReader devices (e.g., iPads and Google devices). However, these apps have limited functionality compared to native eReader devices. Despite this limitation, users are able to connect using the app to access and read current materials without having to use a dedicated eReader. This allows mobile devices such as laptops, smartphones, and tablets to become, in essence, eBook readers making the purchase of a separate eReader unnecessary.

In the health education arena, textbook suppliers are offering electronic texts for students at all levels. Vendors offering electronic textbooks, including Elsevier, Lippincott Williams & Wilkins, McGraw-Hill, and Pearson, often including web-based resources. These books are available in an eReader format such as Kindle and Nook, as well as browser-based format. The browser-based format usually requires a "plug-in" and functions within a LMS software such as Blackboard. The ability to link to web-based resources has appeal for students. Faculty resources are available in a similar fashion in particular, allowing faculty to quiz students via e-textbook-created tests and quizzes. In the last few years, textbook suppliers are also altering the eBook model to allow faculty to purchase or rent (a.k.a. use) needed chapters versus an entire textbook.

The limitations of these eText offerings include cost, availability only as a proprietary publisher eBook or in Adobe Reader file format, reduced print selections, and restricted ability to mark up or highlight text. An early study reported student reluctance to pay for the use of eBooks as well as frustration with the search function within eBooks.[5] In addition, depending on the size of the screen, viewing charts, figures, and other nontext content can be difficult.

The obvious advantages are user mobility and content portability. The ability to integrate graphics, multimedia, and text material is becoming more prominent. eReaders are now able to download files, so the need to maintain online access while reading a text is not required. The prevalence of students interacting with eBooks is increasing, and students are now able to connect to additional resources cited in a text via a URL. Text highlighting is becoming more available. Students may also copy and save, in some cases, text information for later use and/or sharing with others. In the clinical realm, texts, compendiums, and reference materials are now more available to students and other users of this information for patient care at the point of care. However, how these tools can be effectively integrated into the educational process at the point of care is in many ways an unanswered question from both a technical and an academic perspective. For example, if a student is reading a patient's EHR and needs to check a reference for additional information about a drug, lab test, or diagnosis, should the student reference materials be on a separate device, or integrated with the decision support content in the EHR?

A search of the literature using the terms "electronic books" and "nursing education" demonstrates limited information on how these tools are being used. Nonetheless, eBooks, in general, are gaining popularity by users and vendors. Many of the vendor solutions can be integrated with course management software such as Blackboard or Merlot. There is also limited research reported regarding use of such tools by learners. In one study, undergraduate nursing students were very pleased to use eBooks and personal digital assistant (PDA) devices as tools during their clinical rotation.[6]

Smartphones

A smartphone offers a host of additional functionality beyond calling and texting between callers. They have become handheld computers. Some are better at handling graphics (such as movies, pictures, and games), while others offer improved functionality for internet browsing and social media use. Many smartphones are able to take advantage of wireless networks for data transmissions. At this point in time, smartphones with the largest market share operate using either Google's Android or Apple's iOS platform. There are advantages and disadvantages with each operating system and device. Android-based smartphones tend to employ a larger screen size and more powerful chipsets or computer processing units (CPUs) and are able to use additional storage via mini storage disk (SD) cards. iPhones now have variable screen sizes, are not able to take advantage of additional storage, and do not interact well with Adobe Flash–based web applications. However, iPhones do have access to the largest app store, iTunes. Many current smartphones are powered by dual-core low power CPUs. This power, coupled with the size, allows for a large amount of computational horsepower in a small portable device.

Due to their computational power and increasing popularity, the integration of smartphones into both healthcare delivery and education is growing. As of 2014, there were more electronic gadgets (smartphones, cellphones, and tablets) than there are people in the world.[7] In the United States, more than 60% of all adults own a smartphone,[8] with higher rates of ownership in the college setting. In 2014, Pearson reported that 83% of college students regularly use a smartphone. This is up significantly from 72% in 2013.[9] One can expect these numbers to continue growing until they reach almost 100%.

Regardless of the operating system, many smartphones are able to interact with a variety of mainstream educational LMSs, such as Blackboard, Canvas (http://www.canvaslms.com), and Instructure (http://www.instructure.com/). Smartphones can even be "substituted" for handheld classroom interactive devices within CMS software such as Canvas (e.g., i > clicker, http://support.iclicker.com/customer/portal/topics/662688–ic-lms-canvas/articles).

A variety of applications are available for smartphones for health students and practitioners. The more common types are drug reference software such as Davis's Drug Guide and Epocrates. iTunes and Android app stores offer an increasing variety of healthcare applications beyond drug references, including formula calculators, physical assessment guides, protocols such as Advanced Cardiac Life Support (ACLS), Pediatric Advanced Life Support (PALS), and audio assist applications for lung and heart sounds. Many of these apps are free, while others are available for a nominal fee. The free version of an app may not have the full features of the same app with an associated cost. Textbooks and other typically hard copy–only reference manuals are becoming increasingly available for smartphone platforms. There is limited regulation of these types of apps, so one should use caution in assuming every app selected from iTunes and Android app stores will function as described. Testing of apps before using in an educational setting is strongly recommended.

Due to their increasing popularity among students, healthcare providers, and patients, smartphones are increasingly included as requisite tools for education and healthcare practice. Smartphones can interact not only with educational management systems (e.g., Blackboard, Moodle, Joomla) but also with different electronic health record systems. While a wide variety of apps are available, some caution is warranted. Some institutional policies may preclude smartphone use because of potential patient privacy and information security breaches. Every organization has a policy and protocol detailing Health Insurance Portability and Accountability Act (HIPAA) requirements and the use of mobile devices. See Chapters 13 and 26 for additional information on this topic.

Tablets

Tablet computers are another tool available to faculty and students. Tablets are increasing in popularity and use in higher education. Early tablets were bulky and heavy, but the iPad, first available in early 2010, revolutionized widespread tablet use. Lightweight and novel in design, the iPad is a device with strong support from a wide range of software companies. The iPad employs a touch screen user interface that allows users' fingers to maneuver through the internet and documents. A virtual keyboard, with an optional Bluetooth keyboard, provides standard data entry capability. Using almost the same iOS platform as the iPhone, the iPad is rapidly becoming a dominant tablet on the market if not already *the* dominant tablet. However, Windows 10 has succeeded Windows 8, which made it possible to convert a laptop into a tablet computer.

Tablets such as the iPad have proven useful for educators, students, and healthcare providers. Apple has recently released a new version of the iPad to counter the latest version of Microsoft's Surface model. Both are tablets with removable keyboard covers. With the availability of applications similar to the Microsoft Office suite, these devices are becoming increasingly functional for a wide variety of activities. Some current examples include SmartOffice 2 and Documents To Go—Office Suite. The price for these applications can range from free to $50 or more, and they are available only at the App Store run by Apple. Equivalent applications are available for Android platform tablets via the Android App store.

One concern with using these sorts of devices is storage. iPads do not have USB ports for accessing flash storage. Instead users must access online or cloud environments to store and retrieve material. An example of cloud storage is Dropbox (www.dropbox.com), a free service that works on a wide variety of devices and operating systems. The free account for this service includes 2.5 GB of space, which is a fair amount of space for access and storage of a wide variety of documents for educational use. Of a more serious concern is not only reliability and/or accessibility but also security of cloud services. As this storage modality increases in popularity, all too soon preservation of data may require much more than "strong" password accessibility.

Despite the positives, some issues remain. As with any mobile device, battery life varies depending on how the device is used. Simple browsing and word processing will drain the battery at a slower rate than using multiple applications simultaneously. The iPad has a sealed battery, which means that the entire device must be returned to Apple Service for any battery service. Another limitation relates to use. Tablets, for the most part, are not replacements for office computers but rather adjuncts to them. The built-in virtual keyboard is not conducive to long periods of use. Tablets, including the iPad, are more suited to an educational environment than smartphones. Because common eReader devices have applications available for tablets, reading textbooks and accessing course management applications is feasible. Most tablets include a built-in webcam, providing users with the ability to videoconference on many courses and seminars. The physical footprint of these devices makes them more appealing to some users than a laptop.

Laptops and Desktop Computers

Historically, the desktop computer was the mainstay of academic computing; however, desktop computers are declining in popularity. Laptops are now more popular computing devices for educational use. A fairly robust laptop can be purchased for around $500, about the same cost as a comparably equipped or more powerful desktop. The portability of laptops or tablets is often the deciding factor for students and faculty. The increasing availability of broadband access is an additional strong influence for users. Students and faculty are able to access courses and content from anywhere with internet access. Many online courses promote this aspect of their respective programs. For an in-person class, students often bring a computing device with them to take notes, research a topic, and link items for reference at a later time. A subcategory of the laptop category, called ultrabook, is a smaller and lighter device that sacrifices a device drive (typically a DVD) and a spinning hard drive for a solid-state drive (SSD). Most major vendors now offer at least one ultrabook model.

Clickers

A clicker is a device used with an audience response system; however, the term *clicker* is often used to refer to the complete system. These systems provide faculty with real-time feedback from learners during a presentation. The device itself is about the size of a deck of cards or smaller and wirelessly linked, via sensors in the room, to a computer that records the responses. Software is available for those who want to use their own smartphone as the feedback device. Instructors phrase questions as if administering a poll and ask students to respond using the clickers. Questions can be basic ("Do you understand the concept?—Yes or no") or more complex ("What are the best options to solve a stated problem?"). Many users employ a multiple-choice approach, and feedback questions can be embedded in a Microsoft PowerPoint presentation. Real-time feedback can be depicted in graphic format to help the instructor and audience understand the results of the poll. Examples of companies offering this technology include eInstruction (www. einstruction.com), i > clicker (www.iclicker.com), and Turning Technologies (www.turningtechnologies.com).

Audience response systems, also available for conference settings, have been integrated into webinar delivery type products. Uses include determining the winner of a competition, helping the audience understand a concept or information by helping the presenter to shape the presentation to meet the audience's needs, and facilitating interactivity. There are several positive aspects of this technology. No matter the device, responses are typically anonymous, although the system can be set up to tie the response to the user, for example, to take classroom attendance. The anonymity may provide more honest responses. Audience response technology provides course instructors or conference presenters with immediate feedback. The immediacy of the response allows presenters to customize content to clarify audience concerns, meet audience needs, and facilitate user interaction and involvement with the educational content.

Barriers to this technology include instructor resistance to changing a class format; the time commitment to reformat a course; the cost of the devices, sensors, setup time, and software; system maintenance; and possible student resistance to the cost of the technology (i.e., another fee) and the need to learn and use more technology. For some instructors, the device is a novelty, good for occasional use rather than a mainstream method of learning. For many faculty, their respective educational employer provides readily accessible guides, suggestions, and/or evidence-based research regarding use of clicker and other pedagogical technologies in the classroom and beyond. A good example of this can be found at the University of Wisconsin–Milwaukee (http://www4.uwm.edu/ltc/srs/faculty/articles_research.cfm).

Educational Software

Many choices exist for faculty and students, but there are some general considerations when selecting educational software. Many schools provide assistance to their respective faculty regarding the selection and/or use of educational software. This type of software can be proprietary, such as Microsoft Word, or open source, such as OpenOffice. Even though downloading and installing open source software is free, there are costs associated with obtaining support and maintenance for the software. Support and maintenance can also be an additional cost with proprietary software and should be negotiated before signing a contract. In addition, many educational software products have hardware limitations that should be carefully evaluated during the selection process. A number of products are discussed in this section, including learning and content management systems, mind maps, gaming, and ePortfolios.

Learning and Content Management Systems

An LMS is generally defined as software used to address educational functions, ranging from class administration and document and grade tracking to report generation and delivery of online courses.[7] These systems are mainly used as course management systems delivering hybrid or online courses. However, they can also be used for other group activities such as setting up access to online advising or university enrollment services.

LMSs can also provide content management functionality at the program or university level. However, a separate content management system or application can also be used for this purpose. A content management system encompasses the process of content development (create, edit, store, and deliver) and storage of learning materials such as PowerPoint slides, videos, and so forth that can be used in different courses for different purposes. Depending on the vendor, a content management system may be a component of an LMS or can function in a solo capacity with an interface to an LMS.[10] It should be noted that when used in higher education literature, the acronym CMS usually refers to a course management system, as denoted in Chapter 30, but can also refer to a content management system, as described here.

LMSs are increasingly used by higher education institutions for distance education and as a supplement to traditional classroom education. LMSs allow for asynchronous access, online meetings, and remote testing and grading, as well as inline grading of learner assignments. Student assessment is a large component of an LMS. Blackboard, for instance, includes a dashboard for faculty to monitor student progress. Barriers to use of an LMS include the need for a broadband connection by students and the use of certain operating systems, although these barriers are fading over time. The largest barrier is the cost to purchase and maintain an LMS, especially a proprietary system. A detailed discussion of distance education, and the use of LMSs, is provided in Chapter 31.

Mind Maps

Mind maps are graphic or visual representations connecting words, ideas, tasks, or other items to a central core word or idea.[11] This type of activity may also be called a concept map. The visualization provides students with a tool to see how various components are related to a particular core idea or item (e.g., categories of medications and pain management, specific drug side effects related to a specific disease process). An example of a mind map is shown in Fig. 32.2.

While individual students can use mind map software, it can also be used by students collaborating in face-to-face or online groups to create mind maps via an assortment of point devices (from fingers to color-coded digital markers). Maps can be saved and referenced for later review or incorporated into a student's ePortfolio (discussed later) as an example of his or her work. The interactive creation of mind maps or concept maps can also be a tool for educators in healthcare. Studies indicate concept maps facilitate critical thinking as well as student engagement.[12,13] Mind maps are also visually appealing for students. However, software costs may be a barrier, although other hardware platforms such as interactive whiteboards or LMSs can reduce overall costs.

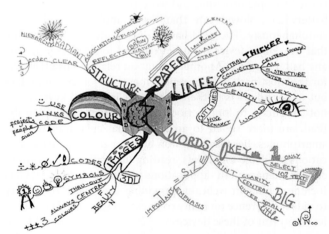

FIG 32.2 An example of a mind map. (From *Litemind*. What is mind mapping? [and how to get started immediately]. Litemind.com. <http://litemind.com/what-is-mind-mapping/>; 2012.)

Digital Portfolios

The electronic portfolio, or ePortfolio, reflects a shift from the pen-and-paper portfolio model to a digital environment. The components of an ePortfolio are basically the same as a traditional portfolio but stored and presented in a digital format. The general structure, with some variation depending on the profession or department, includes a curriculum vita, a personal statement of some sort, a description of personal skills, and examples of the individual's work. The work example category, using the digital format, allows for digitization of pictures, movies, and other similar interactive presentations of personal work. The ePortfolio provides an improved process for an individual to present a detailed picture of his or her work. Examples of commercial software supporting this concept include Google (https://sites.google.com/site/eportfolioapps/overview), Desire 2Learn ePortfolio (https://documentation.desire2learn.com/en/ePortfolio), and Brightspace. (http://www.brightspace.com/products/eportfolio/). In addition, many higher education institutions offer homegrown as well as proprietary products to their users and learners.

Many educational programs require ePortfolios as a component of student learning and evaluation. However, the requirement that students complete an ePortfolio and the procedures for using portfolios and ePortfolios vary greatly from one institution to another. For example, requiring that a student complete an ePortfolio could ensure that students would be able to show future employers examples of their work. However, many institutions do not provide students with access to their ePortfolios after graduation.

A significant advantage of using ePortfolios is that faculty can use them to provide individualized feedback and advice to students. Drawbacks include a lack of quality assurance and the amount of time that ePortfolios consume for both student and faculty.[14] Research on using portfolios (and ePortfolios) in educational applications is limited. Nonetheless, this application facilitates student self-evaluation and continues to be a useful tool in education.

Web-Based Student Testing

Other educational tools include applications that facilitate online, or web-based, student testing. Web-based testing is usually independent of an operating system, and the testing software is accessed using a web browser. Most LMSs (e.g., Blackboard, Moodle) support web-based testing options. Within an application, tests can be customized to question type (e.g., multiple choice, multiple answer, write-in, matching, essay). Common features of online testing solutions include the ability to control student access, length of tests, time available to take the test, feedback customization, and score analyses. Instructors can randomize the order of questions for each person taking the test. Obviously randomization helps discourage screen sharing and easy answer sharing between students. Testing within an LMS is advantageous because the test score is automatically integrated into the LMS

grading module and students receive immediate feedback on their performance. In nursing, web-based NCLEX review content is available. Examples of companies providing this testing include ATI (http://www.atitesting.com/Home.aspx) and Kaplan (http://www.kaptest.com/NCLEX/Home/index.html). Both companies provide materials and tests for faculty to use and integrate in their programs.

Online testing tools usually can be configured to administer surveys to students. Other freestanding survey-specific tools are available for limited, if any, cost (e.g., SurveyMonkey, www.surveymonkey.com). More powerful and costly tools are also available. Proprietary applications often include a free version with limitations, but these are useful for trying out the software. A well-known example is Qualtrics (www.qualtrics.com).

The advantages of web-based testing include faculty control and customization, the ability to incorporate feedback on a question-by-question basis, and immediate scoring available to the student. Faculty may incorporate these tests into mastery learning, where students who have not done well on the test can relearn and retest before moving on to new content.

Security issues can present a major disadvantage for online testing. Students may share tests either visually (sitting next to each other), remotely, or by using a browser with less security (allowing screenshots to be saved and shared); they may even report a power failure to quickly look up answers to a test. Solutions to security issues such as plagiarism and sharing may be found with an application such as Proctorio, a remote software proctoring application (www.proctorio.com). Proctorio can be integrated into the CMS for greater ease of use by faculty and learners. Another software example is Software Secure (www.softwaresecure.com). Each of these examples allows for remote student proctoring, which decreases the need for on-site personal proctoring.

As with all software in academia, the users, such as faculty, should agree on the software as needed, appropriate, and functional for all users, including students, before adoption. Additional concerns for use of this type of software may be how the webcam is placed (for remote viewing), along with the scan intervals of the student learner during the assessment and/or test. In addition, policy and procedure needs should be addressed prior to development and implementation of such software.

Student Journaling Software

Journaling is a methodology to engage students in reflective learning. Reflective journaling is often used to evaluate students' clinical or practicum progress; at the same time, it improves critical thinking by providing students with insight into their own experiences and performance. Paper journals with handwritten faculty comments and questions were cumbersome and have been replaced by digital applications providing easy access for faculty and more timely responses for students. These applications can be as simple as using blog applications to create an online diary. Free services are available, such as Blogger (www.blogger.com) or Google Drive (http://www.google.com/drive/). In both of these examples, the preference section includes the option of adjusting privacy settings to protect the students' work from the general public. Before using these types of free services for class assignments, faculty should review the site's terms and conditions as well as the privacy statement students must accept before use. These documents are legal contracts, and using the site is the same as signing a printed contract. A number of LMSs also include this option but usually do not raise the same legal issues.

Gaming

Learning games, often termed "serious games," are designed to entertain players as they educate, train, or change behavior.[15] They may be used to vary course content delivery and provide students with an active learning environment. As such, they are useful teaching strategies in healthcare.[15] Gaming commonly involves competition (a winner and a loser). This element helps compel students to engage in the content, thereby improving learning. A number of topics can be used for gaming, from learning metabolic pathways to critical care for surgical patients.[16]

Gaming software typically involves the use of a game format, such as Jeopardy, Wheel of Fortune, a board game, or a card game, to engage students. PowerPoint templates of some television games are even available for faculty. Gaming does not always require information technology; it can be very low tech and still work well. Simple gaming formats can be relatively easy and inexpensive to use. In addition, a number of higher complexity computer games have been developed to provide interactive learning for students. Some examples include Critical Decisions (http://virtualheroes.com/portfolio/Medical/Critical-Decisions) and Virtual Pain Manager (http://vpm.glam.ac.uk/).

Other applications use a computer gaming interface without being a game. For instance, one vendor, Anesoft (www.anesoft.com), produces a wide variety of browser-based software targeting for clinical specialties such as critical care and anesthesia. The two-dimensional application simulates patient care by providing the student with a picture of the patient along with vital signs and laboratory results. The student is able to evaluate patient data, make decisions, and view the results of those decisions. These materials can be especially useful in teaching groups of interprofessional students to work together in teams. Regardless of the format, gaming provides active learning and student engagement in an approach that is usually well received by students.

Virtual Worlds

Virtual worlds are computerized settings that simulate a world without traditional boundaries. Typically the setting in a virtual world is viewed as three-dimensional. Avatars (computer-generated objects that may or may not be humanlike) are characters that users adopt and portray as their own personalities in the virtual world. Avatars then interact with each other within the virtual world setting. For example, the setting may be a hospital, a clinic, or a community setting. The virtual environment can provide different experiences for health education students by allowing students to experience different settings and/or different roles via their avatars. They can practice different aspects of care, ranging from communication (since avatars can speak) to clinical skills. This makes the use of virtual worlds an excellent tool for simulation-type learning with groups of students from a variety of disciplines.

One of the earliest well-developed virtual world–based applications is Second Life (http://secondlife.com), a browser-based experience requiring the user to install a viewer on his or her computer. Users create their own avatar or virtual person and experience the environment of Second Life. Another example of a virtual world software application is OpenSimulator (http://opensimulator.org/wiki/Main_Page). OpenSimulator is an open source application used to simulate virtual environments similar to Second Life, with much of the same functionality.

Although there could be several potential advantages to the use of virtual world applications, their use has been limited by four major constrictions:

- *Creativity.* Creating a realistic simulation requires that one is able to conceptualize all of the complex detail and interaction present in an actual healthcare setting. As a result, faculty often find it helpful to select one of these applications and work together in developing learning environments.
- *Time requirements.* Major time commitments can be required for learning the software and developing stimulation.
- *Direct and indirect costs.* For example, access to Second Life is available to the viewer without charge. However, there are costs associated with developing student-learning environments within Second Life. In general, for one private region in Second Life (or what is sometimes called an "island"), the initial one-time set-up fee listed on their website (http://wiki.secondlife.com/wiki/Second_Life_Education/FAQs) on October 15, 2016, was $1000 USD and then $295 USD a month in maintenance costs, per region. Educators can be offered a 50% discount. In addition, indirect costs can increase quickly when one hires an assistant to develop or maintain the virtual environment.
- *Technology limitation.* For example, there is no sensory feedback such as odor or touch (haptics), which can be a barrier for some experiences.

Originally these virtual worlds were designed for fantasy experiences, but they have evolved to support not only education but also others such as those with compromised health. For example, in a virtual world, physically handicapped persons are without limitations and can enjoy activities such as dancing, swimming, and walking. Healthcare sites, created by health professionals, representing hospitals, clinics, and recreational areas, can provide a potential means of engagement and support for patients. However, research suggests that the use of online virtual environments has not yet reached this potential opportunity. Suomi, Mäntymäki, and Söderlund reported in 2014 on the results of a review of the current health-related activity in Second Life. The intent of the study was to determine whether Second Life was a working and functional platform supporting the empowerment of people in health-related issues. They concluded from their research that "For the average user, Second Life offers very little unique value compared to other online health resources."[17]

IMPACT ON THE TEACHING AND LEARNING PROCESS

Today, technology drives a teaching-learning process that is increasingly student centered, faculty facilitated, collaborative, open sourced, and globally focused, using a blend of synchronous and asynchronous modalities focused on contextual learning to enhance the acquisition of new knowledge for both students and faculty. The ripple effects of the paradigm change is evident, with intergenerational differences in teaching and learning styles, the time requirements of teaching, faculty evaluations, and impact on tenure.

The use of technology in education is changing both educators' and students' roles and responsibilities. For example, educational theorists have acknowledged that individuals learn in different ways. Several examples of learning theories are provided in Chapter 2. Perhaps one of the most adopted theoretical approaches used in education to explain these individual differences is Gardner's multiple intelligences. Gardner determined that people learn through nine different intelligences: linguistic, logical-mathematical, spatial, bodily-kinesthetic, musical, interpersonal, intrapersonal, naturalistic, and existentialist. Gardner determined that while everyone uses all nine intelligences with some degree of competence, one or two of the intelligences are more dominant in each individual (Box 32.2).[18]

For several decades, educators have attempted to individualize the process of educating students by creating instructional materials and experiences to address individual students' intelligences or learning styles. Today's technology can make that goal a reality. Matching students' nine intelligences or learning styles through the use of technology allows for more meaningful educational experiences.[19,20] Essentially,

faculty and students are engaged in subtle and not-so-subtle shifts in technology-driven changes that will continue to transform the process of teaching and learning.

Teaching From a Global Perspective

Creating and delivering learning relevant to students is a challenge for educators and education systems worldwide. The advent of twenty-first century technologies and global connectivity offers students who are geographically dispersed the opportunity to enroll in online courses around the world. Busy adults worldwide especially appreciate the predominantly asynchronous format of online courses. Culturally, however, students worldwide are exposed to a variety of different teaching and learning experiences; teachers' expectations of student behavior differ; and communication styles differ; as does the reading, writing, comprehension, speaking and idioms/slang of a foreign language. The need for social presence, patience, cultural context, extra student mentoring, and a designated virtual place for all students to ask questions and discuss course information becomes extraordinarily important. It is essential faculty and instructional designers who create and deliver online courses are mindful of how everyone's personal cultural lens influences learning.[21–23] Brodrick provides several suggestions for managing classes with online global students:

- Learners who may not be used to the specifics of the typical U.S. online classroom. Provide easy, clean, and clear navigability of online courses and content.
- Students who may not have ideal internet connectivity in their locations abroad. Consider accessibility and speed when creating learning experiences.
- Learning groups who may not share time zones, culture, and language. Provide support in complex logistical planning such as identifying and managing student time zones, managing deadlines, and setting up cooperative.
- Provide culturally sensitive imagery, content, and graphics for a global audience.
- Students from a wide variety of language backgrounds may have difficulty hearing or reading the language used in the course. When possible, provide clear text and voice/video recording of course content.

BOX 32.2 **Examples of Learning Activities Using Gardner's Nine Multiple Intelligences**

- Develop podcasts, wikis, or blogs for the expressive linguistic learner.
- Play online strategy games, search databases for information, or use graphics packages for the logical-mathematical learner.
- Create a digital story, develop a digital art project, or create a concept map for the visual creative spatial learner.
- Interact with software programs to write and create music or to create a music video or podcast for the auditory musical learner.
- Create experiences with simulation, virtual field trips, or virtual role-playing games for the bodily-kinesthetic learner.

- Expound on discussion boards or develop embedded audio and video PowerPoint presentations for online class introductions for the interpersonal learner.
- Write a blog, develop online survey tools, and encourage independent exploration of any of the aforementioned activities for the intrapersonal learner.
- Develop photo journals or use mapping and graphic organizing software for the naturalistic learner.
- Use web research, presentation applications, e-mail, and chat to encourage big-picture thinking (questioning, analyzing, and figuring out why things work) for the existentialist learner.

- All students like to make a good impression and can be somewhat uncomfortable in new situations with strangers. Use videoconferencing and live chat to put them at ease and help them to connect with the instructor and fellow students.
- Consider using more smartphones and mobile applications, since not everyone has computer access.
- End the traditional lecture and replace it with easily accessible, open source, short educational videos.
- Use free web tools for course discussions and projects to better prepare students for jobs after college.
- Encourage scholarly associations to set up blog-like online forums to allow scholars to share ideas and openly conduct peer review.

When offering courses on an international stage, there is a need to evaluate the changes in education and consider both student and faculty self-expectations for learning.[24–26] Proponents of interprofessional learning, both nationally and internationally, suggest that students and faculty need to learn with, from, and about each other. As the emphasis on teacher-centered, didactic instruction changes to a student-centered, interdisciplinary, faculty-facilitated, and collaborative approach to learning, shared experiences and collaborative learning have the potential to break down the traditional professional silos that exist both nationally and internationally. The use of information systems and technology strategies, such as online course delivery, could help facilitate shared interprofessional knowledge building and knowledge mobilization and transfer this collaboratively generated new knowledge into practice.[26–28]

IMPACT ON THE FACULTY ROLE

Faculty are now being asked to be proactive in the adoption and integration of technology while maintaining traditional research, practice, and service requirements. The impact of this demand on faculty satisfaction, time related to teaching, student evaluations, and tenure can be dramatic. While many faculty have enthusiastically embraced the use of technology in the classroom, faculty have also expressed concerns about being undervalued, the changing focus of pedagogy, compensation and workload issues (especially the amount of time necessary to create and maintain technology-enhanced courses), the lack of institutional support for these new teaching methods, and the need to continually update their own technology skills without compensation or institutional support.[29,30]

Nelson et al.[1] and Moseley[31] remind us the cultures of technology and academia differ, as demonstrated by a quote from Nelson: "The cultures of information technology and academia are characterized by competing traits. Words like *ubiquitous, youthful, volatile, instantaneous,* and *profitable* are used to define information technology. Conversely, words such as *steadfast, autonomous, venerable, persistence, resistant, patient,* and *non-lucrative* are words we associate with

academia."[1, p. 194] Faculty are now being asked to reach across this divide. Institutions of higher education must help by investing in high levels of support and training for faculty and students who use technology.

Technology-enhanced courses as well as online and hybrid courses have become an integral part of the teaching-learning experiences provided in today's higher educational settings. Historically, the majority of faculty of many disciplines had limited education in the teaching-learning process and had limited knowledge about the process of effectively transitioning from the traditional lecture-based classroom to a technology-enhanced course. In many traditional academic settings, the distance learning infrastructure has only recently been retooled to fully facilitate health professional faculty preparedness to create and teach using current technology. If they have not already developed a formal faculty development program, institutions of higher education may want to consider partnerships with other institutions to develop such programs as well as pair faculty with instructional designers (ID) to provide support and training for creating robust, quality, and pedagogically sound courses.[32–37] Effective collaboration between an ID and health profession faculty member does not occur in a happenstance manner but must be carefully structured. The collaboration requires knowledge of the best practices available to develop, implement, and evaluate an online course, plus the content expertise of health professions faculty. Box 32.3 uses Outlaw's Six-Phase Course Development Model[32] as a framework for demonstrating the process of collaboration between an ID and expert faculty, with the goal of collaboratively developing, reviewing, implementing, and evaluating a quality technology-enhanced course.

Using Best Practices for Technology-Enhanced Course

The phrase *best practice* refers to an industry-wide agreement concerning the most efficient and effective procedure or process to accomplish a desired outcome.[38] The drive toward best practice is increasingly based on professionals' use of evidence-based research to support quality online education.[32,35,40–42,47–50] The following websites, which are excellent examples of toolkits and online references for best practice in online education, are provided for your reference:

- <https://sph.uth.edu/faculty/instructional-development/online-education-best-practice-reference-list/>[51]
- <http://sites.duke.edu/onlineguide/>[52]
- <http://citt.ufl.edu>[50]
- <http://cgsnet.org/best-practices/graduate-education-2020>[47]

Quality may be defined as "how good or bad something is; a characteristic or feature that someone or something has; something that can be noticed as a part of a person or a thing; and/or a high level of value.[43] Quality Matters (QM) is a quality assurance program used inter-institutionally both nationally and internationally. QM is one example, based

Phase	Description
1	This phase involves conducting a comprehensive needs analysis of (1) the subject matter expert, (2) the course, and (3) the audience.
2	In this phase, faculty begin the process of designing the course in its entirety, including readings, lectures, assignments, discussions, assessments. The instructional designer reviews this work, making edits and recommendations concerning instructional strategies and instructions; they also provide guidance where accessibility, copyright, and media are concerned, and design instruction and learning objects.
3	It is at this point in the process the faculty is ready to be trained on the use of the selected technology. This not only includes how to use the technology but also includes pedagogy so that the faculty is prepared to effectively use the technology to support learning.
4	In this phase, the course is built into the technology. Any issues or concerns in design, pedagogy, or technology should be resolved during this phase.
5	The course review and quality assurance phase is where the course as a whole is reviewed in detail to identify and resolve any pending issues across the course or between sections of the course.
6	The phase can be considered a "shakedown cruise" when the course is implemented. The ID should be available to help resolve immediate problems. In addition, a weekly journal should be kept, noting what worked well as well as problems. In addition, faculty should keep notes on new and innovative ideas about how the course may be strengthened in the future.
7	In the last phase, the course will be revised and taught to a new group of students using all that was learned in the first six phases.

on ongoing research evidence and best practice, of how higher education faculty who use a proprietary peer review process for course development and an established rubric are able to continuously enhance the design quality of online and blended courses.[44] There are eight general standards and specific review standards that must be aligned with course components.[44] The eight general standards are (1) course overview and introduction, (2) learning objectives (competencies), (3) assessment and measurement, (4) instructional materials, (5) course activities and learner interaction, (6) course technology, (7) learner support, and (8) accessibility and usability. Course components that are aligned include learning objectives, assessment and measurement, resources and materials, learner engagement, and course technology,

all linked together to support students' course learning objectives.[45]

Courses approved by QM certified peer reviewers are considered to have attained a gold standard in higher education. For further exploration of QM, the contents of *The American Journal of Distance Education* September 2015 edition is dedicated to articles that address the use of research and quality, QM as an ongoing design-based research project, measuring the impact of the QM rubric, small student focused studies to determine the effect of standardization of online course design and peer review, peer review and feedback as an intervention, and the exponential growth of QM used nationally and internationally, plus a vision for the future.[44,46].

A scenario with two short exemplars incorporating best practices is presented next to illustrate a course development partnership between a nursing faculty member and an ID working together at an institution of higher education.

Scenario

A nursing faculty member wanted to create an engaging online course for undergraduate and graduate students participating in an international experience with Japanese faculty and students. Collaboration with an ID facilitated development and use of an online learning environment created in Blackboard for American students. The incorporation of best practices for online experiential teaching and learning by faculty, students, and the ID were shared with a consortium of Japanese school faculty and selected students. Sequelae included multiple presentations at traditional conferences as well as a virtual conference. Tables 32.1 and 32.2 briefly describe the technology tools used, collaborative design partnership roles, and selected best practices for creating an engaging, quality online educational experience for nursing students.

Impact of Technology Enhanced Courses on Faculty Evaluation

While faculty are working to maximize the benefits of technology in the classroom, the inclusion of technology can potentially have a significant impact on student course evaluations. Student evaluations for faculty teaching with technology in general are limited, and as a result, some have looked to research concerning faculty teaching online where more data is available. These findings have been mixed, ranging from lower scores for faculty teaching online versus face to face to no difference in scores.[50,51] In addition, if the students experience a number of technical problems, their overall satisfaction with the course will be decreased, and this dissatisfaction can be reflected in their rating of the teacher. This can be especially troublesome in settings where student evaluations of faculty play a significant role in determining promotion and tenure decisions.

TABLE 32.1 Nursing Faculty Exemplar #1

Technology Tools, Collaboration Between Experts, and Best Practices

Technology Tools	Nursing Faculty Content Expert	Instructional Designer Role	Best-Practices Online Education
Blackboard	Portal to develop and deliver course content. Students required to submit an image and text-based biography for the introductory flipbooks; weekly blogs; submit a reflective evaluation paper and student presentations (incorporating images and/or video).	ID created a course shell that included the announcement, syllabus, gradebook, e-mail, homepage (with the link to the introductory flipbook), blogs, journals, assignments in course drop box (reflective evaluation paper and student presentations), transcultural videos, faculty welcome video, published journal articles from the Japanese faculty, and links to external website.	Using the announcements, syllabus, e-mail, and a well-designed homepage could make for clear instructions on how students get started in a course and where to find various course components (Quality Matters (QM) #1.1).[61] The flipbook and faculty welcome video are appropriate for building community and presence in an online course (QM #1.8, 1.9).[61–63] The assignments (blogs, papers, and presentations) were forms of assessments that were varied and sequenced (QM #3.4), and aligned with the learning objectives (QM #3.1).[61] The course blogs provided the opportunity to continue online community building,[62] and the journal allowed private communications with the faculty, which enhanced faculty presence.[63]
Desktop computers and laptops	Medium used to create, deliver, and access online course as well as collaborate with students and colleagues.	ID operated desktop computer to navigate to geographical locations (using GoogleEarth) during the taping of the introduction video. The desktop was used for the international conference call via Blackboard Collaborate software. Laptops used by faculty and students to access the online course and communicate with peers.	The best practice of ensuring all participants (faculty and students) are aware, and know, which hardware to use to access content. For example, it is not advisable to access a course from a mobile device, as some options and features may not be accessible. The smaller the device, in general, the more restrictive the view.
Google Earth	Faculty described travel from American university to hotel and university in metropolitan Japan.	ID operated desktop computer to navigate to geographical locations during the videotaping of the faculty introduction video. In addition, a storyboard was created to organize and direct the scenes in the introduction video, along with a script to allow faculty to read from the teleprompter.	Incorporating GoogleEarth with the faculty welcome video allowed faculty presence[63] and enhanced student engagement.[58,60] Storyboard.[63] Scripts were used to guide the faculty narration while taping the video[64] and also provided a means to ensure the video met accessibility requirements with closed captioning and transcription (QM #8.2, 8.3, 8.4).[62]

Continued

TABLE 32.1 **Nursing Faculty Exemplar #1—cont'd**

Technology Tools, Collaboration Between Experts, and Best Practices

Technology Tools	Nursing Faculty Content Expert	Instructional Designer Role	Best-Practices Online Education
Green screens (including storyboards and scripts for lectures)	Faculty and ID worked together to create storyboard using PowerPoint and a scripted narration.	The use of GreenScreen allowed the integration of GoogleEarth and other interactive background props (i.e., flying airplane). The ID advised on the proper attire and colors to wear. The green color family makes the user appear transparent and patterns appear as moving dots on the screen in postproduction.	GreenScreen and GoogleEarth aid in producing interactive and engaging multimedia for active learning.[62]
Flipbook	Orientation to faculty and student.	ID used FlipSnack flipbook to have faculty, ID, and students introduce themselves (including an image) to their peers.	Course introductions help build community in a faceless environments and increases presence (Quality Matters #1.8, 1.9).[61–63]
Blackboard Blogging for purposes of class journaling	Students' journaled daily experiences (including images and video).	ID set up the Blackboard Blog tool with instructions and tutorials to correctly use this tool.	Blogging builds community and provides an avenue for students to engage and interact with each other.[47]
Blackboard Journaling for purpose of communicating with faculty regarding any concerns	Students had the option of using the journal tool or e-mail tool to communicate with faculty.	ID set up the Blackboard Journal tool to give students the option to communicate with the faculty through this medium.	The journal option (like e-mail) offers students individual communication with faculty, which promotes faculty presence.[63]
Static or voice over MS-Powerpoint presentations (Screencast-O-Matic)	Student requirements included the completion of a static PowerPoint (undergraduate) and voice-over PowerPoint presentations using Screencast-O-Matic (graduates).	ID created tutorials for using Screencast-O-Matic and how to upload or link the videos and/or PowerPoints in the Blog tool.	Creating assignments requiring integration of multiple technologies provides opportunity for students to engage and interact with the content. The outcome results in a product engaging users.[62]
Image attachments	Students were encouraged to include images of daily experiences and upload them to the Blog tool.	ID posted a video tutorial on how to attach and/or upload images to the Blog tool.	Including images in a blog of text allows the author to break the monotony of text and provides alternatives for readers who have different learning styles.[65]
Blackboard Collaborate	Used for synchronous collaboration between United States and Japan.	ID discussed the ID role in the project and attempted to address questions from the Chiba faculty and students. **International Issues**: Blackboard Collaborate bandwidth issues arose, along with interoperability and software access.	Synchronous communications eliminated the geographical barriers and allowed users to interact in real-time to actively collaborate. This form of delivery also aids in building community,[62] faculty presence,[63] student engagement,[46,62] and possibly increased student retention.[65]

Continued

TABLE 32.1　Nursing Faculty Exemplar #1—cont'd

Technology Tools, Collaboration Between Experts, and Best Practices

Technology Tools	Nursing Faculty Content Expert	Instructional Designer Role	Best-Practices Online Education
AvayaLive Engage: Online submission process for abstracts, uploading PowerPoint presentations creating avatars, presenting content, and polling feature	Opportunity for nursing faculty, undergraduate and graduate students, and the ID to participate in a virtual conference hosted by two institutions of higher education.	ID implemented a polling application within AvayaLive (https://engage.avayalive.com/engage/). ID and faculty created the PowerPoint presentation for the conference, which included data from the Blackboard Chiba course experience of overall summary of user activity.	Polling allows faculty to obtain immediate feedback on student knowledge.[62] Answers can be broadcast to engage with students about how they fared on the assessment.

ID, Instructional designers; *QM,* quality matters.

TABLE 32.2　Nursing Faculty Member Scenario Exemplar #2

A Nursing Faculty Member With the Assistance of an Instructional Designer Incorporates Experiential Learning Activities in Selected Online Graduate Courses

Categories	Technology Tools	Nursing Faculty Content Expert	Instructional Designer Role	Best Practices for Online Education
Matching activities for population health course	Assessment option in Blackboard	Match words to concepts identified in each chapter	Faculty are asked to explain the purpose of the interactivity so the ID can plan how to set it up, which software would be best to use, and how to integrate it with the LMS, especially if grading is involved. At the outcome of the activity, what is expected of the student?	Providing gaming and other types of learning objects; provides students the opportunities to interact and engage with the content. It also provides a means for self-assessment for immediate feedback.[58]
Mind maps/ concept mapping	https://bubbl.us Free software	DNP student assignment used to conceptualize a capstone and/or a healthcare informatics project.	Typically ID researches the tool, compares brands and features, then suggests the most appropriate tool. The ID learns how to use the tool and disseminates the knowledge.	Keywords used to describe the reason, or reasons, for this tool, such as critical thinking, become the keywords the ID uses to search and match up with best practices.
APA format software	https://www.perrla.com Free software to assist students with APA formatting of scholarly papers.	Faculty suggestion or requirement for scholarly papers or assignments.	ID would suggest providing students with a practice assignment to get familiar with using the tool. The feedback would help with the mastery of the writing and the use of the tool.	Practice, feedback, self-assessment[62]
Cloud-based secure testing software	https://proctorio.com Free software demo with a lease/purchase option	Faculty require safe, secure encrypted online examinations for students	Generally an institutional decision made by faculty in consultation with ID or faculty technology experts.	Clarification of the focus is requisite to locate relevant best practices. (Is this about assessments and/or is the purpose for academic integrity?)

Continued

TABLE 32.2   Nursing Faculty Member Scenario Exemplar #2—cont'd

A Nursing Faculty Member With the Assistance of an Instructional Designer Incorporates Experiential Learning Activities in Selected Online Graduate Courses

Categories	Technology Tools	Nursing Faculty Content Expert	Instructional Designer Role	Best Practices for Online Education
Google for Education	Google Docs, Google Hangouts, Desktop Sharing https://www.google.com/edu/	Need faculty input	The ID would generally suggest the use of new tools to be incorporated into an introductory assignment. This gives students the opportunity to get acclimated to the new tool(s) so that they prepare to work on assignments using the tools and they are not struggling to complete them. Doing this eliminates frustration, with the main focus being "the use of the tool" and not the actual outcomes for the assignment.	Open educational resources for file sharing, collaboration/sharing, synchronous contributions, engaging, interactive, and so on.
Typhon	Student tracking systems for nursing and health education programs http://www.typhongroup.com/	Supported for adoption by faculty, administration	May participate in the discussion related to cost, effectiveness, adoption, continued evaluation, and implementation	

APA, American Psychological Association; *ID,* Instructional designer; *LMS,* learning management system.

Other related barriers to the tenure process possibly affected by the implementation of technology include the following:

- Outdated policies and explicit expectations for performance
- Escalating expectations for the quantity and quality of publications, practice, service, and especially funded research
- Lack of or infrequent feedback or formal mentoring by seasoned faculty
- Marrying online education information systems and technology tools with a changing teaching-learning process
- The need for work-life balance[55]

New models may be in order for technology and tenure. The following two examples exemplify technology-driven scholarly activities that may be considered during the tenure process for health professions faculty:

- A collaborative, international, digitally developed, implemented, and evaluated project rather than a written dissertation by one person
- Rewriting scholarly activity guidelines for tenure to include the creation and use of open source resources and publication opportunities available globally and free of charge[56–58]

Teaching, learning, and the tenure process are in a state of flux for faculty and students. How university administrators will factor the impact of technology into faculty promotion and tenure remains a focus for discussion far into the future.

CONCLUSION AND FUTURE DIRECTIONS

Bartholomew wondered whether higher education is really ready for the information revolution.[59] Despite recommendations from a multitude of organizations, government, and the business sector, some institutions of higher education have been slow to adopt and use information management and technology tools and to view technology enhanced learning as a strategic asset.[60] A myriad of reasons are described, including the cost of purchasing technologies; administrative, staff, faculty, and student dislike or fear of change; a parochial view of traditional education; and the need to generate a new model for education other than student credit hours.[58,60,61]

In the United States, there are an estimated 4400 institutions of postsecondary education. Three vendors provide approximately 3000 administrative systems, such as student information systems for managing student records. In addition, many larger research universities have built their own solutions, and others are using a best-of-breed approach to create their administrative information systems.[62] As a result, "colleges and universities are swimming in an ever widening sea of data" and creating pools of big data.[63, p. 11] In the future, analysis of these data with appropriate data mining tools will create a better picture of what does and does not work in education. For example, a number of the health professions require students to complete courses from the physical sciences, such as chemistry, anatomy, or physiology, before they are introduced to the health-related sciences, such as pathophysiology. From an intuitive perspective, this makes sense, but is it possible students may comprehend a chemistry course better if it follows a course such as pathophysiology? In actual practice, this progression rarely happens, but in big data repositories there may be the numbers to answer this question and other questions one currently may not think to ask.

While many universities are now using administrative systems and the technology used to deliver education has become increasingly robust, much of the teaching-learning process is still manually managed. A number of computerized teaching tools have been discussed in this chapter. Currently these tools are being used to provide innovative approaches to delivering content and engaging students in learning the content, but they do not track data related to a student's individual learning process. For example, in most cases, clickers record a student's response and discard that response with the introduction of the next question. A few of these applications, especially in the area of LMS, are beginning to track each student's progress with the assessment tools used in an individual course. For example, LMSs are designed to track a student's amount of participation in various discussion groups.

However, in most university settings, very little data (other than the course grade) about the individual student's learning across educational programs are recorded and maintained. The current system could be compared to a paper patient chart with additional limitations. In the healthcare system, health-related data are maintained in one chart for each patient. In education, the final record of a student's learning is the limited information included on the transcript. In the manual world of education, for the most part, all other data collected by individual faculty or academic departments are maintained, if at all, in file cabinets or individual faculty files. This can be called the ultimate system for creating an island of lost data and information. In the future, with the computerization of the academy, the student record will become rich with data related to individual learning, thereby creating new options for academic success.

Over the next several years, education information systems and technical tools will continue to increase in number and complexity. User interfaces will become more intuitive and learning curves less steep. Increased technical presence will drive increased use. Interactions with applications may become more "natural," using voice and motion recognition. Greater functionality for education is likely for smartphones and tablets. As hardware increases in capacity and shrinks in size, mobile learning (mlearning) will likely become easier and easier. Questions for the future are as follows: How much and what data should be collected about individual administrators, faculty, staff, and students, and why? Do faculty and students want 24/7 learning? Can learning truly become ubiquitous? Should the formal learning process truly become lifelong?

REFERENCES

1. Nelson R, Meyers L, Rizzolo MA, Rutar P, Proto MB, Newbold S. The evolution of education information systems and nurse faculty roles. *Nurs Educ Perspect.* 2006;27(5):189–195.
2. Rocha, R. *SmartBoard Tutorials.* http://www.uticaschools.org/Page/2098. Accessed July 6, 2016.
3. *Privacy Technical Assistance Center.* U.S. Department of Education. Homepage. http://ptac.ed.gov/. Accessed July 6, 2016.
4. Lord R. *Pennsylvania bills aim to protect students' data. Pittsburgh Post-Gazette;* October 14, 2015. http://www.post-gazette.com/news/surveillance-society/2015/10/14/Legislation-introduced-to-protect-student-privacy-pennsylvania/stories/201510140188.
5. Appleton L. The use of electronic books in midwifery education: the student perspective. *Health Info Libr J.* 2004;21:245–252.
6. Williams MG, Dittmer A. Textbooks on tap: using electronic books housed in handheld devices in nursing clinical courses. *Nurs Educ Perspect.* 2009;30(4):220–225.
7. Boren ZD. *There are Officially More Devices than People in the World;* October 7, 2014. http://www.independent.co.uk/life-style/gadgets-and-tech/news/there-are-officially-more-mobile-devices-than-people-in-the-world-9780518.html.
8. Pew Research Center. *Mobile Technology Fact Sheet;* 2014. http://www.pewinternet.org/fact-sheets/mobile-technology-fact-sheet/.
9. Harris P. Pearson Student Mobile Device Survey: College Students; May 16, 2014. http://www.pearsoned.com/wp-content/uploads/Pearson-HE-Student-Mobile-Device-Survey-PUBLIC-Report-051614.pdf.
10. Ellis RK. A Field Guide to Learning Management Systems. *ASTD Learning Circuits;* 2009. http://cgit.nutn.edu.tw:8080/cgit/PaperDL/hclin_091027163029.PDF.
11. Passuello L. *What Is Mind Mapping? (and how to get started immediately)* [Web log post]; 2007. http://litemind.com/what-is-mind-mapping.
12. Atay S, Karabacak U. Care plans using concept maps and their effects on the critical thinking dispositions of nursing students. *Int J Nurs Pract.* 2012;18:233–239.
13. Revell SMH. Concept maps and nursing theory: a pedagogical approach. *Nurse Educ.* 2012;37(3):131–135.
14. Buckley S, Coleman J, Davison I, et al. The educational effects of portfolios on undergraduate student learning: a Best Evidence Medical Education (BEME) systematic review: BEME Guide No. 11. *Med Teach.* 2009;31:340–355.
15. Stokes B. Video games have changed: time to consider "serious games". *Dev Educ J.* 2005;11:108.
16. Akl EA, Pretorius RW, Sackett K, et al. The effect of educational games on medical students' learning outcomes: a systematic review: BEME Guide No 14. *Med Teach.* 2010;32:16–27.
17. Suomi R, Mäntymäki M, Söderlund S. Promoting health in virtual worlds: lessons from second life. *J Med Internet Res.* 2014;16(10):e229. http://dx.doi.org/10.2196/jmir.3177 [PMID: 25313009, PMCID: 4210951].
18. Gardner H. *Frames of Mind: The Theory of Multiple Intelligences.* New York: Basic Books; 1983.
19. Smith MK. *Howard Gardner and Multiple Intelligences.* The Encyclopedia of Informal Education; 2008. http://www.infed.org/thinkers/gardner.htm 2002.
20. Johnson L, Lamb A. *Technology and Multiple Intelligences.* Teacher Tap: Professional Development Resources for Educators & Librarians; 2007.

21. Broderick M. Teaching International Students Online: The Importance of Quality Online Learning Systems [Electronic Version]. *vcamp360 blog*; August 10, 2015. http://www. vcamp360.com/blog/teaching-interational-students-online-the-importance-of-quality-online-learning-systems.

22. Pritchard T. Supporting International Students in the Online Environment. *Faculty Focus Higher Ed Teaching Strategies From Magna Publications [Electronic Version]*; 2011. http://www. facultyfocus.com/articles/online-education/supporting-international-students-in-the-online-environment/.

23. Zhang Z, Kenny R. Learning in an Online Distance Education Course: Experiences of Three International Students. *Int Rev Res Open Dist Learn*. 2010;11(1). [Electronic Version]. http://www. irrodl.org/index.php/irrodl/article/view/775/1481. Accessed July 6, 2016.

24. The Lancet. International Collaboration for Health Professions Education's Commission on Education for Health Professions for the 21st Century. *Lancet*. 2010;376 (9756):1873–1958. http://www.thelancet.com/journals/lancet/issue/vol376no9756/PIIS0140-6736(10)X6159-1. Accessed July 6, 2016.

25. Nicholas P, White T. e-Learning, e-books and virtual reference service: the nexus between the library and education. *J Libr Inf Serv Dist Learn*. 2012;6(1):3–18.

26. Hsieh PH. Globally-perceived experiences of online instructor: a preliminary exploration. *Comput Educ*. 2010;54:27–36.

27. Centre for the Advancement of Interprofessional Education (CAIPE). *Interprofessional Education: A Definition*. CAIPE; 2002. http://www.caipe.org.uk/about-us/the-definition-and-principles-of-interprofessional-education/.

28. Lewis K, Baker R. Expanding the scope of faculty educator development for health care professionals. *J Educ Online*. 2009;6 (1):1–17.

29. Schell G. Universities marginalize online courses: why should faculty members develop online courses if the effort is detrimental to their promotion or tenure? *Commun ACM*. 2004;47(7):53–56.

30. Neely PW, Tucker JP. Unbundling faculty roles in online distance education programs. *Int Rev Res Open Distance Learn*. 2010;11(2).

31. Moseley WL. Student and faculty perceptions of technology's usefulness in community college general education courses. *Open Access Theses and Dissertations from the College of Education and Human Sciences*. Lincoln: University of Nebraska; 2010. Paper 74.

32. Outlaw V, Rice M. Best practices: implementing an online course development & delivery model. *Online Journal of Distance Learning Administration*. 2015;15(3). Fall 2015, University of West Georgia, Distance Education Center. http://www.westga.edu/~distance/ojdla/fall183/outlaw_rice183.html.

33. Chao IT, Saj T, Hamilton D. Using collaborative course development to achieve online course quality standards. *Int Rev Res Open Distance Learn*. 2010;11(3):106–121.

34. Schwier RA, Wilson JR. Unconventional roles and activities identified by instructional designers. *Contemp Educ Technol*. 2010;1(2):134–147.

35. Stevens KB. Contributing factors to a successful online course development process. *J Cont High Educ*. 2013;61(1):2–11.

36. Borgemenke AJ, Holt WC, Fish WW. Universal course shell template design and implementation to enhance student outcomes in online coursework. *Q Rev Distance Educ*. 2013;14 (1):17–23.

37. Chickering AW, Ehrmann SC. Implementing the seven principles: technology as a lever. *AAHE Bull*. 1996;49(2):3–6.

38. *Techopedia Best Practice*. https://www.techopedia.com/definition/14269/best-practice. Accessed July 6, 2016.

39. Reference deleted in proofs.

40. Keengwe J, Kidd T. Toward best practices in online learning and teaching in higher education. *MERLOT J Online Learn Teach*. 2010;6(2). http://jolt.merlot.org/vol6no2/keengwe_0610.htm. Accessed July 6, 2016.

41. U.S. Department of Education. *Office of planning, evaluation, and policy development, evaluation of evidence-based practices in online learning: a meta-analysis and review of online learning studies, Washington, D.C*; 2010. https://www2.ed.gov/rschstat/eval/tech/evidence-based-practices/finalreport.pdf.

42. Reed S, Shell R, Kassis K, et al. Applying adult learning practices in medical education. *Curr Probl Pediatr Adolesc Health Care*. 2014;44(6):170–181. http://dx.doi.org/10.1016/j. cppeds.2014.01.008. http://www.ncbi.nlm.nih.gov/pubmed/24981666. Accessed July 6, 2016.

43. *Merriam-Webster*. Quality. http://www.merriam-webster.com/dictionary/quality. Accessed July 6, 2016.

44. *Quality Matters (QM™)*. Homepage. https://www. qualitymatters.org/. Accessed July 6, 2016.

45. *Quality Matters (QM™)*. Higher Ed Program > Rubric https:// www.qualitymatters.org/rubric. March 22, 2016.

46. *American Journal of Distance Education Special Issue: Quality Matters* http://www.tandfonline.com/toc/hajd20/29/3; September 18, 2015.

47. Council of Graduate Schools. Best Practices. http://cgsnet.org/best-practices. Accessed July 6, 2016.

48. Chickering A, Gamson Z. Seven Principles for Good Practice in Undergraduate Education. *Wingspread J*. 1987;9(2). http://sites. duke.edu/onlineguide/files/2011/12/Chickering-Gamson.pdf. Accessed July 6, 2016.

49. Chickering AW, Ehrmann SC. Implementing the seven principles: technology as a lever. *AAHE Bull*. 1996;49(2):3–6.

50. *Gagne's 9 Events of Instructions*; 2013. http://citt.ufl.edu/tools/gagnes-9-events-of-instruction/#application-to-online–hybrid-courses.

51. *The University of Texas Health Science Center at Houston's School of Public Health*. Online education best practice reference list. https://sph.uth.edu/faculty/instructional-development/online-education-best-practice-reference-list/. Accessed July 6, 2016.

52. *The Duke University*. Online Teaching Guide http://sites.duke. edu/onlineguide/. Accessed July 6, 2016.

53. Reference deleted in proofs.

54. Reference deleted in proofs.

55. *American Association of University Professors (AAUP)*. Academic due process. Recommended institutional regulations on academic freedom and tenure. http://www.aaup.org/file/RIR %202014.pdf. Accessed July 6, 2016.

56. Sorcinelli M. New conceptions of scholarship for a new generation of faculty members. *N Dir Teach Learn*. 2002;90:41–48.

57. Pannapacker W. Invisible gorillas are everywhere. *Chron High Educ*. 2012;24.

58. Pepicello W. University of Phoenix. In: Oblinger DG, ed. *Game Changers Education and Information Technologies*. EDUCAUSE 2012; 2012. http://www.educause.edu/library/resources/chapter-10-university-phoenix. Accessed July 6, 2016.

59. Bartholomew N. Is higher education ready for the information revolution? *Int J Ther Rehabil*. 2011;18(10):558–565.

60. Association of Public and Land-Grant Universities. *APLU-Sloan National Commission on Online Learning. Online Learning as a Strategic Asset. Volume 1: A Resource for Campus Leaders; Volume 2: The Paradox of Faculty Voices: Reviews and Experiences with Online Learning*; 2009.
61. Oblinger DG. IT as a game changer. In: Oblinger DG, ed. *Game Changers: Education and Information Technologies*. Louisville, CO: EDUCAUSE; 2012:37–51.
62. Bonig R. Latest trends in student information systems: driven by competition. *Educ Rev*; May 9, 2012. http://www.educause.edu/ero/article/latest-trends-student-information-systems-driven-competition.
63. Walters J. Big data. *Campus Technol*. 2012;26(2):11–16.
64. *Quality Matters*. https://www.qualitymatters.org/node/2299/download/QM%20Standards%20with%20Point%20Values%20Fifth%20Edition.pdf. Accessed August 1, 2016.
65. Zepke N, Leach L. Improving student engagement: ten proposals for action. *Act Learn High Educ*. 2010;11(3):167–177.

DISCUSSION QUESTIONS

1. How might comprehensive academic information systems affect the work of faculty within an academic setting?
2. What role should faculty play in the selection, implementation, and evaluation of information systems and computerized teaching tools?
3. What are some advantages and disadvantages of the current computerized education tools?
4. How are interprofessional education, the tenure process, and information technology educational tools connected?
5. Describe how computerized teaching tools might be employed in an interdisciplinary environment.
6. What do you think are the key questions one might consider when using big data in health education programs?
7. The future has many pathways. What do you see in the future regarding information systems and technology tools in healthcare education?

CASE STUDY

You are a baccalaureate-prepared health practitioner in the school system and are also certified to teach kindergarten to 12th grade. You are intrigued by the teaching-learning process and decide that you are now interested in teaching new health professionals in an institution of higher education about the importance of school health. You begin your education to obtain the necessary degrees and experience. You select a program with an emphasis on education, teaching, and learning. Through your course work, you acquire knowledge about education's history and learn how cognition processes transform knowledge gained from social, biological, cultural, and historical contexts. You are also introduced to a number of new computer-based technologies designed for educational use. Informatics and its application to education and the process of teaching and learning fascinate you. You eagerly begin to incorporate student-centered learning, technology-related activities in your classes and frequently work collaboratively with interdisciplinary faculty peers and staff in planning, assessing, implementing, and evaluating the addition and adoption of new student-centered learning activities. You and the students learn both individually and collaboratively during, for example, the adoption of online testing, ePortfolio development, the use of videoconferencing, online courses, and other similar activities, including online class chats and discussions with international nursing faculty and their students.

You begin to do research and publish your findings in online journals as well as on a blog that focuses on the use of technology in health education programs. However, in your annual review, you are advised that you now need to take a more traditional approach to teaching, research, and publications. Using technology to create the innovative classes you are teaching is taking up too much of your time, and this is time that would be better spent in developing grants from traditional sources.

Discussion Questions

1. Resistance to change is a formidable foe to progress. What are some possible options to facilitate change in education and the introduction of technology?
2. Suppose that the educational setting in this case study decides to become interdisciplinary. Describe educational technologies and methods that would facilitate the process.
3. If you could collect and track learning data related to individual students across their educational program, what data elements would you consider a priority? For example, would you want to track learning preferences; writing ability, including specific strengths and weaknesses; or clinical strengths and weaknesses?

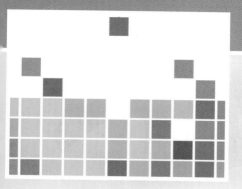

33

Simulation in Healthcare Education

Valerie M. Howard, Kim Leighton, and Teresa Gore

The emergence of technology for educational purposes creates a need for faculty and health science educators to understand how to not only operate the technology but also implement it within the academic and service settings while using sound academic principles.

OBJECTIVES

At the completion of this chapter, the reader will be prepared to:
1. Define the different types of simulation modalities available.
2. Describe the challenges and opportunities inherent to simulation.
3. Apply the 2016 International Nursing Association for Clinical Simulation and Learning (INACSL) Standards

of Best Practice: Simulation[SM] in developing educational experiences.
4. Discuss the use of simulation-based education in interprofessional experiences.
5. Analyze the similarities and differences related to the available simulation resources.
6. Develop evidence-based simulation activities.

KEY TERMS

clinical scenario, 564
debriefing, 566
fidelity, 558
learning environment, 561

simulation, 557
simulation learning environment, 557
standards of best practice: simulation[SM], 561
theory-based debriefing, 564

ABSTRACT ❖

The use of simulated learning experiences has rapidly emerged in healthcare education as a method of training healthcare providers in a safe environment without subjecting patients to harm. Multiple definitions of simulation-related terms exist, so the importance of the use of standardized terminology is stressed. Best practice standards for implementing simulated learning experiences are discussed. These should be provided in a standardized manner while adhering to guidelines to maximize learning. Simulated learning experiences directly correlate with the Core Competencies for Interprofessional Collaborative Practice. Finally, issues, challenges, and opportunities for the future of healthcare education and the use of simulation are outlined.

INTRODUCTION

Simulation is a time-honored method of teaching that has been used in health education for decades. It is defined as the use of "one or more typologies to promote, improve, and/or validate a participant's progression from novice to expert,"[1, p. S9] in which the novice to expert continuum is consistent with that promoted by Benner.[2] Experiential learning

theory is used in health professions education to emphasize the importance of clinical practice in the educational process.[3] Simulation is one method of experiential, hands-on applied learning and can range from a simple activity used to mimic reality (e.g., the process of injecting an orange to create the feel of puncturing skin) to the use of high-fidelity simulation to create the comprehensive experience of interacting with a healthcare team during a clinical emergency. In each case, the simulation-based learning experience includes "an array of structured activities that represent actual or potential situations in education and practice and allow participants to develop or enhance knowledge, skills, and attitudes or analyze and respond to realistic situations in a simulated environment or through an unfolding case study."[1, p. S9]

Types of Simulations

The term **simulation learning environment** refers to the physical set-up, context, and culture in which a simulated learning experience occurs. Virtual simulation in the educational environment involves the use of a device or tool such as an avatar, partial task trainers, or patient simulators and a realistic environment in which to teach cognitive processing, supportive attitudes, and skills. Several types of simulation are used in healthcare education, including written case studies, virtual environments (e.g., Second Life, computerized gaming, virtual reality), standardized patients, partial task trainers, and medium- to high-fidelity patient simulators. "Virtual simulation may be used by educators to enhance lecture or web based courses, replicate high-risk clinical experiences, act as clinical makeup, foster intradisciplinary and interdisciplinary education, and address practical challenges and barriers to contemporary nursing education."[4, p. 412]

Gaming is the use of games designed to teach about a specific subject or specific skills. They can be especially useful in the education of health professionals. Gaming is a type of virtual simulation technique that creates an environment that can meet the needs of millennial learners and has been embraced more fully in the past few years by educators.[5] Both gaming and virtual simulations are examples of experiential learning techniques.

Simulators are used to help students improve critical thinking, clinical judgment, communication, and teamwork skills while assisting learners to meet psychomotor, cognitive, and affective learning objectives. Most of the growth in simulation is with standardized patients, partial task trainers, and simulators.

Standardized patients consistently portray a patient or other individual in a scripted scenario for the purposes of instruction, practice, or evaluation.[6] Standardized patients may be actors who require little training. Others may be people who respond to requests for assistance with healthcare training and require significant resources for training. Still others may actually have the disease, illness, symptom, or injury under study. In most cases, standardized patients are paid for their assistance to the educational process.

Partial task trainers typically represent anatomic parts of the human body and are used to practice skill acquisition.[7] This type of simulator assists learners to meet psychomotor objectives, those accomplished when a student demonstrates the ability to perform a task such as inserting a urinary catheter, giving an injection, or attaching a heart monitor. Partial task trainers can range from low to high levels of realism, also known as fidelity. Examples of low-fidelity partial task trainers are when learners practice giving intradermal injections using a silicone pad that is flexible enough to allow a bleb to form when fluid is injected or using a hot dog with skin for the same purpose. An example of a more realistic partial task trainer is a model that promotes practice of intravenous needle insertion through a virtual model that includes haptic technology. Haptics is a feature allowing tactile sensation, for example, when the needle enters a vein.

Simulators include full-body mannequins and can range from static mannequins that do not respond to any intervention to high-fidelity computerized simulators designed to realistically respond to learner interventions. High-fidelity mannequins can have blinking eyes, a chest that rises and falls with breaths, heart and lung sounds, and palpable peripheral pulses, and can be capable of being intubated, having chest tubes inserted, and having other assessments and procedures performed on them. High-fidelity simulators are particularly useful for interprofessional training on interdisciplinary

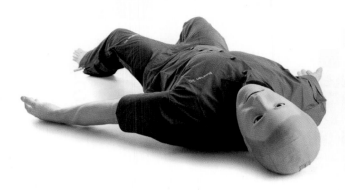

FIG 33.1 Sample high-fidelity simulator. (Photo courtesy of Laerdal Medical Corporation.)

activities such as cardiopulmonary arrest, in which a variety of clinicians have specific roles to enact. An example is the mannequin shown in Fig. 33.1, marketed by Laerdal. These types of simulators are considered the most lifelike compared to human patients. The most realistic simulators in healthcare education are, of course, real persons. Obviously, numerous skills and conditions cannot be recreated for safety reasons. Instead, educators often use a hybrid simulation involving two types of simulators. A student can explain the procedure, risks, and potential complications to the standardized patient while performing the procedure on the partial task trainer. Standardized patients can assist learners to meet objectives while enhancing communication, clinical judgment, critical thinking, and teamwork skills.

Fidelity

Fidelity, also known as realism or authenticity, is "the degree to which a simulated experience approaches reality; as fidelity increases, realism increases."[1, p. S6] There are a variety of ways to create fidelity in the learning experience. It has recently been recognized that fidelity has very little to do with *what* equipment is used and much more to do with *how* that equipment is used. Fidelity can involve a variety of dimensions, including the following[1, p. S6]:

- Physical factors such as environment, equipment, and related tools
- Psychological factors such as the emotions, beliefs, and self-awareness of participants
- Social factors such as participant and instructor motivation and goals
- Culture of the group
- Degree of openness and trust, as well as participants' modes of thinking

On a trajectory from low fidelity to high fidelity, task trainers are considered of lower fidelity than high-fidelity simulators and finally standardized patients. However, this type of classification is not without controversy. Alinier places computer-controlled simulators above standardized patients in his continuum.[8] This continuum may actually depend on how the learning experience is designed. For example, a high-fidelity mannequin used in a cardiopulmonary arrest simulation may not even be turned on, depending on the level of the learner. A low-fidelity task trainer used in a high-fidelity environment may allow the combination to rank higher than the task trainer alone. Other types of simulation (e.g., written, screen-based) fall into the trajectory, depending on how they are used. The decision about the level of fidelity needed for any simulation-based learning experience should always be based on the learning objectives. Thus it is not always necessary to have high fidelity, especially when cost as well as technology needs are considered. The example in Table 33.1 involves inserting a central line.

The most common fidelity consideration is the type of simulator to be used; however, educators have become aware of additional types of fidelity such as environment and holistic dimensions of a person. Fidelity of the environment considers the location in which the simulation-based learning experience takes place. A high-fidelity mannequin may need to be used within a psychomotor skills lab, a classroom, outside environment, or even office space. An environment most similar to where real patient care takes place is highly desirable. Additionally, the equipment, furniture, and supplies should all be as realistic as possible to the traditional clinical environment. Creating methods to add patients' emotions, beliefs, spirituality, culture, and communication are also ways to make the experience more realistic. Table 33.2 outlines ideas for assessing and meeting learning needs in the developmental, spiritual, sociocultural, and psychological dimensions.

Benefits of Simulation

Simulation offers the opportunity for learners to practice in a safe environment without placing patients at risk. Simulation significantly increases learners' knowledge,[9,10] competence,[11] self-efficacy,[12] and confidence[13] at no added risk to patients. While the former are intermediate outcomes, a longer-term outcome of better training is to improve the quality and safety of patient care. Deliberate practice, the process of practicing a skill multiple times until mastery is reached, is facilitated within the simulation environment through the use of task trainers, further reducing the risk of harm to patients.[11] Simulation also offers the opportunity to create standardized learning experiences in a controlled environment and provides exposure to low-occurrence, high-risk situations with opportunities to practice critical thinking skills, problem solving, and decision making.

An evaluation of any educational training program should align with evaluation models of training. Two examples are Kirkpatrick's model[14] and translational science research (TSR).[15] TSR and Kirkpatrick identified the following levels of outcomes of training programs, which were summarized in a review article by Adamson et al.[16]:

- *Level 1 (TSR Level 0): Reaction* measures the learners' reactions to the training program. For example, were the learners satisfied with the program, and how do they plan to use the information provided?
- *Level 2 (TSR Level 1): Learning* measures the amount of knowledge, attitudes, or skills that have changed and the level of the change as a result of the training.
- *Level 3 (TSR Level 2): Behavior or Training Transfer* measures the amount of "on the job" behavior change by the learner following the training sessions, or if

TABLE 33.1 Fidelity Correlated With Objectives

Objective: The Learner Will	Type of Simulator
Accurately place central line catheter	Task trainer
Maintain sterile technique when placing a central line	Task trainer
Clearly communicate risks when obtaining consent from patient	Standardized patient
Use various communication techniques to calm patient's anxiety	Standardized patient
Recognize need for central line insertion during hypotensive crisis	High-fidelity simulator
Insert central line when rapid blood transfusion is required	High-fidelity simulator

TABLE 33.2 Dimensions of Learning and Fidelity

Dimension	Simulated Patient	Improving Fidelity
Developmental	Forty-two-year-old male patient with myocardial infarction (MI); works as laborer	Place frame with picture of young family at bedside. Does the learner recognize that the patient likely will not be able to return to work? Does he or she consider how the family will have their financial needs met?
Spiritual	Patient will be having emergent surgery	Place religious or spiritual book or icon at the bedside. Does the learner recognize the need to ask the patient about his or her beliefs and practices?
Sociocultural	Patient is being discharged with five new prescriptions	Provide discharge instruction sheet. Does the learner determine whether the patient has the resources to get new prescriptions filled?
Psychological	Post-operative knee replacement and patient cannot return home to care for self	The patient reveals that there are 10 steps before entering his home. Does the learner explore how the patient feels about the loss of his or her independence?

MI, Myocardial infarction.

the simulation training translated into behavioral changes in the clinical setting.

- *Level 4 (TSR Level 3): Results* measures the organizational impact of the training program on either performance or cost savings, or, in the case of simulation training, to improved health outcomes.

Much of the research related to simulation has focused on the first levels, measuring the learner's perspective, satisfaction, and knowledge gain related to the experience. However, ultimately simulation researchers will want to demonstrate the benefit of simulation training and its impact on patient outcomes (level 4 or T3). As an example, most recently simulation training has been correlated with lower central line infection rates,[17] decreased complications resulting from shoulder dystocia obstetrical emergencies,[18] and healthcare cost savings related to decreased malpractice claims.[19]

Challenges and Opportunities

While simulation is an ideal environment for creating standardized learning opportunities and applying theoretical knowledge in the practice setting, inherent challenges exist related to the ease of implementation.

Cost

High-fidelity simulation mannequins can be expensive to purchase; however, the costs extend well beyond equipment. A fortunate aspect of technology is that costs tend to decrease over time as technology advances. Many features originally only found in the higher-priced mannequins are now available in lower-cost models. The most commonly overlooked costs include long-term maintenance and replacement costs for equipment and the initial and ongoing training and development of faculty and staff. Table 33.3 outlines some of the major initial and ongoing expenses related to simulation education.

To cover these costs, many health professional programs include student simulation lab fees. Others may seek grant funding from foundations, corporations, or private donors to support these efforts. Funding success can be maximized by developing a relationship with the potential funder, correlating the funding proposal with the mission and vision of the funding agency, and forming collaborative partnerships to demonstrate a unique and sustainable project.

Technology

High-fidelity simulation mannequins can be difficult to operate by faculty who lack technological experience or knowledge. In addition, skills are required to operate the digital audiovisual equipment used to record simulation experiences. Recently, the use of electronic health record (EHR) systems has increased in simulation learning environments. With each layer of technology comes the associated challenges involved in managing multiple systems. One must consider the benefits that come with consolidating purchases to one or two vendors: centralized ordering, management of warranties, and individualized customer service. Also, with volume

TABLE 33.3 Initial and Ongoing Major Expenses Related to Simulation Education

Expense	Initial Costs	Additional Expense
High-fidelity mannequins	$30,000–$250,000	Maintenance and replacement costs, depreciation, upgrades, warranties, insurance
Task trainers	$250 and up	Maintenance and replacement costs
Standardized patients	$12–$40/h	Hire and training costs, vary based on region of country and level of experience
Audiovisual systems	$10,000–$50,000/room	Upgrades, training
Faculty development	$5000 initially, then $1000/year	Training on use of mannequins and systems, ongoing system updates, ongoing development on use of simulation pedagogy, consultants, conference attendance and association dues, journals

purchases, costs are often decreased. However, purchasing from a variety of vendors may result in lower initial purchase prices and the ability to customize to existing spaces; on the other hand, this also increases the number of customer service contacts and cost of individual warranties. The budget allocated toward simulation tends to dictate these decisions.

Partnering with simulation equipment vendors may allow specific training opportunities to enhance understanding of the simulator technology and promote ease of use. Hiring a full-time or part-time simulation technician may be necessary. Generally, previous experience with computers, information technology, and audiovisual systems can enhance the effectiveness of the simulation technology. The Society for Simulation in Healthcare (SSH) offers the opportunity to become a Certified Healthcare Simulation Operations Specialist (CHSOS) for those with a bachelor's degree or equivalent experience and 2 years of experience in an operations role. In a forecast of the importance that this role has taken on, several institutions have announced associate degree programs that teach basic medical knowledge with the skills needed to manage the technology and environment. Box 33.1 offers a sample job description for a simulation technician.

Faculty Development

Simulation is just one example of an experiential teaching and learning strategy, but many faculty lack the understanding of

---

BOX 33.1   Job Description for Simulation Technician

Under the direction of the Simulation Center Director, the technician will provide technical support for all simulation experiences and operations, including preparation, maintenance, and repair of computerized mannequins, task trainers, simulation-related hardware and software systems, audiovisual equipment, administrative website management, and digital recording systems.

---

educational principles related to the best methods for implementing experiential learning strategies within the curriculum. Therefore knowledge of the following educational principles as they apply to experiential learning will assist the simulation facilitator in developing educationally sound experiences:

- Educational theory
- Application of theory to practice
- Development of clear and measurable objectives
- Instructional design
- Facilitation of learning
- Creating a safe learning environment in the simulation lab
- Debriefing strategies
- Formative and summative learner evaluation
- Program evaluation

To maintain a supportive learning environment and ensure commitment to academic principles, each simulation facilitator should have an orientation period to learn the aforementioned principles and observe experienced simulation facilitators, similar to a mentorship model. If schools do not have the appropriate experts within their organizations, resources should be committed to educate the simulation facilitator. Likewise, institutions will need to develop policies that require the simulation facilitator to have appropriate training before interacting with learners in the lab.

As a result of the landmark experimental, longitudinal multisite study of simulation, the National Council of State Boards of Nursing (NCSBN) identified criteria that must be met if undergraduate nursing schools are to consider replacing up to 50% of traditional clinical time with simulation-based learning experiences:

1. Faculty must be formally trained in simulation pedagogy.
2. There must be an adequate number of faculty members to support the student learners.
3. Subject matter experts must conduct theory-based debriefing.
4. Equipment and supplies must be available to create a realistic environment.
5. The INACSL Standards of Best Practice: Simulation[SM] should be incorporated.[20]

These criteria should not be limited to consideration only by undergraduate programs, as the principles of simulation-based education apply across the educational continuum.

Graduate program administrators and faculty should also consider the following recommendations. Due to concern that programs might substitute simulation without adequate preparation, support, and resources, the NCSBN convened an expert panel to provide recommendations intended to assist the individual state boards of nursing and nursing education programs.[21] These guidelines include the following[2, p. 40]:

1. There is commitment on the part of the school for the simulation program.
2. Program has appropriate facilities for conducting simulation.
3. Program has the educational and technological resources and equipment to meet the intended objectives.
4. Lead faculty and simulation lab personnel are qualified to conduct simulation.
5. Faculty are prepared to lead simulations.
6. Program has an understanding of policies and processes that are a part of the simulation experience.

Several organizations, such as the INACSL, the National League for Nursing (NLN), the SSH, and the Association of Standardized Patient Educators (ASPE) offer annual meetings, conferences, and faculty development webinars to assist with this challenge. A group of simulation scholars in the NLN Leadership Development Program has designed a theory-based simulation educator resource that is available through the Simulation Innovation Resource Center (SIRC).[22] In addition, several higher education institutions offer graduate-level certificates with concentrations in simulation. Four scholarly journals are devoted to simulation: *Clinical Simulation in Nursing, Simulation in Healthcare, Advances in Simulation*, and the International Pediatric Simulation Societies' (IPSS) Cureus.com channel, which offers publication opportunities in a new peer-reviewed online journal. Finally, many organizations offer continuing education programs for credit through their ongoing developmental programs.

Organizations

The two largest simulation organizations are the International Nursing Association for Clinical Simulation & Learning (INACSL) and the International Nursing Association for Clinical Simulation & Learning (SSH). INACSL was founded after discussions by several attendees of the annual Learning Resource Center Conference in 2001. The nonprofit organization has grown to more than 1800 members worldwide. The organization's mission statement reads as follows: *advancing the science of healthcare simulation. The vision of INACSL is to be a global leader in transforming practice to improve patient safety through excellence in healthcare simulation.*[23] The majority of members are nurses, although anyone is welcome to become a member. Institutional membership is also available. The organization is affiliated with SSH and a founding member of the Global Network for Simulation in Healthcare (GNSH), an organization composed of the leadership of simulation organizations worldwide. INACSL spearheaded the development of the *Standards of*

Best Practice: Simulation[SM] and offers research grant funding, scholarships for conference attendance, and fellowships for simulation education.

SSH was founded in 2004 and has a membership of approximately 3000 healthcare providers in all specialty areas. Their mission states: "The Society for Simulation in Healthcare is a leading inter-professional society that advances the application of simulation in healthcare through global engagement."[24] SSH is affiliated with numerous multiprofession simulation organizations and is also a founding member of GNSH. SSH offers a simulation center accreditation program and certification for healthcare simulation educators (CHSE), as well as the previously mentioned CHSOS certification.

An additional key organization supporting simulation in nursing education is the National League for Nursing (NLN). The NLN, founded in 1893, boasts over 40,000 individual and 1200 institutional members, focuses on the support of nursing education. The mission of the NLN is to "promote excellence in nursing education to build a strong and diverse nursing workforce to advance the health of our nation and the global community."[25]

Most notably for simulation educators, the NLN has partnered with industry to create simulation products, supports research, and provides ongoing resources. The NLN Jeffries Simulation Theory is one outcome of these endeavors.[26] In addition, unfolding case studies have been developed to help teach concepts related to Alzheimer's patient care and care of the veteran. The SIRC was created as a repository for development opportunities for simulationists of all levels and offers numerous courses of study on various aspects of simulation-based learning experiences.[27] Lastly, the NLN has partnered with Laerdal to develop vSim, a product designed to develop clinical reasoning skills, competence, and confidence in nursing students.

The Association of Standardized Patient Educators (ASPE) is an international organization for simulation educators that focuses on the use of standardized patient methodology. It is their mission to: "promote best practices in the application of standardized patient methodology for education, assessment and research; foster the dissemination of research and scholarship in the field of standardized patient methodology; and to advance the professional knowledge and skills of its members."[28] ASPE offers a mentorship program, recognizes outstanding educators through awards, and offers a scholars certificate program as well as a variety of professional development opportunities.

In the area of gaming, the Games + Learning + Society (GLS) is one of the oldest organizations in the world devoted to game-based learning and research. "GLS investigates how games engage, enrich, and transform, then design great games based on this research."[29] Games are developed strategically, in partnerships with various organizations from conception to finished products. An annual conference is held to provide education opportunities to educators using game-based theory.

There are many additional simulation organizations that have become active around the world, some of which offer support in geographical locations, while others support specialty areas of healthcare or practitioners. Several of these are listed on the website of The Society in Europe for Simulation Applied to Medicine (SESAM; https://www.sesam-web.org/network/nationalsocieties/), including simulation organizations located in the United Kingdom, Australia, Brazil, Latin America, Canada, Holland, France, Italy, Japan, Korea, New Zealand, Poland, Russia, Chile, Portugal, Switzerland, and across Europe. Specialty organizations include those supporting pediatric educators and practitioners, and those who are simulation operators.

Faculty or Administrative Buy-In

The use of simulation modalities to enhance learning can be considered an organizational change, and resistance to change efforts has been widely reported in all disciplines, including business, organizational behavior, psychology, and healthcare. Faculty may be resistant to learning new methods of teaching and technology. Administrators may not understand the importance of dedicating time and resources to the successful implementation of the simulation efforts. Students may be anxious about the possibility of being recorded as they practice in the simulation lab.

Successful change efforts can be facilitated by having a thorough understanding of change theories and using this theoretical knowledge to guide the efforts. One change model useful in healthcare was developed by John Kotter, who suggests following eight steps when leading a change effort (Table 33.4).[30] Creating a mission and vision statement for the simulation program and developing a strategic plan can also guide future efforts related to integrating advanced practice experiences within the simulation program.[31] Evaluating the participants' satisfaction related to the simulation experiences through the use of postsimulation surveys can provide necessary data to share with administrators in an effort to gain support. Faculty members can be given an opportunity to visit the simulation lab and experience firsthand the learners' reaction to this powerful educational tool. It is also helpful to involve faculty in their own simulation-based educational experience and have them perform in the learner role. This immersive experience has been reported to be helpful in increasing understanding of the value of this type of learning. Finally, sharing the positive experiences of students both quantitatively and qualitatively, through reflections and stories, can also generate buy-in.

THE SIMULATION PROCESS
Learning Theories Applied to Simulation

Simulation is often accepted without any validation and based on the technology instead of a theoretical grounding. However, many learning theories are applicable to simulation-based learning, and several are presented below. Kneebone identified the following four concepts to lay the foundation for simulation:

TABLE 33.4 **Kotter's Principles Applied to Simulation**

Kotter's Principle	Application to Simulation Education
Creating a sense of urgency	• Identify the need for simulation-based training within institution. • Share simulation-based research and evidence with stakeholders.
Developing a guiding coalition	• Identify simulation champions and other like-minded individuals in your organization to form your simulation team. • Choose representatives from all stakeholders (faculty, administrators, clinicians, educators, learners, students, staff, patients, families).
Developing a vision	• Develop a mission, vision, name, and strategic plan for your simulation program or center. • Create a business plan. • Include input from all stakeholders.
Communicating that vision	• Share the plan with all stakeholders. • Use a marketing or branding approach for the name of your organization. • Consult with your public relations department.
Empowering stakeholders to act upon that vision	• Develop an organizational structure to support each team member. • Schedule regular meetings for progress updates and document the minutes from each meeting. • Develop clear and concise roles and responsibilities for simulation related activities and ensure accountability. • Seek resources from administration, outside funding agencies, participant fees to support the structure.
Create short term wins	• Develop one or two simulation activities based on sound educational principles and implement according to the best simulation evidence available. • Celebrate the successes of each individual in your simulation team.
Consolidation of improvements	• Collect data on each simulation experience and use the data to improve quality.
Institutionalizing new approaches	• Develop and implement policies and procedures related to simulation (i.e., simulation facilitator, facilitation, simulation design, scheduling, debriefing). • Maximize use of your simulation center. • Continue to share the positive simulation evaluation data, both quantitative and qualitative, with administrators, faculty, clinicians, educators, and all stakeholders.

Adapted From Kotter, JP. Leading Change. Boston, MA: Harvard Business Review Press; 1996.

1. Gaining technical proficiency with psychomotor skills
2. Learning theory with repetitive practice and frequent reinforcement
3. Tailoring support to the individual learner's need using situated learning
4. Addressing the affective domain of emotions with learning[32]

In addition, Kneebone identified the following four criteria for evaluating existing and new simulations. These are discussed further in the next section focused on standards:

1. Allow sustained, repetitive, and purposeful practice in a safe, controlled environment
2. Level interaction with the expert or mentor, depending on the proficiency of the student
3. Simulation should mimic actual life experiences
4. The simulated environment should foster a learner-centered approach that inspires and supports students[32]

The theoretical foundation for simulation can be based on experiential learning theory, as well as several other learning theories, models, and frameworks that are applicable to the use of simulation, as follows:

• *Knowles's adult learning theory.* This theory originally stated that adults learn differently due to andragogy (theory of adult learning).[33] Characteristics of adult learners are that they are self-directed, want to be involved in planning and evaluating their learning experience, use past experiences to build new learning, need to understand the reason for learning, want immediate application of knowledge to solve problems, and are more invested when the learning is associated with a new role. In 1984, Knowles changed his position to recognize that the assumptions about andragogy are situation specific and not unique to adults.[34] In 2010, Clapper expanded on this assumption of what adult learners wanted educators to know, sharing that learners want educators to create a safe learning environment that uses active and collaborative learning experiences, encourage reflection on current and past experiences, and focus more on the assessment of improvements made instead of pure evaluation.[35]

• *Kolb's experiential learning.* This theory refers to a person's ability to transfer knowledge from theory into practice, thereby leading to acquisition of knowledge.[36] Foronda and Bauman[4] discuss how students using gaming are immersed in learning environments with preconceived beliefs and judgments. They reflect on their activities and form abstract conceptualizations. They then will experiment and form new concrete experiences, then beginning again in the learning cycle.[4]

- *Situated cognition.* Learning occurs as a social activity incorporating the mind, the body, the activity, and the tools in a context that is complex and interactive. This incorporates all domains of learning: psychomotor, cognitive, and affective.[37] Wyrostok et al.[38] describe how learning is socially situated so that learning occurs as a result of human interactions and the social context of the situation when teaching end-of-life care to undergraduate nursing students.

- *Lasater's Interactive Model of Clinical Judgment Development.* Four areas of clinical judgment are noticing, interpreting, responding, and reflecting.[39,40] This model can be applied to simulation for noticing and assessing patient situations and conditions, interpreting the assessment findings, responding by developing a plan of care and interventions, and reflecting during the debriefing process.

- *Jeffries/NLN Simulation Theory:* This theory was established as a conceptual framework developed for use in nursing education to design, implement, and evaluate simulation experiences, formerly known as the Jeffries/NLN Simulation Framework.[41] Based on the evidence from literature review and dialogue with simulation researchers and educators, the NLN Jeffries Simulation Framework has progressed to a mid-level theory.[26] This evolution occurred after groups evaluated each of the constructs of the framework and a theorist reviewed and provided additional recommendations for advancing the framework. A literature review was conducted[42] and synthesized to conclude there was enough evidence to progress the framework to a theory with a few minor edits. The major edits occurred within the educational practices of the simulation experience with teacher and student to facilitator and participants to more clearly reflect the current practice in simulation. Within the simulation experience, there must be an environment of trust; it must be experiential, interactive, collaborative, and learner centered. The outcomes of the simulation experience are measured on a system, patient, or participant level. This theory depicts the triadic relationship of participants, facilitators, and educational practices, and their influence on the simulation design and desired outcomes. Five possible outcomes of simulations are increased knowledge, improved skill performance, enhanced learner satisfaction, improved critical-thinking abilities, and increased self-confidence of the participants.

- *Gaba's 11 dimensions of simulation.* Gaba's vision of 2004 remains relevant today, as he outlines various components of simulation-based learning[43, p.13-16]:
  1. The purpose and aims of simulation activity
  2. Unit of participation
  3. Experience level of participants
  4. Healthcare domain in which simulation is applied
  5. Healthcare disciplines of participants
  6. Type of knowledge, skills, attitudes, or behavior addressed in simulation
  7. Age of patient being simulated
  8. Applicable or required technology
  9. Site of simulation participation
  10. Extent of direct participation
  11. Feedback method accompanying simulation

The many aspects of simulation-based education have been studied to determine best practices. A clinical scenario should be developed based on the specific learning objectives of the participants. During the planning and development of a scenario, it is important to construct an experience that is appropriate to the participant's level of learning as well as the participant's objective. Since many simulation experts believe that the majority of learning occurs during the debriefing process, a planned theory-based debriefing strategy should guide the facilitator in the process. A theory-based debriefing is an active discussion that follows a simulation experience. The debriefing is led by a facilitator who is prepared to apply educational principles in guiding the discussion of clinical content underlying the simulation experience. The feedback provided via the discussion should provide the participants with an opportunity to use reflective thinking to analyze their performance and the clinical concepts presented in the stimulation experience. In developing, implementing, and evaluating a simulation, faculty should strive to ensure the identification and application of a theoretical framework proving the theoretical underpinning for that simulation and simulation program.[1,41,44,45] These aspects will be explored further in the next section.

International Nursing Association for Clinical Simulation and Learning Standards of Best Practice: Simulation

The INACSL Standards of Best Practice: Simulation[SM] was developed by the INACSL board of directors at the request of its membership after an extensive needs analysis was conducted via member e-mail and listserv.[1] The purpose of the analysis was to identify, prioritize, and rank the areas of simulation education required standards that would serve to improve this teaching strategy. Top priorities were established as standards and the lower priorities were developed as guidelines. The simulation standards have been developed to assist with developing simulation experiences that will lead to better learning experiences and improved learning outcomes for participants.[1]

The first seven standards were presented at the 2011 conference and published for all members in the fall of 2011 by Elsevier, sponsored by an educational grant from CAE. These initial standards included (1) terminology, (2) professional integrity of the participants, (3) participant objectives, (4) facilitation methods, (5) simulation facilitator, (6) the debriefing process, and (7) evaluation of expected outcomes.

In 2013, guidelines were established and published online by Elsevier. The paper publication of the standards was funded by CAE and Elsevier Simulation. In 2015, two additional standards focused on simulation-enhanced interprofessional education (Sim-IPE) and simulation design were created and published.

In 2016 INACSL Standards of Best Practice: Simulation[SM 46] were again updated. This latest update is based on current practice and incorporated external feedback from 20 professional healthcare organizations. The 2016 INACSL Standards update includes a new format that more effectively reflects the relationship between the standards and describes their non-hierarchical nature. The Standards of Best Practice: Simulation[SM] include:

- Simulation Design[47]
- Debriefing[48]
- Facilitation[49]
- Outcomes and Objectives[50]
- Participant Evaluation[51]
- Professional Integrity[52]
- Simulation-Enhanced Interprofessional Education (Sim-IPE)[53]

For full information about the updates to the 2016 INACSL Standards, visit www.inacsl.org/INACSLStandards.

The major changes that occurred with the revised INACSL Standards include:

- Removal of numeration with each standard
- Revision of the standard template
- Replacement of the terminology standard with a glossary of terms
- Combination of existing standards to reduce duplication

Each standard includes the statement, background, and criteria necessary to meet the standard, as well as the required elements for each criterion.

Glossary[46]

The Terminology Standard from the previous Standards was moved to a Glossary in the 2016 revision.[46] This was accomplished when the INACSL Terminology was incorporated into the Healthcare Simulation Dictionary[54] published in June 2016. The glossary was incorporated into the revised Standards to ensure that those using simulation are speaking a "common language." The definitions in the Glossary were developed using current literature and practice. Standard definitions make it possible for consistent use of educational principles within educational application, clear communication within publications, replication of research, and evidence-based practices.

Professional Integrity of the Participants

This standard states that "professional integrity is demonstrated and upheld by all involved in simulation-based experiences."[52, p. S30] Four criteria are necessary to meet this standard[52, p. S31]:

- Foster and role model attributes of professional integrity at all times.
- Follow standards of practice, guidelines, principles, and ethics of one's profession.
- Create and maintain a safe learning environment.
- Require confidentiality of the performances and scenario content based on institution policy and procedures.

Participant Objectives and Outcomes

This standard states that "all simulation-based experiences begin with the development of measureable objectives designed to achieve expected outcomes."[50, p. S13] The simulated clinical experience should align with course, clinical, or program objectives and should be based on the participants' level of experience rather than on the fidelity, or realism, of the equipment. Clearly stating the objectives and outcomes helps guide the simulation experience toward an end point or goal Two criteria are necessary to meet this standard[50, p. S14]:

- Determine expected outcomes from simulation-based activities and/or programs.
- Construct S.M.A.R.T. objectives based on expected outcomes.

Facilitation

This standard states that "facilitation methods are varied and use of a specific method is dependent on the learning needs of the participants and the expected outcomes. A facilitator assumes responsibility and oversight for managing the entire simulation-based experience."[49, p. S16] Five criteria are necessary to meet this standard[49, p. S17]:

- Effective facilitation requires a facilitator who has specific skills and knowledge in simulation pedagogy.
- The facilitative approach is appropriate to the level of learning, experience, and competency of the participants.
- Facilitation methods prior to the simulation-based experience include preparatory activities and a pre-briefing to prepare participants for the simulation-based experience.
- Facilitation methods during a simulation-based experience involve the delivery of cues (pre-determined and/or unplanned) aimed to assist participants in achieving expected outcomes.
- Facilitation after and beyond the simulation-based experience aims to support participants in achieving expected outcomes.

The facilitation method should be determined by the level of the participant and the type of evaluation for the simulation.[49] Several types of facilitation can be used and must be appropriate to the participants' level of experience. Beginning participants usually require more instructor cueing or prompting. As the level of experience increases, less instructor prompting is required. During a summative evaluation, such as high-stakes testing, minimal to no prompting by the instructor is performed.

The facilitator is the major component that provides the link between the scenario and the participant to provide guidance for meeting the objectives of the simulation. The role of the facilitator is to adjust the scenario to respond to the actions or inactions of the participants according to the objectives of the scenario. The facilitator also leads the participants in the debriefing process in a positive manner to reflect on ways to improve the care provided for better patient outcomes.

The Debriefing Process

This standards states that "all simulation-based experiences include a planned debriefing session aimed at improving

BOX 33.2 Sample Debriefing Questions for a Pediatric Patient in Isolation for Pneumonia With Cystic Fibrosis

Ask at least one question from each section.

Aesthetic Questions

"I would like each of you to talk to me about the problems _____ was experiencing today."

"What was your main objective during this simulation?"

"How did patient safety and isolation issues affect the patient care you provided?" (scenario specific)

Personal Questions

"Was there any point during the scenario when you felt unsure of your decisions? If yes, how did you manage your feelings and focus on the patient's needs?"

"What made you choose the actions, interventions, and focus that you chose for _____?"

Empirical Question

"I would like each of you to talk with me about the knowledge, skills, attitudes, and previous experiences that provided you with the ability to provide evidence-based care to _____."

Ethical Question

"Talk to me about how your personal beliefs and values influenced the care provided to _____."

Reflection Questions

"Please tell me how you knew what to do for a cystic fibrosis patient with pneumonia in isolation and why."

"If we could repeat this scenario now, what would you change and why?"

"How will you use this in your professional practice?"

---

future performance."[48, p. S21] The purpose of a debriefing is to promote reflective thinking by allowing participants to think about and clarify actions that occurred during the simulation (Box 33.2). The debriefing process has been reported as the most important component of simulation because of the learning that occurs when concepts are clarified.[55,56] Literature suggests that debriefing should last at least as long as the simulation scenario, but current practices vary.[57] Five criteria are necessary to meet this standard[48, p. S21–S22]:

- The debrief is facilitated by a person(s) competent in the process of debriefing.
- The debrief is conducted in an environment that is conducive to learning and supports confidentiality, trust, open communication, self-analysis, feedback, and reflection.
- The debrief is facilitated by a person(s) who can devote enough concentrated attention during the simulation to effectively debrief the simulation-based experience.
- The debrief is based on a theoretical framework for debriefing that is structured in a purposeful way.
- The debrief is congruent with the objectives and outcomes of the simulation-based experience.

Participant Evaluation

This standard states that "all simulation-based experiences require participant evaluation."[51, p. S26] The evaluation and assessment of the participants' performance during the simulation should be based on the focus and desired outcomes of the simulation scenario. The participants should be aware of the evaluation or assessment methods being used before beginning the simulation.[44,58] Four criteria are necessary to meet this standard[51, p. S26–S27]:

- Determine the method of participant evaluation prior to the simulation-based experience.
- Simulation-based experiences may be selected for formative evaluation.
- Simulation-based experiences may be selected for summative evaluation.
- Simulation-based experiences may be selected for high-stakes evaluation.

Simulation-Enhanced Interprofessional Education

This standard states that "simulation-enhanced interprofessional education (Sim-IPE) enables participants from different professions to engage in a simulation-based experience to achieve shared or linked objectives and outcomes."[53, p. S34]

Interprofessional education (IPE) in healthcare is essential to produce high-performing, effective teams to improve patient safety and outcomes. The Sim-IPE is designed for the individuals involved to "learn about, from and with each other to enable effective collaboration and improve health outcomes."[59, p. 2] Four criteria are necessary to meet this standard[53, p. S34–S35]:

- Conduct Sim-IPE based on a theoretical or a conceptual framework.
- Utilize best practices in the design and development of Sim-IPE.
- Recognize and address potential barriers to Sim-IPE.
- Devise an appropriate evaluation plan with Sim-IPE.

Simulation Design

This standard states that "simulation-based experiences are purposefully designed to meet identified objectives and optimize achievement of expected outcomes."[47, p. S5] This standard has eleven criteria[47, p. S6]:

- A needs assessment provided the foundational evidence of the need for a well-designed simulation-based experience.
- Measureable objectives are determined.
- The format of a simulation is structured based on the purpose, theory, and modality for the simulation-based experience.
- A scenario or case provides the context for the simulation-based experience.
- Various types of fidelity are used to create the required perception of realism.
- The facilitator/facilitative approach is participant-centered and driven by the objectives, participant's knowledge or level of experience, and the expected outcomes.
- Simulation-based experiences begin with a pre-briefing.
- Simulation-based experiences are followed by a debriefing and/or feedback session.

BOX 33.3 **Steps for the Simulation Process**

1. Assign the pre-simulation or pre-scenario exercises to be completed by the participants
2. Pre-briefing sessions immediately prior to the simulation
3. Simulation scenario with appropriate facilitation by a trained facilitator
4. Debriefing and/or guided reflection
5. Postsimulation exercises

- The evaluation process includes an evaluation/assessment of the participant(s), facilitator(s), the simulation-based experience, the facility, and the support team.
- Participant preparation and resources promote participants' ability to meet identified objectives and achieve expected outcomes of the simulation-based experience.

The simulation process should follow the steps outlined in Box 33.3 in designing the scenario or experience to assist the participants in achieving the objectives.

APPLICATION OF SIMULATION

General Application of Simulation to Education

The use of simulation in undergraduate nursing, graduate schools for advanced practice nurses (especially nurse anesthetists), medical schools, and IPE has been well documented in the literature. However, literature is limited for simulation applied to doctoral education.

Multiple research studies revealed that students have higher satisfaction with higher levels of fidelity.[10,60] However, studies have not shown that high-fidelity simulation increases students' clinical reasoning skills.[10] There is a growing body of health literature evaluating the differences in student outcomes using low- and high-fidelity simulation experiences. Multiple studies indicated no statistically significant differences in student learning outcomes using traditional pencil-and-paper testing scores, compared to varying levels of fidelity teaching strategies.[61-65]

Some studies have demonstrated a statistically significant difference in students' self-perceived improvements, depending on the level of fidelity used in simulation.[66-70] The participants of these studies preferred high-fidelity teaching strategies as compared to low-fidelity strategies.

Several studies recommend that educators need to compare the level of fidelity when considering cost and short- and long-term participant outcomes.[62,63] Some authors have questioned the choice of appropriate evaluation method: an objective structure clinical examination (OSCE) or a paper-and-pencil test.[63,70] However, there have not been consistent results with OSCEs in terms of finding differences in participants' performances to compare acquisition of knowledge and applying that knowledge to clinical practice.[61]

Application of Simulation for Evaluation

Although there is growing interest in the adoption of clinical simulation within educational programs, there is a gap in empirical research to identify valid and reliable tools for

evaluating simulation effectiveness, especially in translating knowledge and skills from simulation experiences to actual clinical practice; research is needed.[45,71,72]

The American Association of Colleges of Nursing (AACN) has published a white paper for re-envisioning clinical education for nurse practitioner programs as a result of a national think tank group.[73] One of the themes identified was the need for standardized preclinical preparation using simulation activities and standardized core content before students enter the clinical environment. These two factors could impact performance and skills in the patient care environment. Another theme identified was incorporating technology into the curriculum to improve the transition into clinical practice. This could include the use of simulation, both mannequins and standardized patients, in the clinical education of nurse practitioner students. However, the National Organization of Nurse Practitioner Faculties (NONPF) sets the standards for nurse practitioner education and does not currently allow any of the nurse practitioner students' 500 mandatory clinical hours to be obtained using simulation. Clinical hours used for simulation activities must be in addition to the required clinical hours. Several published studies regarding nurse practitioner students or advanced practice nursing (APN) students[74-78] and simulation state that simulation was effective, but this was in addition to the mandatory 500 hours for clinical performance.

Types of evaluations include a formative assessment of performance, or summative evaluation. Skills checklists may be used during a skills validation, such as an indwelling catheter or chest tube insertion for students or an endotracheal intubation for respiratory therapy students.

Formative assessments measure a participant's progress toward overall or long-term program objectives. This type of assessment provides the participant with feedback that will aid in professional growth and promote self-reflection.

Summative evaluations are traditionally measured at the end of a learning experience to correlate with the end of the course or program. This type of evaluation may have a grade assigned or use another method to determine student progression. An example of a summative evaluation is an OSCE. An OSCE summative evaluation can be a graduate student's evaluation at the end of the advanced assessment course to determine his or her ability to perform in a traditional clinical setting. Some medical boards require successful completion of an OSCE to become certified. Regardless of the type of evaluation, the instrument used should have reported psychometric data demonstrating reliability and validity.

The evaluation tools currently used in simulation were described in a review by Kardong-Edgren et al. and were categorized within the cognitive, psychomotor, and affective learning domains.[79] The *cognitive domain* focuses on application with thinking, such as performing, identifying, maintaining, communicating, prioritizing, and providing. An example is that the participant will be able to identify the signs and symptoms of congestive heart failure and provide appropriate interventions for best patient outcomes. The *psychomotor domain* focuses on the precision of performing

---

BOX 33.4 **Learning Domains**

Cognitive domain. Simulation evaluation tools included the Basic Knowledge Assessment Tool 6 (paper-and-pencil test); the Outcome Present State Test Model for Debriefing (worksheets that participants complete during the structured debriefing); the Lasater Clinical Judgment Rubric, based on Tanner's Clinical Judgment Model for student evaluation during simulation; and the Simulation Evaluation Instrument, developed to evaluate the AACN core competencies for undergraduate nursing students during simulation.

Psychomotor domain. There were no tools identified for the psychomotor domain for simulation that reported validity and reliability testing.

Affective domain. The evaluation tools identified in this section were developed to measure student satisfaction and perceived effectiveness of the simulated clinical experience. The tools identified included a satisfaction survey, the Emergency Response Performance Tool (ERPT), and the Simulation Design Scale. Other tools were reviewed for group evaluation.

AACN, American Association of Colleges of Nursing; *ERPT,* Emergency Response Performance Tool.

---

the assessment or skill, such as insertion of an intravenous catheter and effective therapeutic communication using situation-background-assessment-recommendation (SBAR) communication. The *affective domain* focuses on the emotion of reflective thinking by responses to and prioritization of patient care (Box 33.4).

The Clinical Learning Environment Comparison Survey (CLECS) was designed to determine how well undergraduate students' learning needs were met in the simulated clinical environment and in the traditional clinical environment.[80] The CLECS was used during the national simulation study by the NCSBN.[20] Psychometric analysis shows this to be a valid and reliable tool.

The Creighton Simulation Evaluation Instrument (C-SEI)—now known as the Creighton Competency Evaluation Instrument (C-CEI)—is a tool that evaluates simulation experiences by measuring assessment skills.[81] C-CEI was the second tool used in the NCSBN's study and also has established reliability and validity.[20] The C-CEI tool was designed to be modifiable to meet the specific outcomes of the simulation. The goal of this tool was to evaluate student assessment skills for improvement. As the assessment skills improve, so will clinical performance.

The Simulation Effectiveness Tool-Modified (SET-M)[82] was updated in 2015. The original SET tool was developed in 2005 to evaluate the effectiveness of the simulation experience. In 2015, the tool was modified to reflect the INACSL Standards of Best Practice: Simulation[SM], the Quality and Safety Educating Nurses (QSEN) practices, and the AACN baccalaureate essentials. This tool remains valid and reliable for evaluating simulations. The modification of this tool demonstrates the importance of reassessing evaluation instruments as our knowledge of best practices in simulation progresses.

Application of Simulation to Interprofessional Education

Many professional medical organizations stated an increasing need for IPE, as evidenced by the newly introduced Core Competencies for Interprofessional Collaborative Practice sponsored by the Interprofessional Education Collaborative (IPEC) (Table 33.5).[59] IPEC was a collaborative effort of multiple associations, including the AACN, American

Association of Colleges of Osteopathic Medicine, American Association of Colleges of Pharmacy, American Dental Education Association, Association of American Medical Colleges, and Association of Schools of Public Health.

To improve patient safety, evidence-based practice, and translational research, more IPE opportunities are needed. New teaching strategies have evolved. Some of these are in response to the changing technology that has proliferated over the past 25 years. The strategies include the following:

1. Communication tools such as SBAR (situation, background, assessment, recommendation) for more effective professional and interprofessional communication.
2. Simulation scenarios to practice skills and techniques, assessment, therapeutic communication, interprofessional collaboration, reflection on actions and inactions of participants, and incorporation of evidence-based practice throughout the curriculum and applying these in simulation.
3. Informatics capabilities to improve patient care with point-of-care access to information through handheld devices and EHRs.

If the interprofessional members of the healthcare team have access to the pertinent information about a patient, healthcare delivery can be more holistic and potentially decrease harm to the patient. Health sciences students can learn the roles and responsibilities of other healthcare team members for collaborative purposes through IPE simulations to ensure the best patient outcomes. For students in the healthcare profession, IPE simulations are an excellent way to learn how to function and adapt practices to achieve the best outcomes.

Simulation is a strategy to assist team members with effective communication and promote collaboration with other professionals. According to an INACSL survey in 2010, only about half of the respondents provided any IPE. Of the programs providing IPE experiences, only a few institutions stated that the practice was used more than occasionally in the simulation community.[56] Challenges to this type of education exist. In particular, the logistics of scheduling multiple professions for simulation is one of the major obstacles for IPE experience.[83-86] The Institute of Medicine (IOM) also called for the federal government and professional organizations to study the approaches and foci to determine their

TABLE 33.5   Core Competencies for Interprofessional Collaborative Practice

Core Competency	Focus	Application With Simulation	Opportunity for IPE
Roles and responsibilities for collaborative practice	Use the knowledge of each profession's role to assess and address the populations served.	Demonstrate collaboration of team members in a scenario to clearly communicate with each other and provide the best holistic care to meet the needs of the individual or population.	• Disaster drill simulation • Prehospital injury requiring ambulance transport to the emergency department
Interprofessional communication	Communicate in a team approach with individuals, families, and communities in a responsive and responsible manner to support well-being and quality of life.	1. Communicate with confidence, clarity, and respect to promote understanding of information and management of issues. 2. Actively listen and encourage sharing or input from others. 3. Recognize one's uniqueness and role within the team and contribute to effective communication, conflict resolution, and positive interprofessional working relationships.	Scenarios that require multiple professions in diagnosis and planning the care of a patient: • Code situation • Respiratory decline of patient with unknown etiology
Interprofessional teamwork and team-based service	Apply relationship-building values and the principles of team dynamics to perform effectively in different team roles to plan and deliver services that are safe, timely, efficient, effective, and equitable.	1. Work with others to develop consensus on the ethical principles to guide all aspects of interaction with individuals and teamwork. 2. Use process improvement strategies. 3. Reflect on individual and team performance for individual as well as team performance improvement.	• Home health scenario that requires collaboration via phone. • Focus the debriefing process on improvement of any interprofessional simulation.
Values and ethics for interprofessional practice	Work with individuals of other professions to maintain a climate of mutual respect and shared values.	1. Provide care for the community. 2. Demonstrate high standards of ethical conduct. 3. Act with honesty and integrity in relationships with all team members and clients. 4. Maintain competence in one's profession.	Complex scenarios that include moral or ethical decision making and counseling with the patient or family: • Organ transplant decisions • Hospice care • Cultural themes

Data from Interprofessional Education Collaborative Expert Panel. *Core Competencies for Interprofessional Collaborative Practice: Report of an Expert Panel.* Washington, DC: Interprofessional Education Collaborative; 2011.
IPE, Interprofessional education.

contribution to improving the workforce.[87,88] The professional organizations have a responsibility to determine the best resources and methods for improving the education of the healthcare workforce, both in initial education and in continuing professional development.

Example

The following scenario was used in a doctorate of nursing practice program to evaluate nurse practitioner students' ability to assess and develop a differential diagnosis for a patient presenting with angina. Students participated in this experience at the end of their clinical diagnostics course, and this was used for summative evaluation purposes. Prior to any simulation experience, a curricular simulation integration form was used to document objectives, evaluation measures, and the specific details related to the scenario (Fig. 33.2). This plan mapped out the specific details related to the simulation experience and contributed to a successful simulation experience for both the faculty and the students. To prepare, the students received the evaluation rubric to review prior to entering the simulation lab for testing (Fig. 33.3). The detailed evaluation rubric (Fig. 33.4) was used by the faculty member to evaluate the students and provide summative feedback. After the scenario, the students completed a Scenario Evaluation Form to evaluate the quality of the learning experience (Fig. 33.5).[9] These evaluation data were reviewed by the simulation facilitators after the scenario activity to ensure that the scenario met the needs of the students and reflected the highest quality and evidence.

<u>Course Title:</u> **Diagnosis and Management of Adults II**

<u>Scenario Topic:</u> Caring for a patient experiencing chest pain progressing to unstable angina

<u>Time Allotment:</u> 15 minutes for scenario

<u>Instructor:</u> Dr. Ross and Dr. Howard

<u>Facilitation Method:</u> No Facilitator Prompting

<u>Student Level (# of participants, role descriptions)</u>
One DNP–NP student per scenario demonstrating the role of the NP

<u>Scenario Objectives and Evaluation Criteria</u>
Upon completion of this scenario, the student will be able to:
  Obtain pertinent subjective and objective data from history related to chest pain
  Perform a focused physical exam related to complaints of cardiac-related chest pain
  Identify clinical manifestations associated with multiple etiologies of chest pain
  Consider differential diagnosis related to chest pain
  Recognize stable angina progressing to unstable angina
  Maintain a safe environment during patient consult
  Initiate an appropriate diagnostic work-up
  Prescribe appropriate pharmacologic therapy
  Provide patient education regarding treatment regimen
  Document appropriate SOAP note regarding clinical consult

<u>Set-up/Equipment</u>
• High fidelity patient simulator   • Stethoscope
• BP cuff   • Thermometer

<u>Prescenario Learning Activities</u>
Attend class lectures and participate in clinical sharing on coronary artery disease (CAD) and chest pain
Review PowerPoint materials and participate in Discussion Board conversation related to cardiac conditions
Review competency evaluation form

<u>Instructions for Starting Scenario</u>
Introduction to Scenario:
Mr. Pat Tassium is a 50 y/o obese male with history of stable angina reports to the office with the following complaints. He recently noticed increased SOB when ambulating up to his second floor bedroom. He noticed that he has to stop one time before reaching the top of the stairs. Mr. Tassium experienced tightness in his chest X 2 last week as he climbed the stairs to bed. What brings him into the office is when he was mowing his lawn he had to stop twice and take SL NTG. This is different than his past action of just resting and the chest pain would subside.

<u>Social History</u>
Married with three children
Works as the dean in the school of business for the local university
Smokes a pack of cigarettes in three days; this is a considerable decrease from a pack a day a year ago
Admits to social drinking only; one to two drinks on weekends
Currently on the following medications:
  ASA a day
  Lopressor 50 mg 1 tablet daily for HTN
  NTG 0.4 mg SL prn for chest pain

FIG 33.2 Simulation integration and planning form. *ASA*, Acetylsalicylic acid; *BP*, blood pressure; *CAD*, coronary artery disease; *DNP*, doctor of nursing practice; *HTN*, hypertension; *NP*, nurse practitioner; *prn*, as needed; *SL NTG*, sublingual nitroglycerin; *SOAP*, subjective, objective, assessment, and plan; *SOB*, shortness of breath. (Developed by C. Ross, PhD, RN, and V. Howard, EdD, RN. Courtesy of RMU Regional RISE Center.)

Simulator Actions (Vital Signs/Simulator Controls)	Expected Student Interventions/Events
Initial State **Pulse:** 62 **BP:** 140/92 **RR:** 16 **Pulse oximeter:** 96% **Heart rhythm:** regular with occasional unifocal PVC	Obtains pertinent subjective and objective data from history related to chest pain Performs focused physical exam related to complaints of cardiac related chest pain Identifies clinical manifestations associated with multiple etiologies of chest pain Considers differential diagnosis related to chest pain Recognizes stable angina progressing to unstable angina Maintains safe environment during patient consult Initiates appropriate diagnostic work-up Prescribes appropriate pharmacologic therapy Provides patient education regarding treatment regimen Documents appropriate SOAP note regarding clinical consult

Relevant Debriefing Points (Event Management)
- Problem Recognition
- Prioritization
- Problem Intervention
- Rationales

Positive Feedback and Areas for Improvement

Application to Clinical Practice

Simulation Evaluation Survey

Procedure
1. Students given copy of competency evaluation form with general categories one week prior to exam
2. Schedule students for 15-minute time frame
3. Arrive at simulation room and conduct scenario 9 times
4. All students return for 30 minutes upon completion for debriefing:
   - Perception of simulation experience
   - Scenario specifics
   - Simulation evaluation form
5. Other NP faculty view scenarios and complete student performance evaluation forms

FIG 33.3 Student evaluation rubric. *BP*, Blood pressure; *NP*, nurse practitioner; *PVC*, premature ventricular contraction; *RR*, respiratory rate; *SOAP*, subjective, objective, assessment, and plan. (Developed by C. Ross PhD, RN, and V. Howard EdD, RN. Courtesy of RMU Regional RISE Center.)

CONCLUSION AND FUTURE DIRECTIONS

The use of simulation is rapidly emerging as a preferred way to train healthcare professionals in a safe, controlled manner with no risk to patients. One of the reasons for its emergence is that simulation can overcome current barriers with traditional clinical experiences. There may be a shortage of clinical sites; patients may have complex conditions that a novice learner is unprepared to manage; and clinical sites may have limited student experiences for EHRs, administering medications to pediatric patients, and other situations. These factors, combined with a nursing and nurse educator shortage and the aging population, will further increase the need to teach healthcare providers in a simulation environment. IPE experiences are essential to the development of healthcare workers that function as an effective team to improve patient safety and outcomes. Educators must seek out IPE collaboration opportunities for students to improve their experiential learning and working in teams.

Newer approaches that reflect the advances in technology are virtual reality computer-based simulations and gaming. Gaming is a type of simulation technique that meets the needs of millennial learners and has been embraced more fully in the past few years by educators.[89] However, gaming faces some of the same challenges as simulation has in its understanding, growth, and acceptance as a teaching strategy. The emergence of technology for educational purposes creates a need for faculty and health science educators to understand how to not only operate the technology but also implement it within the academic and service settings while still using sound academic principles. Standards of Best Practice: Simulation will continue to serve as a foundation for all types of simulation-based teaching methodologies.

Simulation use and guidelines will provide a foundation to build experiential learning experiences, evaluate student performance, and learn to practice as a healthcare team. As the science and technology of simulation advances, so will the learning opportunities. The NCSBN Simulation guidelines

Evaluation Rating			Performance Criteria	Comments
Exceeds Expectations	**Meets Expectations**	**Does Not Meet Expectations**		
			Initial Encounter	2 pts
			Introduces self to patient	
			Checks and verifies patient's identification	
			Validates demographic data	
			Obtains or validates vital signs	
			Assessment/ History Taking/ Differential Diagnosis	8 pts
			Asks important questions to elicit cardiovascular risk factors	
			Asks important questions to characterize chest pain; may use PQRST	
			Able to differentiate between stable and unstable angina	
			Considers differentials related to chest pain	
			Identifies clinical manifestations associated with multiple etiologies of chest pain	
			Informs patient of possible differential diagnosis	
			Physical Examination	5 pts
			General appearance and validation of vital signs	
			Examination of skin, eyes, carotid pulse, & JVD	
			Chest wall examination: heart & lungs	
			Abdomen	
			Lower extremities	
			Neurologic exam for focal deficits	
			Correlates abnormal assessment findings with differential diagnoses	
			Interventions	6 pts
			Ensures patient safety and safe environment by staying with patient or having co-worker stay with patient	
			Orders appropriate immediate interventions	
			Initiates orders for appropriate diagnostic studies: Imaging Laboratory	
			Prescribes appropriate pharmacological therapy	
			Provides patient education and health promotion	
			Evaluation of Patient Responses	2 pts
			Evaluates patient's response to all interventions Follow up & referral	
			Documentation	2 pts
			Writes an appropriate SOAP note from patient encounter	

FIG 33.4 Detailed faculty evaluation rubric. *JVD*, jugular venous distention; *PQRST*, provokes, quality, radiates, severity, time; *SOAP*, subjective, objective, assessment, and plan.

Please circle the best response to each of the following questions.

Please circle the response that best describes how you feel about the simulation experience:

	Strongly Disagree	Disagree	Agree	Strongly Agree
1. The simulation experience helped me to better understand advanced nursing concepts.	1	2	3	4
2. The simulation was a valuable learning experience.	1	2	3	4
3. The simulation helped to stimulate critical thinking abilities.	1	2	3	4
4. The simulation was realistic.	1	2	3	4
5. The knowledge gained through the simulation experiences can be transferred to the advanced practice clinical setting.	1	2	3	4
6. I was nervous during the simulation experience.	1	2	3	4
7. Because of the simulation experience, I will be less nervous in the primary care setting when providing care for similar patients.	1	2	3	4
8. Simulation experiences can be a substitute for clinical experiences in the primary care clinical areas.	1	2	3	4
9. Simulation experiences should be included in our DNP education.	1	2	3	4

10. Now, please add any additional comments regarding the simulation experience:

FIG 33.5 Simulation evaluation. *DNP*, Doctor of nursing practice. (Developed by V. Howard. 2010. Courtesy of RMU Regional RISE Center.)

for prelicensure nursing programs were released in fall 2015 as a guideline for including simulation as part of clinical hours in nursing education. This will impact nursing education and practice depending on how each state adopts the guidelines. One area that will need to be investigated is simulation and the APN degree. Some nursing leaders have stated the NCSBN National Simulation Study results indicate that simulation could be beneficial in the education and training of APNs. This is an area for future research that could require policy change also.[73]

High-stakes testing, such as OSCEs similar to those for medical students, may someday be required for licensure into nursing practice. The NLN has been evaluating the possibility of including a high-stake testing OSCE for licensure to practice nursing for greater than 5 years However, there are many challenges involved with faculty wanting to use high-stakes testing, especially for licensure. Some of these challenges are a lack of trained faculty and quality simulations for validity and reliability, lack of students with enough experience in other types of simulation, and the concept that "no student should be judged via one single test."[90, p. 302] The NCSBN National Simulation Study results and simulation guideline may begin to move this concept forward.

As technology advances, so will healthcare simulations. We do not know the possibilities that await us. Everyday new technology is invented that will assist with the education and training of healthcare providers. The current technology allows for tracking eye movement during simulation and patient care to see where the healthcare provider is focusing. This is accomplished by utilizing glasses, which can be bulky or cumbersome. However, newer technology may advance, and this could become common practice. Newer virtual technology under development is similar to the hologram deck seen in futurist space shows and is beginning to be used in some labs. These include the ability to view the human body on different levels: whole body, muscles, bones, and internal organs. This will provide more learners the ability to apply didactic learning to the clinical setting without the need for cadavers and some simulators.

REFERENCES

1. International Nursing Association for Clinical Simulation and Learning Board of Directors. Standards of best practice: Simulation[SM]. *Clin Simul Nurs.* 2013;9(6S):S1–S32. http://www.inacsl.org/files/journal/Complete%202013%20Standards.pdf.
2. Benner P. *From Novice to Expert: Excellence and Power in Clinical Nursing Practice.* Menlo Park, CA: Addison-Wesley; 1984.
3. Kolb DA. *Experiential Learning.* Englewood Cliffs, NJ: Prentice-Hall; 1984.

4. Foronda C, Bauman EB. Strategies to incorporate virtual simulation in nursing education. *Clin Simul Nurs*. 2014;10: e412–e418. http://dx.doi.org/10.1016/j.ecns.2014.03.005.

5. Smith NT. Physiologic modeling for simulators: get real. In: Kyle RR, Bosseau Murray W, eds. *Clinical Simulation: Operations, Engineering, and Management*. Burlington, VT: Elsevier; 2008:459–467.

6. Guise V, Chambers M, Valimaki M. What can virtual patient simulation offer mental health nursing education? *J Psychiatr Ment Health Nurs*. 2012;19(5):410–418.

7. Paige JB, Morin KH. Simulation fidelity and cueing: a systematic review of the literature. *Clin Simul Nurs*. 2013;9 (11):e481–e489. http://dx.doi.org/10.1016/j.ecns.2013.01.001.

8. Alinier G. A typology of educationally focused medical simulation tools. *Med Teach*. 2007;29(8):1–8. http://dx.doi.org/ 10.1080/01421590701551185.

9. Howard V, Ross C, Mitchell A, Nelson G. Human patient simulators and interactive case studies: a comparative analysis of learning outcomes and student perceptions. *Comput Inform Nurs*. 2010;28(1):42–48.

10. Mariani B, Cantrell MA, Meakim C, Prieto P, Dreifuerst KT. Structured debriefing and students' clinical judgment abilities in simulation. *Clin Simul Nurs*. 2013;9(5):e147–e155. http://dx.doi. org/10.1016/j.ecns.2011.11.009.

11. McGaghie W, Issenberg SB, Petrusa E, Scalese R. A critical review of simulation-based medical education research: 2003–2009. *Med Educ*. 2009;44:50–63.

12. Ozkara San E. Using clinical simulation to enhance culturally competent nursing care: a review of the literature. *Clin Simul Nurs*. 2015;11(4):228–243. http://dx.doi.org/10.1016/j.ecns. 2015.01.004. 2015.

13. Cooper S, Cant R, Porter J, et al. Simulation based learning in midwifery education: a systematic review. *Women Birth*. 2011;25(2):64–78. http://dx.doi.org/10.1016/j. wombi.2011.03.004.

14. Kirkpatrick DL, Kirkpatrick JD. *Evaluating Training Programs*. 3rd ed. San Francisco, CA: Berrett-Koehler Publishers; 2006.

15. McGaghie WC, Draycott TJ, Dunn WF, Lopez CM, Stefanidis D. Evaluating the impact of simulation on translational patient outcomes. *Simul Healthc*. 2011;(6 suppl):S42–S47. http://dx.doi. org/10.1097/SIH.0b013e318222fde9.

16. Adamson K, Kardong-Edgren S, Wilhaus J. An updated review of published simulation evaluation instruments. *Clin Simul Nurs*. 2013;9(9):e393–e400. http://dx.doi.org/10.1016/j.ecns. 2012.09.004.

17. Barsuk JH, Cohen ER, Vozenilek JA, et al. Simulation-based education with mastery learning improves paracentesis skills. *J Grad Med Educ*. 2012;4(1):23–27. http://dx.doi.org/10.4300/ JGME-D-11-00161.

18. Draycott T, Crofts J, Ash J, et al. Improving neonatal outcome through practical shoulder dystocia training. *Obstet Gynecol*. 2008;112(1):14–20.

19. McCarthy J. Malpractice insurance carrier provides premium incentive for simulation-based training and believes it has made a difference. *Anesthesia Patient Safety Foundation Newsletter*; 2007. http://www.apsf.org/newsletters/html/2007/spring/17_ malpractice.htm.

20. Hayden JK, Smiley RA, Alexander M, Kardong-Edgren S, Jeffries PR. The NCSBN national simulation study: a longitudinal, randomized, controlled study replacing clinical hours with simulation in prelicensure nursing education. *J Nurs Regul*. 2014;5(2):C1–S64.

21. Alexander M, Durham CF, Hooper JI, et al. NCSBN simulation guidelines for prelicensure nursing programs. *J Nurs Regul*. 2015;6:39–42.

22. Thomas CM, Sievers LD, Kellgren M, Manning SJ, Rojas DE, Gamblian VC. Developing a theory-based simulation educator resource. *Nurs Educ Perspect*. 2015;36:340–342. http://dx.doi. org/10.5480/15-1673.

23. International Nursing Association for Clinical Simulation and Learning (INACSL). *Welcome to INACSL*; 2015. http://www. inacsl.org/i4a/pages/index.cfm?pageid=1.

24. Society for Simulation in Healthcare (SSH). *Society for Simulation in Healthcare*; 2015. http://www.ssih.org.

25. National League for Nursing. *National League for Nursing (NLN)*; 2015. http://www.nln.org.

26. Jeffries PR, ed. *The NLN Jeffries Simulation Theory*. Philadelphia, PA: Wolters Kluwer; 2016.

27. Simulation Innovation Resource Center (SIRC). *An interactive global simulation community*. http://www.sirc.nln.org; 2015.

28. Association of Standardized Patient Educators (ASPE). *Association of Standardized Patient Educators*; 2015. http:// www.aspeducators.org.

29. Games + Learning + Society. *We research and design games for learning*; 2015. www.gameslearningsociety.org.

30. Kotter JP. *Leading Change*. Boston, MA: Harvard Business Review Press; 1996.

31. Jeffries PR, Battin J, Franklin M, et al. Creating a professional development plan for a simulation consortium. *Clin Simul Nurs*. 2013;9(6):e183–e189. http://dx.doi.org/10.1016/j. ecns.2012.02.003.

32. Kneebone R. Evaluating clinical simulations for learning procedural skills: a theory-based approach. *Acad Med*. 2005;80 (6):549–553.

33. Knowles MS. Andragogy, not pedagogy. *Adult Leadership*. 1968;16(10):350–352. 386.

34. Knowles MS. *The Adult Learner: A Neglected Species*. 3rd ed. Houston, TX: Gulf; 1984.

35. Clapper TC. Beyond Knowles: what those conducting simulation need to know about adult learning theory. *Clin Simul Nurs*. 2010;6(1):e7–e14. http://dx.doi.org/10.1016/j. ecns.2009.07.003.

36. Kolb DA. *Organizational Behavior: An Experiential Approach to Human Behavior in Organizations*. Englewood Cliffs, NJ: Prentice-Hall; 1995.

37. Onda EL. Situated cognition: its relationship to simulation in nursing education. *Clin Simul Nurs*. 2012;8(7):e273–e280. http:// dx.doi.org/10.1016/j.ecns.2010.11.004.

38. Whrostok LJ, Hoffart J, Kelly I, Ryba K. Situated cognition as a learning framework for international end-of-life simulation. *Clin Simul Nurs*. 2014;10:e217–e222. http://dx.doi.org/10.1016/j. ecns.2013.11.005.

39. Lasater K. High-fidelity simulation and the development of clinical judgment: students' experience. *J Nurs Educ*. 2007;46 (6):269–276.

40. Lasater K. Clinical judgment development: using simulation to create an assessment rubric. *J Nurs Educ*. 2007;46(11): 498–503.

41. Jeffries PR. Preface. In: Jeffries PR, ed. *Simulation in Nursing Education: From Conceptualization to Evaluation*. New York: National League for Nursing; 2007:xi–xii.

42. Adamson K. A systematic review of the literature related to the NLN/Jeffries simulation framework. *Nurs Educ Perspect*. 2015;36:281–291. http://dx.doi.org/10.5480/15-1655.

43. Gaba DM. The future vision of simulation in health care. *Qual Saf Health Care.* 2004;13:i2–i10. http://dx.doi.org/10.1136/qshc.2004.009878.
44. Decker S, Gore T, Feken C. Simulation. In: Bristol T, Zerwekh J, eds. *Essentials of e-Learning for Nurse Educators.* Philadelphia, PA: FA Davis; 2011:277–294.
45. Howard VM, Englert N, Kameg K, Perozzi K. Integration of simulation across the undergraduate curriculum: student and faculty perspectives. *Clin Simul Nurs.* 2011;7(1):e1–e10. http://dx.doi.org/10.1016/j.ecns.2009.10.004.
46. INACSL Standards Committee. Standards of best practice simulation^SM. *Clin Simul Nurs.* 2016;12(S):S39–S47. http://dx.doi.org/10.1016/j.ecns.2016.09.012.
47. INACSL Standards Committee. Standards of best practice simulation^SM: Simulation design. *Clin Simul Nurs.* 2016;12(S):S5–S12. http://dx.doi.org/10.1016/j.ecns.2016.09.005.
48. INACSL Standards Committee. Standards of best practice simulation^SM: Debriefing. *Clin Simul Nurs.* 2016;12(S):S21–S25. http://dx.doi.org/10.1016/j.ecns.2016.09.008.
49. INACSL Standards Committee. Standards of best practice simulation^SM: Facilitation. *Clin Simul Nurs.* 2016;12(S):S16–S20. http://dx.doi.org/10.1016/j.ecns.2016.09.007.
50. INACSL Standards Committee. Standards of best practice simulation^SM: Outcomes and objectives. *Clin Simul Nurs.* 2016;12(S):S13–S15. http://dx.doi.org/10.1016/j.ecns.2016.09.006.
51. INACSL Standards Committee. Standards of best practice simulation^SM: Participants evaluation. *Clin Simul Nurs.* 2016;12(S):S26–S29. http://dx.doi.org/10.1016/j.ecns.2016.09.009.
52. INACSL Standards Committee. Standards of best practice simulation^SM: Professional integrity. *Clin Simul Nurs.* 2016;12(S):S30–S33. http://dx.doi.org/10.1016/j.ecns.2016.09.010.
53. INACSL Standards Committee. Standards of best practice simulation^SM: Simulation-enhanced interprofessional education (Sim-IPE). *Clin Simul Nurs.* 2016;12(S):S34–S38. http://dx.doi.org/10.1016/j.ecns.2016.09.011.
54. Lopreiato JO, ed., Downing D, Gammon W, Lioce L, Sittner B, Slot V, Spain AE, Associate eds., and the Terminology & Concepts Working Group. *Healthcare Simulation Dictionary.* 2016. Retrieved from http://www.ssih.org/dictionary.
55. Mariani B, Cantrell MA, Meakim C, Prieto P, Dreifuerst KT. Structured debriefing and students' clinical judgment abilities in simulation. *Clin Simul Nurs.* 2013;9(5):e147–e155. http://dx.doi.org/10.1016/j.ecns.2011.11.009.
56. Gore T, Van Gele P, Ravert P, Mabire C. A 2010 survey of the INACSL membership about simulation use. *Clin Simul Nurs.* 2012;8(4):e125–e133. http://dx.doi.org/10.1016/j.ecns.2012.01.002.
57. Waxman KT. The development of evidence-based clinical simulation scenarios: guidelines for nurse educators. *J Nurs Educ.* 2010;49(1):29–35.
58. Jeffries PR, McNelis AM. Evaluation. In: Nehring WM, Lashley FR, eds. *High-Fidelity Patient Simulation in Nursing Education.* Boston, MA: Jones and Bartlett; 2010:405–424.
59. Interprofessional Education Collaborative Expert Panel. *Core Competencies for Interprofessional Collaborative Practice: Report of an Expert Panel.* Washington, DC: Interprofessional Education Collaborative; 2011.
60. Weaver A. The effect of a model demonstration during debriefing on students' clinical judgment, self-confidence, and satisfaction during a simulated learning experience. *Clin Simul Nurs.* 2015;11(1):20–26. http://dx.doi.org/10.1016/j.ecns.2014.10.009.
61. Gore T, Leighton K, Sanderson B, Wang C-H. Fidelity's effect on student perceived preparedness for patient care. *Clin Simul Nurs.* 2014;10(6):e309–e315. http://dx.doi.org/10.1016/j.ecns.2014.01.003. 2014.
62. Wang AL, Fitzpatrick JJ, Petrini MA. Comparison of two simulation methods on Chinese BSN students' learning. *Clin Simul Nurs.* 2013;9(6):e207–e212. http://dx.doi.org/10.1016/j.ecns.2012.01.007.
63. Rutherford-Hemming T, Simko L, Dusaj TK, Kelsey NC. What moves simulation. *Clin Simul Nurs.* 2015;11:199–200. http://dx.doi.org/10.1016/j.ecns.2014.11.007.
64. Foronda C, Liu S, Bauman EB. Evaluation of simulation in undergraduate nurse education: an integrative review. *Clin Simul Nurs.* 2013;9(10):e409–e416. http://dx.doi.org/10.1016/j.ecns.2012.11.003.
65. Groom JA, Henderson D, Sittner BJ. NLN/Jeffries simulation framework state of the science project: simulation design characteristics. *Clin Simul Nurs.* 2014;10(7):337–344. http://dx.doi.org/10.1016/j.ecns.2013.02.004.
66. Faran JM, Paro JAM, Rodriguez RM, et al. Hand-off education and evaluation: piloting the observed simulated hand-off experience (OSHE). *J Gen Intern Med.* 2010;25(2):129–134.
67. Stroup C. Simulation usage in nursing fundamentals: integrative literature review. *Clin Simul Nurs.* 2014;10(3):e155–e164. http://dx.doi.org/10.1016/j.ecns.2013.10.004.
68. Arnold JJ, Johnson LM, Tucker SJ, Chesak SS, Dierkhising RA. Comparison of three simulation-based teaching methodologies for emergency response. *Clin Simul Nurs.* 2013;9(3):e85–e93. http://dx.doi.org/10.1016/j.ecns.2011.09.004.
69. Goodstone L, Goodstone MS. Use of simulation to develop a medication administration safety assessment tool. *Clin Simul Nurs.* 2013;9(12):e609–e615. http://dx.doi.org/10.1016/j.ecns.2013.04.017.
70. Johnson MP, Hickey KT, Scopa-Goldman J, et al. Manikin versus web-based simulation for advanced practice nursing students. *Clin Simul Nurs.* 2014;10(6):e317–e323. http://dx.doi.org/10.1016/j.ecns.2014.02.004.
71. Hayden J. Use of simulation in nursing education: national survey results. *J Nurs Regul.* 2010;1(3):52–57.
72. Kardong-Edgren S, Willhaus J, Bennett D, Hayden J. Results of the National Council of State Boards of Nursing National Simulation Survey: Part II. *Clin Simul Nurs.* 2012;8(4):e117–e123. http://dx.doi.org/10.1016/j.ecns.2012.01.003.
73. AACN APRN Clinical Training Task Force. *White Paper: Current state of APRN Clinical Education*; 2015; 1–42. http://www.aacn.nche.edu/APRN-White-Paper.pdf.
74. Tiffen J, Graf N, Corbridge S. Effectiveness of a low fidelity simulation experience in building confidence among advanced practice nursing graduate students. *Clin Simul Nurs.* 2009;5(3):e113–e117.
75. Johnson MP, Hickey KT, Scopa-Goldman J, et al. Manikin versus web-based simulation for advanced practice nursing students. *Clin Simul Nurs.* 2014;10(6):e317–e323.
76. Mompoint-Williams D, Brooks A, Lee L, Watts P, Moss J. Using high-fidelity simulation to prepare advanced practice nursing students. *Clin Simul Nurs.* 2014;10(1):e5–e10.
77. Lucisano KE, Talbot LA. Simulation training for advanced airway management for anesthesia and other healthcare providers: a systematic review. *AANA J.* 2012;80(1):25–31.
78. Penprase B, Mileto L, Bittinger A, et al. The use of high fidelity simulation in the admission process: one nurse anesthesia program's experience. *AANA J.* 2012;80(1):43–48.

79. Kardong-Edgren S, Adamson KA, Fitzgerald C. A review of currently published evaluation instruments for human patient simulation. *Clin Simul Nurs.* 2010;6(1):e25–e35. http://dx.doi.org/10.1016/j.ecns.2009.08.004.

80. Leighton KL. Development of the clinical learning environment comparison survey. *Clin Simul Nurs.* 2015;11(1):e44–e51.

81. Parsons ME, Hawkins KS, Hercinger M, Todd M, Manz JA, Fang X. Improvement in scoring consistency for the Creighton Simulation Evaluation Instrument. *Clin Simul Nurs.* 2012;8(6):e233–e238. http://dx.doi.org/10.1015.jecns.2012.02.008.

82. Leighton K, Ravert P, Mudra V, Macintosh C. Updating the simulation effectiveness tool: Item modification and reevluation of psychometric properties. *Nurs Educ Perspect.* 2015;36 (5):317–323.

83. Failla KR, Macauley K. Interprofessional simulation: a concept analysis. *Clin Simul Nurs.* 2014;10(11):574–580. http://dx.doi.org/10.1016/j.ecns.2014.07.006.

84. Angelini DJ. Interdisciplinary and interprofessional education: what are the key issues and considerations for the future? *J Perinat Neonatal Nurs.* 2011;25(2):175–179.

85. Leonard B, Shuhaibar EL, Chen R. Nursing student perceptions of intraprofessional team education using high-fidelity simulation. *J Nurs Educ.* 2010;4(11):628–631. http://dx.doi.org/10.3928/01484834-20100730-06.

86. Reese CE, Jeffries PR, Engum SA. Learning together: using simulations to develop nursing and medical student collaboration. *Nurs Educ Perspect.* 2010;31(1):33–37.

87. Institute of Medicine (IOM). *Health Professions Education: A Bridge to Quality.* Washington, DC: National Academies Press; 2003.

88. Wachter RM. The end of the beginning: patient safety five years after "to err is human" *Health Aff.* 2004;W4-534–W4-545. http://content.healthaffairs.org/content/early/2004/11/30/hlthaff.w4.534.short. 2004.

89. Bauman EB. *Game-Based Teaching and Simulation in Nursing and Healthcare.* New York: Springer; 2012.

90. Rizzolo MA, Kardong-Edgren S, Oermann MH, Jeffries PR. The National League for Nursing project to explore the use of simulation for high-stakes assessment: process, outcomes and recommendations. *Nurs Educ Prospect.* 2015;36 (5):299–303.

DISCUSSION QUESTIONS

1. You are a graduate teaching assistant at the local university. A faculty member approaches you to "do" a simulation for class. What information do you need prior to developing the simulation? Provide a rationale for the information needed.

2. As a faculty member facilitating a debriefing, list five questions that you would ask to promote self-reflection.

3. Provide an example of an interprofessional simulation that would facilitate your graduate-level education. List the specific learning objectives, the team members, the participants' experience level and learning, and the type of facilitation and debriefing to guide this simulation scenario.

4. You are a faculty member struggling with generating support for your simulation program. You are experiencing resistance from faculty members and administration with the implementation of this new technology. What can you do to enhance buy-in?

CASE STUDY

You have been hired to teach in a graduate health program. Your newly developed course has an objective that states: *Upon completion of this course, the learner will be able to demonstrate interprofessional team-building concepts.* As a new educator, you would like to include simulation as a teaching methodology to achieve this and other course objectives.

After you are hired, you find a rarely used, high-fidelity human patient simulator in the corner of your skills lab. You inquire about using it for your course but are met with resistance from other faculty members, who tell you that "There is no reason to use simulation. We tried that approach and it takes much too much time to learn the technology and develop the teaching materials. We've always taught our content using written case scenarios, and the students are doing just fine."

Discussion Questions

1. Use Kotter's eight steps leading to successful change to develop a plan for using simulation to teach team concepts.

2. Which published documents can assist you in clarifying the interprofessional competencies and objectives for a team-building, simulation-based learning experience?

3. What information should you incorporate when developing the scenario?

4. Develop an evaluation plan for determining the effectiveness of the learning experience.

5. Unfortunately, students who experienced the scenario at 8 AM are sharing information with students scheduled later in the day. Which INACSL standard addresses this issue, and how can you deter this behavior?

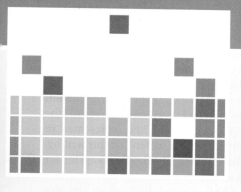

34

International Efforts, Issues, and Innovations

Hyeoun-Ae Park and Nicholas R. Hardiker

The promotion of eHealth internationally requires the engagement of people and organizations in the development of national and regional eHealth initiatives and strategies.

OBJECTIVES

At the completion of this chapter, the reader will be prepared to:
1. Outline key international eHealth initiatives.

2. Describe key organizations that are leading international initiatives to promote eHealth.
3. Discuss global challenges to eHealth.

KEY TERMS

eHealth, 577
information and communication technology (ICT), 577

international standards, 587

ABSTRACT ❖

This chapter highlights international eHealth initiatives, international organizations involved in these initiatives, and the challenges faced by these organizations. Numerous international eHealth-related activities have been initiated across the different regions of the world. Several international organizations are also involved in the development of eHealth, such as the World Health Organization (WHO), the International Medical Informatics Association (IMIA), the International Organization for Standardization (ISO), the International Council of Nurses (ICN), the International Health Terminology Standards Development Organisation (IHTSDO), and Health Level Seven (HL7). These activities and organizations are introduced here, prior to a wider discussion of global challenges to eHealth.

INTRODUCTION

Healthcare is one of the largest sectors of the economy in many parts of the world. As a result, health spending plays a major role in economic policy. The healthcare industry is challenged by economic uncertainty to streamline costs, gain efficiencies, and become more innovative to improve and maintain population health. Today the health industry seeks better ways to provide global healthcare. The use of information and communication technology (ICT) for health, referred to by the World Health Organization (WHO) as eHealth, is seen as key to realizing this aim. The shared goal is to use technology to effectively and efficiently improve the health of individuals, families, and communities.

eHealth faces many international challenges. A coordinated effort is necessary to overcome these challenges. This chapter highlights international eHealth initiatives and describes the work of health professionals such as nurses in meeting these challenges. Throughout the chapter, eHealth and health informatics will be used interchangeably, depending on the context.

KEY INITIATIVES IN WORLD REGIONS

The following sections explore key initiatives to promote eHealth region by region. For each region, government-supported eHealth initiatives are described, along with an overview of the regional groupings of the International Medical Informatics Association (IMIA). These regional initiatives in turn contribute to a coordinated global effort.

eHealth Initiatives in Europe

eHealth emerged in Europe in the late 1950s and early 1960s. The European Union (EU) was formed under the Maastricht Treaty in 1993. The European Commission (EC), through its executive body, provided billions of euros in research funding to develop eHealth tools and systems. These EU-supported projects helped establish Europe as a leader in the use of national and regional health networks and electronic health records (EHRs)—for example, through the deployment of digital health cards in primary care.

In 2004, the EU adopted an eHealth action plan, "Making Healthcare Better for European Citizens: An Action Plan for a European e-Health Area," to facilitate a more harmonious and complementary European approach to eHealth.[1] The action plan covered a range of functions, from electronic prescriptions to new information systems that reduce medical errors, for example, through electronic prescribing. The plan identified actions required for widespread European adoption of eHealth technologies and encouraged individual members to customize strategies based on individual needs. Each member state also developed a national or regional road map for eHealth. The strategies addressed the challenges of providing citizen-centered healthcare services in order to meet rising expectations of Europeans, while concomitantly dealing with issues raised by increasing mobility, aging populations, and budgetary constraints. National and regional strategies currently focus on deploying eHealth systems, ensuring interoperability, using EHRs and reimbursing eHealth.

The revised EU eHealth action plan, "eHealth Action Plan 2012–2020: Innovative Healthcare for the 21st Century,"[2] combines previously implemented actions while looking toward the future of eHealth in Europe. The EU also supports eHealth research programs and projects under Horizon 2020, its Research Framework Programme for Research and Innovation.

The EC created two expert groups, the stakeholder group and a temporary task force (TF), to further the eHealth Action Plan. Details of the groups can be found at https://ec.europa.eu/digital-agenda/en/ehealth-experts. Members of the eHealth stakeholder group are appointed for a 3-year term to contribute to legislation and policy, focusing on patient access to health records, the deployment of telemedicine, health inequality, eHealth workforce, and issues related to interoperability (see https://ec.europa.eu/digital-agenda/interoperability-standardisation-connecting-ehealth-services). TF members—healthcare professionals, patient representatives, representatives of pharmaceutical and ICT industries, legal experts, and policy makers—advise the EC and provide recommendations related to unlocking the eHealth potential (see http://ec.europa.eu/digital-agenda/en/news/eu-task-force-ehealth-redesigning-health-europe-2020).

The work of these two groups is complemented by the eHealth network, a voluntary network of representatives from EU member states that aims to enhance interoperability between electronic health systems to promote continuity of care and to ensure access to safe and quality healthcare. The network meets annually. Health ministers and secretaries of state from EU member states also meet annually at a high-level conference to discuss and move eHealth initiatives forward.

Part of the eHealth Action Plan concerns collaboration between the EC and the United States. The U.S. Department of Health and Human Services (HHS) and the EC's DG CONNECT signed a Memorandum of Understanding (MoU) in 2010 to strengthen transatlantic cooperation in eHealth. The two organizations published a draft road map, which has been the subject of public consultation, with a focus on standards to support transatlantic interoperability and workforce development for both regions (see https://ec.europa.eu/digital-single-market/en/news/transatlantic-ehealthhealth-it-cooperation-roadmap). The road map has subsequently been extended to include innovation.

The European Federation for Medical Informatics

The European Federation for Medical Informatics (EFMI) was created in 1976 with the assistance of the WHO Regional Office for Europe. Its main purpose was and is to enhance European health sciences by encouraging the implementation of information science in the field. Each country within the European Region of WHO is entitled to be represented in EFMI by a suitable health informatics society. At this writing, 32 countries in Europe have joined EFMI. The footprint for these countries can be seen in Fig. 34.1.

The objectives of EFMI (established when it was founded) are to[3]:

- Advance international cooperation and dissemination of information in Medical Informatics on a European basis.
- Promote high standards in the application of medical informatics.
- Promote research and development in medical informatics.
- Encourage high standards in education in medical informatics.
- Function as the autonomous European regional Council of IMIA

For EFMI, the term medical informatics includes health informatics and all disciplines concerned with health and informatics (this would include eHealth). EFMI is a regional member of the International Medical Informatics Association (IMIA) and has formal liaison relations with WHO and the Council of Europe. Activities of EFMI include academic conferences and publications, including the Medical Informatics Europe (MIE) congress, which has been running since 1978. Congress proceedings are published as a series: Lecture Notes in Medical Informatics and Studies in Health Technologies and Informatics. A selection of the best papers from the MIE conferences is published in special volumes of the International Journal of Medical Informatics and Methods of Information in Medicine. Open access to the latest MIE conference proceedings is provided on the EFMI website at https://www.efmi.org/index.php/publications/conference-proceedings. Less well known but important are the Special Topic Conferences. A Special Topic Conference is organized by an EFMI member society in combination with its annual meeting. The topic of the conference is defined by the needs of the member society. Relevant EFMI working groups (WGs) are engaged for content selection. EFMI's WGs also organize their own working conferences or business meetings. Currently there are 17 WGs within EFMI (Box 34.1).

eHealth Initiatives in the Asia-Pacific Economic Cooperation Region

One of the three priorities of the Asia-Pacific Economic Cooperation (APEC) Health Working Group (www.apechwg.org) is "strengthening health systems of economies including health financing, human resources, and health information technologies which would contribute to inclusive and secure growth."[4] Because eHealth has great potential to support healthcare improvements in the APEC region,

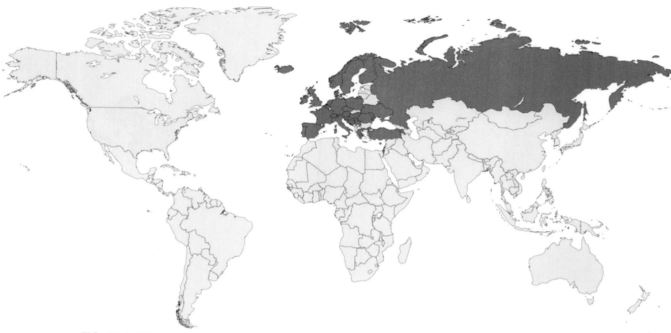

FIG 34.1 EFMI member countries: Armenia, Austria, Belgium, Bosnia Herzegovina, Croatia, Cyprus, Czech Republic, Denmark, Finland, France, Germany, Greece, Hungary, Iceland, Ireland, Israel, Italy, Netherlands, Norway, Poland, Portugal, Republic of Moldova, Romania, Russia, Serbia, Slovenia, Spain, Sweden, Switzerland, Turkey, Ukraine, and United Kingdom.

BOX 34.1 European Federation for Medical Informatics Working Groups

- Education (EDU)
- Electronic Health Records (EHR)
- Assessment of Health Information Systems (EVAL)
- Health Informatics for Interregional Cooperation (HIIC)
- Health Information Management Europe (HIME)
- Human and Organizational Factors of Medical Informatics (HOFMI)
- Information and Decision Support in Biomedicine and Health-care (IDeS)
- Libre/Free and Open Source Software in Health Informatics (LIFOSS)

- Casemix, Resources Management and Outcomes of Care (MCRO/MBDS)
- Medical Image Processing (MIP)
- Natural Languages Understanding (NLU)
- Nursing Informatics in Europe (NURSIE)
- Primary Healthcare Informatics (PCI)
- Personal Portable Devices (PPD)
- Security, Safety and Ethics (SSE)
- Traceability of Supply Chains (TRACE)
- Translational Health Informatics (THI)

---

investing in eHealth could address the health challenges facing the region.

Asia Pacific Association for Medical Informatics

The Asia Pacific Association for Medical Informatics (APAMI) began in 1993 as a regional group within IMIA (www.apami. org) to promote the theory and practice of health informatics within the APEC region. At this writing APAMI has 18 society members, as seen in Fig. 34.2 and listed in Box 34.2.

APAMI activities include biennial conferences and WGs. The inaugural APAMI conference was held in Singapore in 1994. Over the last several years, these conferences have been held in eight different Asian countries. WGs within APAMI have included Standardization, Health Informatics for

Developing Countries, Decision Support, and Nursing Informatics. Each WG has hosted a workshop during the APAMI conference.

APAMI actively promotes telemedicine, bioinformatics, and public health informatics. Because of the large size of its countries, the low specialist-to-population ratio, the affordable cost of technology and telecommunication, and the high penetration rate of eHealth for equitable distribution of healthcare services, telemedicine is an important aspect of eHealth within the Asia-Pacific region. One example is a project called Med@Tel, which began in 2010 and has involved the introduction of telehealth to the Thai Health Care System by the Thai National Health Security Office to revitalize existing telehealth programs in Thailand. This

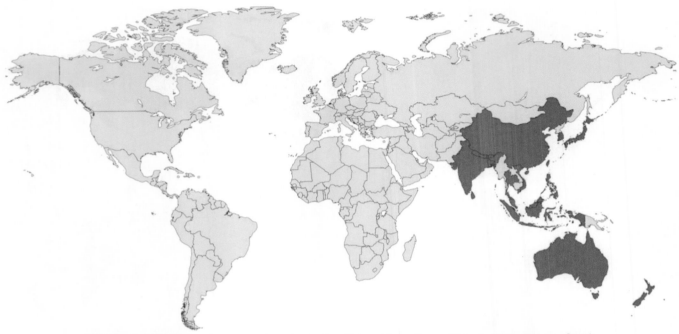

FIG 34.2 APAMI member countries: Australia, China, Hong Kong (China), India, Japan, South Korea, New Zealand, Philippines, Singapore, Sri Lanka, Taiwan (China), Thailand. Via corresponding members: Bangladesh, Bhutan, Indonesia, Malaysia, Nepal, and Vietnam.

BOX 34.2 Asia Pacific Association for Medical Informatics

Member Countries
- Australia
- China
- Hong Kong
- India
- Japan
- South Korea
- New Zealand
- Philippines
- Singapore
- Sri Lanka
- Taiwan
- Thailand

Corresponding Members
- Bangladesh
- Bhutan
- Indonesia
- Malaysia
- Nepal

---

telehealth program supports remote, underserved populations in Southern Thailand. It links hospitals in the region with a videoconferencing system for consultation and education; provides real-time, web-based consultation and education for healthcare providers and patients; provides telehome care using webcams, notebooks, and videophones installed in patients' homes and home care centers; and broadcasts selected tele-consultations, lectures, and presentations on a real-time internet TV.[5]

Another example comes from Japan, where telemedicine practice was strongly promoted by the Japanese government after the Great East Japan Earthquake of March 2011 as an attempt to revive medical services in the disaster area, along with the computer-based patient record network. The earthquake will be marked in history as an important trigger for the spread of telemedicine in Japan. Telemedicine practice in Japan includes telepathology, telemonitoring, telemedicine for cancer therapy, telemedicine for ophthalmology, telemedicine for pregnant women, home telemedicine, telenursing, mobile telemedicine, and telehealth for health promotion.[6] Other Asia-Pacific countries with active telemedicine projects include China, Korea, Australia, India, Bhutan, Malaysia, Singapore, Indonesia, Hong Kong Special Administrative Region (SAR), and New Zealand.

Many countries in the Asia-Pacific region, including Australia, China, Japan, Korea, Singapore, India, Malaysia, Taiwan, Thailand, and New Zealand, are actively promoting bioinformatics. APAMI plays a key role in advancing, developing, and promoting bioinformatics through cooperation within the region.

China, Hong Kong SAR, Singapore, Taiwan, and Korea have been particularly active in public health informatics since the outbreak of severe acute respiratory syndrome (SARS) in early 2003 and Middle East respiratory syndrome (MERS) in mid-2015. The SARS and MERS outbreaks provided an opportunity for APAMI to demonstrate

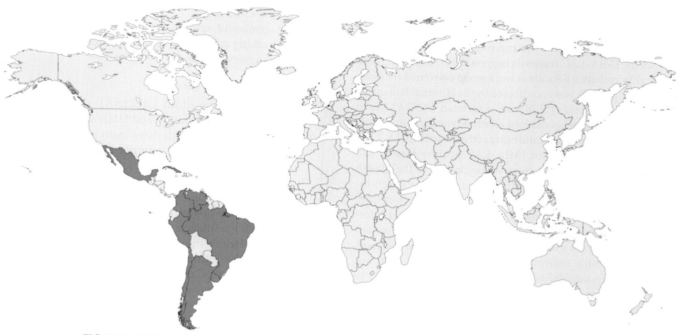

FIG 34.3 IMIA-LAC member countries: Argentina, Brazil, Chile, Columbia, Cuba, Mexico, Peru, Uruguay, and Venezuela.

the importance of a public health informatics approach to population health for each country within the region. APAMI continues to address public health informatics research and development through contact tracing, epidemiologic reporting, and monitoring for acute disease outbreaks.

eHealth Initiatives in the Pan American Health Organization Region

The Pan American Health Organization (PAHO), in conjunction with WHO, initiated the PAHO eHealth Program, a joint effort to increase research, teaching, and technology knowledge and transfer and to improve public health in the Americas and the Caribbean through the use of innovative eHealth tools and methodologies (see www.paho.org/ict4health).[7] The PAHO eHealth Program was a strategic response to the Health Agenda for the Americas presented by the Ministers of Health of the Americas in 2007.[8] The PAHO eHealth Strategy and Plan of Action (2012–2017)[9] describes the following components of eHealth:

- EHRs
- Telehealth
- mHealth (mobile health)
- eLearning
- Continuing education in ICT
- Standardization and interoperability

The eHealth Strategy and Plan of Action is focused around four strategic areas:

1. Policies on the use and implementation of ICT for health
2. Improvements in public health through innovative ICT tools and techniques

3. Cooperation among countries toward development of a digital health agenda for the region
4. Knowledge management, digital literacy, and education in ICT

The overall objective is the development of sustainable health systems. Examples of indicators include the following:

- Extent of funding for health ICT activities
- Strategies for strengthening infrastructure
- A common framework for patient identification
- Use of mobile technologies for electronic disease surveillance
- A common framework for data exchange
- A common framework for the development of portals
- Strategies for the use of social media in emergencies

International Medical Informatics Association for Latin America and the Caribbean

The Regional Federation of Health Informatics for Latin America and the Caribbean (IMIA-LAC) was founded in 1996 to promote theory development and the practice of health informatics within Latin America and the Caribbean (LAC). The IMIA-LAC board proposed the following two goals to develop health informatics within the region and strengthen regional ties[10]:

1. Strengthen the network of health informatics societies in Latin America and the Caribbean
2. Define the main health informatics topics to promote and the best groups to engage in such initiatives

Member societies of IMIA-LAC include Argentina, Brazil, Chile, Columbia, Cuba, Mexico, Peru, Uruguay, and Venezuela, as shown in Fig. 34.3.

Activities include regional congresses, national conferences, and WGs. An inaugural regional congress of IMIA-LAC was held in 2008 in Buenos Aires, Argentina, coordinated by Asociación Argentina de Informática Médica (AAIM). As part of the conference, IMIA held its board meeting, demonstrating its support for the IMIA-LAC regional congress. The IMIA Health and Medical Informatics Education workgroup convened the business meeting, which was coordinated by the Hospital Italiano de Buenos Aires. Spanish (SEIS) and American (AMIA) health informatics societies/associations continue support and participate in regional congresses and other activities with IMIA-LAC.

The major WGs within IMIA-LAC are the Health and Medical Informatics Education workgroup and the Health Information Systems workgroup, coordinated by Argentinean, Brazilian, and Cuban experts, with participation from several countries in the region. The Health and Medical Informatics Education workgroup has devised a work plan, including an assessment of the situation in each country and a coordination of health informatics education. Three additional WGs have been established by experts working in the region:

1. Bioinformatics workgroup
2. Nursing Informatics workgroup
3. Informatics and Quality in Healthcare workgroup

eHealth Initiatives in Africa

Africa is one of the least economically developed areas of the world. The wealth of a nation depends, in part, on the health of its population, making healthcare an area of high priority with regard to economic development. The progress of countries in sub-Saharan Africa in reaching WHO's Millennium Development Goals (MDGs) related to health—reducing child and maternal mortality, improving access to reproductive health, and reducing the spread of HIV/AIDS and tuberculosis—has fallen behind other countries in other regions.[11]

The WHO regional office in Africa predicted that eHealth might play a significant role in strengthening national health systems to accelerate progress toward the MDGs and improving health outcomes in the region.[12] WHO called for strengthened health information systems, public health surveillance systems, mobile devices at the point of care, EHRs, and other applications that provide patient billing, patient scheduling, and the electronic transmission of prescriptions. It is hoped that telehealth will also contribute to improving access to health services for underserved populations in rural areas.

Key challenges impeding the wide-scale implementation of eHealth solutions in Africa include:

- The "digital divide," as demonstrated by the need for increased awareness of eHealth among health professionals and patients
- A cohesive policy environment, providing leadership and coordination with improved financial and human resources
- A technical infrastructure and services within the health sector with monitoring and evaluation systems

More recently, Africa has seen a rapid rise in use of mobile devices and mobile health (mHealth) services across the region and their potential role in the transformation of

maternal care, management of noncommunicable diseases, and management of epidemics such as Ebola, through more effective tracking and reporting and by extending health services to underserved areas.[13]

Health Informatics in Africa

Health Informatics in Africa (HELINA), the Pan African Health Informatics Association and IMIA's African regional arm was created in 1993 with three main goals[14]:

1. To encourage African countries to develop their own National Health Informatics Societies
2. To develop education and research programs adapted to the African context, fostering alliance with government and the private sector
3. To develop a strategic plan for the sustainable development of Health Informatics and eHealth in Africa

The latest available information lists 10 countries as members of HELINA: Burundi, Cameroon, Ghana, Ivory Coast, Kenya, Malawi, Mali, Nigeria, South Africa, and Togo, as shown in Fig. 34.4. Algeria, Democratic Republic of the Congo, Egypt, Kenya, Madagascar, Tanzania, Uganda, Zambia, and Zimbabwe are corresponding members. HELINA organizes health informatics conferences within the African region. The first was held in Nigeria in 1993, and six more conferences have been organized since that inaugural meeting.

The HELINA Education Working Group, established in 2015, provides a platform for the development of initiatives to support health informatics education, training, and research. Activities will be channeled through eight worksets[15]:

- Workset One: Develop health informatics curricula for French-speaking participants.
- Workset Two: Develop a repository of training materials for health informatics.
- Workset Three: Compile a database of health informatics curricula from Africa.
- Workset Four: Develop a repository of tools to enable the development of curricula at a master's level.
- Workset Five: Work with education and training providers to foster the provision of health informatics using Web 2.0 technologies to provide free access to events for African health informatics participants.
- Workset Six: Develop a network of authors within each HELINA country in collaboration with the country representative, to help and advise health informaticians who wish to publish a paper but lack the skills or confidence to do so.
- Workset Seven: Develop a short-term certification program via blended learning for professionals in English- and French-speaking countries.
- People living in different regions of the world face very different challenges. However, the ongoing work around eHealth within these regions and within the IMIA regional bodies has much in common. The various interrelated regional agendas coalesce at an international level through a number of international organizations and standards efforts.

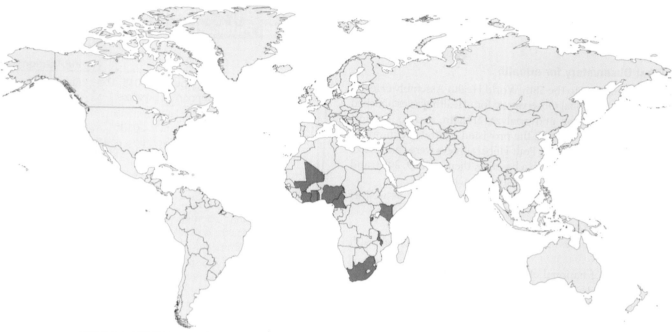

FIG 34.4 HELINA member countries: Burundi, Cameroon, Ghana, Ivory Coast, Kenya, Malawi, Mali, Nigeria, South Africa, and Togo.

INTERNATIONAL ORGANIZATIONS WITH eHEALTH INVOLVEMENT

International health-related organizations have played a major leadership role in the development of eHealth from the outset. This section of the chapter provides an overview of key organizations that are providing that leadership, along with a brief description of their programs and efforts.

eHealth and Health Informatics at the World Health Organization

WHO plays a key role in the development of global eHealth. The vision of WHO's Department of Knowledge Management and Sharing (KMS) is "a world with better and more equitable health outcomes."[16] The mission of KMS is "to improve the understanding and application of knowledge management."[16] One strategic direction is "to promote the use of information and communication technologies to improve health services and systems."[16] WHO has recently taken steps to make eHealth a priority in strengthening health systems worldwide.

The eHealth Resolution

In 2005 the 58th World Health Assembly took a historical step toward supporting eHealth by adopting a resolution for a global movement recognizing the role of the ICT in strengthening health systems and improving the safety, quality, and efficiency of services.[17] The resolution urged member states to do the following:

- Create a lasting plan for eHealth development.
- Create eHealth infrastructure.
- Encourage private and nonprofit collaboration.

- Broaden the reach of eHealth services.
- Encourage universal collaboration to determine eHealth standards supported by evidence-based practice.
- Create centers and networks for sharing best practices, policies, technical innovations, service improvement, communications, capacity building, and surveillance.
- Think about developing national public health information systems.
- Enhance surveillance and response to public health emergencies through increased flow of information.[18]

The 66th World Health Assembly in 2013 recognized the need for health data standardization as part of eHealth systems and services, as well as the importance of proper governance and operation of health-related global top-level internet domain names, including "health."[19] The resolution urged member states to do the following:

1. Consider collaborating with a range of relevant stakeholders in order to draw up a road map for implementation of eHealth and health data standards at national and subnational levels.
2. Consider developing policies and legislative mechanisms to ensure compliance in the adoption of eHealth and health data standards, as well as to ensure the privacy of personal clinical data.
3. Consider ways to coordinate national positions toward the delegation, governance, and operation of health-related global top-level domain names, including ". health."

Information about major eHealth projects at WHO is available at http://www.who.int/ehealth/programmes. These projects cover eLearning on a range of health-related topics, support for eHealth standards development, governance and national strategy development, and the Global Observatory for eHealth.

Global Observatory for eHealth

In direct response to the 58th World Health Assembly eHealth resolution, the Global Observatory for eHealth was established in 2005 to monitor and analyze eHealth and to support national planning through the provision of strategic information in member countries. Four global surveys were conducted, the first in 2005 to establish a baseline, then in 2009, 2013, and 2015. Key findings of the first survey included[20]:

- Acknowledging a digital divide in eHealth as well as other areas
- A willingness to implement eHealth policies
- A need for assistance and guidance in the eHealth domain
- A lack of national eHealth governance mechanisms
- A need to promote public-private partnerships for eHealth projects as effective management practices
- A lack of citizen protection policies to ensure patient data confidentiality
- A need to focus on interoperability issues
- Health information in electronic formats should be provided in relevant community languages.

The second survey, conducted in late 2009, was designed to build on the knowledge base generated by the first survey and identify and analyze trends in eHealth, including[21]:

- Uptake of eHealth foundation policies and strategies
- Deployment of mHealth initiatives
- Application of telehealth solutions and adoption of eLearning for health professionals and students
- Collection, processing, storage, and transfer of patient information
- Legal and ethical frameworks for electronic patient information
- Legislation and initiatives concerning online child safety, internet pharmacies, and health information on the internet
- Governance and organization of eHealth within countries

The second survey proved to be a rich source of data, which has been used to create a series of publications titled the Global Observatory for eHealth series.[22] For example, the third survey (conducted in 2013) focused on the use of eHealth for women's and children's health; the fourth (2015) focused on the use of eHealth in support of universal health coverage.[22] A list of publications from the global surveys is included in Table 34.1. Readers may view the detailed results on the Global Observatory eHealth website at http://www.who.int/goe/data/en/.[22]

World Health Organization Family of International Classifications

WHO is responsible for developing, disseminating, and maintaining international classifications on health, collectively referred to as the WHO Family of International Classifications

TABLE 34.1   Global Observatory for eHealth Publications

Title	Date of Publication
Atlas of eHealth country profiles 2015: The use of eHealth in support of universal health covered	February 1, 2016
Atlas of eHealth country profiles 2013: eHealth and innovation in women's and children's health	May 3, 2014
eHealth and innovation in women's and children's health: A baseline review full report	March 16, 2014
eHealth and innovation in women's and children's health: A baseline review executive summaries	January 13, 2014
Global observatory for eHealth series—Volume 6, Management of patient information: Trends and challenges in member states	November 1, 2012
Global observatory for eHealth series—Volume 5, Legal frameworks for eHealth	February 1, 2012
Global observatory for eHealth series—Volume 4, Safety and security on the internet: Challenges and advances in member states	December 1, 2011
Global Observatory for eHealth series—Volume 3 mHealth: New horizons for health through mobile technologies	June 7, 2011
Global Observatory for eHealth series—Volume 2 Telemedicine: Opportunities and developments in Member States	January 13, 2011
Global Observatory for eHealth series—Volume 1 Atlas: eHealth country profiles	December 22, 2010

From WHO (nd) Global Observatory for eHealth: Publications. <http://www.who.int/goe/publications/en/>. Accessed July 13, 2016.

(WHO-FIC), to promote a consensual, meaningful, and useful framework that governments, healthcare providers, and consumers can use as a common language in health information systems (www.who.int/classifications/). Internationally endorsed classifications facilitate the storage, retrieval, analysis, and interpretation of data as well as allow data within and between populations to be compared (see Chapter 22 for detailed discussions about standard taxonomies).

The classifications within the WHO-FIC fall into three main categories: **reference classifications**, **derived classifications**, and **related classifications.** Reference classifications are classifications of the basic parameters of health. Derived classifications are developed by modifying or rearranging reference classifications. Related classifications are associated with the reference classification at specific levels of structure only. Box 34.3 provides a list of the WHO classifications and their related types.

BOX 34.3 World Health Organization Family of International Classifications

Reference Classifications

Main classifications based on basic parameters of health. These classifications have been prepared by the World Health Organization (WHO) and approved by its governing bodies for international use.

- International Classification of Diseases (ICD)
- International Classification of Functioning, Disability and Health (ICF)
- International Classification of Health Interventions (ICHI)

Derived Classifications

Those based on reference classifications (i.e., ICD and ICF). Derived classifications may be prepared either by adopting the reference classification structure and categories and providing additional detail beyond that provided by the reference classifications or by rearranging or aggregating items from one or more reference classifications.

- International Classification of Diseases for Oncology, 3rd edition (ICD-O-3)
- ICD-10 for Mental and Behavioral Disorders Clinical Descriptions and Diagnostic Guidelines
- ICD-10 for Mental and Behavioral Disorders Diagnostic Criteria for Research
- Application of the International Classification of Diseases to Neurology (ICD-10-NA)
- Application of the International Classification of Diseases to Dentistry and Stomatology, 3rd edition (ICD-DA)

Related Classifications

Those that partially refer to reference classifications or are associated with reference classifications at specific levels of structure only.

- International Classification of Primary Care, Second edition (ICPC-2)
- International Classification of External Causes of Injury (ICECI)
- Technical aids for persons with disabilities—Classification and terminology (ISO9999)
- The Anatomical Therapeutic Chemicals Classification with Defined Daily Doses (ATC/DDD)
- International Classification for Nursing Practice (ICNP)

Adapted from World Health Organization (WHO). *Derived and Related Classifications in the WHO-FIC.* Geneva, Switzerland: WHO. <http://www.who.int/classifications/related/en/index.html>; 2016.

International Medical Informatics Association

IMIA is the world body for health and biomedical informatics (http://www.imia-medinfo.org/new2/), originating in 1967 as Technical Committee (TC) 4 of the International Federation for Information Processing (IFIP; www.ifip.org). It evolved from a special interest group (SIG) of IFIP to its current status in 1979. IMIA is connected with WHO as a nongovernmental organization (NGO) and with the International Federation of Health Information Management Associations (IFHIMA). Membership in IMIA is limited to organizations, societies, and corporations. For example, each country can be represented by only one member society. At this writing, there are 58 member societies. The regional members, with the exception of the North America member countries shown in Fig. 34.5 and the Middle East Association for Health Informatics (MEAHI) member countries included in Fig. 34.6, were discussed earlier in the sections dealing with informatics regions of the world. In a country where no representative society exists, IMIA accommodates involvement through corresponding members, especially within developing economies. At the time of this writing, there were 31 corresponding members.

IMIA is an important player in ensuring that information science and technology are integrated into all fields of healthcare. Its main goals are to[23]:

- Promote informatics in health care and research in health, bio and medical informatics
- Advance and nurture international cooperation
- Stimulate research, development and routine application
- Move informatics from theory into practice in a full range of health delivery settings, from physician's office to acute and long-term care
- Further the dissemination and exchange of knowledge, information and technology
- Promote education and responsible behaviour
- Represent the medical and health informatics field with the World Health Organization and other international professional and governmental organizations."

In its function as a bridge organization, IMIA's goals are[23]:

- "Moving theory into practice by linking academic and research informaticians with caregivers, consultants, vendors, and vendor-based researchers
- Leading the international medical and health informatics communities throughout the 21st century
- Promoting the cross-fertilization of health informatics information and knowledge across professional and geographical boundaries
- Serving as the catalyst for ubiquitous worldwide health information infrastructures for patient care and health research

IMIA provides networking opportunities as well as an international platform for eHealth providers, consultants, and publishers. IMIA organizes a bi-annual conference called the World Congress on Medical and Health Informatics, commonly known as MedInfo. The event provides opportunities to share and exchange ideas and research as well as to hold formal meetings and facilitate informal networking of members.

IMIA also publishes the annual *IMIA Yearbook of Medical Informatics* and additional official journals. Since its inception in 1992, the *IMIA Yearbook of Medical Informatics* has been one of the most valuable products that IMIA provides to its members and to the health informatics community. IMIA's official journals include *Applied Clinical Informatics* (www.aci-journal.org), *International Journal of Medical Informatics* (www.ijmijournal.com/home), and *Methods of Information in Medicine* (www.methods-online.com).

IMIA pursues its scientific activity in specific fields of the wider domain of health and biomedical informatics through

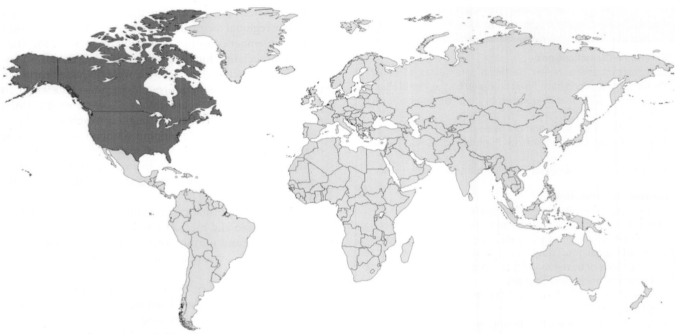

FIG 34.5 IMIA North America member countries: United States and Canada.

BOX 34.4   International Medical Informatics Association Working Groups and Special Interest Groups (SIGs)

- Biomedical Pattern Recognition
- Consumer Health Informatics
- Critical Care Informatics
- Data Mining and Big Data Analytics
- Dental Informatics (inactive)
- Francophone SIG
- Health and Medical Informatics Education
- Health Geographical Information Systems (GIS)
- Health Informatics for Development
- Health Informatics for Patient Safety
- Health Information Systems
- Health Record Banking
- History of BioMedical and Health Informatics
- Human Factors Engineering for Healthcare Informatics
- Informatics in Genomic Medicine (IGM)

- Language and Meaning in Biomedicine
- Mental Health Informatics (inactive)
- Open Source Health Informatics
- Organizational and Social Issues
- Primary Healthcare Informatics
- Security in Health Information Systems
- Nursing Informatics SIG
- Smart Homes and Ambient Assisted Living
- Social Media
- Standards in Healthcare Informatics
- Technology Assessment & Quality Development in Health Informatics
- Telehealth
- Wearable Sensors in Healthcare

Data from IMIA: *Working Groups.* <http://www.imia-medinfo.org/new2/WG>; 2016.

WGs and SIGs. A WG or SIG consists of a group of experts with a specific interest. At this writing there are 28 WGs and SIGs (Box 34.4). Activities of WGs and SIGs include organizing business meetings at IMIA conferences or IMIA regional meetings, publishing papers related to WG activity written by members of WGs and SIGs, and collaborating with other organizations within IMIA or IMIA regional or member societies. The International Medical Informatics Association Nursing Informatics (IMIA-NI) SIG is one of the initial and most consistently active SIGs.

IMIA-NI

The Nursing Informatics component of IMIA, IMIA-NI (see http://www.imia-medinfo.org/new2/node/151), was

originally called WG 8 in 1983. The main goals of IMIA-NI are listed in Box 34.5.

IMIA-NI currently has 33 members from 33 member societies of IMIA. IMIA-NI pursues its scientific activity in specific fields of the wider domain of nursing informatics through WGs. Currently there are four IMIA-NI WGs: Consumer/Client Health Informatics, Education, Evidence-Based Practice, and Health Informatics Standards.

IMIA-NI organizes a biennial International Congress on Nursing Informatics, which provides a scientific exchange of current research and thinking in nursing informatics, formal meetings on nursing informatics topics, and informal networking. The first meeting of IMIA-NI was held in 1982 in London, England, as an international open forum titled "The Impact of

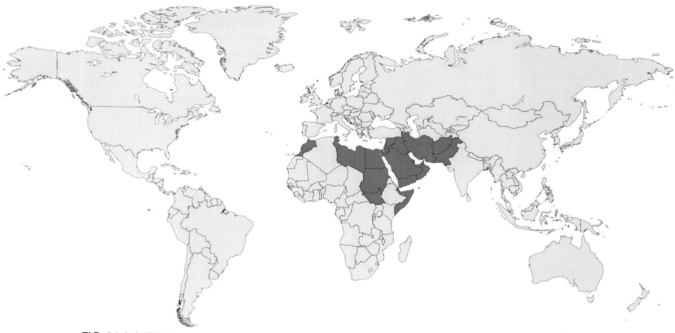

FIG 34.6 MEAHI member countries: Afghanistan, Bahrain, Djibouti, Egypt, Iran, Iraq, Jordan, Kuwait, Lebanon, Libya, Morocco, Oman, Pakistan, Palestine, Qatar, Saudi Arabia, Somalia, South Sudan, Sudan, Syrian Arab Republic, Tunisia, United Arab Emirates, and Yemen.

BOX 34.5   Goals of IMIA-NI

- To foster collaboration among nurses and other professionals who are interested in nursing informatics
- To explore the scope of nursing informatics and its implication for information-handling activities associated with nursing care delivery, nursing administration, nursing research, nursing education, and various relationships with other healthcare information systems
- To support the development of nursing informatics in member countries and worldwide
- To provide appropriate informatics meetings, conferences, and postconferences and to provide opportunities to share knowledge and research to facilitate the communication of developments in the field
- To encourage the publication and dissemination of research and development materials in the field of nursing informatics
- To develop recommendations, guidelines, and courses related to nursing informatics
- To work with patients, families, and communities to implement informatics in healthcare

Adapted from International Medical Informatics Association (IMIA). *SIG NI Nursing Informatics.* Geneva, Switzerland: IMIA. <http://www.imia-medinfo.org/new2/node/151>; 2016.

Computers on Nursing." A list of the IMIA-NI conferences with locations and themes is in Table 34.2.

INTERNATIONAL STANDARDS EFFORTS

Over the past several decades, significant efforts have been made in terminology development and standards. This section summarizes international work in this area, and readers are referred to Chapter 22 for more details.

International Organization for Standardization

The International Organization for Standardization (ISO) is the world's largest developer and publisher of international standards (www.iso.org). It is managed by a Central Secretariat in Geneva, Switzerland, and currently includes national standards institutes of 162 countries. ISO is not affiliated with governments and provides a link between the public and private sectors. Although many member institutes belong to the governmental structure of their countries (or are mandated by their government), others have private sector origins (i.e., they were established through national partnerships of industry associations). Therefore ISO is uniquely able to establish a consensus on standards-related solutions for business and the broader needs of society. Currently there are 238 TCs developing standards in different domains.

ISO TC 215 is the ISO's TC on health informatics. The scope of ISO TC 215 is to achieve compatibility and interoperability between independent systems, achieve compatibility and consistency of data for comparative statistical purposes (classifications), and reduce duplication of effort and redundancies through standardization. Currently there are 32 active participating (P-member) countries and 27 observing (O-member) countries. At this writing, the number of published ISO standards under the direct responsibility of TC 215 (including updates) is 150 (in May 2012, there were just 94). ISO TC 215's current work program comprises 50 items, comprehensively covering the contemporary health

TABLE 34.2 List of Past International Conferences on Nursing Informatics

Series	Year	Hosting City and Country	Theme
1	1982	London, England	The impact of computers on nursing
2	1985	Calgary, Canada	Building bridges to the future
3	1988	Dublin, Ireland	Where caring and technology meet
4	1991	Melbourne, Australia	Nurses managing information in healthcare
5	1994	San Antonio, USA	Nursing in a technological era
6	1997	Stockholm, Sweden	The impact of nursing knowledge on healthcare informatics
7	2000	Auckland, New Zealand	One step beyond: The evolution of technology and nursing
8	2003	Rio de Janeiro, Brazil	Nursing eHealth
9	2006	Seoul, Korea	Consumer-centered computer-supported care for healthy people
10	2009	Helsinki, Finland	Nursing informatics— Connecting health and humans
11	2012	Montreal, Canada	Advancing global health through informatics
12	2014	Taipei, Taiwan	eSmart+
13	2016	Geneva, Switzerland	eHealth for all: Every level collaboration—From project to realization

TABLE 34.3 List of ISO TC 215 Subcommittees/Working Groups

Subcommittee/ Working Group	Scope
ISO/TC 215/CAG 1	Executive council, harmonization, and operations
ISO/TC 215/WG 1	Architecture, frameworks, and models
ISO/TC 215/JWG 1	Joint ISO/TC 215-ISO/TC 249 WG: Traditional Chinese medicine (informatics)
ISO/TC 215/WG 2	Systems and device interoperability
ISO/TC 215/WG 3	Semantic content
ISO/TC 215/WG 4	Security, safety, and privacy
ISO/TC 215/WG 6	Pharmacy and medicines business
ISO/TC 215/JWG 7	Joint ISO/TC 215–IEC/SC 62A WG: Application of risk management to IT networks incorporating medical devices

CAG, Corporate Advisory Group; *IEC*, International Electrotechnical Commission; *ISO*, International Organization for Standardization; *IT*, information technology; *JWG*, joint working group; *TC*, technical committee; *WG*, working group.

information standards spectrum. Table 34.3 presents ISO TC 215's subcommittees and WGs and their activities. Fig. 34.7 illustrates the current structure of ISO TC 215.

Many health professionals are involved in ISO activities. For example, nurses have played an active and important role in different WGs of ISO TC 215 in the development and testing of ISO 18104: Integration of a Reference Terminology Model for Nursing. This provides an agreed structure for statements that represent nursing diagnoses and nursing actions which will make it easier to combine and compare information from different settings in different regions worldwide.[24]

International Council of Nurses

The International Council of Nurses (ICN) is a federation of 136 national nurses associations (NNAs) representing more than 16 million nurses globally.[25] ICN began in 1899 with the goal of encouraging quality healthcare, solid health policies, advanced health knowledge, and a respected global nursing presence.

The aim of the ICN eHealth Programme[24] is to transform nursing through the visionary application of information and communication technologies. The Programme encompasses a range of ICN activities, including the International Classification for Nursing Practice (ICNP), which provides a "standard [nursing terminology] for comparing nursing practice locally, regionally, nationally, and internationally,"[26] and the ICN Telenursing Network, which encourages and assists nurses in the development and use of telehealth. A third workstream is Connecting Nurses, supported by Sanofi, which provides a platform for sharing knowledge and best practice. ICN has also participated in other international terminology standards development activities, such as the ISO reference terminology standard described previously and the International Nursing Minimum Data Set (i-NMDS). The i-NMDS builds on the Nursing Minimum Data Set work of Werley and Lang, explained in more detail in Chapter 22.

International Classification for Nursing Practice

ICNP is a vocabulary system developed by the ICN after the ICN Congress passed a resolution in 1989 (see also Chapter 22 for a discussion on ICNP). ICNP provides a systematic way of describing nursing practice across the world, with the goal of improving communication within nursing and with other disciplines. Using the ICNP, reliable information about nursing practice can be generated to influence decision making, education, and policy; better meet the needs of individuals and groups; deliver more effective interventions; enhance safety and quality; improve health outcomes; and better use resources. ICNP has been implemented and is used in several countries around the world.[27] For example, Paulino Sousa, an NI expert in Portugal, estimated that over 90% of nurses in Portugal use ICNP daily to support their practice.

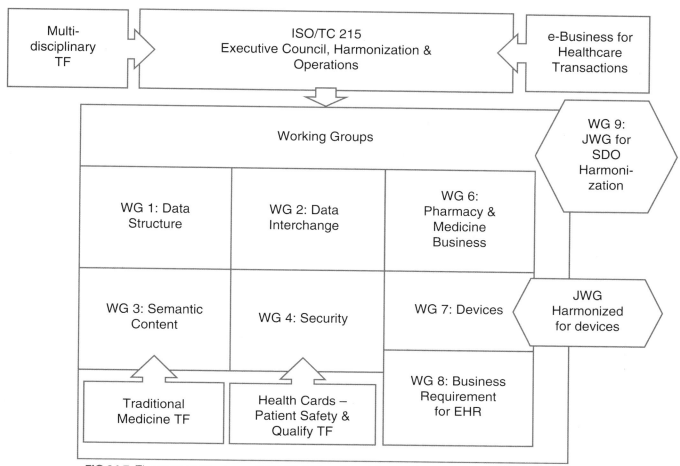

FIG 34.7 The current structure of ISO TC 215 and its eight working groups. *EHR*, Electronic health record; *ISO*, International Organization for Standardization; *JWG*, joint working group; *SDO*, standard development organization; *TC*, technical committee; *TF*, task force; *WG*, working group.

The ICN Telenursing Network

The Telenursing Network is one of 10 networks that ICN introduced as a mechanism to provide opportunities for nurses to communicate and pursue common professional interests (www.icn.ch/networks/telenursing-network/). ICN acknowledges that nurses using eHealth extend nursing's reach and improve access to care. Telenursing represents an advance in healthcare delivery and is ideal for addressing health system challenges (e.g., an ageing population; higher incidence of noncommunicable diseases; community- and home-based care; geographic, social, and financial issues; increased costs and reduced funding; nursing shortages). Telehealth is defined and described in Chapter 8.

The history of the ICN Telenursing Network dates back to early 2000. ICN published a monograph on telenursing in 2000 entitled *Telehealth and Telenursing: Nursing and Technology Advance Together* and in 2001 published *International Professional Standards for Telenursing Programmes*.[28] Through publications like *International Competencies for Telenursing* in 2007, telenursing was recognized as an important contributor to the ICN's mission of advancing nursing and health worldwide.

The Telenursing Network was launched in 2009 with the aim of seeking, educating, supporting, and collaborating with nurses and other telenursing supporters worldwide. The overarching goal of the Telenursing Network is to improve healthcare services for individuals and institutions worldwide.[29]

Connecting Nurses

Connecting Nurses provides a forum for nurses from around the world to share their ideas, advice, and innovations, and contribute to patient empowerment. The aim is simply to bring nurses together. Connecting Nurses provides an online platform for nurses from around the world to share ideas, advice, and innovations, both among themselves and with other health professionals, patients, caregivers, and the general public.[30]

As an integrated part of Connecting Nurses, Care Challenge[31] was created to celebrate the important role the nursing community plays in healthcare provision around the world, while addressing the challenges arising within modern healthcare systems. Taking a social media approach, nurses are able to submit and showcase, on an ongoing basis, a summary of an innovation from their practice. Best projects are supported, for example, through the production of high-quality video to further showcase the innovation.

Health Level Seven

Health Level Seven (HL7) is an international community composed of healthcare subject matter experts and information scientists. Its goal is to create and sustain standards for the exchange, management, and integration of data that facilitate patient care and management, delivery, and evaluation of healthcare services.[32] As explained in Chapters 6 and 22, HL7 encourages the use of such standards within and among healthcare organizations to optimize healthcare delivery for all.

International Health Terminology Standards Development Organisation

International Health Terminology Standards Development Organisation (IHTSDO) (www.ihtsdo.org) is an international nonprofit organization. It owns and administers the rights to Systematized Nomenclature of Medicine—Clinical Terms (SNOMED CT) and related terminology standards. The goal of IHTSDO is to establish and maintain optimum interoperability and harmonization between SNOMED CT and standards produced by other international standards development organizations (e.g., American Academy of Ophthalmology; GS1; HL7; ICN; Institute of Electrical and Electronics Engineers; Logical Observation Identifiers Names and Codes; Nomenclature, Properties and Units; openEHR; WHO; and World Organization of National Colleges, Academies). Additional details on SNOMED CT are included in Chapter 22.

GLOBAL CHALLENGES TO eHEALTH

Multiple challenges face eHealth usage, at the local, national, and international levels. This section explores some of the more important challenges.

Global Interoperability

A key problem in achieving global interoperability in eHealth is the lack of semantic (the meaning of terms) interoperability. Key barriers include issues relating to the terminology used in describing and documenting healthcare such as cost and accessibility, gaps in exhaustiveness, and lack of granularity.[33] Many international efforts are underway to solve this problem, such as the development of international standards to underpin clinical terminologies, the development of clinical data models like HL7 Clinical Document Architecture (CDA) documents, openEHR Archetypes, and integration of standard data models with terminologies such as SNOMED CT.[34] Harmonization activities among international standards development organizations, such as ISO TC 215, HL7, and European Committee for Standardization (CEN) TC251, are ongoing. For example, tables of equivalents have been developed for concepts within ICNP and SNOMED CT under a formal collaboration agreement between ICN and IHTSDO, to ensure that data recorded in one terminology can be easily transformed into the format of the other. This will ensure, for example, that nursing remains connected to a wider health informatics infrastructure.

Human Resources for eHealth

According to the first global survey on eHealth carried out in 2005 by WHO, and described previously in this chapter, all respondents expressed a need for education and training in eHealth. The lack of human resources with the necessary skills and competencies is a problem for the introduction and use of eHealth in many parts of the world. Different types of professionals with an appropriate mix of skills are needed for the best use of ICT in healthcare (e.g., health informatics professionals, health information management professionals, and others with specialized informatics skills). Current shortages of skilled workers in the healthcare profession demand a human resource strategy and long-term plan for the education and training of eHealth personnel to ensure the quality of collected health data and its security and confidentiality and to manage and maintain the systems and data in the future.[35]

Based on the 2005 WHO survey data, eLearning programs and professional development for professional education were recommended in the health sciences. In addition, collaborations were needed that could establish databases of existing eLearning courses. Finally, it was recommended that WHO should advocate for the inclusion of eHealth courses within university curricula.[36] While progress has been made over the last 15 years, there is clearly still some way to go.

eHealth Infrastructure

If eHealth infrastructure or services are missing or deficient, eHealth becomes less effective. The digital divide[37] is the result of a gap in information exchange between different demographics and remains a major problem in terms of internet, and especially broadband, uptake. This divide continues to expand as healthcare systems and providers and citizens increasingly depend on information from the internet to guide day-to-day care. This is most evident in comparing fixed broadband penetration in developed countries (29%) to that in developing countries (7.1%).[38] While the gap may be closing slowly over time, significant differences also exist in the percentage of internet users, ranging from 87.9% in North America to 27% in Africa.[39] The persisting digital divide inspired ICN to publish a position statement on people's right to connect via information and communication technology.[40] As with the solutions to problems caused by a lack of knowledgeable personnel, awareness of the disparity and its impact on healthcare is the first step in narrowing the gap. Education programs will prove beneficial in the attempt to close the digital divide.

On the other hand, developments in the mobile sector have been phenomenal. In 2015, 96.8 mobile phone subscriptions per 100 inhabitants existed worldwide (from 120.6 in developed countries to 91.8 in developing countries). This particular digital divide was reduced due to a high level of competition and a decrease in prices.[38] However, having a tool does not necessarily indicate that functionality is available, and the lack of data communication services prevents isolated mobile phones from being an effective tool for health management. Improved infrastructure to store data and transfer data securely and in a cost-effective manner and full compatibility, interoperability, and possibly integration with other services would help address this challenge.

Legal and Regulatory Framework for eHealth

Patient privacy is a core element of good healthcare practice, and legislation and regulation are key tools in protecting privacy. According to the second global survey on eHealth by WHO, a reasonably high level of legal protection of the general privacy of health-related information exists. However, the number of countries adopting more specific eHealth-related privacy protection legislation is still low.[41]

Legal and regulatory eHealth challenges vary from ambiguous legal frameworks to poor data management (e.g., access to personal data and lack of data security rules). A lack of regulations in the transfer of data leads to any number of challenges at the international level, including the following:

- Misinformation
- Unethical use
- Concealed bias
- Covert self-dealing
- Fraudulent practices
- Evasion of legitimate regulation

Security is another area within eHealth presenting many challenges. eHealth applications using mobile terminals and internet services require authentication methods that are both convenient and highly secure. The increasing use of technology such as biometric authentication for identification is generating new challenges in security, safety, and privacy protection for healthcare providers and consumers alike.

CONCLUSION AND FUTURE DIRECTIONS

Healthcare faces unprecedented challenges: an aging population, greater citizen engagement, unanticipated disasters, new advances in medicine, and increasing public expectations, all within a context of a shrinking healthcare workforce and ongoing financial constraints. While eHealth cannot resolve the underlying causes of these challenges, it has a significant role to play in supporting the transformation of health services in order to make contemporary healthcare sustainable.

Individuals and organizations are working together within countries and across regions on eHealth strategy, capacity and capability, infrastructure, tools, and techniques. However, many of the challenges to healthcare are not confined to particular regions. For example, outbreaks, epidemics, and pandemics such as SARS, MERS, Ebola, Zika, HIV/AIDS, and tuberculosis do not recognize national and regional boundaries. Their effective management requires an international approach. Many eHealth solutions are applicable at a global level.

Several international organizations are helping facilitate greater global collaboration on eHealth between countries and regions. This sharing of knowledge and experience helps strengthen national and regional initiatives, increasing the uptake of eHealth at a local level in order to improve the quality and safety of healthcare while driving efficiency. eHealth is also improving access to scarce healthcare services, thereby establishing a more equitable global healthcare environment.

REFERENCES

1. European Commission. *First ehealth Action Plan*; 2004. http://eur-lex.europa.eu/legal-content/EN/TXT/HTML/?uri=CELEX:52004DC0356&from=EN.
2. European Commission. *Second eHealth Action Plan*; 2012. https://ec.europa.eu/digital-agenda/en/news/ehealth-action-plan-2012-2020-innovative-healthcare-21st-century.
3. EFMI. *Mission and Objectives.* European Federation for Medical Informatics; 2016. https://www.efmi.org/index.php/about/mission-and-history.
4. APEC Health Working Group. *2010-2015 Medium Term Work Goals*; 2016. http://www.apechwg.org/about-hwg/workplan.
5. Rodklai A, Sutheravut P, Nontapan P. Introduction of telehealth to Thai health care system, experience from Southern Thailand. In: Jordanova M, Lievens F, eds. *Proceedings of the International eHealth, Telemedicine and Health ICT Forum for Education, Networking and Business; Basel.* Switzerland: International Society for Telemedicine and eHealth; 2011:787–788.
6. Japanese Telemedicine Telecare Association. *Telemedicine in Japan 2013*; 2013. http://jtta.umin.jp/pdf/telemedicine/telemedicine_in_japan_20131015-2_en.pdf.
7. D'Agostino M, Novillo-Ortiz D. PAHO/WHO: eHealth conceptual model and work programme for Latin America and the Caribbean. In: Novillo-Ortiz D, Jadad AR, eds. *The Global People-Centred eHealth Innovation Forum.* London, England: Affinity; 2011.
8. Pan American Health Organization. Health Agenda for the Americas. In: *Paper Presented at 37th General Assembly of the Organization of American States; Panama City, Panama*; June 2007.
9. Pan American Health Organization (PAHO). *eHealth Strategy and Plan of Action (2012-2017)*; 2011. http://www.paho.org/ict4health/index.php?option=com_content&view=article&id=54&Itemid=146&lang=en.
10. International Medical Informatics Association (IMIA). *IMIA LAC: Regional Federation of Health Informatics for Latin America and the Caribbean*; 2016. http://www.imia-medinfo.org/new2/node/159.
11. African Health Observatory. *Mobile Health: Transforming the Face of Health Service Delivery in the African Region.* World Health Organization; 2015. https://www.aho.afro.who.int/en/blog/2015/03/10/mobile-health-transforming-face-health-service-delivery-african-region.

12. World Health Organization (WHO). *Millennium Development Goals: 2015 Progress Chart*; 2015. http://www.un.org/millenniumgoals/2015_MDG_Report/pdf/MDG%202015%20PC%20final.pdf/.

13. World Health Organization Regional Office for Africa. *eHealth Solutions in the African Region: Current Context and Perspectives*; 2010. http://www.afro.who.int/en/downloads/doc_download/5728-afrrc60r3-ehealth-solutions-in-the-african-region-current-context-and-perspectives.html.

14. International Medical Informatics Association (IMIA). *HELINA African Region*; 2011. http://www.imia-medinfo.org/new2/node/158.

15. International Medical Informatics Association (IMIA). *HELINA Education Working Group*; 2015. http://wg-education.helina-online.org/?page_id=2.

16. World Health Organization (WHO). *What Is Knowledge Management and Sharing?* 2016. http://www.who.int/kms.

17. World Health Organization (WHO). *eHealth Resolutions and Decisions*; 2005. http://www.who.int/healthacademy/media/WHA58-28-en.pdf.

18. Al-Shorbaji N. *eHealth and Health Informatics @ WHO/HQ*. Washington, DC: Pan American Health Organization; 2010. http://new.paho.org/ict4health/index.php?option=com_content&view=article&id=32%3Aehealth-and-health-informatics-whohq-by-najeeb-al-shorbaji-director-of-the-department-of-knowledge-management-and-sharing-world-health-organization-who-&catid=17%3Aentrevistas&Itemid=16&lang=en.

19. World Health Organization (WHO). *eHealth Standardization and Interoperability*; 2013. http://apps.who.int/gb/ebwha/pdf_files/WHA66/A66_R24-en.pdf.

20. World Health Organization (WHO). *Global Observatory for eHealth: 2005 Survey*; 2005. http://www.who.int/goe/data/2005survey/en/.

21. World Health Organization (WHO). *Global Observatory for eHealth: 2009 Survey*; 2009. http://www.who.int/goe/survey/2009/2009survey/en/.

22. World Health Organization (WHO). *Global Observatory for eHealth: Global Surveys*; 2016. http://www.who.int/goe/data/en/.

23. International Medical Informatics Association (IMIA). *Welcome to IMIA!* 2016. http://www.imia-medinfo.org/new2/node/1.

24. International Organization for Standardization (ISO). *ISO 18104:2014 Health Informatics—categorial Structures For Representation of Nursing Diagnoses and Nursing Actions in Terminological Systems*. Geneva, Switzerland: ISO; 2016.

25. International Council of Nurses (ICN). *Who We Are*; 2016. /who-we-are/who-we-are/.

26. International Council of Nurses (ICN). *What We Do*; 2016. http://www.icn.ch/what-we-do/ehealth/.

27. Lee YS, Park KO, Bong MR, Park HA. Development and evaluation of ICNP-based electronic nursing record system. *Stud Health Technol Inform*. 2009;146:498–502.

28. Hunter KM. *International Professional Standards for Telenursing Programmes*. International Council of Nurses: Geneva, Switzerland; 2001.

29. International Council of Nurses (ICN); 2015. *Telenursing Network*; 2015. http://www.icn.ch/networks/telenursing-network/.

30. Connecting Nurses. *About Connecting Nurses*. http://www.connecting-nurses.com/web/about. Accessed August 4, 2016.

31. Connecting Nurses. *Care challenge*. http://www.care-challenge.com. Accessed August 4, 2016.

32. *Health Level 7 International (HL7)*; 2016. http://www.hl7.org/.

33. Hammond W. Semantic interoperability issue of standardizing medical vocabularies. In: Mohammed S, Fiaidhi J, eds. *Ubiquitous Health and Medical Informatics: The Ubiquity 2.0 Trend and Beyond*. IGI Global: Hershey, PA; 2010:19–42.

34. Qamar R. *Semantic Mapping of Clinical Model Data to Biomedical Terminologies to Facilitate Interoperability*. Manchester, UK: University of Manchester; 2008. http://www.cs.man.ac.uk/~qamarr/papers/HealthcareComputing2007_Qamar.pdf.

35. Gibson CJ, Covvey HD. *Demystifying E-Health Human Resources*. Washington, DC: Information Resources Management Association; 2010. http://www.irma-international.org/viewtitle/53656/.

36. World Health Organization (WHO) Global Observatory for eHealth. *eHealth Tools and Services: Needs of the Member States*. Geneva, Switzerland: WHO; 2006. http://www.who.int/kms/initiatives/tools_and_services_final.pdf.

37. Coverdell M, Utley R. The health care information gap: a global and national perspective. *Online J Nurs Inf*. 2005;9(1). http://ojni.org/9_1/coverdell.htm.

38. International Telecommunication Union (ITU). *ICT Data and Statistics (IDS): Global ICT Developments*; 2015. http://www.itu.int/ITU-D/ict/statistics/ict/index.html.

39. Internet World Stats. *Usage and Populations Statistics: 2014. Internet World Stats*; 2014. http://www.internetworldstats.com/.

40. International Council of Nurses. *The Right to Connect via Information and Communication Technology*. Geneva, Switzerland: ICN; 2015. http://www.icn.ch/images/stories/documents/publications/position_statements/E12a_Right_Connect_Information_Communication_Technology.pdf.

41. World Health Organization (WHO). *Legal Frameworks for eHealth*. WHO; 2012. http://whqlibdoc.who.int/publications/2012/9789241503143_eng.pdf.

DISCUSSION QUESTIONS

1. Compare and contrast the aims and activities of eHealth initiatives for two different regions of the world.

2. Discuss two international organizations involved in eHealth initiatives. Describe their roles and provide examples of their activities.

3. What types of international academic organizations exist in different regions of the world? Based on your specialty, choose the conferences most appropriate for you to attend and explain why.

4. What types of roles can a health professional in your specialty play in global eHealth initiatives?

5. How can the different disciplines in health informatics use the current international efforts to work together with an interprofessional approach to improving the health of individuals, families, and communities?

CASE STUDY

You are applying, through a competitive process, for a 3-month internship to the ICN eHealth Programme. According to the call for applications, the internship involves a number of activities, including the development of a strategy to promote collaboration between the major global eHealth organizations on (1) international standards development, (2) initiatives to promote the implementation of eHealth across different regions, and (3) eHealth workforce development.

Discussion Questions

1. Review the ICN goals. Think about what your internship goals might be in relation to the ICN goals.
2. Now consider what ICN hopes to achieve with internships, your knowledge about global eHealth, and your suitability for an internship. What information would be critical for you to include in your application?

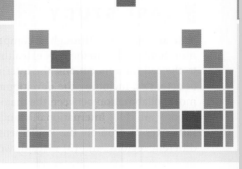

35

The Evolution of Health Informatics

Ramona Nelson

Over time, the collaborative opportunities to create a more effective and efficient healthcare system will become more interesting and motivating than the historical struggles and hierarchical relations of the past.

OBJECTIVES

At the completion of this chapter, the reader will be prepared to:

1. Discuss the development of health informatics as a discipline, profession, and specialty.
2. Analyze how historical events have influenced the definition and current scope of practice of health informatics.
3. Explore informatics-related professional organizations and their contributions to professional development and informatics.
4. Analyze the history and process for naming the specialty and the discipline.

KEY TERMS

biomedical informatics, 606
clinical informatics, 603
computer science, 595
dental informatics, 598
health informatics, 594

informatics, 596
information science, 595
medical informatics, 597
nursing informatics, 598

ABSTRACT ❖

Health informatics has evolved as both a discipline or field of study and an area of specialization within the health professions. This chapter describes the historical progression of that evolution as a basis for understanding the current status of health informatics as both a discipline and a specialty within healthcare. The historical roots within computer and information science are explored. The development of professional organizations, educational programs, and the knowledge base, as documented in conference presentations, proceedings, journals, and books, is described. The history of and process for naming the specialty and the discipline are then analyzed.

INTRODUCTION

Health informatics has evolved as a discipline and an area of specialization within the health professions. It incorporates processes, procedures, theories, and concepts from a number of different health professions and is therefore a unique interprofessional field of study as well as an area of specialization within the different health professions. As both a practice specialty and a field of study, health informatics incorporates processes, procedures, theories, and concepts from computer and information sciences, the health sciences (e.g., nursing and medical science), and the social sciences (e.g., cognitive psychology and organizational science). Health informatics professionals use information technology (IT) tools to collect, store, process, and communicate health data, information, knowledge, and wisdom. IT and related hardware, as well as software, are viewed as tools to be used by consumers, patients, and clients; healthcare providers; and administrators to achieve the goals of health informatics. The goals of health informatics include both supporting healthcare delivery and improving the health status of all people. This chapter explores the evolution of health informatics as both a discipline and a specialty practice within healthcare.

THE ROOTS OF INFORMATICS WITHIN THE COMPUTER AND INFORMATION SCIENCES

Health informatics emerged as a distinct specialty within healthcare over time as nurses, physicians, and other healthcare visionaries applied innovative developments in the computer and information sciences to complex problems in healthcare. Computer science brings to health informatics the technology and software coding required for this specialty, while information science contributes the procedures and processes needed to develop and process data, information, and knowledge. The health professions provide the knowledge and wisdom to use computer and information science effectively in delivering healthcare and improving the health of all people. Understanding the scope and boundaries of health informatics begins with an appreciation of its roots within computer and information sciences.

Computer Science

Computer science is defined as the "systematic study of algorithmic methods for representing and transforming information, including their theory, design, implementation, application, and efficiency. The roots of computer science extend deeply into mathematics and engineering. Mathematics imparts analysis to the field; engineering imparts design."[1] The word *computer* is derived from the Latin word *computare*, which means to count or sum up. The word first appeared in English in 1646, meaning a person who computes or processes mathematical data.

A key problem with these early human computers was that they made errors. In the early 1800s, Charles Babbage, a mathematician, became increasingly concerned with the high error rate in the calculation of mathematical tables. Impressed by existing work completed with calculating machines, he proposed the development of a "difference engine." As a result of his efforts to create a general-purpose, programmable computer employing punch cards, he is often identified as the first person to create a nonhuman computer or a programmable mechanical device aimed at solving problems.[2] While Babbage was not successful in building a functioning computer, the process of using punch cards to input data and obtain output did become an effective technology in other fields, such as rug making.

The Babbage approach to creating a computer included input and output but not storage. Herman Hollerith took this idea a step forward in the late 1800s when he used punch cards for input, processing, creating output, and storing data. Hollerith, like Babbage, was motivated by his concern with laborious, time-consuming, and error-prone human operations. In Hollerith's case, the problems were evident in the processes used for collecting and calculating the 1880 U.S. Census and related data. His invention, which both sorted and tabulated data, "was the first wholly successful information processing system to replace pen and paper."[3, p. 2] In 1896, starting with this and related inventions, Hollerith founded the Tabulating Machine Company. In 1911, the Tabulating Machine Company merged with two other companies, creating the company that is now IBM. Hollerith's technology, developed for completing the U.S. Census for 1890, was used well into the 1960s, by which time automation was becoming part of healthcare, and health informatics was beginning to emerge as a new discipline.

The move from a mechanical to an electronic digital computer is usually dated to the creation of the Electronic Numerical Integrator and Computer (ENIAC) in the 1940s. This was a large machine requiring huge amounts of space, a specialized environment, and specially trained personnel. It initiated the concepts of centralized computing and the information services department. Twenty years after ENIAC began functioning, the first Department of Computer Sciences in the United States was established in 1962 at Purdue University, within the school's Division of Mathematical Sciences.[4] The foundational relationship between the science of mathematics and the development of computer science provides certain benefits for health informatics. The culture of mathematics brings to the study of informatics systematic, logical approaches, processes, and procedures for understanding natural phenomena and solving problems.

In the 1980s, the personal computer (PC) emerged and forever changed the role of the user as well as the organizational infrastructure for supporting computerization within institutions. Computerization within healthcare institutions was no longer totally centralized, and computer use was no longer limited to specially trained personnel. As healthcare providers became direct users of computers, they began to discover a wide range of new uses for the tools contained therein. The increased interest in the value of computers and the increased level of computer literacy among a number of healthcare providers proved a major advantage in the creation of the informatics specialty. These same factors have also created a certain tension between centralized and decentralized infrastructures to support technology within healthcare settings.

Information Science

"Information science is a discipline that investigates the properties and behavior of information, the forces governing the flow of information, and the means of processing information for optimum accessibility and usability. It is concerned with that body of knowledge relating to the origination, collection, organization, storage, retrieval, interpretation, transmission, transformation, and utilization of information. This includes the investigation of information representations in both natural and artificial systems, the use of codes for efficient message transmission, and the study of information processing devices and techniques, such as computers and their programming systems."[5, p. 3]

Establishing the origins of information science is difficult since it emerged from the convergence of various disparate disciplines, including library, computer, communication, and behavioral sciences.[6] However, there are key dates and events that can be used to demonstrate the evolution of information science as a distinct specialty whose roots extend deeply into the profession of library science, including the following:

- 1937: The American Documentation Institute (ADI) was established. The initial organizational focus was the development of microfilm as an aid to information dissemination. Because of the expansion and diversification of its members, ADI changed its name to the American Society for Information Science in 1968 and then to the American Society for Information Science and Technology in 2000.[7]

- 1948: The Royal Society of Great Britain held a conference bringing together "libraries, societies, and institutions responsible for publishing, abstracting, and information services to examine the possibility of improvement in existing methods of collection, indexing, and distribution of scientific literature, and for the extension of existing abstracting services."[8, p. 136] The decision by this prestigious group to hold such a conference demonstrated the growing importance of managing information.
- 1963: The first textbook that treated information science as a discrete discipline was published. The book was titled *Information Storage and Retrieval: Tools, Elements and Theories*.[6]
- 1964: The National Library of Medicine (NLM) began using the computerized Medical Literature Analysis and Retrieval System (MEDLARS) as a mechanism to create *Index Medicus*.[9]
- 1971: The NLM began offering national online access to MEDLINE.
- 1972: The NLM began training physicians and other health scientists in the use of computer technology for medical education and the provision of healthcare. This was the beginning of its informatics training programs.[10] The NLM would go on to play a major role in the development of the health informatics specialty.

The relationship between library science and the development of information science provides certain benefits for health informatics. The culture of library science brings to the study of informatics policies and procedures for managing information, an awareness of the value of the information to the user of that information, and a culture of service. Evidence of this cultural value is demonstrated by the guiding principles of the American Library Association as outlined in Box 35.1.

Health Informatics

The development of health informatics is usually traced to the 1950s, with the beginning uses of computers in healthcare.[11] This early period in the history of informatics extended into the 1960s and was characterized by experimenting with the use of this new technology in medicine and in nursing education.[12] For example, Robert Ledley, a dentist interested in biomedical research, published with Lee Lusted one of the first papers in this field. The paper, titled "Reasoning Foundations of Medical Diagnosis," discussed computer-based medical diagnosis.[13] Ledley went on to invent the computed tomography (CT) scanner in the 1970s. An example from nursing is the work of Connie Settlemeyer, a graduate student in the University of Pittsburgh School of Nursing in the late 1960s. Settlemeyer designed a mainframe-based computer-assisted instruction program for teaching students how to chart using the common problem-oriented format referred to as SOAPE or SOAP. See Table 35.1 for an overview of this format. This program was then used to teach undergraduate nursing students at the University of Pittsburgh throughout the 1970s.

The term *informatics* was established in the late 1960s and into the 1970s. Informatics is actually the English translation of terms used in other languages. Because of differences in language, it is difficult to determine whether the initial use of the word *informatics* was referring to the discipline of informatics, information science, computer science, or a combination of these. A. I. Mikhailov at Moscow State University is credited with first using the Russian terms *informatik* and *informatikii*. In 1968, Mikhailov published the book *Osnovy Informatiki*, which was translated as *Foundations of Informatics*. In 1976, he published a second book, *Nauchnye Kommunikatsii i Informatika*, which was translated as *Scientific Communication and Informatics*. In this book, he defined informatics as the science that "studies the structure and general properties of scientific information and the laws of all processes of scientific communication."[14, p. 39]

In the 1960s, the word *informatique* began to appear in the French literature. *Informatique* translates to English as informatics or computing, data processing, or the handling of information, especially by a computer. During these same years, the German term *informatik* was used. *Informatik* translates as meaning computing, calculating, figuring, or reckoning. The term *medical informatics* began to appear in

TABLE 35.1 Charting Using the SOAPE Format

Letter	Item	Description
S	Subjective data or observations	Data provided by the patient, family, or others that cannot be observed, such as pain
O	Objective data or observations	Data that can be observed, such as the condition of an incision (inflamed, open with purulent drainage)
A	Assessment	The conclusion, diagnosis, or interpretation of the data, such as wound infection
P	Plan	A list of goals and planned interventions
E	Evaluation	A description of the outcomes or responses to the interventions

English publications in the early 1970s. While the term med-ical informatics was not explicitly defined in these initial publications, it was generally accepted to mean the use of a computer to process medical data and information.[14]

While the period before the 1970s was characterized by experimentation and the establishment of the term *informatics*, the next 10 to 15 years were characterized by the beginning use of computers in actual patient care and the development of health informatics as a discipline. Beginning in 1971, El Camino worked in partnership with Lockheed to install the world's first computer-aided medical information system, known as MIS.[15] A number of hospitals followed this example by installing information systems to manage business and inventory data.

At that time, nurses and unit secretaries under the direction of nurses were responsible for completing the paper forms necessary to implement physicians' orders that had been handwritten on patients' charts. These paper forms were used to communicate the orders to other departments and to capture the hospital charges associated with these orders. As a result, "order entry" and "results reporting" were some of the first hospital information system functionalities with direct patient care implications. Nurses, along with employees in specialty departments such as labs and radiology, were some of the first healthcare providers directly affected by the use of this technology in healthcare. During this same decade, computers were beginning to be used in specialty areas. One example is the use of hemodynamic monitoring systems in the cardiac lab. In these environments, computers were used to do calculations, returning accurate results within seconds. By the end of the 1970s, both commercial and academic developments in computers, libraries, and healthcare had created a fertile environment for the growth and development of the new discipline of health informatics.

ESTABLISHING THE SPECIALTY OF HEALTH INFORMATICS

Evidence during the next several decades indicated that a new specialty was being established, as seen in the following:
1. Publications of health informatics books
2. Development of new journals
3. Establishment of professional organizations
4. Number of informatics conferences that are now recurring events
5. Creation of university-level educational programs
6. Development of certification programs
7. Recognition by the U.S. Bureau of Labor Statistics

The history of each of these activities contributed to the development of the knowledge base unique to the discipline. Over time, a result of these activities is an organized body of knowledge that is specific to the discipline. The newest information within the discipline is often presented at conferences. While a conference may have a theme and even subthemes, the focus is on presenting the newest information and not an organized body of knowledge. "The timeliest articles on computer applications in medicine [are] found in proceedings and transactions of meetings sponsored by professional and

commercial organizations."[14, p. 46] As journals develop, the information and knowledge specific to the discipline become more established and organized. As the knowledge increases, the organizational structure of that knowledge is recognized and accepted within the discipline. At this point in the development of any discipline, including health informatics, books play a key role in presenting the knowledge of the discipline in an organized format. For example, scan the table of contents of this book and notice the overall organization of the knowledge specific to this discipline. This general pattern of increasing organization within publications over time is demonstrated in Fig. 35.1. As the discipline matures, these elements intersect with conferences and journal material, coinciding and then feeding more formal material to books.

Books

Books related to computers and healthcare began appearing in the 1960s. Examples of these types of books are included in Box 35.2. However, the use of the word *informatics* in a book title did not appear until 1971, when the International Federation for Documentation published *An Introductory Course on Informatics/Documentation* by A. I. Mikhailov and R. S. Giljarevskij. This was followed in 1977 by *Informatics and Medicine: An Advanced Course*, edited by P. L. Reichertz and G. Goos. In the 1980s, books related to computers and nursing began to appear. The first of these books, *Nursing Information Systems* by Werley and Grier, established

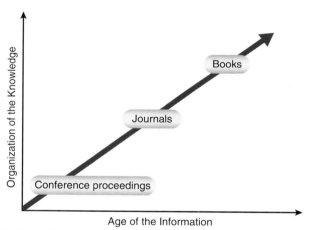

FIG 35.1 General trends in the development of knowledge within a discipline.

BOX 35.2   Early Books on Computers and Healthcare

- *Computer Applications in the Behavioral Sciences* (1962) by Harold Borko
- *Computer Applications in Medicine* (1964) by Edward Eaton Mason and William G. Bulgren
- *Use of Computers in Biology and Medicine* (1965) by Robert Steven Ledley, with the assistance of James Bruce Wilson
- *Computers in Biomedical Research* (1965) by Ralph W. Stacy and Bruce D. Waxman

and explained the minimum dataset in nursing practice.[16] This was quickly followed by one of the classic publications in informatics, *Computers in Nursing* by Rita Zielstorff.[17]

The 1980s were characterized by several publications dealing with computers and nursing. Well-recognized examples include the first edition of *Essentials of Computers* by Virginia Saba and Kathleen McCormick in 1987 and *Guidelines for Basic Computer Education in Nursing* by Diane Skiba and Judith Ronald. In 1988, the first book using the term **nursing informatics** (NI) in its title was published. This book, authored by Ball, Hannah, Newbold, and Douglas, was titled *Nursing Informatics: Where Caring and Technology Meet.*[18] In 1990, one of the first medical informatics textbooks, titled *Medical Informatics: Computer Applications in Health Care and Biomedicine*, was published by Shortliffe, Perreault, Wiederhold, and Fagan.[19] In this same year, the first **dental informatics** book, *Dental Informatics: Strategic Issues for the Dental Profession*, part of the series Lecture Notes in Medical Informatics, was edited and published by John J. Salley, John L. Zimmerman, and Marion Ball. Today most if not all of the major publishers in the healthcare arena publish books related to health informatics. A search of offerings on Amazon or the Books in Print database can result in well over 1000 hits. However, because different editions, as well as hardback and paperback editions, are counted as separate books, it is impossible to get an accurate count of the total number of informatics books now in print. See Table 35.2 for a brief book list.

Journals

Following the same pattern as books, new journals began to be published in the 1960s and used the word *computer* as opposed to *informatics*. Homer Warner at the University of Utah edited the first peer-reviewed journal within the new discipline. This journal, titled *Computers in Biomedical Research*, began publishing in 1967.[14] Table 35.3 includes the names and beginning dates of other initial health informatics journals from this time period.

In 1982, the first edition of the journal *Computers in Nursing* was published as a newsletter. The newsletter became an official journal published by Lippincott in 1984. Today the journal is known as *CIN: Computers Informatics Nursing*. While these journals provided a publishing resource for the evolving discipline, articles were also being published in other professional journals. In 1960, a total of 38 articles were indexed under the subject "computers in medicine."[14] Since that date, close to 15,000 articles have been indexed in MEDLINE and CINAHL using the key word "informatics."

While the term *informatics* began appearing in the titles of articles in the early 1970s, it was not until 1986 that the first journal article using the term *nursing informatics (NI)* was indexed in MEDLINE as well as CINAHL. This article, titled "The NI Pyramid—A Model for Research in Nursing Informatics," presented a model for research in NI.[20] This model is described in Chapter 2 of this book. As with books, the number of journals has expanded significantly. As of January 2016, the NLM catalog of journals included 219

TABLE 35.2   **Examples of Informatics Books**

Title	Authors or Editors	Edition and Date of Copyright
Biomedical Informatics: Computer Applications in Health Care and Biomedicine	Edward H. Shortliffe and James J. Cimino	4th edition, 2013
Health Informatics: Practical Guide for Healthcare and Information Technology Professionals	Robert E. Hoyt, Nora Bailey, and Ann Yoshihashi	6th edition, 2014
Information Technology for the Health Professions	Lillian Burke and Barbara Weill	4th edition, 2012
Essentials of Nursing Informatics	Virginia Saba and Kathleen McCormick	6th edition, 2015
Introduction to Computers for Healthcare Professionals	Irene Joos, Ramona Nelson, and Marjorie J. Smith	6th edition, 2013
Informatics and Nursing: Opportunities and Challenges	Jeanne Sewell	5th edition, 2016

TABLE 35.3   **Early Journals in Health Informatics**

Name	Beginning Date	Publisher
Computers and Medicine	1972	American Medical Association
Journal of Clinical Computing	1972	Gallagher Printing
Journal of Medical Systems	1977	Plenum Press
MD Computing 1983	1983	Springer-Verlag

informatics-related journals. Updated numbers can be seen by searching the database online at http://www.ncbi.nlm.nih.gov/nlmcatalog. Note that not all of the referenced journals are traditional print journals. The *Online Journal of Public Health Informatics* (http://firstmonday.org/htbin/cgiwrap/bin/ojs/index.php/ojphi/index), established in 2009, is and always has been an online journal. The journals in this growing database reflect the overall field of informatics as well as subspecialties within informatics. For example, one of the journals indexed in MEDLINE—*CIN: Computers Informatics Nursing*—is specific to NI. The proceedings from the International Medical Informatics Association (IMIA) NI Conferences were added to this list starting in late 2012.

Professional Organizations

Many of the early practitioners interested in the field of health informatics soon discovered there were no formal education programs or colleagues in their professional associations and local community who were also interested in the growing impact of computers. As a result, beginning in the late 1960s and early 1970s, professional organizations began to emerge, playing a significant role in the development of this specialty and providing a major source of education and networking for these early pioneers.[21] Initially informatics groups formed within other larger professional groups. For example, the American Medical Association (AMA) formed a committee on computers in medicine in 1969.[14] As these initial efforts expanded, professional organizations focused on health informatics began to split off from the larger organizations. At the same time that national and international groups were being established, a number of health informatics groups were established as smaller local groups.

The 1980s was a key decade for these activities. IMIA, which was established in 1967 as a technical committee of the International Federation for Information Processing (IFIP), became an independent organization in 1987. Prior to this, IMIA established Working Group 8 on NI in 1981, with representatives from 25 countries. The IMIA NI group continues to this day as a special interest group within IMIA. In the United States, the Symposium on Computer Applications in Medical Care (SCAMC) merged with the American Association for Medical Systems and Informatics (AAMSI) and the American College of Medical Informatics (ACMI) in 1989 to become the American Medical Informatics Association (AMIA). AMIA established a special interest group, Computers in Nursing, that same year.

In 1986, the Hospital Management Systems Society (HMSS), an affiliate of the American Hospital Association (AHA), became the Healthcare Information and Management Systems Society (HIMSS), reflecting the growing influence of information systems and telecommunications professionals within HIMSS as well as healthcare. In 1993, HIMSS became an independent, not-for-profit corporation.[22]

The American Nurses Association (ANA) established the Council on Computer Applications in Nursing in 1984, and the National League for Nursing (NLN) established the National Forum on Computers in Health Care and Nursing. Beginning in the 1980s and continuing over the next three decades, several local NI groups were formed. One of the largest and best known of these organizations was the Capital Area Roundtable on Informatics in Nursing (CARING), established in 1982. In 2010, the American Nurses Informatics Association (ANIA) from California and CARING from Washington, DC, merged, creating ANIA-CARING, a national NI organization that includes five regions. In 2012, the word CARING was dropped from the name, and today

the group is known as ANIA. ANIA is one of the largest NI organizations in existence.[23] Their membership, as reported on their website, has remained steady at about 3000 members.

Today a number of other local or regional NI groups continue to exist. In 2004, realizing the advantage of collaboration between these different nursing groups, 18 national and regional NI groups established the Alliance for Nursing Informatics (ANI) with the financial and leadership support of AMIA and HIMSS.[24] As of August 2016, there were 32 member groups and two associated organizations listed on their website. Box 35.3 lists examples of ANI's accomplishments.

An additional major informatics organization is the American Health Information Management Association (AHIMA). This association has taken a slightly different path than the other significant informatics-related organizations. In 1928, the Association of Record Librarians of North America (ARLNA) was formed. One of the goals of this new organization was to improve the record of care provided to patients through the use of standards. Professionals within ARLNA were titled as registered record librarians (RRLs). In the mid-1940s the association changed its name to the American Association of Medical Record Librarians (AAMRL). However, this was not the last name change. As medical records were increasingly computerized and as members assumed increasing responsibility within that process, the emphasis on information management became obvious. In 1991, the AAMRL changed its name to AHIMA.[25] Today, AHIMA continues to play "a leadership role in the effective management of health data and medical records needed to deliver quality healthcare to the public."[26] Box 35.4 lists the major health informatics organizations and includes additional information on NI groups.

BOX 35.3 Examples of the Alliance for Nursing Informatics' Accomplishments

- Successfully asked Google to appoint a nurse to the Google Health Advisory Council
- Worked closely with Technology Informatics Guiding Educational Reform (TIGER) initiative to increase the knowledge and awareness of students and practicing nurses concerning informatics
- Provided expert testimony for the Institute of Medicine and the Robert Wood Johnson forum on the Future of Nursing
- Recommended numerous nursing experts for service on national committees and expert panels
- Submitted comments to the National Institute of Standards and Technology (NIST) on the Usability Framework as well as a number of other such documents
- Created a 2-year program to enhance leadership skills and competencies in (1) communication and networking, (2) strategic planning, (3) negotiation and persuasion, as well as (4) leading and managing change for emerging leaders in NI
- Created a Consumer eHealth toolkit for use by nurses and other health professional

NI, Nursing informatics.

Given the number of health informatics–related professional organizations with similar names, it is not surprising that there is sometimes confusion, even among specialists in the field, concerning the missions and goals of the different groups. For example, because of the overlapping and complementary interests of AMIA and AHIMA, members of these organizations have at times expressed confusion about how the interests and activities of these organizations relate to one another. In response to this, AMIA and AHIMA jointly developed a document addressing potential questions about the two professional associations and their relationship: "AMIA is the professional home for informatics professionals who are concerned with basic research in the field or any of the biomedical or health application domains, either as researchers or practitioners. AHIMA is the professional home for health information management professionals, with a focus on those elements of informatics that fall under the health informatics area of applied research and practice."[27] The need for such a statement and the wide range of professional organizations focused on informatics reflect the interprofessional nature of informatics and the evolution of health informatics as a distinct area of specialization within the different health professions.

Educational Programs

During the 1950s, selected medical schools at major universities began to fund medical computer centers to support the computing requirements of a variety of new biomedical

---

BOX 35.4   Major Health Informatics and Nursing Informatics Groups

Health-Related Informatics Associations With Special Interest Groups

AMIA: www.amia.org

- "AMIA leads the way in transforming health care through trusted science, education, and the practice of informatics, a scientific discipline."
- Regular member dues are $350.
- A significant number of members are involved in academic settings.
- Publishes a monthly peer-reviewed journal: *Journal of the American Medical Informatics Association (JAMIA)*
- Is the official American representative to the IMIA
- Includes a special interest group in nursing located at https://www.amia.org/programs/working-groups/nursing-informatics. This group is responsible for appointing the nursing representative to the IMIA—Nursing Informatics Special Interest Group.

HIMSS: http://www.himss.org/ASP/index.asp

- "Advancing the best use of information and management systems for the betterment of health care"
- Regular individual member dues are $199.
- A significant number of members are involved in the practice setting or work for IT vendors.
- HIMSS North America includes 61,000 individual members, 640 corporate members, and over 450 nonprofit organizations as of January 2016.
- Includes a NI community located at http://www.himss.org/get-involved/community/nursing-informatics

Health-Related Informatics Associations With Specific Areas of Interest

American Telemedicine Association (ATA): www.americantelemed.org

- "Telemedicine will be fully integrated into healthcare systems to improve quality, access, equity and affordability of healthcare throughout the world."
- Regular member dues are $235.
- Members include individuals and organizations interested in telemedicine, including healthcare and academic institutions

and corporations that provide products and services supporting remote healthcare.

- Includes a telehealth nursing special interest group located at http://www.americantelemed.org/members/ata-members/ata-member-groups/special-interest-groups/telehealth-nursing#.VqvgM1I7Lws

AHIMA: www.ahima.org

- "Leading the advancement and ethical use of quality health information to promote health and wellness worldwide."
- Regular dues are $175.
- Members are employed mainly in medical records management.

College of Healthcare Information Management Executives (CHIME): www.cio-chime.org

- "CHIME was created as a complement to HIMSS, intending to provide a specific focus for healthcare CIOs."
- Regular dues are $498 for joint CHIME-HIMSS membership or $375 for CHIME-only membership.
- Members are the highest-ranking IT executives within their organizations.

Nursing Informatics Associations

ANI: www.allianceni.org

- "Transform health and health care through NI"
- The organization is jointly sponsored by AMIA and HIMSS; there are no dues for members.
- Regular membership is open to NI-related organizations. A list of the members with links to each organization is located at http://www.allianceni.org/members.asp. A comprehensive list of the local NI groups can be found in this list.

ANIA: www.ania.org

- "To provide education, networking, and information resources that enrich and strengthen the roles in the field of NI"
- Regular membership dues are $79.
- Membership is open to individuals interested in NI and includes around 3000 members in 15 countries.

AHIMA, American Health Information Management Association; *AMIA*, American Medical Informatics Association; *ANI*, Alliance for Nursing Informatics; *ANIA*, American Nursing Informatics Association; *HIMSS*, Healthcare Information and Management and Systems Society; *IMIA*, International Medical Informatics Association; *IT*, information technology; *NI*, nursing informatics.

research projects. During the 1960s and 1970s, the federal government, mainly via the National Institutes of Health (NIH), played a major role in supporting these efforts. In 1962, NIH was authorized to spend an additional $2 million to fund regional biomedical instrumental centers. By 1968, there were 48 fully operational biomedical computer centers. By introducing medical students, interns, and residents to informatics, these centers were fertile ground for the future development of medical informatics as a specialty. Individual lectures, elective courses, and, in time, medical informatics programs began to develop. In 1968, James Sweeney at Tulane University became the first professor of computer medicine in the United States.[14] One of the earliest departments of medical informatics was established in 1964 at the University of Utah.[28]

Beginning in the 1980s, the NLM became more active in supporting medical informatics education through its extramural grants program. In 1984, the NLM began the Integrated Advanced Information Management Systems (IAIMS) grant program, with the goal of helping health science institutions and medical centers integrate information systems to support patient healthcare, health professions education, and basic and clinical research. By 1986, the NLM was supporting five academic sites, training a total of 29 students.[29] Two decades later, the NLM was supporting 18 sites around the nation, with 270 students.[29] While most of these informatics-related educational programs were located in medical schools and attracted mainly physicians, a number of programs offered master's and doctoral degrees that were interprofessional in their recruitment of students.

The early acceptance of other professions in these programs may have supported the position that medical informatics programs are interprofessional and that the term *medical* was meant to be inclusive of all health-related professions in the same way that the term *man* can refer to both men and women. However, a number, if not most, of the health professions did not and still do not consider the term *medical* as inclusive of all health-related specialties. This is especially true for nurses who continued to develop their own university-based educational programs and be recognized as a separate profession in their own right. By 2012, AMIA took a formal position that medical informatics and NI are both subspecialties; medical informatics is not an inclusive name for both.[30]

In 1977, the State University of New York at Buffalo offered the first computer-related course in a nursing program, a three-credit elective. Just one decade later, in 1988, the University of Maryland offered the first master's program in NI. Within just a few years, a doctoral degree with a focus in NI was offered. This was followed in 1990 by a master's program at the University of Utah and in 1995 by a graduate program at New York University.[31] Over the next several years, a number of educational programs in NI were established. These programs reflected their unique setting as well as the strengths and interests of their individual faculty and varied from postbaccalaureate certificate programs to doctoral programs. Because of the wide variation in programs and the lack of any organization

tracking them, it is impossible to determine how many NI programs have actually existed over the years.

In 2002, the AMIA Nursing Informatics Working Group (AMIA NI-WG) established a task force on NI curriculum that was charged with developing a working document on the status of graduate curricula in NI. The goal was to achieve a consensus on the requirements for a master's level informatics program. The task force identified 18 graduate programs that had been in existence for at least 2 years and issued their report in 2004, which concluded the following:

> Despite several attempts, the task force did not reach consensus on a model that would represent the underlying themes and concepts, yet be flexible. The need for flexibility is important so that individual programs can determine the depth and breadth of the underlying themes and concepts, as well as the development of niche informatics areas, such as consumer informatics, telehealth, or educational applications. Such a model was deemed premature at this time. So a narrative organization of the concepts and themes and content was selected to represent the work of this task force.[32]

Today, as the number of NI educational programs and other informatics educational programs expand, a variety of degrees and certificates are offered. While nursing and medicine make up the largest groups within the healthcare specialties, a number of other healthcare disciplines have developed informatics programs specific to each discipline. For example, in 1996, Temple University established the nation's first department of dental informatics.[33]

The Health Information Technology for Economic and Clinical Health (HITECH) Act of 2009 included funding for workforce development through health IT education. Funding ran from 2010 until 2013 and included the following four programs:

- The creation or expansion of university-based health IT training programs
- The development or improvement of nondegree health IT training programs at 81 community colleges in 50 different states
- The development at five universities of health IT educational materials for use in community college–based health IT programs. These materials were also made freely available to other schools outside of the workforce development program.
- The development of the Certified Healthcare Technology Specialist (CHTS) Exam administered by AHIMA for individuals completing the nondegree training[34]

In 2015, the Office of the National Coordinator (ONC) again funded workforce development grants. With this funding, seven grantees received a total of $6.7 million to both update training materials from the original curriculum development program funded and train 6000 incumbent healthcare workers to use new health information technologies. Through this funding, the HITECH act has established a new educational program for health informatics specialists, a certificate (nondegree) program. Recognizing the shortage of informatics specialists, the designers of this program wanted to provide beginning formal education to health professionals to quickly increase the numbers of available informatics specialists. The creation of these community college–based programs means that additional avenues of informatics education are available; however, it is unclear how these different levels of education will relate to each other and to the needs of healthcare. Chapter 30 includes additional information on this program.

Accreditation for Health Informatics Education Programs

By the turn of the century, a number of health informatics related educational programs had been established. The first professional association to express interest in accreditation for these emerging programs was AHIMA. In 2003, the AHIMA House of Delegates determined that the profession of health information management was strong, unique, and should be able to conduct and confirm final accreditation actions for all health information management (HIM) programs. As part of this process, they incorporate within their scope the field of health informatics.[35] In March 2005, the Council on Accreditation for Health Information and its sponsoring organization, AHIMA, left the Commission on Accreditation of Allied Health Education Programs to form a freestanding accrediting body, the Commission on Accreditation for Health Informatics and Information Management Education (CAHIIM).[36] Only a small number of health informatics programs obtained accreditation through CAHIIM over the next few years. In September 2014, AMIA joined (CAHIIM) as an organizational member, thereby becoming an equal partner with AHIMA in CAHIIM's governance. AMIA brought to this union the involvement of the AMIA Academic Forum. The AMIA Academic Forum is a membership unit within AMIA with close to 60 full, emerging, and affiliate members who are responsible for the management of educational and research programs in universities and colleges. This group is "dedicated to serving the needs of post-baccalaureate biomedical and health informatics training programs."[37] With AMIA's involvement, CAHIIM has established a new health informatics accreditation council, with the goal of revising the accreditation standards for masters' degree programs in health informatics. The revised standards are now under development.

Certification

While attempts to create a consistent and systematic approach to educating health informatics professionals have not been successful, some level of success has been achieved in informatics specialty recognition, developing certification processes and identifying competencies within a scope of practice.

Nursing was the first group to develop a certification process within health informatics. As a result, other groups have looked to nursing's process as a model. In 1992, the ANA designated NI a specialty within the practice of nursing. Subsequently, an ANA task force developed a monograph outlining the scope of practice and describing the specialty attributes of NI.[38] The scope of practice was followed a year later by a second monograph

outlining the standards of practice and professional performance for NI.[39] These resources defining the scope and standards of practice provided the necessary groundwork for the development of a certification process. In 1995, a certification examination was created at the generalist practitioner level by the American Nurses Credentialing Center (ANCC). A baccalaureate degree in nursing (BSN) was and still is required to sit for the certification exam.

In 2001, a new task force was established to update and combine the scope and standards documents. That document was updated and revised again in 2008[40] and again in 2015.[41]

The NI certification examination is revised on a 3-year schedule to reflect evolving practice. Nurses who successfully complete the certification process include the letters RN-BC after their names to indicate they are registered nurses with board certification. In 2010, 15 years after certification was first available, the ANCC reported that there were only 779 nurses certified in informatics. In January 2013, there were 1039.[42] By December of that same year, the ANA reported there were 1326 nurses certified in informatics.[41] Clearly the AANC certification is being increasingly recognized by NI nurses as an important credential.

While the AANC offers only one level of certification for the informatics nurse, the ANA scope and standards of practice makes a clear distinction between an informatics nurse and an informatics nurse specialist. An informatics nurse specialist requires graduate preparation, while the informatics nurse does not require this level of preparation. However, with only one level of certification, this distinction is not always clear. For example, in 2002 Johnson & Johnson launched a campaign to deal with the predicted nursing shortage. The website DiscoverNursing.com is an online extension of that campaign. As of 2016, the site included 104 specialties, including Informatics Nurse. The educational requirement listed on the site is a BSN, with a diagram showing a path that includes ANCC certification. Internet searches for available NI positions frequently show a requirement of a nurse with a BSN, or baccalaureate in a related field such as computer science, with a master's degree preferred.

The 2015 ANA task force that wrote the current scope and standards of practice followed the 2008 task group in recognizing the wide variation in job titles, broad scope of responsibilities, and wide range of roles of informatics nurses. Rather than focus on roles and titles, they identified twelve functional areas within the NI scope of practice:

- Administration, leadership, and management
- Systems analysis and design
- Compliance and integrity management
- Consultation
- Coordination, facilitation, and integration
- Development of systems, products, and resources
- Educational and professional development
- Genetics and genomics
- Information management and operational architecture
- Policy development and advocacy
- Quality and performance improvement
- Research and evaluation

NI specialists employed in research, administration, or education employ each of these functional areas to varying degrees, depending on the specific task at hand. The task force's conclusion was further supported by a national informatics nurse role delineation and job analysis survey completed by ANCC in 2013 as a basis for updating the certification examination. This survey included 412 informatics-certified nurses from across the United States. The majority of certified informatics nurse specialists are employed in healthcare settings, providing leadership and support during the life cycle of a healthcare information system within healthcare institutions.[42] This is reflected in the content areas of the certification examination (Box 35.5).

The next group to develop a certification examination was HIMSS. In 2002, HIMSS launched Certified Professional in Healthcare Information and Management Systems (CPHIMS). The "certification examination is designed to test a well-defined body of knowledge representative of professional practice in healthcare information and management systems. Successful completion of a certification examination is an indicator of broad-based knowledge in healthcare information and management systems."[41, p. 2] As with ANCC, the content tested on the CPHIMS examination was developed by conducting a role delineation study. However, with this exam, IT professionals were surveyed to identify tasks that were performed routinely and considered important to competent practice. The content developed from the survey is divided into three major topics with subsections. Box 35.6 outlines the topic areas tested on this examination. A detailed outline is provided in the Candidate Handbook.[43]

HIMSS's publications concerning the development of the certification examination do not describe how the IT professionals were selected. However, the qualifications to sit for the exam do indicate how the term *IT professional* is defined. These qualifications include (1) a baccalaureate degree, or global equivalent, plus 5 years of associated information and management systems experience, with 3 of those years in healthcare; or (2) a graduate degree, or global equivalent, plus 3 years of associated information and management systems experience, with 2 of those years in healthcare. Associated information and management systems experience is defined as including experience in administration or management, clinical information systems, eHealth, information systems, or management engineering.

As with the ANCC exam, there is a heavy emphasis on systems life cycle. In addition, both certifications require recertification (including fees). ANCC has a 5-year period of certification, and CPHIMS requires recertification in 3 years. As of 2011, there were 1651 individuals with CPHIMS certification. Of these individuals, 251 were healthcare providers, divided as follows:

- 68.5% registered nurses
- 18.3% medical doctors
- 8.8% registered pharmacists
- 4.4% other[44]

AMIA is the third group to begin the process of formally recognizing an area of specialization related to informatics. A town hall discussion in 2005 at the AMIA annual meeting concluded the following:

1. Informatics as a discipline is more than clinical informatics.
2. Clinical informatics is an interprofessional domain.
3. There is social value in formal clinical informatics training and certification.[45]

While the town hall discussion described clinical informatics as an interprofessional domain and AMIA adopted this as formal policy, the actual process for recognizing clinical informatics as a specialty since then has limited this recognition to clinical informatics as a medical specialty for physicians only. In 2007, AMIA was awarded a grant to develop two documents that are required by the American Board of Medical Specialties (ABMS) to establish a medical subspecialty. In 2009, the core content for the subspecialty of clinical informatics[46] and the program requirements for fellowship education in clinical informatics[47] were published. In July 2009, the American Board of Preventive Medicine (ABPM) agreed to

---

BOX 35.5 Content Areas in the American Nurses Credentialing Center Certification Examination for Nursing Informatics

I. Foundations of Practice (47.33%)
 A. Professional Practice
 B. Models and Theories
 C. Rules, Regulations, and Requirements
II. System Design Life Cycle (26.00%)
 A. Planning and Analysis
 B. Designing and Building
 C. Implementing and Testing
 D. Evaluating, Maintaining, and Supporting
III. Data Management and Health Care Technology (26.67%)
 A. Data Standards
 B. Data Management
 C. Data Transformation
 D. Hardware, Software, and Peripherals

BOX 35.6 Content Areas in the Certified Professional in Healthcare Information and Management Systems Certification Exam for Information Technology Professionals

1. General
 a. Healthcare Environment
 b. Technology Environment
2. Systems
 a. Analysis
 b. Design
 c. Selection, Implementation, Support, and Maintenance
 d. Testing and Evaluation
 e. Privacy and Security
3. Administration
 a. Leadership
 b. Management

sponsor the specialty application, and in March 2010, ABPM submitted the application to ABMS. After an extensive review, the proposal was approved by the ABMS Board in a vote on September 21, 2011.[48] While the proposal was sponsored by ABMS, all 24 American Board of Medical Specialties boards agreed that diplomates in good standing with their primary boards can sit for this subspecialty certificate.[49] As of December 2015, there were 1105 board-certified clinical informatics diplomates.[50]

The Accreditation Council for Graduate Medical Education (ACGME) accredits training programs in clinical informatics for physicians. In February, 2014, ACGME released its program requirements for graduate medical education in clinical informatics. Initially a grandfathering process was used for physicians who had not completed a formal fellowship in clinical informatics. Beginning in 2018, the board exam will be available only for those physicians who have completed an ACGME-accredited fellowship in clinical informatics.[47]

As mentioned earlier in this chapter, AHIMA is the fourth group to offer certification. In 2010, the ONC for Health Information Technology awarded a $6 million grant to Northern Virginia Community College to support the development of a competency examination program for individuals who complete the community college–based certificate (nondegree) for training in IT Professionals in Health Care. The HIT Pro competency exam, developed through this grant, laid the groundwork for the establishment of a competency examination for health IT professionals who have completed the HITECH-funded nondegree community college program. As of July 29, 2013, the HIT Pro exam was transitioned to the AHIMA CHTS credentials.[34] The six exams currently offered include:

- Clinician/Practitioner Consultant
- Implementation Manager
- Implementation Support Specialist
- Practice Workflow and Information Management Redesign Specialist
- Technical/Software Support Staff
- Trainer

As of 2016 two additional certification exams and certification processes in health informatics is currently under development. In February 2012, the AMIA Academic Forum created a Task Force on Advanced Interprofessional Informatics Certification (AIIC). This task force issued a consensus statement (1) supporting the development of a certification process for individuals not eligible for the subspecialty certification offered to physicians, (2) recommending the certification process focus on core informatics content that is relevant to all professions, and (3) recommending that the interprofessional informatics certification should be at the graduate level. As of 2015, AMIA was in the process of collecting data to inform the development of recommended eligibility pathways. The goal is to provide recommendations for the core content, eligibility pathways, and an approach for creating a neutral organization to administer the new certification process.[51]

In April 2016 AHIMA announced that they were in the process of developing two new informatics-related certifications: "By December of this year, AHIMA and CCHIIM plan to make the beta exam available for an AHIMA health informatics credential."[51a] Following this announcement, a brochure outlining the exam content topics and the cost to take the beta version of the exam was posted on the AHIMA website.[51b] In July 2016 Tom Payne, AMIA Board Chair, sent a "special message" to the membership of AMIA entitled *AMIA Board of Directors Action on AHIMA Health Informatics Certification Efforts*. This message described the AMIA Board of Directors concern with AHIMA's announcement of the new health informatics certification exam and process: "Development of a certification process with a very similar name—Certification for Health Informatics and Information Management—that does not collaborate with AMIA's clinical and health informatics certification efforts will confuse our colleagues and key stakeholders about the role of informatics and information management."[51c] A meeting between the two professional associations was then scheduled for August 2016.

As demonstrated by this review of events from published books to the development of credentialing processes, health informatics evolved as a fragmented interprofessional specialty from a variety of disciplines having their own histories, cultures, and established structures. Books are written with "nursing informatics" or "medical informatics" in their titles, suggesting that these are texts for different health-related disciplines; however, core informatics domain knowledge spans these disciplines. Credentialing exams with overlapping content are developed by different informatics-related professional organizations and are targeted to select specialties within health informatics. The next section explores the implications of the history of health informatics.

Recognition by the U.S. Bureau of Labor Statistics

For several years the professional associations concerned with health informatics have lobbied for health informatics to be included as a recognized occupation by the U.S. Bureau of Labor Statistics and included in the Standard Occupation Classification (SOC) system. The SOC was established by the Office of Management and Budget (OMB) for use in the federal statistical system. The SOC and the statistics generated by use of this standard classification system are widely used by individuals, businesses, researchers, educators, and public policy makers.[51d]

In 2012 the SOC Policy Committee (SOCPC) began to revise the 2010 occupations and definitions in order to develop the 2018 SOC occupations and definitions. Public input was solicited in 2014, and in 2016 the SOCPC posted the draft document and requested public comments on the SOCPC recommendations.[51e] Health informatics was included for the first time, but the SOCPC recommendations proposed a single code and a definition that included health information management (HIM) and health IT occupations along with health informatics. In September 2016, 39 health informatics–related organizations sent a joint response strongly recommending separate codes for health

BOX 35.7   **Response From 39 Organizations to SOCPC Concerning Recommended Definitions for Health Informatics and Related Occupations**

- **Health informatics professionals:** Design, develop, select, test, implement, and evaluate new or modified informatics solutions, data structures, and clinical decision support mechanisms to support patients, healthcare professionals, and improved usability of such systems for patient safety within healthcare contexts.
- **HIM professionals:** Acquire, analyze, and protect digital and traditional medical information vital to the daily operations management of health information and electronic health records (EHRs).
- **Health IT professionals:** Apply knowledge of healthcare and information systems to assist in the design, development, and continued modification of computerized health care systems.

From American Medical Informatics Association (AMIA). *AMIA Responds to Proposed Updates to Standard Occupational Classification Codes.* https://www.amia.org/public-policy/amia-responds-proposed-updates-standard-occupational-classification-codes; September 2016.

BOX 35.8   **Naming Health Informatics: Related Disciplines**

- Biomedical imaging informatics
- Biomedical pattern recognition
- Clinical informatics
- Clinical research informatics
- Consumer health informatics
- Critical care informatics
- Dental informatics
- Global health informatics
- Health and medical informatics education
- Informatics in genomic medicine (IGM)
- Intensive care informatics
- Mental health informatics
- Nursing informatics
- Open source health informatics
- Pediatric health informatics and technology (PHIT)
- Pharmacoinformatics or pharmacy informatics
- Primary care informatics or primary healthcare informatics
- Public health informatics
- Public health / population informatics
- Telemedicine and mobile computing informatics
- Translational bioinformatics
- Veterinary informatics

information management professionals, health informatics, and health IT.[51f] Their posed definitions are included in Box 35.7. The final version of the 2018 SOP codes, occupations, and definitions is scheduled to be released in spring 2017.

RECOGNITION OF THE SPECIALTY

While health informatics has evolved as an interprofessional informatics specialty with a focus on healthcare, combining the words *interprofessional* and *specialty* may have created an oxymoron. First, the study of informatics is not limited to healthcare. Informatics as a field of study has been combined with a number of other professions. For example, Indiana University–Purdue University Indianapolis (http://informatics.iupui.edu/) has established a School of Informatics, which offers, along with a number of other programs, an undergraduate degree in informatics with the opportunity to specialize in biology, business, computer IT, computer science, health science, human-computer interaction, or legal informatics, among other options. Purdue also offers a graduate program in bioinformatics that prepares students to design and execute translational research linking data to medicine and drug discoveries, as well as a separate graduate program in health informatics prepares students to analyze and protect patient data, increase healthcare efficiencies, and produce quality patient care.[52]

Second, while health informatics is considered an area of specialization with a focus on healthcare, the question of which discipline it falls within has never been established. In other words, is health informatics (1) a specialty within computer science, (2) a specialty within information science, (3) a specialty within each of the various healthcare disciplines, (4) an interdisciplinary healthcare specialty with students from the different healthcare specialties combined, or (5) a new specialty distinct from its historical roots in the other disciplines? Currently, examples of educational programs representing each of these approaches can be found in colleges and universities across the United States. These programs vary, offering certificates, associate degrees, and postdoctoral fellowships. As a result, the type and amount of previous education required for admission to these different health informatics programs can vary widely. In addition, there is limited consistency in the number of credits and types of courses required in programs of the same type. In recognition of these issues, key leaders within the professional organizations have attempted to establish the appropriate name of this specialty, describe the relationship of the specialty to other related fields of study, and develop a scope of practice with core competencies for the specialty.

NAMING THE SPECIALTY—NAMING THE DISCIPLINE

Earliest references in the late 1950s used the term *bioengineering*. However, as the computer emerged as integral to health informatics, a number of terms combining the disciplines of medicine and computing, including *medical computer science, medical computing,* and *computer medicine,* were used to reflect the new specialty.[14] As other healthcare disciplines continue to develop a focus on informatics, using the terms *medicine* or *medical* to include all specialties has become more controversial, as noted earlier in this chapter. Many disciplines solved this problem by combining the name of their field of practice with the word *informatics.* Box 35.8 provides several examples. This approach is consistent with the strong division of labor, often called scope of practice, and hierarchical structures in healthcare education and healthcare delivery. This approach is also based on the assumption that informatics is a subspecialty within a specific health-related profession. However, the approach of modifying the term *informatics* with a specific health-related discipline, area of interest, or specialization does not provide a name and definition for the discipline as a whole. As pointed out previously, over the years, some have argued that *medicine* was an inclusive term covering all aspects, including all healthcare roles in preventing, diagnosing, and treating health problems, including disease. This is demonstrated by the current names of the international and national associations: the IMIA and the AMIA. These are interdisciplinary informatics associations with members from various healthcare disciplines. The 5000+ members of AMIA include individual members such as physicians, nurses, dentists, biomedical engineers, medical librarians, those in IT, and other health professionals and institutional or corporate members such as nonprofit organizations, universities, hospitals, libraries, and corporations with an interest in biomedical and health informatics.[53] Many educational programs changed their names to **biomedical informatics** to solve this issue, and there have been suggestions to change the names of the IMIA and AMIA to use *biomedical* in place of the term *medical*[30]; however, not all members may consider the term *biomedical* as more inclusive than *medical informatics*.

Others have pointed out that the practice of medicine defines the scope of practice for a physician and therefore have suggested that *health* or *healthcare* is a more inclusive term, since it includes all levels of wellness as well as disease and other health problems. For example, the HIMSS can be described as an interprofessional informatics association but uses the term *healthcare*.

The challenge has been and may still be to select a name that describes the discipline as a whole and yet acknowledges the different informatics disciplines and their relationship with the broader field of study. In 2002, Englebardt and Nelson used the term *health informatics* but presented two different "interdisciplinary" models in response to these issues. Fig. 35.2 shows an umbrella model that recognizes the clear boundaries between the different health informatics disciplines at the same time as it demonstrates that it is the connections between the boundaries or the frame of the umbrella that create the discipline. Fig. 35.3 uses a Venn diagram to describe health informatics as overlapping the different health informatics disciplines yet being distinct. However, neither model suggests a name that would be inclusive of the different health informatics specialties and their relationships.

In 2006, Shortliffe and Blois recommended the term *biomedical informatics* (BMI) in the first chapter of a book that was retitled for the third edition, *Biomedical Informatics: Computer Applications in Health Care and Biomedicine*. "In an effort to be more inclusive and to embrace the biological applications with which many medical informatics groups had already been involved, the name medical informatics has gradually given way to BMI. Several academic groups

have already changed their names, and a major medical informatics journal *Computers and Biomedical Research* was reborn as *The Journal of Biomedical Informatics*."[19, p. 23] In arriving at this position, Shortliffe and Blois explain within the chapter why they believe the terms *health* and *health informatics* are not inclusive but rather exclude key groups:

> Many observers have expressed concern that the adjective "medical" is too focused on physicians and fails to appreciate the relevance of this discipline to other health and life science professionals, although most people in the field do not intend that the word "medical" be viewed as being specifically physician-oriented or even illness-oriented. Thus, the term health informatics, or healthcare informatics, has gained some popularity, even though it has the disadvantage of tending to exclude applications to biology . . . and, as we will argue shortly, it tends to focus the field's name on an application domain (public health and prevention) rather than the basic discipline and its broad range of applicability.[19, p. 23]

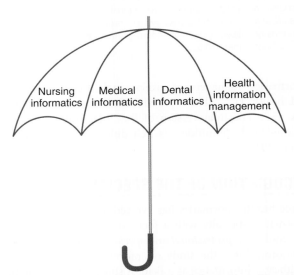

FIG 35.2 Umbrella model of health informatics. (Copyright Ramona Nelson. Reprinted with permission. All rights reserved.)

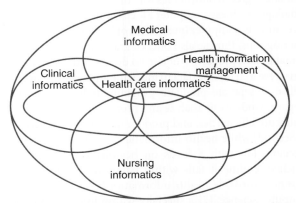

FIG 35.3 Venn Diagram Model. (Copyright Ramona Nelson. Reprinted with permission. All rights reserved.)

The term *biomedical* and the rationale for selecting it resonated with a number of other leaders within AMIA. Six years later, the AMIA Board white paper, *Definition of BMI and Specifications of Core Competencies for Graduate Education in the Discipline*, was formally approved by the AMIA Board on April 17, 2012, and published online in June 2012.[30] With the acceptance of this paper, AMIA now defined BMI as "the interdisciplinary field that studies and pursues the effective uses of biomedical data, information, and knowledge for scientific inquiry, problem solving and decision making, motivated by efforts to improve human health."[30, p. 3] The areas of research and application within BMI range from molecules to populations and societies.

In selecting the term *biomedical informatics*, the authors of the paper noted that they had adopted the newer position that the term *medical informatics* refers solely to the "component of research and practice in clinical informatics that focuses on disease and predominantly involves the role of physicians. Thus AMIA now uses *medical informatics* primarily as a parallel notion to other subfields of clinical informatics such as NI or dental informatics."[30, pp. 2–3] The term *health informatics* is also seen as limited in scope: "BMI is the core scientific discipline that supports applied research and practice in several biomedical disciplines, including health informatics, which is composed of clinical informatics (including subfields such as medical, nursing, and dental informatics) and public health informatics."[30, p. 3] Fig. 35.4 demonstrates the relationships of these previously used terms, now under the broad definition of BMI. The distinction between BMI and health informatics is further clarified in a slide set on the AMIA website. Fig. 35.5 is a slide taken from the slide set demonstrating this distinction.

However, the authors of the AMIA paper may have realized that the term *biomedical informatics* may not have sounded inclusive to all health-related informatics disciplines in stating that "the phrase 'biomedical *and* health informatics' is often used to describe the full range of application and research topics for which BMI is the pertinent underlying scientific discipline" (emphasis added).[30, p. 1]

Not all groups within healthcare identify biomedical as the inclusive term, in that it contains the term *medical* as opposed to *health*. However, combining the terms *health* and *BMI*, as in the previous quote, may be more acceptable. For example, the Northwestern University Feinberg School of Medicine, Department of Preventive Medicine, chose to name its program the Department of Health and Biomedical Informatics. This was after careful consideration of the evolution of the names for the discipline. A summary of this consideration is posted at http://www.preventivemedicine.northwestern.edu/divisions/hbmi/about-us/biomedical-informatics.html and is illustrated in Fig. 35.6. As can be seen in these two figures, a common consensus has not yet been achieved, but there are more similarities than there are differences. In both diagrams, informatics is the broader or parent discipline, and nursing, medicine, dentistry, and so forth are subspecialties within that broader field.

CONCLUSION AND FUTURE DIRECTIONS

This chapter has traced the evolution of informatics as a specialty within healthcare and as a discipline. The history of health informatics has been strongly influenced by the history of the health professions and their current infrastructures, such as the educational systems, professional

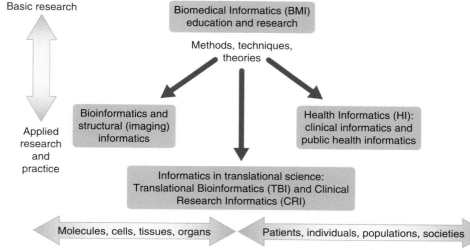

FIG 35.4 AMIA position: BMI and its areas of application and practice. *AMIA,* American Medical Informatics Association. *BMI,* biomedical informatics; *CRI,* clinical research informatics; *HI,* health informatics; *TBI,* translational bioinformatics. (Redrawn from Kulikowski CA, Shortliffe EH, Currie LM, et al. AMIA Board white paper: definition of biomedical informatics and specification of core competencies for graduate education in the discipline. *J Am Med Inform Assoc.* 2012;19(6):931-938. With permission from BMJ Publishing Group Ltd.)

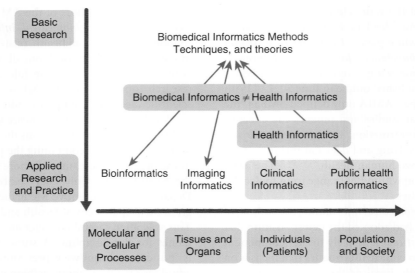

FIG 35.5 Biomedical informatics in perspective. (Used with permission from the American Medical Informatics Association.)

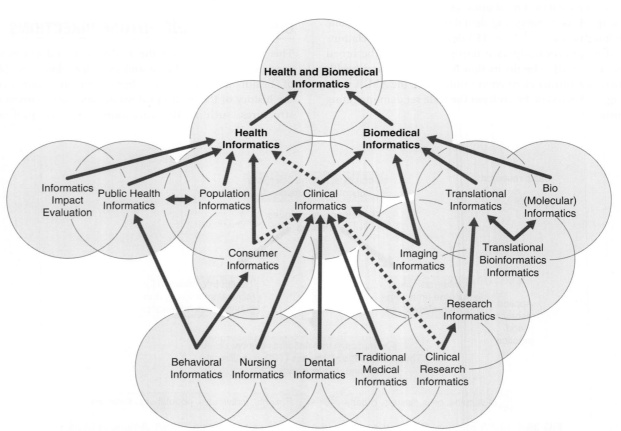

FIG 35.6 Hierarchy of informatics. This diagram shows the relationships between various subdomains of Health and BMI. The domains are shown as blobs rather than as discrete boxes to emphasize the high degree of overlap among the domains. This hierarchy should be considered a snapshot in time rather than as a definitive final solution. (Northwestern University Feinberg School of Medicine, Department of Preventive Medicine.)

organizations, and professional cultures. As informatics-related education among the professions becomes more consistent and as computerization becomes more integrated into every aspect of healthcare, these historical struggles will become yesterday's story. The emphasis will move from defining the differences and establishing boundaries between the professions to creating an interprofessional approach to meet the health-related needs of individuals and societies. Within this environment, one can expect the healthcare-related specialties to move forward in reaching a working consensus on their individual roles as well as their ever-changing scope of practice within health informatics as well as BMI. The focus will evolve to shared core competencies, knowledge, and skills rather than emphasizing differences. Over time, the collaborative opportunities to create a more effective and efficient healthcare system will become more interesting and motivating than the historical struggles and hierarchical relations of the past.

REFERENCES

1. UB School of Engineering and Applied Sciences. *Computer science vs computer engineering.* University at Buffalo School of Engineering and Applied Sciences. http://www.eng.buffalo.edu/undergrad/academics/degrees/cs-vs-cen. Accessed July 5, 2016.
2. Cesnik B, Kidd MR. History of health informatics: a global perspective. *Stud Health Technol Inform.* 2010;151:3–8.
3. da Cruz F. *Herman Hollerith.* Columbia University, Computing History; 2011. http://www.columbia.edu/cu/computinghistory/hollerith.html.
4. Rice J, Rosen S. *History of the Department of Computer Sciences at Purdue University.* Purdue University, Department of Computer Science; 1994. http://www.cs.purdue.edu/history/history.html.
5. Borko H. Information science: what is it? *Am Doc.* 1968;19(1):3–5.
6. Herner S. Brief history of information science. *J Am Soc Inform Sci.* 1984;35:157–163.
7. American Society for Information Science and Technology (ASIS&T). *History of ASIS&T.* ASIS&T. http://www.asist.org/history.html. Accessed July 5, 2016.
8. McNinch JH. The Royal Society Scientific Information Conference, London, June 21–July 2, 1948. *Bull Med Libr Assoc.* 1949;37(2):136–141.
9. U.S. National Library of Medicine. *OLDMEDLINE Data.* U.S. National Library of Medicine; 2012. http://www.nlm.nih.gov/databases/databases_oldmedline.html.
10. U.S. National Library of Medicine. *United States National Library of Medicine 1836–2011.* U.S. National Library of Medicine; 2011. http://apps.nlm.nih.gov/175/milestones.cfm.
11. Dezelic G. A short review of medical informatics history. *Acta Inform Med.* 2007;15:43–48.
12. Masic L. A review of informatics and medical informatics history. *Acta Inform Med.* 2007;15(3):178–188.
13. Ledley R, Lusted LB. Reasoning foundations of medical diagnosis. *Science.* 1959;130(3366):9–21.
14. Collen MF. *A History of Medical Informatics in the United States.* Washington, DC: American Medical Informatics Association; 1995.
15. El Camino Hospital. *About El Camino Hospital: History & Milestones.* El Camino Hospital. http://www.elcaminohospital.org/About_El_Camino_Hospital/History_Milestones. Accessed July 5, 2016.
16. Werley H, Grier MR. *Nursing Information Systems.* New York: Springer-Verlag; 1980.
17. Zielstorff R. *Computers in Nursing.* Rockville, MD: Aspen Systems Corp; 1982.
18. Ball M, Hannah K, Newbold S, Douglas J. *Nursing Informatics: Where Caring and Technology Meet.* New York: Springer-Verlag; 1988.
19. Shorttliffe E, Perreault LE, Wiederhold G, Fagan L. *Medical Informatics: Computer Applications in Health Care and Biomedicine.* Boston, MA: Addison-Wesley; 1990.
20. Schwirian PM. The NI, pyramid: a model for research in nursing informatics. *Comput Nurs.* 1986;4(3):134–136.
21. Nelson R, Joos I. Resources for education in nursing informatics. In: Arnold JM, Pearson GA, eds. *Computer Applications in Nursing Education and Practice.* New York: National League for Nursing; 1992:9–23.
22. HIMSS Legacy Workgroup: Chair Berry Ross. *A History of the Healthcare Information and Management Systems Society.* HIMSS; 2007. http://www.himss.org/content/files/HIMSS_HISTORY.pdf.
23. CIN: News Release. Leading nursing informatics organizations merge. *CIN—Comput Inform Nu.* 2010;28(2):126.
24. Greenwood K. The alliance for nursing history informatics: a history. *CIN—Comput Inform Nu.* 2010;28(2):124–127.
25. Abdelhak M, Grostick S, Hanken M. *Health Information: Management of a Strategic Resource.* 4th ed. St. Louis: Elsevier; 2012.
26. American Health Information Management Association (AHIMA). *AHIMA Facts.* AHIMA; 2012. http://www.ahima.org/about/facts.aspx.
27. American Medical Informatics Association (AMIA), American Health Information Management Association (AHIMA). *Joint AMIA/AHIMA Summary of their Relationship and Links to the Informatics Field.* AMIA; 2012. http://www.amia.org/joint-amia-ahima-summary.
28. University of Utah School of Medicine. *Biomedical Informatics: About Us—An Introduction.* School of Medicine, Department of Biomedical Informatics; 2010. http://medicine.utah.edu/bmi/about/index.php.
29. U.S. National Library of Medicine (NLM). *1986–2006: Two Decades of Progress: A Brief Report: Major Elements of NLM's Work since Its Long Range Plan of 1986.* NLM; 2007. http://www.nlm.nih.gov/pubs/plan/lrp06/report/decadesofprogress.html#18.
30. Kulikowski CA, Shortliffe EH, Currie LM, et al. AMIA Board white paper: definition of biomedical informatics and specification of core competencies for graduate education in the discipline. *J Am Med Inform Assoc.* 2012;19(6):931–938.
31. Saba V, McCormick K. *Essentials of Nursing Informatics.* 5th ed. Columbus, OH: McGraw-Hill; 2012.
32. American Medical Informatics Association. *Nursing Informatics Working Group. Educational Think Tank. Report of the Nursing Informatics Working Group Think Tank.* Bethesda, MD: AMIA; 2007.
33. University of Pittsburgh School of Dental Medicine, Center for Dental Informatics. *University of Pittsburgh School of Dental Medicine establishes Center for Dental Informatics.* University of Pittsburgh School of Dental Medicine. http://www.dental.pitt.edu/informatics/cdipr021402.html. Accessed July 5, 2016.

34. NORC at the University of Chicago. *Final Report: Evaluation of the Information Technology Professionals in Health Care ("workforce") Program.* Office of the National Coordinator; 2014. https://www.healthit.gov/providers-professionals/workforce-development-programs.

35. *Commission on Accreditation of Health Informatics Information Management (CAHIIM).* Accreditation history in health information management. http://www.cahiim.org/about%20us/history.html. Accessed July 5, 2016.

36. *Commission on Accreditation of Allied Health Education Programs.* Annual report: July 1, 2004–June 30, 2005. http://www.caahep.org/documents/file/Publications-And-Governing-Documents/2004-05AnnualReport.pdf. Accessed July 5, 2016.

37. American Medical Informatics Association (AMIA): News Releases. *AMIA Joins CAHIIM to Lead Informatics Program Accreditation;* 2014. https://www.amia.org/news-and-publications/press-release/amia-joins-cahiim-lead-informatics-program-accreditation.

38. American Nurses Association. *Scope of Practice for Nursing Informatics.* Silver Spring, MD: Nursesbooks.org; 1994.

39. American Nurses Association. *Standards of Practice for Nursing Informatics.* Silver Spring, MD: Nursesbooks.org; 1995.

40. American Nurses Association. *Nursing Informatics: Scope & Standards of Practice.* Silver Spring, MD: Nursesbooks.org; 2008.

41. American Nurses Association. *Nursing Informatics: Scope & Standards of Practice.* 2nd ed. Silver Spring, MD: Nursesbooks.org; 2015.

42. American Nurses Credentialing Center (ANCC). *2013 Role Delineation Study: Informatics Nurse: National Survey Results.* ANCC; 2013. http://www.nursecredentialing.org/Documents/Certification/RDS/2010RDSSurveys/Informatics-RDS2012.aspx. http://www.nursecredentialing.org/Certification/NurseSpecialties/Informatics/RELATED-LINKS/Informatics-2013RDS.pdf.

43. HIMSS, CPHIMS Technical Committee. *Candidate Handbook and Application.* HIMSS; 2015. http://www.himss.org/health-it-certification/cphims/handbook.

44. HIMSS, CPHIMS. *CPHIMS Statistics: January 27, 2002 thru December 15, 2011.* HIMSS; 2012. http://www.himss.org/content/files/CPHIMS_Statistics.pdf.

45. Detmer D, Lumpkin JR, Williamson J. Defining the medical subspecialty of clinical informatics. *J Am Med Inform Assoc.* 2009;16(2):167–168.

46. Gardner R, Overhage J, Steen E, et al. Core content for the subspecialty of clinical informatics. *J Am Med Inform Assoc.* 2009;16(2):153–157.

47. Safran C, Shabot MM, Munger B, et al. Program requirements for fellowship education in the subspecialty of clinical informatics. *J Am Med Inform Assoc.* 2009;16(2):158–166.

48. American Medical Informatics Association (AMIA): News Releases. *Clinical Informatics Becomes a Board-Certified Medical Subspecialty Following ABMS Vote.* AMIA; 2011. http://www.amia.org/news-and-publications/press-release/ci-is-subspecialty.

49. American Medical Informatics Association (AMIA). *Frequently asked questions (FAQ): Clinical informatics subspecialty.* https://www.amia.org/clinical-informatics-board-review-course/faq. Accessed July 5, 2016.

50. American Medical Informatics Association (AMIA). *2015 Clinical informatics diplomates.* https://www.amia.org/clinical-informatics-board-review-course/2015-diplomates. Accessed July 5, 2016.

51. American Medical Informatics Association (AMIA). *Advanced interprofessional informatics certification (AIIC): current status.* https://www.amia.org/advanced-interprofessional-informatics-certification; https://www.amia.org/faq-clinical-informatics-medical-subspecialty. Accessed July 5, 2016.

51a. American Health Information Management Association (AHIMA). Under construction: two new certifications. *Certification Connection;* April 2016. http://bit.ly/2cBw4om.

51b. American Health Information Management Association (AHIMA). *Informatics and Data Analytics: Certification.* http://www.ahima.org/topics/ida?tabid=certification. Accessed September 28, 2016.

51c. American Medical Informatics Assocation (AMIA). *AMIA Board of Directors Action on AHIMA Health Informatics Certification Efforts.* Email communication to AMIA members. July 26, 2016.

51d. U.S. Bureau of Labor Statistics. *Revising the Standard Occupational Classification;* March 2014. http://www.bls.gov/soc/revising_the_standard_occupational_classification_2018.pdf.

51e. U.S. Bureau of Labor Statistics. 2018 SOC Revision Process (n.d.). http://www.bls.gov/soc/revisions.htm. Accessed September 28, 2016.

51f. American Medical Informatics Assocation (AMIA). *AMIA Responds to Proposed Updates to Standard Occupational Classification Codes;* September 2016. https://www.amia.org/public-policy/amia-responds-proposed-updates-standard-occupational-classification-codes.

52. Purdue University Indianapolis School of Informatics. *School of Informatics: Degrees & Courses.* Indiana University Purdue University Indianapolis School of Informatics; 2016. http://informatics.iupui.edu/degrees/.

53. American Medical Informatics Association (AMIA). *Homepage.* AMIA; 2016. http://www.amia.org.

DISCUSSION QUESTIONS

1. Healthcare as a professional field of practice is often traced to the Middle Ages. Its historical roots are tied to the hierarchical structure of the church and the military. How does this history influence the current structure and relationships among the subspecialties within health informatics?

2. Which professional associations would be most appropriate for professionals interested in nursing informatics, pharmacy informatics, or public health informatics? Explain the combination selected and the rationale for each choice.

3. Is health informatics a discipline or is this an area of sub-specialization of interest to health professionals such as nurses, physicians, dentists, and so forth?

4. Should there be one certification process and set of credentials for all health informatics specialists, or should each of the health professions develop a certification process specific to that specialty?

5. What interprofessional name would you recommend and why?

CASE STUDY

In this case study, you, as the reader, will need to fill in a number of the details. The case study begins at the point when you return to school for a graduate degree. Details related to your previous education, professional experience in healthcare, and goals in returning to school should be filled in from your own life story.

The program of study for your graduate degree includes an Introduction to Informatics course. This is a required course for all students in the program. One of the first course requirements is that you join an informatics organization and complete a short paper explaining why and how you selected that specific organization. Be sure to explain how you analyzed the options and narrowed your choice to the one organization.

Discussion Questions

1. Talk to several faculty members or others with an interest in informatics to see what organizations they belong to and why. Ask how they became interested in informatics and see if you can match their history with informatics to what you learned about the history of informatics in this chapter.

2. Review the organization websites in Box **35.4** to determine which organization fits best with your interests. Explain how you matched your areas of interest to the information on the website of your chosen organization.

3. Discuss how you would use the information from questions 1 and 2 in selecting appropriate mentors.

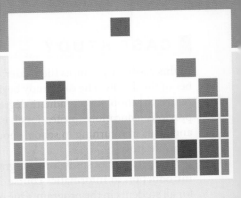

36

Future Directions and Future Research in Health Informatics

Nancy Staggers, Ramona Nelson, and David E. Jones*

Health informatics can be described as an interprofessional discipline that is grounded in the present while planning for the future.

OBJECTIVES

At the completion of this chapter, the reader will be prepared to:

1. Explore major trends and their implications for future developments in healthcare, health informatics, and informatics research.
2. Analyze techniques and challenges of planning for future directions and trends.
3. Apply futurology methodologies in identifying trends and possible, probable, and preferred futures.
4. Describe the fields of nanomaterials and nanoinformatics, the role of these fields in healthcare, and implications for the future.
5. Analyze the advantages and disadvantages of nanotechnology in health and health informatics.

KEY TERMS

ABSTRACT ❖

This chapter expands on the future directions sections included in the individual chapters and provides broad guidance about the future of health informatics. First, healthcare trends in society are outlined. Second, futures studies or futurology (methods to analyze probable future directions in any field) is discussed. Third, an overview of future directions in healthcare and informatics is given: (1) person-centered health, the fusion of health information technology (health IT) into healthcare and concomitant implications for health informatics; (2) technical trends in health IT, such as the internet of things (IoT) and cybersecurity issues; and (3) clinical informatics trends, including analytics, data visualization, and improving the user experience (UX). Last, this chapter offers a section on nanotechnology and nanoinformatics. The last topics are discussed in more detail because of their likely profound impacts on society, healthcare, and health informatics in the future.

INTRODUCTION

Health informatics can be described as an interprofessional discipline grounded in the present while planning for the future. Health professionals and informatics specialists are implementing today's health information technology (health IT), while creating the foundation for the technology of tomorrow. By reviewing current trends and predictions, as well as employing tools for predicting and managing the future, health professionals and informatics specialists can prepare for their leadership roles in planning effective and innovative future healthcare information systems.

Clearly, health IT and informatics will play integral roles in the future of all aspects of healthcare. Precisely which informatics trends will prevail is not completely clear; however, emerging areas can be seen. In each of the chapters in this book, authors outlined evolving areas of influence. This final chapter offers material on healthcare trends in society, methods for

*Acknowledgment: David E. Jones's contribution was supported by Grant Number T15LM007124 from the National Library of Medicine.

predicting the future, directions in health informatics and, finally, a section on nanomaterials and nanoinformatics.

To understand the future of health informatics, healthcare providers and informaticians need to be aware of societal trends. Examples of trends in society include the following:

- *Healthcare costs.* Analysts initially predicted continual increases in healthcare costs at about 6% annually through 2020.[1,2] Although costs are predicted to still rise over time, current spending projections are now $2.5 trillion less due to the Affordable Care Act in the United States and the economic recession that occurred in the late 2000s.[3]
- *Aging populations.* From 2000 to 2050, the global population of those aged 60 years or older will rise from 600 million to more than 2 billion.[4]
- *Increasing numbers of patients with chronic diseases.* By 2030, chronic diseases will be the leading cause of deaths worldwide.[5] The rate for diabetes alone across the globe is predicted to increase from 382 million in 2013 to 592 million by 2035.[6]
- *Predicted shortage of healthcare providers.* By 2025, the United States will have a shortage of nurses in 16 states[7] and a national shortage of 46,000 to 90,000 physicians, mostly in primary care and surgical specialties.[8]

These trends clearly have implications for the future practice of health informatics. But how does one determine and plan for these implications? Futures research, or futurology, the method used to determine future directions and trends in any field, can help answer this question.

FUTURES RESEARCH (FUTUROLOGY)

This section introduces readers to levels of change that can be anticipated in future trends. By analyzing methodologies and tools for predicting, planning for, and managing the future, health professionals and informatics specialists are able to prepare for the leadership roles they will play in planning future healthcare information systems. With a better understanding of the potential future, healthcare providers and informatics professionals can make better decisions today.

Defining Futures Research (Futurology)

Futures research is the rational and systematic study of the future, with the goal of identifying possible, probable, and preferable futures. The focus can be anywhere from 5 to 50 years in the future. The formal study of the future goes by a number of names, including *foresight and futures studies, strategic foresight, prospective studies, prognostic studies,* and *futurology.* Using a research approach to study the future formally began after World War II. Initially this field of study aroused skepticism. Since that time, a number of institutes, foundations, and professional associations have been established supporting the field of futures studies. Examples of these are included in Box 36.1. In addition, a number of educational programs related to futures studies now use the various futurology terms to describe their programs. Box 36.2 includes examples of university programs in futures studies. Researchers and corporate strategists are also using numerous concepts, theories, principles, and methods based on the field

---

| BOX 36.1 | **Futures Studies: Selected Associations, Institutes, and Foundations** |

- Acceleration Studies Foundation, http://accelerating.org/index.html
- Copenhagen Institute for Future Studies, http://cifs.dk/about-us/
- Foresight Canada, http://www.foresightcanada.ca
- Fullerton and Cypress Colleges, and School of Continuing Education: Center for the Future, http://fcfutures.fullcoll.edu
- The Arlington Institute, http://www.arlingtoninstitute.org
- Association of Professional Futurists, http://www.profuturists.org

- The Institute for Alternative Futures (IAF) http://www.altfutures.org/home
- The Club of Rome, http://www.clubofrome.org
- *The Futurist,* http://www.wfs.org/futurist/about-futurist
- Institute for the Future, http://www.iftf.org/home
- The Millennium Project, http://www.millennium-project.org
- World Future Society, http://www.wfs.org/node/920
- World Futures Studies Federation (WFSF), http://www.wfsf.org

IAF, Institute for Alternative Futures; *WFSF,* World Futures Studies Federation.

| BOX 36.2 | **Selected University Programs in Futures Studies** |

- University of Southern California (USC) Annenberg Center for the Digital Future http://www.digitalcenter.org
- Regent University: School of Business and Leadership, http://www.regent.edu/acad/global/degree_programs/masters/strategic_foresight/home.cfm
- TamKang University: Graduate Institute of Futures Studies, http://future.tku.edu.tw/en/
- University of Advanced Technology, http://majors.uat.edu/Emerging-Tech

- University of Hawaii: Hawaii Research Center for Futures Studies, http://www.futures.hawaii.edu/academic-offerings.html
- University of Houston: College of Technology, http://www.houstonfutures.org/program.html
- University of Stellenbosch: Institute for Futures Research, http://www.ifr.sun.ac.za/Pages/Welcome.aspx
- University of Turku: Finland Futures Research Centre (FFRC), http://www.utu.fi/en/units/ffrc/Pages/home.aspx/

FFRC, Finland Futures Research Centre; *USC,* University of Southern California.

of futures research. Despite the initial skepticism today, the futures studies techniques are accepted, educational programs are available, and these methods can be very useful for healthcare providers and informaticians.

Health and informatics professionals can use traditional forecasting and planning methods in combination with futures studies methods. Strategic planning in health informatics typically focuses on projects 1 to 3 years in the future. Institutional long-range planning tends to focus on 5 to 10 years in the future. Vendor contracts for major healthcare informatics systems often cover a 10-year period, spanning both strategic and long-range planning.

There are some differences between forecasting and futures studies. First, forecasters focus on incremental changes from existing trends, while futurists focus on systemic, transformational change. Second, futurists do not offer a single prediction. Rather, they describe alternative, possible, and preferable futures, keeping in mind that the future will be created, in most part, by decisions made today. The technical, political, and sociocultural infrastructure being built today will have a major impact on the choices of tomorrow. Both traditional forecasting and futures studies methods are key to planning health informatics projects.[9] Understanding the impact of future trends and using this information for planning begins by understanding the degree and scope of change that occurs over time.

Future Directions and Scope of Change

Degrees or the scope of change can be divided into three levels.[10] First-level change does not really change the process being used or the goal one might want to achieve. This level of change makes the process in use more effective and efficient. Replacing a typewriter with a word processor is an example of a first-level change. The user is still producing a document, but the technology makes the process more effective and efficient. Within the levels of change, first-level change is the least disruptive and the most comfortable. In many ways, requests that new technology be designed to fit the workflow of healthcare providers is, in reality, a request, or perhaps a demand, for first-level change only. In fact, if the equipment and related procedures do not support the current roles and responsibilities of the healthcare providers, they quickly develop workarounds to meet their requirement that the degree of change be limited to a first-level change.

A second-level change involves changing how a specific outcome is achieved. For example, historically the peer review process used by professional journals involved sending a submitted manuscript to a limited number of selected experts for anonymous opinions. The goal was to ensure that only the highest quality articles were published. The process of review and revision could take several weeks or months. In addition, with a limited number of experts screening what was published, some degree of professional censorship existed. Articles representing a paradigm shift in thinking risked being rejected by this limited set of reviewers. Today, professional online journals and journals that prepublished online versions of an article usually offer all readers the opportunity to comment. Opening up the opportunity for all readers to comment is now changing who is ultimately involved in peer review and how the peer review process is completed.

Another example of second-level change is demonstrated by patient groups within social media applications. These are changing what and how patients learn about their health problems. Groups of patients help each other read and interpret the latest research to create a new level of health literacy within these groups. Social media interactions not only change the process for achieving an outcome, but also change the relationships between the participants. As patients become organized and knowledgeable, they take a more active role in their own care and move from the role of patients needing education about their diseases into more of a collegial role, even sharing new and innovative findings with healthcare providers.

The scope of change at this level creates both excitement and anxiety within professional groups and among individual healthcare providers. The scope of practice, policies, procedures, and established professional customs, such as professional boundaries, are challenged, and resistance to this challenge can be expected. For example, in healthcare, the goals of improved health for individuals, families, groups, and communities have not changed, but technology is changing the roles and responsibilities related to how these goals might be achieved.

A third-level change alters the process and can also refocus the goal. For example, a hyperlinked multimedia journal, with a process for adding reader comments and linking to related publications, may change not only the definition of an expert but also the historical gold standard for review of new information and knowledge.

Another example is the use of knowledge discovery and data mining in the research process. In the traditional approach to scientific research, the researcher begins with a theory and a theoretically based hypothesis. This foundation is used to determine what variables or data are collected and how those data are analyzed. With knowledge discovery and data mining, the goal is to discover clusters and relationships among existing data with no preconceived concept of theories, data collection, or how these data are related, redefining (or at least expanding) the concept of the research process.

Third-level change involves changes at the societal and institutional level, typically occurring over long periods of time. For instance, the evolving role of the nurse from a handmaiden for the physician to a leader in healthcare delivery can be seen as a third-level change. Both the goal of nursing, from an efficient and effective handmaiden to a leader, is changing, as well as the activities that make up the nursing process.

Today, innovations in healthcare and computer technology are interactively creating first-, second-, and third-level changes, creating the future of healthcare within a society that is also undergoing change in most other society based institutions. Informatics experts are among the key leaders managing and guiding these change processes within healthcare. However, they face a number of challenges in achieving these goals.

The Challenge of Anticipating Future Directions

Almost 50 years ago in 1970, Toffler published the book *Future Shock*.[11] One of the themes in the book was "what happens to people when they are overwhelmed by change. It is about how we adapt or fail to adapt to the future."[11, p. 1] Interestingly, *Future Shock* was written long before the widespread use of personal computers or the internet. As Toffler identified many decades ago in a slower-paced world, the degree and speed of change was overwhelming for many. Today, this includes both providers and consumers of healthcare who are in the midst of exponential knowledge growth and must adapt to the overwhelming changes in healthcare.

While there are no research methods for predicting the future with absolute certainty, techniques can be used to rationally predict future directions and trends. A historical example of this is the publication of the book *Megatrends* by Naisbitt,[12] well before the general population was aware of the internet or the potential of owning a computer. Megatrends are trends that affect all aspects of society. The 10 trends identified by Naisbitt are listed in Box 36.3. These trends, identified many years ago, continue to have a major influence on health informatics today.

While health providers and health informatics specialists clearly recognize the importance of planning and the long-term implications of building today's healthcare information systems, immediate challenges exist in thinking about the future. First, present issues are often more pressing and take a higher priority over tasks that can wait for another day. This type of thinking is sometimes referred to as "putting out fires." For example, a health informatics specialist may spend an afternoon answering users' questions, but as the number of communications increases, the notes documenting these calls can become increasingly sparse. Trends and patterns that could be used as a basis for a new education and training program, or for upgrading functions in the current healthcare informatics system, can be lost in the pressing demands of the moment.

Second, small rates of growth often seem insignificant. However, major trends start from small, persistent rates of growth. This is especially true when dealing with exponential growth. A few years ago, very few patients asked for copies of their health reports, and a very small percentage of those patients would have considered accessing their healthcare data via the internet. As of October 2015, the Office of the National Coordinator (ONC) reported that over 90% of hospitals provide patients the option of viewing their health data online. See Table 36.1 for additional details about how hospitals and providers are engaging patients in their own healthcare via the internet and personal health records (PHRs).

Third, there are intellectual, imaginative, and emotional limits to the amount of change that individuals and organizations can anticipate. The imagined future is built on assumptions developed in the past and therefore includes gaps and misinterpretations. Future predictions can seem vague, and the further one looks into the future, the more disconnects exist between the present and the significance of the future. For example, nurses educated in small diploma schools in the 1950s and 1960s usually called a physician to restart an intravenous (IV). If nurses from that era were asked to predict the future of nursing, they would have struggled to anticipate the high levels of responsibility common in today's staff nurse role, where starting an IV is a common task.

BOX 36.3 Naisbitt's Megatrends for the 1980s

- Industrial society → Information society
- Forced technology → High tech/High touch
- National economy → World economy
- Short term → Long term
- Centralized → Decentralized
- Institutional help → Self-help
- Representative democracy → Participatory democracy
- Hierarchies → Networking
- North → South
- Either/Or → Multiple options

TABLE 36.1 Extent of Patient Engagement Functions in Hospitals

Online Patient Engagement Functionality	PERCENT OF HOSPITALS WITH CAPABILITY			
	2012	2013	2014	2015
Online Capabilities Incentivized by Federal Policy				
View information from health/medical record	24	39.8	90.8	95.1
Download information from health/medical record	14.3	27.8	82.2	86.8
Transmit care/referral summaries to a third party	N/A*	11.6	66.4	71.5
View, download, and transmit health information	N/A*	10	64	68.8
Secure messaging with health care provider†	N/A*	N/A*	51.3	63
Online Capabilities Not Incentivized by Federal Policy				
Request to update health/medical record	30.9	32.8	72.4	77.1
Pay bills	49.3	55.4	66.9	74.1
Schedule appointments	21.6	29.8	41.4	43.6
Request prescription refills	19.3	27	39.4	42.1
Submit patient-generated data	7.3	12.5	32.5	37.1

From Office of the National Coordinator for Health Information Technology. *U.S. hospital adoption of patient engagement functionalities: Health IT Quick-Stat #24.* dashboard.healthit.gov/quickstats/pages/FIG-Hospital-Adoption-of-Patient-Engagement-Functionalities.php; September 2016.
*Measure was not collected in survey year.
†Secure messaging was added to survey in 2014.

Approaches for Predicting

Qualitative and quantitative methods are used in traditional forecasting and planning as well as by futurists to foresee, manage, and create the future. The use of established research methods separates these researchers from soothsayers. Multiple methods used in concert are needed to identify and address future challenges. Selected examples of methods used in conduction futures research are presented here. In addition, Box 36.4 includes resources for exploring a number of other methodologies used in this field of study.

Trend Analysis and Extrapolation

Trend analysis involves looking at historical data to identify trends over time. For example, a log of help desk calls demonstrates that over the past 2 months, there has been an increasing number of calls from clinical managers and department heads concerning the institution's newly introduced budget software. This new software offers a number of options and levels of analysis that are more robust and complex than the software that was used in the past. Initially several calls occurred from three managers who work in the same division. However, these managers are now making very few calls. Instead, the majority of the calls are coming from a different division. Extrapolation consists of extending these historical data into the future. For example, if the trend line is sloping upward, one would continue this line at the same degree of slope into future time periods. Needless to say, this historical upward trend line will not continue forever. Eventually the growth will start to slow and an S curve will develop. With an S curve, the growth is initially slow but then becomes very rapid. Once the event begins to reach its natural limit, the rate of growth slows again, creating an S-shaped curve.

A potential example of this pattern is the future use of PHRs by the general public. Initially only a small number of people were using this resource. Google, an early entrant in PHR development, withdrew from this market because of lack of

interest by the general public. However, the current Blue Button data from the Veterans Health Administration (VHA) suggests that the use of PHRs may be at the beginning of an S curve, with the possibility of very rapid growth in the next few years. The expected patterns of growth can be used to plan educational programming as well as support services. The need for these services can be expected to grow and then level off.

While trend analysis and extrapolation demonstrate using numerical data or quantitative methods to foresee the future, qualitative methods are also important. One example of qualitative methods is content analysis.

Content Analysis

Content analysis was the major research approach used to identify the trends in the book *Megatrends*.[12] Content analysis within the futures research realm involves reviewing a number of information resources and noting what topics are discussed, what is being said about these topics, and what topics are not discussed. A current example of this type of analysis can be seen in the website created as an informational tool for public health. This application searches open-source Twitter data for health topics and delivers an analysis of that data for both a specified geographic area and the national level, thereby serving as an indicator of potential health issues emerging in the population, building a baseline of trend data, and engaging the public on trending health topics. A screenshot showing the types of data being tracked is provided in Fig. 36.1. The assumptions made in identifying resources, topics, and trends to monitor can have a major impact on determining the forecasts produced. This is one of the reasons it is important that informatics specialists review several different resources from several different perspectives in analyzing trends.

Scenarios

Scenarios involve asking individuals to envision possible futures within a certain context. For example, people may be asked to describe the electronic health record (EHR) they might expect to see 10 to 15 years in the future. This can be done as a group process or individually. Participants should be encouraged to envision scenarios that are multifaceted and holistic, internally consistent, and free of personal bias. Elements in the scenario should not be contradictory or improbable. A well-constructed scenario may suggest events and conditions not presently being considered.

The following three major approaches can be used to construct a scenario:

1. The Delphi method can be used to elicit expert forecasts for a specific time frame. A combination or synthesis of opinions is used to develop the scenario.
2. Experts develop scenarios that reflect the viewpoint of their disciplines. These are modified and combined to produce an overall scenario.
3. A cross-impact technique is used to test the effect of one aspect of the scenario on all of its contributing parts.

The creation of scenarios can be used in concert with backcasting.

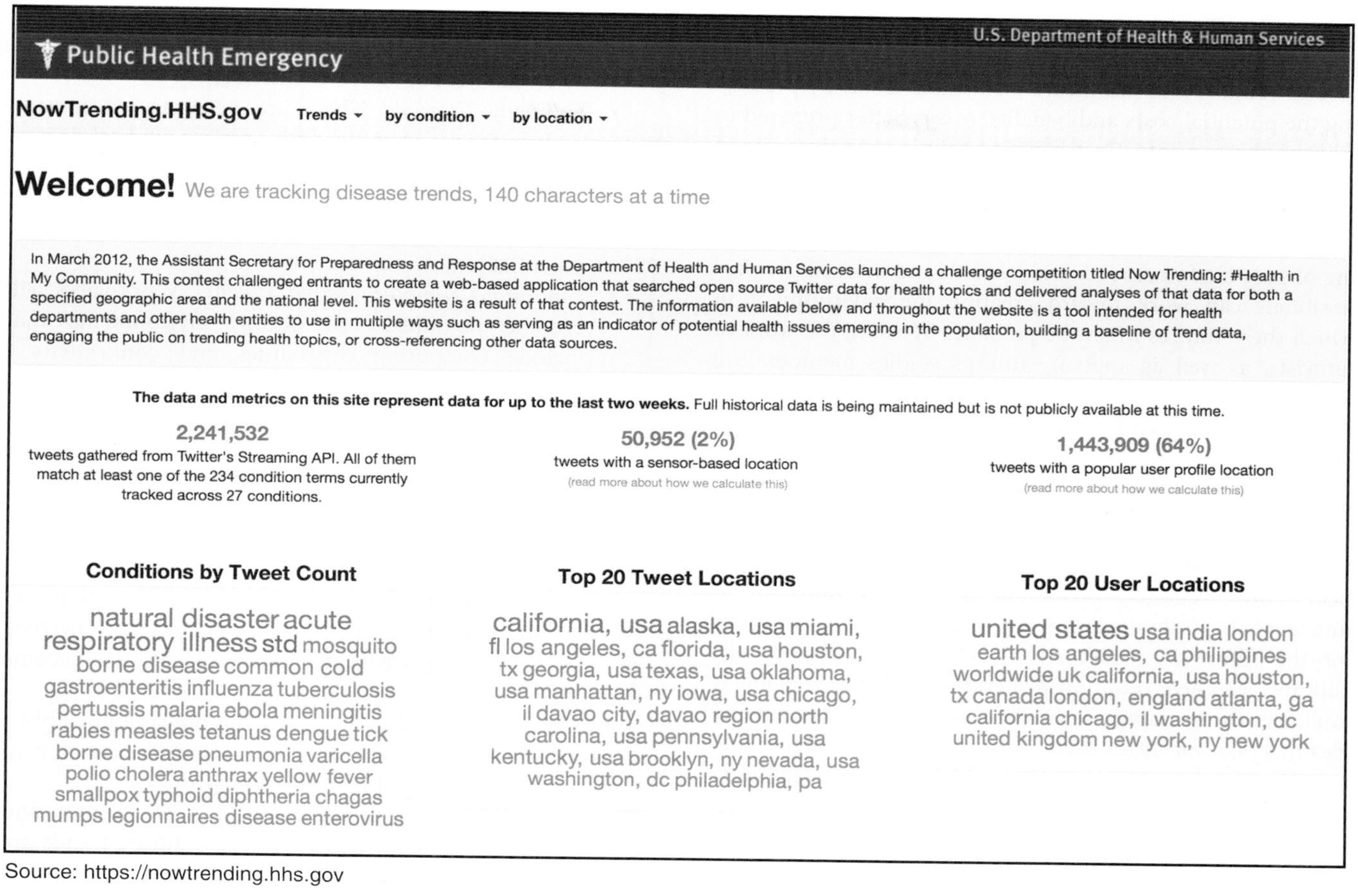

Source: https://nowtrending.hhs.gov

FIG 36.1 What is now trending. Following disease trends 140 characters at a time. (From *U.S. Department of Health and Human Services.* <https://nowtrending.hhs.gov/>.)

Backcasting

With **backcasting,** one envisions a desired future end point and then works backward to determine what activities and policies would be required to achieve that future. Backcasting involves the following six steps:

1. Determine goals or the desired future state.
2. Specify objectives and constraints.
3. Describe the present system.
4. Specify exogenous variables.
5. Undertake scenario analysis.
6. Undertake impact analysis.

The end result of backcasting is to develop alternative images of the future, thoroughly analyzed as to their feasibility and consequences.[13]

With the rapid changes in informatics, the use of futures research methods is likely to increase. Informatics specialists concentrated on implementation and change issues during first generation of EHRs, data warehouses, and mHealth. For the next generations of health IT products, futurology can more readily be incorporated in the health professional or informatician's suite of skills.

Application of Futures Research

Health and informatics professionals can use methodologies and strategies from futures studies in two primary ways. First is foreseeing or predicting future trends and directions. For example, in the 1970s and 1980s, much of healthcare was financed via fee-for-service funding approaches. Health information systems were designed to capture charges but not to measure the cost of care. A number of items, including nursing and other services, are included in the patient's charge for a hospital room. In a fee-for-service approach, the contribution of nursing and other services to the total cost was irrelevant. Cost and charges did not need to correlate. The charge could be whatever the market would bear.

The introduction of the prospective payment system in the 1980s and managed care in the 1990s is now followed by the current value-based approach, Merit-Based Incentive Payment System (MIPS), included with the Medicare Access and CHIP Reauthorization Act (MACRA) of 2015. These initiatives require that healthcare institutions capture costs and quality rather than just charges. Existing information systems were never designed to facilitate capturing discrete costs (versus charges). The ability to predict these kinds of major changes in healthcare delivery could be a significant advantage to vendors and healthcare institutions alike. By predicting the potential costs and benefits, one is better prepared to manage these events. Cost-benefit analysis is an example of using futures studies for management.

Creating the future is the second way in which health informatics specialists use futures studies methods. By thinking of possible futures scenarios, health and informatics professionals can work toward creating the environment in which these futures might be possible. By using the work of futurists, as well as applying futures studies methods and tools, it is feasible to imagine possible future trends and directions and thereby work to create preferable future directions.

THE FUTURE OF HEALTH INFORMATICS

Health informatics is and will remain a dynamic and complex field. Thus accurately predicting precise directions for its future is inherently uncertain. To determine likely directions for the future in healthcare and health informatics, the authors searched traditional literature databases, publicly available white papers such as the National Institute of Health's plan for 2016–2020,[14] and reports from major analytic firms such as Manatt's Megatrends Shaping Healthcare 2016–2020[15] and Pricewaterhouse Coopers' (PwC) Top Health Industry Issues,[16] as well as less formal sources such as futures presentations by national and regional experts.

Formal literature does not provide consensus about emerging or future directions for informatics. Authors in the past wrote about the future of academic biomedical informatics,[17] created a nursing informatics research agenda for 2008–2018,[18] and provided an analysis of the past, present, and future of medical informatics[19]; however, none of these was published recently. Within informatics and nursing, major past efforts internationally centered on terminology development.[20] Future trends will certainly include this emphasis but likely will expand into new areas, as outlined in the following discussion.

Looking further into the future can influence thinking about near-term trends. Outside the field of healthcare, contemporary issues of *The Futurist* (http://www.wfs.org/futurist) list annual outlooks. A sampling of trends pertinent to healthcare include the following:

- *Tiny chips.* Computer chips will shrink to the size of dust and be ubiquitous.[21]
- *Huge amounts of transmitted personal health data.* Embedded or swallowed sensors will collect and transmit an array of personal data.[22]
- *New leader skills.* These will be shaped by those with social networking, content management, data mining, and data meaning skills. New job titles will include Chief Content Officer and Chief Data Scientist.[23]
- *Nanotechnology products.* Buckypaper is composed of industrial-grade carbon nanotubes and is 100 times stronger than steel per unit of weight. It conducts electricity like copper and disperses heat like steel or brass.[24]

- *Nanorobots or nanobots.* These carry molecule-sized elements, can detect cancer, and are being developed by researchers at Harvard University.[25]
- *Full-body firewalls.* These are necessary to prevent hackers from tampering with wireless medical devices and internal drug delivery systems. Researchers at Purdue and Princeton Universities are developing a medical monitor (MedMon) designed to identify potentially malicious activity.[26]
- *Ubiquitous computing environments.* Workplaces will become ubiquitous computing environments that include computing capabilities and connectivity.[27] Likewise, homes and personal devices will provide constant communication and computing outside work.
- *Image-driven communication.* Graphics and images will be more heavily relied on for communication, allowing faster comprehension and possibly new ways of thinking, but at the cost of eloquence and precision.[28]
- *Living data.* Connectivity will expand to millions of devices, and sensors will gather more data that will be processed by more computers. Data may become too big, so channeling the power of data will become important.[29]
- *The intelligent "cloud."* This will become not just a place to store data but will evolve into an active resource, providing analysis and contextual advice.[30]

These more futuristic trends are important to monitor, and some inform near-term trends. Near-term future trends are (1) person-centered health and concomitant implications for health informatics; (2) technical trends in health IT such as the internet of things (IoT) and cybersecurity issues; and (3) clinical informatics trends, including what is beyond traditional EHRs, improving the user experience (UX), predictive analytics, and data visualization.

Person-Centered Health and Informatics

An obvious shift has occurred away from provider-centric healthcare toward person-centered health.[31,32] The importance of this shift is underscored in a number of chapters of this book: Chapter 8 (Telehealth), Chapter 9 (Home Health), Chapter 12 (ePatients), Chapter 13 (Social Media), Chapter 14 (Personal Health Records) and Chapter 15 (mHealth). This direction will continue to accelerate over time, although healthcare and informatics will likely see the fusion of several of these separate areas in the future.

The term person-centered health is used as a generic term to encompass ideas about the various terms in use today: person-centered care, patient-centered care, precision medicine, and consumer-centered care. Person-centered care embodies personal choice and autonomy in healthcare decision making.[33] More specifically, this newer term most frequently includes these six principles: (1) whole-person care, (2) respect and value, (3) choice, (4) dignity, (5) self-determination, and (6) purposeful living. They are being applied to the care of older adults in particular.[33] Precision (or personalized) medicine includes a central premise that health interventions are tailored to specific individual differences such as genome, environments, and lifestyle.[34] For example, therapeutics would be tailored specifically to individuals' genetic tumor compositions and their responses to previous interventions. In support of research for precision medicine, an initial $215 million investment was recently included in the U.S. budget.[34] No matter the current term, the shift is toward tailoring care to and improved support of health decision making for individuals. This shift has substantial implications for informatics because these areas are highly data-centric. Demiris and Kneale[35] outlined initial informatics support for the move toward person- and patient-centric care (e.g., improvements in clinical decision support, e-tools to support care transitions, PHRs, and telehealth). Two other near-term informatics trends are outlined in support of person-centered health in the future: (1) care anywhere and everywhere and (2) personal data integration.

Care Anywhere

EHRs by design are organization- and provider-focused. The movement toward person-centered health requires rethinking the design of disparate health data into a person-centric format. Aspects of traditional care settings, supported by EHRs and to a lesser extent by PHRs, are evolving into remote, on-demand services for many nonemergent services. Through informatics tools, consumers are supported as they assume more responsibility for their own care, especially consumers with chronic diseases. Informatics support via apps and the internet is expanding at an enormous rate. From 2013 to 2015 alone, mHealth applications expanded fourfold from 40,000 to over 165,000,[36] and on-demand services are easily accessible via the internet (e.g., dermatology).[37] Although the care models of the future are not precisely clear, the move is toward care anytime, anywhere for areas such as primary care and chronic care.

The design of tailored, person-centered applications provides a wealth of opportunities for research and development, including the following:

- Theory-based studies on the impact of person-centered health IT products
- The effectiveness of changing care models on care collaboration for individuals focused on person-centered health

Personal Data Integration

As information in Chapter 8 points out, simple personal monitoring tools such as electronic scales and remote blood glucose monitors are already expanding into a suite of robust biometric sensor technologies. One source indicated that by 2018, 130 million wearable sensors will be acquired by the public.[38] Smart textiles and other personal devices such as smart contact lenses and smart homes in the future could provide constant monitoring of individuals' health and chronic conditions. No doubt many people will be actively monitoring and interpreting their own data from these devices.

Care anywhere and the increase in personal data mandates an amalgamation of pertinent health data beyond a casual level and away from informal personal records or users keeping data in their heads. Instead, these will need to include data integration across disparate sources for an interpretable individual view. Today, mHealth apps and online services result in stand-alone data viewed primarily by patients and families. Thus the challenge will be to effect data integration across diverse sources and to provide monitoring with appropriate interventions for any acute changes. Future research and evaluation might include the following:

- Evaluating the impact of role changes from provider-centric to patient-centric data
- Exploring outcomes of the new digital divide among individuals who cannot or choose not to be "quantified" by personal data

Technical Trends

Technical aspects of health informatics are trending toward cloud computing and remote application services, as indicated in Chapter 5. Two other important technical trends are especially relevant for the near future: the IoT and increased cybersecurity threats.

The Internet of Things

Simply put, the IoT refers to a network of connected devices.[39] Currently, the IoT might be used to remotely monitor a patient after discharge[40] or to track equipment or people inside health facilities. In the future, the IoT has broader applications. With multiple devices and people connected via the internet, new applications are possible. A simple application might involve improved remote physiologic monitoring using sensors. For example, flexible and wearable sensors, which adhere to skin better, and silicon-based materials, which conduct signals better, can combine with the IoT to allow improved, remote physiologic monitoring for patients.[41] More complex IoT applications in a facility might include a suite of interacting devices and applications, including:

- Physiologic monitoring across hospital units and areas without equipment changes
- Inpatient assignments coordinated with nurses' experience levels due to the integration of smart staffing and scheduling applications with patient conditions
- Consumable supplies and medications automatically creating their own charges on patients' bills
- Consumable supplies automatically reordering themselves when supplies run low
- Durable medical equipment that automatically appears on units when a discharge order is written

In fact, Gartner estimates that by the year 2020, nearly 26 billion devices will be on the IoT.[42] Trends in healthcare informatics will likely mirror the increase in connectivity via the IoT. Imagine the potential of this kind of capability combined with care anywhere, personal device data, and EHRs. Future research might include the following:

- Evaluation of the timeliness of diagnoses with newer models of data availability
- Changes in provider and patient treatment adherence and monitoring with the IoT data

However, with this expanded connectivity, the available health data increases but so do the risks to health data privacy and security.

Cybersecurity Threats and Mitigation

One of the most ominous risks in health informatics now and in the future is the increase in cybersecurity threats (see Chapter 26). With the proliferation of devices, their connectivity to the IoT, the increased use of mHealth apps, and the increase in health data posted on social media, cybersecurity threats will only increase in volume and severity. New threats are emerging. For example, hackers cut off health data access at a California hospital and demanded a $3.5 million ransom.[43] All data were affected, from prescriptions to CT scans and even e-mails, forcing the staff to revert to paper methods and potentially compromising patient care. The hospital executives decided to pay a $17,000 ransom in bitcoins to end the incident. These incidences will likely be more prevalent in the future.

The informatics future will surely include more emphasis on health IT security, improved security using thorough risk assessments, and increased fiscal allocations for cybersecurity. A particular emphasis will be on improving the cybersecurity of personal health devices and preparing for the IoT connections. Policies, procedures, and code will be developed to prevent hacking and to avert paying ransoms in the future. Future research might include the following:

- The impact of threats on patients' willingness to share private data such as mental health concerns
- National efforts to combat cybersecurity threats

CLINICAL INFORMATICS

Beyond EHRs 1.0

With EHR adoption rates rising, especially for ambulatory practices,[44] leaders and informaticians are shifting the focus away from basic implementations to other issues such as system optimization and data science (discussed in Chapter 23 and later in this chapter). One of the most common foci is system optimization. The term *optimization* is used for both initial and postimplementation efforts. Users can benefit from applying known principles for project management and systems implementation (Chapters 17 and 19), as well as by using available guides such as Strategies for Optimizing an EHR System[45] from the ONC for Health IT. Optimization, more importantly, includes post-implementation evaluations, ongoing training, and system re-tailoring where needed. Installations obviously do not end with go-live. Many institutions consider EHR installations as continual transformation instead.

Unfortunately, the Health Information Technology for Economic Clinical Health (HITECH) Act did not include funding for research to evaluate the impact of EHRs,[17] so this type of research constitutes a future direction for informatics practice and research. In an editorial for *The New England Journal of Medicine*, Mandl and Kohane argue that vendors propagated a myth of complexity that precludes innovation and that EHRs are different than more flexible and robust consumer technology.[46] The authors' impatience and health IT leaders could drive needed changes for EHRs in the future.

One change might be that vendors no longer are full-service providers of EHRs. Instead, they may become smaller service and application providers, allowing sites to pick and choose best options among vendors, including among nontraditional vendors such as Google or Microsoft.

Another approach is described by Celi et al.,[47] who propose the construction of what they call optimal data systems. They recommend a focus on clinical decision making through the collection of data from various sources (Box 36.5). Although UX and data visualization issues would need to be central to development, this approach certainly provides an interesting vision beyond EHRs 1.0.

Newer infrastructures, such as cloud computing, middleware, and mobile applications, could allow more robust integration efforts at the healthcare provider and consumer end of computing. Facilities are already incorporating mHealth apps into their suite of applications, although current statistics indicate only about 2% of patients are using them currently.[48] User demands may force vendors to incorporate newer tools in their offerings, such as more robust clinical documentation tools with integrated graphics and drawing capabilities and even a basic spell-checker, currently lacking in today's EHRs. Previous authors indicated that disruptive technologies for EHRs are needed to displace the current model of EHRs.[46]

EHR interoperability efforts will continue, especially in the United States, where the diversity of products and components has caused the nation to lag behind others in creating integrated, person-centered, and longitudinal EHRs. Regional integration efforts have helped in the effort to share data, although interoperability beyond regions will be a continuous, costly future direction for the U.S. informatics research,

---

BOX 36.5   Elements of an Optimal Data System[46]

- Automatic collection and display of new data (real-time data), including alternative sources such as prehospital and personal device data
- Capture and integration of new data with historical to visualize trends and determine the current clinical state of the patient
- Integration of clinical decision support systems and Watson capabilities for diagnostic, therapeutic, and prognosis activities
- Use of machine learning to improve the quality of information
- User-tailored views of data
- Data sharing for population management
- Reports on adherence to best practice management
- Flexible system architecture to allow importing new modalities for decision support
- Prioritization of information types to allow urgent information to be incorporated (e.g., epidemics, disaster information)
- Use of user-centered design techniques (prototyping)

Source: Celi LA, Csete M, Stone D. Optimal data systems: the future of clinical predictions and decision support. *Curr Opin Crit Care*. 2014;20 (5):573-580.

and operational efforts on ontologies will continue to facilitate this work. What is urgently needed in the short term is a decision about the use of one or two specific ontologies, versus an endorsement of a suite of competing ontologies, especially for nursing. A more long-term solution may be found in the current research on national language processing and semantic mapping, where the process of mapping concepts can be automated. An early example of this can be seen with the diagnostic reasoning of IBM Watson, where analysis occurs at the cognitive level and does not require consistent use of the exact same terminology.

As is being seen with care anywhere efforts already, the traditional view of EHRs may fade. EHRs may be less organization- and site-specific and may become dispersed with data owners related to their roles (patient, healthcare provider, insurer, lab, pharmacy, etc.). In this case, data are pulled and integrated from geographic or other defined areas. A particular need for the future is more team-based, interdisciplinary views, and collaborations based on EHR data. New visions for EHRs are needed to be more patient-centric (beyond initial PHRs) and to serve as communication hubs.[49] Given the importance of teams in healthcare, the next generation of EHRs, no matter how they are instantiated, should offer collaborative workflow tools and methods for synthesizing data and information for "at-a-glance" views across disciplines, sites, types of agencies, and traditional modules.

Potential areas for future research include the following:

- Evaluative research on the impacts of EHRs from various viewpoints of consumers, healthcare providers, teams, care outcomes, and quality of care
- Impacts of integrative views of patient-centered data across traditional EHR modules and disciplines
- Cost-effectiveness research and comparative effectiveness for EHR designs

IMPROVING THE USER EXPERIENCE FOR HEALTH INFORMATION TECHNOLOGY

Efforts to improve the UX for health IT have now begun after years of relative neglect. More are needed. Leaders are recognizing that UX issues can affect patient safety as well as user efficiency and satisfaction. Healthcare providers deplore the poor usability of today's EHRs. Improving the UX for health IT is an obvious future trend. As noted in Chapter 21, the American Medical Association (AMA) and 30 physician groups wrote to the ONC for health IT about poor EHR usability and its impact on physician productivity and reimbursements.[50] In late 2015, the AMA held two town hall meetings to outline usability issues and subsequently released a framework for sites to gauge the effectiveness of a vendor's user-centered design techniques.[51] Other professions need similar efforts to improve the UX. Within nursing, Staggers et al. issued a recent call to action to improve the UX for health IT for nurses. UX efforts are needed, especially for vexing designs such as care transitions, medication management (Electronic Medication Administration Recordsor [eMARs]), and clinical documentation.[52]

On a more hopeful note, some large health IT vendors have hired UX professionals and are beginning to employ user-centered design techniques like those discussed in Chapter 21. These efforts were incentivized by Meaningful Use requirements. Whether these efforts continue as robustly remains to be seen. At this writing, UX improvements are occurring more slowly for nurses and allied health professionals than for physicians.

What is needed in the future are repositories for excellent designs and solutions to current UX issues. Typically, each site grapples with problems *de novo*, meaning wasted effort across the nation. Excellent, generic designs should be constructed and shared for common applications such as assessments, eMARs, and the like.

Due to current complaints by users, federal UX requirements will likely expand (beyond medical devices regulated by the U.S. Food and Drug Administration), and vendors will have to respond to the need for improved products. Organizations will need to increase their knowledge about and skills for improving the UX. Excellent resources for meeting this challenge are the Healthcare Information and Management Systems Society (HIMSS) Usability Maturity Model,[53] the ONC's SAFER (Safety Assurance Factors for EHR Resilience) guides,[54] and documents from the National Institute for Standards and Technology (NIST).[55] Research directions for improving the UX are many. Examples include the following:

- Comparative effectiveness research on EHR and device designs, especially for complex patient views, such as clinical summaries, care transitions, and eMARs.
- Developing and implementing best design practices agnostic of vendors. Perhaps decoupling user views from underlying code could occur so that optimal designs could be downloaded by healthcare providers and layered onto their local data.
- Determining outcomes for varying application designs. For instance, improved displays can positively affect clinicians' situation awareness and performance in intensive care units (ICUs).[56–58] Similar studies for other applications could be completed.

ANALYTICS (BIG DATA) AND DATA VISUALIZATION

The world is generating mass amounts of data. IBM estimates that 2.5 quintillion bytes of information are generated each day. That is three times the equivalent of the Library of Congress each second.[59] In the life sciences, genomic data have created large datasets for analyses. Bioinformatics efforts are underway to integrate data across disparate fields. For example, the National Center for Integrative Biomedical Informatics from the National Institutes of Health is developing interactive, integrated, analytic, and modeling technologies from molecular biology, experimental data, and the published literature.[60]

Within healthcare, data warehouses combine longitudinal, administration, and financial data into a searchable database, although typically at the local or healthcare enterprise level. Now, the boundaries are blurring among personal health data sources: mHealth, social media, wearable and sensor devices, and PHRs,[61] so opportunities for increased data collection are manifest. Thus data from personal devices such as sensor data and mobile and remote technologies could be integrated with EHR data in the near future. Personalized medicine efforts, including genomic data and nanotechnology, promise the expansion of these kinds of databases even further.

With these super-sized datasets, an unparalleled opportunity exists to examine data and issues across thousands of data points integrated across fields (population data, genomics, etc). The challenge is that the ability *to collect* these types of data has outstripped the ability *to analyze* them.[62] Data science was discussed in Chapter 23, and as readers recall, data analytics help in sense making by revealing patterns in datasets. A current trend is the shift from retrospective to predictive analytics.

PREDICTIVE ANALYTICS

According to current national and regional presentations, Chief Information Officers (CIOs) and health IT leaders are moving their foci to predictive analytics. As mentioned in Chapter 23, predictive analytics is the use of past data to predict future trends. The goal is to present data to decision makers as close to real time as possible. A simple example might be the real-time analysis of vital sign trends in a patient on a medical-surgical unit to predict the need to call a rapid response team and prevent a code. On a more complex level, the description about the optimal data system for EHRs discussed previously would rely on predictive analytics for decision making about intensive care patients—that is, the system would amass near real-time data from traditional sources like physiologic monitoring and less traditional sources including IBM Watson, analyzing them and displaying data in near real time for care decisions across complex datasets.

From an analytics tools perspective, Shameer et al.[63] depict a model for data integration and subsequent analyses at the individual level (Fig. 36.2). Here, data from different sources would be integrated for uses in person-centered health and precision medicine to provide individualized predictive analytics. This type of real-time analysis is a marriage of EHRs, decision support, and computer science and is being proposed for clinical settings, although it is not yet actualized.[63] As this type of real time analysis becomes available at the individual level, healthcare providers will be challenged to integrate yet more information into their cognitive processes and workflow.

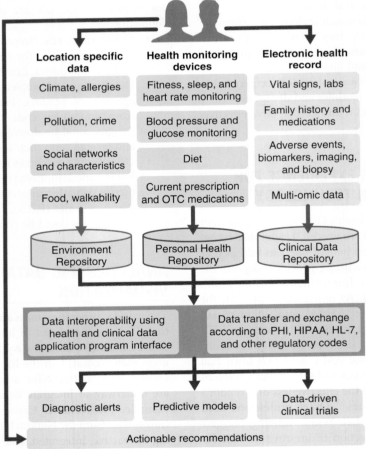

FIG 36.2 Healthcare and wellcare data model. (From Shameer K, Badgeley MA, Glicksberg BS, Morgan JW, Dudley JT. Translational bioinformatics in the era of real-time biomedical health care and wellness data streams. *Brief Bioinform.* 2016, pii: bbv118. Reprinted with permission from Oxford University Press.)

In other examples, predictive analytics could be useful at the population level in detecting global diseases such as the Zika virus or even in real-time fraud detection for someone attempting to use information to cheat on insurance coverage, much like credit card fraud detection is done today. These kinds of advanced applications are predicated on having quality source data, standards for integration and appropriate integrated data, and a capability of being able to interpret data using tools like data visualization.

DATA VISUALIZATION

One of the pressing issues with analytics is making sense of vast amounts of stored data. Unlike traditional graphs and charts, new methods are being developed outside healthcare. Fig. 36.3 provides an example from biology and computer science. At the intersection of science, design, and data, **data visualization** involves understanding principles of human perception, design, and computing capabilities.[64]

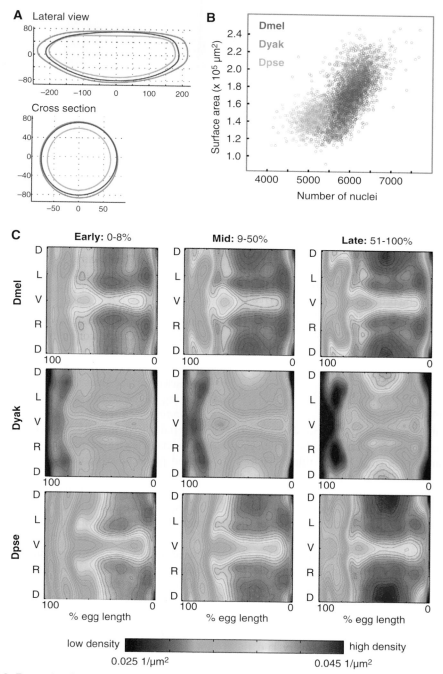

FIG 36.3 Example of visualization tools used to compare fruit fly attributes. (From Fowlkes CC, Eckenrode KB, Bragdon MD, et al. A conserved developmental patterning network produces quantitatively different output in multiple species of Drosophila. *PLoS Genet.* 2011;7(10):e1002346.)

In the life sciences, interdisciplinary teams of biologists and computer scientists developed interactive visualization tools like MulteeSum to compare genes in fruit flies.[65] In healthcare, analytic tools for searching data warehouses are emerging, but data visualization tools like those from the life sciences are still very limited in their application to health data, and they do not yet exist at the point of care. Because analyzing data and making conclusions from stored data can affect organizational and patient care decisions, data visualization efforts for healthcare will be an important future trend.

Research directions for analytics and data visualization include the following:

- Developing and implementing at the key decision points and interactive visualization tools for health practitioners, especially for nursing, pharmacy, and other healthcare providers whose analytic and decision support needs are often neglected.
- Developing big datasets, combining published literature, population data, and regional data warehouses.
- Detecting patterns for interventions and outcomes in national databases, including databases that incorporate include newer data such as sleep monitoring, metabolic values such as pO_2, and patient-generated fitness data with more traditional EHR data.

Nanotechnology

Nanotechnology is the study of controlling and altering matter at the atomic or molecular level.[66] The focus of the field is the creation of materials, devices, and other structures at the nanoscale (1 to 1000 nm). The produced items are referred to as nanomaterials, which are composed of smaller subunits called nanoparticles. Nanotechnology is a diverse field that requires a collaborative environment across multiple domains (e.g., surface engineering, physics, organic chemistry, molecular biology, and materials science).

History of Nanotechnology

Even though the majority of research in the field of nanotechnology was conducted in the past few decades, the field began in 1959 when Feynman presented a lecture titled "There's Plenty of Room at the Bottom."[67] In this talk, he discussed being able to manipulate individual atoms, which would allow for more flexibility and use in synthetic chemistry.

The field expanded in the 1980s with the invention of the scanning tunneling microscope and the discovery of fullerenes, a carbon molecule. With the scanning tunneling microscope, scientists could visualize particles at the nanoscale. In 1985, Kroto and his collaborators discovered a molecule composed solely of carbon, which they named Buckminsterfullerene.[68] Buckminsterfullerene is a spherical molecule composed of 60 carbon atoms. This gives the molecule a high structural integrity and makes it very stable. This discovery laid the foundation for the development of a well-recognized nanoparticle, the carbon nanotube. A carbon nanotube is a nanoparticle composed of carbon atoms bound to one another to form a tubelike structure (Fig. 36.4). Thus carbon nanotubes

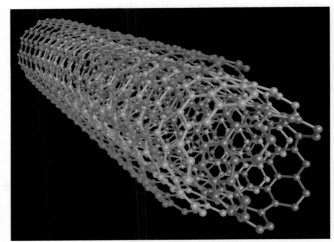

FIG 36.4 A carbon nanotube. (Copyright Owen Thomas/123RF Stock Photo. Reprinted with permission.)

are a member of the fullerene family of molecules. They have a unique combination of thermal conductivity, mechanical properties, and electrical properties that makes them useful in the development of structural materials like steel.

Nanofabrication and Nanomedicine

Nanomaterials and nanoparticles are used in electronics, biomaterials, and healthcare. Some claim that this area of science and technology has the opportunity to revolutionize our world. Manipulation of particles at the nanoscale allows the creation of unique materials with special properties (e.g., unique chemical, physical, or biologic properties, such as increased electrical conductivity or strength). The special properties are due to the particles' incredibly small size, which allows absorption or unique movement, and also due to increased surface areas that interact with their environments, creating increased interactions among materials.

Nanofabrication. Nanofabrication is the development of materials used in structures, electronics, and commercial products. Fabricated nanoparticles are typically added to larger physical structures to enhance them, resulting in increased strength, elasticity, conductivity, or antimicrobial properties. Much work has been done with carbon nanotubes, because the tubelike structure provides increased material strength. Carbon nanotubes are now commonly used in electronics as wiring for electrical components. For example, a research group at Rice University bound carbon nanotubes to Kevlar fibers to make durable, conductive wires that can be used in wearable electronics and battery-heated body armor.[69] Quantum dots, semiconductor devices whose elements move in all three dimensions, are another nanoparticle often used in electronics as semiconductors.

The number of commercially available items containing nanoparticles has increased at an aggressive pace over the past two decades. When the Project on Emerging Nanotechnologies (PEN) began its inventory in 2005, 212 products were listed. The latest inventory in 2015 estimates that more than 1800 manufactured, nanotechnology-enabled products have entered the commercial marketplace; the majority are in the health and fitness category.[70] Items containing nanoparticles are very diverse, ranging from everyday items such as nonstick cookware and lotions to unique items such as self-cleaning window treatments. Probably the most commonly used and commercially available product is silver nanoparticles, due to its antimicrobial properties.

Nanomedicine. Nanomedicine centers on the application of nanoparticles and nanoscience techniques to healthcare and clinical research.[71] Its primary goal is the use of nanotechnology for the diagnosis, treatment, and prevention of diseases. Applications include nanoparticles as delivery devices for pharmaceutics, diagnostic devices, and tissue replacement.[72] Nanoparticles, due to their size and structure, behave differently than traditional particles because they avoid the body's immune defense mechanisms, avoid filtration by the body, and interact more with tissues. Antibodies and a variety of other surface-engineered materials can be conjugated to the surface of nanoparticles, increasing their specificity for individual cell types (e.g., tumors). Importantly, the use of nanomaterials reduces medication dosages and effects on nontargeted tissues. Current research focuses on exploiting the highly soluble, targeting properties of nanoparticles to improve the delivery of cancer drugs to tumor-containing tissues[73] and on using nanoparticles to deliver nonviral genes and small interfering ribonucleic acid (RNA) to combat viruses and cancer.[74]

Another very intriguing area of nanomedicine research is advanced imaging and thermotherapy. Quantum dot nanoparticles are used in conjunction with magnetic resonance imaging (MRI) techniques to produce exceptional images of tumorous tissues. Chemical or physical groups can be attached to these nanoparticles via surface engineering, so that they seek out tumor cells and increase the resolution of images.[75] These same nanoparticles can then be used in the treatment of tumor cells using techniques such as thermotherapy. The process aggregates nanoparticles in tumorous tissues and then excites the nanoparticles using targeted radio waves, lasers, or focused magnetic waves. The excitation causes the metals in these nanoparticles to heat up, raising the temperature of nearby tissues (localized hyperthermia) and causing targeted cell death.[76]

Work is being done to develop in vitro early disease detection methods using nanoparticles. Thus nanoparticles are being used as diagnostic tools. One example is the use of a dime-sized microfluidic device containing a network of carbon nanotubes coated with tumor-specific antibodies.[77] A patient's blood sample passes through the device, and any tumor cells are bound to the nanotubes. Another sensor includes chips containing thousands of nanowires able to detect proteins and other biomarkers produced by cancerous cells. These types of advances could, in the future, enable the widespread detection and diagnosis of cancer in very early stages.

Cautions About Nanotechnology

Even though nanoparticles are incredibly effective and useful, caution is warranted. Unintended consequences of nanomaterials are due to secondary effects, such as cytotoxicity. For the same reasons that nanoparticles are effective (i.e., their size and increased surface interactions), they also can cause toxicity to the environment and humans. This is a key area of concern and current research in the nanoscience and nanomedicine community.[78,79] Many authors discuss inherent toxicity due to nanomaterials' surface charge.[78-81] This surface charge is necessary for cellular uptake. However, if the charge is too high, it can create holes within the cell membranes, resulting in membrane degradation, erosion, and ultimately cell lysis. Clearance of nanoparticles from the human body is another key area of concern, because nanoparticles may be rapidly eliminated by the kidneys or, alternatively, remain in circulation for long periods of time, increasing exposure and potential toxicity.

Synthetic methods such as the use of surface engineering and biodegradable components to construct nanoparticles are being employed to counteract the inherent toxicity of nanoparticles. These processes are used to alter the cationic surface charge of most nanoparticles by reducing the cationic charge, making it neutral or completely changing it to an anionic charge. However, if the surface charge of nanoparticles is reduced too much, the bioavailability of the nanoparticles is also decreased. Because of potential toxicity, nanoparticles must be evaluated carefully before they are approved for routine use in the clinical arena.[81,82]

Nanoinformatics

Nanoinformatics was created in an effort to help manage the large volumes of data being produced by the field of nanotechnology. The foundations for nanoinformatics began in 2007 at the U.S. National Science Foundation. The focus of nanoinformatics is the use of biomedical informatics techniques and tools for nanoparticle data and information. In October 2011, the U.S. National Nanotechnology Initiative (NNI) document was developed, which outlined the following three major goals for nanoinformatics:

1. Enhance the quality and availability of data about nanoparticles.
2. Expand nanotechnology theory, modeling, and simulation.
3. Develop an informatics infrastructure.[83]

The first goal has received the most attention to date. A number of groups are standardizing nanotechnology terms and developing ontologies to represent the relationships among the terms. The two most recognized standards organizations in nanotechnology are the Nanotechnology Standards Panel of the American National Standards Institute and the Nanotechnology Technical Committee of the International Organization for Standardization. The National Cancer Institute leads one of the most well-recognized ontology programs in nanotechnology, the NanoParticle Ontology.

Some progress has been made on the second and third NNI goals. The U.S. National Science Foundation hosts a site named nanoHUB that offers a wide variety of nanotechnology simulation tools for use by the general public and researchers. Recently, 10 federal organizations formed the

Nanotechnology Knowledge Infrastructure Signature Initiative, or NKI. Its purpose is to create a knowledge infrastructure to speed nanotechnology innovations by developing a cyber toolbox, models, and an information infrastructure.[84] The latest collection of nanotechnology cybertools are shown at http://www.nano.gov/NKIPortal/CyberToolbox. Also, many different research groups have been working on the development of predictive models to determine a number of different properties of nanoparticles. Overall, good progress has been made in the young field of nanoinformatics. However, the future will include much more work in this area.

In the future, one of the most pressing goals is to create an available public database of easily computable, nanoparticle data. To accomplish this, the extensive available literature on nanoparticles needs to be mined for relevant properties matched to existing standards systems or ontologies. This type of database could then be used for future data mining and model development. Beyond that, a next goal could be to develop predictive modeling software for developing quantitative structure activity relationships for nanoparticles. This would allow researchers to develop computer-generated structural images of nanoparticles and test them in a simulated environment, allowing toxicity, bioavailability, and many other functional property predictions for nanoparticles.

Issues in Regulation and Ethics

Previous authors are debating the regulatory and ethical implications of nanomaterials because of the unique properties and potential toxicity inherent in these materials. While some indicate that current frameworks are adequate to allow regulatory and ethical assessments,[85,86] pressing considerations are evident. For example, current cosmetic products such as sunscreens are seldom labeled as containing nanomaterials,[87,88] leaving consumers uninformed. No regulations require such labeling as yet.

Scientists can manufacture completely new materials with nanoscience, yet reliable information about the safety of nanomaterials lags behind their fabrication.[88] Exact risks for patients, employees, and scientists are not yet known. The potential applications for nanomaterials are enormous; likewise, their risks and regulatory and ethical implications are equally grand. Future applications could enhance oxygen storage in blood. This would, of course, be a boon to patients with illnesses such as emphysema or chronic anemia, but it has implications for ethics and regulation of sports competitions, as well as general use in humans.[89]

More alarming findings are emerging. For instance, researchers found that nanoparticle uptake by salmon negatively altered feeding behavior and lipid metabolism.[90] This finding is of particular concern because this kind of nanoparticle ingestion mimics typical feeding activity in the world's food chain. Whether regulatory controls will keep pace with discoveries such as these is an issue.

Once nanomaterials are more commonplace in healthcare, ethical issues will arise for the workplace related to hazards, risks, and projected controls.[91] Ethically, workers will need

to be informed about potential exposure to nanomaterials and risks related to inhalation, skin absorption, or unintended ingestion. This implies a responsibility for accurate assessment by employers, communication about risks, and perhaps even a form of informed consent by workers. For patients, expanded informed consent may be needed for nano-based medications, because all interactions are unlikely to be identified during testing.[72,92] Clearly, safety, regulatory, and ethical concerns are paramount for nanomaterials.

The field of nanotechnology is exciting, but caution is warranted. By virtue of the rapid advancements, nanotechnology is a major future direction for informatics, informatics research, commercial product development, health products, and impact assessment.

CONCLUSION AND FUTURE DIRECTIONS

Health professionals, informatics specialists, and leaders cannot afford to leave the future to chance. They must proactively and systematically identify future trends and directions in society, healthcare, technology, and informatics. This information and knowledge can provide the foundation for designing and building health information systems of the future. The methods and trends discussed in this chapter provide tools and ideas for health professional informaticians to use in identifying important future trends locally, regionally, and nationally.

As the rate of change continues to expand, it is expected that healthcare providers and informaticians will increase their use of e-tools and methods of futures research to predict and plan for an informatics-supported future in healthcare.

REFERENCES

1. Chantrill C. US health care spending history from 1900. http://www.usgovernmentspending.com/healthcare_spending; Accessed February 11, 2016.
2. Centers for Medicare and Medicaid Services. *National Health Expenditures Projections 2014–2024*. Centers for Medicare & Medicaid Services; 2014. https://www.cms.gov/Research-Statistics-Data-and-Systems/Statistics-Trends-and-Reports/NationalHealthExpendData/Downloads/proj2014.pdf.
3. Holahan J, McMorrow S. *The widespread slowdown in health spending growth: urban Institute*; April 8, 2015. http://www.urban.org/research/publication/widespread-slowdown-health-spending-growth.
4. World Health Organization (WHO). *What Are the Public Health Implications of Global Ageing?* WHO; 2011. http://www.who.int/features/qa/42/en/index.html.
5. Pellerin C. *Global Causes of Death Move from Infectious to Chronic Diseases*. America.gov; June 12, 2008. http://iipdigital.usembassy.gov/st/english/article/2008/06/20080612141457lcnirellep0.7136347.html#axzz4GCOYoMFZ.
6. Guariguata L, Whiting DR, Hambleton I, Beagley J, Linnenkamp U, Shaw JE. Global estimates of diabetes prevalence for 2013 and projections for 2035. *Diabetes Res Clin Pract.* 2014;103(2):137–149.
7. Staffing Industry Analysts. *No more nursing shortage: surplus projected for 2025. Healthcare staffing report*; January 8, 2015. http://www.staffingindustry.com/eng/Editorial/Healthcare-

Staffing-Report/Jan.-8-2015/No-more-nurse-shortage-Surplus-projected-for-2025.

8. Association of American Medical Colleges. *New physician workforce projections show the doctor shortage remains significant.* Association of American Medical Colleges; March 3, 2015. https://www.aamc.org/newsroom/newsreleases/426166/20150303.html.

9. Nordlund G. Time-scales in futures research and forecasting. *Futures.* 2012;44(4):408–414.

10. Nelson R. Future directions in health care informatics. In: Nelson SER, ed. *Health Informatics: An Interdisciplinary Approach.* St. Louis: Mosby; 2002:505–518.

11. Toffler A. *Future Shock.* New York, NY: Bantam Books; 1970.

12. Naisbitt J. *Megatrends.* New York: Warner Communication Company; 1982.

13. Goertzel T. *Methods and Approaches of Future Studies.* Camden Computing Services, Rutgers Camden. http://crab.rutgers.edu/~goertzel/futuristmethods.htm; Accessed July 13, 2016.

14. NIH. *NIH-Wide Strategic Plan: Fiscal Years 2016–2020.* National Institutes of Health. http://www.nih.gov/sites/default/files/about-nih/strategic-plan-fy2016-2020-508.pdf. Accessed July 13, 2016.

15. Glaudemans J, Morin A. *The Megatrends Reshaping Healthcare: Managing Change and Maximizing Opportunity.* Manatt, Phelps & Phillips, LLP; December 2015. https://www.manatt.com/uploadedFiles/Content/5_Insights/White_Papers/MEGATRENDS2015WhitePaper.pdf.

16. Pricewaterhouse Coopers. *Top health industry issues of 2016: thriving in the new health economy*; December 2015. http://www.pwc.com/us/en/health-industries/top-health-industry-issues/assets/2016-us-hri-top-issues.pdf.

17. Shortliffe EH. The future of biomedical informatics: a perspective from academia. *Stud Health Technol Inform.* 2012;180:19–24.

18. Bakken S, Stone PW, Larson EL. A nursing informatics research agenda for 2008–2018: contextual influences and key components. *Nurs Outlook.* 2012;60(5):280–288. e283.

19. Haux R. Medical informatics: past, present, future. *Int J Med Inform.* 2010;79(9):599–610.

20. Hovenga EJ. Milestones of the IMIA-NI history and future directions. *Stud Health Technol Inform.* 2009;146:3–10.

21. Yonck R. Connecting with our connected world. *Futurist.* 2013.47(6):17. http://www.wfs.org/futurist/2014-issues-futurist/november-december-2014-vol-48-no-6/outlook-2015.

22. Mesko B. Rx disruption: technology trends in medicine and healthcare. *Futurist.* 2014;48(3):31. https://www.questia.com/magazine/1G1-370319925/rx-disruption-technology-trends-in-medicine-and-health.

23. Colon J. Shakeups in the "C suite": hail to the new chiefs. *Futurist.* 2012;46(4):6–7.

24. Bisk T. Unlimiting energy's growth. *Futurist.* 2012;46(3):31.

25. World Future Society. World trends & forecasts. *Futurist.* 2012;46(3):15–16.

26. World Future Society. Blocking bodyhackers. *Futurist.* 2012;46(4):2.

27. World Future Society. The best predictions of 2011. *Futurist.* 2012;46(1):30.

28. Baines L. A future of fewer words?: five trends shaping the future of language. *Futurist.* 2012;46(2):46.

29. Johnson BD. The secret life of data in the year 2020. *Futurist.* 2012;46(4):21–23.

30. Carbone C, Nauth K. From smart house to networked home. *Futurist.* 2012;46(4):30.

31. Forum LE. *The Future of Healthcare: It's Health, Then Care.* Falls Church, VA: Computer Sciences Corporation; 2010.

32. Voros S, Moreau-Gaudry A. How sensor, signal and imaging informatics may impact patient centered care and care coordination. *IMIA Yearb Med Inform.* 2015;10(1):102–105.

33. Kogan AC, Wilber K, Mosqueda L. Person-centered care for older adults with chronic conditions and functional impairment: A systematic literature review. *J Am Geriatr Soc.* 2016;64(1):e1–e7.

34. The White House. *FACTSHEET: President Obama's Precision Medicine Initiative.* https://www.whitehouse.gov/the-press-office/2015/01/30/fact-sheet-president-obama-s-precision-medicine-initiative; 2015.

35. Demiris G, Kneale L. Informatics systems and tools to facilitate patient-centered care coordination. *IMIA Yearb Med Inform.* 2015;10(1):15–21.

36. IMS. *Patient Adoption of mHealth. Use, Evidence and Remaining Barriers to Mainstream Acceptance.* IMS Institute for Healthcare Informatics; 2015. http://www.imshealth.com/en/thought-leadership/ims-institute.

37. iDoc24. *Ask an online dermatologist*; 2016. https://www.idoc24.com/.

38. Sopher J. *Hot Health Care Trends for 2015: Eye Imaginations*; 2014. https://blog.eyemaginations.com/hot-health-care-technology-trends-2015/.

39. Morgan J. *A Simple Explanation of the "Internet of Things".* Forbes; May 13, 2014. http://www.forbes.com/sites/jacobmorgan/2014/05/13/simple-explanation-internet-things-that-anyone-can-understand/#11e461cc6828.

40. Harpham B. *How the Internet of Things is Changing Healthcare and Transportation.* CIO; July 2, 2016. http://www.cio.com/article/2981481/healthcare/how-the-internet-of-things-is-changing-healthcare-and-transportation.html.

41. Khan Y, Ostfeld AE, Lochner CM, Pierre A, Arias AC. Monitoring of vital signs with flexible and wearable medical devices. *Adv Mater.* 2016;28(22):4373–4395. http://dx.doi.org/10.1002/adma.201504366.

42. Gartner, Inc. *Gartner Says the Internet of Things Installed Base Will Grow to 26 Billion Units by 2020.* Press Release: Gartner Newsroom; December 12, 2013. http://www.gartner.com/newsroom/id/2636073.

43. Siwicki B. *Hollywood Presbyterian Declares Emergency after Hackers Cut Off Data, Demand $3.$ Million Ransom.* Health IT News; February 16, 2016. http://www.healthcareitnews.com/news/hollywood-presbyterian-declares-emergency-after-hackers-cut-data-demand-34-million-ransom?mkt_tok=3RkMMJWWfF9wsRonua7Leu%2FhmjTEU5z16ewsXaayg4kz2EFye%2BLIHETpodcMTcFhMrzYDBceEJhqyQJxPr3MLtINwNlqRhPrCg%3D%3D.

44. CDC. *Adoption of Certified Electronic Health Record System and Electronic Information Sharing in Physician Offices: United States, 2013 and 2014.* Centers for Disease Control; January 2016. NCHS Data Brief No. 236, http://www.cdc.gov/nchs/data/databriefs/db236.htm.

45. NLC. *Strategies for Optimizing an EHR System.* National Learning Consortium. Office of the National Coordinator for Health IT; 2014. http://www.bing.com/search?q=EHR+optimization&form=PRHPR1&src=IE11TR&pc=EUPP_HRTS.

46. Mandl KD, Kohane IS. Escaping the EHR trap—the future of health IT. *New Engl J Med.* 2012;366(24):2240–2242.

47. Celi LA, Ceste M, Stone D. Optimal data systems: the future of clinical predictions and decision support. *Curr Opin Crit Care.* 2014;20(5):573–580.

48. Accenture. *Losing Patience: Why Healthcare Providers Need to Up Their Mobile Game.* Accentureconsulting; 2015. https://www.accenture.com/t20151112T042615__w__/us-en/_acnmedia/Accenture/Conversion-Assets/DotCom/Documents/Global/PDF/Dualpub_24/Accenture-Losing-Patience.pdf.

49. Staggers N, Elias B, Makar E, Hunt J, Alexander G. *Identifying nurses' health IT pain points and solutions: Preliminary findings.* Paper presented at 10th International Conference UACHI 2016. Human-Computer Interaction International 2016; Toronto, ON, Canada.

50. American Medical Association (AMA). *AMA Board Chair: HHS should Address EHR Usability Issues Immediately.* American Medical Association; 2014. http://www.ama-assn.org/ama/pub/news/news/2014/2014-09-16-solutions-to-ehr-systems.page.

51. Bresnick J. *AMA Tackles EHR Usability, Physician Burnout, Meaningful Use.* HealthIT analytics; November 19, 2015. http://healthitanalytics.com/news/ama-tackles-ehr-usability-physician-burnout-meaningful-use.

52. Staggers N, Elias BL, Hunt JR, Makar E, Alexander GL. Nursing-centric technology and usability: a call to action. *Comput Inform Nurs.* 2015;33(8):325–332.

53. Healthcare Information and Management Systems Society (HIMSS). *Promoting Usability in Health Organizations: Initial Steps and Progress toward a Healthcare Usability Maturity Model.* Chicago, IL: HIMSS; 2011. http://www.himss.org/ResourceLibrary/ResourceDetail.aspx?ItemNumber=6920.

54. ONC. *SAFER: Safety Assurance Factors for EHR Resilience.* Washington D.C: Office of the National Coordinator for Health IT; 2014. https://www.healthit.gov/sites/safer/files/guides/safer_highprioritypractices_sg001_form_0.pdf.

55. NIST. *Technical Evaluation, Testing and Validation of Electronic Health Records.* NISTIR 7804. Gaitherburg, MD: National Institutes of Standards and Technology; 2011. http://www.nist.gov/healthcare/usability/.

56. Koch SH, Weir C, Haar M, et al. Intensive care unit nurses' information needs and recommendations for integrated displays to improve nurses' situation awareness. *J Am Med Inform Assoc.* 2012;19(4):583–590.

57. Gorges M, Staggers N. Evaluations of physiological monitoring displays: a systematic review. *J Clin Monit Comput.* 2008;22(1):45–66.

58. Drews FA, Westenskow DR. The right picture is worth a thousand numbers: data displays in anesthesia. *Hum Factors.* 2006;48(1):59–71.

59. McBurney V. *The origin and growth of big data buzz*; Toolbox for IT/Topics/Business Intelligence/Blogs; 2012. http://it.toolbox.com/blogs/infosphere/the-origin-and-growth-of-big-data-buzz-51509.

60. Athey BD, Cavalcoli JD, Jagadish HV, et al. The NIH National Center for Integrative Biomedical Informatics (NCIBI). *J Am Med Inform Assoc.* 2012;19(2):166–170.

61. Fernandiz-Luque L, Bau T. Health and social media: perfect storm of information. *Heathc Inform Res.* 2015;21(2):67–73.

62. Holland CM, Foley KT, Asler AL. Can big data bridge the chasm? Issues, opportunities, and strategies for the evolving value-based health care environment. *Neurosurg Focus.* 2015;39(6):E2.

63. Shameer K, Badgeley MA, Miotto R, Glicksberg BS, Morgan JW, Dudley JT. Translational bioinformatics in the era of real-time biomedical health care and wellness data streams. *Brief Bioinform.* 2016. pii: bbv118 [e-pub ahead of print].

64. Meyer M. *Visualizing Data: Why an (Interactive) Picture is Worth 1000 Numbers. Gould Lecture Series: Technology and the Quality of Life.* University of Utah, USA; September 5, 2012.

65. Meyer M, Munzner T, DePace A, Pfister H. MulteeSum: a tool for comparative spatial and temporal gene expression data. *IEEE Trans Vis Comput Graph.* 2010;16(6):908–917.

66. National Nanotechnology Initiative. *What is Nanotechnology?* Nano.gov; 2012. http://www.nano.gov/nanotech-101/what/definition.

67. Feynman RP. There's plenty of room at the bottom. *Caltech Eng Sci.* 1960;23(5):22–36.

68. Kroto HW, Heath JR, O'Brien SC, Curl RF, Smalley RE. C60: buckminsterfullerene. *Nature.* 1985;318(6042):162–163.

69. Xiang C, Lu W, Zhu Y, et al. Carbon nanotube and graphene nanoribbon-coated conductive Kevlar fibers. *ACS Appl Mater Interfaces.* 2012;4(1):131–136.

70. Vance ME, Kuiken T, Vejerano EP, et al. Nanotechnology in the real world: redeveloping the nanomaterial consumer products inventory. *Beilstein J Nanotechnol.* 2015;6: 1769–1780.

71. de la Iglesia D, Maojo V, Chiesa S, et al. International efforts in nanoinformatics research applied to nanomedicine. *Methods Inf Med.* 2011;50(1):84–95.

72. Staggers N, McCasky T, Brazelton N, Kennedy R. Nanotechnology: the coming revolution and its implications for consumers, clinicians, and informatics. *Nurs Outlook.* 2008;56(5):268–274.

73. Zhao P, Wang H, Yu M, et al. Paclitaxel loaded folic acid targeted nanoparticles of mixed lipid-shell and polymer-core: in vitro and in vivo evaluation. *Eur J Pharm Biopharm.* 2012;81(2):248–256.

74. Zhou J, Liu J, Cheng CJ, et al. Biodegradable poly(amine-coterpolymers) for targeted gene delivery. *Nat Mater.* 2012;11(1):82–90.

75. Pericleous P, Gazouli M, Lyberopoulou A, Rizos S, Nikiteas N, Efstathopoulos EP. Quantum dots hold promise for early cancer imaging and detection. *Int J Cancer.* 2012;131(3): 519–528.

76. Ma M, Chen H, Chen Y, et al. Au capped magnetic core/mesoporous silica shell nanoparticles for combined photothermo-/chemo-therapy and multimodal imaging. *Biomaterials.* 2012;33(3):989–998.

77. Veetil JV, Ye K. Development of immunosensors using carbon nanotubes. *Biotechnol Prog.* 2007;23(3):517–531.

78. Elsaesser A, Howard CV. Toxicology of nanoparticles. *Adv Drug Deliv Rev.* 2012;64(2):129–137.

79. Fadeel B, Garcia-Bennett AE. Better safe than sorry: understanding the toxicological properties of inorganic nanoparticles manufactured for biomedical applications. *Adv Drug Deliv Rev.* 2010;62(3):362–374.

80. Mukherjee SP, Davoren M, Byrne HJ. In vitro mammalian cyto-toxicological study of PAMAM dendrimers—towards quantitative structure activity relationships. *Toxicol In Vitro.* 2010;24(1):169–177.

81. Adiseshaiah PP, Hall JB, McNeil SE. Nanomaterial standards for efficacy and toxicity assessment. *Wiley Interdiscip Rev Nanomed Nanobiotechnol.* 2010;2(1):99–112.

82. Blobel B. Architectural approach to ehealth for enabling paradigm changes in health. *Methods Inf Med.* 2010;49 (2):123–134.
83. National Nanotechnology Initiative (NNI). *NNI 2011 Environmental, Health, and Safety Research Strategy*; October 20, 2011. http://www.nano.gov/node/681.
84. U.S. National Nanotechnology Initiative. *Introduction to nanoinformatics*; Webinar October 2, 2015, http://www.nano. gov/sites/default/files/nki_2015_webinar_1_with_transcript_-_ final5.pdf.
85. Litton P. "Nanoethics"? What's new? *Hastings Cent Rep.* 2007;27 (1):22–27.
86. Godman M. But is it unique to nanotechnology?: reframing nanoethics. *Sci Eng Ethics.* 2008;14(3):391–403.
87. White GB. Missing the boat on nanoethics. *Am J Bioeth.* 2009;9 (10):18–19.
88. Hristozov DR, Gottardo S, Critto A, Marcomini A. Risk assessment of engineered nanomaterials: a review of available data and approaches from a regulatory perspective. *Nanotoxicology.* 2012;6:880–898.
89. Toth-Fejel T. Nanotechnology will change more than just one thing. *Am J Bioeth.* 2009;9(10):12–13.
90. Cedervall T, Hansson LA, Lard M, Frohm B, Linse S. Food chain transport of nanoparticles affects behaviour and fat metabolism in fish. *PLoS One.* 2012;7(2):e32254.
91. Schulte PA, Salamanca-Buentello F. Ethical and scientific issues of nanotechnology in the workplace. *Environ Health Perspect.* 2007;115(1):5–12.
92. Resnik DB, Tinkle SS. Ethical issues in clinical trials involving nanomedicine. *Contemp Clin Trials.* 2007;28(4):433–441.

DISCUSSION QUESTIONS

1. In your work setting, which future trend(s) are likely to have the largest effect on patient care and related information systems?
2. Select one of the chapter topics in this book. For example, you might select mHealth in Chapter 15. Use the three levels of change to describe how your selected area of informatics might evolve over the next several years.
3. Use Box 36.4 to access and explore a futures research methodology that was not discussed in this chapter. Describe the methodology and how it could be used in health informatics.
4. Compare and contrast the trends of EHR directions and personal healthcare informatics. Where do they overlap and where do they differ?
5. Describe how nanomaterials might affect your own life in the near future. Consider the consumer products you use and your role in healthcare.
6. Using futures research methods, identify how you think nanotechnology might impact both health IT and health informatics.

CASE STUDY

You have just been hired as a clinical informatics leader for a new health system. The health system has 23 acute care facilities and 36 outpatient clinics. It serves as a regional referral center for three states in the Midwest. Your installed base includes a vendor-supplied EHR from a national vendor. Work on the data warehouse is being rethought. Your site has more than 300 varying applications across sites, including everything from a stand-alone pharmacy application for drug interactions to a cancer registry. Your goal is to provide IT support for the organizational vision of being the premier health organization in patient safety for the region. Your goal is also to provide predictive analytics for patient care for your ICUs. One of the first things you want to do is to plan for the future of IT.

Discussion Questions

1. Given the future directions discussed in this chapter, select the two directions you want to emphasize. Provide rationale for your choices.
2. Discuss how you can use methodologies from futures research to plan for your preferred future with the future directions you selected in Question 1.
3. Outline steps to introduce the chief executive officer to nanotechnology and its potential impact on the organization.
4. You want to increase collaborative work with a local university. What future directions for education do you think are most important as CIO?

   CIO, Chief information officer; *ICU,* intensive care units.

GLOSSARY

Academy Higher education in general with an emphasis on the institution as a society of scholars, scientists, and artists.

Accountable Care Organization A network of doctors and hospitals that share responsibility for providing care to a specific group of patients and in return receive bonuses when these providers keep costs down and meet specific quality benchmarks.

Accounts payable The monies that are owed to companies such as vendors and suppliers for items purchased on credit.

Accounts receivable The monies that are owed to the institution.

Accreditation A form of recognition provided to a healthcare or educational institution by an accrediting agency indicating that the institution has meet the standards of that agency.

Advanced practice nurse Nurses educated at the graduate level and authorized to practice as a specialist with advanced expertise in a specialty of nursing.

Adverse event An unintended and unfavorable event associated with the provision of medical care, use of a medical product, or treatment protocol.

American Recovery and Reinvestment Act (ARRA) Federal legislation, commonly referred to as the Stimulus or The Recovery Act, that was enacted in 2009 to help the United States economy recover.

Analytics Techniques for managing and processing data.

Analytics Maturity Model A model depicting how organizations mature over time in their use of data science and analytics by moving from descriptive to prediction to prescription.

Ancillary systems Software applications used by patient care support departments such as laboratory, radiology, and pharmacy.

Anti-Kickback Statute A criminal statute that prohibits the exchange or offer to exchange anything of value in an effort to induce referral of a federal healthcare program beneficiary.

Application A software program designed to help the user perform specific tasks.

Application service provider (ASP) A company, located remotely, that hosts an electronic health record or departmental system solution for a healthcare enterprise and provides access to the application via a secure network.

Architecture The formal description and design of information technology components, the relationships among them, and their implementation guide.

Assets Property items that can be converted easily into cash.

Attributes The characteristics or properties of the components of a system. Attributes are used to describe a system.

Automated system A computer system that responds to an event with little or no human intervention.

Availability A general term used to describe the amount of time that computer system resources are available to users. This is usually calculated for a 1-year period.

Avatar A graphic image representing a person or other entity, usually on the internet or in a video game.

Backcasting A technique for predicting the future by envisioning a desired future end point and then working backward to determine what activities and policies would be required to achieve that future.

Bar Code Medication Administration (BCMA) A method for administering medications using medication administration software, barcodes, and scanners, with the goal of reducing errors during the medication administration process.

Basic literacy The ability to identify, understand, interpret, create, communicate, and compute, using printed and written materials in a variety of settings and context.

Bayesian knowledge base A knowledge base built using decision trees and a branch of statistical inference that permits the use of prior knowledge in assessing the probability of an event in the presence of new data. For example, if a patient has a fever and increased white blood cells, the Bayesian knowledge base provides the probability that the patient has an infection versus another disorder that also creates an inflammatory process.

Best of breed An approach to selecting applications involving reviewing vendors' products to determine the "best" for a department or setting. When this approach is used, each department selects the "best" and the organization is tasked with achieving interoperability among them all.

Big bang A go-live approach in which all applications or modules are implemented at once.

Big data Very large datasets.

Biomedical informatics The interdisciplinary scientific field that studies and pursues the effective uses of biomedical data, information, and knowledge for scientific inquiry, problem solving, and decision making, motivated by efforts to improve human health (AMIA); http://www.amia.org/biomedical-informatics-core-competencies.

Bolt-on system A software program or application that is used in association with a larger application to give users their full required functionality. Users often require interfaces between the primary and bolt-on system. An example is an application for U.S. Mail address verification used in conjunction with a billing system.

Boundary The demarcation between a system and the environment of the system.

Business associate An organization supporting the work of a covered entity and having access to personal health information.

Business continuity The process created to ensure that essential functions and services continue during an adverse event.

Business intelligence Automated tools for analyzing massive amounts of data with the goal of improved decision making, typically at the organizational or departmental level.

Certification Commission for Health Information Technology (CCHIT) CCHIT tested and certified new EHR software applications in cooperation with the ONC from 2006 to 2015.

Change theory The study of change in individuals or social systems such as organizations.

Channel A physical element that carries a message between a sender and a receiver. Examples of channels are radio waves, fiber optic lines, and paper.

Chaos theory The qualitative study of unstable aperiodic behavior in deterministic, nonlinear dynamical systems.

Charge description master file A list of all prices for services (e.g., diagnosis-related group, Healthcare Common Procedure Coding, and Current Procedural Terminology 4) or goods provided to patients that serves as the basis for billing.

Children's Health Insurance Program (CHIP) Provides health coverage to eligible children, through both Medicaid and separate CHIP programs. CHIP is administered by states, according to federal requirements.

Citizen science People who volunteer to help scientists with their research.

Claims denial management The tracking and follow-up of denials for payment from insurance companies.

Claims processing and management The submission of an insurance claim or bill to a third-party payer, either manually or electronically, and the follow-up on the payment from the payer.

Classification A single hierarchical terminology that aggregates data at a prescribed level of abstraction for a particular domain.

Clicker A device that is part of a classroom or audience response system that allows real-time feedback to an instructor on, for example, comprehension of presented material.

Clinical application A software program used to perform specific tasks supporting the clinical aspects of healthcare—for example, documentation or orders management.

Clinical data repository The storage component for all patient clinical records data.

Clinical decision support (CDS) Tools and applications that assist the healthcare provider with some aspect of clinical decision making.

Clinical documentation Software that provides a medium for recording, managing, and reporting patient care activities by a variety of disciplines.

Clinical informatics The application of informatics and information technology to deliver healthcare services.

Clinical practice guidelines (CPGs) Statements and recommendations created from evidence-based practice or consensus-based processes and used to guide patient care.

Clinical scenario The plan of an expected and potential course of events for a simulated clinical experience. The clinical scenario provides the context for the simulation and can vary in length and complexity, depending on the objectives.

Closed system A system that is enclosed in an impermeable boundary and does not interact with the environment.

Cloud-based license A license for software that resides and runs on the vendor's server (s). The licensee remotely accesses and uses that software through the internet (e.g., via a web browser).

Cloud computing A model for enabling convenient, on-demand network access to a shared pool of computing resources that can be rapidly provisioned and released with minimal management effort or service provider interaction.

Cold site A relocation site for a company pending a disaster (e.g., fire, flood, terrorist event). It usually does not include backed-up copies of data from the original location. Hardware may be available but may need to be configured.

Comparative effectiveness research Studies designed to determine which methods to prevent, diagnose, treat, and monitor a health condition work best in terms of both benefit and harm, for which patients, and under what circumstances.

Complex adaptive systems (CAS) An entity consisting of many diverse and autonomous parts that are interrelated, interdependent, linked through many interconnections, and behave as a unified whole in learning from experience and in adjusting to changes in the environment.

Complexity theory Complexity theory builds on chaos theory using a qualitative approach to the study of dynamic nonlinear social systems that change with time and demonstrate complex relationships.

Comprehensive educational information system The hardware, applications, data, and integrated functionality designed for managing an academic setting such as a university.

Computer science The "systematic study of algorithmic methods for representing and transforming information, including their theory, design, implementation, application, and efficiency…. The roots of computer science extend deeply into mathematics and engineering. Mathematics imparts analysis to the field; engineering imparts design" (University at Buffalo School of Engineering and Applied Sciences; http://www.eng.buffalo.edu/undergrad/academics/degrees/cs-vs-cen).

Computerized provider order entry (CPOE) Software designed to allow clinicians to enter and manage a variety of patient care orders, such as medications, laboratory, nutrition care, and other diagnostic tests, via the computer.

Concept A term that represents a group of ideas or items. It may represent an abstract idea, such as love, or be concrete, such as fruit.

Conceptual framework A description and explanation of concepts and their relationships and interactions related to a specific phenomenon. Conceptual frameworks can be used to propose theories and generate research questions. A conceptual framework can also be used to develop a conceptual model.

Confidentiality Ensuring that data or information is disclosed only to authorized personnel.

Configuration management database (CMDB) A data repository containing all related components of an information system or information technology (IT) environment. A CMDB represents the authorized configuration of the significant components of the IT environment. A key goal of a CMDB is to help an organization understand the relationships between these components and track their configuration.

Connected health Healthcare that is provided remotely through the use of technology.

Contextual inquiry A method of usability testing that involves interacting with users in their actual sites or setting.

Course delivery system Software programs or applications that permit the development and delivery of a course or training program without requiring knowledge of programming code.

Course management systems/Learning management systems (CMS/LMS) Software programs or applications that permit a faculty member to deliver a course without knowing any programming code. Students use the programs to learn the concepts/skills being taught.

Covered entity A health plan, a healthcare clearinghouse, or a healthcare provider that transmits health information in electronic form.

Critical (key) application Defined by the stakeholders as an application that must be recovered first in the case of a disaster or downtime, as it is critical to some aspect of the organization and its operations (business).

Crowdsourcing The process of tapping into the collective intelligence of a group to complete business-related tasks that a company would normally either perform itself or outsource to a third-party provider.

Cytotoxicity The property of an agent being toxic to cells.

D

Dashboard An application designed to provide a visual display of specific data points, for example, for organizational performance data.

Data Uninterpreted elements such as a person's name, weight, or age. Because they are uninterpreted, they do not have meaning.

Data center A housing facility for computer systems, applications, and related components (e.g., servers and storage systems).

Data dictionary Stores standard terms for healthcare. Defines the terms and structure in a database and is used to control and maintain integration in large databases. It records (1) what data is stored, (2) the description and characteristics of the data, (3) relationships among data elements, and (4) access rights and frequency of terms.

Data exchange The sharing of data among systems using an agreed-upon standard electronic communication, convention, or "rule."

Data governance Formal mechanisms within an organization for determining who has authority over data-related matters and decision-making procedures.

Data integrity The accuracy and consistency of stored and transmitted data. Data integrity can be compromised when information is entered incorrectly or deliberately altered or when the system protections are not working correctly or suddenly fail.

Data mining A step in the knowledge discovery process of finding correlations or patterns among dozens of fields in large relational databases.

Data science The science of extracting knowledge or insights from data in various forms, either structured or unstructured.

Data standards Data processes that have been approved by a recognized body and provide for common and repeated use, rules, guidelines, or characteristics for activities or their results, aimed at achieving the optimum degree of order in a given context.

Data visualization Using software tools to detect visual patterns in large datasets.

Debriefing A review and self-reflection activity led by a facilitator following a simulation or other IT-related experience.

Decision making The process of considering available data and information, which is then matched with available knowledge to reach a conclusion or to make a judgment.

Dental informatics The application of computer and information sciences to improve dental practice, research, education, and management.

Derivative works A work based upon one or more preexisting works, including software application.

Derived classifications World Health Organization classifications based on reference classifications but adapted by either providing additional detail or becoming a compilation of multiple reference classifications.

Design thinking A formal process of addressing ill-defined problems through creative design, using an iterative process of creating and testing multiple designs, as in UCD, to evaluate their fit as an appropriate solution.

Digital divide The gap between groups of users in the adoption and use of personal electronic devices and the internet.

Digital health The use of a wide range of technologies such as smartphones, social networks, and internet applications to both obtain and provide healthcare, including health-related information.

Digital literacy The ability to operate and understand digital devices of all types, including the technical skills to operate these devices, the conceptual knowledge to understand their functionality, and the ability to creatively and critically use these devices to access, manipulate, evaluate, and apply data, information, knowledge, and wisdom in activities of daily living.

Disaster recovery Plans and procedures that organizations use when essential services or systems will not be available for an extended period of time or when it is expected that the disaster or event will have a significant impact on operations. Includes plans for response during the event or disaster, as well as plans for recovery.

Discount usability evaluations Cost-effective methods to determine usability issues for applications. These methods require minimal human resources and time, yet still find about 80% of critical design issues.

Discount usability methods A set of usability methods that offer economies of time, effort, and cost and can be completed at any point in the system's life cycle.

Disruptive technology An innovation that replaces long-held traditional ideas and ways of doing things. A technology that abruptly causes a change in thinking or direction.

Distance education Instruction and learning that takes place when the teacher and the learner are in two different settings and possibly teaching and learning at two different times.

Distance learning The process of learning using distance education technology, which separates the learner in time and space from his or her peers and instructor.

Distributed learning Learning that occurs through the use of technologies (such as video and Web 2.0 tools) and interactive activities and that may include augmented classrooms, hybrid courses, or distance education courses.

Distributive education A change in pedagogy where the course developer uses technology to customize the learning environment to the learning styles of the learners; the learners may be taking distance, hybrid (combination of online and face to face), or on-site courses. Includes interactive activities using available technologies.

Downtime A time during which a computer or software is not available or not functioning due to hardware, operating system, or application program failure.

Dynamic homeostasis The constantly changing processes used by a system to maintain a steady state or balance. The normal fluctuations seen in body chemistry levels demonstrate dynamic homeostasis.

Dynamic system A system that is in a constant state of change in response to a reiterative feedback loop.

E

e-books Books in a digital format that may or may not require a proprietary device to read (e.g., Kindle, Nook).

Education games Games that engage students in active learning. They generally include some sort of competition related to teams and winning a contest.

eHealth Refers to the broad use of information and communication technologies (ICT) to support health and health related fields; electronic communication and information technology related to health information and processes accessible through online means.

eHealth initiatives Efforts and programming implemented to standardize and transform the use of technology in healthcare, with the goal of improving patient care.

EHR adoption The depth and breadth of use or penetration of electronic health records in healthcare provider organizations and practices.

EHR donation A program whereby a healthcare institution underwrites the cost of an EHR for a physician or group of physicians who are independent practitioners from the hospital.

elatrogenesis Patient harm caused at least in part by the use of health IT.

eLearning A change in the learner's knowledge and/or skills that is attributable to an experience with an electronic device.

Electronic data interchange (EDI) The standards or act of transferring data via computer technology between organizations (trading partners).

Electronic health record (EHR) A longitudinal electronic record of patient health information produced by encounters in one or more care settings.

Electronic medical record (EMR) Electronic information resource used in a single healthcare setting to capture patient data. Term often used interchangeably with electronic health record.

Electronic Medication Administration Record (eMAR) Software used to view and document patient medications.

Eligible professionals Healthcare professionals who meet the eligibility criteria defined by law to receive incentive payments from the CMS for implementing electronic health records.

Enterprise resource planning (ERP) Facilitates the flow of data or information for business functions inside an organization and manages the connections to outside vendors or stakeholders. Most often associated with the supply chain functions.

Entropy A measure of the disorder or unavailability of energy within a system.

ePatient A person who uses technology to actively engage in his or her healthcare and manages the responsibility for his or her own health and wellness.

ePatient movement A movement in which patients play an increasing role in their own healthcare and contribute to the care of others.

ePortfolio A portfolio that is maintained in a digital format.

Equifinality The tendency of open systems to reach a characteristic final state from different initial conditions and in different ways.

Ergonomics In the United States, this focuses on the physical design and implementation of equipment, tools, and products as they relate to human safety, comfort, and convenience. The term is used interchangeably with human factors in Europe and elsewhere.

Evaluation A systematic collection of information about the activities, characteristics, and results of programs to make judgments about the program, improve or further develop program effectiveness, inform decisions about future programming, and/or increase understanding.

Evidence-based practice (EBP) The use of research, data, and scientific evaluation as a basis for clinical decision making and the provision of patient care.

Expert system A computer system that uses knowledge and a set of rules or procedures to interpret data and information and make decisions. Such a system differs from a decision support system in that the final decision is made by the computer as opposed to the provider. This term has also been used to refer to a type of clinical decision support system that provides diagnostic or therapeutic advice in a manner consistent with a clinical domain expert.

Exploratory data analysis An approach to analyzing datasets to summarize their main characteristics

Extrapolation Extending historical data to create future predictions and trend lines.

F

Fat client A personal computer with full functionality and disk storage that exists in a client–server environment. It contrasts with a thin client that is, in essence, solely a terminal with no embedded software (e.g., a dummy terminal).

Fidelity Believability or the degree to which a simulated experience approaches reality; as fidelity increases, realism increases.

Financial information system (FIS) A system that records, stores, and manages financial operations within an organization for the purposes of reporting and decision making.

FIT persons People who are fluent with information technology. FIT people go beyond proficiency in using a computer; they are able to express themselves creatively, reformulate knowledge, and synthesize new information using a wide range of information technology.

Fixed asset management The management of objects that cannot be easily converted to cash or sold or used for the care of a patient.

Focused ethnographies Research methods borrowed from anthropology and sociology in which the focus is on the person's point of view and his or her experiences and interactions in social settings.

Formative evaluation Feedback provided with the goal of improving a program or a person's performance, typically given in the early or middle portion of the program.

Fractal type patterns Irregular geometric shapes that are repeatedly subdivided into parts that are a smaller copy of the whole (e.g., a snowflake).

Framework A basic conceptual structure for organizing ideas.

Futures research A rational and systematic approach to identifying possible, probable, and preferable futures. The formal study of the future is also called foresight and futures studies, strategic foresight, prospective studies, prognostic studies, and futurology.

G

General ledger A listing of all financial transactions made by the healthcare organization.

Generalist nurse A professional nurse educated at the undergraduate level for the broad practice of nursing in primary, secondary, and tertiary healthcare.

Guided discovery A process by which clinicians engage ePatients in developing a shared hypothesis and plan of care based on data and reported experiences.

H

Harmonization The process of adjusting for differences and inconsistencies among different measurements, terms, methods, procedures, schedules, specifications, or systems to make them uniform or mutually compatible.

Health 1.0 Use of the internet to search for health-related information. The user can read but cannot interact in any way with the website or the information.

Health 2.0 Internet-based healthcare resources that allow interactive communication with other patients and healthcare resources across the country and around the world.

Health 3.0 Anticipated internet-based healthcare resources that learn from a user's behaviors and search activities.

Health advocacy Supports and promotes patient's healthcare rights as well as enhances community health and policy initiatives that focus on the availability, safety, and quality of care.

Health communication A process whereby practitioners create social change by changing people's attitudes and external structures, modify or eliminate certain behaviors using multiple behavioral and social learning theories and models to advance program planning, and identify steps to influence audience attitudes and behavior.

Health informaticians The title of a professional who whose proactive is focused on the discipline of health informatics. Other spellings or titles include *informaticist or informatician* and *informaticien*.

Health informatics An interdisciplinary specialty and scientific discipline focused on integrating the health sciences, computer science, and information science to discover, manage, and communicate data, information, knowledge, and wisdom supporting the provision of healthcare for individuals, families, and communities.

Health information exchange (HIE) The process of reliable and interoperable electronic health-related information sharing conducted in a manner that protects the confidentiality, privacy, and security of the information.

Health information organization (HIO) An organization that oversees and governs the exchange of health-related information among organizations according to nationally recognized standards.

Health information technology (health IT) The use of electronic methods for managing health-related date and information.

Health Information Technology for Economic and Clinical Health (HITECH) Act A law that established programs designed to improve healthcare quality, safety, and efficiency using health information technology.

Health IT Capability Maturity Assessment A qualitative model that can be used to assess an organization's capabilities with respect to five dimensions, measured on a scale of 1 (basic) to 5 (innovative).

Health IT governance The process of establishing an overarching structure for health IT in organizations, including establishing goals and objectives; creating policies, standards, and services; and developing mechanisms and processes for the oversight, enforcement, and coordination of the policies, standards, and services.

Health IT support personnel Individuals who assist in the design, development, implementation, ongoing support, and maintenance of the health IT hardware and software.

Health literacy The degree to which individuals have the capacity to obtain, process, and understand basic health information and services needed to make appropriate health decisions.

Health policy Includes the decisions, plans, and actions that guide the achievement of healthcare goals within a society.

Heuristic evaluations Assessments of a device or product against accepted guidelines or published usability principles.

High availability Processes that allow full functioning of systems during downtimes. Includes a redundant system in place, configured and waiting in standby mode if the primary production node fails. Requires manual intervention for end users to access it.

Home health Healthcare and social services provided by free-standing and facility-based community agencies at patients' residences, work sites, or other locations.

Hospice Item Set (HIS) A set of quality measures that must be reported by hospice programs to the Secretary of Health and Human Services under the Affordable Care Act of 2010.

Hot site An alternative site that is an exact duplication of the original site with real-time synchronization to allow an organization to relocate with minimal losses.

Human factors The scientific discipline concerned with the understanding of interactions among humans and other elements of a system. The term also refers to the profession that applies theory, principles, data, and methods to product design to optimize human well-being and overall system performance.

Human resources information system (HRIS) A computerized information system and applications used to record, store, and manage human resource data and information.

Human–computer interaction (HCI) The study of how people design, implement, and evaluate interactive computer systems in the context of users' tasks and work. Used interchangeably with the term ergonomics in Europe and elsewhere.

Human-made disaster A disaster created by humans that results in significant injuries, deaths, or damage to property.

I

Immunization information system (IIS) A confidential, population-based, computerized database that records all immunization-related data and information, such as doses administered by participating healthcare providers to persons residing within a given geopolitical area. Can be used at the healthcare provider, patient, and population level.

Incentive management Use of monetary and point-based rewards for staff who volunteer to meet institutional needs, such as staffing needs.

Incident response team (IRT) A group of people from the organization who prepare for and respond to incidents, downtimes, or other emergencies.

Informatics The study and use of information processes and technology in the arts, sciences, and the professions.

Informatics nurse specialist A nurse formally educated at the graduate level in nursing informatics, health informatics, or biomedical informatics.

Informatics researcher and innovator A nurse educated in a doctoral-level education program who uses health data, information, knowledge, and wisdom to generate new knowledge and best practices or to develop new technologies to continuously improve health outcomes.

Information A collection of data that has been processed to produce meaning.

Information and communication technology (ICT) Includes any communication device or application such as radio, television, cellular phones, computer networks, and the services and applications associated with these devices. The term is more commonly used outside of the United States and usually used within a context such as ICTs in education or healthcare.

Information ecology A science that studies the laws governing the influence of information summary on the formation and functioning of biosystems, including those of individuals, human communities, and humanity in general, and on the health and psychological, physical, and social well-being of the human being, and that undertakes to develop methodologies to improve the information environment.

Information literacy A set of abilities requiring individuals to recognize when information is needed and have the ability to locate, evaluate, and effectively use the needed information.

Information science The discipline that investigates the properties and the means of processing information for optimum accessibility and usability. It is concerned with the origination, collection, organization, storage, retrieval, interpretation, transmission, transformation, and use of information.

Information supply chain A full set of elements (technology based, process specific, and organizational in nature) that is necessary to support logistics and supplies in organizations. It includes (1) collecting information from discrete processes, (2) transforming this information from data to knowledge, and (3) distributing this information efficiently and in a timely manner to the appropriate data consumers.

Information system A combination of information technology, data, and human activities or processes that support operations and decision making.

Information theory Two theoretical models dealing with information, the Shannon-Weaver information-communication model and the Nelson data-information-knowledge-wisdom model.

Informed consent Permission given by an individual who has been provided with an understanding of the risks, benefits, limitations, and potential implications of consent.

Infrastructure The hardware and software used to connect computers and users, including cables; equipment such as routers, repeaters, and other devices that control transmission paths; software used to send, receive, and manage the signals that are transmitted; and often the computers themselves, although this component is not consistently considered infrastructure.

Integrated system A fully integrated health information system or a fully interoperable system. It may be monolithic (from one vendor) or best of breed.

Integrity Data are complete and have not been altered in an unauthorized manner.

Interactive whiteboard An interactive display controlled by a computer, typically with a touch screen, videoconferencing, and note-taking functionality.

Interface engine Software that transforms or maps data from one application to a receiving application's (or system's) requirements while a message is in transit to allow it to be accepted. The software is built with one-to-many concepts in mind. These import-export modules then are connected to an interface engine so that the mapping, routing, and monitoring are managed by this system.

Interface terminology A set of designations or representations structured to support representation of concepts for data entry and display on the graphical user interface.

International standards Terms, definitions, and/or information transmission guidelines adopted by international organizations and made available to the public.

Interoperability The ability for systems to reliably exchange data and operate in a coordinated, seamless manner.

Interprofessional education (IPE) An environment in which students from two or more disciplines learn from, with, and about each other to enable effective collaboration and improve health outcomes.

Intervention scheme A comprehensive, hierarchical taxonomy designed to organize patient assessment.

Intrusion detection Involves software, policies, and procedures used to detect attempted entry or inappropriate access to a computer or network.

J

Joint cognitive systems Systems in which information is shared or distributed among humans and technology.

K

Knowledge Created when data and information are identified and the relationships between the data and information are formalized.

Knowledge base A component, typically within an electronic health record, that stores and organizes a healthcare enterprise's information and knowledge used by the enterprise for clinical operations.

Knowledge discovery and data mining (KDDM) An approach to identifying patterns in large datasets that entails methods such as statistical analysis, machine learning methods, and data visualization. In some literature, the terms knowledge discovery and data mining are used interchangeably. Also, the terms knowledge discovery and knowledge discovery in data are sometimes used to refer to the broad process of finding knowledge in data.

Knowledge transformation Converting knowledge from research results, to evidence summary, to practice guidelines, to integration, and then evaluation of the impact.

L

Lead part The unit of a system that plays the dominant role in the operation of the system.

Learning An increase in knowledge, a change in attitude or values, or the development of new skills.

Learning environment An atmosphere that is created by the facilitator to allow for sharing and discussion of participant experiences without fear of humiliation or punitive action. The goals of the simulation learning environment are to promote trust and foster learning.

Learning health system (LHS) A health system in which science, informatics, incentives, and culture are aligned for continuous improvement and innovation, with best practices seamlessly embedded in the delivery process and new knowledge captured as a by-product of the delivery experience.

Learning theory Provides a framework for understanding how patients and healthcare providers as open learning systems take in, process, and output data, information, knowledge, and wisdom.

Liability Something (typically monetary) for which an organization or person is legally responsible.

Limitations and exclusions of liability The specific contractual exceptions and specifications for liabilities (i.e., something [typically monetary] for which an organization or person is legally responsible).

Logic model A graphical depiction of the logical relationships between the resources, activities, outputs, and outcomes of a program.

M

Machine learning Adjustment of a computer model or algorithm based on exposure to training examples.

Man-made disaster A disaster created by humans that results in significant injuries, deaths, or damage to property.

Master person index (MPI) The information used to uniquely identify each person, patient, and customer of a healthcare enterprise. Synonyms for this term include master patient index, master member index, and patient master index.

Material management The storage, inventory control, quality control, and operational management of supplies, pharmaceuticals, equipment, and other items used in the delivery of patient care or the management of the patient care system. Material management is a subset of the larger function of supply chain management; the supply chain also includes the acquisition of materials of care and the logistics or movement of those materials to caregiving facilities and organizations.

Meaningful Use Sets of specific objectives that must be achieved to qualify for federal incentive payments. Meaningful Use means that healthcare providers must show that they are using certified electronic health record technology in ways that can be measured using specific criteria.

Meaningful Use Objectives Specific targets that must be achieved for providers and/or hospitals to qualify for incentive payments under the HITECH Act. These include the use of certified EHRs and specific usage such as ePrescribing, CPOE, medication reconciliation, information exchange and patient electronic access, and clinical decision support.

Medical informatics The branch of informatics that focuses on disease diagnosis and management.

Medicine 2.0 The evolution of healthcare across seven themes: technology, patients, professionals, social networking, health information and content, collaboration, and change of healthcare.

mHealth Medical and public health practice supported by mobile devices, such as mobile phones, patient monitoring devices, personal digital assistants (PDAs), and other wireless devices.

Microblogging A form of blogging (online journaling of an author's thoughts) in which entries are kept brief using character limitations (e.g., Twitter).

Mobile applications Applications (apps) on mobile devices.

Modified Stage 2 (Meaningful Use) Specific Meaningful Use Stage 2 requirements updated in 2015 that provide a consolidated list of objectives.

N

Nanofabrication The development of nanomaterials used in structures, electronics, and commercial products.

Nanoinformatics The use of informatics techniques and tools for nanomaterial or nanoparticle data management and storage; information to improve research in the field of nanotechnology.

Nanomaterials Materials, devices, and other structures at the subatomic level, specifically the nanoscale of 1 to 1000 nm.

Nanomedicine A subspecialty of nanotechnology, centering on the application of nanoparticles and nanoscience techniques to healthcare and clinical research.

Nanotechnology The study of controlling and altering matter at the atomic or molecular level.

Nationwide Health Information Network (NwHIN) A set of standards, services, and policies that enable secure health information exchange over the internet and across diverse settings.

Natural disaster A disaster created by nature.

Natural language processing Computer processing of text written or spoken by humans.

Negentropy A measure of energy that can be used by a system for maintenance as well as growth.

Networked personal health record A personal health record that is electronically linked to multiple data sources (e.g., electronic health records, pharmacies, labs). Entities that are linked to the networked record may provide services to the user (e.g., secure messaging). These systems also allow for the storage of personally entered data.

Niche applications Specialty software applications created to address the requirements of specific departments and groups of users.

Noise Anything that is not part of a message but occupies space on the channel and is transmitted with the message.

Nurse-managed health center A site that primarily offers outpatient clinic and primary healthcare and social services provided by nurses.

Nursing informatics A specialty that integrates nursing science, computer science, and information science to manage and communicate data, information, knowledge, and wisdom in nursing practice, education, research, and administration.

O

Omaha System A research-based taxonomy designed to support documenting client care from admission to discharge in various settings. It exists in the public domain and can be used without licensing fees. Its primary application has been in the home health arena.

Online education A version of distance education that requires the use of the internet to deliver the educational materials.

Ontology A model of a domain that defines the concepts existing in that domain as well as taxonomic and other relationships existing between the concepts. Within health informatics, an ontology would be a formal, computer-understandable description of a domain.

Open shift management A web-based self-scheduling solution in which the manager uses a variety of instant communication tools to announce openings in the schedule and staff members respond by tendering schedule and shift requests for consideration and approval.

Open system A system that is enclosed in a semipermeable boundary and interacts with the environment.

Open-source software Source code are typically made available to the public.

Outcome and Assessment Information Set (OASIS) A standardized assessment tool and core dataset mandated by the Centers for Medicare and Medicaid Services, for use by Medicare-certified home health agencies.

Outcomes-based quality improvement (OBQI) A risk-adjusted outcome reporting tool that is based on Outcome and Assessment Information Set and mandated by the Centers for Medicare and Medicaid Services for use by Medicare-certified home health agencies.

P

P4 Medicine Medicine that is predictive, preventive, personalized, and participatory.

Palliative care and hospice Healthcare and social services provided to those with life-threatening or terminal illnesses.

Participatory healthcare A healthcare model that includes patients, caregivers, and healthcare professionals working together in all aspects of a patient's health.

Participatory medicine A cooperative model of healthcare that encourages and expects active involvement by all connected parties, including patients, caregivers, and healthcare professionals, as integral to the full continuum of care.

Patient accounting A process for collecting and tracking debits and credits for patient care provided by clinicians that is billed to insurance companies and/or the patient.

Patient generated data (PGD) Data input or uploaded from patients, such as into a PHR or from wearable devices.

Patient safety Freedom from accidental injury due to healthcare, medical care, or medical errors, where error is defined as the failure of a planned action to be completed safely or as intended or the use of a wrong plan to achieve an aim.

Patient-centered care An essential partnership between interprofessional care providers and the individuals, families, and communities that are the recipients of care.

Pay for performance (P4P) A strategy to pay healthcare providers for high-quality care, as measured by selected evidence-based standards and procedures. A network of doctors and hospitals share responsibility for providing care to a specific group of patients and in return receive bonuses when these providers keep costs down and meet specific quality benchmarks.

Payroll system An application that creates and disburses compensation payments to employees. This is also referred to as a disbursement system.

Phased go-live A gradual go-live approach within an institution by service line, selected areas, or departments.

Phenomenon An observable fact or event.

Picture archiving and communication system (PACS) A combination of hardware and software configured to provide for the storage, retrieval, management, distribution, and presentation of radiological images.

Point of care Patient care and procedures that are performed at or near the patient care site.

Portfolio management Common programs and projects that are not necessarily related but are important to combine and view as a whole, such as a clinical portfolio in which all projects and programs that directly affect patient care are managed or aligned in a common category.

Practice-based evidence A specific research design using observations and cohorts of patients. Used to answer questions of treatment effectiveness that involves meticulous prospective data collection in a naturalistic clinical setting of multiple interventions and outcomes, with rigorous statistical control of relevant patient differences.

Practice management system (PMS) An application designed to assist in the management of a practice by collecting patient demographic information, insurance information, appointment scheduling, reason for the visit, patient care procedures done for the patient, charging information for the billing process, and collection and follow-up.

Predictive analytics The development of analytic models that predict future probabilities or trends based on the analysis of retrospective or real-time data.

Predictive scheduling Resource scheduling based on a predictive model used to forecast bed demand changes in patient acuity, workload distribution, and variability caused by shift, day of the week, month, and seasonality.

Preprocessing (of data) Preparation of data for data mining (e.g., data cleaning, transformation, replacement of missing values).

Prescriptive analytics The use of models to evaluate and determine new ways of operating in a health system. The models predict system output under a range of system configurations, allowing decision makers to choose the best of potential alternatives.

Privacy The capacity to control when, how, and to what degree information about oneself is communicated to others.

Problem classification scheme A comprehensive, hierarchical taxonomy designed to identify diverse patients' health-related concerns.

Problem rating scale for outcomes A comprehensive, recurring evaluation framework designed to measure patient progress.

Program evaluation The systematic collection of information about the activities, characteristics, and results of programs to make judgments about the program, improve or further develop program effectiveness, inform decisions about future programming, and increase understanding.

Program management Multiple, aligned projects affecting many teams or departments that are coordinated and managed in concert.

Project management A temporary endeavor undertaken to create a unique product, service, or result. The project has specific boundaries, including initialization and a defined end.

Protected health information (PHI) Personally identifiable health information, such as name, birth date, and social security number, created or received by a covered entity.

Public health The science and art of protecting and improving the health of communities through education, promotion of healthy lifestyles, and research for disease and injury prevention.

Public health informatics The application of informatics in areas of public health, including disease or condition surveillance, reporting, and health promotion. Public health informatics and its corollary, population informatics, are concerned with groups rather than individuals.

Public health surveillance Collecting, analyzing, and interpreting health-related data for the planning, implementation, and evaluation of public health.

Q

Quality of care The degree to which health services for individuals and populations increase the likelihood of desired health outcomes and are consistent with current professional knowledge.

Quantified self A person invested in using tools and data to quantify and monitor his or her daily experiences using personal metrics.

R

Radio frequency identification (RFID) Technology that uses electronic tags to track and monitor equipment and activities. Typically used in patient bands, lab specimens, or surgical sponges.

Randomized controlled trial A specific research design involving random assignment of subjects to experimental and control groups and other design features to assure as much variable control as possible. With this research design approach, the differences between the groups are most likely related to the treatment each group received.

Receiver A device or individual that receives a message that has been sent over a channel.

Reference classifications Main terminology classifications based on basic parameters of health.

Reference terminology A set of atomic level designations, representing a domain knowledge of interest, structured to support representations of both simple and compositional concepts independent of human language (within machine) that facilitates data collection, processing, and aggregation.

Regional Health Information Organization (RHIO) Characterized as a quasi-public, nonprofit organization whose goal is to share secure health-related data within a region.

Reiterative feedback loops Feedback loops where the effect of the system's actions or output is continuously returned to the system as input, thereby effecting the system's future output.

Related classifications World Health Organization classifications that partially refer to reference classifications, or are associated with the reference classification at specific levels of structure only.

Remote hosting An application hosted off site, typically by a vendor, at a site with vendor-owned hardware.

Request for information (RFI) A document that is developed and sent to vendors requesting basic or overview information to determine which vendors are most likely to meet the institution's requirements for a new information system. Not as formal as a request for proposal (RFP). Both RFP and RFI are used as part of the purchasing process.

Request for proposal (RFP) A detailed document developed and sent to vendors outlining the institution's requirements to request a proposal describing the vendors' capabilities to meet the listed requirements and the related costs. RFPs and requests for information (RFIs) are used as part of the purchasing process.

Requirements definition The process of determining the specific needs that the organization has for an information system and the specific functionality that is desired.

Revenue cycle All business components (administrative and clinical) dealing with patient service revenue.

Reverberation The process of change throughout a system that occurs in response to change in one part of a system.

Risk A person or situation that poses a threat to the security of an information system.

Risk analysis or assessment A systematic process for examining an information system to identify the security vulnerabilities and potential risks to an information system or organization. Also referred to as risk assessment.

S

SaaS (software as a service) A software distribution model where applications are hosted by a vendor and made available to customers over a network, typically the internet.

Safeguard In cybersecurity, this refers to three processes to lessen or alleviate threats to security: administrative, technical, and physical.

Scope creep Occurs when requirements are added on after the initial project was defined and approved. Added requirements are substantial enough to affect the project costs and/or timeline.

Security The administrative, technical, and physical safeguards in an organization or information system to prevent privacy breaches.

Sender The originator of a message to be sent over a channel.

Service level agreement (SLA) An agreement made between information technology and a key stakeholder where the level of service is formally defined and agreed upon. This can include uptime guarantees, response time to issues, and even disaster recovery timelines.

Service-oriented architecture (SOA) An architecture design configuration where services are business oriented, loosely coupled with other services and system components, vendor and platform independent, message based, and encapsulated with internal architecture and program flow that are hidden from the service user.

Simulation A pedagogy, or instructional method, using one or more teaching strategies to promote, improve, and validate a participant's progression from novice to expert.

Simulation experience A term often used synonymously with simulated clinical experience or scenario.

Simulation learning environment An atmosphere that is created by the facilitator to allow for sharing and discussion of participant experiences without fear of humiliation or punitive action. The goals of the simulation learning environment are to promote trust and foster learning.

Social media An application used to create an online environment that is established for the purpose of mass collaboration.

Social networking The use of social media and online platforms that enable groups and individuals to connect with others sharing similar interests.

Sociotechnical Refers to complex systems recognizing the interaction between people and technology in work settings, particularly settings such as healthcare.

Software escrow A neutral third-party company holds the source code, programming documentation, and other items needed for maintenance and modification of the software.

Software license agreements Contracts for software.

Software warranty A written guarantee from a vendor promising repair or replacement within a specific time period.

Stakeholders People affiliated with an organization (internal and external) who share a vested interest in the outcomes produced by that organization.

Stand-alone personal health record A personal health record that is not electronically linked to other data sources and can serve as a portable electronic store of personally entered data.

Standardized terminology Terms and definitions adopted by a national or international standardizing and standards organization and made available to the public.

Standards development organizations (SDO) Entities whose primary activities are developing, coordinating, disseminating, and maintaining standards addressing a large group of users. Also called *standards setting organizations*.

Standards of Best Practice: Simulation Seven sets of definitions and principles developed by the International Nursing Association for Clinical Simulation and Learning that should be considered and incorporated when developing all simulation-based learning experiences for learners (terminology, professional integrity, participants' objectives, facilitation methods, facilitator, debriefing process, and evaluation of outcomes).

Standards setting organizations (SSO) Entities whose primary activities are developing, coordinating, disseminating, and maintaining standards addressing a large group of users. Also called *standards developing organizations*.

Stark A law passed in 1992 that governs physician self-referral for Medicare and Medicaid patients. It generally prohibits a physician from referring patients for certain designated health services (DHS) to entities where the physician has a financial relationship.

Strategic alignment The process of matching two or more organizational strategies to ensure that they synergistically support the organization's goals and vision.

Strategic vision The desired future state of an organization or institution.

Subsystem Any system within the target system.

Summative evaluation An evaluation that determines the effects or outcomes of a person's, program's, or organization's performance; a program's impact; or a technology's effectiveness. The goal is to determine the merit of the evaluation target.

Supersystem The overall system in which the target system exists.

Supply chain management (SCM) The acquisition, movement of, storage, inventory control, quality control, and operational management of supplies, pharmaceuticals, equipment, and other items used in the delivery of patient care or the management of the patient care system.

Supply item master file A list (hard copy or electronic) of all items used in the delivery of care for a health organization that can be requested by healthcare providers and managers. This file typically contains between 30,000 and 100,000 items.

Systems life cycle A conceptual model or framework used to describe each stage in the life of a living or nonliving system, such as an information system.

T

Tall Man lettering The use of mixed case lettering, allowing easy differentiation of similar terms such as look-alike medication names.

Target system The system of interest.

Task analysis A suite of well-known usability methods to decompose and understand users' actions and behaviors. Composed of more than 100 different methods, it is used to determine goals, tasks, issues with interactions, the flow of work, and other activities in sociotechnical systems.

Telehealth The use of telecommunication methods to provide patient care and education as well as public health and health administration.

Telehealth competency Having and using knowledge, understanding, and judgment when providing telehealth.

Telemedicine The use of medical information exchanged from one site to another via electronic communications for the health and education of the patient or healthcare provider and for the purpose of improving patient care, treatment, and services.

Telenursing The use of telehealth technology to deliver nursing care and conduct nursing practice.

Terminology cross-mapping Assigning an element or concept in one set to an element or concept in another set through semantic correspondence.

Terminology harmonization A process of ensuring consistency of terms and the definitions of those terms within and across different terminologies.

Tethered personal health record A personal health record that is electronically linked to the clinical information systems of a given healthcare provider or organization. It may include functions such as secure messaging and online scheduling as well as storage of personally entered data.

Theoretical model A visual representation of a theoretical framework, a relationship among concepts.

Theory A scientifically acceptable explanation of a phenomenon.

Thin client A centrally managed computer workstation without a hard drive that has its operating system and application delivered from a central server via the network and all data stored on network storage. This is in contrast to a fat client, which has software embedded in the client.

Think-aloud protocol A usability method in which users talk aloud about what they are doing as they interact with a product. These interactions are observed or recorded and then analyzed.

Threat An act of man or nature that has the potential to cause harm to an informational asset.

Transaction history file A running log of all material transactions of the healthcare organization.

Transparency Indicates that the policies, procedures, and technologies affecting health information use for individuals' health information are easily accessed and understood.

Trend analysis The process of analyzing historical data and identifying trends over time.

U

uHealth Ubiquitous health technologies that integrate core components of computers, wireless networks, sensors, and other modalities, such as mHealth (mobile) devices, to create an environment that can monitor, respond to, and assist in meeting healthcare needs of individuals.

Unintended consequences Unplanned and unexpected consequences from a device, process, or event such as the adoption of health IT.

Untethered personal health record A personal health record that is not electronically linked to other data sources, such as a host EHR.

Usability The extent to which a product can be utilized by specific users in a specific context to achieve specific goals with effectiveness, efficiency, and satisfaction.

User interface A boundary between users and products, typically a display or computer screen or interaction device. It allows humans and products to cooperatively perform tasks.

User-centered design A structured application development process with three primary emphases: an early and central focus on users in the design and development of products, iterative design, and systematic measures of the interactions between users and products.

V

Vendor A person or business that sells products, goods, or services to a company or institution.

Vendor master file A list of all manufacturers and distributors (vendors) who provide materials needed for the healthcare organization that also contains the associated contract terms and prices for specific items. This file typically contains between 200 and 500 different vendors and suppliers.

Virtual community An online community that shares many characteristics with traditional social groups.

Vulnerability A weakness in an information system, system security procedures, internal controls, or implementation that could be exploited.

W

Wearable devices Accessories, sensors, or clothing that have embedded computers or advanced technologies. Examples are activity trackers.

Web 2.0 Sophisticated web functionality with social engagement, interaction, and networking capabilities.

Web 3.0 Emerging functionality in which browsers learn from user search behavior and adapt accordingly.

Wisdom The appropriate use of knowledge in managing or solving human problems. It involves knowing when and how to use knowledge in managing a client need or problem.

Workaround A temporary and potentially unsafe fix for a problem which fails to provide a genuine solution to the problem.

INDEX

Note: Page numbers followed by *f* indicate figures, *t* indicate tables, and *b* indicate boxes.